Concise Colour
Medical Dictionary

Editor
Elizabeth A. Martin MA

Contributors and Advisers
Rajesh Aggarwal BM, MRCP,
  FRCS, FRCOphth
W. Leslie Alexander FRCS,
  FRCOphth
J. A. D. Anderson MA, MD,
  FRCP, FFPHM, FFOM, FRCGP
J. H. Angel MD, FRCP
Dr Andrea Atherton MA,
  MSc, MRCP(UK)
John R. Bennett MD, FRCP
Stuart Anthony Bentley MB,
  BS
Dr J. N. Bowles BSc, MRCP,
  FRCR
Dr Peter Bradbury FRCP
Bruce M. Bryant MB, ChB,
  MRCP
Robert E. Coleman
Patrick Collins MD, MRCP
J. A. Cullen BSc, MSc
W. J. Dinning FRCS, MRCP
Ivan T. Draper MB, ChB,
  FRCPEd
J. C. Gingell MB, BCh, FRCSEd,
  FRCS
John M. Goldman DM, FRCP,
  FRCPath

Dr Helen K. Gordon MRCOG,
  MMFP
W. J. Gordon MD, FRCS(G),
  FRCOG
Michael Klaber MA, MB, FRCP
Alexander J. Lewis BSc, MB,
  BS, MRCPsych
D. J. McFerran MA, FRCS
Gordon Macpherson MB, BS
Charles V. Mann MA, MCh,
  FRCS
J. E. Nicholl MA, FRCS(Orth)
Heather E. Pitt Ford FDS
T. R. Pitt Ford PhD, BDS, FDS
D. L. Phillips FRCR, FRCOG
Helen Phillips MBBS, MRCGP,
  DCH, DRCOG
Dr John R. Sewell MA, MB,
  MRCP
Dr Mary Sibellas MD, FFPHM,
  DTM&H
Dr Tony Smith MA, BM, BCh
Eric Taylor MA, MB, MRCP,
  MRCPsych
William F. Whimster MRCP,
  MRCPath
Robert M. Youngson MB,
  ChB, DRM&H, DO, FRCOpthal

Oxford Paperback Reference

The most authoritative and up-to-date reference books for both students and the general reader.

Concise Colour

Medical Dictionary

SECOND EDITION

Oxford New York

OXFORD UNIVERSITY PRESS

OXFORD
UNIVERSITY PRESS

Great Clarendon Street, Oxford OX2 6DP

Oxford University Press is a department of the University of Oxford.
It furthers the University's objective of excellence in research, scholarship,
and education by publishing worldwide in

Oxford New York

Athens Auckland Bangkok Bogotá Buenos Aires Calcutta
Cape Town Chennai Dar es Salaam Delhi Florence Hong Kong Istanbul
Karachi Kuala Lumpur Madrid Melbourne Mexico City Mumbai
Nairobi Paris São Paulo Singapore Taipei Tokyo Toronto Warsaw

with associated companies in Berlin Ibadan

Oxford is a registered trade mark of Oxford University Press
in the UK and in certain other countries

© Market House Books Ltd, 1980, 1985, 1990, 1994, 1998

This colour edition first published as an
Oxford University Press paperback 1996.
Second edition, which uses the text of the fifth edition
of the *Concise Medical Dictionary*, 1998

Reprinted with corrections

British Library Cataloguing in Publication Data

Data available

ISBN 0-19-280085-X

10 9 8 7

Typeset by Market House Books Ltd
Printed in Great Britain by
The Bath Press
Bath

Preface

This dictionary provides full coverage of all the important terms and concepts used in medicine today. Written by a distinguished team of practising specialists and medical writers, it is intended primarily for workers in the paramedical fields: pharmacists, physiotherapists, speech therapists, social workers, hospital secretaries, administrators, technicians, and so on. It will also be invaluable for medical students and practising doctors. Each entry contains a basic definition, followed – where appropriate – by a more detailed explanation or description. A feature of the dictionary is that the articles are written in clear and concise English without the use of unnecessary technical jargon. For this reason the book will also be of both interest and value to the general reader who needs a home medical dictionary.

The dictionary defines terms in anatomy, physiology, biochemistry, and pharmacology, as well as in all the major medical and surgical specialties. Its coverage of psychology and psychiatry, public health medicine, and dentistry is unusually comprehensive, and this edition includes many new entries for imaging and surgical techniques, infertility treatments, accident and emergency medicine, and recently developed drugs. To make room for this additional material, many of the more obscure and obsolescent terms found in the larger medical dictionaries have been omitted. The inclusion of these terms in a dictionary reflecting the practice of modern medicine is of questionable value, and their meanings can be readily derived from definitions of the medical prefixes and suffixes, which are included in this book. To avoid cluttering the entry list with derivative words (e.g. adjectival forms of nouns that are defined), these words are listed at the end of the definitions of the words from which they are derived. Where necessary, articles are supplemented by clear and fully labelled line drawings An asterisk against a word used in a definition indicates that this term has its own entry in the dictionary and that additional information can be found there. Some entries simply refer the reader to another entry, indicating either that they are synonyms or abbreviations or that they – together with related terms – are most conveniently explained in one of the dictionary's longer articles. Synonyms and abbreviations are shown in brackets after the defined term.

E. A. M.
1998

a- (an-) *prefix denoting* absence of; lacking; not. Examples: **amastia** (absence of breasts); **amorphic** (lacking definite form); **atoxic** (not poisonous).

A and E medicine accident and emergency medicine: an important specialty dealing with the immediate problems of the acutely ill and injured.

ab- *prefix denoting* away from. Example: **abembryonic** (away from or opposite the embryo).

abarticulation *n.* **1.** the dislocation of a joint. **2.** a synovial joint (*see* DIARTHROSIS).

abasia *n.* an inability to walk for which no physical cause can be identified. *See also* ASTASIA.

abbreviated injury scale a quick method for determining the severity of a case of serious trauma. It can be used for purposes of *triage and *medical (clinical) audit.

abdomen *n.* the part of the body cavity below the chest (*see* THORAX), from which it is separated by the *diaphragm. The abdomen contains the organs of digestion – stomach, liver, intestines, etc. – and excretion – kidneys, bladder, etc.; in women it also contains the ovaries and uterus. The

regions of the abdomen are shown in the illustration. —**abdominal** *adj.*

abdomin- (abdomino-) *combining form denoting* the abdomen. Examples: **abdominalgia** (pain in the abdomen); **abdomino-thoracic** (relating to the abdomen and thorax).

abducens nerve the sixth *cranial nerve (VI), which supplies the lateral rectus muscle of each eyeball, responsible for turning the eye outwards.

abduct *vb.* to move a limb or any other part away from the midline of the body. —**abduction** *n.*

abductor *n.* any muscle that moves one part of the body away from another or from the midline of the body.

aberrant *adj.* abnormal: usually applied to a blood vessel or nerve that does not follow its normal course.

aberration *n.* (in optics) a defect in the image formed by a lens. In **chromatic aberration** the image formed by a lens has coloured fringes as a result of the different extent to which light of different colours is refracted by glass. It is corrected by using an *achromatic lens. In **spherical aberration**, the image is blurred because rays from the object

right hypochondrium — epigastrium — left hypochondrium

right lumbar — umbilical — left lumbar

right inguinal — hypogastrium — left inguinal

Regions of the abdomen

come to a focus in slightly different positions as a result of the curvature of the lens: the rays passing more peripherally through the lens are bent more than those passing through centrally. This occurs even with monochromatic light.

abiotrophy *n.* degeneration or loss of function without apparent cause; for example, **retinal abiotrophy** is progressive degeneration of the retina leading to impaired vision, occurring in genetic disorders such as *retinitis pigmentosa.

ablatio *n.* separation; abruptio. *See* RETINAL DETACHMENT (ABLATIO RETINAE).

ablation *n.* the removal of tissue, a part of the body, or an abnormal growth, usually by cutting. *See also* ENDOMETRIAL ABLATION.

ablepharia *n.* absence of or reduction in the size of the eyelids.

ablepsia *n.* an obsolete term for *blindness.

abortifacient *n.* a drug that induces abortion or miscarriage. *See* MIFEPRISTONE, PROSTAGLANDIN.

abortion *n.* the expulsion or removal of an embryo or fetus from the uterus at a stage of pregnancy when it is incapable of independent survival (i.e. at any time between conception and the 24th week of pregnancy). In **threatened abortion** there may be abdominal pain and bleeding from the uterus but the fetus is still alive; once the fetus is dead abortion becomes **inevitable**. Abortion is **incomplete** so long as the uterus still contains some of the fetus or its membranes. Abortion may be **spontaneous** or it may be **induced** for medical or social reasons (**termination of pregnancy**). **Habitual** (or **recurrent**) **abortion** is the occurrence of three consecutive pregnancy losses before 20 weeks' gestation, with fetuses weighing under 500 grams. The presence of a uterine abnormality, such as *bicornuate uterus or *cervical incompetence, may account for 10–15% of recurrent abortions.

Procuring or attempting to procure abortion are both criminal offences in the UK unless carried out within the terms of the Abortion Act 1967 and the subsequent Abortion Regulations 1991. Two doctors must agree that termination of pregnancy

is necessary for one of the reasons specified in the Regulations, and the procedure must be carried out in an approved hospital or clinic. Methods in current use include the administration of drugs, e.g. *mifepristone with or without the addition of prostaglandins (e.g. *gemeprost). The surgical methods of termination of pregnancy include vacuum aspiration of the products of conception through an intrauterine cannula, *dilatation and curettage, and uterine evacuation by ovum forceps. Termination carries little risk early in pregnancy, but complications are more likely to occur after the 13th week of pregnancy.

Nonmedical people make a distinction between abortion and **miscarriage**, the former being a procedure deliberately carried out to end the pregnancy, the latter being an accidental occurrence. The medical profession increasingly recognizes this useful distinction.

abortus *n.* a fetus, weighing less than 500 g, that is expelled from the uterus either dead or incapable of surviving.

ABO system *see* BLOOD GROUP.

abrasion *n.* **1.** a graze: a minor wound in which the surface of the skin or a mucous membrane is worn away by rubbing or scraping. **2.** the wearing of the teeth, particularly at the necks by overvigorous brushing. It is frequently enhanced by *erosion. **3.** any rubbing or scraping action that produces surface wear.

abreaction *n.* the release of strong emotion associated with a buried memory. While this can happen spontaneously, it is usually deliberately produced by a therapist using psychotherapy, hypnosis, or drugs such as *thiopentone. The technique is used as a treatment for conversion disorder, anxiety state, and other neurotic conditions, especially when they are thought to be caused by *repression of memories or emotions.

abruptio (ablatio) *n.* separation.

abruptio placentae bleeding from a normally situated placenta causing its complete or partial detachment from the uterine wall after the 24th week of gestation. There may be varying degrees of shock; *hypofibrinogenaemia (a blood coagulation defect) is a further complication. Abruptio placentae is often associated with hypertension and pre-eclampsia.

abscess *n.* a localized collection of pus anywhere in the body, surrounded and walled off by damaged and inflamed tissues. A *boil is an example of an abscess within the skin. The usual cause is local bacterial infection, often by staphylococci, that the body's defences have failed to overcome. In a **cold abscess**, due to tubercle organisms, there is swelling, but little pain or inflammation (as in acute abscesses). Antibiotics, aided by surgical incision to release pus where necessary, are the usual forms of treatment.

The brain and its meninges have a low resistance to infection and a **cerebral abscess** is liable to follow any penetration of these by microorganisms. The condition is fatal unless relieved by aspiration or surgical drainage.

absence *n.* (in neurology) *see* EPILEPSY.

Absidia *n.* a genus of fungi that sometimes cause disease in man (*see* PHYCOMYCOSIS).

absorption *n.* (in physiology) the uptake of fluids or other substances by the tissues of the body. Digested food is absorbed into the blood and lymph from the alimentary canal. Most absorption of food occurs in the small intestine – in the jejunum and ileum – although alcohol is readily absorbed from the stomach. The small intestine is lined with minute finger-like processes (*see* VILLUS), which greatly increase its surface area and therefore the speed at which absorption can take place. *See also* ASSIMILATION, DIGESTION.

abulia *n.* absence or impairment of will power. The individual still has desires but they are not put into action; initiative and energy are lacking. It is commonly a symptom of *schizophrenia.

abutment *n.* (in dentistry) a component of a dental *bridge or *implant.

acalculia *n.* an acquired inability to make simple mathematical calculations. It is a symptom of disease in the *parietal lobe of the brain. *See* GERSTMANN'S SYNDROME.

acantha *n.* **1.** a spine projecting from a *vertebra. **2.** the *backbone.

Acanthamoeba *n.* a genus of amoebae that are commonly found in soil and contaminated water and cause painful corneal infection and ulcers in man, usually resulting from improper sterilization of contact lenses. Acanthamoebae are the most common cause of human corneal infections.

acanthion *n.* the tip of the spine formed where projecting processes of the upper jaw bones (maxillae) meet at the front of the face.

acanthosis *n.* an increase in the number of *prickle cells in the innermost layer of the epidermis, leading to thickening of the epidermis. **Acanthosis nigricans** is believed to be associated with insulin resistance; it is characterized by papillomatous growths, mainly in the armpits, giving the skin a pigmented appearance and a velvety texture. It may be benign or malignant. **Pseudoacanthosis nigricans** is more common and is associated with obesity.

acapnia (hypocapnia) *n.* a condition in which there is an abnormally low concentration of carbon dioxide in the blood. This may be caused by breathing that is exceptionally deep in relation to the physical activity of the individual.

acardia *n.* congenital absence of the heart. The condition may occur in conjoined twins; the twin with the heart controls the circulation for both.

acariasis *n.* an infestation of mites and ticks and the symptoms, for example allergy and dermatitis, that their presence may provoke.

acaricide *n.* any chemical agent used for destroying mites and ticks.

acarid *n.* a *mite or *tick.

Acarina *n.* the group of arthropods that includes the *mites and *ticks.

Acarus (Tyroglyphus) *n.* a genus of mites. The flour mite, *A. siro (T. farinae)*, is nonparasitic, but its presence in flour can cause a severe allergic dermatitis in flour-mill workers.

acatalasia *n.* an inborn lack of the enzyme *catalase, leading to recurrent infections of the gums (gingivitis) and mouth. It is most common in the Japanese.

acceptor *n.* (in biochemistry) a substance that helps to bring about oxidation of a reduced *substrate by accepting hydrogen ions.

accessory nerve (spinal accessory nerve) the eleventh *cranial nerve (XI), which arises from two roots, cranial and spinal. Fibres from the cranial root travel with the nerve for only a short distance before branching to join the vagus and then forming the recurrent laryngeal nerve, which supplies the internal laryngeal muscles. Fibres from the spinal root supply the sternomastoid and trapezius muscles, in the neck region (front and back).

accident *n.* a traumatic incident involving any part of the body. **Accident and emergency (A and E) medicine** is evolving as a specialized area of patient care.

accommodation *n.* adjustment of the shape of the lens to change the focus of the eye. When the ciliary muscle (*see* CILIARY BODY) is relaxed, suspensory ligaments attached to the ciliary body and holding the lens in position are stretched, which causes the lens to be flattened. The eye is then able to focus on distant objects. To focus the eye on near objects the ciliary muscles contract and the tension in the ligaments is thus lowered, allowing the lens to become rounder.

accommodation reaction (convergence reaction) the constriction of the pupil that occurs when an individual focuses on a near object.

accouchement *n.* delivery of a baby. *See also* HYDROSTATIC ACCOUCHEMENT.

acebutolol *n.* a *beta blocker drug commonly used to treat high blood pressure, angina pectoris, and irregular heart rhythms. It is administered by mouth. Possible side-effects include breathing difficulty, especially in asthmatics, and cold hands and feet. Trade name: **Sectral**.

ACE inhibitor angiotensin-converting enzyme inhibitor: any one of a group of drugs used in the treatment of raised blood pressure and heart failure. ACE in-

hibitors act by interfering with the action of the enzyme that converts the inactive *angiotensin I to the powerful artery constrictor angiotensin II. The absence of this substance allows arteries to widen and the blood pressure to drop. ACE inhibitors are administered by mouth; they include *captopril and *enalapril. Possible side-effects include weakness, dizziness, loss of appetite, and skin rashes.

acentric *n.* (in genetics) a chromosome or fragment of a chromosome that has no *centromere. Since acentrics cannot attach to the *spindle they are usually lost during cell division. They are often found in cells damaged by radiation. —**acentric** *adj.*

acephalus *n.* a fetus without a head.

acervulus cerebri a collection of granules of calcium-containing material that is sometimes found within the *pineal gland as its calcification proceeds (normally after the 17th year): 'brain sand'.

acetabulum (cotyloid cavity) *n.* either of the two deep sockets, one on each side of the *hip bone, into which the head of the thigh bone (femur) fits at the *hip joint.

acetaminophen *n. see* PARACETAMOL.

acetazolamide *n.* a *diuretic used in the treatment of glaucoma to reduce the pressure inside the eyeball and also as a preventative for altitude sickness. Side-effects include drowsiness and numbness and tingling of the hands and feet. Trade name: **Diamox**.

acetoacetic acid an organic acid produced in large amounts by the liver under metabolic conditions associated with a high rate of fatty acid oxidation (for example, in starvation). The acetoacetic acid thus formed is subsequently converted to acetone and excreted. *See also* KETONE.

acetohexamide *n.* a *sulphonylurea oral hypoglycaemic drug used in the treatment of noninsulin-dependent *diabetes mellitus. It is administered by mouth; side-effects include headache, dizziness, and nervousness.

acetone *n.* an organic compound that is an intermediate in many bacterial fermentations and is produced by fatty acid oxidation. In certain abnormal conditions (for example, starvation) acetone and other *ketones may accumulate in the blood (see KETOSIS). Acetone is a volatile liquid that is miscible with both fats and water and therefore of great value as a solvent. It is used in chromatography and in the preparation of tissues for enzyme extraction.

acetone body (ketone body) *see* KETONE.

acetonuria *n.* *see* KETONURIA.

acetylcholine *n.* the acetic acid ester of the organic base choline: the *neurotransmitter released at the synapses of parasympathetic nerves and at *neuromuscular junctions. After relaying a nerve impulse, acetylcholine is rapidly broken down by the enzyme *cholinesterase. *Atropine and curare cause muscular paralysis by blocking the action of acetylcholine at muscle membranes; physostigmine and other *anticholinesterases prolong the activity of acetylcholine by blocking cholinesterase.

acetylcysteine *n.* a drug used to break down thick mucous secretions. It is administered as an aerosol, primarily for the treatment of respiratory diseases, such as bronchitis and cystic fibrosis; it is also used to prevent liver damage in paracetamol overdosage. Side effects may include spasm of the bronchial muscles, nausea, vomiting, and fever. Trade names: **Fabrol, Parvolex**.

acetylsalicylic acid *see* ASPIRIN.

achalasia (cardiospasm) *n.* a condition in which the normal muscular activity of the oesophagus (gullet) is disturbed, especially failure of an abnormally strong sphincter at the lower end, which delays the passage of swallowed material. It may occur at any age: symptoms include difficulty in swallowing liquids and solids, slowly increasing over years; sometimes regurgitation of undigested food; and occasionally severe chest pain caused by spasm of the oesophagus. Diagnosis is by a barium X-ray examination and sometimes manometric studies (see MANOMETRY). Treatment is by forceful stretching of the tight lower end of the oesophagus (cardia), by surgical splitting of the muscular ring

in that area (**cardiomyotomy** or **Heller's operation**), or by injecting *botulinum toxin into the sphincter.

Achilles tendon the tendon of the muscles of the calf of the leg (the *gastrocnemius and soleus muscles), situated at the back of the ankle and attached to the calcaneus (heel bone).

achlorhydria *n.* absence of hydrochloric acid in the stomach. Achlorhydria that persists despite large doses of histamine is associated with atrophy of the lining (mucosa) of the stomach. In this condition there is usually an absence of secretion of *intrinsic factor, which will lead to *pernicious anaemia. In some people, however, achlorhydria is not associated with any disease, produces no ill-effects, and needs no treatment.

acholia *n.* absence or deficiency of bile secretion or failure of the bile to enter the alimentary canal (for example, because of an obstructed bile duct).

acholuria *n.* absence of the *bile pigments from the urine, which occurs in some forms of jaundice (**acholuric jaundice**). —**acholuric** *adj.*

achondroplasia *n.* a disorder, inherited as a *dominant characteristic, in which the bones of the arms and legs fail to grow to normal size due to a defect in both cartilage and bone. It results in a type of *dwarfism characterized by short limbs, a normal-sized head and body, and normal intelligence. —**achondroplastic** *adj.*

achromatic *adj.* without colour.

achromatic lenses lenses that are specially designed for use in the eyepieces of microscopes and other scientific instruments. They give clear images, unblurred by the coloured fringes that are produced with ordinary lenses (caused by splitting of the light into different wavelengths).

achromatopsia *n.* the inability to perceive colour. Such complete *colour blindness is very rare and is usually associated with poor *visual acuity; it is usually determined by hereditary factors.

achylia *n.* absence of secretion. The term is usually applied to a nonsecreting stomach (**achylia gastrica**) whose lining (mucosa) is atrophied (*see* ACHLORHYDRIA).

acidaemia *n.* abnormally high blood acidity. This condition may result from an increase in the concentration of acidic substances and/or a decrease in the level of alkaline substances in the blood. *See also* ACIDOSIS. *Compare* ALKALAEMIA.

acid-base balance the balance between the amount of carbonic acid and bicarbonate in the blood, which must be maintained at a constant ratio of 1:20 in order to keep the hydrogen ion concentration of the plasma at a constant value (pH 7.4). Any alteration in this ratio will disturb the acid-base balance of the blood and tissues and cause either *acidosis or *alkalosis. The lungs and the kidneys play an important role in the regulation of the acid-base balance.

acid-etch technique a technique for bonding resin-based materials to the enamel of teeth; it is used to retain and seal the margins of *fillings, to retain brackets of fixed *orthodontic appliances, and to retain resin-based *fissure sealants and adhesive bridges. A porous surface is created by applying phosphoric acid for one minute or less.

acid-fast *adj.* **1.** describing bacteria that have been stained and continue to hold the stain after treatment with an acidic solution. For example, tuberculosis bacteria are acid-fast when stained with a *carbol fuchsin preparation. **2.** describing a stain that is not removed from a specimen by washing with an acidic solution.

acidophil (acidophilic) *adj.* **1.** (in histology) describing tissues, cells, or parts of cells that stain with acid dyes (such as eosin). **2.** (in bacteriology) describing bacteria that grow well in acid media.

acidosis *n.* a condition in which the acidity of body fluids and tissues is abnormally high. This arises because of a failure of the mechanisms responsible for maintaining a balance between acids and alkalis in the blood (*see* ACID-BASE BALANCE). In **gaseous acidosis** more than the normal amount of carbon dioxide is retained in the body, as in drowning. In **renal acidosis**, kidney failure results in excessive loss of bicarbonate or retention of phosphoric

and sulphuric acids. Patients with diabetes mellitus suffer from a form of acidosis in which sodium, potassium, and *ketone bodies are lost in the urine.

acinus *n.* (*pl.* **acini**) **1.** a small sac or cavity surrounded by the secretory cells of a gland. Some authorities regard the term as synonymous with *alveolus, but others distinguish an acinus by the possession of a narrow passage (lumen) leading from the sac. **2.** (in the lung) the tissue supplied with air by one terminal *bronchiole. *Emphysema is classified by the part of the acinus involved (i.e. **centriacinar, panacinar,** or **periacinar**). —**acinous** *adj.*

acitretin *n.* *see* RETINOID.

aclarubicin *n.* an *antimitotic drug administered by injection in the treatment of leukaemia and other cancers. It is an *anthracycline antibiotic; possible side-effects include nausea and vomiting, loss of hair, and damage to bone marrow. Trade name: **Aclacin**.

aclasis *n.* *see* DIAPHYSIAL ACLASIS.

acne (acne vulgaris) *n.* a common inflammatory disorder of the sebaceous glands. These grease-producing glands are under androgen control, but the cause of acne is unknown. It involves the face, back, and chest and is characterized by the presence of blackheads with papules, pustules, and – in more severe cases – cysts and scars. Acne is readily treatable. Mild cases respond to topical therapy with *benzoyl peroxide, while more refractory conditions require treatment with long-term antibiotics or (for treating women only) *anti-androgens, such as Dianette (cyproterone and ethinyloestradiol); severe or cystic acne can be treated with *isotretinoin.

aconite *n.* the dried roots of the herbaceous plant *Aconitum napellus* (monkshood or wolfbane), containing three *analgesic substances: **aconine, aconitine,** and **picraconitine**. Aconite was formerly used to prepare liniments for muscular pains and a tincture for toothache, but is regarded as too toxic for use today.

acoustic *adj.* of or relating to sound or the sense of hearing.

acoustic holography a technique of

building up a three-dimensional picture of structures within the body using *ultrasound waves. Two separate sound sources cause ultrasound waves to be transmitted through and reflected from the organs being examined. The interference patterns produced on a liquid surface are illuminated by laser light and photographed to form a **hologram**.

acoustic nerve *see* VESTIBULOCOCHLEAR NERVE.

acquired *adj.* describing a condition or disorder contracted after birth and not attributable to hereditary causes. *Compare* CONGENITAL.

acquired immune deficiency syndrome *see* AIDS.

acrania *n.* congenital absence of the skull, either partial or complete, due to a developmental defect.

acriflavine *n.* a dye used in antiseptic skin preparations and to disinfect contaminated wounds. It may cause sensitivity of the skin to sunlight.

acrivastine *n.* an *antihistamine drug used to treat hay fever and urticaria (nettle rash). It is administered by mouth. Possible side-effects include drowsiness. Trade name: **Semprex**.

acro- *prefix denoting* **1.** extremity; tip. Example: **acrohypotharmy** (abnormal coldness of the extremities (hands and feet)). **2.** height; promontory. Example: **acrophobia** (morbid dread of heights). **3.** extreme; intense. Example: **acromania** (an extreme degree of mania).

acrocentric *n.* a chromosome in which the *centromere is situated at or very near one end. —**acrocentric** *adj.*

acrocyanosis *n.* bluish-purple discoloration of the hands and feet due to slow circulation of the blood through the small vessels in the skin.

acrodermatitis *n.* inflammation of the skin of the feet or hands. A diffuse chronic variety produces swelling and reddening of the affected areas, followed by atrophy. The cause is unknown and there is no treatment.

acrodynia *n. see* PINK DISEASE.

acromegaly *n.* increase in size of the hands, feet, and the face due to excessive production of *growth hormone (somatotrophin) by a tumour of the anterior pituitary gland. The tumour can be treated with X-rays or surgically removed. *See also* GIGANTISM.

acromion *n.* an oblong process at the top of the spine of the *scapula, part of which articulates with the clavicle (collar bone) to form the **acromioclavicular joint**. —**acromial** *adj.*

acroparaesthesiae *pl. n.* tingling sensations in the hands and feet. *See* PARAESTHESIAE.

acrosclerosis *n.* a skin disease thought to be a type of generalized *scleroderma. It also has features of *Raynaud's disease, with the hands, face, and feet being mainly affected.

acrosome *n.* the caplike structure on the front end of a spermatozoon. It breaks down just before fertilization (the **acrosome reaction**), releasing a number of enzymes that assist penetration between the follicle cells that still surround the ovum. Failure of the acrosome reaction is a cause of male infertility (*see also* ANDROLOGY).

acrylic resin one of a group of polymeric materials used for making denture teeth, denture bases, and formerly as a dental filling material.

ACTH (adrenocorticotrophic hormone, adrenocorticotrophin, corticotrophin) a hormone synthesized and stored in the anterior pituitary gland, large amounts of which are released in response to any form of stress. ACTH controls the secretion of *corticosteroid hormones from the adrenal gland. It is administered by injection to test adrenal function and to treat conditions such as rheumatic diseases (especially in children) and asthma.

actin *n.* a protein, found in muscle, that plays an important role in the process of contraction. *See* STRIATED MUSCLE.

Actinobacillus *n.* a genus of Gram-negative nonmotile aerobic bacteria that are characteristically spherical or rodlike in shape but occasionally grow into branching filaments. Actinobacilli cause disease in animals that can be transmitted to man.

Actinomyces *n.* a genus of Gram-positive nonmotile fungus-like bacteria that cause disease in animals and man. The species *A. israelii* is the causative organism of human *actinomycosis.

actinomycin *n.* a *cytotoxic drug, produced by *Streptomyces* bacteria, that inhibits the growth of cancer cells. There are two forms, both of which are administered by injection. Actinomycin C may damage bone marrow. Actinomycin D (Cosmegen, Lyovac) may cause nausea, vomiting, diarrhoea, blood disorders, and bone-marrow damage.

actinomycosis *n.* a noncontagious disease caused by the bacterium *Actinomyces israelii*, which most commonly affects the jaw but may also affect the lungs, brain, or intestines. The bacterium is normally present in the mouth but it may become pathogenic following an *apical abscess or extraction of a tooth. It is characterized by multiple sinuses that open onto the skin. Treatment is by drainage of pus and a prolonged course of antibiotics.

actinotherapy *n.* the treatment of disorders with *infrared or *ultraviolet radiation.

action potential the change in voltage that occurs across the membrane of a nerve or muscle cell when a *nerve impulse is triggered. It is due to the passage of charged particles across the membrane (*see* DEPOLARIZATION) and is an observable manifestation of the passage of an impulse.

active transport (in biochemistry) an energy-dependent process in which certain substances (including ions, some drugs, and amino acids) are able to cross cell membranes against a concentration gradient. The process is inhibited by substances that interfere with cellular metabolism (e.g. high doses of digitalis).

actomyosin *n.* a protein complex formed in muscle between actin and myosin during the process of contraction. *See* STRIATED MUSCLE.

acupuncture *n.* a traditional Chinese system of healing in which symptoms are relieved by thin metal needles inserted into selected points beneath the skin. The needles are stimulated either by rotation or, more recently, by an electric current. Hypotheses suggest that the needling activates deep sensory nerves, which cause the pituitary and midbrain to release *endorphins – the brain's natural pain-killers. Acupuncture is widely used in the Far East for the relief of pain and in China itself it has become an alternative to anaesthesia for some major operations. Acupuncturists in the West may be medically qualified but many are not.

acute *adj.* **1.** describing a disease of rapid onset, severe symptoms, and brief duration. *Compare* CHRONIC. **2.** describing any intense symptom, such as severe pain.

acute abdomen an emergency surgical condition caused by damage to one or more abdominal organs following injury or disease. The patient is in severe pain and often in shock. Perforation of a peptic ulcer or a severely infected appendix, or rupture of the liver or spleen following a crushing injury, all produce an acute abdomen requiring urgent treatment.

acute retinal necrosis (ARN) severe inflammation and necrosis of the retina associated with inflammation and blockage of retinal blood vessels, haemorrhage and death of retinal tissue, and retinal detachment. It may affect both eyes (**bilateral acute retinal necrosis, BARN**), and visual prognosis is poor. ARN is thought to be due to viral infection.

acute rheumatism *see* RHEUMATIC FEVER.

acyclovir *n.* an antiviral drug that inhibits DNA synthesis in cells infected by *herpesviruses. Administered topically, by mouth, or intravenously, it is used in patients whose immune systems are disturbed and also in the treatment of herpes zoster, genital herpes, herpetic eye disease, and herpes encephalitis. Trade name: **Zovirax**.

ad-.*prefix denoting* towards or near. Examples: **adaxial** (towards the main axis); **adoral** (towards or near the mouth).

ADA deficiency *see* ADENOSINE DEAMINASE DEFICIENCY.

Adam's apple (laryngeal prominence) a projection, lying just under the skin, of the thyroid cartilage of the *larynx.

Adams-Stokes syndrome see STOKES-ADAMS SYNDROME.

adaptation n. the phenomenon in which a sense organ shows a gradually diminishing response to continuous or repetitive stimulation. The nose, for example, may become adapted to the stimulus of an odour that is continuously present so that in time it ceases to report its presence. Similarly, the adaptation of touch receptors in the skin means that the presence of clothes can be forgotten a few minutes after they have been put on.

ADD see ATTENTION DEFICIT DISORDER.

addiction n. a state of *dependence produced by the habitual taking of drugs. Strictly speaking, the term implies the state of physical dependence induced by such drugs as morphine, heroin, and alcohol, but it is also used for the state of psychological dependence, produced by drugs such as barbiturates. Treatment is aimed at gradual withdrawal of the drug and eventually total abstention. See also ALCOHOLISM, TOLERANCE.

Addison's disease a syndrome due to inadequate secretion of corticosteroid hormones by the *adrenal glands, sometimes as a result of tuberculous infection. Symptoms include weakness, loss of energy, low blood pressure, and dark pigmentation of the skin. Formerly fatal, the disease is now treatable by replacement hormone therapy. [T. Addison (1793–1860), British physician]

adduct vb. to move a limb or any other part towards the midline of the body. —**adduction** n.

adductor n. any muscle that moves one part of the body towards another or towards the midline of the body.

aden- (adeno-) prefix denoting a gland or glands. Examples: **adenalgia** (pain in); **adenogenesis** (development of); **adenopathy** (disease of).

adenine n. one of the nitrogen-containing bases (see PURINE) that occurs in the nucleic acids DNA and RNA. See also ATP.

adenitis n. inflammation of a gland or group of glands (or glandlike structures). For example, **mesenteric adenitis** affects the lymph nodes (formerly called lymph glands) in the membranous support of the intestines (the mesentery); **cervical adenitis** affects the lymph nodes in the neck.

adenocarcinoma n. a malignant epithelial tumour arising from glandular structures, which are constituent parts of most organs of the body. The term is also applied to tumours showing a glandular growth pattern. These tumours may be subclassified according to the substances that they produce, for example **mucussecreting** and **serous adenocarcinomas**, or to the microscopic arrangement of their cells into patterns, for example **papillary** and **follicular adenocarcinomas**. They may be solid or cystic (**cystadenocarcinomas**). Each organ may produce tumours showing a variety of histological types; for example, the ovary may produce both mucinous and serous cystadenocarcinomas.

adenohypophysis n. the anterior lobe of the *pituitary gland.

adenoidectomy n. surgical removal of the *adenoids in patients who suffer from either *glue ear or difficulty in breathing through the nose.

adenoids (nasopharyngeal tonsil) n. the collection of lymphatic tissue at the rear of the nose. Enlargement of the adenoids can cause obstruction to breathing through the nose and can block the Eustachian tubes, causing *glue ear.

adenolymphoma n. see WARTHIN'S TUMOUR.

adenoma n. a benign tumour of epithelial origin that is derived from glandular tissue or exhibits clearly defined glandular structures. Adenomas may undergo malignant change (see ADENOCARCINOMA). Some show recognizable tissue elements, such as fibrous tissue (**fibroadenomas**), while others, such as some bronchial adenomas, produce active compounds giving rise to clinical syndromes (see ARGENTAFFINOMA). Tumours in certain organs, including the pituitary gland, are often classified by their histological staining affinities, for example **eosinophil, basophil,** and **chromophobe adenomas.**

adenomyosis *n. see* ENDOMETRIOSIS.

adenosine *n.* a compound containing adenine and the sugar ribose: it occurs in ATP. *See also* NUCLEOSIDE.

adenosine deaminase deficiency (ADA deficiency) a genetic disorder affecting about one baby in 25,000 and characterized by a defect in **adenosine deaminase (ADA),** an enzyme that is involved in purine metabolism. Deficiency of this enzyme results in selective damage to the antibody-producing lymphocytes; this in turn leads to a condition known as *severe combined immune deficiency (SCID), in which the affected baby has no resistance to infection and must be entirely isolated from birth. Such children have only about a 50% chance of surviving for six months. *See also* GENE THERAPY.

adenosine diphosphate *see* ADP.

adenosine monophosphate *see* AMP.

adenosine triphosphate *see* ATP.

adenosis *n.* (*pl.* **adenoses**) **1.** excessive growth or development of glands. **2.** any disease of a gland or glandlike structure, especially of a lymph node.

adenovirus *n.* one of a group of DNA-containing viruses causing infections of the upper respiratory tract that produce symptoms resembling those of the common cold.

Adept *n.* antibody-directed enzyme prodrug therapy: a method under development for the treatment of cancer. It involves the patient being injected first with an antibody-enzyme complex that binds specifically to tumour cells, and later with a **pro-drug,** which is inactive until it comes into contact with the antibody-enzyme complex. The enzyme converts the pro-drug into a *cytotoxic form, which is concentrated around the tumour and can therefore destroy the cancer cells without damaging normal tissue.

adhesion *n.* **1.** the union of two normally separate surfaces, such as the moving surfaces of joints, by fibrous connective tissue developing in an inflamed or damaged region. (The fibrous

tissue itself is also called an adhesion.) Adhesions between loops of intestine often occur following abdominal surgery but only rarely cause symptoms, such as intestinal obstruction. If the pericardial sac is affected by adhesion, the movements of the heart may be restricted. **2.** a healing process in which the edges of a wound fit together. In **primary adhesion** there is very little *granulation tissue; in **secondary adhesion** the two edges are joined together by granulation tissue.

adhesion molecules *cell-surface molecules that are important for binding cells to neighbouring cells (**intercellular adhesion molecules, ICMA**) and tissues. Absence or weakening of intercellular binding facilitates the local spread of cancer.

adiadochokinesis *n. see* DYSDIADOCHOKINESIS.

Adie's pupil *see* TONIC PUPIL. [W. J. Adie (1886–1935), British physician]

Adie's syndrome (Holmes-Adie syndrome) an abnormality of the pupils of the eyes, often affecting only one eye. The affected pupil is dilated and reacts slowly to light; the response on convergence of the eyes is also slow (*see* TONIC PUPIL). One or more tendon reflexes may be absent. The condition is almost entirely restricted to women. [W. J. Adie; Sir G. M. Holmes (1876–1965), British neurologist]

adipocere *n.* a waxlike substance, consisting mainly of fatty acids, into which the soft tissues of the body can be converted after death. This usually occurs when the body is buried in damp earth or is submerged in water. Adipocere delays post-mortem decomposition and is a spontaneous form of preservation without mummification.

adipocyte *n. see* ADIPOSE TISSUE.

adipose tissue fibrous *connective tissue packed with masses of fat cells (**adipocytes**). It forms a thick layer under the skin and occurs around the kidneys and in the buttocks. It serves both as an insulating layer and an energy store; food in excess of requirements is converted into fats and stored within these cells.

adiposis (liposis) *n.* the presence of abnormally large accumulations of fat in the body. The condition may arise from overeating, hormone irregularities, or a metabolic disorder. In **adiposis dolorosa**, a condition affecting women more commonly than men, painful fatty swellings are associated with defects in the nervous system. *See also* OBESITY.

aditus *n.* an anatomical opening or passage; for example, the opening of the tympanic cavity (middle ear) to the air spaces of the mastoid process.

adjuvant *n.* any substance used in conjunction with another to enhance its activity. Aluminium salts are used as adjuvants in the preparation of vaccines from the toxins of diphtheria and tetanus: by keeping the toxins in precipitated form, the salts increase the efficacy of the toxins as antigens.

adjuvant therapy *cytotoxic drug treatment given to patients after surgical removal of, or radiotherapy to, their primary tumour when there is known to be a high risk of future tumour recurrence arising from *micrometastases. Adjuvant therapy is aimed at destroying these secondary tumours and is recommended for patients with breast cancer, colorectal cancer, and other types of cancer. *Compare* NEOADJUVANT CHEMOTHERAPY.

adnexa *pl. n.* adjoining parts. For example, the **uterine adnexa** are the Fallopian tubes and ovaries (which adjoin the uterus).

adolescence *n.* the stage of development between childhood and adulthood. It begins with the start of *puberty, which in girls is usually at the age of about 12 and in boys about 14.

ADP (adenosine diphosphate) a compound containing adenine, ribose, and two phosphate groups. ADP occurs in cells and is involved in processes requiring the transfer of energy (*see* ATP).

adrenal glands (suprarenal glands) two triangular *endocrine glands, each of which covers the superior surface of a kidney. Each gland has two parts, the **medulla** and **cortex**. The medulla forms the grey core of the gland; it consists mainly of *chromaffin tissue and is stimulated by the sympathetic nervous system to produce *adrenaline and *noradrenaline. The cortex is a yellowish tissue surrounding the medulla. It is derived embryologically from mesoderm and is stimulated by pituitary hormones (principally *ACTH) to produce three kinds of *corticosteroid hormones, which affect carbohydrate metabolism (e.g. *cortisol), electrolyte metabolism (e.g. *aldosterone), and the sex glands (oestrogens and androgens).

adrenaline (epinephrine) *n.* an important hormone secreted by the medulla of the adrenal gland. It has the function of preparing the body for 'fright, flight, or fight' and has widespread effects on circulation, the muscles, and sugar metabolism. The action of the heart is increased, the rate and depth of breathing are increased, and the metabolic rate is raised; the force of muscular contraction improves and the onset of muscular fatigue is delayed. At the same time the blood supply to the bladder and intestines is reduced, their muscular walls relax, and the sphincters contract. *Sympathetic nerves were originally thought to act by releasing adrenaline at their endings, and were therefore called **adrenergic** nerves. In fact the main substance released is the related substance *noradrenaline, which also forms a portion of the adrenal secretion.

Adrenaline given by injection is valuable for the relief of bronchial asthma, because it relaxes constricted airways. It is also used during surgery or by injection through an endoscope to reduce blood loss by constricting vessels in the skin or mucous membranes. It is included in some local anaesthetic solutions, particularly those used in dentistry, to prolong anaesthesia.

adrenergic *adj.* **1.** describing nerve fibres that release *noradrenaline as a neurotransmitter. **2.** describing *receptors at which noradrenaline acts to pass on messages from sympathetic nerves. *Compare* CHOLINERGIC.

adrenocorticotrophic hormone (adrenocorticotrophin) *see* ACTH.

adrenogenital syndrome a hormonal disorder resulting from abnormal steroid production by the adrenal cortex, due to a genetic fault. It may cause masculinization in girls, precocious puberty in boys, and adrenocortical failure (see ADDISON'S DISEASE) in both sexes. Treatment is by lifelong steroid replacement.

adrenoleukodystrophy n. a genetically determined condition of neurological degeneration with childhood and adult forms. It is characterized by progressive *spastic paralysis of the legs and sensory loss, associated with adrenal gland insufficiency and small gonads. The demonstration of abnormal fatty-acid metabolism has implications for future possible drug therapies. *Prenatal diagnosis is possible.

adrenolytic adj. inhibiting the activity of *adrenergic nerves. Adrenolytic activity is opposite to that of *adrenaline.

adult respiratory distress syndrome (ARDS) a form of acute respiratory failure that occurs after a precipitating event, such as trauma, aspiration, or inhalation of a toxic substance; it is particularly associated with septic shock. Lung injury is characterized by reduced oxygen in the arteries, reduced lung volume, and decreased lung compliance, and diffuse infiltrates are seen on a chest X-ray. Treatment is correction of the original cause, volume replacement, diuretics, oxygen, and mechanical ventilation.

advancement n. the detachment by surgery of a muscle, musculocutaneous flap, or tendon from its normal attachment site and its reattachment at a more advanced (anterior) point. The technique is used, for example, in the treatment of squint and extensively in plastic surgery to cover large defects (see also PEDICLE).

adventitia (tunica adventitia) n. **1.** the outer coat of the wall of a *vein or *artery. It consists of loose connective tissue and networks of small blood vessels, which nourish the walls. **2.** the outer covering of various other organs or parts.

adventitious adj. **1.** occurring in a place other than the usual one. **2.** relating to the adventitia.

Aëdes n. a genus of widely distributed mosquitoes occurring throughout the tropics and subtropics. Most species are black with distinct white or silvery-yellow markings on the legs and thorax. Aëdes species are not only important as vectors

of *dengue, *yellow fever, *filariasis, and Group B viruses causing encephalitis but also constitute a serious biting nuisance. A. aegypti is the principal vector of dengue and yellow fever.

aegophony n. see VOCAL RESONANCE.

-aemia suffix denoting a specified biochemical condition of the blood. Example: **hyperglycaemia** (excess sugar in the blood).

aer- (aero-) prefix denoting air or gas. Examples: **aerogastria** (gas in the stomach); **aerogenesis** (production of gas).

aerobe n. any organism, especially a microbe, that requires the presence of free oxygen for life and growth. See also ANAEROBE, MICROAEROPHILIC.

aerobic adj. **1.** of or relating to aerobes: requiring free oxygen for life and growth. **2.** describing a type of cellular *respiration in which foodstuffs (carbohydrates) are completely oxidized by atmospheric oxygen, with the production of maximum chemical energy from the foodstuffs.

aerobic exercises see EXERCISE.

aerodontalgia n. pain in the teeth due to change in atmospheric pressure during air travel or the ascent of a mountain.

aeroneurosis n. a syndrome of anxiety, agitation, and insomnia found in pilots flying unpressurized aircraft and attributed to *anoxia.

aerophagy n. the swallowing of air. This may be done voluntarily to stimulate belching, accidentally during rapid eating or drinking, or unconsciously as a habit. Voluntary aerophagy is used to permit oesophageal speech after surgical removal of the larynx (usually for cancer).

aerosol n. a suspension of extremely small liquid or solid particles (about 0.001 mm diameter) in the air. Drugs in aerosol form may be administered by inhalation.

aetiology (etiology) n. **1.** the study or science of the causes of disease. **2.** the cause of a specific disease.

afebrile adj. without, or not showing any signs of, a fever.

affect n. (in psychiatry) **1.** the predominant emotion in a person's mental state. **2.** the emotion associated with a particular idea. —**affective** adj.

affective disorder any psychiatric disorder featuring abnormalities of mood or emotion (*affect). The most serious of these are *depression and *mania. Other affective disorders include *SADS (seasonal affective disorder syndrome).

afferent adj. **1.** designating nerves or neurones that convey impulses from sense organs and other receptors to the brain or spinal cord, i.e. any sensory nerve or neurone. **2.** designating blood vessels that feed a capillary network in an organ or part. **3.** designating lymphatic vessels that enter a lymph node. *Compare* EFFERENT.

afibrinogenaemia n. complete absence of the coagulation factor *fibrinogen in the blood. *Compare* HYPOFIBRINOGENAEMIA.

aflatoxin n. a poisonous substance produced in the spores of the fungus *Aspergillus flavus*, which infects peanuts. The toxin is known to produce cancer in certain animals and is suspected of being the cause of liver cancers in human beings living in warm and humid regions of the world, where stored nuts and cereals are contaminated by the fungus.

afterbirth n. the placenta, umbilical cord, and ruptured membranes associated with the fetus, which normally become detached from the uterus and expelled within a few hours of birth.

aftercare long-term surveillance as an adjunct or supplement to formal medical treatment of those who are chronically sick or disabled, including those with mental illness or learning disability. Aftercare includes the provision of special aids and the adaptation of homes to improve daily living.

after-image n. an impression of an image that is registered by the brain for a brief moment after an object is removed from in front of the eye, or after the eye is closed.

afterpains pl. n. pains caused by uterine contractions after childbirth, especially during breast feeding, due to release of the hormone *oxytocin. The contractions help restore the uterus to its nonpregnant

size and are more common in women who have given birth twice or more.

agammaglobulinaemia n. a total deficiency of the plasma protein *gammaglobulin. *Compare* HYPOGAMMAGLOBULIN-AEMIA.

agar n. an extract of certain seaweeds that forms a gel suitable for the solidification of liquid bacteriological *culture media. **Blood agar** is nutrient agar containing 5–10% horse blood, used for the cultivation of certain bacteria or for detecting haemolytic (blood-destroying) activity.

Age Concern (in Britain) a voluntary agency with particular interest in the problems of the aged.

agenesis n. absence of an organ, usually due to total failure of its development in the embryo.

age-related macular degeneration (AMD, ARMD) *see* MACULAR DEGENERATION.

agglutination (clumping) n. the sticking together, by serum antibodies called **agglutinins**, of such microscopic antigenic particles as red blood cells or bacteria so that they form visible clumps. Any substance that stimulates the body to produce an agglutinin is called an **agglutinogen**. Agglutination is a specific reaction: in the laboratory, sera containing different known agglutinins provide an invaluable means of identifying unknown bacteria. When blood of different groups is mixed, agglutination occurs because serum contains natural antibodies (**isoagglutinins**) that attack red cells of a foreign group, whether previously encountered or not. This is not the same process as occurs in *blood coagulation.

agglutinin n. an antibody that brings about the *agglutination of bacteria, blood cells, or other antigenic particles.

agglutinogen n. any antigen that provokes formation of an agglutinin in the serum and is therefore likely to be involved in *agglutination.

aglossia n. congenital absence of the tongue.

agnathia *n.* congenital absence of the lower jaw, either partial or complete.

agnosia *n.* a disorder of the brain whereby the patient cannot interpret sensations correctly although the sense organs and nerves conducting sensation to the brain are functioning normally. It is due to a disorder of the *association areas in the parietal lobes. In **auditory agnosia** the patient can hear but cannot interpret sounds (including speech). A patient with **tactile agnosia (astereognosis)** retains normal sensation in his hands but cannot recognize three-dimensional objects by touch alone. In **visual agnosia** the patient can see but cannot interpret symbols, including letters (*see* ALEXIA).

agonal *adj.* describing or relating to the phenomena, such as cessation of breathing or change in the ECG or EEG, that are associated with the moment of death.

agonist *n.* **1. (prime mover)** a muscle whose active contraction causes movement of a part of the body. Contraction of an agonist is associated with relaxation of its *antagonist. **2.** a drug or other substance that acts at a cell-receptor site to produce an effect that is the same as, or similar to, that of the body's normal chemical messenger. Cholinergic drugs (*see* PARASYMPATHOMIMETIC) are examples.

agoraphobia *n.* a morbid fear of public places and/or of open spaces. *Compare* CLAUSTROPHOBIA. *See also* PHOBIA.

agranulocytosis *n.* a disorder in which there is a severe acute deficiency of certain blood cells (*neutrophils) as a result of damage to the bone marrow by toxic drugs or chemicals. It is characterized by fever, with ulceration of the mouth and throat, and may lead rapidly to prostration and death. Treatment is by the administration of antibiotics in large quantities. When feasible, transfusion of white blood cells may be life-saving.

agraphia (dysgraphia) *n.* an acquired inability to write, although the strength and coordination of the hand remain normal. It is related to the disorders of language and it is caused by disease in the *parietal lobe of the brain. *See* GERSTMANN'S SYNDROME.

agromania *n.* a pathologically strong impulse to live alone in open country.

ague *n. see* MALARIA.

AIDS (acquired immune deficiency syndrome) a syndrome first identified in Los Angeles in 1981; a description of the causative virus – the human immunodeficiency virus (HIV) – was available in 1983. The virus destroys a subgroup of lymphocytes, the *helper T-cells (or *CD4 lymphocytes), resulting in suppression of the body's immune response (*see* IMMUNITY). AIDS is essentially a sexually transmitted disease, either homosexually or heterosexually. The two other main routes of spread are via infected blood or blood products (current processing of blood for transfusion and for haemophiliacs has virtually eliminated this danger) and by the maternofetal route. The virus may be transmitted from an infected mother to the child in the uterus or it may be acquired from maternal blood during parturition; it may also be transmitted in breast milk.

Acute infection following exposure to the virus results in the production of antibodies (seroconversion), their presence indicating that infection has taken place. However, not all those who *seroconvert progress to chronic infection. For those who do enter a chronic stage there may be illness of varying severity, including persistent generalized involvement of the lymph nodes; what is termed **AIDS-related complex (ARC)**, including intermittent fever, weight loss, diarrhoea, fatigue, and night sweats; and AIDS itself, presenting as opportunistic infections (especially pneumonia caused by the protozoan *Pneumocystis carinii*) and/or tumours, such as *Kaposi's sarcoma.

HIV has been isolated from semen, cervical secretions, plasma, cerebrospinal fluid, tears, saliva, urine, and breast milk but the concentration shows wide variations. Moreover HIV is a fragile virus and does not survive well outside the body. It is therefore considered that ordinary social contact with HIV-positive subjects involves no risk of infection. However, high standards of clinical practice are required by all health workers in order to avoid inadvertent infection via blood, blood products, or body fluids from HIV-positive people. Staff who become HIV-positive are expected to declare their status and will be counselled.

Until recently, AIDS has been considered to be universally fatal, although the type and length of illness preceding death varies considerably. The development of antiviral drugs, initially used singly but more recently used in dual or triple combinations, may well modify the gloomy outlook. These drugs include *zidovudine (AZT), *didanosine (ddI), *zalcitabine (ddC), lamivudine (3TC), stavudine (D4T), and the recently developed *protease inhibitors.

AIH see ARTIFICIAL INSEMINATION.

ainhum n. loss of one or more toes due to slow growth of a fibrous band around the toe that eventually causes a spontaneous amputation. The condition is found in Black Africans and is associated with going barefoot.

air bed a bed with a mattress whose upper surface is perforated with thousands of holes, through which air is forced under pressure. The patient is thus supported, like a hovercraft, on a cushion of air. This type of bed is invaluable for the treatment of patients with large areas of burns.

air embolism an air lock that obstructs the outflow of blood from the right ventricle of the heart. Air may gain access to the circulation as a result of surgery, injury, or intravenous infusions. The patient experiences breathlessness and chest discomfort and develops acute heart failure. Tipping the patient head down, lying on the left side, may move the air lock.

air sickness see MOTION SICKNESS.

akathisia n. a pattern of involuntary movements induced by antipsychotic drugs, such as *phenothiazines. An affected person is driven to restless overactivity, which can be confused with the agitation for which the drug was originally prescribed.

akinesia n. a loss of normal muscular tonicity or responsiveness. In **akinetic epilepsy** there is a sudden loss of muscular tonicity, making the patient fall with momentary loss of consciousness. **Akinetic mutism** is a state of complete physical unresponsiveness although the patient's eyes

remain open and appear to follow movements. It is a consequence of damage to the base of the brain. —**akinetic** adj.

ala n. (pl. **alae**) (in anatomy) a winglike structure; for example, either of the two lateral flared portions of the external nose or the winglike expansion of the ilium.

alactasia n. absence or deficiency of the enzyme lactase, which is essential for the digestion of milk sugar (lactose). All babies have lactase in their intestines, but the enzyme disappears during childhood in about 10% of northern Europeans, 40% of Greeks and Italians, and 80% of Africans and Asians. Alactasia causes symptoms only if the diet regularly includes raw milk, when the undigested lactose causes diarrhoea and abdominal pain.

alanine n. see AMINO ACID.

alastrim n. a mild form of smallpox, causing only a sparse rash and low-grade fever. Medical name: **variola minor**.

albendazole n. an *anthelmintic drug used to get rid of roundworms, hookworms, and other worm parasites. It is administered by mouth. Possible side-effects include headache, dizziness, fever, skin rashes, and loss of hair. Trade name: **Eskazole**.

Albers-Schönberg disease see OSTEO-PETROSIS. [H. E. Albers-Schönberg (1865–1921), German radiologist]

albinism n. the inherited absence of pigmentation in the skin, hair, and eyes, resulting in white hair and pink skin and eyes. The pink colour is produced by blood in underlying blood vessels, which are normally masked by pigment. Ocular signs are reduced visual acuity, sensitivity to light (see PHOTOPHOBIA), and involuntary side-to-side eye movements.

albino n. an individual lacking the normal body pigment (melanin). See ALBINISM.

albumin n. a protein that is soluble in water and coagulated by heat. An example is **serum albumin**, which is found in blood plasma and is important for the maintenance of plasma volume. Albumin is synthesized in the liver; the inability to synthesize it is a prominent feature of chronic liver disease (*cirrhosis).

albuminuria (proteinuria) *n.* the presence of serum albumin, serum globulin, or other serum proteins in the urine. This may be associated with kidney or heart disease. Albuminuria is not always associated with disease: it may occur after strenuous exercise or after a long period of standing (**orthostatic albuminuria**).

albumose *n.* a substance, intermediate between albumin and peptones, produced during the digestion of proteins by pepsin and other endopeptidases (*see* PEPTIDASE).

alcaptonuria (alkaptonuria) *n.* the congenital absence of an enzyme, homogentisic acid oxidase, that is essential for the normal breakdown of the amino acids tyrosine and phenylalanine. Accumulation of *homogentisic acid causes dark brown discoloration of the skin and eyes (**ochronosis**) and progressive damage to the joints, especially of the spine. The gene responsible for the condition is recessive, so that a child is affected only if both parents are carriers of the defective gene.

alclometazone *n.* a *corticosteroid drug administered externally as a cream or ointment to treat inflammatory skin disorders. Possible side-effects include skin thinning and allergic reactions. Trade name: **Modrasone**.

alcohol *n.* any of a class of organic compounds formed when a hydroxyl group (–OH) is substituted for a hydrogen atom in a hydrocarbon. The alcohol in alcoholic drinks is **ethyl alcohol** (**ethanol**), which has the formula C_2H_5OH. It is produced by the fermentation of sugar by yeast. 'Pure' alcohol contains not less than 94.9% by volume of ethyl alcohol. It is obtained by distillation. A solution of 70% alcohol can be used as a preservative or antiseptic. When taken into the body ethyl alcohol depresses activity of the central nervous system (*see also* ALCOHOLISM). *Methyl alcohol (methanol) is extremely poisonous.

Alcoholics Anonymous a voluntary agency of self-help that is organized and operated locally among those with alcoholic dependency and has national and international support. Members are expected to admit to their drink problems, discuss these openly and frankly at the regular meetings of the group, and also to take part in efficient family support schemes to help those members who have lapses.

alcoholism *n.* the syndrome due to physical *dependence on alcohol, such that sudden deprivation may cause withdrawal symptoms – tremor, anxiety, hallucinations, and delusions (*see* DELIRIUM TREMENS). The risk of alcoholism for an individual and its incidence in a society depend on the amount drunk. Countries such as France, where heavy drinking is socially acceptable, have the highest incidence. Usually several years' heavy drinking is needed for addiction to develop, but the range is from one to 40 years. Alcoholism impairs intellectual function, physical skills, memory, and judgment: social skills, such as conversation, are preserved until a late stage. Heavy consumption of alcohol also causes *cardiomyopathy, peripheral *neuritis, *cirrhosis of the liver, and enteritis. Treatment is usually given in a psychiatric hospital, where the alcoholic is first 'dried out' and then helped to understand the psychological pressures that led to his heavy drinking. Drugs such as *disulfiram (Antabuse), which cause vomiting if alcohol is taken, may help in treatment.

alcuronium *n.* a drug causing profound relaxation of voluntary muscles (*see* MUSCLE RELAXANT). Used during anaesthesia, it is administered by injection and may delay the resumption of spontaneous breathing, so that artificial ventilation is needed. Trade name: **Alloferin**.

aldesleukin *n.* *interleukin 2 produced by recombinant DNA technology (genetic engineering). It enhances the function of the immune system by prompting T-lymphocytes to become *natural killer cells, active against cancer cells. It is administered by injection. The results against certain cancers, including melanomas and kidney-cell cancer, have been encouraging. Trade name: **Proleukin**.

Aldomet *n.* *see* METHYLDOPA.

aldosterone *n.* a steroid hormone (*see* CORTICOSTEROID) that is synthesized and released by the adrenal cortex and acts on the kidney to regulate salt (potassium and sodium) and water balance. It may be given by injection as replacement therapy when the adrenal cortex secretes insufficient amounts of the hormone and also to treat shock.

aldosteronism n. overproduction of aldosterone, one of the hormones secreted by the adrenal cortex, leading to abnormalities in the amounts of sodium, potassium, and water in the body. It is one cause of raised blood pressure (hypertension). *See also* CONN'S SYNDROME.

alendronate n. *see* BIPHOSPHONATES.

Aleppo boil *see* ORIENTAL SORE.

aleukaemic *adj.* describing a stage of *leukaemia in which there is no absolute increase in the number of white cells in the blood. The stage is usually followed by one in which excessive numbers of white cells are produced, as typical in leukaemia.

alexia n. an acquired inability to read. It is due to disease in the left hemisphere of the brain in a right-handed person. In **agnosic alexia (word blindness)** the patient cannot read because he is unable to identify the letters and words, but he retains the ability to write and his speech is normal. This is a form of *agnosia. A patient with **aphasic alexia (visual asymbolia)** can neither read nor write and often has an accompanying disorder of speech. This is a form of *aphasia. *See also* DYSLEXIA.

alexin n. a former name for the serum component now called *complement.

alexithymia n. a lack of psychological understanding of one's own emotions and moods. It is considered by some psychiatrists to be a way in which people develop *psychosomatic symptoms.

alfacalcidol n. a synthetic form of vitamin D that is used to raise blood calcium levels in *osteomalacia and bone disorders caused by kidney disease. It is administered by mouth or by injection. Trade name: **One-Alpha**.

alfentanil hydrochloride a narcotic *analgesic drug used to relieve severe pain. It is administered by injection. Trade name: **Rapifen**.

ALG antilymphocyte globulin. *See* ANTILYMPHOCYTE SERUM.

algesimeter n. a piece of equipment for determining the sensitivity of the skin to various touch stimuli, especially those causing pain.

-algia *suffix denoting* pain. Example: **neuralgia** (pain in a nerve).

algid *adj.* cold: usually describing the cold clammy skin associated with certain forms of malaria.

alginic acid an *antacid drug used to treat heartburn caused by acid reflux into the gullet and hiatus hernia. It is administered by mouth. Trade names: **Gastrocote, Gastron**.

algodystrophy n. a specific post-traumatic syndrome after nerve injury, in which a limb remains exquisitely sensitive to any stimulus and later develops disuse *atrophy. Overactivity of sympathetic nerves may contribute to the syndrome.

algorithm n. a complex mathematical formula used in computers to form the final images from the data acquired by CT or MRI scanners.

alienation n. (in psychiatry) **1.** the experience that one's thoughts are under the control of somebody else, or that other people participate in one's thinking. It is a symptom of *schizophrenia. **2.** insanity.

alimentary canal the long passage through which food passes to be digested and absorbed (see illustration). It extends from the mouth to the anus and each region is specialized for a different stage in the processing of food, from mechanical breakdown in the mouth to chemical *digestion and *absorption in the stomach and small intestine and finally to faeces formation and water absorption in the colon and rectum.

alizarin (alizarin carmine) n. an orange-red dye derived from coal tar and originally isolated from the plant madder (*Rubia tinctorum*). Alizarin is insoluble in water but dissolves in alkalis, alcohol, and ether. It is used as a pH indicator and as a histochemical reagent for calcium, thallium, titanium, and zirconium.

ALK *see* AUTOMATED LAMELLAR KERATECTOMY.

alkalaemia n. abnormally high blood alkalinity. This may be caused by an increase in the concentration of alkaline substances and/or a decrease in that of

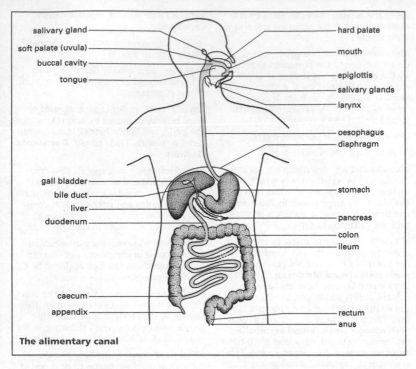

salivary gland — hard palate
soft palate (uvula) — mouth
buccal cavity — epiglottis
tongue — salivary glands
— larynx
— oesophagus
— diaphragm
gall bladder — stomach
bile duct — pancreas
liver — colon
duodenum — ileum
caecum — rectum
appendix — anus

The alimentary canal

acidic substances in the blood. *See also* AL-
KALOSIS. *Compare* ACIDAEMIA.

alkaloid *n.* one of a diverse group of nitrogen-containing substances that are produced by plants and have potent effects
on body function. Many alkaloids are important drugs, including *morphine, *quinine, *atropine, and *codeine.

alkalosis *n.* a condition in which the alkalinity of body fluids and tissues is abnormally high. This arises because of a
failure of the mechanisms that usually
maintain a balance between alkalis and
acids in the arterial blood (*see* ACID-BASE
BALANCE). Alkalosis may be associated with
loss of acid through vomiting or with excessive sodium bicarbonate intake.
Breathing that is abnormally deep in relation to the amount of physical exercise
may lead to **respiratory alkalosis**.
Alkalosis may produce symptoms of muscular weakness or cramp.

alkaptonuria *n. see* ALCAPTONURIA.

alkylating agents a class of drugs used
in chemotherapy that includes *cyclophosphamide and *melphalan. These drugs
bind to DNA and prevent complete separation of the two DNA chains during cell division.

allantois *n.* the membranous sac that
develops as an outgrowth of the embryonic hindgut. Its outer (mesodermal) layer
carries blood vessels to the *placenta and
so forms part of the *umbilical cord. Its
cavity is small and becomes reduced further in size during fetal development (*see*
URACHUS). —**allantoic** *adj.*

allele (allelomorph) *n.* one of two or
more alternative forms of a *gene, only
one of which can be present in a chromosome. Two alleles of a particular gene occupy the same relative positions on a pair
of *homologous chromosomes. If the two
alleles are the same, the individual is

*homozygous for the gene; if they are different he is *heterozygous. *See also* DOMINANT, RECESSIVE. **—allelic** *adj.*

allelomorph *n. see* ALLELE.

allergen *n.* any *antigen that causes *allergy in a hypersensitive person. Allergens are diverse and affect different tissues and organs. Pollens, fur, feathers, mould, and dust may cause hay fever; house mites have been implicated in some forms of asthma; drugs, dyes, cosmetics, and a host of other chemicals can cause rashes and dermatitis; some food allergies may cause diarrhoea or constipation or simulate acute bacterial food poisoning. When a patient's allergen has been identified (*see* PATCH TEST), it may be possible to attempt *desensitization to alleviate or prevent allergic attacks. **—allergenic** *adj.*

allergy *n.* a disorder in which the body becomes hypersensitive to particular antigens (called *allergens), which provoke characteristic symptoms whenever they are subsequently inhaled, ingested, injected, or otherwise contacted. Normally antibodies in the bloodstream and tissues react with and destroy specific antigens without further trouble. In an allergic person, however, the allergens provoke the release of a class of antibodies (IgE) that become bound to *mast cells in the body's tissues. The subsequent reaction of allergen with tissue-bound antibody (*see* REAGIN) also leads, as a side-effect, to cell damage, release of *histamine and *serotonin (5-hydroxytryptamine), inflammation, and all the symptoms of the particular allergy. Different allergies afflict different tissues and may have either local or general effects, varying from asthma and hay fever to severe dermatitis or gastroenteritis or extremely serious shock (*see* ANAPHYLAXIS). **—allergic** *adj.*

allodynia *n.* extreme tenderness of the skin. It results from nerve damage causing hypersensitivity of the pain receptors in that area, such as occurs in shingles (postherpetic neuralgia – *see* HERPES).

allogeneic *adj.* describing grafted tissue derived from a donor of the same species as the recipient but with different *histocompatibility.

allograft *n. see* HOMOGRAFT.

alloisoleucine *n.* one of the isomers of the amino acid isoleucine.

allopathy *n.* (in homeopathic medicine) the orthodox system of medicine, in which the use of drugs is directed to producing effects in the body that will directly oppose and so alleviate the symptoms of a disease. *Compare* HOMEOPATHY.

allopurinol *n.* a drug used in the treatment of chronic gout. It acts by reducing the level of uric acid in tissues and blood. It is administered by mouth; side-effects include nausea, vomiting, diarrhoea, headache, fever, stomach pains, and skin rashes. Occasionally, nerve damage and enlargement of the liver may occur. Trade names: **Hamarin, Zyloric.**

allylestrenol (allyloestrenol) *n.* a synthetic female sex hormone (*see* PROGESTOGEN) that is used in the treatment of abnormal bleeding from the uterus. It is administered by mouth. Trade name: **Gestanin.**

almoner *n.* a former name for a *medical social worker.

alopecia (baldness) *n.* absence of hair from areas where it normally grows. **Non-scarring alopecias** include common baldness in men, which is familial, and **androgenetic alopecia** in women, in which the hair loss is associated with increasing age. Acute hair fall (**telogen effluvium**), in which much or all of the hair is shed but starts to regrow at once, may occur after pregnancy or a serious illness. **Alopecia areata** consists of bald patches that may regrow; it is an example of an organ-specific *autoimmune disease. In **scarring** (or **cicatricial**) **alopecias** the hair does not regrow; examples include *lichen planus and discoid *lupus erythematosus. **Alopecia totalis** is loss of all the hair, due to an autoimmune condition; in some 70% of cases it regrows within a few years.

aloxiprin *n.* a compound made from aluminium oxide and *aspirin. Its actions and uses are similar to those of aspirin, but it is said to be more stable and less liable to cause irritation and bleeding of the stomach.

alpha blocker (alpha-adrenergic

blocker) a drug that prevents the stimulation of alpha-adrenergic receptors at the nerve endings of the sympathetic nervous system by adrenaline-like hormones: it therefore causes widening of arteries (vasodilatation) and a drop in blood pressure. Alpha blockers include *doxazosin, *phentolamine, *phenoxybenzamine, *thymoxamine, *indoramin, and *prazosin. Overdosage causes a severe drop in blood pressure, a rapid pulse, nausea and vomiting, diarrhoea, a dry mouth, flushed skin, convulsions, drowsiness, and coma.

alpha-fetoprotein (afp) *n.* a protein that is formed in the liver and yolk sac of the fetus and is present in the *amniotic fluid and secondarily in maternal blood. The level of afp can be detected by a maternal blood test performed between the 16th and 18th weeks of pregnancy to aid *prenatal diagnosis of certain fetal conditions. Levels are elevated in open *neural tube defects (e.g. spina bifida), twins and triplets, open abdominal wall defects (e.g. *gastroschisis), and fetal death. Levels of afp are decreased in *Down's syndrome. However, afp levels are affected by the length of gestation and the mother's weight, and these factors must be considered when interpreting the results. When levels are unexpectedly high or low, further investigations (for example *ultrasound scanning) are indicated.
Alpha-fetoprotein is also produced by certain tumours (*see* TUMOUR MARKER).

Alport's syndrome a hereditary disease that causes *nephritis accompanied by deafness. Affected males usually develop end-stage renal failure and, unless treated with a kidney transplant, die before the age of 40. Females have a better prognosis. [A. C. Alport (1880–1959), South African physician]

alprazolam *n.* a *tranquillizer of the benzodiazepine class used to relieve anxiety and as a sedative. It is administered by mouth; side-effects include drowsiness and lightheadedness. Trade name: **Xanax.**

alprostadil *n.* a *prostaglandin drug (PGE$_1$) administered by infusion to improve lung blood flow in newborn babies with congenital heart defects who are awaiting surgery; it acts by preventing the closure of the blood vessel connecting the aorta to the pulmonary artery (*see* DUCTUS ARTERIOSUS). Possible side-effects include diminished respiratory efforts. Alprostadil is also administered by injection into the corpora cavernosa of the penis to treat erectile *impotence in men; side-effects may include dizziness and headache. Trade names: **Caverject, Prostin VR.**

ALS **1.** *see* ANTILYMPHOCYTE SERUM.
2. amyotrophic lateral sclerosis. *See* MOTOR NEURONE DISEASE.

ALT argon laser *trabeculoplasty.

alteplase *n.* a *tissue plasminogen activator made by recombinant DNA technology (genetic engineering). Alteplase is used to dissolve blood clots (*see* FIBRINOLYTIC), especially in the coronary arteries of the heart. It is administered by injection. Possible side-effects include local bleeding, cerebral haemorrhage, nausea, and vomiting. Trade name: **Actilyse.**

alternative medicine (complementary medicine, fringe medicine) the various systems of healing, including *homeopathy, herbal remedies, *hypnosis, and faith healing, that are not regarded as part of orthodox treatment by the medical profession, especially when offered by unregistered practitioners. Most of the treatments are of unproven benefit but are tried by sufferers of chronic or incurable conditions when orthodox treatment has failed. Many alternative therapies are ridiculed by the medical profession, but *acupuncture and *osteopathy are now generally accepted to be of value in some circumstances. The extent to which individual registered practitioners indulge in or spurn these therapies varies enormously but is governed by the overriding principle (laid down by the General Medical Council) that shared care is only permitted if the registered practitioner remains in overall control; this is often unacceptable to those practising alternative medicine. *See also* CHIROPRACTIC, HOLISTIC, NATUROPATHY.

altitude sickness (mountain sickness) the condition that results from unaccustomed exposure to a high altitude (4500 m or more above sea level). Reduced atmospheric pressure and shortage of oxygen cause deep rapid breathing (*hyperventilation), which lowers the concentration of carbon dioxide in the blood (see ALKALOSIS). Symptoms include nausea, exhaustion, and anxiety. In severe cases there may be acute shortness of breath due to fluid collecting in the lungs (pulmonary *oedema), which requires treatment by diuretics and return to a lower altitude.

aluminium hydroxide a safe slow-acting antacid and *laxative. It is administered by mouth as a gel in the treatment of indigestion, gastric and duodenal ulcers, and reflux *oesophagitis. Trade name: **Aludrox.**

alveolitis n. inflammation of an *alveolus or alveoli. Chronic inflammation of the walls of the alveoli of the lungs is usually caused by inhaled organic dusts (**external allergic alveolitis**; see BIRD-FANCIER'S LUNG, FARMER'S LUNG) but may occur spontaneously (**cryptogenic fibrosing alveolitis**). The latter may be associated with connective tissue diseases, such as rheumatoid arthritis or systemic sclerosis. Both types of alveolitis may progress slowly to a state of fibrosis, and both types usually respond to corticosteroid therapy.

alveolus n. (pl. **alveoli**) **1.** (in the *lung) a blind-ended air sac of microscopic size. About 30 alveoli open out of each **alveolar duct**, which leads from a respiratory *bronchiole. The **alveolar walls**, which separate alveoli, contain capillaries. The alveoli are lined by a single layer of *pneumocytes, which thus form a very thin layer between air and blood so that exchange of oxygen and carbon dioxide is normally rapid and complete. Children are born with about 20 million alveoli. The adult number of about 300 million is reached around the age of eight. **2.** the part of the upper or lower jawbone that supports the roots of the teeth (see also MANDIBLE, MAXILLA). After tooth extraction it is largely absorbed. **3.** the sac of a *racemose gland (see also ACINUS). **4.** any other small cavity, depression, or sac. —**alveolar** adj.

alverine citrate a bulking agent and *antispasmodic drug used to treat the *irritable bowel syndrome and other colonic disorders. It is administered by mouth. Possible side-effects include occasional

mild distension of the bowel. Trade names: **Alvercol, Spasmonal.**

alveus n. a cavity, groove, or canal. The **alveus hippocampi** is the bundle of nerve fibres in the brain forming a depression in which the hippocampus lies.

Alzheimer's disease a progressive form of *dementia occurring in middle age or later, characterized by loss of short-term memory, deterioration in behaviour and intellectual performance, and slowness of thought. The condition may be mimicked by severe depression. The demonstration of damage to the cholinergic pathways in the brain has led to great interest in drug treatments (e.g. *anticholinesterases and vasodilators) but to date none have proved successful. The anticholinesterase drug Aricept has now been granted a limited licence for use in some cases, but its benefit would seem to be restricted. Pathological studies have revealed excess *amyloid protein in the brains of Alzheimer's patients. A genetic locus on chromosome 21 has been found for some inherited forms of Alzheimer's disease. [A. Alzheimer (1864–1915), German physician]

amalgam n. any of a group of alloys containing mercury. In dentistry amalgam fillings are made by mixing a silver-tin alloy with mercury in a machine known as an **amalgamator.**

Amanita n. a genus of fungi that contains several species of poisonous toadstools, including A. phalloides (death cap), A. pantherina (panther cap), and A. muscaria (fly agaric). They produce toxins that cause abdominal pain, violent vomiting, and continuous diarrhoea. In the absence of treatment death occurs in approximately 50% of cases, due to severe liver damage.

amantadine n. an antiviral drug that probably acts by preventing the penetration of the virus into the host cell and is used in the treatment of influenza infections. Because it stimulates an increase in the concentration of *dopamine in the brain, it is also used to treat parkinsonism. Common side-effects include nervousness, loss of muscular coordination, and insomnia. Trade name: **Symmetrel.**

amaurosis n. partial or complete blindness. For example, **amaurosis fugax** is a condition in which loss of vision is transient. See also LEBER'S CONGENITAL AMAUROSIS. —**amaurotic** adj.

amaurotic familial idiocy see TAY-SACHS DISEASE.

ambivalence n. (in psychology) the condition of holding opposite feelings (such as love and hate) for the same person or object. Excessive and prevalent ambivalence was thought by Bleuler to be a feature of schizophrenia.

Amblyomma n. a genus of hard *ticks, several species of which are responsible for transmitting tick *typhus. The bite of this tick can also give rise to a serious and sometimes fatal paralysis.

amblyopia n. poor sight, not due to any detectable disease of the eyeball or visual system. In practice this strict definition is not always obeyed. For example, in **toxic amblyopia**, caused by tobacco, alcohol, certain other drugs, and vitamin deficiency, there is a disorder of the *optic nerve. The commonest type is **amblyopia ex anopsia**, in which factors such as squint (see STRABISMUS), cataract, and other abnormalities of the optics of the eye (see REFRACTION) impair its normal use in early childhood by preventing the formation of a clear image on the retina.

amblyoscope (orthoptoscope, synoptophore) n. an instrument for measuring the angle of a squint and assessing the degree to which a person uses both eyes together. It consists of two L-shaped tubes, the short arms of which are joined by a hinge so that the long arms point away from each other. The subject looks into the short end and each eye sees, via a system of mirrors and lenses, a different picture, which is placed at the other end of each tube. If a squint is present, the tubes may be adjusted so that the short arms line up with the direction of each eye.

AMD age-related *macular degeneration.

amelia n. congenital total absence of the arms or legs due to a developmental defect. It is one of the fetal abnormalities induced by the drug *thalidomide taken early in pregnancy. See also PHOCOMELIA.

ameloblast n. a cell that forms the enamel of a tooth and disappears before tooth eruption.

ameloblastoma n. a locally malignant tumour in the jaw. It is considered to develop from ameloblasts although it does not contain enamel.

amelogenesis n. the formation of enamel by *ameloblasts, a process that is completed before tooth eruption. **Amelogenesis imperfecta** is a hereditary condition in which enamel formation is disturbed. The teeth have an unusual surface but may not be more prone to decay.

amenorrhoea n. the absence or stopping of the menstrual periods. It is normal for the periods to be absent before puberty, during pregnancy and milk secretion, and after the end of the reproductive period (see MENOPAUSE). In **primary amenorrhoea** the menstrual periods fail to appear at puberty. This may be due to absence of the uterus or ovaries, a genetic disorder (e.g. *Turner's syndrome), or hormonal imbalance. In **secondary amenorrhoea** the menstrual periods stop after establishment at puberty. Causes include disorders of the hypothalamus (a part of the brain), deficiency of ovarian, pituitary, or thyroid hormones, mental disturbance, depression, anorexia nervosa, or a major change of surroundings or circumstances.

amentia n. failure of development of the intellectual faculties. See MENTAL RETARDATION.

amethocaine n. a potent local anaesthetic. It is applied to skin or mucous membranes for eye, ear, nose and throat surgery, but it has also been employed for *spinal anaesthesia.

ametropia n. any abnormality of *refraction of the eye, resulting in blurring of the image formed on the retina. See ASTIGMATISM, HYPERMETROPIA, MYOPIA. Compare EMMETROPIA.

amiloride n. a potassium-sparing *diuretic that causes the increased excretion of sodium and chloride; it is often combined with a thiazide diuretic (e.g. hydrochlorothiazide in **Moduretic**) to reduce the potassium loss that occurs with these drugs. Amiloride may produce dizziness and weakness and its continued use may lead to an excessive concentration of potassium in the blood. Trade name: **Midamor**.

amino acid an organic compound containing an amino group ($-NH_2$) and a carboxyl group ($-COOH$). Amino acids are fundamental constituents of all *proteins. Breakdown of proteins found in the body yields the following amino acids: alanine, arginine, asparagine, aspartic acid, cysteine, cystine, glutamic acid, glutamine, glycine, histidine, isoleucine, leucine, lysine, methionine, phenylalanine, proline, serine, threonine, tryptophan, tyrosine, and valine. Some of these amino acids can be synthesized by the body; others, the *essential amino acids, must be obtained from protein in the diet. Certain amino acids present in the body are not found in proteins; these include *citrulline, *ornithine, *taurine, and *gamma-aminobutyric acid.

aminobenzoic acid see PARA-AMINOBENZOIC ACID.

aminoglutethimide n. a drug used in the treatment of advanced breast cancer. It inhibits synthesis of adrenal steroids (medical adrenalectomy) and the peripheral conversion of androgens to oestrogens. It is administered by mouth, usually with corticosteroid replacement therapy. Side-effects, which are largely dose-related, may include drowsiness, dizziness and a transient skin rash. Trade name: **Orimeten**.

aminoglycosides pl. n. a group of antibiotics active against a wide range of bacteria. Included in the group are *gentamicin, *kanamycin, *neomycin, and *streptomycin. Because of their toxicity (side-effects include ear and kidney damage), they are used only when less toxic antibacterials are ineffective or contraindicated. They are usually administered by injection.

aminopeptidase n. any one of several enzymes in the intestine that cause the breakdown of a *peptide, removing an amino acid.

aminophylline n. a drug that relaxes smooth muscle and stimulates respiration. It is widely used to dilate the air passages in the treatment of asthma and emphysema, to dilate the coronary arteries in angina pectoris, and as a *diuretic, particularly in cases of *oedema. Administered by injection or in suppositories, it may cause nausea, vomiting, dizziness, and fast heart rate. See also THEOPHYLLINE. Trade name: **Pecram**.

amiodarone n. an *anti-arrhythmic drug used to control a variety of abnormal heart rhythms, including atrial *fibrillation and abnormally rapid heartbeat. It is administered by mouth or by injection. Side-effects are uncommon. Trade name: **Cordarone X**.

amitosis n. division of the nucleus of a cell by a process, not involving *mitosis, in which the nucleus is constricted into two.

amitriptyline n. a tricyclic *antidepressant drug that has a mild tranquillizing action. Common side-effects include drowsiness, dizziness, numbness, and tingling of limbs. Trade names: **Elavil**, **Tryptizol**.

amlodipine n. a *calcium antagonist used to treat angina pectoris. It is administered by mouth. Possible side-effects include headache, dizziness, fatigue, nausea, and fluid retention. Trade name: **Istin**.

amnesia n. total or partial loss of memory following physical injury, disease, drugs, or psychological trauma (see CONFABULATION, FUGUE, REPRESSION). **Anterograde amnesia** is loss of memory for the events following some trauma; **retrograde amnesia** is loss of memory for events preceding the trauma. Some patients experience both types.

amnihook n. a small plastic hooked instrument for performing *amniotomy. The hook is introduced through the cervix.

amniocentesis n. withdrawal of a sample of the fluid (amniotic fluid) surrounding an embryo in the uterus by piercing the amniotic sac through the abdominal wall. As the amniotic fluid contains cells from the embryo (mostly shed from the skin), cell cultures enable chromosome patterns to be studied so that *prenatal diagnosis of chromosomal abnormalities (such as *Down's syndrome) can be made. Metabolic errors and other diseases, such as *spina bifida, can also be diagnosed pre-natally from the biochemistry of the cells or that of the fluid (see ALPHA-FETOPROTEIN). Although the risks of amniocentesis, in skilled hands, are extremely low, there is no point in undertaking it unless the parents agree to a termination of the pregnancy if a serious abnormality is discovered.

amnion n. the membrane that forms initially over the dorsal part of the embryo but soon expands to enclose it completely within the *amniotic cavity; it is connected to the embryo at the umbilical cord. It expands outwards and fuses with the chorion, obliterating virtually all the intervening cavity. The double membrane (**amniochorion**) normally ruptures at birth. —**amniotic** adj.

amnioscopy n. examination of the inside of the amniotic sac by means of an instrument (**amnioscope**) that is passed through the abdominal wall. This allows the developing fetus in the cavity to be viewed directly. **Cervical amnioscopy**, performed late in pregnancy, enables the amniotic sac to be inspected through the cervix (neck) of the uterus, using a different instrument (a fetoscope). When transilluminated, its fluid volume can be appraised without puncture of the amnion and any meconium observed.

amniotic cavity the fluid-filled cavity between the embryo and the *amnion. It forms initially within the inner cell mass of the *blastocyst and later expands over the back of the embryo, eventually enclosing it completely. See also AMNIOTIC FLUID.

amniotic fluid the fluid contained within the *amniotic cavity. It surrounds the growing fetus, protecting it from external pressure. The fluid is initially secreted from the *amnion and is later supplemented by urine from the fetal kidneys. Some of the fluid is swallowed by the fetus and absorbed through its intestine. See also AMNIOCENTESIS.

amniotomy (artificial rupture of membranes, ARM) n. a method of surgically inducing labour by puncturing the *amnion surrounding the baby in the uterus using an *amnihook or similar instrument.

amodiaquine n. an antimalarial drug with effects and uses similar to those of *chloroquine. It has also been used for the treatment of lupus erythematosus, leprosy, and rheumatoid arthritis. Doses used to treat malaria have almost no side-effects, but prolonged use may cause blue-grey deposits on the cornea of the eye, fingernails, and hard palate.

amoeba n. (pl. **amoebae**) any protozoan of jelly-like consistency and irregular and constantly changing shape. Found in water, soil and other damp environments, they move and feed by means of flowing extensions of the body (see PSEUDOPODIUM). Some amoebae cause disease in man (see ACANTHAMOEBA, ENTAMOEBA). —**amoebic** adj.

amoebiasis n. see DYSENTERY.

amoebocyte n. a cell that moves by sending out processes of its protoplasm in the same way as an amoeba.

amoeboma n. a tumour that occurs in the rectum or caecum of the large intestine and is caused by the parasite *Entamoeba histolytica, a protozoan that invades and destroys the walls of the gut. Tumours may ulcerate and become infected with pus-forming (pyogenic) bacteria, causing severe inflammation of the bowel wall. The tumours usually harden and may even obstruct the bowel.

amok n. a sudden outburst of furious and murderous aggression, directed indiscriminately at everybody in the vicinity. It is encountered particularly in certain cultures, such as that of the Malays.

amorolfine n. an antifungal drug used to treat ringworm, candidosis, and other fungal infections of the skin and nails. It is applied externally as a cream or nail lacquer; possible side-effects include itching and a transient burning sensation. Trade name: **Loceryl**.

amoxapine n. a tricyclic antidepressant drug similar to *imipramine. It is administered by mouth. Overdosage may cause acute kidney failure, convulsions, and coma. Trade name: **Asendis**.

amoxicillin n. an antibiotic used to treat infections caused by a wide range of bacteria and other microorganisms. It is administered by mouth. Side-effects include nausea, vomiting, diarrhoea, rashes, and anaemia. Sensitivity to penicillin prohibits its use. Trade name: **Amoxil, Galenamox, Rimoxallin**.

AMP (adenosine monophosphate) a compound containing adenine, ribose, and one phosphate group. AMP occurs in cells and is involved in processes requiring the transfer of energy (see ATP).

ampere n. the basic *SI unit of electric current. It is equal to the current flowing through a conductor of resistance 1 ohm when a potential difference of 1 volt is applied between its ends. The formal definition of the ampere is the current that when passed through two parallel conductors of infinite length and negligible cross section, placed 1 metre apart in a vacuum, produces a force of 2×10^{-7} newton per metre between them. Symbol: A.

amphetamine n. a *sympathomimetic drug that has a marked stimulant action on the central nervous system. It alleviates fatigue and produces a feeling of mental alertness and well-being. The drug has been used in the treatment of *narcolepsy, mild depressive neuroses, and obesity, but the chief indication is for the treatment of *attention deficit disorder in children. It is administered by mouth; side-effects include insomnia and restlessness. *Tolerance to amphetamine develops rapidly, and prolonged use may lead to *dependence.

amphiarthrosis n. a slightly movable joint in which the bony surfaces are separated by fibrocartilage (see SYMPHYSIS) or hyaline cartilage (see SYNCHONDROSIS).

amphoric breath sounds see BREATH SOUNDS.

amphotericin n. an *antibiotic, derived from the bacterium *Streptomyces nodosus*, that is used to treat deep-seated fungal infections; it is inactive against bacteria and viruses. It can be administered by mouth, but is usually given by intravenous injection. Common side-effects include headache, fever, muscle pains, and diarrhoea. In some cases kidney damage may occur. Trade names: **Fungilin, Fungizone**.

ampicillin n. an *antibiotic used to treat a variety of infections, including those of the urinary, respiratory, biliary, and intestinal tracts. It is inactivated by *penicillinase and therefore cannot be used against organisms producing this enzyme. It is given by mouth or injection; side-effects include nausea, vomiting, and diarrhoea, and some allergic reactions may occur. Trade names: **Amfipen, Penbritin**.

ampoule (ampule) n. a sealed glass or plastic capsule containing one dose of a drug in the form of a sterile solution for injection.

ampulla n. (pl. **ampullae**) an enlarged or dilated ending of a tube or canal. The semicircular canals of the inner ear are expanded into ampullae at the point where they join the vestibule. The **ampulla of Vater** is the dilated part of the common bile duct where it is joined by the pancreatic duct.

amputation n. the removal of a limb, part of a limb, or any other portion of the body (such as a breast or the rectum). The term is customarily modified by an adjective showing the particular type of amputation. Once a common operation in surgery, it is now usually performed only in cases of severe injury to limbs or, particularly in elderly people, when circulation to a limb is inadequate and gangrene develops. In planning an amputation the surgeon takes account of the patient's work and the type of artificial part (prosthesis) that will be fitted.

amsacrine n. a *cytotoxic drug administered by injection to treat various forms of cancer. Possible side-effects include nausea, vomiting, hair loss, and interference with bone marrow blood-cell production. Trade name: **Amsidine**.

Amsler grid a chart usually consisting of a grid of black lines on a white background. It is used to detect and monitor problems of central vision, for example in macular disease. [M. Amsler (1891–1968), Swiss ophthalmologist]

amygdala (amygdaloid nucleus) n. one of the *basal ganglia: a roughly almond-shaped mass of grey matter deep inside each cerebral hemisphere. It has extensive connections with the olfactory system and sends nerve fibres to the hypothalamus; its functions are apparently concerned with mood, feeling, instinct, and possibly memory for recent events.

amylase *n.* an enzyme that occurs in saliva and pancreatic juice and aids the digestion of starch, which it breaks down into glucose, maltose, and dextrins. Amylase will also hydrolyse *glycogen to yield glucose, maltose, and dextrins.

amyl nitrite a drug that relaxes smooth muscle, especially that of blood vessels. Given by inhalation, amyl nitrite is used mainly in the treatment of angina pectoris. It is rapidly absorbed and acts quickly, producing a fall in arterial blood pressure. Side-effects include flushing, faintness, and headache. High doses may cause restlessness, vomiting, and blue coloration of the skin.

amylobarbitone *n.* an intermediate-acting *barbiturate. Prolonged use may lead to *dependence and overdosage has serious toxic effects (*see* BARBITURISM). Trade name: **Amytal**.

amyloid *n.* a *glycoprotein, resembling starch, that is deposited in the internal organs in amyloidosis. β-amyloid protein has been found in the brains of Alzheimer's patients but the significance of this is unclear.

amyloidosis *n.* infiltration of the liver, kidneys, spleen, and other tissues with amyloid, a starchlike substance. In **primary amyloidosis** the disorder arises without any apparent cause; **secondary amyloidosis** occurs as a late complication of such chronic infections as tuberculosis or leprosy and also in *Hodgkin's disease. Amyloidosis is also very common in the genetic disease familial Mediterranean fever (*see* POLYSEROSITIS).

amylopectin *n.* *see* STARCH.

amylose *n.* *see* STARCH.

amyotonia congenita (floppy baby syndrome) a former diagnosis for various conditions, present at birth, in which the baby's muscles are weak and floppy (i.e. hypotonic). The term is becoming obsolete as more specific diagnoses are discovered to explain the cause of floppiness in babies.

amyotrophy *n.* a progressive loss of muscle bulk associated with weakness of these muscles. It is caused by disease of the nerve that activates the affected muscle. Amyotrophy is a feature of any chronic *neuropathy and it may be the most prominent neurological symptom of diabetes mellitus and meningovascular syphilis. A combination of amyotrophy and spasticity may be found in the different forms of *motor neurone disease.

an- *prefix. see* A-.

anabolic *adj.* promoting tissue growth by increasing the metabolic processes involved in protein synthesis. Anabolic agents are usually synthetic male sex hormones (*see* ANDROGEN); they include *ethyloestrenol, *nandrolone, *oxymetholone, and *stanozolol. They have been used to help weight gain in underweight patients, such as the elderly and those with serious illnesses, and to stimulate the production of blood cells by the bone marrow. Some anabolic steroids cause virilization in women and liver damage.

anabolism *n.* the synthesis of complex molecules, such as proteins and fats, from simpler ones by living things. *See also* ANABOLIC, METABOLISM.

anacidity *n.* a deficiency or abnormal absence of acid in the body fluids.

anacrotism *n.* the condition in which there is an abnormal curve in the ascending line of a pulse tracing. It may be seen in cases of aortic stenosis. —**anacrotic** *adj.*

anaemia *n.* a reduction in the quantity of the oxygen-carrying pigment *haemoglobin in the blood. The main symptoms are excessive tiredness and fatigability, breathlessness on exertion, pallor, and poor resistance to infection.

There are many causes of anaemia. It may be due to loss of blood (**haemorrhagic anaemia**), resulting from an accident, operation, etc., or from chronic bleeding, as from an ulcer or haemorrhoids. **Iron-deficiency anaemia** results from lack of iron, which is necessary for the production of haemoglobin (*see* SIDEROPENIA). **Haemolytic anaemias** result from the increased destruction of red blood cells (which contain the pigment). This can be caused by toxic chemicals; *autoimmunity; the action of parasites, especially in *malaria; or conditions such as *thalassaemia and *sickle-cell disease, associated with abnormal forms of haemoglobin, or *spherocytosis, which is associated with abnormal red blood cells. (*See also* HAEMOLYTIC DISEASE OF THE NEWBORN.) Anaemia can also be caused by the impaired production of red blood cells, as in *leukaemia (when red-cell production in the bone marrow is suppressed) or *pernicious anaemia.

Anaemias can be classified on the basis of the size of the red cells, which may be large (**macrocytic anaemias**), small (**microcytic anaemias**), or normal-sized (**normocytic anaemias**). (*See also* MACROCYTOSIS, MICROCYTOSIS.) The treatment of anaemia depends on the cause. —**anaemic** *adj.*

anaerobe *n.* any organism, especially a microbe, that is able to live and grow in the absence of free oxygen. A **facultative anaerobe** is a microorganism that grows best in the presence of oxygen but is capable of some growth in its absence. An **obligate anaerobe** can grow only in the absence of free oxygen. *Compare* AEROBE, MICROAEROPHILIC.

anaerobic *adj.* **1.** of or relating to anaerobes. **2.** describing a type of cellular respiration in which foodstuffs (usually carbohydrates) are never completely oxidized because molecular oxygen is not used. *Fermentation is an example of anaerobic respiration.

anaesthesia *n.* loss of feeling or sensation in a part or all of the body. Anaesthesia of a part of the body may occur as a result of injury to or disease of a nerve; for example in leprosy. The term is usually applied, however, to the technique of reducing or abolishing an individual's sensation of pain to enable surgery to be performed. This is effected by administering drugs (*see* ANAESTHETIC) or by the use of other methods, such as *acupuncture or hypnosis.

General anaesthesia is total unconsciousness, usually achieved by administering a combination of injections and gases (the latter are inhaled through a mask). **Local anaesthesia** abolishes pain in a limited area of the body and is used for minor operations, particularly many dental procedures. It may be achieved by injections of substances such as lignocaine

(commonly used in dentistry) close to a local nerve, which deadens the tissues supplied by that nerve. Local anaesthesia may be combined with intravenous sedation. An appropriate injection into the spinal column produces *spinal anaesthesia in the lower limbs or abdomen. **Regional anaesthesia**, usually of a limb, is achieved by encircling local anaesthetic solutions and is used in situations where general anaesthesia is not appropriate.

anaesthetic 1. *n.* an agent that reduces or abolishes sensation, affecting either the whole body (**general anaesthetic**) or a particular area or region (**local anaesthetic**). General anaesthetics, used for surgical procedures, depress activity of the central nervous system, producing loss of consciousness. *Anaesthesia is induced by short-acting *barbiturates (such as thiopentone) and maintained by inhalation anaesthetics (such as *halothane). Local anaesthetics inhibit conduction of impulses in sensory nerves in the region where they are injected or applied; they include *amethocaine, *bupivacaine, and *lignocaine. **2.** *adj.* reducing or abolishing sensation.

anaesthetist *n.* a medically qualified doctor who administers an anaesthetic to induce unconsciousness in a patient before a surgical operation.

anagen *n.* the growth phase of a hair follicle, lasting two to three years. It is followed by a transitional stage, called **catagen**, and then a resting phase, **telogen**, each of which lasts for about two weeks. On average about 85% of hairs are in anagen and hence growing actively. There are about 100,000 hairs on the human scalp and up to 100 may be shed each day.

anákhré *n. see* GOUNDOU.

anal *adj.* of, relating to, or affecting the anus; for example an anal *fissure or an anal *fistula.

anal canal the terminal portion of the large intestine, which is surrounded by the muscles of defecation (**anal sphincters**). The canal ends on the surface at the anal orifice (*see* ANUS).

analeptic *n.* a drug that restores consciousness to a patient in a coma or faint; for example, *doxapram, *nikethamide, or *naloxone. Analeptics stimulate the central nervous system to counteract the effects of large doses of narcotic drugs, which depress the central nervous system.

anal fissure a break in the skin lining the anal canal, usually causing pain during bowel movements and sometimes bleeding. Anal fissures occur as a consequence of constipation or sometimes of diarrhoea. Treatment is by soothing ointments, but if the condition is severe the operation of **lateral sphincterotomy** (cutting the muscle of the anal sphincter) is required.

analgesia n. reduced sensibility to pain, without loss of consciousness and without the sense of touch necessarily being affected. The condition may arise accidentally, if nerves are diseased or damaged, or be induced deliberately by the use of pain-killing drugs (see ANALGESIC). Strictly speaking, local *anaesthesia should be called **local analgesia**. See also RELATIVE ANALGESIA.

analgesic **1.** n. a drug that relieves pain. Mild analgesics, such as *aspirin and *paracetamol, are used for the relief of headache, toothache, and mild rheumatic pain. More potent **narcotic analgesics**, such as *morphine and *pethidine, are used only to relieve severe pain since these drugs may produce *dependence and *tolerance (see also NARCOTIC, OPIATE). Some analgesics, including aspirin, *indomethacin, and *phenylbutazone, also reduce fever and inflammation and are used in rheumatic conditions (see also NSAID). **2.** adj. relieving pain.

analogous adj. describing organs or parts that have similar functions in different organisms although they do not have the same evolutionary origin or development. Compare HOMOLOGOUS.

analogue n. a drug that differs in minor ways in molecular structure from its parent compound. Examples are *calcipotriol (an analogue of vitamin D), *betahistine (an analogue of histamine), and the *LHRH analogues. Useful analogues of existing drugs are either more potent or cause fewer side-effects. *Carboplatin, for example, is a less toxic analogue of *cisplatin.

analysand n. a person undergoing *psychoanalysis.

analysis n. (in psychology) any means of understanding complex mental processes or experiences. There are several systems of analysis used by different schools of psychology; for example, *psychoanalysis; **transactional analysis**, in which people's relationships are explained in psychoanalytic terms; and **functional analysis**, in which a particular kind of behaviour is thoroughly described with reference to its frequency, its antecedents, and its consequences.

anamnesis n. memory, particularly the recollection by a patient of the symptoms that he noticed at the time when his disease was first contracted.

anankastic adj. describing a collection of longstanding personality traits, including stubbornness, meanness, an overmeticulous concern to be accurate in small details, a disposition to check things unnecessarily, severe feelings of insecurity about personal worth, and an excessive tendency to doubt evident facts. See PERSONALITY DISORDER, OBSESSION.

anaphase n. the third stage of *mitosis and of each division of *meiosis. In mitosis and anaphase II of meiosis the chromatids separate, becoming daughter chromosomes, and move apart along the spindle fibres towards opposite ends of the cell. In anaphase I of meiosis the pairs of homologous chromosomes separate from each other. See DISJUNCTION.

anaphylaxis n. an abnormal reaction to a particular *antigen, in which histamine is released from tissues and causes either local or widespread symptoms. An allergic attack (see ALLERGY) is an example of localized anaphylaxis. Rarer, but much more serious, is **anaphylactic shock**: an extreme and generalized allergic reaction in which widespread release of histamine causes swelling (oedema), constriction of the bronchioles, heart failure, circulatory collapse, and sometimes death. —**anaphylactic** adj.

anaplasia n. a loss of normal cell characteristics or differentiation, which may be to such a degree that it is impossible to define the origin of the cells. Anaplasia is typical of rapidly growing malignant tumours.

anasarca *n.* massive swelling of the legs, trunk, and genitalia due to retention of fluid (*oedema): found in congestive heart failure and some forms of renal failure.

anastomosis *n.* **1.** (in anatomy) a communication between two blood vessels without any intervening capillary network. *See* ARTERIOVENOUS ANASTOMOSIS. **2.** (in surgery) an artificial connection between two tubular organs or parts, especially between two normally separate parts of the intestine. *See also* SHUNT.

anatomy *n.* the study of the structure of living organisms. In medicine it refers to the study of the form and gross structure of the various parts of the human body. The term **morphology** is sometimes used synonymously with anatomy but it is usually used for **comparative anatomy**: the study of differences in form between species. *See also* CYTOLOGY, HISTOLOGY, PHYSIOLOGY. —**anatomical** *adj.* —**anatomist** *n.*

anatoxin *n.* a former name for *toxoid.

anconeus *n.* a muscle behind the elbow that assists in extending the forearm.

Ancylostoma (Ankylostoma) *n.* a genus of small parasitic nematodes (*see* HOOKWORM) that inhabit the small intestine and are widely distributed in Europe, America, Asia, and Africa. The worms suck blood from the gut wall, to which they are attached by means of cutting teeth. Man is the principal and optimum host for *A. duodenale.*

ancylostomiasis *n.* an infestation of the small intestine by the parasitic hookworm *Ancylostoma duodenale. See* HOOKWORM DISEASE.

ANDI an acronym for *a*bnormal *d*evelopment and *i*nvolution, used to tabulate benign disorders of the breast.

andr- (andro-) *prefix denoting* man or the male sex. Example: **androphobia** (morbid fear of).

androblastoma (arrhenoblastoma) *n.* a tumour of the ovary, composed of Sertoli cells, Leydig cells, or both. It can produce male or female hormones and may give rise to *masculinization; in chil-

dren it may cause precocious puberty. Up to 30% of these tumours are malignant, but probably as many as 85% of all cases are cured by surgery alone.

androgen *n.* one of a group of steroid hormones, including **testosterone** and **androsterone**, that stimulate the development of male sex organs and male secondary sexual characteristics (e.g. beard growth, deepening of the voice, and muscle development). The principal source of these hormones is the testis (production being stimulated by *luteinizing hormone) but they are also secreted by the adrenal cortex and ovaries in small amounts. In women excessive production of androgens gives rise to *masculinization.

Naturally occurring and synthetic androgens are used in replacement therapy (to treat such conditions as delayed puberty in adolescent boys, *hypogonadism, and impotence due to testicular insufficiency); as *anabolic agents; and in the treatment of breast cancer. Side-effects include salt and water retention, increased bone growth, and masculinization in women. Androgens should not be used in patients with cancer of the prostate gland or in pregnant women. —**androgenic** *adj.*

andrology *n.* **1.** the study of male infertility and impotence. *Seminal analysis reveals the presence of gross abnormalities in the shape and motility of spermatozoa, as well as their concentration in the semen, but further procedures are required to diagnose the underlying causes of the sperm dysfunction. These include the diagnosis of abnormalities in the genital tract (e.g. varicocele, obstruction of the vas deferens), which may be corrected surgically, and testing for the presence of antisperm antibodies in the semen and for the ability of the sperm to penetrate the cervical mucus, as well as for the presence of hormonal disorders. More sophisticated techniques include computer-assisted quantitative motility measurements, which monitor the precise speed and motility patterns of individual sperm; biochemical tests for the production of free oxygen radicals, which cause damage to developing sperm; and *acrosome-reaction assays, which reveal the ability of the sperm to penetrate the barriers surrounding the ovum. The development of all these techniques has enabled the identification of several previously undiagnosed causes of infertility and the selection of treatments most likely to succeed in remedying them. **2.** the study of androgen production and the relationship of plasma androgen to androgen action. This study is necessary to understand *hirsutism and other conditions caused by abnormal androgen production.

androsterone *n.* a steroid hormone (*see* ANDROGEN) that is synthesized and released by the testes and is responsible for controlling male sexual development.

anencephaly *n.* partial or complete absence of the bones of the rear of the skull and of the cerebral hemispheres of the brain. It occurs as a developmental defect, and most affected infants are stillborn; if born live they do not survive for more than a few hours. Anencephaly is often associated with other defects of the nervous system, such as *spina bifida. Prenatal screening tests for anencephaly include *amniocentesis, detection of alpha-fetoprotein levels, and ultrasound scanning.

anergy *n.* **1.** lack of response to a specific antigen or allergen. **2.** lack of energy. —**anergic** *adj.*

aneuploidy *n.* the condition in which the chromosome number of a cell is not an exact multiple of the normal basic (haploid) number. *See* MONOSOMY, TRISOMY; *compare* EUPLOIDY. —**aneuploid** *adj., n.*

aneurine *n. see* VITAMIN B_1.

aneurysm *n.* a balloon-like swelling in the wall of an artery. This may be due to degenerative disease or syphilitic infection, which damages the muscular coats of the vessel, or it may be the result of congenital deficiency in the muscular wall. An **aortic aneurysm** may develop anywhere in the aorta. A **dissecting aneurysm** usually affects the first part of the aorta and results from a degenerative condition of its muscular coat. This weakness predisposes to a tear in the lining of the aorta, which allows blood to enter the wall and track along (dissect) the muscular coat. A dissecting aneurysm may rupture or it may compress the blood vessels arising from the aorta and produce infarction (lo-

calized necrosis) in the organs they supply. The patient complains of severe chest pain that has a tearing quality and often spreads to the back or abdomen. Surgical repair may help in some cases. A **ventricular aneurysm** may develop in the wall of the left ventricle after myocardial infarction. A segment of myocardium becomes replaced by scar tissue, which expands to form an aneurysmal sac. Heart failure may result or thrombosis within the aneurysm may act as a source of embolism.

Most aneurysms within the brain are congenital: there is a risk that they may burst, causing a *subarachnoid haemorrhage. **Berry aneurysms** are small saccular aneurysms most commonly occurring in the branches of the *circle of Willis. Usually associated with congenital weakness of the vessels, these aneurysms are a cause of fatal intracranial haemorrhage in young adults. **Charcot-Bouchard aneurysms** are small aneurysms found on tiny arteries within the brain of elderly and hypertensive subjects. These aneurysms may rupture, causing cerebral haemorrhage. *See also* ARTERIOVENOUS ANEURYSM. —**aneurysmal** *adj.*

angi- (angio-) *prefix denoting* blood or lymph vessels. Examples: **angiectasis** (abnormal dilation of); **angiopathy** (disease of); **angiotomy** (cutting of).

angiitis (vasculitis) *n.* a patchy inflammation of the walls of small blood vessels. It may result from a variety of conditions, including *polyarteritis nodosa, acute nephritis, and serum sickness. Symptoms include skin rashes, arthritis, purpura, and kidney failure. In some cases treatment with cortisone derivatives may be beneficial.

angina *n.* a sense of suffocation or suffocating pain. *See* ANGINA PECTORIS, LUDWIG'S ANGINA.

angina pectoris pain in the centre of the chest, which is induced by exercise and relieved by rest and may spread to the jaws and arms. Angina pectoris occurs when the demand for blood by the heart exceeds the supply of the coronary arteries and it usually results from coronary artery *atheroma. It may be prevented or relieved by such drugs as *glyceryl trinitrate and *propranolol. If drug treatment proves ineffective, *coronary angioplasty or *coronary bypass grafts may be required, the former being less invasive than the latter.

angiocardiography n. X-ray examination of the chambers of the heart after introducing a *radiopaque contrast medium into the blood in the heart. The contrast medium (e.g. Cardioconray) is injected directly into the atria, ventricles, or great vessels of the heart by means of a slim sterile flexible tube (**cardiac catheter**), which is manipulated into position from an accessible point, such as a vein or artery in a limb (see (CARDIAC) CATHETERIZATION). A recording is made by a rapid-sequence digital subtraction technique, which can be viewed subsequently via a TV monitor (see DIGITAL SUBTRACTION ANGIOGRAPHY). The recording is called an **angiocardiogram**. Angiocardiography is used in diagnosing and planning the surgical repair of heart defects and demonstrating coronary artery disease.

angiodysplasia n. an abnormal collection of small blood vessels in the wall of the bowel, which may bleed. It is diagnosed by *colonoscopy, enteroscopy (see ENTEROSCOPE), or *angiography and may be treated by *diathermy coagulation or by surgical removal.

angiogenesis n. the formation of new blood vessels. This process is essential for the development of a tumour and is promoted by *growth factors.

angiography n. X-ray examination of blood vessels. A *contrast medium is injected into the artery and a rapid series of X-ray recordings is made, commonly using *digital subtraction angiography (see also ARTERIOGRAPHY). **Fluorescein angiography** is a common method of investigation in ophthalmology. *Fluorescein sodium is injected into a vein in the arm, from which it circulates throughout the body. Light of an appropriate wavelength is shone into the eye, causing the dye in the retinal blood vessels to fluoresce. This allows the circulation through the retinal blood vessels to be observed and photographed. However, **indocyanine green (ICG) angiography**, using a newer dye, indocyanine green, gives much better

visualization of the choroidal circulation. It is particularly useful for visualization and treatment of choroidal neovascular membranes (see NEOVASCULARIZATION).

angioid streaks reddish to dark-brown irregular streaks radiating outwards from the optic disc underneath the retinal vessels. They represent irregular linear cracks in *Bruch's membrane and can be the site for the development of new vessels from the choroid that leak. They are seen in such systemic conditions as pseudoxanthoma elasticum, Paget's disease, and sickle-cell anaemia.

angiokeratoma n. a localized collection of thin-walled blood vessels covered by a cap of warty material. It is most often seen as an isolated malformation in the genital skin of the elderly or on the hands and feet of children. It is not malignant and its cause is unknown. Angiokeratomas may be removed surgically. Multiple angiokeratomas affecting the viscera and skin are seen as a rare inherited and fatal disease (**Fabry's disease**).

angioma n. a benign tumour composed of blood vessels or lymph vessels. **Cherry angiomas** (or **Campbell de Morgan spots**) are small red spots on the trunk in middle-aged or elderly people. They are completely harmless and consist of a minor vascular malformation. An **arteriovenous angioma** (or **malformation**) is a knot of distended blood vessels overlying and compressing the surface of the brain. It may cause epilepsy, or one of the vessels may burst, causing a *subarachnoid haemorrhage. This type of angioma may be suitable for surgical removal or stereotactic radiotherapy. It may be associated with a purple birthmark on the face: this is called the **Sturge-Weber syndrome**. See also HAEMANGIOMA, LYMPHANGIOMA.

angio-oedema (angioneurotic oedema) n. see URTICARIA.

angioplasty n. surgical repair or reconstruction of narrowed or completely obstructed arteries (or rarely veins). In **percutaneous transluminal angioplasty (PTA; balloon angioplasty)** an inflatable balloon, mounted on the tip of a flexible catheter, is placed within the lumen of the affected artery, at the site of the disease, under X-ray screening control (see

CATHETERIZATION). On inflation of the balloon the lumen is enlarged, disrupting the *intima (which reduces the chance of stenosis recurring). Common sites for PTA are the coronary, iliac, femoral, and popliteal arteries. *See also* CORONARY ANGIOPLASTY.

angiospasm *n. see* RAYNAUD'S DISEASE.

angiotensin *n.* either of two peptides: **angiotensin I** or **angiotensin II**. Angiotensin I is derived, by the action of the enzyme *renin, from a protein (alpha globulin) secreted by the liver into the bloodstream. As blood passes through the lungs, another enzyme acts on angiotensin I to form angiotensin II. This peptide causes constriction of blood vessels and stimulates the release of the hormones *vasopressin and *aldosterone, which increase blood pressure. *See also* ACE INHIBITOR.

angle *n.* **1.** (in anatomy) a corner. For example, the **angle of the eye** is the outer or inner corner of the eye; the **angle of the mouth** is the site where the upper and lower lips join on either side. **2.** the degree of divergence of two lines or planes that meet each other; the space between two such lines. The **carrying angle** is the obtuse angle formed between the forearm and the upper arm when the forearm is fully extended and the hand is supinated.

angstrom *n.* a unit of length equal to one ten millionth of a millimetre (10^{-10} m). It is not a recommended *SI unit but is sometimes used to express wavelengths and interatomic distances: the *nanometre (1 nm = 10 Å) is now the preferred unit. Symbol Å.

anhedonia *n.* total loss of the feeling of pleasure in acts that normally give pleasure.

anhidrosis *n.* the absence of sweating in the presence of an appropriate stimulus for sweating, such as heat. A reduction in sweating is known as **hypohidrosis**. Anhidrosis and hypohidrosis may accompany disease or occur as a congenital defect.

anhidrotic **1.** *n.* any drug that inhibits sweating, such as a *parasympatholytic drug. **2.** *adj.* inhibiting sweating.

anhydraemia *n.* a decrease in the proportion of water, and therefore plasma, in the blood.

anhydrase *n.* an enzyme that catalyses the removal of water from a compound.

anima *n.* (in Jungian psychology) an *archetype that is the feminine component of a male's personality.

animus *n.* the *archetype that is the masculine component of a female's personality.

anion *n.* an ion of negative charge, such as a bicarbonate ion (HCO_3^-) or a chloride ion (Cl^-) (*see also* ELECTROLYTE). The **anion gap** is the difference between the concentrations of cations (positively charged ions) and anions, calculated from the formula:

$$(Na^+ + K^+) - (HCO_3^- + Cl^-)$$

It is used to estimate the unaccounted-for anions in the blood in cases of metabolic disturbance. The normal anion gap is 10–16 mmol/l.

aniridia *n.* congenital absence of the iris (of the eye). In some cases it is caused by a *deletion on the short arm of chromosome no. 11, in which case it is associated with other abnormalities and a predisposition to develop nephroblastoma (the **WAGR syndrome**).

aniseikonia *n.* a condition in which the image of an object differs markedly in size or shape in each eye.

anisocytosis *n.* an excessive variation in size between individual red blood cells. Anisocytosis may be noted on microscopical examination of a blood film; from this a graph of the numbers of cells of different sizes may be drawn. Anisocytosis may be a feature of almost any disease affecting the blood.

anisomelia *n.* a difference in size or shape between the arms or the legs.

anisometropia *n.* the condition in which the power of *refraction in one eye differs from that in the other.

anistreplase *n.* a *fibrinolytic drug consisting of a complex of *streptokinase and *plasminogen. It is administered by injection in the treatment of coronary thrombosis. Possible side-effects include local bleeding, slowing of the heart, flushing, low blood pressure, fever, nausea, vomiting, and allergic reactions. Trade name: **Eminase**.

ankle *n.* **1.** the hinge joint between the leg and the foot. It consists of the *talus (ankle bone), which projects into a socket formed by the lower ends of the *tibia and *fibula. **2.** the whole region of the ankle joint, including the *tarsus and the ends of the tibia and fibula.

ankyloblepharon *n.* an abnormal fusion (partial or complete) of the upper and lower eyelid margins.

ankylosing spondylitis *see* SPONDYLITIS.

ankylosis *n.* fusion of the bones across a joint space, either by bony tissue (**bony ankylosis**) or by shortening of connecting fibrous tissue (**fibrous ankylosis**). Ankylosis is a complication of prolonged joint inflammation, as may occur in chronic infection (e.g. tuberculosis) or rheumatic disease (e.g. ankylosing *spondylitis).

Ankylostoma *n.* *see* ANCYLOSTOMA.

annulus *n.* (in anatomy) a circular opening or ring-shaped structure. —**annular** *adj.*

anodontia *n.* absence of the teeth because they have failed to develop. It is more common for only a few teeth to fail to develop (*see* HYPODONTIA).

anodyne *n.* any treatment or drug that soothes and eases pain.

anomaloscope *n.* an instrument for testing colour discrimination. By adjusting the controls the subject has to produce a mixture of red and green light to match a yellow light. The matching is done on a brightly illuminated disc viewed down a telescope.

anomalous pulmonary venous drainage a congenital abnormality in which the pulmonary veins enter the right atrium or vena cava instead of draining into the left atrium. The features are those of an *atrial septal defect.

anomaly *n.* any deviation from the normal, especially a congenital or developmental defect.

anomia *n.* **1.** a form of *aphasia in which the patient is unable to give the names of objects, although retaining an understanding of their use and the ability to put words together into speech. **2.** absence of respect for laws and established customs, which is a feature of *psychopathy and *dyssocial personality disorder.

anonychia *n.* congenital absence of one or more nails.

Anopheles *n.* a genus of widely distributed mosquitoes, occurring in tropical and temperate regions, with some 350 species. The malarial parasite (*see* PLASMODIUM) is transmitted to man solely through the bite of female *Anopheles* mosquitoes. Some species of *Anopheles* may transmit the parasites of bancroftian *filariasis.

anophthalmos *n.* congenital absence of the eye.

anoplasty *n.* a surgical technique used to repair a weak or injured anal sphincter.

anorchism *n.* congenital absence of one or both testes.

anorexia *n.* loss of appetite.

anorexia nervosa a psychological illness, most common in female adolescents, in which the patients starve themselves or use other techniques, such as vomiting or taking laxatives, to induce weight loss. They are motivated by a false perception of their bodies as fat and/or a *phobia of becoming fat. The result is severe loss of weight, often with *amenorrhoea, and sometimes even death from starvation. The cause of the illness is complicated – problems within the family and rejection of adult sexuality are often factors involved. Patients must be persuaded to eat enough to maintain a normal body weight and their emotional disturbance is usually treated with *psychotherapy. *See also* BULIMIA.

anosmia *n.* a loss of the sense of smell. This is most often due to a head cold but it may be caused by a fracture through the anterior fossa of the skull or a frontal brain tumour.

anovular (anovulatory) *adj.* not associated with the development and release of a female germ cell (ovum) in the ovary, as in **anovular menstruation**.

anoxaemia *n.* a condition in which there is less than the normal concentration of oxygen in the blood. *See also* ANOXIA, HYPOXAEMIA.

anoxia *n.* a condition in which the tissues of the body receive inadequate amounts of oxygen. This may result from low atmospheric pressure at high altitudes; a shortage of circulating blood, red blood cells, or haemoglobin; or disordered blood flow, such as occurs in heart failure. It can also result from insufficient oxygen reaching the blood in the lungs due to poor breathing movements or because disease, such as pneumonia, is reducing the effective surface area of lung tissue. *See also* HYPOXIA. —**anoxic** *adj.*

ansa *n.* (in anatomy) a loop; for example, the **ansa hypoglossi** is the loop formed by the descending branch of the hypoglossal nerve.

ansiform *adj.* (in anatomy) shaped like a loop. The term is applied to certain lobules of the cerebellum.

ant- (anti-) *prefix denoting* opposed to; counteracting; relieving. Examples: **antarthritic** (relieving arthritis); **antibacterial** (destroying or stopping the growth of bacteria).

Antabuse *n.* *see* DISULFIRAM.

antacid *n.* a drug that neutralizes the hydrochloric acid secreted in the digestive juices of the stomach. Antacids, which include aluminium hydroxide, calcium carbonate, magnesium hydroxide, and sodium bicarbonate, are used to relieve pain and discomfort in disorders of the digestive system, including peptic ulcer.

antagonist *n.* **1.** a muscle whose action (contraction) opposes that of another muscle (called the **agonist** or **prime mover**). Antagonists relax to allow the agonists to effect movement. **2.** a drug or other substance with opposite action to that of another drug or natural body chemical, which it inhibits. Examples are the *anti-metabolites. —**antagonism** *n.*

antazoline *n.* a short-acting *antihistamine drug, given by mouth to relieve the symptoms of allergic reactions. It is less irritating than the other antihistamines, but it produces their characteristic side-effects, such as drowsiness, dizziness, and incoordination. Trade name: **Otrivine-Antistin**.

ante- *prefix denoting* before. Examples: **antenatal** (before birth); **anteprandial** (before meals).

anteflexion *n.* the bending forward of an organ. A mild degree of anteflexion of the uterus is considered to be normal.

ante mortem before death. *Compare* POST MORTEM.

antenatal diagnosis *see* PRENATAL DIAGNOSIS.

antepartum *adj.* occurring before the onset of labour.

antepartum haemorrhage bleeding from the genital tract after the 24th week of pregnancy until the birth of the baby.

anterior *adj.* **1.** describing or relating to the front (ventral) portion of the body or limbs. **2.** describing the front part of any organ. For example, the **anterior chamber** of the eye is that part of the eye between the cornea and the lens, which is filled with aqueous humour.

anteversion *n.* the forward inclination of an organ, especially the normal forward inclination of the uterus.

anthelmintic **1.** *n.* any drug or chemical agent used to destroy parasitic worms (helminths), e.g. tapeworms, roundworms, and flukes, and/or remove them from the body. Anthelmintics include *albendazole, *bephenium hydroxynaphthoate, *mebendazole, *niclosamide, *piperazine, and *praziquantel. **2.** *adj.* having the power to destroy or eliminate helminths.

anthracosis *n.* *see* COAL-WORKER'S PNEUMOCONIOSIS.

anthracycline *n.* any of 500 or so antibiotics synthesized or isolated from species of *Streptomyces*. *Doxorubicin is the most important member of this group of compounds, which have wide activity against tumours.

anthrax *n.* an acute infectious disease of farm animals caused by the bacterium *Bacillus anthracis*, which can be transmitted to man by contact with animal hair, hides, or excrement. In man the disease attacks either the lungs, causing pneumonia, or the skin, producing severe ulceration (known as **malignant pustule**).

Woolsorter's disease is a serious infection of the skin or lungs by *B. anthracis*, affecting those handling wool or pelts (*see* OCCUPATIONAL DISEASE). Untreated anthrax can be fatal but administration of large doses of penicillin or tetracycline is usually effective.

anthrop- (anthropo-) *prefix denoting* the human race. Examples: **anthropogenesis** or **anthropogeny** (origin and development of); **anthropoid** (resembling); **anthropology** (science of).

anthropometry *n.* the taking of measurements of the human body or its parts. Comparisons can then be made between individuals of different sexes, ages, and races to determine the difference between normal and abnormal development. —**anthropometric** *adj.*

anthropozoonosis *n.* a disease that is transmissible from an animal to man, or vice versa, under natural conditions. Diseases that are found primarily in animals and sometimes affect man include *leptospirosis, *anthrax, and *rabies.

anti-androgen *n.* any one of a group of drugs that block the cellular uptake of testosterone by the prostate gland and are therefore used in the treatment of prostate cancer, which is an androgen-dependent tumour, and various sexual disorders in men. Anti-androgens include *cyproterone.

anti-arrhythmic *n.* any of a group of drugs used to correct irregularities in the heartbeat (*see* ARRHYTHMIA). They include *atropine, *amiodarone, *verapamil, *quinidine, *disopyramide, and *lignocaine.

antibacterial *adj.* describing an antibiotic that is active against bacteria.

antibiotic *n.* a substance, produced by or derived from a microorganism, that destroys or inhibits the growth of other microorganisms. Antibiotics are used to treat infections caused by organisms that are sensitive to them, usually bacteria or fungi. They may alter the normal microbial content of the body (e.g. in the intestine, lungs, bladder) by destroying one or more groups of harmless or beneficial organisms, which may result in infections (such as thrush in women) due to overgrowth of resistant organisms. These side-effects are most likely to occur with **broad-spectrum antibiotics** (those active against a wide variety of organisms). Resistance may also develop in the microorganisms being treated; for example, through incorrect dosage or overprescription (*see also* SUPERINFECTION). Antibiotics should not be used to treat minor infections, which will clear up unaided. Some antibiotics may cause allergic reactions. *See also* AMINOGLYCOSIDES, ANTIFUNGAL, ANTIVIRAL DRUG, CEPHALOSPORIN, CHLORAMPHENICOL, PENICILLIN, QUINOLONE, STREPTOMYCIN, TETRACYCLINE.

antibody *n.* a special kind of blood protein that is synthesized in lymphoid tissue in response to the presence of a particular *antigen and circulates in the plasma to attack the antigen and render it harmless. The production of specific antibodies against antigens as diverse as invading bacteria, inhaled pollen grains, and foreign red blood cells is the basis of both *immunity and *allergy. Antibody formation is also responsible for tissue or organ rejection following transplantation. Chemically, antibodies are proteins of the globulin type; they are classified according to their structure and function (*see* IMMUNOGLOBULIN)

anticholinergic *adj.* inhibiting the action of *acetylcholine. *Parasympatholytic drugs are anticholinergic.

anticholinesterase *n.* any substance that inhibits the action of *cholinesterase, the enzyme that is responsible for the breakdown of the neurotransmitter acetylcholine, and therefore allows acetylcholine to continue transmitting nerve impulses. Drugs with anticholinesterase activity include *distigmine, *neostigmine, *pyridostigmine, and *physostigmine; their uses include the diagnosis and treatment of *myasthenia gravis. *See also* PARASYMPATHOMIMETIC.

anticoagulant *n.* an agent that prevents the clotting of blood. The natural anticoagulant *heparin directly interferes with blood clotting and is active both within the body and against a sample of blood in a test tube. Synthetic drugs, such as *phenindione and *warfarin, are effective only within the body, since they act by affecting blood *coagulation factors. They take longer to act than heparin. Anticoagulants are used to prevent the formation of blood clots or to break up clots in blood vessels in such conditions as thrombosis and embolism. Incorrect dosage may result in haemorrhage. See also FIBRINOLYTIC.

anticonvulsant *n.* a drug that prevents or reduces the severity and frequency of seizures in various types of epilepsy; the term **antiepileptic drug** is now preferred since not all seizures involve convulsions. The choice of drug is dictated by the type of seizure and the patient's response, and the dosage must be adjusted carefully as individuals vary in their response to these drugs and side-effects may be troublesome. Commonly used antiepileptic drugs include *carbamazepine, *lamotrigine, *phenytoin, *sodium valproate, **topiramate**, **gabapentin**, and **vigabatrin**.

antidepressant *n.* a drug that alleviates the symptoms of depression. The most widely prescribed antidepressants are a group of drugs with a basic chemical structure of three benzene rings, called **tricyclic antidepressants**, which include *amitriptyline and *imipramine. These drugs are useful in treating a variety of different depressive symptoms. Side-effects commonly include dry mouth, blurred vision, constipation, drowsiness, and difficulty in urination. Other antidepressants include the *MAO inhibitors, which have more severe side-effects, and the serotonin-specific reuptake inhibitors (see SSRI), e.g. *fluoxetine and *fluvoxamine, which generally have less sedative effects than the tricyclic antidepressants.

antidiuretic hormone (ADH) *see* VASOPRESSIN.

antidote *n.* a drug that counteracts the effects of a poison or of overdosage by another drug. For example, *dimercaprol is an antidote to arsenic, mercury, and other heavy metals.

antidromic *adj.* describing impulses travelling 'the wrong way' in a nerve fibre. This is rare but may happen in shingles, when the irritation caused by the virus in the spinal canal initiates impulses that travel outwards in normally afferent nerves. The area of skin that the sensory nerves supply (usually a strip on the trunk) becomes painfully blistered. Antidromic impulses cannot pass *synapses, which work in one direction only.

antiemetic *n.* a drug that prevents vomiting. Various drugs have this effect, including some *antihistamines (e.g. cyclizine, promethazine) and *anticholinergic drugs. They are used for such conditions as motion sickness and vertigo; drugs used to counteract nausea and vomiting caused by other drugs include *domperidone, *metoclopramide, and *ondansetron.

antiepileptic drug *see* ANTICONVULSANT.

antifibrinolytic *adj.* describing an agent that inhibits the dissolution of blood clots (see FIBRINOLYSIS). Antifibrinolytic drugs include *aprotinin and *tranexamic acid.

antifungal (antimycotic) *adj.* describing a drug that kills or inactivates fungi and is used to treat fungal (including yeast) infections. Antifungal drugs include *amphotericin, *griseofulvin, the *imidazoles, *nystatin, *terbinafine, and *tolnaftate.

antigen *n.* any substance that the body regards as foreign or potentially dangerous and against which it produces an *antibody. Antigens are usually proteins, but simple substances, even metals, may become antigenic by combining with and modifying the body's own proteins. These are called **haptens**. —**antigenic** *adj.*

antigen-presenting cell *see* APC, HELPER T-CELL.

antihelix (anthelix) *n.* the curved inner ridge of the *pinna of the ear.

antihistamine *n.* a drug that inhibits the action of *histamine in the body by blocking the receptors for histamine, of which there are two types: H_1 and H_2. When stimulated by histamine, H_1 receptors may produce such allergic reactions as hay fever, pruritus (itching), and urticaria (nettle rash). Antihistamines that block H_1 receptors (**H_1-receptor antagonists**), for example *acrivastine, *astemizole, *azatadine, and *chlorpheniramine, are used to relieve these conditions. Many H₁-receptor antagonists, e.g. *cyclizine and *promethazine, also have strong *antiemetic activity and are used to prevent motion sickness. The most common side-effect of these drugs is drowsiness and because of this they are sometimes used to promote sleep. Other side-effects include dizziness, blurred vision, tremors, digestive upsets, and lack of muscular coordination.

H₂ receptors are found mainly in the stomach, where stimulation by histamine causes secretion of acid gastric juice. **H₂ antagonists** (e.g. *cimetidine, *ranitidine) block these receptors and reduce gastric acid secretion; they are used in the treatment of *peptic ulcers and *gastro-oesophageal reflux disease.

anti-inflammatory 1. *adj.* describing a drug that reduces *inflammation. The various groups of anti-inflammatory drugs act against one or more of the mediators that initiate or maintain inflammation. Some groups suppress only certain aspects of the inflammatory response. The main groups of anti-inflammatory drugs are the *antihistamines, the glucocorticoids (*see* CORTICOSTEROID), and the nonsteroidal anti-inflammatory drugs (*see* NSAID). **2.** *n.* an anti-inflammatory drug.

antiketogenic *n.* an agent that prevents formation of *ketones in the body.

antilymphocyte serum (antilymphocyte globulin, ALS, ALG) an *antiserum, containing antibodies that suppress lymphocytic activity, prepared by injecting an animal with lymphocytes. ALS may be given to a patient to prevent the immune reaction that causes tissue rejection following transplantation of such organs as kidneys. Administration naturally also impairs other immunity mechanisms, making infection a serious hazard.

antimetabolite *n.* any one of a group of drugs that interfere with the normal metabolic processes within cells by combining with the enzymes responsible for them. Some drugs used in the treatment of cancer, e.g. *fluorouracil, *methotrexate, and *mercaptopurine, are antimetabolites that prevent cell growth by interfering with enzyme reactions essen-

tial for nucleic acid synthesis. Side-effects of antimetabolites can be severe, involving blood cell disorders and digestive disturbances. *See also* CHEMOTHERAPY, CYTOTOXIC DRUG.

antimitotic *n.* any one of a group of drugs that inhibit cell division and growth, e.g. *doxorubicin, *aclarubicin. The drugs used to treat cancer are mainly antimitotics. *See also* ANTIMETABOLITE, CYTOTOXIC DRUG.

antimutagen *n.* a substance that can either reduce the spontaneous production of mutations or prevent or reverse the action of a *mutagen.

antimycotic *adj. see* ANTIFUNGAL.

anti-oestrogen *n.* one of a group of drugs that oppose the action of *oestrogen. The most important of these drugs is currently *tamoxifen, which antagonizes the action of oestrogens at the tissue receptors and is used in the treatment of breast cancers dependent on oestrogen. Because they stimulate the production of pituitary *gonadotrophins, some anti-oestrogens (e.g. *clomiphene) are used to induce or stimulate ovulation in infertility treatment. Side-effects of anti-oestrogens include hot flushes, itching of the vulva, nausea, vomiting, fluid retention, and sometimes vaginal bleeding.

antioxidant *n.* a substance capable of neutralizing oxygen free radicals, the highly active and damaging atoms and chemical groups produced by various disease processes and by poisons, radiation, smoking, and other agencies. The body contains its own natural antioxidants but there is growing medical interest in the possibility of controlling cell and tissue damage by means of supplementary antioxidants. Those most commonly used are *vitamin C (ascorbic acid), *vitamin E (tocopherols), and beta *carotene. Evidence is accumulating that these substances can reduce the incidence of a number of serious diseases.

antiperistalsis *n.* a wave of contraction in the alimentary canal that passes in an oral (i.e. upward or backwards) direction (*compare* PERISTALSIS). It was formerly thought that antiperistalsis occurred in vomiting but modern physiological studies indicate that it never takes place in man.

antipruritic *n.* an agent that relieves itching (*pruritus). Examples are *calamine and *crotamiton, applied in creams or lotions, and some *antihistamine drugs (e.g. *trimeprazine), used if the itching is due to an allergy.

antipsychotic *adj.* describing a group of drugs used to treat severe mental disorders (psychoses), including schizophrenia and mania; some are administered in small doses to relieve anxiety. Formerly known as **major tranquillizers**, antipsychotic drugs include the *phenothiazines (e.g. *chlorpromazine), *butyrophenones (e.g. *haloperidol), and **thioxanthenes** (e.g. *flupenthixol). The **atypical antipsychotics** are a group of more recently developed drugs that may be helpful in those who do not respond to treatment with other antipsychotics. They include *clozapine, *risperidone, **olanzapine**, and **sertindole**. Side-effects of many antipsychotics at high doses include abnormal involuntary movements.

antipyretic *n.* a drug that reduces fever by lowering the body temperature. Several analgesic drugs have antipyretic activity, including *aspirin, *paracetamol, *phenylbutazone, and *mefenamic acid.

antisecretory drug any drug that reduces the normal rate of secretion of a body fluid, usually one that reduces acid secretion into the stomach. Such drugs include anticholinergic drugs (*see* PARASYMPATHOLYTIC), H_2-receptor antagonists (*see* ANTIHISTAMINE), and *proton-pump inhibitors.

antisepsis *n.* the elimination of bacteria, fungi, viruses, and other microorganisms that cause disease by the use of chemical or physical methods.

antiseptic *n.* a chemical that destroys or inhibits the growth of disease-causing bacteria and other microorganisms and is sufficiently nontoxic to be applied to the skin or mucous membranes to cleanse wounds and prevent infections or to be used internally to treat infections of the intestine and bladder. Examples are *cetrimide, *chlorhexidine, *dequalinium, and *hexamine.

antiserum *n.* (*pl.* **antisera**) a serum that contains antibodies against antigens of a particular kind; it may be injected to treat, or give temporary protection (passive *immunity) against, specific diseases. Antisera are prepared in large quantities in such animals as horses. In the laboratory, they are used to identify unknown organisms responsible for infection (*see* AGGLUTINATION).

antispasmodic *n.* a drug that relieves spasm of smooth muscle. *See* SPASMOLYTIC. *Compare* ANTISPASTIC.

antispastic *n.* a drug that relieves spasm of skeletal muscle. *See also* MUSCLE RELAXANT. *Compare* ANTISPASMODIC.

antitoxin *n.* an antibody produced by the body to counteract a toxin formed by invading bacteria or from any other source.

antitragus *n.* a small projection of cartilage above the lobe of the ear, opposite the tragus. *See* PINNA.

antitussive *n.* a drug, such as *dextromethorphan or *pholcodine, that suppresses coughing, possibly by reducing the activity of the cough centre in the brain and by depressing respiration. Some analgesic drugs also have antitussive activity, e.g. *codeine, diamorphine (*see* HEROIN), and *methadone.

antivenene (antivenin) *n.* an *antiserum containing antibodies against specific poisons in the venom of such an animal as a snake, spider, or scorpion.

antiviral drug a drug effective against viruses that cause disease. Antiviral drugs include *acyclovir, *ganciclovir, *vidarabine, *idoxuridine, **trifluridine** (**Viroptic**), *foscarnet, *zidovudine, *amantadine, and *ribavirin.

antrectomy *n.* **1.** surgical removal of the bony walls of an *antrum. *See* ANTROSTOMY. **2.** a surgical operation in which a part of the stomach (the antrum) is removed. Most secretions of acid, pepsin, and the hormone gastrin occur in the antrum and the operation may be required (usually combined with *vagotomy) in the treatment of peptic ulcers that have recurred after vagotomy and are resistant to H_2-blocking drugs (*see* ANTIHISTA-MINE).

antroscopy *n.* inspection of the inside of the maxillary sinus (*see* PARANASAL SINUSES) using an *endoscope (called an **antroscope**).

antrostomy *n.* a surgical operation to produce a permanent or semipermanent artificial opening to an *antrum in a bone, so providing drainage for any fluid. The operation is sometimes carried out to treat infection of the *paranasal sinuses.

antrum *n.* **1.** a cavity, especially a cavity in a bone. The **mastoid** (or **tympanic**) **antrum** is the space connecting the air cells of the *mastoid process with the chamber of the inner ear. **2.** the part of the *stomach adjoining the pylorus (**pyloric** or **gastric antrum**).

anuria *n.* failure of the kidneys to produce urine. This can occur in a variety of conditions that produce a sustained drop in blood pressure. Urgent assessment is required to differentiate lack of production of urine from an obstruction to the flow of urine from the kidneys, which can readily be relieved. Anuria is associated with increasing *uraemia and may require *haemodialysis.

anus *n.* the opening at the lower end of the alimentary canal, through which the faeces are discharged. It opens out from the *anal canal and is guarded by two sphincters. The anus is closed except during defecation. —**anal** *adj.*

anvil *n.* (in anatomy) *see* INCUS.

anxiety *n.* generalized pervasive *fear. **Anxiety state** is a condition in which anxiety dominates the patient's life; neuroses are now usually called **anxiety disorders** (*see* NEUROSIS, PANIC DISORDER, POST-TRAUMATIC STRESS DISORDER. *See also* GENERALIZED ANXIETY DISORDER.

A-O Association for Osteosynthesis: denoting a widely used system for treating fractures by metal inserts.

aorta *n.* (*pl.* **aortae** or **aortas**) the main artery of the body, from which all others derive. It arises from the left ventricle (**ascending aorta**), arches over the top of the heart (*see* AORTIC ARCH) and descends in front of the backbone (**descending aorta**),

giving off large and small branches and finally dividing to form the right and left *iliac arteries. The part of the descending aorta from the aortic arch to the diaphragm is called the **thoracic aorta**; the part below the diaphragm is the **abdominal aorta**. —**aortic** *adj.*

aortic aneurysm *see* ANEURYSM.

aortic arch that part of the aorta that extends from the ascending aorta, upward over the heart and then backward and down as far as the fourth thoracic vertebra. *Stretch receptors in its outer wall monitor blood pressure and form part of the system maintaining this at a constant level.

aortic regurgitation reflux of blood from the aorta into the left ventricle during diastole. Aortic regurgitation most commonly follows scarring of the aortic valve as a result of previous acute rheumatic fever, but it may also result from other conditions, such as syphilis or dissecting aneurysm. Mild cases are symptom-free, but patients more severely affected develop breathlessness, angina pectoris, and enlargement of the heart; all have a diastolic murmur. A badly affected valve may be replaced surgically with a prosthesis.

aortic replacement a surgical technique used to replace a diseased length of aorta, most often the abdominal aorta. It usually involves inserting into the aorta a flexible tube of artificial material, which functions as a substitute for the diseased section.

aortic stenosis narrowing of the opening of the aortic valve due to fusion of the cusps that comprise the valve. It may result from previous rheumatic fever, or from calcification and scarring in a valve that has two cusps instead of the normal three, or it may be congenital. Aortic stenosis obstructs the flow of blood from the left ventricle to the aorta during systole. Breathlessness on effort, angina pectoris, and fainting may follow. The patient has a systolic murmur. When symptoms develop the valve should be replaced surgically with a mechanical prosthesis (such as a Starr-Edwards ball-cage valve) or with an aortic valve graft.

aortic valve a valve in the heart, lying between the left ventricle and the aorta. It consists of three pockets, shaped like half-moons, that prevent blood returning to the ventricle from the aorta. *See also* SEMILUNAR VALVE.

aortitis *n.* inflammation of the aorta, which most commonly occurs as a late complication of syphilis. Aortitis principally affects the ascending thoracic aorta and may result in the formation of an aneurysm and obstruction to the coronary blood flow. Chest pain may occur from pressure on surrounding structures or from the reduced blood supply to the heart. *Aortic regurgitation may be found. The syphilitic infection is treated with penicillin but surgical repair to the aortic aneurysm or valve may be needed.

aortography *n.* X-ray examination of the aorta, which involves the injection into it of a *radiopaque contrast medium, after which a series of X-rays is taken (*see* ANGIOCARDIOGRAPHY). Aortography is undertaken to reveal the extent and site of diseases such as atheromatous obstruction or aneurysm; it is an essential aid to the planning of surgical treatment.

APC (antigen-presenting cell) a macrophage that processes antigen for presentation to T-lymphocytes (*see* HELPER T-CELL, KILLER CELL).

aperient *n.* a mild *laxative.

apex *n.* the tip or summit of an organ; for example the heart or lung. The apex of a *tooth is the tip of the root, where there is a small hole (the **apical foramen**) through which vessels and nerves pass from the pulp to the periapical tissues. —**apical** *adj.*

apex beat the impact of the heart against the chest wall during *systole. It can be felt or heard to the left of the breastbone, in the space between the fifth and sixth ribs.

apexification *n.* a procedure to allow the end of the root of an immature tooth to form a hard tissue barrier following traumatic injury that has caused the pulp to die.

apexogenesis *n.* a procedure that allows the root tip to continue forming

when an immature tooth has sustained limited injury following trauma.

Apgar score a method of rapidly assessing the general state of a baby immediately after birth. A maximum of 2 points is given for each of the following signs, usually measured at one minute and five minutes after delivery: type of breathing, heart rate, colour, muscle tone, and response to stimuli. Thus an infant scoring 10 points would be in optimum condition. When the score is low, the test is repeated at intervals as a guide to short-term progress. [V. Apgar (1909–74), US anaesthetist]

aphakia *n.* absence of the lens of the eye: the state of the eye after a cataract has been removed.

aphasia (dysphasia) *n.* a disorder of language affecting the generation and content of speech and its understanding (it is not a disorder of articulation: *see* DYSARTHRIA). It is caused by disease in the left half of the brain (the dominant hemisphere) in a right-handed person. It is commonly accompanied by difficulties in reading and writing. *See also* DYSLALIA. —**aphasic** *adj.*

aphonia *n.* absence or loss of the voice caused by disease of the larynx or mouth or by disease of the nerves and muscles involved in the generation and articulation of speech. If loss of speech is due to a defect in the cerebral hemispheres, the disorder is *aphasia.

aphrenia *n.* failure of development of the intellectual faculties. *See* MENTAL RETARDATION.

aphrodisiac *n.* an agent that stimulates sexual excitement.

aphtha *n.* (*pl.* **aphthae**) a small ulcer, occurring singly or in groups in the mouth as white or red spots. Their cause is unknown and only palliative treatment is available. —**aphthous** *adj.*

apical abscess an abscess in the bone around the apex of a tooth. An acute abscess is extremely painful, causing swelling of the jaw and sometimes also the face. A chronic abscess may cause no pain or swelling. An abscess invariably results from damage to and infection of the pulp of the tooth. Treatment is drainage and *root canal treatment or extraction of the tooth; antibiotics may give temporary relief.

apicectomy n. (in dentistry) surgical removal of the apex of the root of a tooth. It is usually accompanied by placement of a filling in the root end and is carried out when *root canal treatment has failed and cannot be redone.

aplasia n. total or partial failure of development of an organ or tissue. See also AGENESIS. —**aplastic** adj.

APMPPE acute posterior multifocal placoid *pigment epitheliopathy.

apneusis n. a state in which prolonged inhalation occurs. It occurs when the appropriate inhibitory influences are prevented from reaching the inspiratory centre of the brain.

apnoea n. temporary cessation of breathing from any cause. Attacks of apnoea are common in newborn babies and should be taken seriously although they do not necessarily indicate serious illness. See also SLEEP APNOEA. —**apnoeic** adj.

apnoea monitor an electronic alarm that is activated by a sensor that responds to a baby's respiratory movements. It can be used at home to monitor babies thought to be at risk of *cot death.

apocrine adj. **1.** describing sweat glands that occur only in hairy parts of the body, especially the armpit and groin. These glands develop in the hair follicles and appear after puberty has been reached. The strong odours associated with sweating result from the action of bacteria on the sweat produced by apocrine glands. Compare ECCRINE. **2.** describing a type of gland that loses part of its protoplasm when secreting. See SECRETION.

apocrinitis n. inflammation of the *apocrine glands (found in the armpits, groin, and perineum), characterized by chronicity and subcutaneous septic tracks. See HIDRADENITIS SUPPURATIVA.

apomorphine n. an *emetic that produces its effect by direct action on the vomiting centre in the brain. It is given by subcutaneous injection and acts within a few minutes. It is employed in the treatment of poisoning by noncorrosive substances that have been taken by mouth. In nonemetic (lower) dosage, apomorphine has sedative, hypnotic, and expectorant actions.

aponeurosis n. a thin but strong fibrous sheet of tissue that replaces a *tendon in muscles that are flat and sheetlike and have a wide area of attachment (e.g. to bones). —**aponeurotic** adj.

apophysis n. **1.** a protuberance of bone to which a tendon is attached. It ossifies separately from the rest of the bone and fuses with it at maturity. **2.** a projection of any other part, e.g. of the brain (**apophysis cerebri**: the *pineal gland).

apophysitis n. inflammation, with pain and swelling, caused by excessive pull of a tendon on the *apophysis to which it is attached. It occurs, for example, in *Osgood-Schlatter disease and *Sever's disease.

apoplexy n. see STROKE.

apoptosis n. programmed cell death, which results in the ordered removal of cells and occurs naturally as part of the normal development, maintenance, and renewal of cells, tissues, and organs. During embryonic development, for example, the fingers are 'sculpted' from the embryonic spadelike hand by apoptosis of the cells between them. Failure of apoptosis has been implicated in the uncontrolled cell division that occurs in cancer. Abnormal apoptosis, due to failure of the mechanisms that control it, may be a causative factor in autoimmune disease.

apotreptic adj. describing *response prevention therapy for obsessional neurosis.

appendectomy n. the usual US term for *appendicectomy.

appendicectomy n. surgical removal of the vermiform appendix. See also APPENDICITIS.

appendicitis n. inflammation of the vermiform *appendix. **Acute appendicitis**, which has become common this century, usually affects young people. The chief symptom is abdominal pain, first central and later (with tenderness) in the right lower abdomen, over the appendix. Unusual positions of the appendix may cause pain in different sites, leading to difficulty in diagnosis. Vomiting and diarrhoea sometimes occur, but fever is slight. If not treated by surgical removal (appendicectomy) the condition usually progresses to cause an abscess or generalized *peritonitis. Conditions that mimic appendicitis include mesenteric *lymphadenitis, acute ileitis (*see* CROHN'S DISEASE), *pyelonephritis, and pneumonia. **Chronic appendicitis** was a popular diagnosis 20–50 years ago to explain recurrent pains in the lower abdomen. It is rare, and appendicectomy will not usually cure such pains.

appendicostomy *n.* an operation in which the vermiform appendix is brought through the abdominal wall and opened in order to drain or decompress the intestine. It is now rarely performed, *ileostomy, *caecostomy, or *colostomy being preferred.

appendicular *adj.* **1.** relating to or affecting the vermiform appendix. **2.** relating to the limbs: the **appendicular skeleton** comprises the bones of the limbs.

appendix (vermiform appendix) *n.* the short thin blind-ended tube, 7–10 cm long, that is attached to the end of the caecum (a pouch at the start of the large intestine). It has no known function in man and is liable to become infected and inflamed, especially in young adults (*see* APPENDICITIS).

apperception *n.* (in psychology) the process by which the qualities of an object, situation, etc., perceived by an individual are correlated with his/her preexisting knowledge.

appestat *n.* a region in the brain that controls the amount of food intake. Appetite suppressants probably decrease hunger by changing the chemical characteristics of this centre.

applanation *n.* a method of flattening the cornea that is used to determine the intraocular pressure in applanation tonometry (*see* OPHTHALMOTONOMETER).

applicator *n.* any device used to apply medication or treatment to a particular part of the body.

apposition *n.* the state of two structures, such as parts of the body, being in close contact. For example, the fingers are brought into apposition when the fist is clenched, and the eyelids when the eyes are closed.

apraclonidine *n.* a *sympathomimetic drug administered in the form of eyedrops to reduce or prevent raised intraocular pressure after laser surgery. Trade name: **Iopidine**.

apraxia (dyspraxia) *n.* an inability to make skilled movements with accuracy. This is a disorder of the *cerebral cortex resulting in the patient's inability to organize the movements rather than clumsiness due to weakness, sensory loss, or disease of the *cerebellum. It is most often caused by disease of the *parietal lobes of the brain and sometimes by disease of the frontal lobes.

aproctia *n.* congenital absence of the anus or its opening. *See* IMPERFORATE ANUS.

aprosexia *n.* inability to fix the attention on any subject, due to poor eyesight, defective hearing, or mental weakness.

aprotinin *n.* a drug that prevents the breakdown of blood clots (*see* FIBRINOLYSIS) by blocking the action of the enzyme plasmin, i.e. it is an *antifibrinolytic drug. It is administered by injection to control the severe bleeding that may occur in certain cancers and with *fibrinolytic treatments. Trade name: **Trasylol**.

APUD cells cells that share the metabolic property of *a*mine-*p*recursor *u*ptake and *d*ecarboxylation. They have a wide distribution, especially in the mucosa of the gastrointestinal tract and pancreas, and are able to form a large variety of peptide hormonal substances; they are often known as the **diffuse endocrine system**.

apudoma *n.* a tumour that contains *APUD cells and may give rise to symptoms caused by excessive production of the hormones and other peptides that these cells produce. *Argentaffinomas are a good example of this group of tumours, but there are many others (e.g. *gastrinomas, *somatostatinomas, and *vipomas).

apyrexia *n.* the absence of fever.

aqueduct *n.* (in anatomy) a canal containing fluid. For example, the **aqueduct of the midbrain** (**cerebral aqueduct, aqueduct of Sylvius**) connects the third and fourth *ventricles.

aqueous humour the watery fluid that fills the chamber of the *eye immediately behind the cornea and in front of the lens. It is continually being formed – chiefly by capillaries of the ciliary processes – and it drains away into Schlemm's canal, at the junction of the cornea and sclera.

arachidonic acid *see* ESSENTIAL FATTY ACID.

arachnidism *n.* poisoning from the bite of a spider. Toxins from the less venomous species of spider cause only local pain, redness, and swelling. Toxins from more venomous species, such as the black widow (*Lactrodectus mactans*), cause muscular pains, convulsions, nausea, and paralysis.

arachnodactyly *n.* abnormally long and slender fingers: usually associated with excessive height and congenital defects of the heart and eyes in *Marfan's syndrome.

arachnoid (arachnoid mater) *n.* the middle of the three membranes covering the brain and spinal cord (*see* MENINGES), which has a fine, almost cobweb-like, texture. Between it and the pia mater within lies the subarachnoid space, containing cerebrospinal fluid and large blood vessels; the membrane itself has no blood supply.

arachnoiditis *n.* an inflammatory process causing thickening and scarring (fibrosis) of the membranous linings (*meninges) of the spinal canal. The resulting entrapment of nerve roots may result in weakness, pain, and numbness in the affected area. The condition may result from infection of the meninges, surgery, or as a response to the oil-based dyes previously used in *myelography. The reaction to myelography is prevented by the current use of water-soluble dyes.

arachnoid villus one of the thin-walled projections outwards of the arachnoid membrane into the blood-filled sinuses of the dura, acting as a one-way valve for the flow of cerebrospinal fluid from the subarachnoid space into the bloodstream. Large villi, known as **arachnoid granulations** (or **Pacchionian bodies**), are found

in the region of the superior sagittal sinus. They may be so distended as to cause pitting of the adjacent bone.

arbor *n.* (in anatomy) a treelike structure. **Arbor vitae** is the treelike outline of white matter seen in sections of the cerebellum; it also refers to the treelike appearance of the inner folds of the cervix (neck) of the uterus.

arbovirus *n.* one of a group of RNA-containing viruses that are transmitted from animals to man by insects (i.e. arthropods; hence *arthropod-borne* viruses) and cause diseases resulting in encephalitis or serious fever, such as dengue and yellow fever.

ARC AIDS-related complex: *see* AIDS.

arc-eye *n.* a painful condition of the eyes caused by damage to the surface of the cornea by ultraviolet light from arc welding. It usually resolves if the eyes are padded for 24 hours. It is similar to *snow blindness and the condition caused by overexposure of the eye to sun-tanning lamps.

arch- (arche-, archi-, archo-) *prefix denoting* first; primitive; ancestral. Example: **archinephron** (first-formed embryonic kidney).

archenteron *n.* a cavity that forms in the very early embryo as the result of gastrulation (*see* GASTRULA). In man it forms a tubular cavity, the **archenteric canal**, which connects the amniotic cavity with the yolk sac. —**archenteric** *adj.*

archetype *n.* (in Jungian psychology) an inherited idea or mode of thought supposed to be present in the *unconscious mind and to derive from the experience of the whole human race, not from the life experience of the individual.

archipallium *n.* the *hippocampal formation of the cerebrum. The term is seldom used.

arcuate keratotomy a curved incision made in the periphery of the cornea. It is usually performed in the region of greatest curvature of the cornea in order to flatten it and hence reduce *astigmatism.

arcus *n.* (in anatomy) an arch; for example the **arcus aortae** (*aortic arch).

arcus senilis a greyish line in the periphery of the cornea, concentric with the edge but separated from it by a clear zone. It begins above and below but may become a continuous ring. It consists of an infiltration of fatty material and is common in the elderly. When it occurs in younger people it may indicate abnormal fat metabolism, but there is great racial variation in its incidence. It never affects vision.

ARDS *see* ADULT RESPIRATORY DISTRESS SYNDROME.

areola *n.* **1.** the brownish or pink ring of tissue surrounding the nipple of the breast. **2.** the part of the iris that surrounds the pupil of the eye. **3.** a small space in a tissue. —**areolar** *adj.*

areolar tissue loose *connective tissue consisting of a meshwork of collagen, elastic tissue, and reticular fibres interspersed with numerous connective tissue cells. It binds the skin to underlying muscles and forms a link between organs while allowing a high degree of relative movement.

Argasidae *n. see* TICK.

argentaffin cells cells that stain readily with silver salts. Such cells occur, for example, in the crypts of Lieberkühn in the intestine.

argentaffinoma (carcinoid) *n.* a tumour of the *argentaffin cells in the glands of the intestine (*see* APUDOMA). Argentaffinomas typically occur in the tip of the appendix and are among the commonest tumours of the small intestine. They may also occur in the rectum and other parts of the digestive tract and in the bronchial tree (**bronchial carcinoid adenoma**). Argentaffinomas sometimes produce 5-hydroxytryptamine (serotonin), prostaglandins, and other physiologically active substances, which are inactivated in the liver. If the tumour has spread to the liver excess amounts of these substances are released into the systemic circulation and the **carcinoid syndrome** results – flushing, headache, diarrhoea, asthma-like attacks, and in some cases damage to the right side of the heart.

arginine *n.* an *amino acid that plays an important role in the formation of *urea by the liver.

argon laser a type of *laser that produces a beam of intense light, used especially in eye surgery to treat disease of the retina (e.g. diabetic retinopathy) or glaucoma (as in argon laser *trabeculoplasty). *See also* PHOTOCOAGULATION.

Argyll Robertson pupil a disorder of the eyes, common to several diseases of the central nervous system, in which the *pupillary (light) reflex is absent. Although the pupils contract normally for near vision, they fail to contract in bright light. [D. Argyll Robertson (1837–1909), Scottish ophthalmologist]

argyria (argyrosis) *n.* the deposition of silver in the skin and other tissues, either resulting from industrial exposure or following ingestion or long-term administration of silver salts. A slate-grey pigmentation develops slowly; this is accentuated in areas exposed to light. Deposition of silver in the conjunctiva, corneal epithelium, stroma, and Descemet's membrane is usually due to chronic exposure to silver compounds or instillation of eye drops containing silver.

ariboflavinosis *n.* the group of symptoms caused by deficiency of riboflavin (vitamin B_2). These symptoms include inflammation of the tongue and lips and sores in the corners of the mouth.

ARMD age-related *macular degeneration.

ARN *see* ACUTE RETINAL NECROSIS.

Arnold-Chiari malformation a congenital disorder in which there is distortion of the base of the skull with protrusion of the lower brainstem and parts of the cerebellum through the opening for the spinal cord at the base of the skull. It is commonly associated with *neural tube defects and *hydrocephalus. [J. Arnold (1835–1915) and H. Chiari (1851–1916), German pathologists]

arousal *n.* **1.** a state of alertness and of high responsiveness to stimuli. It is produced by strong motivation, by anxiety, and by a stimulating environment. **2.** physiological activation of the *cerebral cortex by centres lower in the brain, such as the *reticular activating system, resulting in wakefulness and alertness. It is hypothesized that unduly high or low degrees of arousal lead to neuropsychiatric problems, such as *narcolepsy and *mania.

arrhenoblastoma n. see ANDROBLASTOMA.

arrhythmia n. any deviation from the normal rhythm (sinus rhythm) of the heart. The natural pacemaker of the heart (the sinoatrial node), which lies in the wall of the right atrium, controls the rate and rhythm of the whole heart under the influence of the autonomic nervous system. It generates electrical impulses that spread to the atria and ventricles, via specialized conducting tissues, and cause them to contract normally. Arrhythmias result from a disturbance of the generation or the conduction of these impulses and may be intermittent or continuous. They include *ectopic beats (extrasystoles), ectopic *tachycardias, *fibrillation, and *heart block (which is often associated with slow heart rates). Symptoms include palpitations, breathlessness, and chest pain. In more serious arrhythmias the *Stokes-Adams syndrome or *cardiac arrest may occur. Arrhythmias may result from most heart diseases but they also occur without apparent cause.

arsenic n. a poisonous greyish metallic element producing the symptoms of nausea, vomiting, diarrhoea, cramps, convulsions, and coma when ingested in large doses. Drugs used as antidotes to arsenic poisoning include *dimercaprol. Arsenic was formerly readily available in the form of rat poison and in fly-papers and was the poisoner's first choice during the 19th century, its presence in a body being then difficult to detect. Today detection is relatively simple. Arsenic was formerly used in medicine, the most important arsenical drugs being **arsphenamine (Salvarsan)** and **neoarsphenamine**, used in the treatment of syphilis and dangerous parasitic diseases. Symbol: As.

artefact n. see ARTIFACT.

arter- (arteri-, arterio-) prefix denoting an artery. Examples: **arteriopathy** (disease of); **arteriorrhaphy** (suture of); **arteriovenous** (relating to arteries and veins).

arteriectomy n. surgical excision of an artery or part of an artery. This may be performed as a diagnostic procedure (for example, to take an arterial biopsy in the diagnosis of arteritis) or during reconstruction of a blocked artery when the blocked segment is replaced by a synthetic graft.

arteriogram n. **1.** The final display, on either photographic film or a TV monitor, of the images produced during arteriography. **2.** a tracing of the wave form of an arterial pulse. This can be made directly, by means of an arterial needle puncture and pressure recording, or indirectly, by a recorder placed on the skin over an artery. The tracing may be recorded on a paper strip or on a screen (oscilloscope). Some heart defects produce characteristic pulse wave forms.

arteriography n. X-ray examination of an artery that has been outlined by the injection of a *radiopaque contrast medium. The major uses of arteriography are to demonstrate the site and extent of atheroma, especially in the coronary arteries (**coronary angiography**) and leg arteries (**femoral angiography**), and to reveal the site of aneurysms within the skull or cerebral tumours (**carotid** and **vertebral artery angiography**). See also MUGA SCAN.

arteriole n. a small branch of an *artery, leading into many smaller vessels – the *capillaries. By their constriction and dilation, under the regulation of the sympathetic nervous system, arterioles are the principal controllers of blood flow and pressure.

arteriolitis n. inflammation of the arterioles (the smallest arteries), which may complicate severe hypertension. This produces **necrotizing arteriolitis**, which may result in kidney failure. A similar condition may affect the lung in pulmonary hypertension.

arterioplasty n. surgical reconstruction of an artery; for example, in the treatment of *aneurysms.

arteriosclerosis n. an imprecise term used for any of several conditions affecting the arteries. The term is often used as a synonym for atherosclerosis (see ATHEROMA). It may also be used for **Mönckeberg's degeneration**, in which calcium is deposited in the arteries as part of the ageing process, and **arteriosclero-**

sis, in which the walls of small arteries become thickened due to ageing or hypertension.

arteriotomy *n.* an incision into, or a needle puncture of, the wall of an artery. This is most often performed as a diagnostic procedure in the course of *arteriography or cardiac *catheterization. It may also be required to remove an embolus (*see* EMBOLECTOMY).

arteriovenous anastomosis a thick-walled blood vessel that connects an arteriole directly with a venule, thus bypassing the capillaries. Arteriovenous anastomoses are commonly found in the skin of the lips, nose, ears, hands and feet; their muscular walls can constrict to reduce blood flow or dilate to allow blood through to these areas.

arteriovenous aneurysm a direct communication between an artery and vein, without an intervening capillary bed. It can occur as a congenital abnormality or it may be acquired following injury or surgery. It may affect the limbs, lungs, or viscera and may be single or multiple. If the connection is large, the short-circuiting of blood may produce heart failure. Large isolated arteriovenous aneurysms may be closed surgically.

arteriovenous malformation *see* ANGIOMA.

arteritis *n.* an inflammatory disease that affects the muscular walls of the arteries. It may be part of a *connective-tissue disease or it may be due to an infection, such as syphilis. The affected vessels are swollen and tender and may become blocked. **Temporal** (or **giant-cell**) **arteritis** occurs in the elderly and most commonly affects the arteries of the scalp. The patient complains of severe headache, and double vision or scalp tenderness may be present; blindness may result from thrombosis of the arteries to the eyes. Treatment with cortisone derivatives is rapidly effective.

artery *n.* a blood vessel carrying blood away from the heart. All arteries except the *pulmonary artery carry oxygenated blood. The walls of arteries contain smooth muscle fibres (see illustration), which contract or relax under the control

of the sympathetic nervous system. *See also* AORTA, ARTERIOLE.

Transverse section through an artery

labels: lumen — endothelium — tunica intima — elastic lamina — tunica media — tunica adventitia

arthr- (arthro-) *prefix denoting* a joint. Examples: **arthrology** (science of); **arthrosclerosis** (stiffening or hardening of).

arthralgia *n.* pain in a joint, without swelling or other signs of arthritis. *Compare* ARTHRITIS.

arthrectomy *n.* surgical excision of a joint. It is usually performed on a painful joint that has ceased to function, as may result from intractable infection, or after a failed joint replacement. *See also* (EXCISION) ARTHROPLASTY.

arthritis *n.* inflammation of one or more joints, characterized by swelling, warmth, redness of the overlying skin, pain, and restriction of motion. Over 200 diseases may cause arthritis, including *rheumatoid arthritis, *osteoarthritis, *gout, *tuberculosis, and other infections. Diagnosis is assisted by examination of the pattern of distribution of affected joints, X-rays, blood tests, and examination of synovial fluid obtained by *aspiration of a swollen joint. **Mono-** or **oligoarthritis** is inflammation of one joint, **pauciarthritis** of a few (four or less), and **polyarthritis** of many joints, either simultaneously or in sequence. Any disease involving the synovial membranes or causing degeneration of cartilage may cause arthritis. Treatment of arthritis depends on the cause, but aspirin and similar analgesics are often used to suppress inflammation, and hence reduce pain and swelling. *See also* PSORIATIC ARTHRITIS, SEPTIC ARTHRITIS, HAEMARTHROSIS, PYARTHROSIS, HYDRARTHROSIS. —**arthritic** *adj.*

The principal arteries of the body

arthrodesis *n.* fusion of bones across a joint space by surgical means, which eliminates movement. This operation is performed when a joint is very painful, highly unstable, grossly deformed or chronically infected, or when an *arthroplasty would be inadvisable or impossible. *See also* CHARNLEY CLAMPS.

arthrodic joint (gliding joint) a form of *diarthrosis (freely movable joint) in which the bony surfaces slide over each other without angular or rotational movement. Examples are the joints of the carpus and tarsus.

arthrography *n.* an X-ray technique for examining joints. A *contrast medium (either air or a liquid opaque to X-rays) is injected into the joint space, allowing its outline and contents to be traced accurately. Arthrography has now largely been replaced by *magnetic resonance imaging (MRI).

arthrogryposis *n.* *contracture of soft tissues that causes fixed deformities of the joints if untreated. **Arthrogryposis multiplex congenita** is a congenital disease with multiple causes in which there are contractures, stiff joints, and absent skin creases, as a result of the muscles being replaced by fibrous tissue. Treatment is by manipulation and splintage of deformed joints; surgical correction is sometimes required.

arthropathy *n.* any disease or disorder involving a joint.

arthroplasty *n.* surgical remodelling of a diseased joint. To prevent the ends of the bones fusing after the operation, a large gap may be created between them (**gap** or **excision arthroplasty**), a barrier of artificial material may be inserted (**interposition arthroplasty**), or one or both bone ends may be replaced by a *prosthesis of metal or plastic (**replacement arthroplasty**). This operation may replace both joint surfaces (**total arthroplasty**) or only one (*see* HEMIARTHROPLASTY). *See also* HIP REPLACEMENT.

arthropod *n.* any member of a large group of animals that possess a hard external skeleton and jointed legs and other appendages. Many arthropods are of medical importance, including the *mites, *ticks, and *insects.

arthroscope *n.* a telescope for insertion into a joint through a small incision in order to inspect its contents (*see* ARTHROSCOPY).

arthroscopy *n.* inspection of a joint cavity with an *arthroscope, enabling percutaneous surgery (such as *meniscectomy) and *biopsy to be performed.

arthrotomy *n.* a surgical incision to open a joint in order to inspect the contents or to drain pus in *septic arthritis.

articulation *n.* (in anatomy) the point or type of contact between two bones. *See* JOINT.

articulator *n.* (in dentistry) an apparatus for relating the upper and lower models of a patient's dentition in a fixed position, usually with maximum tooth contact. Some articulators can reproduce jaw movements. They are used in the construction of crowns, bridges, and dentures.

artifact (artefact) *n.* (in microscopy) a structure seen in a tissue under a microscope that is not present in the living tissue. Artifacts, which are produced by faulty *fixation or staining of the tissue, may give a false impression that disease or abnormality is present in the tissue when it is not.

artificial heart a titanium pump that is implanted into the body to take over the function of a failing left ventricle in patients with heart disease. This allows the diseased ventricle time to recover its function. The pump is powered by an external battery, strapped to the patient's body, to which it is connected by wires passed through the patient's skin. Originally pumps were implanted into the abdomen, but the most recent devices are small enough to fit into the heart itself.

artificial insemination instrumental introduction of semen into the vagina in order that a woman may conceive. Insemination is timed to coincide with the day on which the woman is expected to ovulate (*see* MENSTRUAL CYCLE). The semen specimen may be provided by the husband (**AIH** – **artificial insemination husband**), for example in cases of *impotence, or by an anonymous donor (**DI – donor insemination**), usually in cases where the husband is sterile.

artificial kidney (dialyser) *see* HAEMODIALYSIS.

artificial lung *see* RESPIRATOR.

artificial respiration an emergency procedure for maintaining a flow of air into and out of a patient's lungs when the natural breathing reflexes are absent or insufficient. This may occur after drowning, poisoning, etc., or during a surgical operation on the thorax or abdomen when muscle-relaxing drugs are administered. The simplest and most efficient method is *mouth-to-mouth respiration (the 'kiss of life'). In hospital the breathing cycle is maintained by means of a *respirator.

artificial rupture of membranes (ARM) *see* AMNIOTOMY.

artificial sphincter an apparatus designed to replace or support a *sphincter that is either absent or ineffective. *See also* NEOSPHINCTER.

arytenoid cartilage either of the two pyramid-shaped cartilages that lie at the back of the *larynx next to the upper edges of the cricoid cartilage.

arytenoidectomy *n.* surgical excision of the arytenoid cartilage of the larynx in the treatment of paralysis of the vocal folds.

asbestosis *n.* a lung disease – a form of *pneumoconiosis – caused by fibres of asbestos inhaled by those who are exposed to the mineral. The incidence of lung cancer is high in such patients, particularly if they smoke cigarettes. *See also* MESOTHELIOMA.

asbestos-related pleural disease any one of a variety of conditions involving the *pleura, but not the lungs (*see* ASBESTOSIS), in subjects exposed to asbestos. These include the formation of pleural plaques, diffuse pleural thickening, and pleural effusions (*see* OEDEMA).

A-scan *n.* examination of ocular tissue, including measurement of the length of the eye (axial length), by means of a high-frequency ultrasound machine. *See also* B-SCAN.

ascariasis *n.* a disease caused by an infestation with the parasitic worm *Ascaris lumbricoides*. Adult worms in the intestine can cause abdominal pain, vomiting, constipation, diarrhoea, appendicitis, and peritonitis; in large numbers they may cause obstruction of the intestine. The presence of the migrating larvae in the lungs can provoke pneumonia. Ascariasis occurs principally in areas of poor sanitation; it is treated with *piperazine.

Ascaris *n.* a genus of parasitic nematode worms. *A. lumbricoides*, widely distributed throughout the world, is the largest of the human intestinal nematodes – an adult female measures up to 35 cm in length. Eggs, passed out in the stools, may be transmitted to a new host in contaminated food or drink. Larvae hatch out in the intestine and then undergo a complicated migration, via the hepatic portal vein, liver, heart, lungs, windpipe, and pharynx, before returning to the intestine where they later develop into adult worms (*see also* ASCARIASIS).

ascites (hydroperitoneum) *n.* the accumulation of fluid in the peritoneal cavity, causing abdominal swelling. Causes include infections (such as tuberculosis), heart failure, *portal hypertension, *cirrhosis, and various cancers (particularly of the ovary and liver). Obstruction to the drainage of lymph from the abdomen results in **chylous ascites** (*see* CHYLE). *See also* OEDEMA.

ascorbic acid *see* VITAMIN C.

ASD *see* ATRIAL SEPTAL DEFECT.

-ase *suffix denoting* an enzyme. Examples: **lactase**; **dehydrogenase**.

asepsis *n.* the complete absence of bacteria, fungi, viruses, or other microorganisms that could cause disease. Asepsis is the ideal state for the performance of surgical operations and is achieved by using *sterilization techniques. —**aseptic** *adj.*

Asherman syndrome a condition in which *amenorrhoea and infertility follow a major haemorrhage in pregnancy. It may result from overvigorous curettage of the uterus in an attempt to control the bleeding. This removes the lining, the walls adhere, and the cavity is obliterated to a greater or lesser degree. Some 50% of such patients are subsequently infertile, and of those who become pregnant, only a minority achieve an uncomplicated delivery. Compare SHEEHAN'S SYNDROME. [J. G. Asherman (20th century), Czechoslovakian gynaecologist]

asparaginase n. an enzyme that inhibits the growth of certain tumours and is used almost exclusively in the treatment of acute lymphoblastic leukaemia. It may cause allergic reactions and *anaphylaxis. Trade name: **Erwinase**.

asparagine n. see AMINO ACID.

aspartic acid (aspartate) see AMINO ACID.

Asperger's syndrome a condition, often considered to be a mild form of *autism, characterized by social aloofness, lack of interest in other people, stilted and pedantic styles of speech, and an excessive preoccupation with a very specialized interest (such as timetables). Intelligence can be normal or enhanced. [H. Asperger (20th century)]

aspergillosis n. a group of conditions caused by fungi of the genus Aspergillus, usually Aspergillus fumigatus. These conditions nearly always arise in patients with pre-existing lung disease and fall into three categories. The allergic form most commonly affects asthmatic patients and may cause collapse of segments or lobes of a lung. The colonizing form leads to formation of a fungus ball (**aspergilloma**), usually within a pre-existing cavity in the lung (such as an emphysematous *bulla or a healed tuberculous cavity). Similar fungus balls may be found in other cavities, such as the eye or the sinuses around the nose. The third form of aspergillosis, in which the fungus spreads throughout the lungs and may even disseminate throughout the body, is rare but potentially fatal. It is usually associated with deficiency in the patient's immunity.

Aspergillus n. a genus of fungi, including many common moulds, some of which cause infections of the respiratory system in man. The species A. fumigatus causes *aspergillosis. A. niger is commonly found in the external ear and can become pathogenic.

aspermia n. strictly, a lack or failure of formation of semen. More usually, however, the term is used to mean the total absence of sperm from the semen (see AZOOSPERMIA).

asphyxia n. suffocation: a life-threatening condition in which oxygen is prevented from reaching the tissues by obstruction of or damage to any part of the respiratory system. Drowning, choking, and breathing poisonous gas all lead to asphyxia. Unless the condition is remedied by removing the obstruction (when present) and by artificial respiration if necessary, there is progressive *cyanosis leading to death. Brain cells cannot live for more than about four minutes without oxygen.

aspiration n. the withdrawal of fluid from the body by means of suction using an instrument called an **aspirator**. There are various types of aspirator: some employ hollow needles for removing fluid from cysts, inflamed joint cavities, etc.; another kind is used to suck debris and water from the patient's mouth during dental treatment.

aspiration cytology the *aspiration of specimens of cells from tumours or cysts through a hollow needle, using a syringe, and their subsequent examination under the microscope after suitable preparation (by staining, etc.). The technique is now used widely, especially for superficial cysts or tumours, and has become a specialized branch of diagnostic pathology. See also FINE-NEEDLE ASPIRATION CYTOLOGY.

aspirin (acetylsalicylic acid) n. a widely used drug that relieves pain and also reduces inflammation and fever. It is taken by mouth – alone or in combination with other analgesics – for the relief of the less severe types of pain, such as headache, toothache, neuralgias, and the pain of rheumatoid arthritis. It is also taken to reduce fever in influenza and the common cold. Daily doses of aspirin are used in the prevention of coronary thrombosis and strokes in those at risk, and it has been shown to have a protective effect against a range of other conditions, including cataracts, colorectal cancer, and Behçet's syndrome. Aspirin works by inhibiting the production of *prostaglandins; it may irritate the lining of the stomach, causing nausea, vomiting, pain, and bleeding. Tablets should not be held on the gum adjacent to a painful tooth as ulceration may occur. High doses cause dizziness, disturbed hearing, mental confusion, and overbreathing (*see* SALICYLISM). Aspirin has been implicated as a cause of *Reye's syndrome and should therefore not be given to children below the age of 12 unless specifically indicated. *See also* ANALGESIC.

assay *n.* a test or trial to determine the strength of a solution, the proportion of a compound in a mixture, the potency of a drug, or the purity of a preparation. *See also* BIOASSAY.

assimilation *n.* the process by which food substances are taken into the cells of the body after they have been digested and absorbed.

association area an area of *cerebral cortex that lies away from the main areas that are concerned with the reception of sensory impulses and the start of motor impulses but is linked to them by many neurones known as **association fibres**. The areas of association are thought to be responsible for the elaboration of the information received by the primary sensory areas and its correlation with the information fed in from memory and from other brain areas. They are thus responsible for the maintenance of many higher mental activities. *See also* BODY IMAGE.

association of ideas (in psychology) linkage of one idea to another in a regular way according to their meaning. In **free association** the linkage of ideas arising in dreams or fantasy may be used to discover the underlying motives of the individual. In **word association tests** stimulus words are produced to which the subject has to respond as quickly as possible.

astasia *n.* an inability to stand for which no physical cause can be found. **Astasia-abasia** is an inability to stand or walk in the absence of any recognizable physical illness. The patient's attempts are bizarre and careful examination reveals contradictory features. It is most commonly an expression of *conversion disorder.

astemizole *n.* an *antihistamine drug

used to treat hay fever and allergic skin conditions. It is administered by mouth. Possible side-effects include weight gain and, on very high dosage, disordered heart rhythm. Trade name: **Hismanal**.

aster *n.* a star-shaped object in a cell that surrounds the *centrosome during mitosis and meiosis and is concerned with the formation of the *spindle.

astereognosis *n. see* AGNOSIA.

asteroid hyalosis a degenerative condition, formerly known as **asteroid hyalitis**, in which tiny deposits of calcium are suspended in the vitreous humour. They are more commonly seen in the elderly and cause no decrease in vision.

asthenia *n.* weakness or loss of strength.

asthenic *adj.* describing a personality disorder characterized by low energy, susceptibility to physical and emotional stress, and a diminished capacity for pleasure.

asthenopia *n. see* EYESTRAIN.

asthenospermia *n. see* OLIGOSPERMIA.

asthma *n.* the condition of subjects with widespread narrowing of the bronchial airways, which changes in severity over short periods of time (either spontaneously or under treatment) and leads to cough, wheezing, and difficulty in breathing. **Bronchial asthma** may be precipitated by exposure to one or more of a wide range of stimuli, including *allergens, drugs (such as aspirin and other NSAIDs and beta blockers), exertion, emotion, infections, and air pollution. The onset of asthma is usually early in life and in atopic subjects (*see* ATOPY) may be accompanied by other manifestations of hypersensitivity, such as hay fever and dermatitis; however, the onset may be delayed into adulthood or even middle or old age. Treatment is with *bronchodilators, with or without corticosteroids, usually administered via aerosol or dry-powder inhalers, or – if the condition is more severe – via a nebulizer. Oral corticosteroids are reserved for those patients who fail to respond adequately to these measures. Severe asthmatic attacks may need large doses of oral corticosteroids (*see* STATUS ASTHMATICUS). Avoidance of known allergens, especially the house dust mite, allergens arising from domestic pets, and food additives, will help to reduce the frequency of attacks, as will the discouragement of smoking.

Cardiac asthma occurs in left ventricular heart failure and must be distinguished from bronchial asthma, as the treatment is quite different. —**asthmatic** adj.

astigmatism n. a defect of vision in which the image of an object is distorted, usually in either the vertical or the horizontal axis, because not all the light rays come to a focus on the retina. Some parts of the object may be in focus but light from other parts may be focused in front of or behind the retina. This is usually due to abnormal curvature of the cornea and/or lens (see REFRACTION), whose surface resembles part of the surface of an egg (rather than a sphere). The defect can be corrected by wearing **cylindrical lenses**, which produce exactly the opposite degree of distortion and thus cancel out the distortion caused by the eye itself. —**astigmatic** adj.

astragalus n. see TALUS.

astringent n. a drug that causes cells to shrink by precipitating proteins from their surfaces. Astringents are used in lotions to harden and protect the skin and to reduce bleeding from minor abrasions. They are also used in mouth washes, throat lozenges, eye drops, etc., and in antiperspirants.

astrocyte (astroglial cell) n. a type of cell with numerous sheet-like processes extending from its cell body, found throughout the central nervous system. It is one of the several different types of cell that make up the *glia. The cells have been ascribed the function of providing nutrients for neurones and possibly of taking part in information storage processes.

astrocytoma n. a brain tumour derived from non-nervous cells (*glia), which – unlike the neurones – retain the ability to reproduce themselves by mitosis. All grades of malignancy occur, from slow-growing tumours whose histological structure resembles normal glial cells, to rapidly growing highly invasive tumours whose cell structure is poorly differentiated (see GLIOBLASTOMA). In adults astrocytomas are usually found in the cerebral hemispheres but in children they also occur in the cerebellum.

asymbolia n. see ALEXIA.

asymptomatic adj. not showing any symptoms of disease, whether disease is present or not.

asynclitism n. tilting of the fetal skull towards one or other shoulder causing the top of the skull to be either nearer to the sacrum (**anterior asynclitism** or **Naegele's obliquity**) or nearer to the pubis (**posterior asynclitism** or **Litzmann's obliquity**). These mechanisms enable the fetal head to pass more easily through the maternal pelvis.

asyndesis n. a disorder of thought, in which the normal *association of ideas is disrupted so that thought and speech become fragmentary. It is a symptom of schizophrenia, dementia, or confusion.

asynergia n. see DYSSYNERGIA.

asystole n. a condition in which the heart no longer beats, accompanied by the absence of complexes in the electrocardiogram. The clinical features, causes, and treatment are those of *cardiac arrest.

atacurium besylate a *muscle relaxant administered by injection during anaesthesia. Trade name: **Tracrium**.

ataraxia n. a state of calmness and freedom from anxiety, especially the state produced by tranquillizing drugs.

atavism n. the phenomenon in which an individual has a character or disease known to have occurred in a remote ancestor but not in his parents.

ataxia n. the shaky movements and unsteady gait that result from the brain's failure to regulate the body's posture and the strength and direction of limb movements. It may be due to disease of the sensory nerves or the *cerebellum. In **cerebellar ataxia** there is clumsiness of willed movements. The patient staggers when walking; he cannot pronounce words properly and may have *nystagmus. **Cerebellar** (or **Nonne's**) **syndrome** is a form of cerebellar ataxia. **Friedreich's ataxia** is an inherited disorder appearing first in adolescence. It has the features of cerebellar ataxia, together with spasticity of the limbs. The unsteady movements of **sensory ataxia** are exaggerated when the patient closes his eyes (*see* ROMBERG'S SIGN). *See also* ATAXIA TELANGIECTASIA, TABES DORSALIS (LOCOMOTOR ATAXIA). —**ataxic** *adj.*

ataxia telangiectasia an inherited (autosomal *recessive) neurological disorder. *Ataxia is usually noted early in life. Mental retardation, growth retardation, abnormal eye movements, skin lesions, and immune deficiency may be found. Affected individuals may develop malignant disease. A raised level of *alpha-fetoprotein is found in the blood.

atel- (atelo-) *prefix denoting* imperfect or incomplete development. Examples: **atelencephaly** (of the brain); **atelocardia** (of the heart).

atelectasis *n.* failure of part of the lung to expand. This occurs when the cells lining the air sacs (alveoli) are too immature, as in premature babies, and unable to produce the wetting agent (surfactant) with which the surface tension between the alveolar walls is overcome. It also occurs when the larger bronchial tubes are blocked from within by retained secretions, inhaled foreign bodies, or bronchial cancers, or from without by enlarged lymph nodes, such as are found in patients with tuberculosis and lung cancers. The lung can usually be helped to expand by physiotherapy and removal of the internal block (if present) via a *bronchoscope, but prolonged atelectasis becomes irreversible.

ateleiosis *n.* failure of sexual development owing to lack of *pituitary hormones. *See* INFANTILISM, DWARFISM.

atenolol *n.* a drug (*see* BETA BLOCKER) used to treat angina and high blood pressure. It is taken by mouth and the commonest side-effects are fatigue, depression, and digestive upsets. Trade name: **Tenormin**.

atheroma *n.* degeneration of the walls of the arteries due to the formation in them of fatty plaques and scar tissue. This limits blood circulation and predisposes to thrombosis. It is common in adults in Western countries. A diet rich in animal fats (*see* CHOLESTEROL) and refined sugar,

cigarette smoking, obesity, and inactivity are the principal causes. It may be symptomless but often causes complications from arterial obstruction in middle and late life (such as angina pectoris, heart attack, stroke, and gangrene). Treatment is by prevention, but some symptoms may be ameliorated by drug therapy (e.g. angina by glyceryl trinitrate) or by surgical bypass of the arterial obstruction. —**atheromatous** *adj.*

atherosclerosis *n.* a disease of the arteries in which fatty plaques develop on their inner walls, with eventual obstruction of blood flow. *See* ATHEROMA.

athetosis *n.* a writhing involuntary movement especially affecting the hands, face, and tongue. It is usually a form of *cerebral palsy. It impairs the child's ability to speak or use his hands; intelligence is often unaffected. Such movements may also be caused by drugs used to treat *parkinsonism or by the withdrawal of phenothiazines (*see also* DYSKINESIA). —**athetotic** *adj.*

athlete's foot a fungus infection of the skin between the toes: a type of *ringworm. Medical name: **tinea pedis**.

athyreosis *n.* absence of or lack of function of the thyroid gland, causing *cretinism in infancy and *myxoedema in adult life.

atlas *n.* the first *cervical vertebra, by means of which the skull is articulated to the backbone.

ATLS advanced trauma life support, which comprises the treatment programmes for patients who have been subjected to major trauma (e.g. serious road traffic accidents, missile injuries). Doctors, nurses, and paramedical personnel involved in ATLS receive special training for dealing with such emergencies.

atony *n.* a state in which muscles are floppy, lacking their normal elasticity. —**atonic** *adj.*

atopen *n.* any substance responsible for *atopy.

atopy *n.* a form of *allergy in which there is a hereditary or constitutional tendency to develop hypersensitivity reactions (e.g. hay fever, allergic asthma, atopic *eczema) in response to allergens (**atopens**). Individuals with this predisposition – and the conditions provoked in them by contact with allergens – are described as **atopic**.

ATP (adenosine triphosphate) a compound that contains adenine, ribose, and three phosphate groups and occurs in cells. The chemical bonds of the phosphate groups store energy needed by the cell, for muscle contraction; this energy is released when ATP is split into ADP or AMP. ATP is formed from ADP or AMP using energy produced by the breakdown of carbohydrates or other food substances. *See also* MITOCHONDRION.

atresia *n*. **1.** congenital absence or abnormal narrowing of a body opening. *See* BILIARY ATRESIA, DUODENAL ATRESIA, TRICUSPID ATRESIA. **2.** the degenerative process that affects the majority of ovarian follicles. Usually only one Graafian follicle will ovulate in each menstrual cycle. —**atretic** *adj*.

atri- (atrio-) *prefix denoting* an atrium, especially the atrium of the heart. Example: **atrioventricular** (relating to the atria and ventricles of the heart).

atrial septal defect (ASD) a congenital defect of the heart in which there is a hole in the partition (septum) separating the two atria (*see* SEPTAL DEFECT). There are two kinds of ASD – **ostium primum** and **ostium secundum**. Ostium primum defects are rarer but more serious as the defect lies low down near the valves of the heart. Affected children often have heart failure, although in some a heart murmur detected at routine medical examinations is the only indication of the defect. Ostium secundum defects lie away from the valves and most children have no symptoms; the defect is most commonly indicated by the detection of a heart murmur, and may not be apparent until adulthood. Small defects may close spontaneously. Moderate and large ostium secundum and all ostium primum defects require surgery.

Intrauterine surgical techniques now enable a fetus in which an ASD has been detected to proceed to full term by using the placental circulation as a substitute for the *extracorporeal circulation that would otherwise be required.

atrioventricular bundle (AV bundle, bundle of His) a bundle of modified heart muscle fibres (**Purkinje fibres**) passing from the *atrioventricular (AV) node forward to the septum between the ventricles, where it divides into right and left bundles, one for each ventricle. The fibres transmit contraction waves from the atria, via the AV node, to the ventricles.

atrioventricular node (AV node) a mass of modified heart muscle situated in the lower middle part of the right atrium. It receives the impulse to contract from the *sinoatrial node, via the atria, and transmits it through the *atrioventricular bundle to the ventricles.

atrium *n*. (*pl.* **atria**) **1.** either of the two upper chambers of the *heart. Their muscular walls are thinner than those of the ventricles; the left atrium receives oxygenated blood from the lungs via the pulmonary vein; the right atrium receives deoxygenated blood from the venae cavae. *See also* AURICLE. **2.** any of various anatomical chambers into which one or more cavities open. —**atrial** *adj*.

Atromid-S *n*. *see* CLOFIBRATE.

atrophy *n*. the wasting away of a normally developed organ or tissue due to degeneration of cells. This may occur through undernourishment, disuse, or ageing. Forms of atrophy peculiar to women include the shrinking of the ovary at the menopause and of the *corpus luteum during the menstrual cycle. **Muscular atrophy** is associated with various diseases, such as poliomyelitis.

atropine *n*. a drug extracted from deadly nightshade (*see* BELLADONNA) that inhibits the action of certain nerves of the autonomic nervous system (*see* PARASYMPATHOLYTIC). Atropine relaxes smooth muscle and is used to treat biliary colic and renal colic. It also reduces secretions of the bronchial tubes, salivary glands, stomach, and intestines and is used before general *anaesthesia and to relieve peptic ulcers. It is also used to dilate the pupil of the eye. Atropine is administered by mouth, injection, or as eyedrops; common side-effects include dryness of the throat, thirst, and impaired vision. Trade name: **Minims Atropine**.

attachment n. **1.** (in psychology) the process of developing the first close selective relationship of a child's life, most commonly with the mother. The relationship acts to reduce anxiety in strange settings and forms a base from which children develop further relationships. **2.** (in the National Health Service) working arrangements by which workers employed by public bodies (such as *district nurses and *social workers) are engaged in association with specific general practitioners, caring for their registered patients rather than working solely on a geographical or district basis.

attachment disorder a psychiatric disorder in infants and young children resulting from *institutionalization, emotional neglect, or *child abuse. Affected children are either withdrawn, aggressive, and fearful or attention-seeking and indiscriminately friendly. Treatment requires the provision of stable caring adults as parents over a long period of time.

attention deficit disorder (ADD, hyperkinetic disorder) a mental disorder, usually of children, characterized by a grossly excessive level of activity and a marked impairment of the ability to attend. Learning is impaired as a result, and behaviour is disruptive and may be defiant or aggressive. The disorder is more common in the intellectually subnormal, the epileptic, and the brain-damaged. Treatment usually involves drugs (such as amphetamines and *methylphenidate) and behaviour therapy; the family needs advice and practical help.

attenuation n. reduction of the disease-producing ability (virulence) of a bacterium or virus by chemical treatment, heating, drying, by growing under adverse conditions, or by passing through another organism. Treated (**attenuated**) bacteria or viruses are used for many *immunizations.

atticotomy n. a surgical operation to remove *cholesteatoma from the ear. It is a form of limited *mastoidectomy.

attrition n. (in dentistry) the wearing of tooth surfaces by the action of opposing teeth. A small amount of attrition occurs

with age but accelerated wear may occur in *bruxism and with certain diets.

atypical antipsychotics see ANTIPSY-CHOTIC.

atypical facial pain a *neuralgia that has no known cause and is typified by pain in the face that does not fit the distribution of nerves. It may be stress-related, and in some cases appears to be associated with defective metabolism of *tyramine. Treatment may involve the use of antidepressants.

atypical mole syndrome (dysplastic naevus syndrome) a condition in which affected patients have numerous moles, some of which are relatively large and irregular in shape or pigmentation. There may be a family history of this syndrome or of malignant *melanoma.

atypical pneumonia any one of a group of community-acquired *pneumonias that do not respond to penicillin but do respond to such antibiotics as tetracycline and erythromycin. They include infection with *Mycoplasma pneumoniae*, *Chlamydia psittaci* (see PSITTACOSIS), and *Coxiella burnetii* (see Q FEVER).

audi- (audio-) prefix denoting hearing or sound.

audiogram n. the graphic record of a test of hearing carried out on an audiometer.

audiology n. the study of disorders of hearing.

audiometer n. an apparatus for measuring hearing at different sound frequencies, so helping in the diagnosis of deafness. —**audiometry** n.

audit n. see MEDICAL AUDIT.

auditory adj. relating to the ear or to the sense of hearing.

auditory canal (auditory meatus) the canal leading from the pinna to the eardrum.

auditory nerve see VESTIBULOCOCHLEAR NERVE.

Auerbach's plexus (myenteric plexus) a collection of nerve fibres – fine branches of the *vagus nerve – within the walls of the intestine. It supplies the muscle layers and controls the movements of *peristalsis. [L. Auerbach (1828–97), German anatomist]

aura *n.* the forewarning of an epileptic or migrainous attack. An **epileptic aura** may take many forms. The **migrainous aura** may affect the patient's eyesight with brilliant flickering lights or blurring of vision, but it may also result in numbness or weakness of the limbs.

aural *adj.* relating to the ear.

auranofin *n.* a *gold preparation administered by mouth to treat rheumatoid arthritis. Side-effects include nausea, abdominal pain, diarrhoea, and mouth ulcers. Trade name: **Ridaura**.

Aureomycin *n.* *see* CHLORTETRACYCLINE.

auricle *n.* **1.** a small pouch in the wall of each *atrium of the heart: the term is also used incorrectly as a synonym for *atrium. **2.** *see* PINNA.

auriscope (otoscope) *n.* an apparatus for examining the eardrum and the passage leading to it from the ear (external meatus). It consists of a funnel (speculum), a light, and lenses.

light
lens and viewing aperture
speculum
switch
battery case and handle

An auriscope

auscultation *n.* the process of listening, usually with the aid of a *stethoscope, to sounds produced by movement of gas or liquid within the body. Auscultation is an aid to diagnosis of abnormalities of the heart, lungs, intestines, and other organs according to the characteristic changes in sound pattern caused by different disease processes. —**auscultatory** *adj.*

auscultatory gap a silent period in the knocking sounds heard with a stethoscope over an artery, between the systolic and diastolic blood pressures, when the blood pressure is measured with a *sphygmomanometer.

Australia antigen another name for the *hepatitis B antigen, which was first discovered in the blood of an Australian aborigine. This disease is caused by a virus of which the Australia antigen forms part.

aut- (auto-) *prefix denoting* self. Example: **autokinesis** (voluntary movement).

autism *n.* **1. (Kanner's syndrome, infantile autism)** a rare psychiatric disorder of childhood, with an onset before the age of 2½ years. It is marked by severe difficulties in communicating and forming relationships with other people, in developing language, and in using abstract concepts; repetitive and limited patterns of behaviour (*see* STEREOTYPY); and obsessive resistance to tiny changes in familiar surroundings. Autistic children find it hard to understand how other people feel, and so tend to remain isolated even into adult life. About 50% have learning disabilities, but some are very intelligent and may even be gifted in specific areas (*see* IDIOT SAVANT). The cause is unknown, but genetic factors and brain damage may be important. The condition often progresses into adulthood, and independent living is uncommon. Treatment is not specific, but lengthy specialized education is usually necessary. Behaviour problems and anxiety can be controlled with behaviour therapy and drugs (such as *phenothiazines). **2.** the condition of retreating from realistic thinking to self-centred fantasy thinking: a symptom of personality disorder and schizophrenia. —**autistic** *adj.*

autoagglutination *n.* the clumping together of the body's own red blood cells by antibodies produced against them, which occurs in acquired haemolytic anaemia (an *autoimmune disease).

autoantibody *n.* an antibody formed

against one of the body's own components in an *autoimmune disease.

autochthonous adj. **1.** remaining at the site of formation. A blood clot that has not been carried in the bloodstream from its point of origin is described as autochthonous. **2.** originating in an organ without external stimulus, like the beating of the heart.

autoclave 1. n. a piece of equipment for sterilizing surgical instruments, dressings, etc. It consists of a chamber, similar to a domestic pressure cooker, in which the articles are placed and treated with steam at high pressure. **2.** vb. to sterilize in an autoclave.

autocrine adj. describing the production by a cell of substances, such as hormones or *growth factors, that can influence the growth of the cell that produces them.

autofluorescence n. true *fluorescence of structures within the retina, such as optic disc *drusen. Fluorescence of the tissue is seen when it is stimulated by cobalt blue light in the absence of fluorescein dye. This examination is usually performed at the beginning of fluorescein *angiography.

autogenous vaccine see AUTOVACCINE.

autograft n. a tissue graft taken from one part of the body and transferred to another part of the same individual. The repair of burns is often done by grafting on strips of skin taken from elsewhere on the body, usually the upper arm or thigh. Unlike *homografts, autografts are not rejected by the body's immunity defences. See also SKIN GRAFT, TRANSPLANTATION.

autoimmune disease one of a number of otherwise unrelated disorders caused by inflammation and destruction of tissues by the body's own antibodies (**autoantibodies**). These disorders include acquired haemolytic anaemia, pernicious anaemia, rheumatic fever, rheumatoid arthritis, glomerulonephritis, systemic lupus erythematosus, myasthenia gravis, Sjögren's syndrome, and several forms of thyroid dysfunction, including Hashimoto's disease. It is not known why the body should lose the ability to distinguish between substances that are 'self' and those that are 'non-self'.

autoimmunity n. a disorder of the body's defence mechanisms in which antibodies (**autoantibodies**) are produced against certain components or products of its own tissues, treating them as foreign material and attacking them. See AUTOIMMUNE DISEASE, IMMUNITY.

autoinoculation n. the accidental transfer of inoculated material from one site in the body to another. Following vaccination against smallpox, for example, satellite lesions may occur around the site of inoculation. Sometimes the conjunctiva is affected.

autointoxication n. poisoning by a toxin formed within the body.

autologous adj. denoting a graft that is derived from the recipient of the graft.

autolysis n. the destruction of tissues or cells brought about by the actions of their own enzymes. See LYSOSOME.

automated lamellar keratectomy (ALK) excision of the outer layers of the cornea using an automated *keratome. It is usually used as part of a surgical procedure, to alter the shape of the cornea to correct errors of refraction.

automated perimeter see PERIMETER.

automatism n. behaviour that may be associated with *epilepsy, in which the patient performs well-organized movements or tasks while unaware of doing so. The movements may be simple and repetitive, such as hand clapping, or they may be so complex as to mimic a person's normal conscious activities.

autonomic nervous system the part of the *nervous system responsible for the control of bodily functions that are not consciously directed, including regular beating of the heart, intestinal movements, sweating, salivation, etc. The autonomic system is subdivided into **sympathetic** and **parasympathetic nervous systems**. Sympathetic nerves lead from the middle section of the spinal cord and parasympathetic nerves from the brain and lower spinal cord. The heart, smooth muscles, and most glands receive fibres of both kinds: the interplay of sympathetic and parasympathetic reflex activity (the actions are often antagonistic) governs their working. Sympathetic nerve endings liberate *noradrenaline as a neurotransmitter; parasympathetic nerve endings release *acetylcholine.

autoploidy n. the normal condition in cells or individuals, in which each cell has a chromosome set consisting of *homologous pairs, enabling cells to divide normally. —**autoploid** adj., n.

autopsy (necropsy, post mortem) n. dissection and examination of a body after death in order to determine the cause of death or the presence of disease processes.

autoradiography (radioautography) n. a technique for examining the distribution of a radioactive *tracer in the tissues of an experimental animal. The tracer is injected into the animal, which is killed after a certain period. Thin sections of its organs are placed in close contact with a radiation-sensitive material, such as a photographic emulsion, and observed under a microscope. Blackening of the film indicates a high concentration of radioactive material.

autorefractor n. a machine that automatically determines the required correction for a spectacle lens. See also OPTOMETER.

autoscopy n. the experience of seeing one's whole body as though from a vantage point some distance away. It can be a symptom in *epilepsy. See also OUT-OF-THE-BODY EXPERIENCE.

autosomal dominant see DOMINANT.

autosomal recessive see RECESSIVE.

autosome n. any chromosome that is not a *sex chromosome and occurs in pairs in diploid cells. —**autosomal** adj.

autosuggestion n. self-suggestion or self-conditioning that involves repeating ideas to oneself in order to change psychological or physiological states. Autosuggestion is used primarily in **autogenic training**, a technique used to help patients control their anxiety or their habits. See SUGGESTION.

autotransfusion n. reintroduction into a patient of blood that has been lost from the patient's circulation during surgical operation. The blood is collected by suction during the operation, filtered to remove bubbles and small blood clots, and returned into one of the patient's veins through a drip.

autotrophic (lithotrophic) adj. describing organisms (known as **autotrophs**) that synthesize their organic materials from carbon dioxide and nitrates or ammonium compounds, using an external source of energy. **Photoautotrophic** organisms, including green plants and some bacteria, derive their energy from sunlight; **chemoautotrophic** (or **chemosynthetic**) organisms obtain energy from inorganic chemical reactions. All autotrophic bacteria are nonparasitic. Compare HETEROTROPHIC.

autovaccination n. the use of an *autovaccine.

autovaccine (autogenous vaccine) n. a *vaccine prepared by isolating specimens of bacteria from an infected patient, culturing them, and killing them. By injecting this vaccine back into the patient, it was hoped that the body's resistance to the infection would be stimulated. Although such vaccines were once much favoured for the treatment of boils, there is no good evidence that the dead bacteria are any more likely to stimulate immunity than the living and dead bacteria already present in the body.

aux- (auxo-) prefix denoting increase; growth. Example: **auxocardia** (enlargement of the heart).

auxotroph n. a strain of a microorganism, derived by mutation, that requires one or more specific factors for growth not needed by the parent organism.

avascular adj. lacking blood vessels or having a poor blood supply. The term is usually used with reference to cartilage.

aversion therapy a form of *behaviour therapy that is used to reduce the occurrence of undesirable behaviour, such as sexual deviations or drug addiction. *Conditioning is used, with repeated pairing of some unpleasant stimulus with a stimulus related to the undesirable behaviour. An example is pairing the taste of beer with electric shock in the treatment of alcoholism. Aversion therapy is little used nowadays. *See also* SENSITIZATION.

avitaminosis *n.* the condition caused by lack of a vitamin. *See also* DEFICIENCY DISEASE.

AVM arteriovenous malformation (*see* ANGIOMA).

avoidant *adj.* describing a personality type characterized by self-consciousness, hypersensitivity to rejection and criticism from others, avoidance of normal situations because of their potential risk, high levels of tension and anxiety, and consequently a restricted life.

AVPU a system for assessing the depth of unconsciousness: A = alert; V = voice responses present; P = pain responses present; U = unresponsive. It is useful for judging the severity of head injury and the need for specialized neurosurgical assistance.

avulsion *n.* **1.** the tearing or forcible separation of part of a structure. For example, a tendon may be torn from the bone to which it attaches or the skin of the scalp may be torn from the underlying tissue and bone. **2.** (in dentistry) the knocking out of a tooth by trauma. The tooth may be replanted (*see* REPLANTATION).

axilla *n.* (*pl.* **axillae**) the armpit. —**axillary** *adj.*

axis *n.* **1.** a real or imaginary line through the centre of the body or one of its parts or a line about which the body or a part rotates. **2.** the second *cervical vertebra, which articulates with the atlas vertebra above and allows rotational movement of the head.

axolemma *n.* the fine cell membrane, visible only under the electron microscope, that encloses the protoplasm of an *axon.

axon *n.* a nerve fibre: a single process extending from the cell body of a *neurone and carrying nerve impulses away from it. An axon may be over a metre in length in certain neurones. In large nerves the axon has a sheath (**neurilemma**) made of *myelin; this is interrupted at intervals by gaps called **nodes of Ranvier**, at which branches of the axon leave. An axon ends by dividing into several branches called

telodendria, which make contact with other nerves or with muscle or gland membranes.

axonotmesis *n.* rupture of nerve fibres (axons) within an intact nerve sheath. This may result from prolonged pressure or crushing and it is followed by degeneration of the nerve beyond the point of rupture. The prognosis for *nerve regeneration is good. *Compare* NEURAPRAXIA, NEUROTMESIS.

axoplasm *n.* the semifluid material of which the *axon of a nerve cell is composed. It flows slowly outwards from the cell body.

azapropazone *n.* an anti-inflammatory drug (*see* NSAID) used to treat rheumatoid arthritis, osteoarthritis, ankylosing spondylitis, and gout. It is administered by mouth. Possible side-effects include sensitivity of skin to light, fluid retention, and bleeding from the bowel. Trade name: **Rheumox**.

azatadine *n.* an *antihistamine drug used to treat hay fever, urticaria, itching, and stings. It is administered by mouth. Possible side-effects include drowsiness, headache, nausea, and loss of appetite. Trade name: **Optimine**.

azathioprine *n.* an *immunosuppressive drug, used mainly to aid the survival of organ or tissue transplants. It has also been used in the treatment of acute and chronic leukaemias and inflammatory bowel disease (e.g. ulcerative colitis). Azathioprine may damage bone marrow, causing blood disorders. It may also cause muscle wasting and skin rashes. Trade name: **Imuran**.

azelaic acid an antibacterial drug applied externally as a cream in the treatment of acne. Possible side-effects include local irritation and light sensitivity. Trade name: **Skinoren**.

azelastine *n.* an *antihistamine drug administered as a metered-dose nasal spray for the treatment of hay fever. Possible side-effects include nasal irritation and disturbances of taste sensation. Trade name: **Rhinolast**.

azithromycin *n.* an *antibiotic used to treat respiratory, skin, soft-tissue, and other infections, especially those caused by the organism *Chlamydia trachomatis*. It is administered by mouth. Possible side-effects include allergic reactions, nausea, and vomiting. Trade name: **Zithromax**.

azlocillin *n.* a penicillin-type antibiotic used especially to treat infections caused by *Pseudomonas aeruginosa*. It is administered by intravenous infusion; possible side-effects include allergic reactions, nausea, and vomiting. Trade name: **Securopen**.

azo- (azoto-) *prefix denoting* a nitrogenous compound, such as urea. Example: **azothermia** (raised temperature due to nitrogenous substances in the blood).

azoospermia (aspermia) *n.* the complete absence of sperm from the seminal fluid. This is due either to failure of formation of sperm by the seminiferous tubules within the testes or to a blockage in the ducts that conduct sperm from the testes. A biopsy of the testis is necessary in order to differentiate these two causes

of azoospermia; if a blockage is present it may be possible to relieve it surgically (*see* EPIDIDYMOVASOSTOMY).

azotaemia *n.* a former name for *uraemia.

azoturia *n.* the presence in the urine of an abnormally high concentration of nitrogen-containing compounds, especially urea.

aztreonam *n.* an antibiotic administered by injection used to treat infections of the lungs, bones, skin, and soft tissues caused by Gram-negative organisms (*see* GRAM's STAIN). It is especially useful for treating lung infections in children with cystic fibrosis. Possible side-effects include skin rashes, diarrhoea, and vomiting. Trade name: **Azactam**.

azygos vein an unpaired vein that arises from the inferior vena cava and drains into the superior vena cava, returning blood from the thorax and abdominal cavities.

Babinski reflex *see* PLANTAR REFLEX. [J. F. Babinski (1857–1932), French neurologist]

baby blues a colloquial name for the fleeting misery and tearfulness that affects about half of all pregnant women, especially those having their first baby. The state should not be confused with the condition of *puerperal depression.

bacillaemia *n.* the presence of bacilli in the blood, resulting from infection.

bacille Calmette-Guérin *see* BCG. [A. L. C. Calmette (1863–1933) and C. Guérin (1872–1961), French bacteriologists]

bacilluria *n.* the presence of bacilli in the urine, resulting from a bladder or kidney infection. *See* CYSTITIS.

bacillus *n.* (*pl.* **bacilli**) any rod-shaped bacterium. *See also* BACILLUS, LACTOBACILLUS, STREPTOBACILLUS.

Bacillus *n.* a large genus of Grampositive spore-bearing rodlike bacteria. They are widely distributed in soil and air (usually as spores). Most feed on dead organic material and are responsible for food spoilage. The species *B. anthracis*, which is nonmotile, causes *anthrax, a disease of farm animals transmissible to man. *B. polymyxa*, commonly found in soil, is the source of the *polymyxin group of antibiotics. *B. subtilis* may cause conjunctivitis in man; it also produces the antibiotic *bacitracin.

bacitracin *n.* an antibiotic produced by certain strains of bacteria and effective against a number of microorganisms. It is usually applied externally, to treat infections of the skin, eyes, or nose, but can be given by mouth as an intestinal antiseptic or by injection. The principal toxic effect is on the kidneys. Trade names: **Cicatrin**, **Polybactrin**.

backbone (spinal column, spine, vertebral column) *n.* a flexible bony column extending from the base of the skull to the small of the back. It encloses and protects the spinal cord, articulates with the skull (at the atlas), ribs (at the thoracic vertebrae), and hip girdle (at the sacrum), and provides attachment for the muscles of the back. It is made up of individual bones (*see* VERTEBRA) connected by discs of fibrocartilage (*see* INTERVERTEBRAL DISC) and bound together by ligaments. The backbone of a newborn baby contains 33 vertebrae: seven cervical (neck), 12 thoracic (chest), five lumbar (lower back), five sacral (hip), and four coccygeal. In the adult the sacral and coccygeal vertebrae become fused into two single bones (sacrum and coccyx, respectively); the adult vertebral column therefore contains 26 bones (see illustration). Anatomical name: **rachis**.

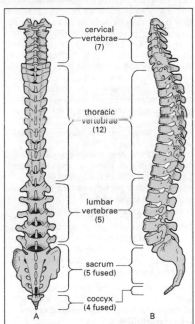

The backbone, seen from the back (A) and left side (B)

baclofen *n.* a skeletal *muscle relaxant drug administered orally to relieve spasm resulting from injury or disease of the brain or spinal cord, including cerebral palsy and multiple sclerosis. Side-effects include dizziness, drowsiness, and nausea. Trade names: **Baclospas, Lioresal**.

bacteraemia *n.* the presence of bacteria in the blood: a sign of infection.

bacteri- (bacterio-) *prefix denoting* bacteria. Example: **bacteriolysis** (dissolution of).

bacteria *pl. n.* (*sing.* **bacterium**) a group of microorganisms all of which lack a distinct nuclear membrane (and hence are considered more primitive than animal and plant cells) and have a cell wall of unique composition (many antibiotics act by destroying the bacterial cell wall). Most bacteria are unicellular; the cells may be spherical (*coccus), rod-shaped (*bacillus), spiral (*Spirillum), comma-shaped (*Vibrio) or corkscrew-shaped (*spirochaete). Generally, they range in size between 0.5 and 5 μm. Motile species bear one or more fine hairs (flagella) arising from their surface. Many possess an outer slimy *capsule, and some have the ability to produce an encysted or resting form (*endospore). Bacteria reproduce asexually by simple division of cells; incomplete separation of daughter cells leads to the formation of *colonies consisting of different numbers and arrangements of cells. Some colonies are filamentous in shape, resembling those of fungi. Some bacteria may reproduce sexually by *conjugation.

Bacteria are very widely distributed. Some live in soil, water, or air; others are parasites of man, animals, and plants. Many parasitic bacteria do not harm their hosts; some cause diseases by producing poisons (*see* ENDOTOXIN, EXOTOXIN).

bactericidal *adj.* being capable of killing bacteria. Substances with this property include antibiotics, antiseptics, and disinfectants; they are known as **bactericides**. *Compare* BACTERIOSTATIC.

bacteriology *n.* the science concerned with the study of bacteria. It is a branch of *microbiology. —**bacteriological** *adj.* —**bacteriologist** *n.*

bacteriolysin *n.* *see* LYSIN.

bacteriophage (phage) *n.* a virus that attacks bacteria. In general, a phage consists of a head, tail, and tail fibres, all composed of protein molecules, and a core of DNA. The tail and tail fibres are responsible for attachment to the bacterial surface and for injection of the DNA core into the host cell. The phage grows and replicates in the bacterial cell, which is eventually destroyed with the release of new phages. Each phage acts specifically against a particular species of bacterium. This is utilized in **phage typing**, a technique of identifying bacteria by the action of known phages on them. *See also* LYSOGENY.

bacteriostatic *adj.* capable of inhibiting or retarding the growth and multiplication of bacteria. Erythromycin is bacteriostatic. *Compare* BACTERICIDAL.

bacterium *n.* *see* BACTERIA.

Bacteroides *n.* a genus of Gram-negative, mostly nonmotile, anaerobic rod-like bacteria. They are normally present in the alimentary and urinogenital tracts of mammals and are found in the mouth, particularly in dental plaque associated with periodontal disease. Some species have now been classified into new genera, *Porphyromonas* and *Prevotella*.

Bactrim *n.* *see* CO-TRIMOXAZOLE.

bagassosis *n.* a form of external allergic *alveolitis caused by exposure to the dust of mouldy bagasse, the residue of sugar cane after the sugar has been extracted, which is used in the production of hardboard and other thermal boards. Symptoms usually appear in the evening after exposure during the day and include fever, malaise, irritant cough, and respiratory distress.

Baghdad boil *see* ORIENTAL SORE.

BAHA *see* BONE-ANCHORED HEARING AID.

Baker's cyst a cyst behind the knee resulting from a protrusion of the synovial membrane from a knee joint affected by osteoarthritis. [W. M. Baker (1839–96), British surgeon]

BAL 1. *see* BRONCHOALVEOLAR LAVAGE. 2. British Anti-Lewisite (*see* DIMERCAPROL).

balanced salt solution (BSS) a solution made to a physiological pH and having physiological concentrations of salts, including sodium, potassium, calcium, magnesium, and chloride. Such fluids are used during intraocular surgery and to replace intraocular fluids.

balanitis *n.* inflammation of the glans penis, usually associated with tightness of the foreskin (*phimosis). It is more common in childhood than in adult life. An acute attack is associated with redness and swelling of the glans. Treatment is by antibiotics, and further attacks are prevented by *circumcision. In **Zoon's plasma cell balanitis** persistent shiny red patches develop on the glans; the cause is unknown. **Balanitis xerotica obliterans** is an autoimmune condition characterized by ivory-white patches on the glans.

balanoposthitis *n.* inflammation of the foreskin and the surface of the underlying glans penis. It usually occurs as a consequence of *phimosis and represents a more extensive local reaction than simple *balanitis. The affected areas become red and swollen, which further narrows the opening of the foreskin and makes passing urine difficult and painful. Treatment of an acute attack is by administration of antibiotics, and further attacks are prevented by *circumcision.

balantidiasis *n.* an infestation of the large intestine of man with the parasitic protozoan *Balantidium coli. Man usually becomes infected by ingesting food or drink contaminated with cysts from the faeces of a pig. The parasite invades and destroys the intestinal wall, causing ulceration and *necrosis, and the patient may experience diarrhoea and dysentery. Balantidiasis is a rare cause of dysentery, mainly affecting farm workers; it is treated with various antibiotics, carbarsone, and *diiodohydroxyquinoline.

Balantidium *n.* a genus of one of the largest parasitic *protozoans affecting man (70 μm or more in length). The oval body is covered with threadlike cilia (for locomotion). *B. coli*, normally living in the gut of pigs as a harmless *commensal, occasionally infects man (*see* BALANTIDIASIS).

baldness *n.* *see* ALOPECIA.

Balkan nephropathy a type of kidney failure that is prevalent in the former Yugoslavia. The cause is unknown. It is associated with a high incidence of carcinoma of the epithelium of the proximal renal tubules.

ball-and-cage valve a form of prosthesis commonly used for replacing damaged heart valves.

ball-and-socket joint *see* ENARTHROSIS.

ballistocardiograph *n.* an instrument for recording the displacement of the whole body produced by the ejection of blood with each heartbeat. The normal record produced by such an instrument (**ballistocardiogram**) may be altered by disease of the heart or aortic valve (*see* AORTIC REGURGITATION, AORTIC STENOSIS).

balloon *n.* an inflatable plastic cylinder of variable size that is mounted on a thin tube and used for dilating narrow areas in blood vessels (*see* ANGIOPLASTY) or in the alimentary tract (*strictures). It is also used to prevent the reflux of solutions being injected, e.g. into a vessel during *angiography.

ballottement *n.* the technique of examining a fluid-filled part of the body to detect a floating object. During pregnancy, a sharp tap with the fingers, applied to the uterus through the abdominal wall or the vagina, causes the fetus to move away and then return to impart an answering tap to the examiner's hand as it floats back to its original position. This confirms that swelling of the uterus is due to a fetus rather than a tumour or other abnormality.

balneotherapy *n.* the treatment of disease by bathing, usually in the mineral-containing waters of hot springs. The once fashionable 'water cures', taken at spas, certainly had a more psychological than physical effect. Today, specialized remedial treatment in baths, under the supervision of physiotherapists, is used to alleviate pain and improve blood circulation and limb mobility in arthritis and in nerve and muscle disorders.

bandage *n.* a piece of material, in the form of a pad or strip, applied to a wound or used to bind around an injured or diseased part of the body.

bandage lens *see* CONTACT LENSES.

band keratopathy the deposition of calcium in the superficial layers of the cornea, usually as a horizontal band starting peripherally and moving centrally. It is associated with chronic eye disease, e.g. chronic *uveitis.

Bandl's ring *see* RETRACTION RING. [L. Bandl (1842–92), German obstetrician]

Banti's syndrome a disorder in which enlargement and overactivity of the spleen occurs as a result of increased pressure within the splenic vein. The commonest cause is *cirrhosis of the liver. [G. Banti (1852–1925), Italian pathologist]

barbiturate *n.* any of a group of drugs, derived from barbituric acid, that depress activity of the central nervous system and were formerly used as sedatives and hypnotics. They are classified into three groups according to their duration of action – short, medium, and long. Because they produce *tolerance and psychological and physical *dependence, have serious toxic side-effects (*see* BARBITURISM), and can be fatal following large overdosage, barbiturates have been largely replaced in clinical use by safer drugs. The main exceptions are the very short-acting drug *thiopentone, which is still used to induce anaesthesia, and the long-acting *phenobarbitone, used to control some forms of epilepsy.

barbiturism *n.* addiction to drugs of the barbiturate group. Signs of intoxication include confusion, slurring of speech, yawning, sleepiness, loss of memory, loss of balance, and reduction in muscular reflexes. Withdrawal of the drugs must be undertaken slowly, over 1–3 weeks, to avoid the withdrawal symptoms of tremors and convulsions, which can prove fatal.

barefoot doctor *see* MEDICAL ASSISTANT.

baritosis *n.* a lung disease – a form of *pneumoconiosis – caused by inhaling barium dust. It gives dramatic shadows on chest X-rays but no respiratory disability.

barium sulphate a barium salt, insoluble in water, that is opaque to X-rays and is used as a contrast medium in radiography of the stomach and intestines. *See also* ENEMA.

Barlow's sign (Von Rosen's sign) a test for *congenital dislocation of the hip that detects whether or not a hip can be readily dislocated. With the baby lying supine and the pelvis steadied with one hand, the hip being tested is gently *adducted and backward pressure is applied to the head of the femur. If the hip is dislocatable, a clunk will be felt and sometimes heard. If the hip is gently *abducted, it will usually relocate. [T. Barlow (1845–1945), British physician]

BARN bilateral *acute retinal necrosis.

baroreceptor (baroceptor) *n.* a collection of sensory nerve endings specialized to monitor changes in blood pressure. The main receptors lie in the *carotid sinuses and the *aortic arch; others are found in the walls of other large arteries and veins and some within the walls of the heart. Impulses from the receptors reach centres in the medulla; from here autonomic activity is directed so that the heart rate and resistance of the peripheral blood vessels can be adjusted appropriately.

barotitis *n.* disease of the ear caused by changing air pressure, as experienced during air travel.

barotrauma *n.* damage to the ear, *Eustachian tube, or paranasal sinuses caused by changes in ambient pressure, as experienced during air flight or deep-sea diving.

Barr body *see* SEX CHROMATIN. [M. L. Barr (1908–), Canadian anatomist]

Barrett's oesophagus (columnar-lined oesophagus, CLO) a condition in which the normal squamous *epithelium lining the oesophagus is replaced by columnar epithelium because of damage caused by *gastro-oesophageal reflux or (occasionally) corrosive *oesophagitis. The condition may be associated with an ulcer (**Barrett's ulcer**), and the epithelium has an abnormally high likelihood of undergoing malignant change. [N. R. Barrett (1903–79), British surgeon]

barrier cream a preparation used to protect the skin against water-soluble irritants (e.g. detergents, breakdown products of urine). Usually applied in the form of a cream or ointment and often containing a silicone (such as *dimethicone), barrier creams are useful in the alleviation of various skin disorders, including napkin rash and bedsores.

Barron's banding apparatus an apparatus for treating haemorrhoids in which a tight elastic band is applied across their base.

bartholinitis *n.* inflammation of *Bartholin's glands. In **chronic bartholinitis** cysts may form in the glands as a result of blockage of their ducts. In **acute bartholinitis** abscess formation may occur (**Bartholin's abscess**).

Bartholin's glands (greater vestibular glands) a pair of glands that open at the junction of the vagina and the external genitalia (vulva). Their secretions lubricate the vulva and so assist penetration by the penis during coitus. The **lesser vestibular glands**, around the vaginal opening, perform the same function. [C. Bartholin (1655–1748), Danish anatomist]

Bartonella (Haemobartonella) *n.* a genus of parasitic rod-shaped or rounded microorganisms, usually regarded as rickettsiae. They occur in the red blood cells and cells of the lymphatic system, spleen, liver, and kidneys. *B. bacilliformis* causes *bartonellosis in man.

bartonellosis *n.* an infectious disease, confined to high river valleys in Peru, Ecuador, and Colombia, caused by the rickettsia *Bartonella bacilliformis*. The parasite, present in red blood cells and cells of the lymphatic system, is transmitted to man by sandflies. There are two clinical types of the disease: **Oroya fever** (**Carrion's disease**), whose symptoms include fever, anaemia, and enlargement of the liver, spleen, and lymph nodes; and **verruga peruana**, characterized by wartlike eruptions on the skin that can bleed easily and ulcerate. Oroya fever accounts for nearly all fatalities. Bartonellosis can be treated successfully with penicillin and other antibiotics and blood transfusions may be given to relieve the anaemia.

basal cell carcinoma (BCC) the commonest form of skin cancer. Although classified as a malignant tumour, it grows very slowly. BCC usually occurs on the central area of the face, especially in fair-skinned people; the prevalence increases greatly with exposure to sunlight. The initial sign is a spot or lump that fails to heal, enlarging to a diameter of 1 cm over five years or so. Treatment is straightforward, using *curettage and cautery, surgical excision, *cryotherapy, or *radiotherapy. Only if neglected for decades does a BCC eventually become a so-called **rodent ulcer** and destroy the surrounding tissue. However, the term 'rodent ulcer' is still sometimes used to mean any basal cell carcinoma.

basal ganglia several large masses of grey matter embedded deep within the white matter of the *cerebrum (see illustration). They include the **caudate** and **lenticular nuclei** (together known as the **corpus striatum**) and the **amygdaloid nucleus**. The lenticular nucleus consists of the **putamen** and **globus pallidus**. The basal ganglia have complex neural connections with both the cerebral cortex and thalamus: they are involved with the regulation of voluntary movements at a subconscious level.

The basal ganglia and neighbouring parts (seen from the front)

basal metabolism the minimum amount of energy expended by the body to maintain vital processes, e.g. respiration, circulation, and digestion. It is expressed in terms of heat production per unit of body surface area per day (**basal metabolic rate** – **BMR**), and for an average man the BMR is 1.7 Calories (7.115 kilojoules) per day. BMR may be determined by the direct method, in which the subject is placed in a respiratory chamber and the amount of heat evolved is measured, or (more normally) by the indirect method, based on the *respiratory quotient. Measurements are best taken during a period of least activity, i.e. during sleep and 12–18 hours after a meal, under controlled temperature conditions. Various factors, such as age, sex, and particularly thyroid activity, influence the value of the BMR.

basement membrane the thin delicate membrane that lies at the base of an *epithelium. It is composed of mucopolysaccharide and fibres of protein.

base pairing the linking of the two strands of a DNA molecule by means of hydrogen bonds between the bases of the nucleotides. Adenine always pairs with thymine and cytosine with guanine. *See* DNA.

basilar artery an artery in the base of the brain, formed by the union of the two vertebral arteries. It extends from the lower to the upper border of the pons Varolii and then divides to form the two posterior cerebral arteries.

basilar membrane a membrane in the *cochlea of the ear that separates two of the three channels (scalae) that run the length of the spiral cochlea. The organ of Corti is situated on the basilar membrane, inside the scala media.

basilic vein a large vein in the arm, extending from the hand along the back of the forearm, then passing forward to the inner side of the arm at the elbow.

basion *n.* the midpoint of the anterior border of the large hole (foramen magnum) at the base of the *skull.

basophil *n.* a variety of white blood cell distinguished by the presence in its cytoplasm of coarse granules that stain purple-black with *Romanowsky stains. The

function of basophils is poorly understood, but they are capable of ingesting foreign particles and contain *histamine and *heparin. There are normally $30-150 \times 10^6$ basophils per litre of blood.

basophilia *n.* **1.** a property of a microscopic structure whereby it shows an affinity for basic dyes. **2.** an increase in the number of certain white blood cells (*basophils) in the blood, which may occur in a variety of blood diseases.

basophilic *adj.* readily stainable by basic dyes: showing *basophilia.

bathyaesthesia *n.* sensation experienced in the deeper parts of the body, such as the joints and muscles.

Batten's disease one of a group of rare hereditary disorders (known as the **neuronal ceroid lipofuscinoses**) that also includes *Tay-Sachs disease. Fatty substances accumulate in the cells of the nervous system, causing progressive dementia, epilepsy, spasticity, and visual failure. The condition starts in late infancy or childhood. There is no treatment. [F. E. Batten (1865–1918), British neurologist]

battered baby syndrome *see* NONACCIDENTAL INJURY.

Bazin's disease a rare disease of young women in which tender nodules develop under the skin in the calves. The nodules may break down and ulcerate though they may clear up spontaneously. The cause is unknown. Medical name: **erythema induratum**. [A. P. E. Bazin (1807–78), French dermatologist]

BCC *see* BASAL CELL CARCINOMA.

B-cell *n.* *see* LYMPHOCYTE.

BCG (bacille Calmette-Guérin) a strain of tubercle bacillus that has lost the power to cause tuberculosis but retains its antigenic activity; it is therefore used to prepare a vaccine against the disease.

bear tracks (in ophthalmology) areas of hypertrophy of retinal pigment epithelium (*see* RETINA) that clinically resemble the prints of bears' paws.

Beau's lines transverse depressions on the nails appearing some weeks after a severe illness, such as pneumonia or a heart attack. [J. H. S. Beau (1806–65), French physician]

Becker muscular dystrophy a *sex-linked (X-linked) disorder in which affected males develop an increase in muscle size followed by weakness and wasting. It usually starts between the ages of 5 and 15, and 25 years after onset most patients are wheelchair-bound. Although most men become severely disabled, life expectancy is close to normal. The disorder is similar to Duchenne *muscular dystrophy but less severe. [P. E. Becker (20th century), German geneticist]

beclomethasone n. a *corticosteroid drug that is administered by inhaler to treat hay fever and asthma and is applied externally in the treatment of inflammatory skin disorders. Possible side-effects include nasal irritation and hoarseness. Trade names: **Beconase**, **Becotide**, **Propaderm**.

becquerel n. the *SI unit of activity of a radioactive source, being the activity of a radionuclide decaying at a rate of one spontaneous nuclear transition per second. It has replaced the curie. Symbol: Bq.

bed bug a bloodsucking insect of the genus *Cimex*. *C. hemipterus* of the tropics and *C. lectularius* of temperate regions have reddish flattened bodies and vestigial wings. They live and lay their eggs in the crevices of walls and furniture and emerge at night to suck blood; although bed bugs are not known vectors of disease their bites leave a route for bacterial infection. Premises can be disinfested with appropriate insecticides.

bed occupancy the number of hospital beds occupied by patients expressed as a percentage of the total beds available in the ward, specialty, hospital, area, or region. It may be recorded in relation to a defined point in time or more usefully for a period, when the calculation is based on bed-days. It is used with other indices (such as *discharge rate) to assess the demands for hospital beds in relation to diseases, specialties, or populations and hence to gauge an appropriate balance between health needs and residential (hospital) resources.

bedsore (decubitus ulcer, pressure sore) n. an ulcerated area of skin caused by continuous pressure on part of the body: a hazard to be guarded against in all bedridden (especially unconscious) patients. Healing is hindered by the reduced blood supply to the area, and careful nursing is necessary to prevent local gangrene. The patient's position should be changed frequently, and the buttocks, heels, elbows, and other regions at risk kept dry and clean.

bedwetting n. see ENURESIS.

behaviourism n. an approach to psychology postulating that only observable behaviour need be studied, thus denying any importance to unconscious processes. Behaviourists are concerned with the laws regulating the occurrence of behaviour (see CONDITIONING). —**behaviourist** n.

behaviour modification the use of the methods of behaviourist psychology (see BEHAVIOURISM) – especially operant *conditioning – to alter people's behaviour. Behaviour modification has wider applications than *behaviour therapy, since it is also used in situations in which the client is not ill; for example, in education. See also CHAINING, PROMPTING.

behaviour therapy treatment based on the belief that psychological problems are the products of faulty learning and not the symptoms of an underlying disease. Treatment is directed at the problem or target behaviour and is designed for the particular patient, not for the particular diagnostic label that has been attached to him. See also AVERSION THERAPY, CONDITIONING, DESENSITIZATION, EXPOSURE, RESPONSE PREVENTION.

Behçet's syndrome a recurrent multisystem disease characterized by aphthous ulcers in the mouth (see APHTHA), genital ulcers, severe inflammation of the iris and other parts of the uveal tract of the eye (see UVEITIS), and *retrobulbar neuritis. It may also involve the joints and cause inflammation of the veins; skin lesions occur in the majority of patients. The condition, the cause of which is unknown, occurs more often in men than women. Treatment is with *azathioprine. [H. Behçet (1889–1948), Turkish dermatologist]

bejel (endemic syphilis) n. a long-lasting nonvenereal form of *syphilis that occurs in the Balkans, Turkey, eastern Mediterranean countries, and the dry savannah regions of North Africa; it is particularly prevalent where standards of personal hygiene are low. The disease is spread among children and adults by direct body contact. Early skin lesions are obvious in the moist areas of the body (mouth, armpits, and groin) and later there may be considerable destruction of the tissues of the skin, nasopharynx, and long bones. Wartlike eruptions in the anal and genital regions are common. Bejel, which is rarely fatal, is treated with penicillin.

bel *n.* see DECIBEL.

belladonna *n.* **1.** deadly nightshade (*Atropa belladonna*): the plant from which the drug atropine is obtained. **2.** the poisonous alkaloid derived from deadly nightshade, from which atropine is extracted. Preparations of belladonna are used as an anticholinergic drug (*see* PARASYMPATHOLYTIC). Trade names: **Alophen, Bellocarb.**

bell and pad a psychological method of treating bed-wetting in children and adults. When the subject starts to pass urine it is detected by a pad (or by sheets of metallic mesh) and this sets off a bell (or loud buzzer). The modern form of the apparatus has a small electronic sensor worn under the underclothes and produces a loud bleep. The purpose of the alarm is to waken the subject, who then empties the bladder fully. A process of conditioning leads to the subject learning to be dry. It is effective in about 80% of cases.

belle indifference a symptom of *conversion disorder in which an apparently grave physical affliction (which has no physical cause) is accepted in a smiling and calm fashion.

Bell's palsy paralysis of the *facial nerve causing weakness of the muscles of one side of the face and an inability to close the eye. In some patients hearing may be affected so that sounds seem abnormally loud, and a loss of taste sensation may occur. The cause of this condition is unknown and recovery nor-

mally occurs spontaneously. [Sir C. Bell (1774–1842), Scottish physiologist]

belly *n.* **1.** the *abdomen or abdominal cavity. **2.** the central fleshy portion of a muscle.

Bence-Jones protein (Bence-Jones albumose) a protein of low molecular weight found in the urine of patients with multiple *myeloma and rarely in patients with *lymphoma, *leukaemia, and *Hodgkin's disease. [H. Bence-Jones (1814–73), British physician]

bendrofluazide (bendroflumethazide) *n.* a potent thiazide *diuretic used in the treatment of conditions involving retention of fluid, such as congestive heart failure, hypertension, and *oedema. Its actions and side-effects are similar to those of *chlorothiazide. Trade names: **Aprinox, Contyl.**

bends *n.* see COMPRESSED AIR ILLNESS.

Benedict's test a test for the presence of sugar in urine or other liquids. A few drops of the test solution are added to **Benedict's solution,** prepared from sodium or potassium citrate, sodium carbonate, and copper sulphate. The mixture is boiled and shaken for about two minutes, then left to cool. The presence of up to 2% glucose is indicated by the formation of a reddish, yellowish, or greenish precipitate, the highest levels corresponding to the red coloration, the lowest (about 0.05%) to the green. [S. R. Benedict (1884–1936), US surgeon]

benethamine penicillin an antibiotic effective against most Gram-positive bacteria (streptococci, staphylococci, and pneumococci). A derivative of *penicillin G, it can be administered by mouth but is usually given as an intramuscular injection, from which it liberates penicillin G slowly. Patients hypersensitive to penicillins may suffer allergic reactions.

benign *adj.* **1.** describing a tumour that does not invade and destroy the tissue in which it originates or spread to distant sites in the body, i.e. a tumour that is not cancerous. **2.** describing any disorder or condition that does not produce harmful effects. *Compare* MALIGNANT.

benign intracranial hypertension

(pseudotumour cerebri) a syndrome of raised pressure within the skull caused by impaired reabsorption of cerebrospinal fluid. The symptoms include headache, vomiting, double vision, and *papilloedema. It normally subsides spontaneously but drug therapy or neurosurgical treatment may be required to protect the patient's vision.

benign prostatic hypertrophy (BPH) *see* PROSTATE GLAND.

benorylate *n.* a compound of *aspirin and *paracetamol that relieves pain, inflammation, and fever. It is an alternative to aspirin, particularly in the treatment of rheumatoid arthritis. Side-effects may include drowsiness, noises in the ears, and skin rashes. Trade name: **Benoral**.

benperidol *n.* a *butyrophenone antipsychotic drug used mainly to treat deviant and antisocial sexual behaviour. It is administered by mouth. Trade name: **Anquil**.

benserazide *n.* a drug that prevents the breakdown of *levodopa to dopamine outside the brain by inhibiting the enzyme dopa decarboxylase. Administered by mouth in combination with levodopa (as **Madopar**), it is used to treat parkinsonism following encephalitis (post-encephalitic parkinsonism). Possible side-effects include nausea, vomiting, loss of appetite, involuntary movements, and faintness on standing up.

benzalkonium *n.* a detergent disinfectant with the same uses and effects as *cetrimide.

benzathine penicillin a long-acting antibiotic, given by mouth or intramuscular injection, that is slowly absorbed and effective against most Gram-positive bacteria (streptococci, staphylococci, and pneumococci). Patients hypersensitive to the penicillins suffer allergic reactions. Trade name: **Penidural**. *See also* PENICILLIN.

benzhexol *n.* a drug that has actions and side-effects similar to those of *atropine. Taken by mouth, it is used mainly to reduce muscle spasm in parkinsonism. Trade names: **Artane, Broflex**.

benzocaine *n.* a local anaesthetic used in the form of an ointment, suppository, or aerosol to relieve painful conditions of the skin and mucous membranes. Virtually non-toxic, it can also be taken by mouth in the form of lozenges to treat such conditions as lacerations of the mouth or tongue and gastric ulcers.

benzodiazepines *n.* a group of pharmacologically active compounds used as minor *tranquillizers and hypnotics. The group includes *bromazepam, *chlordiazepoxide, *diazepam, and *oxazepam.

benzoic acid an antiseptic, active against fungi and bacteria, used as a preservative in foods and pharmaceutical preparations, as well as for the treatment of fungal infections of the skin.

benzoyl peroxide a preparation used in the treatment of acne and other skin conditions. It acts by removing the surface layers of the epidermis and unblocking skin pores and has an antiseptic effect on skin bacteria. It is administered as a cream, lotion, or gel. Side-effects include skin irritation, excessive peeling, and (occasionally) blistering. Trade names: **Acetoxyl, Acnegel, Benoxyl**.

benzthiazide *n.* a *diuretic used in the treatment of conditions involving fluid retention, such as congestive heart failure, *oedema, and hypertension. Trade name: **Dytide**.

benztropine *n.* a drug that is similar to *atropine but also acts as an antihistamine, local anaesthetic, and sedative. Given by mouth, it is used mainly in the treatment of parkinsonism to reduce rigidity and muscle cramps. It is well tolerated, but produces drowsiness and confusion.

benzydamine hydrochloride an anti-inflammatory drug (*see* NSAID) used to treat muscle pain. It is administered as a cream for external use. Trade name: **Difflam**.

benzyl benzoate an oily aromatic liquid that is applied to the body – in the form of a lotion – for the treatment of scabies. It is also useful in treating pediculosis. Trade name: **Ascabiol**.

benzylpenicillin *n.* *see* PENICILLIN.

bephenium hydroxynaphthoate an *anthelmintic drug used to get rid of hookworms and other nematodes. It is administered by mouth. Possible side-effects include stomach irritation. Trade name: **Alcopar**.

beriberi *n.* a nutritional disorder due to deficiency of vitamin B₁ (thiamin). It is widespread in rice-eating communities in which the diet is based on polished rice, from which the seed coat (which is rich in thiamin) has been removed. Beriberi takes two forms: **wet beriberi**, in which there is an accumulation of tissue fluid (*oedema), and **dry beriberi**, in which there is extreme emaciation. There is nervous degeneration in both forms of the disease and death from heart failure is often the outcome.

berry aneurysm *see* ANEURYSM.

berylliosis *n.* poisoning by beryllium or its compounds, either by inhalation or by skin contamination. Inhalation of fumes from molten beryllium causes an acute *alveolitis and is usually fatal. Subacute and chronic forms can result from extremely low levels of exposure to the powder and can produce granulomata in the skin or lungs very similar to those seen in *sarcoidosis. In the lungs, these lead to fibrosis, which can, however, be prevented by prompt use of oral corticosteroids. Although the incidence of berylliosis has been greatly reduced since the use of beryllium compounds in the manufacture of fluorescent light tubes was discontinued in Britain in 1948, new cases are still occurring.

Best's disease *see* VITELLIFORM DEGENERATION. [F. Best (1878–1920), German physician]

beta blocker a drug that prevents stimulation of the beta-adrenergic receptors at the nerve endings of the sympathetic nervous system and therefore decreases the activity of the heart. Beta blockers include *acebutolol, *betaxolol, *bisoprolol, *oxprenolol, *propranolol, and *sotalol; they are used to control abnormal heart rhythms, to treat angina, and to reduce high blood pressure. Blockade of beta receptors may cause constriction of air passages in the lungs and care has to be taken with the use of beta blockers in patients with any bronchial conditions. *See also* SYMPATHOLYTIC.

betahistine *n.* a drug that is an *analogue of *histamine and increases blood flow through the inner ear. It is administered by mouth to treat *Ménière's disease. A common side-effect is nausea. Trade name: **Serc**.

beta-lactam antibiotic one of a group of drugs that includes the *penicillins and the *cephalosporins. All have a four-membered **beta-lactam** ring as part of their molecular structure. Beta-lactam antibiotics function by interfering with the growth of the cell walls of multiplying bacteria. Bacteria become resistant to these antibiotics by producing **beta-lactamases**, enzymes (such as *penicillinase) that disrupt the beta-lactam ring.

betamethasone *n.* a synthetic corticosteroid drug with effects and uses similar to those of *prednisolone. The side-effects are those of *cortisone. Trade names: **Betnelan, Betnesol, Betnovate**.

betatron *n.* a device used to accelerate a stream of electrons (**beta particles**) into a beam of radiation that can be used in *radiotherapy.

betaxolol *n.* a *beta blocker drug used to treat high blood pressure and chronic simple *glaucoma. It is administered by mouth and as eye drops. Possible side-effects include breathing difficulty, fatigue, cold extremities, and sleep disturbances. Trade names: **Kerlone, Betoptic**.

bethanechol *n.* a cholinergic drug (*see* PARASYMPATHOMIMETIC) that acts mainly on the bowel and bladder, stimulating these organs to empty. It is administered by mouth. Possible side-effects include nausea, vomiting, and abdominal cramps. Trade name: **Myotonine**.

bethanidine *n.* a drug that lowers blood pressure. It is given by mouth and acts by blocking the sympathetic nerves that supply the blood vessels. Common side-effects include dizziness, fainting, oedema, and breathlessness.

bezafibrate *n.* a drug that reduces blood *cholesterol levels and is used to treat hypercholesterolaemia that fails to respond to diet. It is administered by mouth. Possible side-effects include skin rashes, nausea and vomiting, and muscle pain. Trade name: **Bezalip**.

bezoar *n.* a mass of swallowed foreign material within the stomach. The material, which is usually swallowed by psychiatrically disturbed patients, accumulates and ultimately causes gastric obstruction. Its removal often requires a surgical operation. *See also* TRICHOBEZOAR.

bi- *prefix denoting* two; double. Examples: **biciliate** (having two cilia); **binucleate** (having two nuclei).

biceps *n.* a muscle with two heads. The **biceps brachii** extends from the shoulder joint to the elbow (see illustration). It flexes the arm and forearm and supinates the forearm and hand. The **biceps femoris** is situated at the back of the thigh and is responsible for flexing the knee, extending the thigh, and rotating the leg outwards.

scapula

biceps brachii short head

biceps brachii long head

radius

The biceps muscle of the arm

biconcave *adj.* having a hollowed surface on both sides. Biconcave lenses are used to correct short-sightedness. *Compare* BICONVEX.

biconvex *adj.* having a surface on each side that curves outwards. Biconvex lenses are used to correct long-sightedness. *Compare* BICONCAVE.

bicornuate *adj.* having two hornlike processes or projections. The term is applied to an abnormal uterus that is divided into two separate halves at the upper end.

bicuspid **1.** *adj.* having two *cusps, as in the premolar teeth and the mitral valve of the heart. **2.** *n.* (in the USA) a premolar tooth.

bicuspid valve *see* MITRAL VALVE.

Bielschowsky head tilt a test used mainly to differentiate between a weakness of the superior oblique muscle and a weakness of the contralateral superior rectus muscle (*see* EXTRINSIC MUSCLE). Tilting the head to the same side as the affected eye causes upward rotation of that eye. [A. Bielschowsky (1871–1940), German ophthalmologist]

bifid *adj.* split or cleft into two parts.

bifocal lenses glasses in which the upper part of the lens gives a sharp image of distant objects and the lower part is for near vision, such as reading. *See also* TRIFOCAL LENSES, MULTIFOCAL LENSES.

bifurcation *n.* (in anatomy) the point at which division into two branches occurs; for example in blood vessels or in the trachea.

bigeminal body one of the two swellings that develop in the roof of the midbrain during its development in the embryo.

bigeminy *n.* the condition in which alternate *ectopic beats of the heart are transmitted to the pulse and felt as a double pulse beat (**pulsus bigeminus**). It is a common manifestation of digitalis poisoning.

biguanide *n.* one of the group of drugs including *metformin, which is used to treat noninsulin-dependent (Type II) diabetes mellitus. Biguanides are *oral hypoglycaemic drugs: they act by reducing the release of glucose from the liver and increasing glucose uptake by muscles.

bilateral *adj.* (in anatomy) relating to or affecting both sides of the body or of a tissue or organ or both of a pair of organs (e.g. the eyes, breasts, or ovaries).

bile *n.* a thick alkaline fluid that is secreted by the *liver and stored in the *gall bladder, from which it is ejected intermittently into the duodenum via the common *bile duct. Bile may be yellow, green, or brown, according to the proportions of the *bile pigments (excretory products) present; other constituents are lecithin, cholesterol, and *bile salts. The bile salts help to emulsify fats in the duodenum so that they can be more easily digested by pancreatic *lipase into fatty acids and glycerol. Bile salts also form compounds with fatty acids, which can then be transported into the *lacteals. Bile also helps to stimulate *peristalsis in the duodenum.

bile acids the organic acids in bile; mostly occurring as bile salts (sodium glycocholate and sodium taurocholate). They are cholic acid, deoxycholic acid, glycocholic acid, and taurocholic acid.

bile duct any of the ducts that convey bile from the liver. Bile is drained from the liver cells by many small ducts that unite to form the main bile duct of the liver, the **hepatic duct**. This joins the **cystic duct**, which leads from the *gall bladder, to form the **common bile duct**, which drains into the duodenum.

bile pigments coloured compounds – breakdown products of the blood pigment *haemoglobin – that are excreted in *bile. The two most important bile pigments are **bilirubin**, which is orange or yellow, and its oxidized form **biliverdin**, which is green. Mixed with the intestinal contents, they give the brown colour to the faeces (*see* UROBILINOGEN).

bile salts sodium glycocholate and sodium taurocholate – the alkaline salts of *bile – necessary for the emulsification of fats. After they have been absorbed from the intestine they are transported to the liver for reuse.

Bilharzia *n. see* SCHISTOSOMA.

bilharziasis *n. see* SCHISTOSOMIASIS.

bili- *prefix denoting* bile.

biliary *adj.* relating to or affecting the bile duct or bile. *See also* FISTULA.

biliary atresia a congenital or acquired condition in which the bile ducts do not drain. Babies usually present within the first few weeks of life with jaundice that does not improve with time. Some forms of biliary atresia can be corrected surgically, but if diagnosis has been delayed the condition may lead to irreversible liver damage.

biliary colic pain resulting from obstruction of the gall bladder or common bile duct, usually by a stone. The pain, which is very severe, is usually felt in the upper abdomen (in the mid-line or to the right). It often occurs about an hour after a meal (particularly if fatty), may last several hours, and is usually steady in severity (unlike other forms of *colic). Vomiting often occurs simultaneously.

bilious *adj.* **1.** containing bile; for example **bilious vomiting** is the vomiting of bile-containing fluid. **2.** a lay term used to describe attacks of nausea or vomiting.

bilirubin *n. see* BILE PIGMENTS.

bilirubinaemia *n.* an excess of the *bile pigment bilirubin in the blood. Normally there is under 0.8 mg bilirubin per 100 ml blood (17 µmol/l); when the concentration of bilirubin is above 1–1.5 mg per 100 ml (20–30 µmol/l), visible *jaundice occurs. *See also* VAN DEN BERGH'S TEST.

biliuria (choluria) *n.* the presence of bile in the urine: a feature of certain forms of jaundice.

biliverdin *n. see* BILE PIGMENTS.

Billings method a method of planning pregnancy, now rarely used, involving the daily examination of cervical mucus in the vagina, which varies in consistency and colour throughout the menstrual cycle. Use of a **Billings mucus observation chart** to help identify the type of mucus enables the woman (in about 50% of cases) to have six days' warning of impending ovulation. It is a rather unreliable method of contraception. [J. and E. Billings (20th century)]

bimanual *adj.* using two hands to perform an activity, such as a gynaecological examination.

binaural *adj.* relating to or involving the use of both ears.

binder *n.* a bandage that is wound around a part of the body, usually the abdomen, to apply pressure or to give support or protection.

binge–purge syndrome *see* BULIMIA.

binocular adj. relating to or involving the use of both eyes.

binocular vision the ability to focus both eyes on an object at the same time, so that a person sees one image of the object he is looking at. It is not inborn, but acquired during the first few months of life. Binocular vision enables judgment of distance and perception of depth. See also STEREOSCOPIC VISION.

bio- prefix denoting life or living organisms. Example: **biosynthesis** (formation of a compound within a living organism).

bioassay n. estimation of the activity or potency of a drug or other substance by comparing its effects on living organisms with effects of a preparation of known strength. Bioassay is used to determine the strength of preparations of hormones or other material of biological origin when other physical or chemical methods are not available.

bioavailability n. the proportion of a drug that is delivered to its site of action in the body. This is usually the amount entering the circulation and may be low when the drugs are given by mouth.

biochemistry n. the study of the chemical processes and substances occurring in living things. —**biochemical** adj. —**biochemist** n.

bioengineering n. the application of biological and engineering principles to the development and manufacture of equipment and devices for use in biological systems. Examples of such products include orthopaedic prostheses and heart pacemakers.

biofeedback n. the giving of immediate information to a subject about his bodily processes (such as heart rate), which are usually unconscious. These processes can then be subject to operant *conditioning. This is an experimental treatment for disturbances of bodily regulation, such as hypertension.

biological response modifier a therapeutic agent, such as *interferon or *interleukin, that influences the body's defence mechanisms to act against a cancer cell. These substances are normally produced in small amounts by the body; relatively large doses are being studied for cancer treatment.

biology n. the study of living organisms – plants, animals, and microorganisms – including their structure and function and their relationships with one another and with the inanimate world. —**biological** adj.

biometry n. the measurement of living things and the processes associated with life, including the application of mathematics, particularly statistics, to problems in biology.

bionics n. the science of mechanical or electronic systems that function in the same way as, or have characteristics of, living systems. Compare CYBERNETICS. —**bionic** adj.

bionomics n. see ECOLOGY.

biophysical profile a physiological assessment of fetal wellbeing, including ultrasound scans, cardiotocograms, and fetal movements.

biopsy n. the removal of a small piece of living tissue from an organ or part of the body for microscopic examination. Biopsy is an important means of diagnosing cancer from examination of a fragment of tumour. It is often carried out with a special hollow needle, inserted into the liver, kidney, or other organ, with relatively little discomfort to the patient.

biostatistics n. statistical information and techniques used with special reference to studies of health and social problems. It embraces, overlaps, and is to some extent synonymous with the fields of **vital statistics** (e.g. *fertility and *mortality rates) and *demography.

biotechnology n. the development of techniques for the application of biological processes to the production of materials of use in medicine and industry. For example, the production of many antibiotics relies on the activity of various fungi and bacteria. Recent techniques of *genetic engineering, in which human genes are cloned in bacterial cells, have enabled the large-scale production of hormones (notably insulin), vaccines, interferon, and other useful products.

biotin n. a vitamin of the B complex that

is essential for the metabolism of fat, being involved in fatty acid synthesis and *gluconeogenesis. A biotin deficiency is extremely rare in man; it can be induced by eating large quantities of raw egg white, which contains a protein – avidin – that combines with biotin, making it unavailable to the body. Rich sources of the vitamin are egg yolk and liver.

biperiden *n.* a drug with effects similar to those of atropine, used in the treatment of parkinsonism, certain forms of spasticity, and to control the muscular incoordination that may result from the use of some tranquillizers. It is given by mouth; side-effects are those of *atropine. Trade name: **Akineton**.

biphosphonates *pl. n.* a group of drugs that inhibit the resorption of bone by blocking the action of *osteoclasts. They include *etidronate and **pamidronate** (**Aredia**), which are used to treat various disorders of bone metabolism, including Paget's disease; and **alendronate** (**Fosamax**), which has been successful in the treatment of osteoporosis by preventing bone loss and increasing bone density.

bipolar *adj.* (in neurology) describing a neurone (nerve cell) that has two processes extending in different directions from its cell body.

bipolar disorder *see* MANIC-DEPRESSIVE PSYCHOSIS.

bird-fancier's lung a form of external allergic *alveolitis caused by the inhalation of avian proteins present in the droppings and feathers of certain birds, especially pigeons and caged birds (such as budgerigars). As in *farmer's lung, there is an acute and a chronic form.

birefringence *n.* the property possessed by some naturally occurring substances (such as cell membranes) of doubly refracting a beam of light, i.e. of bending it in two different directions. —**birefringent** *adj.*

birth *n.* (in obstetrics) *see* LABOUR.

birth control the use of *contraception or *sterilization (male or female) to prevent unwanted pregnancies.

birthing chair a chair specially adapted to allow childbirth to take place in a sitting position. Its recent introduction in the Western world followed the increasing demand by women for greater mobility during labour. The chair is electronically powered and can be tilted back quickly and easily should the need arise.

birthmark *n.* a skin blemish or mark present at birth. The cause is unknown but most birthmarks grow before the baby is born. *See* NAEVUS.

birth rate the number of live births occurring in a year per 1000 total population (the **annual crude birth rate**). *See* FERTILITY RATE.

bisacodyl *n.* a *laxative that acts on the large intestine to cause reflex movement and bowel evacuation. Bisacodyl is administered by mouth or in a suppository. The commonest side-effect is the development of abdominal cramps. Trade name: **Dulcolax**.

bisexual *adj.* **1.** describing an individual who is sexually attracted to both men and women. **2.** describing an individual who possesses the qualities of both sexes.

Bismarck brown a basic aniline dye used for staining and counterstaining histological and bacterial specimens. [O. von Bismarck (1815–98), German statesman]

bismuth carbonate a drug used to treat peptic ulcer, especially cases in which the organism *Helicobacter pylori* is a causal agent. It is administered by mouth. Trade name: **APP**.

bisoprolol *n.* a *beta blocker drug used to treat angina pectoris. It is administered by mouth. Possible side-effects include breathing difficulty, fatigue, cold extremities, and sleep disturbances. Trade names: **Emcor, Monocor**.

Types of bistoury

bistoury *n.* a narrow surgical knife, with a straight or curved blade (see illustration).

bite-raiser *n.* an appliance to prevent normal closure of the teeth in orthodontic treatment and in the treatment of the *temporomandibular joint syndrome.

bite-wing *n.* a dental X-ray film that provides a view of the crowns of the teeth in part of both upper and lower jaws. This view is used in the diagnosis of caries and periodontal disease.

Bitot's spots cheesy foamy greyish spots that form on the surface of dry patches of conjunctiva at the sides of the eyes. They consist of fragments of keratinized epithelium. A common cause is vitamin A deficiency. [P. A. Bitot (1822–88), French physician]

bivalent *n.* (in genetics) a structure consisting of homologous chromosomes attached to each other by *chiasmata during the first division of *meiosis. —**bivalent** *adj.*

blackdamp (chokedamp) *n.* (in mining) the poisonous gas containing carbon dioxide, carbon monoxide, or other suffocating material, sometimes found in pockets in underground workings. *Compare* FIREDAMP.

Black Death *see* PLAGUE.

black eye bruising of the eyelids.

black fly a small widely distributed bloodsucking insect of the genus *Simulium*. Black flies are also known as buffalo gnats from their humpbacked appearance. Female flies can inflict painful bites and constitute a serious pest to man at certain times of the year. *S. damnosum* in Africa and *S. ochraceum* in Central America and Venezuela transmit the parasites causing *onchocerciasis.

blackhead *n.* a plug formed of fatty material (sebum and keratin) in the outlet of a *sebaceous gland in the skin. *See also* ACNE. Medical name: **comedo**.

black heel a black area, usually over the Achilles tendon, resulting from the rupture of capillaries in the skin in those who play basketball, squash, etc. It may be mistaken for malignant melanoma.

blackwater fever a rare and serious complication of malignant tertian (falciparum) *malaria in which there is massive destruction of the red blood cells, leading to the presence of the blood pigment haemoglobin in the urine. The condition is probably brought on by inadequate treatment with *quinine; it is marked by fever, bloody urine, jaundice, vomiting, enlarged liver and spleen, anaemia, exhaustion, and – in fatal cases – a reduced flow of urine resulting from a blockage of the kidney tubules. Treatment involves rest, administration of alkaline fluids and intravenous glucose, and blood transfusions.

bladder *n.* **1.** (**urinary bladder**) a sac-shaped organ that has a wall of smooth muscle and stores the urine produced by the kidneys. Urine passes into the bladder through the *ureters; the release of urine from the bladder is controlled by a sphincter at its junction with the *urethra. The **bladder neck** is the outlet of the bladder where it joins the urethra and in males it is in contact with the *prostate gland; it is under the control of the autonomic nerves of the pelvis. The neck of the bladder is the commonest site for *retention of urine, usually by an enlarged prostate or a urethral *stricture. **2.** any of several other hollow organs containing fluid, such as the *gall bladder.

bladder augmentation (bladder enhancement) a surgical method of increasing the capacity of the bladder. This is usually achieved by ileocaecocystoplasty (*see* CYSTOPLASTY).

bladder replacement *see* CYSTECTOMY.

bladderworm *n.* *see* CYSTICERCUS.

blast *n.* an important cause of serious soft-tissue injury that is associated with explosions or high-velocity missiles. The eardrums, lungs, and gastrointestinal tract are especially vulnerable to the indirect effects of the blast wave.

-blast *suffix denoting* a formative cell. Example: **osteoblast** (formative bone cell).

blastema *n.* any zone of embryonic tissue that is still differentiating and growing into a particular organ. The term is usually applied to the tissue that develops into the kidneys and gonads.

blasto- *prefix denoting* a germ cell or embryo. Example: **blastogenesis** (early development of an embryo).

blastocoele *n.* the fluid-filled cavity that develops within the *blastocyst. The cavity increases the surface area of the embryo and thus improves its ability to absorb nutrients and oxygen.

blastocyst *n.* an early stage of embryonic development that consists of a hollow ball of cells with a localized thickening (the **inner cell mass**) that will develop into the actual embryo; the remainder of the blastocyst is composed of *trophoblast (see illustration). At first the blastocyst is unattached, but it soon implants in the wall of the uterus. *See also* IMPLANTATION.

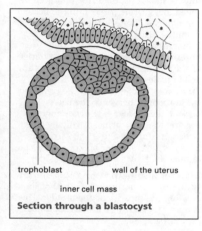

trophoblast   wall of the uterus
inner cell mass
Section through a blastocyst

blastomere *n.* any of the cells produced by *cleavage of the zygote, comprising the earliest stages of embryonic development until the formation of the *blastocyst. Blastomeres divide repeatedly without growth and so decrease in size.

blastomycosis *n.* any disease caused by parasitic fungi of the genus *Blastomyces*, which may affect the skin (forming wart-like ulcers and tumours on the face, neck, hands, arms, feet, and legs) or involve various internal tissues, such as the lungs, bones, liver, spleen, and lymphatics. There are two principal forms of the disease: **North American blastomycosis** (**Gilchrist's disease**), caused by *B. dermati-*

tidis; and **South American blastomycosis**, caused by *B. brasiliensis*. Both diseases are treated with antifungal drugs (such as amphotericin).

blastopore *n.* the opening that forms as a result of invagination of the surface layer of the early embryo (*gastrula). It is very much reduced in man, in which it gives rise to the archenteric canal (*see* ARCHENTERON).

blastula *n.* an early stage of the embryonic development of many animals. The equivalent stage in mammals (including man) is the *blastocyst.

bleb *n.* a blister or large vesicle. A **filtering bleb** is a blister-like cyst underneath the conjunctiva resulting from *trabeculectomy, a surgical procedure commonly used in the treatment of glaucoma.

bleeding *n.* *see* HAEMORRHAGE.

blenn- (blenno-) *prefix denoting* mucus. Example: **blennorrhagia** (excessive production of).

blennophthalmia *n.* *Obsolete.* *conjunctivitis in which there is a sticky yellow discharge from the eye.

blennorrhagia *n.* a copious discharge of mucus, particularly from the urethra. This usually accompanies *urethritis and sometimes occurs with acute *prostatitis. Treatment is directed to clearing the underlying causative organism by antibiotic administration.

blennorrhoea *n.* a profuse watery discharge from the urethra. This, like *blennorrhagia, is associated with either prostatitis or urethritis, and is cleared by the usual measures undertaken in the treatment of these conditions.

bleomycin *n.* an antibiotic with action against cancer cells, used in the treatment of Hodgkin's disease and other lymphomas and in squamous cell carcinoma. It is administered by injection and can cause toxic side-effects in the skin and lungs; it should not be used in patients with impaired kidney function or lung disease.

blephar- (blepharo-) *prefix denoting* the eyelid. Example: **blepharotomy** (incision into).

blepharitis n. inflammation of the eyelids. In **squamous blepharitis**, often associated with dandruff of the scalp, white scales accumulate among the lashes. **Chronic ulcerative blepharitis** is characterized by yellow crusts overlying ulcers of the lid margins. The lashes become matted together and tend to fall out or become distorted. **Allergic blepharitis** may occur in response to drugs or cosmetics put in the eye or on the eyelids.

blepharochalasis n. excessive eyelid skin resulting from recurrent episodes of oedema and inflammation of the eyelid. It occurs in young people, causing drooping of the lid. *Compare* DERMATOCHALASIS.

blepharoconjunctivitis n. inflammation involving the eyelid margins and conjunctiva.

blepharon n. *see* EYELID.

blepharophimosis n. a small aperture between the eyelids. It is usually congenital.

blepharoplasty (tarsoplasty) n. any operation to repair or reconstruct the eyelid. It involves either rearrangement of the tissues of the lid or the use of tissue from other sites (e.g. skin or mucous membrane).

blepharoptosis n. *see* PTOSIS.

blepharospasm n. involuntary tight contraction of the eyelids, either in response to painful conditions of the eye or as a form of *dystonia.

blind loop syndrome (stagnant loop syndrome) a condition of stasis of the small intestine allowing the overgrowth of bacteria, which causes *malabsorption and the passage of fatty stools (*see* STEATORRHOEA). It is usually the result of chronic obstruction (resulting, for example, from *Crohn's disease, a *stricture, or intestinal tuberculosis), or surgical bypass operations producing a stagnant length of bowel, or conditions (e.g. a jejunal *diverticulum) in which a segment of intestine is out of continuity with the rest.

blindness n. the inability to see. Lack of all light perception constitutes total blindness but there are degrees of visual impairment far less severe than this that may be classed as blindness for adminis-

trative or statutory purposes. For example, marked reduction in the *visual field is classified as blindness, even if objects are still seen sharply. The commonest causes of blindness worldwide are *trachoma, *onchocerciasis, and vitamin A deficiency (*see* NIGHT BLINDNESS) but there is wide geographic variation. In Great Britain the commonest causes are age-related *macular degeneration, *glaucoma, *cataract, myopic retinal degeneration, and diabetic *retinopathy.

blind register (in Britain) a list of persons who are technically blind due to reduced visual acuity or who have severely restricted fields of vision (*see* BLINDNESS). Such people are entitled to special education and to financial and other social benefits. *See also* PARTIALLY SIGHTED REGISTER.

blind spot the small area of the *retina of the eye where the nerve fibres from the light-sensitive cells (*see* CONE, ROD) lead into the optic nerve. There are no rods or cones in this area and hence it does not register light. Anatomical name: **punctum caecum**.

blind trial *see* INTERVENTION STUDY.

blinking n. the action of closing and opening the eyelids, which wipes the front of the eyeball and helps to spread the *tears. Reflex blinking may be caused by suddenly bringing an object near to the eye: the eyelids close involuntarily in order to protect the eye.

blister n. a swelling containing watery fluid (serum) and sometimes also blood (**blood blister**) or pus, within or just beneath the skin. Blisters commonly develop as a result of unaccustomed friction on the hands or feet or at the site of a burn. Blisters may be treated with antiseptics and dressings. An unduly painful blister may be punctured with a sterile needle so that the fluid is released.

block n. any interruption of physiological or mental function, brought about intentionally (as part of a therapeutic procedure) or by disease. *See also* HEART BLOCK, NERVE BLOCK.

blocking n. (in psychiatry) **1.** a sudden halting of the flow of thought or speech. Blocking of thought, accompanied by the sensation of thoughts being removed from the mind, is a symptom of *schizophrenia. Blocking of speech may be a consequence of thought block or a result of a mechanical impediment in speech, such as *stammering. **2.** the failure to recall a specific event, or to explore a specific train of thought, because of its unpleasant associations.

blood *n.* a fluid that circulates throughout the body, via the arteries and veins, providing a vehicle by which an immense variety of different substances are transported between the various organs and tissues. It is composed of *blood cells, which are suspended in a liquid medium, the *plasma. An average individual has approximately 70 ml of blood per kilogram body weight (about 5 litres in an average adult male).

blood bank a department within a hospital or blood transfusion centre in which blood collected from donors is stored prior to transfusion. Blood must be kept at a temperature of 4°C and may be used up to four weeks after collection.

blood-brain barrier the mechanism whereby the circulating blood is kept separate from the tissue fluids surrounding the brain cells. It is a semipermeable membrane allowing solutions to pass through it but excluding solid particles and large molecules.

blood cell (blood corpuscle) any of the cells that are present in the blood in health or disease. The cells may be subclassified into three major categories, namely red cells (*erythrocytes); white cells (*leucocytes), which include granulocytes, lymphocytes, and monocytes; and *platelets (see illustration). The blood cells account for approximately 40% of the total volume of the blood in health; red cells comprise the vast majority.

blood clot a solid mass formed as the result of *blood coagulation, either within the blood vessels and heart or elsewhere (*compare* THROMBUS). A blood clot consists of a meshwork of the protein *fibrin in which various blood cells are trapped.

blood clotting *see* BLOOD COAGULATION.

blood coagulation (blood clotting) the process whereby blood is converted from a liquid to a solid state. The process

may be initiated by contact of blood with a foreign surface (**intrinsic system**) or with damaged tissue (**extrinsic system**). These systems involve the interaction of a variety of substances (*coagulation factors) and lead to the production of the enzyme thrombin, which converts the soluble blood protein *fibrinogen to the insoluble protein *fibrin. Blood coagulation is an essential mechanism for the arrest of bleeding (*haemostasis).

Types of blood cells

blood corpuscle *see* BLOOD CELL.

blood count the numbers of different blood cells in a known volume of blood, usually expressed as the number of cells per litre. A sample of blood at known dilution is passed through a narrow opening in an electronic counting device. Blood-count investigations are important in the diagnosis of blood diseases. *See also* DIFFERENTIAL LEUCOCYTE COUNT.

blood donor a person who gives blood

blue baby

Donor's blood group	Blood group of people donor can receive blood from	Blood group of people donor can give blood to
A	A, O	A, AB
B	B, O	B, AB
AB	A, B, AB, O	AB
O	O	A, B, AB, O

for storage in a *blood bank. The blood can then be used for *transfusion into another patient. In Britain collection is organized by the National Blood Transfusion Services, but the armed forces have their own services. See also BLOOD GROUP.

blood group any one of the many types into which a person's blood may be classified, based on the presence or absence of certain inherited antigens on the surface of the red blood cells. Blood of one group contains antibodies in the serum that react against the cells of other groups.

There are more than 30 blood group systems, one of the most important of which is the **ABO system**. This system is based on the presence or absence of antigens A and B: blood of groups A and B contains antigens A and B, respectively; group AB contains both antigens and group O neither. Blood of group A contains antibodies to antigen B; group B blood contains anti-A antibodies or *isoagglutinins; group AB has neither antibody and group O has both. A person whose blood contains either (or both) of these antibodies cannot receive a transfusion of blood containing the corresponding antigens. The table illustrates which blood groups can be used in transfusion for each of the four groups.

blood plasma see PLASMA.

blood poisoning the presence of either bacterial toxins or large numbers of bacteria in the bloodstream causing serious illness. See PYAEMIA, SEPTICAEMIA, TOXAEMIA.

blood pressure the pressure of blood against the walls of the main arteries. Pressure is highest during *systole, when the ventricles are contracting (**systolic pressure**), and lowest during *diastole, when the ventricles are relaxing and refilling (**diastolic pressure**). Blood pres-

sure is measured – in millimetres of mercury – by means of a *sphygmomanometer at the brachial artery of the arm, where the pressure is most similar to that of blood leaving the heart. The normal range varies with age, but a young adult would be expected to have a systolic pressure of around 120 mm and a diastolic pressure of 80 mm. These are recorded as 120/80.

Individual variations are common. Muscular exertion and emotional factors, such as fear, stress, and excitement, all raise systolic blood pressure (see HYPERTENSION). Systolic blood pressure is normally at its lowest during sleep. Severe shock may lead to an abnormally low blood pressure and possible circulatory failure (see HYPOTENSION). Blood pressure is adjusted to its normal level by the *sympathetic nervous system and hormonal controls.

blood serum see SERUM.

blood sugar the concentration of glucose in the blood, normally expressed in millimoles per litre. The normal range is 3.5–5.5 mmol/l. Blood-sugar estimation is an important investigation in a variety of diseases, most notably in diabetes mellitus. See also HYPERGLYCAEMIA, HYPOGLYCAEMIA.

blood test any test designed to discover abnormalities in a sample of a person's blood, such as the presence of alcohol, drugs, or bacteria, or to determine the *blood group.

blood transfusion see TRANSFUSION.

blood vessel a tube carrying blood away from or towards the heart. Blood vessels are the means by which blood circulates throughout the body. See ARTERY, ARTERIOLE, VEIN, VENULE, CAPILLARY.

blue baby an infant suffering from

congenital cyanotic heart disease, the commonest forms of which are *tetralogy of Fallot and *transposition of the great vessels, in which the circulation is misdirected. Both of these conditions result in the presence of partially deoxygenated blood (which is blue in colour) in the peripheral circulation, which gives the skin and lips a characteristic purple colour. Surgical correction is often possible at an early stage. If untreated, infants may survive months or years with persistent *cyanosis.

B-lymphocyte *n.* see LYMPHOCYTE.

Boari flap an operation in which a tube of bladder tissue is constructed to replace the lower third of the ureter when this has been destroyed or damaged or has to be removed because of the presence of a tumour. *See also* URETEROPLASTY. [A. Boari (19th century), Italian surgeon]

Boas's sign excessive sensitivity in the region of the wing of the right scapula, associated with *cholecystitis. [I. I. Boas (1858–1938), German gastroenterologist]

body *n.* **1.** an entire animal organism. **2.** the trunk of an individual, excluding the limbs. **3.** the main or largest part of an organ (such as the stomach or uterus). **4.** a solid discrete mass of tissue; e.g. the carotid body. *See also* CORPUS.

body image (body schema) the individual's concept of the disposition of his limbs and the identity of the different parts of his body. It is a function of the *association areas of the brain. *See also* GERSTMANN'S SYNDROME.

body temperature the intensity of heat of the body, as measured by a thermometer. Body temperature is accurately controlled by a small area at the base of the brain (the *hypothalamus); in normal individuals it is maintained at about 37°C (98.4°F). Heat production by the body arises as the result of vital activities (e.g. respiration, heartbeat, circulation, secretion) and from the muscular effort of exercise and shivering. A rise in body temperature occurs in fever.

body type (somatotype) the characteristic anatomical appearance of an individual, based on the predominance of the structures derived from the three germ layers (ectoderm, mesoderm, endoderm). The three types are described as *ectomorphic, *mesomorphic, and *endomorphic.

Boeck's disease *see* SARCOIDOSIS. [C. P. M. Boeck (1845–1913), Norwegian dermatologist]

boil *n.* a tender inflamed area of the skin containing pus. The infection is usually caused by the bacterium *Staphylococcus aureus* entering through a hair follicle or a break in the skin, and local injury or lowered constitutional resistance may encourage the development of boils. Boils usually heal when the pus is released or with antibiotic treatment, though occasionally they may cause more widespread infection. Medical name: **furuncle**.

bolus *n.* a soft mass of chewed food or a pharmaceutical preparation that is ready to be swallowed.

bonding *n.* **1.** (in psychology) the development of a close and selective relationship, such as that of *attachment. **Mother-child bonding** is the supposed process in which physical contact between mother and child in the child's first hours of life promotes the mother's loving and caring for her baby. **2.** (in dentistry) the attachment of dental restorations, sealants, and orthodontic brackets to teeth. Bonding may be mechanical (*see* ACID-ETCH TECHNIQUE) or chemical, by the use of adhesive *cements or resins. Bonding agents are increasingly used to attach dental fillings to dentine as well as to enamel. In certain artificial *crowns porcelain is bonded to a metal substructure to produce a bonded porcelain crown.

bone *n.* the hard extremely dense connective tissue that forms the skeleton of the body. It is composed of a matrix of collagen fibres impregnated with bone salts (chiefly calcium carbonate and calcium phosphate; *see* HYDROXYAPATITE), in which are embedded bone cells (*see* OSTEOCYTE). **Compact** (or **cortical**) **bone** forms the outer shell of bones; it consists of a hard virtually solid mass made up of bony tissue arranged in concentric layers (**Haversian systems**). **Spongy** (or **cancellous**) **bone**, found beneath compact bone, consists of a meshwork of bony bars (**trabeculae**) with many interconnecting spaces containing marrow. (See illustration.)

Individual bones may be classed as long, short, flat, or irregular. The outer layer of a bone is called the *periosteum. The **medullary cavity** is lined with *endosteum and contains the marrow. Bones not only form the skeleton but also act as stores for mineral salts and play an important part in the formation of blood cells.

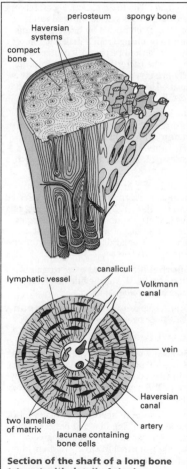

Section of the shaft of a long bone (above) with detail of single Haversian system (below)

Labels (top figure): periosteum, spongy bone, Haversian systems, compact bone

Labels (bottom figure): canaliculi, lymphatic vessel, Volkmann canal, vein, Haversian canal, artery, two lamellae of matrix, lacunae containing bone cells

bone-anchored hearing aid (BAHA) a specialized form of *hearing aid for patients with certain forms of conductive *deafness. A small titanium screw is surgically fixed into the bone of the skull behind the external ear using a process called *osseointegration. Sound energy is passed from a miniature microphone and amplifier to the screw, through the bone, to the *cochlea.

bone graft *see* GRAFT.

bone growth factor any of a group of *growth factors that act to regulate the stages of bone growth and development. An example is **bone morphogenetic protein**, which has been manufactured by genetic engineering techniques and used in trials to stimulate bone formation and fracture healing.

bone marrow (marrow) the tissue contained within the internal cavities of the bones. At birth, these cavities are filled entirely with blood-forming **myeloid tissue (red marrow)** but in later life the marrow in the limb bones is replaced by fat (**yellow marrow**). Samples of bone marrow may be obtained for examination by *aspiration through a stout needle or by *trephine biopsy. *See also* HAEMOPOIESIS.

bony labyrinth *see* LABYRINTH.

BOO bladder outflow obstruction, usually by an enlarged *prostate gland.

BOOP *see* BRONCHIOLITIS OBLITERANS ORGANIZING PNEUMONIA.

borax *n.* a mild astringent with a weak antiseptic action, applied externally to skin and mucous membranes. Borax and boric acid are used in mouth and nasal washes, gargles, eye lotions and contact-lens solutions, and in dusting powder. Side-effects from external application are rare; most reported cases of poisoning are in infants.

borborygmus *n.* (*pl.* **borborygmi**) an abdominal gurgle due to movement of fluid and gas in the intestine. Excessive borborygmi occur when intestinal movement is increased, for example in the *irritable bowel syndrome and in intestinal obstruction, or when there is more intestinal gas than normal.

borderline *adj.* **1.** describing a personality disorder characterized by unstable and intense relationships, exploiting and manipulating other people, rapidly changing moods, recurrent suicidal or self-injuring acts, and a pervasive inner feeling of emptiness and boredom. **2.** *see* SCHIZOTYPAL.

Bordetella *n.* a genus of tiny Gram-negative aerobic bacteria. *B. pertussis* causes *whooping cough, and all the other species are able to break down red blood cells and cause diseases resembling whooping cough.

boric acid *see* BORAX.

borneol *n.* an essential oil used, in preparations with other essential oils, such as menthol, menthone, and camphene, to disperse gallstones and kidney stones. It is administered by mouth. Trade names: **Rowachol**, **Rowatinex**.

Bornholm disease (devil's grip, epidemic myalgia, epidemic pleurodynia) a disease caused by *Coxsackie viruses, named after the Danish island where the first documented cases occurred. It is spread by contact and epidemics usually occur during warm weather in temperate regions and at any time in the tropics. Symptoms include fever, headache, and attacks of severe pain in the lower chest. The illness lasts about a week and is rarely fatal. There is no specific treatment.

Borrelia *n.* a genus of large parasitic *spirochaete bacteria. The species *B. duttonii*, *B. persica*, and *B. recurrentis* cause *relapsing fever in Africa, Asia, North America, and Europe. The species *B. burghdorferi* causes *Lyme disease.

bottom shuffling a normal variant of crawling in which babies sit upright and move on their bottoms, usually by pulling forward on their heels. Babies who bottom-shuffle tend to walk slightly later. There is often a family history of bottom shuffling.

botulinum toxin a powerful nerve toxin, produced by the bacterium *Clostridium botulinum*, that has proved effective, in minute dosage, for the treatment of various conditions of muscle overaction, such as strabismus (squint) and various dystonic conditions (*see* DYSTONIA), including spasm of the orbicularis muscle

in patients with *blepharospasm; it is administered by injection. It is also used to treat *achalasia, being injected through an endoscope into the gastro-oesophageal sphincter, and for relieving the spastic paralysis associated with cerebral palsy. Side-effects include prolonged local muscle paralysis. Trade names: **Botox**, **Dysport**.

botulism *n.* a serious form of *food poisoning from foods containing the toxin produced by the bacterium *Clostridium botulinum*. The toxin selectively affects the central nervous system; in fatal cases, death is often caused by heart and lung failure resulting from a malfunction of the cardiac and respiratory centres of the brain. The bacterium thrives in improperly preserved foods, typically canned raw meats. The toxin, being rather unstable to heat, is invariably destroyed in cooking.

Bouchard's node a bony thickening arising at the proximal interphalangeal joint of a finger in osteoarthritis. It is often found together with *Heberden's nodes. [J. C. Bouchard (1837–1915), French physician]

bougie *n.* a hollow or solid cylindrical instrument, usually flexible, that is inserted into tubular passages, such as the oesophagus (gullet), rectum, or urethra. Bougies are used in diagnosis and treatment, particularly by enlarging *strictures (for example, in the urethra).

Bourneville's disease *see* TUBEROUS SCLEROSIS. [D.-M. Bourneville (1840–1909), French neurologist]

bovine spongiform encephalopathy (BSE) *see* SPONGIFORM ENCEPHALOPATHY.

bowel *n.* *see* INTESTINE.

Bowen's disease a type of carcinoma of the squamous epidermal cells of the skin that does not spread to the basal layers. [J. T. Bowen (1857–1941), US dermatologist]

bow-legs *pl. n.* abnormal out-curving of the legs, resulting in a gap between the knees on standing. A certain degree of bowing is normal in small children, but persistence into adult life, or later development of this deformity, results from abnormal growth of the *epiphysis or arthritis. The condition can be corrected by *osteotomy. Medical name: **genu varum**.

Bowman's capsule the cup-shaped end of a *nephron, which encloses a knot of blood capillaries (**glomerulus**). It is the site of primary filtration of the blood into the kidney tubule. [Sir W. P. Bowman (1816–92), British physician]

BPH benign prostatic hypertrophy. *See* PROSTATE GLAND.

brachi- (brachio-) *prefix denoting* the arm. Example: **brachialgia** (pain in).

brachial *adj.* relating to or affecting the arm.

brachial artery an artery that extends from the axillary artery, at the armpit, down the side and inner surface of the upper arm to the elbow, where it divides into the radial and ulnar arteries.

brachialis *n.* a muscle that is situated at the front of the upper arm and contracts to flex the forearm (see illustration). It works against the triceps brachii.

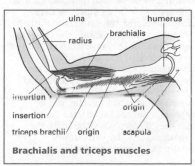

Brachialis and triceps muscles

brachial plexus a network of nerves, arising from the spine at the base of the neck, from which arise the nerves supplying the arm, forearm and hand, and parts of the shoulder girdle (see illustration). *See also* RADIAL NERVE.

brachiocephalic artery *see* INNOMINATE ARTERY.

brachium *n.* (*pl.* **brachia**) the arm, especially the part of the arm between the shoulder and the elbow.

brachy- *prefix denoting* shortness.

Example: **brachydactylia** (shortness of the fingers or toes).

brachycephaly *n.* shortness of the skull, with a *cephalic index of about 80. —**brachycephalic** *adj.*

brachytherapy *n.* radiotherapy administered by implanting radioactive wires or grains into or close to a tumour. This technique is used in the treatment of many accessible tumours (e.g. breast cancer).

bracket *n.* (in dentistry) the component of a fixed *orthodontic appliance that is bonded to the tooth.

brady- *prefix denoting* slowness. Example: **bradylalia** (abnormally slow speech).

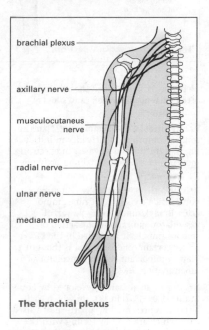

The brachial plexus

bradycardia *n.* slowing of the heart rate to less than 50 beats per minute. **Sinus bradycardia** is often found in healthy individuals, especially athletes, but it is also seen in some patients with reduced thyroid activity, jaundice, hypothermia, or *vasovagal attacks. Bradycardia may also result from *arrhythmias, especially com-

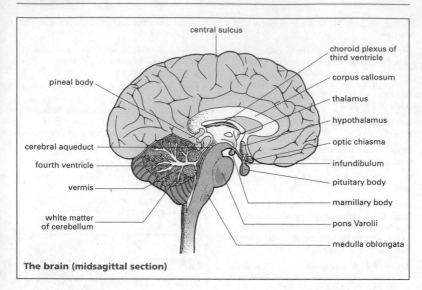

central sulcus

choroid plexus of
third ventricle

corpus callosum

thalamus

hypothalamus

optic chiasma

infundibulum

pituitary body

mamillary body

pons Varolii

medulla oblongata

pineal body

cerebral aqueduct

fourth ventricle

vermis

white matter
of cerebellum

The brain (midsagittal section)

plete *heart block, when the slowing is often extreme and often causes loss of consciousness.

bradykinesia *n.* a symptom of *parkinsonism comprising a difficulty in initiating movements and slowness in executing movements and in maintaining body posture.

bradykinin *n.* a naturally occurring polypeptide consisting of nine amino acids. Bradykinin is a very powerful vasodilator and causes contraction of smooth muscle; it is formed in the blood under certain conditions and is thought to play an important role as a mediator of inflammation. *See* KININ.

braille *n.* an alphabet, developed by Louis Braille (1809–1852) in 1837, in which each letter is represented by a pattern of raised dots, which are read by feeling with the finger tips. It is the main method of reading used by the blind today.

brain *n.* the enlarged and highly developed mass of nervous tissue that forms the upper end of the *central nervous system (see illustration). The average adult human brain weighs about 1400 g (approximately 2% of total body weight) and is

continuous below with the spinal cord. It is invested by three connective tissue membranes, the *meninges, and floats in *cerebrospinal fluid within the rigid casing formed by the bones of the skull. The brain is divided into the hindbrain (rhombencephalon), consisting of the *medulla oblongata, *pons Varolii, and *cerebellum; the *midbrain (mesencephalon); and the forebrain (prosencephalon), subdivided into the *cerebrum and the *diencephalon (including the *thalamus and *hypothalamus). Anatomical name: **encephalon**.

brain death *see* DEATH.

brainstem *n.* the enlarged extension upwards within the skull of the spinal cord, consisting of the medulla oblongata, the pons, and the midbrain. The pons and medulla are together known as the **bulb**, or **bulbar area**. Attached to the midbrain are the two cerebral hemispheres. *See* BRAIN.

brain tumour *see* CEREBRAL TUMOUR.

branchial arch *see* PHARYNGEAL ARCH.

branchial cleft *see* PHARYNGEAL CLEFT.

branchial cyst a cyst that arises at the

site of one of the embryonic *pharyngeal pouches due to a developmental anomaly.

branchial pouch *see* PHARYNGEAL POUCH.

Brandt Andrews method a technique for expelling the placenta from the uterus. Upward pressure is applied to the uterus through the abdominal wall while holding the umbilical cord taut. When the uterus is elevated in this way, the placenta will be in the cervix or upper vagina and is then expelled by applying pressure below the base of the uterus. [T. Brandt (1819–95), Swedish obstetrician; H. R. Andrews (1872–1942), British gynaecologist]

breakbone fever *see* DENGUE.

breast *n.* **1.** the mammary gland of a woman: one of two compound glands that produce milk. Each breast consists of glandular lobules – the milk-secreting areas – embedded in fatty tissue (see illustration). The milk passes from the lobules into ducts, which join up to form 15–20 **lactiferous ducts**. Near the front of the breast the lactiferous ducts are dilated into **ampullae**, which act as reservoirs for the milk. Each lactiferous duct discharges through a separate orifice in the nipple. The dark area around the nipple is called the **areola**. *See also* LACTATION. Anatomical name: **mamma**. **2.** the front part of the chest (thorax).

breastbone *n. see* STERNUM.

breast cancer a malignant tumour of the breast, usually a *carcinoma, rarely a *sarcoma. It is unusual in men but is the commonest form of cancer in women, in some cases involving both breasts. Despite extensive research the cause is not yet known, but it would appear to have a familial link.

The classic sign is a lump in the breast, which is often noticed after minor local injury; bleeding or discharge from the nipple may occur infrequently. Sometimes the first thing to be noticed is a lump in the armpit, which is due to spread of the cancer to the drainage lymph nodes. The tumour may also spread to the bones, lungs, and liver. Current treatment of a localized tumour is usually by surgery (*see* LUMPECTOMY, MASTECTOMY), with or without radiotherapy; cytotoxic drugs and hormone therapy are used as *adjuvant ther-

apy and for widespread (metastatic) disease. *Tamoxifen is the hormonal treatment of choice for breast cancer in postmenopausal women with metastatic disease; it is also increasingly used as a first-line treatment for premenopausal women.

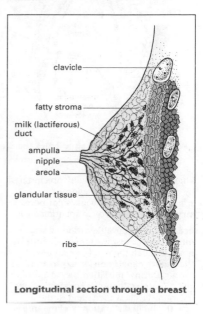

Longitudinal section through a breast

breast implant a prosthesis to replace breast tissue that has been removed surgically during a simple *mastectomy in the treatment of breast cancer. The type of implant in current use is a silicone sac filled with silicone gel; it has recently been found that coating the sac with polyurethane to give a textured surface reduces the incidence of fibrosis around the implant and consequent hardening of breast tissue. Alternatively, an implant with a soya-oil filling may be used. The implant is inserted subcutaneously at the time of operation (the skin and nipple are retained), and follow-up radiotherapy is not normally required. Implants are also used to augment existing breast tissue.

breath-holding attacks episodes in which a child (usually aged between one and five) cries, holds its breath, and goes

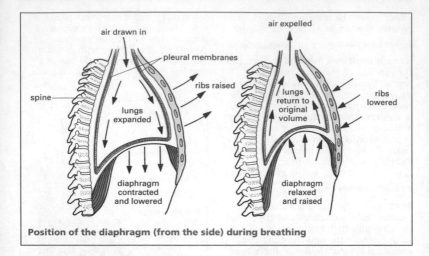

air drawn in

pleural membranes

ribs raised

spine

lungs expanded

air expelled

lungs return to original volume

ribs lowered

diaphragm contracted and lowered

diaphragm relaxed and raised

Position of the diaphragm (from the side) during breathing

blue. Such attacks are usually precipitated by temper and may cause loss of consciousness. Drug treatment is not necessary and the attacks cease spontaneously.

breathing n. the alternation of active **inhalation** (or **inspiration**) of air into the lungs through the mouth or nose with the passive **exhalation** (or **expiration**) of the air. During inhalation the *diaphragm and *intercostal muscles contract, which enlarges the chest cavity and draws air into the lungs. Relaxation of these muscles forces air out of the lungs at exhalation. (See illustration.) Breathing is part of *respiration and is sometimes called external respiration. There are many types of breathing in which the rhythm, rate, or character is abnormal. See also APNOEA, BRONCHOSPASM, CHEYNE-STOKES RESPIRATION, DYSPNOEA, STRIDOR.

breathlessness n. see DYSPNOEA.

breath sounds the sounds heard through a stethoscope placed over the lungs during breathing. Normal breath sounds are soft and called **vesicular** – they may be increased or decreased in disease states. The sounds heard over the larger bronchi are louder and harsher. Breath sounds transmitted through consolidated lungs in pneumonia are louder and harsher; they are similar to the sounds heard normally over the larger

bronchi and are termed **bronchial breath sounds**. *Crepitations and *rhonchi are sounds added to the breath sounds in abnormal states of the lung. **Amphoric** or **cavernous** sounds have a hollow quality and are heard over cavities in the lung; the amphoric quality may also be heard in voice sounds and on percussion.

breech presentation the position of a baby in the uterus such that it will be delivered buttocks first (instead of the normal head-first position). This type of delivery increases the risk of damage to the baby. See also CEPHALIC VERSION, LØVSET'S MANOEUVRE.

bregma n. the point on the top of the skull at which the coronal and sagittal *sutures meet. In a young infant this is an opening, the anterior *fontanelle.

Breslow's measurement (or thickness) the distance (in millimetres) between the surface and the deepest extent of a malignant *melanoma. The measurement correlates with prognosis; tumours that are less than 0.76 mm thick have a good prognosis. [A. Breslow (1928–80), US pathologist]

bretylium tosylate a drug used in patients with cardiac arrest to reverse ventricular *fibrillation that has failed to respond to electrical *defibrillation. It is administered by intravenous injection. Trade name: **Bretylate**.

bridge *n.* (in dentistry) a fixed replacement for missing teeth. The artificial tooth is attached to one or more natural teeth, usually by a crown. Bridges may also be fitted on dental *implants. The supporting teeth (or implants) are referred to as **abutments**, and the artificial teeth that fit over them are referred to as **retainers**. The replacements of missing teeth are known as **pontics**. **Adhesive bridges** are attached to one or more adjacent teeth by a metal plate that adheres to the enamel on the tooth surface prepared by the *acid-etch technique; these bridges require minimal tooth preparation compared with conventional types of bridges.

Bright's disease *see* NEPHRITIS. [R. Bright (1789–1858), British physician]

Briquet's syndrome *see* SOMATIZATION DISORDER. [P. Briquet (1796–1881), French psychiatrist]

British Anti-Lewisite (BAL) *see* DIMERCAPROL.

British thermal unit a unit of heat equal to the quantity of heat required to raise the temperature of 1 pound of water by 1° Fahrenheit. 1 British thermal unit = 1055 joules. Abbrev.: Btu.

Broca's area the area of cerebral motor cortex responsible for the initiation of speech. It is situated in the left frontal lobe in most (but not all) right-handed people, in the region of *Brodmann areas 44 and 45. [P. P. Broca (1824–80), French surgeon]

Brodie's abscess a chronic abscess of bone that develops from acute bacterial *osteomyelitis. Treatment is by surgical drainage and antibiotics. [Sir B. C. Brodie (1783–1862), British surgeon]

Brodmann areas the numbered areas (1–47) into which a map of the *cerebral cortex may conveniently be divided for descriptive purposes, based upon the arrangement of neurones seen in stained sections under the microscope. On the map area 4, for example, corresponds to primary motor cortex, while the primary visual cortex comes into area 17. [K.

Brodmann (1868–1918), German neurologist]

bromazepam *n.* a long-acting *benzodiazepine drug used in the short-term treatment of disabling anxiety. It is administered by mouth. Trade name: **Loxetan**.

bromism *n.* a group of symptoms caused by excessive intake of bromides, formerly widely used as sedatives. Overuse for long periods leads to mental dullness, weakness, drowsiness, loss of sensation, slurred speech, and sometimes coma. A form of acne may also develop.

bromocriptine *n.* a drug, derived from ergot, that has effects similar to those of *dopamine. It is used in the treatment of *parkinsonism and to prevent lactation by inhibiting the secretion of the hormone *prolactin by the pituitary gland. It is also used to treat *acromegaly as it suppresses the release of growth hormone. The drug is administered by mouth. Fairly common side-effects are dizziness and confusion. Trade name: **Parlodel**.

brompheniramine *n.* an *antihistamine given by mouth to relieve the symptoms of allergic reactions, especially hay fever and rhinitis. Common side-effects include drowsiness, dizziness, dryness of the throat, and digestive upsets. Trade name: **Dimotane**.

Brompton cocktail a mixture of alcohol, morphine, and cocaine sometimes given to control severe pain in terminally ill people, especially those dying of cancer. The mixture was first tried at the Brompton Hospital, London, and has given relief to thousands.

bromsulphthalein *n.* a blue dye used in tests of liver function. A small quantity of the dye is injected into the bloodstream, and its concentration in the blood is measured after 5 and then 45 minutes. The presence of more than 10% of the dose in the circulation after 45 minutes indicates that the liver is not functioning normally.

bronch- (broncho-) *prefix denoting* the bronchial tree. Examples: **bronchoalveolar** (relating to the bronchi and alveoli); **bronchopulmonary** (relating to the bronchi and lungs).

bronchial carcinoma cancer of the bronchus, one the commonest causes of death in smokers. *See also* LUNG CANCER, OAT CELL.

bronchial tree a branching system of tubes conducting air from the trachea (windpipe) to the lungs: includes the bronchi (*see* BRONCHUS) and their subdivisions and the *bronchioles.

bronchiectasis *n.* widening of the bronchi or their branches. It may be congenital or it may result from infection (especially whooping cough or measles in childhood) or from obstruction, either by an inhaled foreign body or by a growth (including cancer). Pus may form in the widened bronchus so that the patient coughs up purulent sputum, which may contain blood. Diagnosis is on the clinical symptoms and by X-ray and CT scan. Treatment consists of antibiotic drugs to control the infection and physiotherapy to drain the sputum. Surgery may be used if only a few segments of the bronchi are affected.

bronchiole *n.* a subdivision of the bronchial tree that does not contain cartilage or mucous glands in its wall. Bronchioles open from the fifth or sixth generation of bronchi and extend for up to 20 more generations before reaching the **terminal bronchioles**. Each terminal bronchiole divides into a number of **respiratory bronchioles**, from which the *alveoli open. Each terminal bronchiole conducts air to an acinus in the *lung. —**bronchiolar** *adj.*

bronchiolitis *n.* inflammation of the small airways in the lungs (the *bronchioles) due to viral infection, usually the *respiratory syncytial virus. Bronchiolitis occurs in epidemics and is commonest in infants of less than one year. The bronchioles become swollen, the lining cells die, and the tubes become blocked with debris and mucopus. This prevents air reaching the alveoli and the child becomes short of oxygen (hypoxic) and breathless. In mild cases no treatment is necessary; more severe cases require treatment – administration of oxygen and supportive feeding via a nasogastric tube. Antibiotics are indicated only if there is evidence of a secondary infection. If the child is particularly vulnerable, specific treatment with *ribavirin may be beneficial. Recurrent attacks of bronchiolitis may herald the onset of *asthma.

bronchiolitis obliterans organizing pneumonia (BOOP) a disease entity characterized clinically by a flulike illness with cough, fever, shortness of breath, and late inspiratory crackles; there are specific histological features and patchy infiltrates on X-ray. It is sometimes the result of a viral infection, but may follow medication with certain drugs or be associated with connective-tissue disease, such as rheumatoid arthritis. The condition usually responds to oral corticosteroids; however, if a drug is implicated, it must be withdrawn.

bronchitis *n.* inflammation of the bronchi (*see* BRONCHUS). **Acute bronchitis** is caused by viruses or bacteria and is characterized by coughing, the production of mucopurulent sputum, and narrowing of the bronchi due to spasmodic contraction (*see* BRONCHOSPASM). In **chronic bronchitis** the patient coughs up excessive mucus secreted by enlarged bronchial mucous glands; the bronchospasm cannot always be relieved by bronchodilator drugs. It is not primarily an inflammatory condition, although it is frequently complicated by acute infections. The disease is particularly prevalent in Britain in association with cigarette smoking, air pollution, and *emphysema.

bronchoalveolar lavage (BAL) a method of obtaining cellular material from the lungs that is used particularly in the investigation and monitoring of interstitial lung disease and in the investigation of pulmonary infiltrates in immunosuppressed patients. Examination of the cells in the lavage fluid may help to identify the cause of interstitial lung disease. The combination of cytological and microbiological examination can lead to a very high rate of diagnostic accuracy in such conditions as *Pneumocystis carinii* pneumonia.

bronchoconstrictor *n.* a drug that causes narrowing of the air passages by producing spasm of bronchial smooth muscle.

bronchodilator *n.* an agent that causes

widening of the air passages by relaxing bronchial smooth muscle.

*Sympathomimetic drugs that stimulate beta-receptors, such as *isoprenaline, *salbutamol, and *terbutaline, are potent bronchodilators and are used for relief of bronchial asthma and chronic bronchitis. These drugs are often administered as aerosols, giving rapid relief, but at high doses they may stimulate the heart.

bronchography *n.* X-ray examination of the bronchial tree after it has been made visible by the injection of *radiopaque dye or contrast medium. It was used particularly in the diagnosis of *bronchiectasis, but has now been largely superseded by CT scanning.

bronchophony *n. see* VOCAL RESONANCE.

bronchopneumonia *n. see* PNEUMONIA.

bronchopulmonary dysplasia a chronic lung disease of newborn babies, particularly low birth-weight infants, usually caused by trauma resulting from artificial ventilation of the lungs with oxygen under pressure. It often occurs after recovery from the *respiratory distress syndrome. Treatment is with ventilator support and supplemental oxygen. Long-term diuretic therapy is necessary to prevent pulmonary congestion. Recovery is slow, generally taking several months.

bronchoscope *n.* an instrument used to look into the trachea and bronchi. In addition to the rigid tubular metal type, used for many years, there is now a narrower flexible *fibreoptic instrument with which previously inaccessible bronchi can be inspected. With either instrument the bronchial tree can be washed out (*see* BRONCHOALVEOLAR LAVAGE) and samples of tissue and foreign bodies can be removed with long forceps. —**bronchoscopy** *n.*

bronchospasm *n.* narrowing of bronchi by muscular contraction in response to some stimulus, as in *asthma and *bronchitis. The patient can usually inhale air into the lungs, but exhalation may require visible muscular effort and is accompanied by expiratory noises that are clearly audible (*see* WHEEZE) or detectable with a stethoscope. The condition in which bronchospasm can usually be relieved by bron-

chodilator drugs is known as **reversible obstructive airways disease** and includes asthma; that in which bronchodilator drugs usually have no effect is **irreversible obstructive airways disease** and includes chronic bronchitis.

bronchus *n.* (*pl.* **bronchi**) any of the air passages beyond the *trachea (windpipe) that has cartilage and mucous glands in its wall (see illustration). The trachea divides into two main bronchi, which divide successively into five **lobar bronchi**, 20 **segmental bronchi**, and two or three more divisions. *See also* BRONCHIOLE. —**bronchial** *adj.*

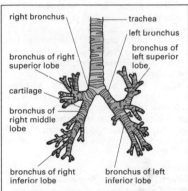

The **bronchi and their principal (lobar) branches**

brown fat a form of fat in adipose tissue that is a rich source of energy and can be converted rapidly to heat. There is speculation that a rapid turnover of brown fat occurs to balance excessive intake of food and unnecessary production of white fat (making up the bulk of adipose tissue). Some forms of obesity may be linked to lack of – or inability to synthesize – brown fat.

Brown-Séquard syndrome the neurological condition resulting when the spinal cord has been partly cut through. In those parts of the body supplied by the damaged segment there is a flaccid weakness and loss of feeling in the skin. Below the lesion there is a spastic paralysis on the same side and a loss of pain and temperature sensation on the opposite side. [C. E. Brown-Séquard (1818–94), French physiologist]

Brucella *n.* a genus of Gram-negative aerobic spherical or rodlike parasitic bacteria responsible for *brucellosis (undulant fever) in humans and contagious abortion in cattle, pigs, sheep, and goats. The principal species are *B. abortus* and *B. melitensis*. **Brucella ring test** is a diagnostic test for brucellosis involving the clumping together of a standard *Brucella* strain by antibodies in an infected person's serum.

brucellosis (Malta fever, Mediterranean fever, undulant fever) *n.* a chronic disease of farm animals caused by bacteria of the genus *Brucella*, which can be transmitted to humans either by contact with an infected animal or by drinking nonpasteurized contaminated milk. Symptoms include headache, fever, aches and pains, sickness, loss of appetite, and weakness; occasionally a chronic form develops, with recurrent symptoms. Untreated the disease may last for years but prolonged administration of tetracycline antibiotics or streptomycin is effective.

Bruch's membrane the transparent innermost layer of the *choroid, which is in contact with the retinal pigment epithelium (*see* RETINA). [K. W. L. Bruch (1819–84), German anatomist]

Brufen *n.* *see* IBUPROFEN.

Brugia *n.* a genus of threadlike parasitic worms (*see* FILARIA). *B. malayi* infects man throughout southeast Asia, causing *filariasis and *elephantiasis (especially of the feet and legs). *B. pahangi*, a parasite of wild cats and domestic animals, produces an allergic condition in humans, with coughing, breathing difficulty, and an increase in the number of *eosinophils in the blood. *Brugia* undergoes part of its development in mosquitoes of the genera *Anopheles* and *Mansonia*, which transmit the parasite from host to host.

bruise (contusion) *n.* an area of skin discoloration caused by the escape of blood from ruptured underlying vessels following injury. Initially red or pink, a bruise gradually becomes bluish, and then greenish yellow, as the haemoglobin in the tissues breaks down chemically and is absorbed. It may be necessary to draw off blood from very severe bruises through a needle, to aid healing.

bruit *n.* *see* MURMUR.

Brunner's glands compound glands of the small intestine, found in the *duodenum and the upper part of the jejunum. They are embedded in the submucosa and secrete mucus. [J. C. Brunner (1856–1927), Swiss anatomist]

brush border *see* MICROVILLUS.

Brushfield spots greyish-brown spots seen in the iris of the eye. They can be found in normal individuals but are usually associated with *Down's syndrome. [T. Brushfield (1858–1937), British physician]

bruxism *n.* a habit in which an individual grinds his teeth, which may lead to excessive wear. This usually occurs during sleep.

B-scan examination of the tissues of the eye in cross section by means of a high-frequency ultrasound machine. It is useful in the diagnosis of eye disease, especially in the posterior segment of the eye when direct viewing is obscured (e.g. by dense cataracts). *See also* A-SCAN.

BSE bovine *spongiform encephalopathy. *See also* CREUTZFELDT-JAKOB DISEASE.

BSS *see* BALANCED SALT SOLUTION.

bubo *n.* a swollen inflamed lymph node in the armpit or groin, commonly developing in some sexually transmitted diseases (e.g. soft sore), bubonic plague, and leishmaniasis.

bubonic plague *see* PLAGUE.

buccal *adj.* **1.** relating to the mouth or the hollow part of the cheek. **2.** describing the surface of a tooth adjacent to the cheek.

buccal cavity the cavity of the mouth, which contains the tongue and teeth and leads to the pharynx. Here food is tasted, chewed, and mixed with saliva, which begins the process of digestion.

buccal glands small glands in the mucous membrane lining the mouth. They secrete material that mixes with saliva.

buccinator *n.* a muscle of the cheek that has its origin in the maxilla and mandible (jaw bones). It is responsible for compressing the cheek and is important in mastication.

buclizine *n.* an *antihistamine with marked sedative properties. Given by mouth, it is used (combined with codeine and paracetamol in **Migraleve**) to treat migraine and is also used to relieve mild anxiety states and tension. Side-effects include drowsiness, dizziness, dryness of the throat, and gastrointestinal upsets. Occasionally it may cause teratogenic effects.

Budd-Chiari syndrome a rare condition that follows obstruction of the hepatic vein by a blood clot or tumour. It is characterized by ascites and cirrhosis of the liver. [G. Budd (1808–82), British physician; H. Chiari (1851–1916), German pathologist]

budesonide *n.* a *corticosteroid drug used in a nasal spray to treat hay fever or as an inhalant for asthma. It is also administered as a cream or ointment for the treatment of eczema, psoriasis, and similar conditions. Trade names: **Pulmicort**, **Preferid**.

Buerger's disease an inflammatory condition of the arteries, especially in the legs, that predominantly affects young male cigarette smokers. Intermittent *claudication (pain due to reduced blood supply) and gangrene of the limbs may develop. Coronary thrombosis may occur and venous thrombosis is common. The treatment is similar to that of *atheroma but cessation of smoking is essential to prevent progression of the disease. Medical name: **thromboangiitis obliterans**. [L. Buerger (1879–1943), US physician]

bufexamac *n.* an anti-inflammatory drug (*see* NSAID) administered externally in the form of a cream for the treatment of skin inflammation and to relieve itching.

buffer *n.* a solution whose hydrogen ion concentration (pH) remains virtually unchanged by dilution or by the addition of acid or alkali. The chief buffer of the blood and extracellular body fluids is the

bicarbonate (H_2CO_3/HCO_3^-) system. *See also* ACID-BASE BALANCE.

bulb *n.* (in anatomy) any rounded structure or a rounded expansion at the end of an organ or part.

bulbar *adj.* **1.** relating to or affecting the medulla oblongata. **2.** relating to a bulb. **3.** relating to the eyeball.

bulbourethral glands *see* COWPER'S GLANDS.

bulimia *n.* insatiable overeating. This symptom may be psychogenic, occurring, for example, as a phase of *anorexia nervosa (**bulimia nervosa** or the **binge–purge syndrome**); or it may be due to neurological causes, such as a lesion of the *hypothalamus.

bulla *n.* (*pl.* **bullae**) **1.** a large blister, containing serous fluid. **2.** (in anatomy) a rounded bony prominence. **3.** a thin-walled air-filled space within the lung, arising congenitally or in *emphysema. It may cause trouble by rupturing into the pleural space (*see* PNEUMOTHORAX), by adding to the air that does not contribute to gas exchange, and/or by compressing the surrounding lung and making it inefficient. —**bullous** *adj.*

bullous keratopathy a pathological condition of the cornea of the eye due to failure in the functioning of its endothelium. It results in corneal oedema, seen as small blisters in the cornea that cause blurring of vision. *See* FUCHS' ENDOTHELIAL DYSTROPHY.

bullous pemphigoid *see* PEMPHIGOID.

bull's-eye maculopathy *see* MACULOPATHY.

bumetanide *n.* a quick-acting *diuretic used to relieve the fluid retention (oedema) occurring in heart failure, kidney disease, and cirrhosis of the liver. It is administered by mouth or by injection. A possible side-effect is dizziness. Trade name: **Burinex**.

bundle *n.* a group of muscle or nerve fibres situated close together and running in the same direction; e.g. the *atrioventricular bundle.

bundle branch block a defect in the specialized conducting tissue of the heart (*see* ARRHYTHMIA) that is recognized as an electrocardiographic abnormality. Left or right bundle branch blocks, affecting the respective ventricles, may be seen. Occasionally both left and right bundle branch blocks occur simultaneously and the patient develops complete *heart block. The causes are similar to those of complete heart block.

bundle of His *see* ATRIOVENTRICULAR BUNDLE. [W. His (1863–1934), Swiss anatomist]

bunion *n.* a swelling of the joint between the great toe and the first metatarsal bone. A *bursa often develops over the site and the great toe becomes displaced towards the others (hallux valgus). Bunions are usually caused by ill-fitting shoes and may require surgical treatment.

buphthalmos (hydrophthalmos) *n.* infantile or congenital glaucoma: increased pressure within the eye due to a defect in the development of the tissues through which fluid drains from the eye. Since the outer coat (sclera) of the eyeball of children is distensible, the eye enlarges as the inflow of fluid continues. It usually affects both eyes and may accompany congenital abnormalities in other parts of the body. Treatment is by surgical operation, e.g. *goniotomy, to improve drainage of fluid from the eye. Spontaneous arrest of buphthalmos may occur before vision is completely lost.

bupivacaine *n.* a potent local anaesthetic, used mainly for regional *nerve block. It is significantly longer acting than many other local anaesthetics. It has been used in childbirth, but may cause slowing of the baby's heart, with a risk of death. Trade name: **Marcain.**

buprenorphine *n.* a powerful synthetic *opiate painkilling drug; it acts for 6–8 hours and is administered by mouth. Side-effects include drowsiness, nausea, dizziness, and sweating. Trade name: **Temgesic.**

bur *n.* **1.** a cutting drill that fits in a dentist's handpiece. It may be made from hardened steel, stainless steel, or tungsten carbide or be coated with diamond particles. Burs are mainly used for cutting cavities in teeth. **2.** (**burr**) a surgical drill for cutting through bone.

bur hole a circular hole drilled through the skull to release intracranial tension (due to blood, pus, or cerebrospinal fluid) or to facilitate such procedures as needle aspiration or biopsy.

Burkitt's lymphoma (Burkitt's tumour) a malignant tumour of the lymphatic system, most commonly affecting children and largely confined to tropical Africa in a zone 15° north and south of the equator. It is the most rapidly growing malignancy, with a tumour doubling time of about five days. It can arise at various sites, most commonly the facial structures, such as the jaw, and in the abdomen. The *Epstein-Barr virus plays a role in the origin and growth of the tumour. Complications affecting the nervous system occur in up to 50% of cases. Non-African Burkitt's lymphoma is increasingly being recognized. All forms are very sensitive to cytotoxic drug therapy but cure is uncommon. [D. P. Burkitt (1911–93), Irish surgeon]

burn *n.* tissue damage caused by such agents as heat, chemicals, electricity, sunlight, or nuclear radiation. A **first-degree burn** affects only the outer layer (epidermis) of the skin. In a **second-degree burn** both the epidermis and the underlying dermis are damaged. A **third-degree burn** involves damage or destruction of the skin to its full depth and damage to the tissues beneath. Burns cause swelling and blistering, due to loss of plasma from damaged blood vessels. In serious burns, affecting 15% or more of the body surface in adults (10% or more in children), this loss of plasma results in severe *shock and requires immediate transfusion of blood or saline solution. Burns may also lead to bacterial infection, which can be prevented by administration of antibiotics. Third-degree burns may require skin grafting.

burr *n.* *see* BUR.

bursa *n.* (*pl.* **bursae**) a small sac of fibrous tissue that is lined with *synovial membrane and filled with fluid (synovia). Bursae occur where parts move over one another; they help to reduce friction. They are normally formed round joints and in places where ligaments and tendons pass over bones. However, they may be formed in other places in response to unusual pressure or friction.

bursitis *n.* inflammation of a *bursa, resulting from injury, infection, or rheumatoid *synovitis. It produces pain and tenderness and sometimes restricts movement at a nearby joint; for example, at the shoulder. Treatment of bursitis not due to infection is by rest and corticosteroid injection. *See also* HOUSEMAID'S KNEE.

buserelin *n.* an *LHRH analogue that is administered as a nasal spray for the treatment of endometriosis and to help in the management of advanced cancer of the prostate gland. Possible side-effects include hot flushes, headache, emotional upset, and loss of libido. Trade names: **Suprecur, Suprefact**.

buspirone *n.* a *tranquillizer used to relieve the symptoms of anxiety. It is administered by mouth; common side-effects are headache, nausea, dizziness, and nervousness. Trade name: **Buspar**.

busulphan *n.* a drug that destroys cancer cells by acting on the bone marrow. It is administered by mouth, mainly in the treatment of chronic myeloid leukaemia.

It may cause blood disorders producing bleeding. Trade name: **Myleran**.

butobarbitone (butobarbital) *n.* an intermediate-acting *barbiturate, used for the treatment of insomnia and for sedation. It produces sleep within 30 minutes when given by mouth and its sedative effect lasts for about six hours. Prolonged administration may lead to *dependence and its use with alcohol should be avoided; overdosage has serious effects (*see* BARBITURISM). Trade name: **Soneryl**.

butriptyline *n.* a tricyclic *antidepressant drug administered by mouth. Possible side-effects include difficulty in urination.

butyrophenone *n.* one of a group of chemically related *antipsychotic drugs that includes *haloperidol, *droperidol, and *benperidol. Butyrophenones inhibit the effects of *dopamine by occupying dopamine receptor sites in the body.

byssinosis *n.* an industrial disease of the lungs caused by inhalation of dusts of cotton, flax, hemp, or sisal. The patient characteristically has chest tightness and *wheeze after the weekend break, which wears off during the working week. The causal agent has not been identified.

C

CABG coronary artery bypass graft. *See* CORONARY BYPASS GRAFT.

cac- (caco-) *prefix denoting* disease or deformity. Example: **cacosmia** (unpleasant odour).

cachet *n.* a flat capsule containing a drug that has an unpleasant taste. The cachet is swallowed intact by the patient.

cachexia *n.* a condition of abnormally low weight, weakness, and general bodily decline associated with chronic disease. It occurs in such conditions as cancer, pulmonary tuberculosis, and malaria.

cacosmia *n.* a disorder of the sense of smell in which scents that are inoffensive to most people are objectionable to the sufferer or in which a bad smell seems to be perpetually present. The disorder is usually due to damage to pathways within the brain rather than in the nose or olfactory nerve.

cadmium *n.* a silvery metallic element that can cause serious lung irritation if the fumes of the molten metal are inhaled. Long-term exposure may also cause kidney damage. Symbol: Cd.

caecostomy *n.* an operation in which the caecum is brought through the abdominal wall and opened in order to drain or decompress the intestine, usually when the colon is obstructed or injured.

caecum *n.* a blind-ended pouch at the junction of the small and large intestines, situated below the *ileocaecal valve. The upper end is continuous with the colon and the lower end bears the vermiform appendix. *See* ALIMENTARY CANAL.

caeruloplasmin *n.* a copper-containing protein present in blood plasma. Congenital deficiency of caeruloplasmin leads to abnormalities of the brain and liver (*see* WILSON'S DISEASE).

Caesarean section a surgical operation for delivering a baby through the abdominal wall. The operation most commonly performed is **lower uterine segment**

Caesarean section (LUSCS), carried out through an incision (usually transverse) in the lower segment of the uterus. **Classical Caesarean section**, in which the upper segment of the uterus is incised vertically, is now rarely performed. In addition to its use in cases of obstructed labour, *malpresentation (breech, brow, and shoulder), and in severe *antepartum haemorrhage, Caesarean section is being performed increasingly when the baby is at risk and is exhibiting signs of distress. Because of improved techniques in perinatal care, particularly of the preterm baby, the operation may be performed, if necessary, as soon as the child is viable.

caesium-137 *n.* an artificial radioactive isotope of the metallic element caesium. The radiation given off by caesium-137 is employed in the technique of *radiotherapy. Symbol: ^{137}Cs. *See also* TELECURIETHERAPY.

café au lait spots well-defined pale-brown patches on the skin. They are present in up to 20% of the normal population, but the presence of six or more in an individual is strongly suggestive of *neurofibromatosis.

caffeine *n.* an alkaloid drug, obtained from coffee and tea, that has a stimulant action, particularly on the central nervous system. It is used to promote wakefulness and increase mental activity; it also possesses diuretic properties and will help relieve certain forms of headache. It is often administered with aspirin or codeine in analgesic preparations.

Caffey's disease *see* HYPEROSTOSIS. [J. Caffey (1895–1966), US paediatrician]

caisson disease *see* COMPRESSED AIR ILLNESS.

calamine *n.* a preparation of zinc carbonate used as a mild astringent on the skin in the form of a lotion, cream, or ointment.

calc- (calci-, calco-) *prefix denoting* calcium or calcium salts. •

calcaneus (heel bone) n. the large bone in the *tarsus of the foot that forms the projection of the heel behind the foot. It articulates with the cuboid bone in front and with the talus above.

calcar n. a spurlike projection. The **calcar avis** is the projection in the medial wall of the lateral ventricle of the brain.

calcicosis n. *pneumoconiosis in marble cutters. The term is not in current use.

calciferol n. see VITAMIN D.

calcification n. the deposition of calcium salts in tissue. This occurs as part of the normal process of bone formation (see OSSIFICATION).

calcinosis n. the abnormal deposition of calcium salts in the tissues. This may occur only in the fat layer beneath the skin or it may be more widespread.

calcipotriol n. a vitamin D analogue administered as an ointment, cream, or scalp lotion for the treatment of psoriasis. Possible side-effects include skin irritation and facial dermatitis. Trade name: **Dovonex**.

calcitonin (thyrocalcitonin) n. a hormone, produced by *C cells in the thyroid gland, that lowers the levels of calcium and phosphate in the blood. Calcitonin is given by injection to treat hypercalcaemia and Paget's disease of the bone. Compare PARATHYROID HORMONE.

calcium n. a metallic element essential for the normal development and functioning of the body. Calcium is an important constituent of bones and teeth: the matrix of *bone, consisting principally of calcium phosphate, accounts for about 99% of the body's calcium. It is present in the blood at a concentration of about 10 mg/100 ml, being maintained at this level by hormones (see CALCITONIN, PARATHYROID HOR MONE). It is essential for many metabolic processes, including nerve function, muscle contraction, and blood clotting.

The normal dietary requirement of calcium is about 1 g per day: dairy products (milk and cheese) are the principal sources. Its uptake by the body is facilitated by *vitamin D; a deficiency of this vitamin may therefore result in such conditions as *rickets, *osteoporosis, and *osteomalacia.

A deficiency of calcium in the blood may lead to *tetany. Excess calcium may be deposited in the body as *calculi (stones), especially in the gall bladder and kidney. Symbol: Ca.

calcium antagonist a drug that inhibits the influx of calcium ions into cardiac and smooth-muscle cells; it therefore reduces the strength of heart-muscle contraction, reduces conduction of impulses in the heart, and causes vasodilatation. Calcium antagonists include *amlodipine, *diltiazem, *nicardepine, *nifedipine, and *verapamil, which are used to treat angina and high blood pressure.

calculosis n. the presence of multiple calculi (stones) in the body. See CALCULUS.

calculus n. (pl. **calculi**) **1.** a stone: a hard pebble-like mass formed within the body, particularly in the gall bladder (see GALL-STONE) or anywhere in the urinary tract (see CYSTOLITHIASIS, NEPHROLITHIASIS, STAGHORN CALCULUS). Calculi in the urinary tract are commonly composed of calcium oxalate and are usually visible on X-ray examination. Most of these stones cause pain, whether sited in the kidney, ureter, or bladder; stones passing down a duct (such as the ureter) cause severe colicky pain. Such stones are usually removed surgically, either by crushing (see LITHOLA-PAXY) or by *lithotripsy to prevent or cure urinary obstruction and infection. Calculi may also occur in the ducts of the salivary glands. **2.** a calcified deposit that forms on the surfaces of teeth. **Supragingival calculus** forms above the *gingivae (gums), principally in relation to the openings of the salivary gland ducts. **Subgingival calculus** forms beneath the crest of the gingivae. Calculus hinders the cleaning of teeth and its presence contributes to *gingivitis and *periodontal disease.

calibrator n. **1.** an instrument used for measuring the size of a tube or opening. **2.** an instrument used for dilating a tubular part, such as the gullet.

caliectasis (hydrocalycosis) n. dilatation or distension of the calyces of the kidney, which is mainly associated with *hydronephrosis and usually demonstrated by ultrasound or IVP (see INTRA-VENOUS PYELOGRAM).

calliper (caliper) n. **1.** an instrument with two prongs or jaws, used for measuring diameters: used particularly in obstetrics for measuring the diameter of the pelvis. **2.** (also called **calliper splint**) a surgical appliance (see ORTHOSIS) that is used to correct or control deformity of a joint in the leg. It consists of a metal bar that is fixed to the shoe and held to the leg by means of straps.

callosity (callus) n. a hard thick area of skin occurring in parts of the body subject to pressure or friction. The soles of the feet and palms of the hands are common sites, and if much hard dead skin develops a callosity can become painful. A *corn is a type of callosity.

callotasis n. the process of stretching the callus that forms between the ends of a bone that has been divided. It is achieved by means of an external fixator attached to the bone in the procedure for *limb lengthening. The elongated callus consolidates to form new bone.

callus n. **1.** the tissue formed between bone ends when a fracture is healing. It initially consists of bloodclot and *granulation tissue, which develops into cartilage and then calcifies to form bone. Callus formation is an essential part of the process of healthy union in a fractured bone. **2.** see CALLOSITY.

calor n. heat: one of the classical signs of inflammation in a tissue, the other three being *rubor (redness), *dolor (pain), and *tumor (swelling). An inflamed region has a higher temperature than normal because of the distended blood vessels, which allow an increased flow of blood.

calorie n. a unit of heat equal to the amount of heat required to raise the temperature of 1 gram of water from 14.5°C to 15.5°C (the 15° calorie). One Calorie (also known as the **kilocalorie** or **kilogram calorie**) is equal to 1000 calories; this unit is used to indicate the energy value of foods. Except in this context, the calorie has largely been replaced by the *joule (1 calorie = 4.1855 joules).

calorimeter n. any apparatus used to measure the heat lost or gained during various chemical and physical changes. For example, calorimeters may be used to determine the total energy values of different foods in terms of calories. —**calorimetry** n.

calvaria n. the vault of the *skull.

calyx n. (pl. **calyces**) a cup-shaped part, especially any of the divisions of the pelvis of the *kidney. Each calyx receives urine from the urine-collecting tubes in one sector of the kidney.

Campbell de Morgan spots see ANGIOMA. [C. G. de Morgan (1811–76), British physician]

camphor n. a crystalline substance obtained from the tree *Cinnamomum camphora* that has been used to treat flatulence. It is used in the form of **camphorated oil** (camphor in cottonseed oil) in liniments as a counterirritant.

campimetry n. a method of assessing the central part of the *visual field. The patient fixes his gaze with one eye at a target in the centre of a black screen two metres away. A small object on the end of a black rod is moved onto the screen and the patient tells the examiner when he sees it. This is repeated many times from different directions until a map is built up of the area in front of the eye in which such an object can be seen. Campimetry allows examination only of that part of the field of vision within 30° in all directions from the centre.

camptodactyly n. congenital forward bending of a finger, most commonly the little finger. It often affects both hands and is first noticed at the age of about ten; no treatment is needed.

Campylobacter n. a genus of spiral motile Gram-negative bacteria. Species of *Campylobacter* are a common cause of food poisoning, producing headache, nausea, diarrhoea, and vomiting lasting for 3–5 days. See also HELICOBACTER.

canal n. a tubular channel or passage; e.g. the *alimentary canal and the auditory canal of the ear.

canaliculitis n. inflammation of a canaliculus, especially a lacrimal canaliculus (see LACRIMAL APPARATUS).

canaliculus n. (pl. **canaliculi**) a small channel or canal. Canaliculi occur, for example, in compact bone, linking lacunae containing bone cells. **Bile canaliculi** are minute channels within the liver that transport bile to the bile duct. **Lacrimal canaliculi** drain tears into the lacrimal sac (*see* LACRIMAL APPARATUS).

cancellous *adj.* lattice-like: applied to the bony tissue laid down by *osteoblasts during development of *bone and in the *consolidation stage of fracture repair. In a mature bone cancellous bone has a low density and is surrounded by denser cortical bone.

cancer *n.* any *malignant tumour, including *carcinoma and *sarcoma. It arises from the abnormal and uncontrolled division of cells that then invade and destroy the surrounding tissues. Spread of cancer cells (*metastasis) may occur via the bloodstream or the lymphatic channels or across body cavities such as the pleural and peritoneal spaces, thus setting up secondary tumours at sites distant from the original tumour. Each individual primary tumour has its own pattern of local behaviour and metastasis; for example, bone metastasis is very common in breast cancer and in cancer of the ovary, but less common in other tumours.

There are probably many causative factors, some of which are known; for example, cigarette smoking is associated with lung cancer, radiation with some bone sarcomas and leukaemia, and several viruses are known to cause tumours (*see* ONCOGENIC). A genetic element is implicated in the development of many cancers. In more than half of all cancers a gene called *p53* is deleted or impaired: its normal function is to prevent the uncontrolled division of cells (*see* TUMOUR NECROSIS FACTOR).

Treatment of cancer depends on the type of tumour, the site of the primary tumour, and the extent of spread.

cancer phobia a personality disorder of the phobic type leading to compulsively performed rituals, especially repeated hand-washing, changing of clothes that have been touched by others, avoidance of air breathed by others, and even avoidance of any contact with other persons. Minor symptoms are interpreted as signs of cancer and panic attacks may occur. As with any other phobic disorder, cancer phobia cannot be treated by appeals to reason. Some success has been achieved by various forms of *behaviour therapy.

cancrum oris ulceration of the lips and mouth. *See also* NOMA.

candela *n.* the *SI unit of luminous intensity, equal to the intensity in a given direction of a source that emits monochromatic radiation of frequency 540×10^{12} Hz and has a radiant intensity in that direction of 1/683 watt per steradian. Symbol: cd.

Candida *n.* a genus of *yeasts (formerly called *Monilia*) that inhabit the vagina and alimentary tract and can – under certain conditions – cause *candidosis. The species *C. albicans*, a small oval budding fungus, is primarily responsible for candidosis.

candidosis (candidiasis) *n.* a common *yeast infection of moist areas of the body, usually caused by *Candida albicans*. It is especially common in the vagina, where it is known as **thrush**, but is also found in the mouth and skin folds. On the skin the lesions are bright red with small satellite pustules, while in the mouth candidosis appears as white patches on the tongue or inside the cheeks. In the vagina it produces itching and sometimes a thick white discharge. Candidosis may develop in patients receiving broad-spectrum antibiotics as well as in those who are *immunocompromised. Topical, intravaginal, or oral therapy with *imidazoles is effective; oral *nystatin helps to reduce candidal infection of the bowel.

canine *n.* the third tooth from the midline of each jaw. There are thus four canines, two in each jaw, in both the permanent and primary (deciduous) *dentitions. It is known colloquially as the **eye tooth**.

canities *n.* loss of pigment in the hair, which causes greying or whitening. It is usually part of the ageing process, when it starts at the temples. White patches may occur as a result of *alopecia areata or *vitiligo.

cannabis *n.* a drug prepared from the Indian hemp plant (*Cannabis sativa*), also known as **pot**, **marijuana**, **hashish**, and **bhang**. Smoked or swallowed, it produces euphoria and hallucinations and affects perception and awareness, particularly of time. Cannabis has little therapeutic value and its nonmedical use is illegal: there is evidence that prolonged use may cause brain damage and lead the user onto 'hard' drugs, such as heroin. *See also* DEPENDENCE.

cannula *n.* a hollow tube designed for insertion into a body cavity, such as the bladder, or a blood vessel. The tube contains a sharp pointed solid core (**trocar**), which facilitates its insertion and is withdrawn when the cannula is in place.

cantharidin *n.* the active principle of **cantharides**, or **Spanish fly** (the dried bodies of a blister beetle, *Lytta vesicatoria*). A toxic and irritant chemical, cantharidin causes blistering of the skin and was formerly used in veterinary medicine as a counterirritant and vesicant. If swallowed it causes nausea, vomiting, and inflammation of the urinary tract, the latter giving rise to its reputation as an aphrodisiac. It is very dangerous and may cause death.

cantholysis *n.* a surgical procedure to divide the attachment of the *canthus (corner of the eye) from its underlying bone and tendon. It is performed as part of some operations on the eyelid.

canthoplasty *n.* a surgical procedure to reconstruct the *canthus (corner of the eye).

canthus *n.* either corner of the eye; the angle at which the upper and lower eyelids meet. —**canthal** *adj.*

cap *n.* a covering or a cover-like part. The **duodenal cap** is the superior part of the duodenum as seen on X-ray after a barium meal.

CAPD chronic ambulatory peritoneal dialysis: a method of treating renal failure on an out-patient basis. *See* HAEMODIALYSIS.

Capgras' syndrome (illusion of doubles) the delusion that a person closely involved with the patient has been replaced by an identical-looking impostor. It is often, but not necessarily, a form of paranoid *schizophrenia. [J. M. J. Capgras (1873–1950), French psychiatrist]

capillary *n.* an extremely narrow blood vessel, approximately 5–20 μm in diameter. Capillaries form networks in most

tissues; they are supplied with blood by arterioles and drained by venules. The vessel wall is only one cell thick, which enables exchange of oxygen, carbon dioxide, water, salts, etc., between the blood and the tissues (see illustrations).

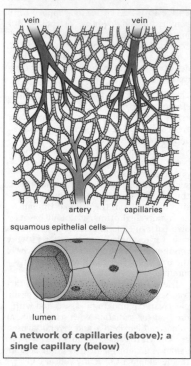

A network of capillaries (above); a single capillary (below)

capitate *adj.* head-shaped; having a rounded extremity.

capitate bone the largest bone of the wrist (*see* CARPUS). It articulates with the scaphoid and lunate bones behind, with the second, third, and fourth metacarpal bones in front, and with the trapezoid and hamate laterally.

capitellum *n. see* CAPITULUM.

capitulum *n.* the small rounded end of a bone that articulates with another bone. For example, the **capitulum humeri** (or **capitellum**) is the round prominence at the elbow end of the humerus that articulates with the radius.

capping *n.* (in dentistry) **1.** a colloquial term for crowning: the technique of fitting a tooth with an artificial *crown. **2.** *see* PULP CAPPING.

capreomycin *n.* an antibiotic, derived from the bacterium *Streptomyces capreolus*, that is used in the treatment of tuberculosis. It is given with other antituberculosis drugs to reduce the development of resistance by the infective bacteria. Capreomycin is poorly absorbed from the gastrointestinal tract and therefore must be administered by intramuscular injection. The more serious side-effects include ear and kidney damage. Trade name: **Capastat**.

capsule *n.* **1.** a membrane, sheath, or other structure that encloses a tissue or organ. For example, the kidney, adrenal gland, and lens of the eye are enclosed within capsules. A **joint capsule** is the fibrous tissue, including the synovial membrane, that surrounds a freely movable joint. **2.** a soluble case, usually made of gelatin, in which certain drugs are administered. **3.** the slimy substance that forms a protective layer around certain bacteria, hindering their ingestion by phagocytes. It is usually made of *polysaccharide.

capsulitis *n.* inflammation of the capsule surrounding a joint.

capsulorrhexis *n.* a surgical procedure in which a continuous circular tear is made in the lens capsule of the eye. In **anterior capsulorrhexis**, performed during cataract surgery, the tear is made in the anterior surface of the capsule. It has the advantage over a *capsulotomy in making the residual capsule much more resilient to being torn during surgery.

capsulotomy *n.* an incision into the capsule of the lens. In modern operations for cataract the lens capsule is not removed and tends, after months or years, to become opaque. Before the advent of laser surgery a tiny knife (**cystitome**) was inserted into the eye and a hole cut in the centre of the capsule, thus providing a clear path for light rays to reach the retina. Currently this procedure is routinely performed with a *YAG laser at an out-patient clinic.

captopril *n.* a drug used in the treatment of heart failure and hypertension; it acts by inhibiting the action of angiotensin (*see* ACE INHIBITOR). Side-effects include rash, *neutropenia or *agranulocytosis, hypotension, and loss of taste. Trade names: **Acepril, Capoten**.

caput succedaneum a temporary swelling of the soft parts of the head of a newly born infant that occurs during birth, due to compression by the muscles of the cervix (neck) of the uterus.

carbachol *n.* a *parasympathomimetic drug that is used after surgical operations to restore the function of inactive bowels or bladder. It is also (but now infrequently) used as a treatment for glaucoma. Side-effects may include sweating, nausea, and faintness.

carbamazepine *n.* an *anticonvulsant drug used in the treatment of epilepsy and to relieve the pain of trigeminal neuralgia. Common side-effects include drowsiness, dizziness, and muscular incoordination; abnormalities of liver and bone marrow may occur with long-term treatment. Trade name: **Tegretol**.

carbaryl *n.* a drug administered in the form of a lotion or shampoo to kill head and pubic lice. Trade names: **Carylderm, Clinicide**.

carbenicillin *n.* a synthetic penicillin: an antibiotic that is effective against a wide range of bacterial infections. It is poorly absorbed from the gastrointestinal tract and must be given by intramuscular injection. Allergic reactions are common side-effects. Trade name: **Pyopen**.

carbenoxolone *n.* a drug that reduces inflammation, used mainly to promote healing in the treatment of gastric ulcers or ulcers of the mouth. It is given by mouth; side-effects include the retention of salt and water (*see* OEDEMA), weight gain, and raised blood pressure. Trade names: **Bioplex, Bioral**.

carbimazole *n.* a drug used to reduce the production of thyroid hormone in cases of overactivity of the gland (thyrotoxicosis). It is administered by mouth; some allergic reactions may occur and high dosage may cause enlargement of the thyroid gland, which may obstruct the windpipe. Trade name: **Neo-Mercazole**.

carbohydrate *n.* any one of a large group of compounds, including the *sugars and *starch, that contain carbon, hydrogen, and oxygen and have the general formula $C_x(H_2O)_y$. Carbohydrates are important as a source of energy: they are manufactured by plants and obtained by animals and man from the diet, being one of the three main constituents of food (*see also* FAT, PROTEIN). All carbohydrates are eventually broken down in the body to the simple sugar *glucose, which can then take part in energy-producing metabolic processes. Excess carbohydrate, not immediately required by the body, is stored in the liver and muscles in the form of *glycogen. In plants carbohydrates are important structural materials (e.g. cellulose) and storage products (commonly in the form of starch). *See also* DISACCHARIDE, MONOSACCHARIDE, POLYSACCHARIDE.

carbol fuchsin a red stain for bacteria and fungi, consisting of carbolic acid and *fuchsin dissolved in alcohol and water.

carbolic acid *see* PHENOL.

carbon dioxide a colourless gas formed in the tissues during metabolism and carried in the blood to the lungs, where it is exhaled (an increase in the concentration of this gas in the blood stimulates respiration). Carbon dioxide occurs in small amounts in the atmosphere; it is used by plants in the process of *photosynthesis. It forms a solid (dry ice) at $-75°C$ (at atmospheric pressure) and in this form is used as a refrigerant. Formula: CO_2.

carbon monoxide a colourless almost odourless gas that is very poisonous. When breathed in it combines with haemoglobin in the red blood cells to form *carboxyhaemoglobin, which is bright red in colour. This compound is chemically stable and thus the haemoglobin can no longer combine with oxygen. Carbon monoxide is present in coal gas and motor exhaust fumes. Formula: CO.

carbon tetrachloride a pungent volatile fluid used as a dry-cleaner. When inhaled or swallowed it may severely damage the heart, liver, and kidneys, causing cirrhosis and nephrosis, and it can also affect the optic nerve and other nerves. Treatment is by administration of oxygen. Formula: CCl_4.

carboplatin *n.* a derivative of platinum that is used in the treatment of certain types of cancer. It is similar to *cisplatin but has fewer side-effects.

carboxyhaemoglobin *n.* a substance formed when carbon monoxide combines with the pigment *haemoglobin in the blood. Carboxyhaemoglobin is incapable of transporting oxygen to the tissues and this is the cause of death in carbon monoxide poisoning. Large quantities of carboxyhaemoglobin are formed in carbon monoxide poisoning, and low levels are always present in the blood of smokers and city dwellers.

carboxylase *n.* an enzyme that catalyses the addition of carbon dioxide to a substance.

carbuncle *n.* a collection of *boils with multiple drainage channels. The infection is usually caused by *Staphylococcus aureus* and may result in an extensive slough of skin. Treatment is with antibiotics and sometimes also by surgery.

carcin- (carcino-) *prefix denoting* cancer or carcinoma. Example: **carcinogenesis** (development of).

carcino-embryonic antigen (CEA) a protein produced in the fetus but not in normal adult life. It may be produced by carcinomas, particularly of the colon, and is a rather insensitive marker of malignancy. It is an example of an *oncofetal antigen that is used as a *tumour marker.

carcinogen *n.* any substance that, when exposed to living tissue, may cause the production of cancer. Known carcinogens include ionizing radiation and many chemicals, e.g. those found in cigarette smoke and those produced in certain industries. They cause damage to the DNA of cells that may persist if the cell divides before the damage is repaired. Damaged cells may subsequently develop into a cancer (*see* CARCINOGENESIS). An inherent susceptibility to cancer is probably necessary for a carcinogen to promote the development of cancer. *See also* ONCOGENIC. —**carcinogenic** *adj.*

carcinogenesis n. the evolution of an invasive cancer cell from a normal cell. Intermediate stages, sometimes called **premalignant, preinvasive**, or **noninvasive** may be recognizable.

carcinoid n. see ARGENTAFFINOMA.

carcinoma n. *cancer that arises in epithelium, the tissue that lines the skin and internal organs of the body. It may occur in any tissue containing epithelial cells. In many cases the site of origin of the tumour may be identified by the nature of the cells it contains. Organs may exhibit more than one type of carcinoma; for example, an adenocarcinoma and a squamous carcinoma may be found in the cervix (but not usually concurrently). Treatment depends on the nature of the primary tumour, different types responding to different drug combinations. —**carcinomatous** adj.

carcinoma in situ (CIS) the earliest stage of cancer spread, in which the tumour is confined to the epithelium and surgical removal of the growth should lead to cure. See also CERVICAL CANCER, CERVICAL INTRAEPITHELIAL NEOPLASIA.

carcinomatosis n. carcinoma that has spread widely throughout the body. Spread of the cancer cells occurs via the lymphatic channels and bloodstream and across body cavities, for example the peritoneal cavity.

carcinosarcoma n. a malignant tumour of the cervix, uterus, or vagina containing a mixture of *adenocarcinoma, sarcoma cells, and stroma. It may be bulky and polypoid, with grapelike fronds (**sarcoma botryoides**). Tissues of mesodermal origin, such as bone, cartilage, or striated muscle, may also be present.

cardi- (cardio-) prefix denoting the heart. Examples: **cardiomegaly** (enlargement of); **cardiopathy** (disease of).

cardia n. **1.** the opening at the upper end of the *stomach that connects with the oesophagus (gullet). **2.** the heart.

cardiac adj. **1.** of, relating to, or affecting the heart. **2.** of or relating to the upper part of the stomach (see CARDIA).

cardiac arrest the cessation of effective pumping action of the heart, which most commonly occurs when the muscle fibres of the ventricles start to beat rapidly without pumping any blood (ventricular *fibrillation) or when the heart stops beating completely (*asystole). There is abrupt loss of consciousness, absence of the pulse, and breathing stops. The most common cause is *myocardial infarction. Unless treated promptly, irreversible brain damage and death follow within minutes. Some patients may be resuscitated by massage of the heart, artificial respiration, and *defibrillation.

cardiac cycle the sequence of events between one heartbeat and the next, normally occupying less than a second. The atria contract simultaneously and force blood into the relaxed ventricles. The ventricles then contract very strongly and pump blood out through the aorta and pulmonary artery. During ventricular contraction, the atria relax and fill up again with blood. See DIASTOLE, SYSTOLE.

cardiac muscle the specialized muscle of which the walls of the *heart are composed. It is composed of a network of branching elongated cells (fibres) whose junctions with neighbouring cells are marked by irregular transverse bands known as **intercalated discs**.

cardiac reflex reflex control of the heart rate. Sensory fibres in the walls of the heart are stimulated when the heart rate increases above normal. Impulses are sent to the cardiac centre in the brain, stimulating the vagus nerve and leading to slowing of the heart rate.

cardinal veins two pairs of veins in the embryo that carry blood from the head (**anterior cardinal veins**) and trunk (**posterior cardinal veins**); they unite to form the **common cardinal vein**, which drains into the sinus venosus of the heart.

cardiology n. the science concerned with the study of the structure, function, and diseases of the heart. See also NUCLEAR CARDIOLOGY. —**cardiologist** n.

cardiomyopathy n. any chronic disorder affecting the muscle of the heart. It may be inherited but can be caused by various conditions, including virus infections, alcoholism, beriberi (vitamin B_1 deficiency), and amyloidosis. The cause is often unknown. It may result in enlargement of the heart, *heart failure, *arrhythmias, and embolism. There is often no specific treatment but patients improve following the control of heart failure and arrhythmias.

cardiomyoplasty n. a recent surgical technique to replace or reinforce damaged cardiac muscle with skeletal muscle.

cardiomyotomy n. see ACHALASIA.

cardioplegia n. a technique in which the heart is stopped by injecting it with a solution of salts, by hypothermia, or by an electrical stimulus. This has enabled complex cardiac surgery and transplants to be performed safely.

cardiopulmonary bypass a method by which the circulation to the body is maintained while the heart is deliberately stopped during heart surgery. The function of the heart and lungs is carried out by a pump-oxygenator (see HEART-LUNG MACHINE) until the natural circulation is restored.

cardiospasm n. see ACHALASIA.

cardiotocograph n. the instrument used in *cardiotocography to produce a **cardiotocogram**, the graphic printout of the measurements obtained.

cardiotocography n. the electronic monitoring of the fetal heart rate and rhythm, either by an external microphone or transducer or by applying an electrode to the fetal scalp, recording the fetal ECG and hence the heart rate. The procedure also includes a measurement of the strength and frequency of uterine contractions by means of an external transducer or an intrauterine catheter.

cardiotomy syndrome (postcardiotomy syndrome) a condition that may develop weeks or months after surgery to the heart and the membrane surrounding it (pericardium) and is characterized by fever and also *pericarditis. Pneumonia and pleurisy may form part of the syndrome. It is thought to be an *autoimmune condition and may be recurrent. A similar syndrome (**Dressler's syndrome**) may follow myocardial infarction. It may respond to anti-inflammatory drugs.

cardiovascular system (circulatory system) the heart together with two networks of blood vessels – the *systemic circulation and the *pulmonary circulation (see illustration). The cardiovascular system effects the circulation of blood around the body, which brings about transport of nutrients and oxygen to the tissues and the removal of waste products.

cardioversion (countershock) n. a method of restoring the normal rhythm of the heart in patients with increased heart rate due to arrhythmia. A controlled direct-current shock, synchronized with the R wave of the electrocardiograph, is given through electrodes placed on the chest wall of the anaesthetized patient. The apparatus is called a **cardiovertor** and is a modified defibrillator (see DEFIBRILLATION).

care assistant a person who assists with the general care of a patient, usually assisting a nurse or social worker with care of the vulnerable elderly in the community. Care assistants include home helps.

caries n. decay and crumbling of the substance of a tooth (see DENTAL CARIES) or a bone. —**carious** adj.

carina n. a keel-like structure, such as the keel-shaped cartilage at the bifurcation of the trachea into the two main bronchi.

cariogenic adj. causing caries, particularly dental caries: refers especially to the sugar in food and drinks.

cariology n. the branch of dentistry concerned with the study of tooth decay (see DENTAL CARIES).

carminative n. a drug that relieves flatulence, used to treat gastric discomfort and colic.

carmustine (BCNU) n. a drug (an *alkylating agent) used in the treatment of certain cancers, including lymphomas and brain tumours.

carneous mole a fleshy mass in the uterus consisting of pieces of placenta and products of conception that have not been expelled after abortion.

carotenaemia n. see XANTHAEMIA.

deoxygenated blood   **oxygenated blood**

veins from upper body

head, upper limbs

arteries to upper body

pulmonary veins

lungs (oxygenation)

aorta

pulmonary artery

veins from lower body

right atrium

left atrium

right ventricle

left ventricle

hepatic artery

liver

spleen, gastrointestinal tract

portal vein

kidneys

trunk, lower limbs

Diagram of the cardiovascular system

carotene *n.* a yellow or orange plant pigment – one of the carotenoids – that occurs in four forms: alpha (α), beta (β), gamma (γ), and delta (δ). The most important form is β-carotene, which is an *antioxidant and can be converted in the body to retinol (vitamin A). Foods containing β-carotene (for example, milk and some vegetables) are therefore a source of the vitamin.

carotenoid *n.* any one of a group of about 100 naturally occurring yellow to red pigments found mostly in plants. The group includes the *carotenes.

carotid artery either of the two main arteries in the neck whose branches supply the head and neck. The **common carotid artery** arises on the left side directly from the aortic arch and on the right from the innominate artery. They ascend the neck on either side as far as the thyroid cartilage (Adam's apple), where they each divide into two branches, the **internal carotid**, supplying the cerebrum, forehead, nose, eye, and middle ear, and the **external carotid**, sending branches to the face, scalp, and neck.

carotid-artery stenosis (carotid

stenosis) narrowing of the carotid artery, which reduces the supply of blood to the brain and is a cause of strokes. Sometimes the condition is due to a tumour of the *carotid body. Many cases can be treated by surgical excision or bypass of the narrowed segment (*see also* ENDARTERECTOMY).

carotid body a small mass of tissue in the carotid sinus containing *chemoreceptors that monitor levels of oxygen, carbon dioxide, and hydrogen ions in the blood. If the oxygen level falls, the chemoreceptors send impulses to the cardiac and respiratory centres in the brain, which promote increases in heart and respiration rates.

carotid sinus a pocket in the wall of the carotid artery, at its division in the neck, containing receptors that monitor blood pressure (*see* BARORECEPTOR). When blood pressure is raised, impulses travel from the receptors to the vasomotor centre in the brain, which initiates a reflex *vasodilatation and slowing of heart rate to lower the blood pressure to normal.

carp- (carpo-) *prefix denoting* the wrist (carpus).

carpal 1. *adj.* relating to the wrist. **2.** *n.* any of the bones forming the carpus.

carpal tunnel the space between the carpal bones of the wrist and the connective tissue (retinaculum) over the flexor tendons. It contains the flexor tendons and the median nerve.

carpal tunnel syndrome a combination of *paraesthesiae (pins and needles), numbness, and pain affecting all of the hand except the little finger. There may be weakness of the thumb. It is caused by pressure on the median nerve as it passes through the wrist (*see* CARPAL TUNNEL). Treatment is by surgical release of the nerve.

carphology (floccillation) *n.* plucking at the bedclothes by a delirious patient. This is often a sign of extreme exhaustion and may be the prelude to death.

carpopedal spasm *see* SPASM.

carpus *n.* the eight bones of the wrist (see illustration). The carpus articulates with the metacarpals distally and with the ulna and radius proximally.

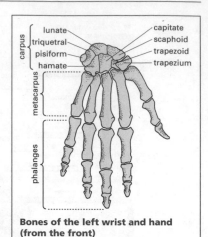

Bones of the left wrist and hand (from the front)

carrier *n.* **1.** a person who harbours the microorganisms causing a particular disease without experiencing signs or symptoms of infection and who can transmit the disease to others. **2.** (in genetics) a person who bears a gene for an abnormal trait without showing any signs of the disorder; the carrier is usually *heterozygous for the gene concerned, which is *recessive. **3.** an animal, usually an insect, that passively transmits infectious organisms from one animal to another or from an infected animal to a human being. *See also* VECTOR.

cartilage *n.* a dense connective tissue composed of a matrix produced by cells called **chondroblasts**, which become embedded in the matrix as **chondrocytes**. It is a semiopaque grey or white substance, consisting chiefly of *chondroitin sulphate, that is capable of withstanding considerable pressure. There are three types: *hyaline cartilage, *elastic cartilage, and *fibrocartilage (see illustration). In the fetus and infant cartilage occurs in many parts of the body, but most of this cartilage disappears during development. In the adult, hyaline cartilage is found in the costal cartilages, larynx, trachea, bronchi, nose, and covering the surface of bones at joints, where wear and damage results in *osteoarthritis. Elastic cartilage occurs in the external ear, and fibrocartilage in the intervertebral discs and tendons. Cartilage is the precursor of bone following a fracture (*see* CALLUS).

fibrocytes
perichondrium
chondrocytes
hyaline
matrix

Hyaline cartilage

chondrocytes

elastic fibres

Elastic cartilage

chondrocytes

collagen fibres

Fibrocartilage

Types of cartilage

caruncle *n.* a small red fleshy swelling. The **lacrimal caruncle** is the red prominence at the inner angle of the eye. **Hymenal caruncles** occur around the mucous membrane lining the vaginal opening.

caseation *n.* the breakdown of diseased tissue into a dry cheeselike mass: a type of degeneration associated with tubercular lesions.

case control study comparison of a group of people who have a disease with another group free from that disease, in terms of *variables in their backgrounds (e.g. cigarette smoking in those who have died from lung cancer and in those dying from other causes). In the more precise **matched pair study** every individual with the disease is paired with a control matched on the basis of (say) age, sex, and/or occupation in order to place greater emphasis on a factor for which the pairs have not been matched. *Compare* COHORT STUDY, CROSS-SECTIONAL STUDY.

case fatality ratio the number of fatalities from a specified disease in a given period per 100 episodes of the disease arising in the same period. Unless all such deaths occur rapidly after the onset of the disease (e.g. cholera) they are likely to be the outcome of episodes that started in an earlier period (hence the term **ratio** rather than **rate**). Comparison of the annual number of admissions and fatalities in a given hospital in respect of a specific disease is known as the **hospital fatality ratio**.

casein *n.* a milk protein. Casein is precipitated out of milk in acid conditions or by the action of rennin: it is the principal protein of cheese. Casein is very easily prepared and is useful as a protein supplement, particularly in the treatment of malnutrition.

case work *see* SOCIAL SERVICES.

cassette *n.* (in radiography) a thin lightproof box in which a piece of X-ray film is placed during the taking of an X-ray. It usually contains special screens that fluoresce under the influence of X-rays and so intensify the image that is formed on the film.

cast *n.* **1.** a rigid casing for a limb or other part of the body, made of plastic or with open-woven bandage impregnated with plaster of Paris and applied while wet. A plaster cast is designed to protect a broken bone and prevent movement of the aligned bone ends until healing has progressed sufficiently. **2.** a mass of dead cellular, fatty, and other material that forms within a body cavity and takes its shape. It may then be released and appear elsewhere. For example, *granular casts appearing in the urine indicate kidney disease.

castor oil *see* LAXATIVE.

castration *n.* removal of the sex glands (the testes or the ovaries). Castration in childhood causes failure of sexual development but when done in adult life (usually as part of hormonal treatment for cancer) it produces less marked physical changes in both sexes. Castration inevitably causes sterility but it need not cause impotence or loss of sexual desire.

CAT computerized axial tomography, now referred to as *computerized tomography (CT).

cata- *prefix denoting* downward or against.

catabolism *n.* the chemical decomposition of complex substances by the body to form simpler ones, accompanied by the release of energy. The substances broken down include nutrients in food (carbohydrates, proteins, etc.) as well as the body's storage products (such as glycogen). *See also* METABOLISM. —**catabolic** *adj.*

catagen *n.* *see* ANAGEN.

catalase *n.* an enzyme, present in many cells (including red blood cells and liver cells), that catalyses the breakdown of hydrogen peroxide.

catalepsy *n.* the abnormal maintenance of postures or physical attitudes, occurring in *catatonia. These may have arisen spontaneously or they may be induced by the examiner.

catalyst *n.* a substance that alters the rate of a chemical reaction but is itself unchanged at the end of the reaction. The catalysts of biochemical reactions are the *enzymes.

cataphoresis *n.* the introduction into the tissues of positively charged ionized substances (cations) by the use of a direct electric current. *See* IONTOPHORESIS.

cataplasia *n.* degeneration of tissues to an earlier developmental form.

cataplexy *n.* a recurrent condition in which the patient suddenly collapses to the ground without loss of consciousness. Laughter or any strong emotion can provoke an attack. It is usually associated with *narcolepsy.

cataract *n.* any opacity in the lens of the eye that results in blurred vision. Cataracts may be congenital or due to metabolic disease (such as *diabetes), direct or indirect injury to the lens, or prolonged exposure of the eye to infrared rays (e.g. **glass-blowers' cataract**) or ionizing radiation, but they are most commonly a result of age (**senile cataract**). A type commonly related to ageing is **nuclear sclerotic cataract**, which results from increasing density and yellowing of the centre of the lens. A **posterior subcapsular cataract**, which develops at the rear surface of the lens within the lens capsule, is also related to ageing but occurs in addition with prolonged use of steroids and chronic ocular inflammation. **Brunescent cataracts** are dark brown and very dense, and a **cortical cataract** is one in which the opacity occurs in the soft outer part (cortex) of the lens. A **Morgagnian cataract** is a longstanding very opaque cataract in which the cortex has started to shrink and liquefy, leaving a central shrunken nucleus. Minor degrees of cataract do not necessarily impair vision seriously.

Cataract is treated by removal of the affected lens (*see* CATARACT EXTRACTION, PHACOEMULSIFICATION); patients may wear a contact lens or appropriate spectacles to compensate for the missing lens but in modern practice a plastic **intraocular lens implant** is routinely placed inside the eye after surgery.

cataract extraction surgical removal of a cataract from the eye. In **extracapsular cataract extraction** the cataract alone is removed, leaving the lens capsule behind to support the remaining lens tissue. **Intracapsular cataract extraction** is the removal of the whole lens, including the capsule that surrounds it.

catarrh *n.* the excessive secretion of thick phlegm or mucus by the mucous membrane of the nose, nasal sinuses, nasopharynx, or air passages. The term is not used in any precise or scientific sense.

catatonia *n.* a state in which a person becomes mute or stuporous or adopts bizarre postures. The features include **flexibilitas cerea**, in which the limbs may be moved passively by another person into positions that are then retained for hours on end. Catatonia was once a noted feature of *schizophrenia but is now hardly ever seen in developed countries. It remains common in Third World countries. —**catatonic** *adj.*

catchment area the geographic area from which a hospital can expect to receive patients and on which in Britain the designated population of the hospital is based. There is no statutory requirement forcing patients to use the hospital(s) of their area, but a code of zoning practice exists for some specialties (e.g. mental illness). A hospital may have a smaller catchment area (e.g. a National Health Service District) for common specialties than for rarer ones, which may be shared between several districts (**regional specialty**) or regions (**supraregional specialty**). *See also* INDEPENDENT CONTACT.

catecholamines *pl. n.* a group of physiologically important substances, including *adrenaline, *noradrenaline, and *dopamine, having various different roles (mainly as *neurotransmitters) in the functioning of the sympathetic and central nervous systems. Chemically all contain a benzene ring with adjacent hydroxyl groups (catechol) and an amine group on a side chain. Catecholamines act at both alpha (α) and beta (β) *adrenergic receptor sites.

catgut *n.* a natural fibrous material prepared from the tissues of animals, usually from the walls of sheep intestines, twisted into strands of different thicknesses and used to sew up wounds (*see* SUTURE) and tie off blood vessels during surgery. The catgut gradually dissolves and is absorbed by the tissues, so that the stitches do not have to be removed later. This also minimizes the possibility of long-term irritation at the site of operation. Some catgut is treated with chromic acid for different periods during manufacture (**chromic catgut**). This gives catguts that last for longer lengths of time before absorption is complete.

catharsis *n.* purging or cleansing out of the bowels by giving the patient a *laxative (cathartic) to stimulate intestinal activity.

cathartic *n. see* LAXATIVE.

cathepsin *n.* one of a group of enzymes found in animal tissues, particularly the spleen, that digest proteins.

catheter *n.* a flexible tube for insertion into a narrow opening so that fluids may be introduced or removed. **Urinary catheters** are passed into the bladder through the urethra to allow drainage of urine in certain disorders and to empty the bladder before abdominal operations.

catheterization *n.* the introduction of a *catheter into a hollow organ. This is most often performed as **urethral catheterization**, when a catheter is introduced into the bladder to relieve obstruction to the outflow of urine (*see also* INTERMITTENT SELF-CATHETIZATION). **Cardiac catheterization** entails the introduction of special catheters into the arteries and veins of the arms or legs through which their tips are manipulated into the various chambers of the heart. Cardiac catheterization provides data on pressures and blood flow within the various chambers of the heart. It permits *angiocardiography. **Arterial catheterization** enables the introduction into the arteries of dyes for radiographic purposes, of drugs to constrict or expand the vessels for treatment purposes, and of insoluble microspheres to block the vessel and arrest haemorrhage or necrose tumours.

cation *n.* an ion of positive charge, such as a sodium ion (Na^+). *Compare* ANION. *See* ELECTROLYTE.

cation-exchange resins complex insoluble chemical compounds that may be administered with the diet to alter the *electrolyte balance of the body in the treatment of heart, kidney, and metabolic disorders. For example, in patients on a strict low-sodium diet such resins combine with sodium in the food so that it cannot be absorbed and passes out in the faeces.

cat-scratch fever an infectious disease, possibly viral in origin, transmitted to man following injury to the skin by a cat scratch, splinter, or thorn. The injury becomes inflamed and mild fever and swelling of the lymph nodes (usually those closest to the wound) develop about a week after infection. In some cases, especially in immunocompromised patients, serious abscess formation occurs, but generally recovery is complete.

cauda n. a tail-like structure. The **cauda equina** is a bundle of nerve roots from the lumbar, sacral, and coccygeal spinal nerves that descend nearly vertically from the spinal cord until they reach their respective openings in the vertebral column.

caudal adj. relating to the lower part or tail end of the body.

caul n. **1.** (in obstetrics) the *amnion, either as a piece of membrane that covers an infant's head at birth, or the entire unruptured sac that encloses the fetus during pregnancy. **2.** (in anatomy) see OMENTUM.

causal agent a factor associated with the definitive onset of an illness (or other response, including an accident). Examples are bacteria and trauma. The relationship is more direct than in the case of a *risk factor, in general the ill health only occurs if the agent is a precursor.

causalgia n. an intensely unpleasant burning pain felt in a limb where there has been partial damage to the sympathetic and somatic sensory nerves.

caustic n. an agent, such as silver nitrate, that destroys tissue. Caustic agents may be used to remove dead skin, warts, etc., but care must be taken not to damage the surrounding area.

caustic soda see SODIUM HYDROXIDE.

cauterize vb. to destroy tissues by direct application of a heated instrument (known as a **cautery**): used for the removal of small warts or other growths.(see also CURETTAGE) and also to stop bleeding from small vessels. —**cautery** n.

Caverject n. see ALPROSTADIL.

cavernitis n. inflammation of the corpora cavernosa of the *penis or the corpus cavernosum of the clitoris.

cavernosography n. a radiological examination of the penis that entails the in-

fusion of a radiopaque contrast material into the corpora cavernosa of the penis via a small butterfly needle. X-rays taken during the infusion give information regarding the veins draining the penis.

cavernosometry n. the measurement of pressure within the corpora cavernosa of the penis during infusion. The flow rate required to produce an erection is recorded and also the flow necessary to maintain the induced erection. The examination is important in the investigation of failure of erection and impotence.

cavernous breathing see BREATH SOUNDS.

cavernous sinus one of the paired cavities within the *sphenoid bone, at the base of the skull behind the eye sockets, into which blood drains from the brain, eye, nose, and upper cheek before leaving the skull through connections with the internal jugular and facial veins. Through the sinus, in its walls, pass the internal carotid artery and the abducens, oculomotor, trochlear, ophthalmic, and maxillary nerves.

cavity n. **1.** (in anatomy) a hollow enclosed area; for example, the abdominal cavity or the buccal cavity (mouth). **2.** (in dentistry) **a.** the hole in a tooth caused by *caries or abrasion. **b.** the hole shaped in a tooth by a dentist to retain a filling.

cavity varnish (in dentistry) a solution of natural or synthetic resin in an organic solvent. It is used as a sealer for amalgam fillings or as a coating over newly inserted cement fillings.

CBW (chemical and biological warfare) the use of poisonous gases and other chemicals, bacteria, viruses, and toxins during war.

CCDC see CONSULTANT IN COMMUNICABLE DISEASE CONTROL.

C cells parafollicular cells of the thyroid gland, which are derived from neural crest tissue. They produce *calcitonin. *Medullary carcinoma of the thyroid has its origin in the C cells.

CCST Certification of Completion of Specialist Training. See CONSULTANT.

CD cluster of differentiation: a numeri-

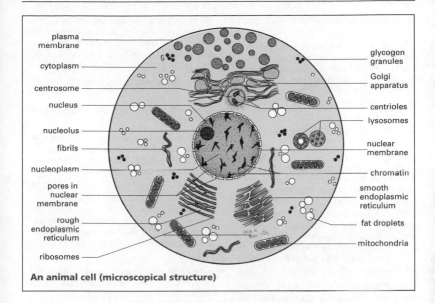

plasma membrane
cytoplasm
centrosome
nucleus
nucleolus
fibrils
nucleoplasm
pores in nuclear membrane
rough endoplasmic reticulum
ribosomes

glycogen granules
Golgi apparatus
centrioles
lysosomes
nuclear membrane
chromatin
smooth endoplasmic reticulum
fat droplets
mitochondria

An animal cell (microscopical structure)

cal system for classifying antigens expressed on the surface of lymphocytes. *See also* CD4.

CD4 a surface antigen on *helper T-cells that is particularly important for immune resistance to viruses; progressive reduction of CD4-bearing T-cells reflects the progression of *AIDS.

CDH *see* CONGENITAL DISLOCATION OF THE HIP.

cefaclor *n.* a *cephalosporin antibiotic used in the treatment of otitis media, upper and lower respiratory-tract infections, urinary-tract infections, and skin infections. It is administered by mouth; side-effects include diarrhoea and skin eruptions. Trade name: **Distaclor**.

cefadroxil *n.* a *cephalosporin antibiotic used in the treatment of urinary-tract infections, skin infections, pharyngitis, and tonsillitis. It is administered by mouth; side-effects include skin rash and generalized itching. Trade name: **Baxan**.

-cele (-coele) *suffix denoting* swelling, hernia, or tumour. Example: **gastrocele** (hernia of the stomach).

cell *n.* the basic unit of all living organisms, which can reproduce itself exactly (*see* MITOSIS). Each cell is bounded by a **cell membrane** of lipids and protein, which controls the passage of substances into and out of the cell. Cells contain *cytoplasm, in which are suspended a *nucleus and other structures (*organelles) specialized to carry out particular activities in the cell (see illustration).

Complex organisms such as man are built up of millions of cells that are specially adapted to carry out particular functions. The process of cell differentiation begins early on in the development of the embryo and cells of a particular type (e.g. blood cells, liver cells) always give rise to cells of the same type. Each cell has a particular number of *chromosomes in its nucleus. The sex cells (sperm and ova) always contain half the number of chromosomes of all the other cells of the body (*see* MEIOSIS); at fertilization a sperm and ovum combine to form a cell with a complete set of chromosomes that will develop into the embryo.

cell body (perikaryon) the enlarged portion of a *neurone (nerve cell), containing the nucleus. It is concerned more with the nutrition of the cell than with propagation of nerve impulses.

cell division reproduction of cells by division first of the chromosomes (karyokinesis) and then of the cytoplasm (cytokinesis). Cell division to produce more body (somatic) cells is by *mitosis; cell division during the formation of gametes is by *meiosis.

cellophane maculopathy see EPIRETINAL MEMBRANE.

cell-surface molecules molecules on the surface of cell membranes that are responsible for most cellular functions directly related to their immediate environment. Many have very precise functions of adhesion (see ADHESION MOLECULES), metabolic exchange, hormone reception, respiration, and immune reactions. Cell-to-cell exchanges involve specialized surface structures (junctions), which form a communicating nexus.

cellulitis n. an infection of the deep dermis of the skin by β-haemolytic streptococci. It is most common on the lower legs and there may be associated *lymphangitis and *lymphadenitis. It is otherwise similar to *erysipelas, but the margins are less clearly defined because the infection is deeper. Penicillin is the antibiotic of choice for treatment.

cellulose n. a carbohydrate consisting of linked glucose units. It is an important constituent of plant cell walls. Cellulose cannot be digested by man and is a component of *dietary fibre (roughage).

Celsius temperature (centigrade temperature) temperature expressed on a scale in which the melting point of ice is assigned a temperature of 0° and the boiling point of water a temperature of 100°. For many medical purposes this scale has superseded the Fahrenheit scale (see FAHRENHEIT TEMPERATURE). The formula for converting from Celsius (C) to Fahrenheit (F) is: $F = 9/5C + 32$. [A. Celsius (1701–44), Swedish astronomer]

cement n. **1.** any of a group of materials used in dentistry either as fillings or as *lutes for crowns. Glass ionomer cements are used for filling, and zinc phosphate, zinc polycarboxylate, and glass ionomer cements are used for luting. Zinc

oxide–eugenol cements are widely used as temporary fillings or as an impression material. **2.** a fast-setting material used to fix prostheses (e.g. artificial hips) in place. **3.** see CEMENTUM.

cementocyte n. a cell found in cementum.

cementoma n. a benign overgrowth of cementum.

cementum (cement) n. a thin layer of hard tissue on the surface of the root of a *tooth. It attaches the fibres of the periodontal membrane to the tooth.

censor n. (in psychology) the mechanism, postulated by Freud, that suppresses or modifies desires that are inappropriate or feared. The censor is usually regarded as being located in the *superego but was also described by Freud as being in the *ego itself.

-centesis suffix denoting puncture or perforation. Example: **amniocentesis** (surgical puncture of the amnion).

centi- prefix denoting one hundredth or a hundred.

centigrade temperature see CELSIUS TEMPERATURE.

centile chart a graph with lines showing average measurements of height, weight, and head circumference compared with age and sex, against which a child's physical development can be assessed. The lines of growth on the graph are called **centiles**, and the number of a centile predicts the percentage of children who are below that measurement for a given age; for example, the 10th centile means that 10% of the age- and sex-matched population will be smaller and 90% will be bigger. A child will normally follow a particular centile, but if growth crosses centiles or lies outside the 97th or 3rd centiles, further investigation may be warranted.

centoxin n. a *monoclonal antibody that neutralizes the effects of bacterial *endotoxins. It is administered by injection in cases of dangerous bacterial infection with overwhelming toxicity.

central nervous system (CNS) the *brain and the *spinal cord, as opposed to the cranial and spinal nerves and the *autonomic nervous system, which together form the **peripheral nervous system**. The CNS is responsible for the *integration of all nervous activities.

central serous chorioretinopathy shallow *retinal detachment in the area of the macula due to leakage through the retinal pigment epithelium (*see* RETINA) into the subretinal space. The cause is unknown. It affects young adult males, causing reduced or distorted vision that usually settles in a few months.

central venous pressure (CVP) the pressure of blood within the right atrium. Measurement of CVP is obtained by *catheterization of the right side of the heart; the catheter is attached to a manometer. CVP measurements are used to estimate circulatory function and blood volume in cases of shock or severe haemorrhage and to monitor blood replacement. In a recumbent patient, with the zero point of the manometer level with the mid-axilla (centre of the armpit), CVP should measure between 5 and 8 cm saline under normal conditions.

centre *n.* (in neurology) a collection of neurones (nerve cells) whose activities control a particular function. The **respiratory** and **cardiovascular centres**, for example, are regions in the lower brainstem that control the movements of respiration and the functioning of the circulatory system, respectively.

centrencephalic *adj.* (in electroencephalography) describing discharges that can be recorded synchronously from all parts of the brain. The source of this activity is in the *reticular formation of the midbrain. **Centrencephalic epilepsy** is associated with a congenital predisposition to seizures.

centri- *prefix denoting* centre. Example: **centrilobular** (in the centre of a lobule (especially of the liver)).

centrifugal *adj.* moving away from a centre, as from the brain to the peripheral tissues.

centrifuge *n.* a device for separating components of different densities in a liquid, using centrifugal force. The liquid is placed in special containers that are spun at high speed around a central axis.

centriole *n.* a small particle found in the cytoplasm of cells, near the nucleus. Centrioles are involved in the formation of the *spindle and aster during cell division. During interphase there are usually two centrioles in the *centrosome; when cell division occurs these separate and move to opposite sides of the nucleus, and the spindle is formed between them.

centripetal *adj.* moving towards a centre, as from the peripheral tissues to the brain.

centromere (kinetochore) *n.* the part of a chromosome that joins the two *chromatids to each other and becomes attached to the spindle during *mitosis and *meiosis. When chromosome division takes place the centromeres split longitudinally.

centrosome (centrosphere) *n.* an area of clear cytoplasm, found next to the nucleus in nondividing cells, that contains the *centrioles.

centrosphere *n.* **1.** an area of clear cytoplasm seen in dividing cells around the poles of the spindle. **2.** *see* CENTROSOME.

centrum *n.* (*pl.* **centra**) the solid rod-shaped central portion of a *vertebra.

cephal- (cephalo-) *prefix denoting* the head. Example: **cephalalgia** (pain in).

cephalad *adj.* towards the head.

cephalexin *n.* a *cephalosporin antibiotic used in the treatment of respiratory-tract and genitourinary-tract infections, bone and skin infections, and otitis media. It is administered by mouth; diarrhoea is the most common side-effect. Trade names: **Ceporex**, **Keflex**.

cephalhaematoma *n.* a swelling on the head caused by a collection of bloody fluid between one or more of the skull bones (usually the *parietal bone) and its covering membrane (periosteum). It is most commonly seen in newborn infants delivered with the aid of forceps or subjected to pressures during passage through the birth canal. No treatment is necessary and the swelling disappears in a few months. If it is extensive, the blood in the fluid may break down, releasing bilirubin into the bloodstream and causing *jaundice. A cephalhaematoma in an older baby or child is evidence of some recent injury to the head; occasionally an unsuspected fracture is revealed on X-ray.

cephalic *adj.* of or relating to the head.

cephalic index a measure of the shape of a skull, commonly used in *craniometry: the ratio of the greatest breadth, multiplied by 100, to the greatest length of the skull. *See also* BRACHYCEPHALY, DOLICHOCEPHALY.

cephalic version a procedure for turning a fetus that is lying in a breech or transverse position so that its head will enter the birth canal first. It may give rise to complications and is therefore only carried out in selected cases.

cephalin *n.* one of a group of *phospholipids that are constituents of cell membranes and are particularly abundant in the brain.

cephalocele *n. see* NEURAL TUBE DEFECTS.

cephalogram *n.* a special standardized X-ray picture that can be used to measure alterations in the growth of skull bones.

cephalometry *n.* the study of facial growth by examination of standardized lateral radiographs of the head. It is used mainly for diagnosis in *orthodontics.

cephalosporin *n.* any one of a group of semisynthetic *beta-lactam antibiotics, derived from the mould *Cephalosporium*, which are effective against a wide range of microorganisms and are therefore used in a variety of infections (*see* CEFACLOR, CEFADROXIL, CEPHALEXIN, CEPHAZOLIN). Cross-sensitivity with penicillin may occur and the principal side-effects are allergic reactions and irritation of the digestive tract.

cephazolin *n.* a semisynthetic antibiotic, given by intramuscular or intravenous injection in the treatment of a number of infections. *See* CEPHALOSPORIN. Trade name: **Kefzol**.

CEPOD Confidential Enquiry into Peri-Operative Deaths: an influential enquiry by the Royal College of Surgeons of England that is used to monitor standards of surgical treatment.

cercaria *n.* (*pl.* **cercariae**) the final larval stage of any parasitic trematode (*see* FLUKE). The cercariae, which have tails but otherwise resemble the adults, are released into water from the snail host in which the parasite undergoes part of its development. Several thousand cercariae may emerge from a single snail in a day.

cerebellar syndrome (Nonne's syndrome) *see* (CEREBELLAR) ATAXIA.

cerebellum *n.* the largest part of the hindbrain, bulging back behind the pons and the medulla oblongata and overhung by the occipital lobes of the cerebrum. Like the cerebrum, it has an outer grey cortex and a core of white matter. Three broad bands of nerve fibres – the inferior, middle, and superior cerebellar peduncles – connect it to the medulla, the pons, and the midbrain respectively. It has two hemispheres, one on each side of the central region (the **vermis**), and its surface is thrown into thin folds called **folia** (see illustration). Within lie four pairs of nuclei.

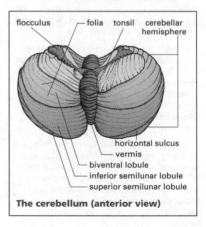

flocculus — folia   tonsil   cerebellar hemisphere

horizontal sulcus
vermis
biventral lobule
inferior semilunar lobule
superior semilunar lobule

The cerebellum (anterior view)

The cerebellum is essential for the maintenance of muscle tone, balance, and the synchronization of activity in groups of muscles under voluntary control, converting muscular contractions into smooth coordinated movement. It does not, however, initiate movement and plays no part in the perception of conscious sensations or in intelligence. —**cerebellar** *adj.*

cerebr- (cerebri-, cerebro-) *prefix denoting* the cerebrum or brain.

cerebral abscess *see* ABSCESS.

cerebral aqueduct (aqueduct of Sylvius) the narrow channel, containing cerebrospinal fluid, that connects the third and fourth *ventricles of the brain.

cerebral cortex the intricately folded outer layer of the *cerebrum, making up some 40% of the brain by weight and composed of an estimated 15 thousand million neurones (*see* GREY MATTER). This is the part of the brain most directly responsible for consciousness, with essential roles in perception, memory, thought, mental ability, and intellect, and it is responsible for initiating voluntary activity. It has connections, direct or indirect, with all parts of the body. The folding of the cortex provides a large surface area, the greater part lying in the clefts (**sulci**), which divide the upraised convolutions (**gyri**). On the basis of its microscopic appearance in section, the cortex is mapped into *Brodmann's areas; it is also divided into functional regions; including *motor cortex, *sensory cortex, and *association areas. Within, and continuous with it, lies the *white matter, through which connection is made with the rest of the nervous system.

cerebral haemorrhage bleeding from a cerebral blood vessel into the tissue of the brain. It is commonly caused by degenerative disease of the arteries and high blood pressure but it may result from bleeding from congenital abnormalities of blood vessels. The extent and severity of the symptoms depend upon the site and volume of the haemorrhage; they vary from a transient weakness or numbness to profound coma and death. *See also* ATHEROMA, HYPERTENSION, STROKE.

cerebral hemisphere one of the two paired halves of the *cerebrum.

cerebral palsy a nonprogressive disorder of movement resulting from damage to the brain before, during, or immediately after birth. It is often associated with other neurological and mental problems. The underlying brain damage is permanent. There are many causes, including birth injury, *hypoxia, *hypoglycaemia,

jaundice, and infection. The most common disability is a *spastic paralysis. Sensation is often affected, leading to a lack of balance, and intelligence, posture, and speech are frequently impaired. Contractures of the limbs may cause fixed abnormalities. Other associated features include epilepsy, visual impairment, squint, reduced hearing, and behavioural problems.

Management of cerebral palsy requires a multidisciplinary approach, the mainstays of which are physiotherapy, speech therapy, and appropriate appliances. Surgery may be necessary to relieve the contractures.

cerebral tumour an abnormal multiplication of brain cells. This forms a swelling that compresses or destroys the healthy brain cells and – because of the rigid nature of the skull – increases the pressure on the brain tissue. Malignant tumours, which include *medulloblastomas and *gliomas, grow rapidly, spreading through the otherwise normal brain tissue and causing progressive neurological disability. Benign tumours, such as *meningiomas, grow slowly and compress the brain tissue. Both benign and malignant tumours commonly cause fits. Benign tumours are often cured by total surgical resection. Malignant tumours may be treated by neurosurgery, chemotherapy, and radiotherapy, but a complete cure is uncommon.

cerebration *n.* **1.** the functioning of the brain as a whole. **2.** the unconscious activities of the brain.

cerebroside *n.* one of a group of compounds occurring in the *myelin sheaths of nerve fibres. They are *glycolipids, containing *sphingosine, a fatty acid, and a sugar, usually galactose (in **galactocerebrosides**) or glucose (in **glucocerebrosides**).

cerebrospinal fever (spotted fever) *see* MENINGITIS.

cerebrospinal fluid (CSF) the clear watery fluid that surrounds the brain and spinal cord. It is contained in the *subarachnoid space and circulates in the *ventricles of the brain and in the central canal of the spinal cord. The brain floats in the fluid (its weight so being reduced from about 1400 g to less than 100 g) and is cushioned by it from contact with the skull when the head is moved vigorously. The CSF is secreted by the *choroid plexuses in the ventricles, circulates through them to reach the subarachnoid space, and is eventually absorbed into the bloodstream through the *arachnoid villi. Its normal contents are glucose, salts, enzymes, and a few white cells, but no red blood cells.

cerebrovascular disease any disorder of the blood vessels of the brain and its covering membranes (meninges). Most cases are due to atheroma and/or hypertension, clinical effects being caused by rupture of diseased blood vessels (*cerebral or *subarachnoid haemorrhage) or inadequacy of the blood supply to the brain (ischaemia), due to cerebral thrombosis or embolism. The term **cerebrovascular accident** is given to the clinical syndrome accompanying a sudden and sometimes severe attack, which leads to a *stroke.

cerebrum (telencephalon) *n.* the largest and most highly developed part of the brain, composed of the two **cerebral hemispheres**, separated from each other by the **longitudinal fissure** in the midline (see illustration). Each hemisphere has an outer layer of grey matter, the *cerebral cortex, below which lies white matter containing the *basal ganglia. Connecting the two hemispheres at the bottom of the longitudinal fissure is the **corpus callosum**, a massive bundle of nerve fibres. Within each hemisphere is a crescent-shaped fluid-filled cavity (lateral *ventricle), connected to the central third ventricle in the *diencephalon. The cerebrum is responsible for the initiation and coordination of all voluntary activity in the body and for governing the functioning of lower parts of the nervous system. The cortex is the seat of all intelligent behaviour. —**cerebral** *adj.*

cerumen (earwax) *n.* the waxy material that is secreted by the sebaceous glands in the external auditory meatus of the outer ear. Its function is to protect the delicate skin that lines the inside of the meatus.

cervic- (cervico-) *prefix denoting* **1.** the neck. Example: **cervicodynia** (pain in). **2.** the cervix, especially of the uterus.

Example: **cervicectomy** (surgical removal of).

cervical *adj.* **1.** of or relating to the neck. **2.** of, relating to, or affecting the cervix (neck region) of an organ, especially the cervix of the uterus.

parieto-occipital fissure
parietal lobe
central sulcus
frontal lobe
lateral sulcus
temporal lobe
occipital lobe

Lobes of the cerebrum (from the right side)

cervical cancer (cervical carcinoma) cancer of the neck (cervix) of the uterus. The tumour may develop from the surface epithelium of the cervix (squamous carcinoma) or from the epithelial lining of the cervical canal (adenocarcinoma). In both cases the tumour is invasive, spreading to involve surrounding tissue and subsequently to neighbouring lymph nodes and adjacent organs, such as the bladder and rectum. In carcinoma in situ (*see* CERVICAL INTRAEPITHELIAL NEOPLASIA) the tumour is confined to the epithelium: there is no invasion of surrounding tissue but, if untreated, it can become malignant. Cancer of the cervix can be detected in an early stage of development (*see* CERVICAL SMEAR). Features of cervical cancer include vaginal discharge, often foul-smelling and usually blood-stained. Treatment is by irradiation or surgery, or a combination of both, and cytotoxic drugs may also be used. *See also* HUMAN PAPILLOMAVIRUS.

cervical cerclage a procedure to help prevent *preterm delivery. It involves placing a stitch around the cervix of the uterus to keep it closed and reduce the possibility of preterm cervical dilatation and rupture of membranes.

cervical fracture a fracture of a vertebra in the neck (see CERVICAL VERTEBRAE). Cervical fractures range from minor, requiring no treatment, to those associated with paralysis and instant death. Treatment can be support with a collar, skull traction, an *orthosis attached to the skull, or surgery, depending on the severity of the fracture.

cervical incompetence unnatural spontaneous dilatation of the cervix of the uterus during the second trimester of pregnancy. The membranes bulge and subsequently rupture, and the fetus is expelled prematurely. It may be caused by forcible dilatation of the cervix during the operation of *dilatation and curettage or it may be related to laceration of the cervix during a previous confinement.

cervical intraepithelial neoplasia (CIN) cellular changes in the cervix of the uterus preceding the invasive stages of *cervical cancer. The CIN grading system distinguishes three stages: **CIN 1** (mild dysplasia); **CIN 2** (moderate dysplasia); and **CIN 3** (severe dysplasia, *carcinoma in situ). CIN is uncommon after the menopause. Treatment may be by *laser beam, which destroys the tissue, or by large loop excision of the *transformation zone of the cervix, a procedure performed through a colposcope, under local anaesthetic, using diathermy.

cervical smear (Papanicolaou (Pap) test) a specimen of cellular material scraped from the neck (cervix) of the uterus that is stained and examined under a microscope in order to detect cell changes indicating the presence of cancer. The *transformation zone of the cervix is most likely to produce evidence of *cervical intraepithelial neoplasia if present. Routine cervical smears are taken to detect precancerous and early cancerous changes.

cervical vertebrae the seven bones making up the neck region of the *backbone. The first cervical vertebra – the

atlas – consists basically of a ring of bone that supports the skull by articulating with the occipital condyles (see OCCIPITAL BONE). The second vertebra – the **axis** – has an upward-pointing process (the **odontoid process** or **dens**) that forms a pivot on which the atlas can rotate, enabling the head to be turned. See also VERTEBRA.

cervicitis n. inflammation of the neck (cervix) of the uterus.

cervix n. a necklike part, especially the **cervix uteri** (neck of the uterus), which projects into the vagina. The cervical canal passes through it, linking the cavity of the uterus with the vagina; the canal normally contains mucus, the viscosity of which changes throughout the menstrual cycle. The cervix is capable of wide dilation during childbirth.

cestode n. see TAPEWORM.

cetrimide n. a detergent disinfectant, used for cleansing skin surfaces and wounds, sterilizing surgical instruments and babies' napkins, and in shampoos. There are few adverse reactions from external application; most toxic effects are due to poisoning from ingestion. Trade name: **Cetavlon**.

cetylpyridinium n. a detergent disinfectant, used for the disinfection of skin, wounds, and burns, as a mouthwash, and in the form of throat lozenges. Trade name: **Merocet**.

Chagas' disease a disease caused by the protozoan parasite *Trypanosoma cruzi. It is transmitted to man when the trypanosomes, present in the faeces of nocturnal bloodsucking *reduviid bugs, come into contact with wounds and scratches on the skin or the delicate internal tissues of the nose and mouth. The presence of the parasite in the heart muscles and central nervous system results in serious inflammation and lesions, which can prove fatal. The disease, limited to poor rural areas of South and Central America, is especially prevalent in children and young adults. It may be treated with nifurtimox. See also TRYPANOSOMIASIS. [C. Chagas (1879–1934), Brazilian physician]

chaining n. a technique of *behaviour modification in which a complex skill is taught by being broken down into its separate components, which are gradually built up into the full sequence. Usually the last component in the sequence is taught first, because it is this component that is followed by *reinforcement: this is termed **backwards chaining**.

chalazion (meibomian cyst) n. a swollen sebaceous gland in the eyelid, caused by chronic inflammation following blockage of the gland's duct. The gland becomes converted into a jelly-like mass, producing disfigurement of the lid. It may become secondarily infected, when it will be painful and may discharge. Treatment is by application of antibiotic ointments or surgical incision and curettage of the gland.

chalcosis n. the deposition of copper in the tissues of the eye, usually resulting from the presence of a copper foreign body within the eye.

chancre n. a painless ulcer that develops at the site where infection enters the body, e.g. on the lips, penis, urethra, or eyelid. It is the primary symptom of such infections as sleeping sickness and syphilis.

chancroid n. see SOFT SORE.

Charcot-Leyden crystals fine colourless sharp-pointed crystals seen in the sputum of asthmatics. [J. M. Charcot (1825–93), French neurologist; E. V. von Leyden (1832–1910), German physician]

Charcot-Marie-Tooth disease (peroneal muscular atrophy) a group of inherited diseases of the peripheral nerves, now more commonly known as **hereditary sensorimotor neuropathics**, causing a gradually progressive weakness and wasting of the muscles of the legs and the lower part of the thighs. The hands and arms are eventually affected. [P. Marie (1853–1940), French physician; H. H. Tooth (1856–1925), British physician]

Charcot's joint a damaged, swollen, and deformed joint resulting from repeated minor injuries of which the patient is unaware because the nerves that normally register pain are not functioning. The condition may occur in syphilis, diabetes mellitus, and syringomyelia.

Charcot's triad the combination of fever, rigors, and jaundice that indicates acute *cholangitis.

Charnley clamps an apparatus used to encourage *arthrodesis between the ends of two bones on either side of a joint. Parallel pins driven through the bone ends are connected on each side of the joint by bolts bearing wing nuts; tightening of the screw arrangements forces the surfaces of the bones together. When the two bones have joined, by growth and reshaping, the clamps can be removed. [Sir J. Charnley (1911–82), British orthopaedic surgeon]

Chart n. continuous hyperfractionated accelerated radiotherapy: a recently developed radiotherapeutic technique aimed at the rapid destruction of tumour cells when they are actively proliferating and therefore most sensitive to radiation. The technique is currently being evaluated at research level.

Chediak-Higashi syndrome a rare fatal hereditary disease in children, inherited as an autosomal *recessive condition, causing enlargement of the liver and spleen, albinism, and abnormalities of the eye. The cause is unknown but thought to be due to a disorder of glycolipid metabolism. [A. Chediak (20th century), Cuban physician; O. Higashi (20th century) Japanese paediatrician]

cheil- (cheilo-) prefix denoting the lip(s). Example: **cheiloplasty** (plastic surgery of).

cheilitis n. inflammation of the lips. **Angular cheilitis** affects the angles of the lips and is often caused by a staphylococcal-candidal infection.

cheiloplasty n. see LABIOPLASTY.

cheiloschisis n. see CLEFT LIP.

cheilosis n. swollen cracked bright-red lips. This is a common symptom of many nutritional disorders, including ariboflavinosis (vitamin B_2 deficiency).

cheir- (cheiro-) prefix denoting the hand(s). Examples: **cheiralgia** (pain in); **cheiroplasty** (plastic surgery of).

cheiropompholyx n. a type of *eczema affecting the palms and fingers. The thickness of the skin in these areas prevents the pinhead vesicles from breaking and eventually the skin peels after a period of intense itching. *See* POMPHOLYX.

chelating agent a chemical compound that forms complexes by binding metal ions. Some chelating agents, including *desferrioxamine and *penicillamine, are drugs used to treat metal poisoning: the metal is bound to the drug and excreted safely. Chelating agents often form the active centres of enzymes.

chem- (chemo-) *prefix denoting* chemical or chemistry.

chemodectoma *n.* a tumour arising from tissues that are rich in chemoreceptors (such as the *carotid body and the *glomus jugulare). Chemodectomas are also known as 'potato tumours' because of their appearance.

chemoreceptor *n.* a cell or group of cells that responds to the presence of specific chemical compounds by initiating an impulse in a sensory nerve. Chemoreceptors are found in the taste buds and in the mucous membranes of the nose. *See also* RECEPTOR.

chemosis *n.* swelling (oedema) of the *conjunctiva. It is usually due to inflammation but may occur if the drainage of blood and lymph from around the eye is obstructed.

chemotaxis *n.* movement of a cell or organism in response to the stimulus of a gradient of chemical concentration.

chemotherapy *n.* the prevention or treatment of disease by the use of chemical substances. The term is sometimes restricted to the treatment of infectious diseases with antibiotics and other drugs or to the control of cancer with antimetabolites and similar drugs (in contrast to *radiotherapy).

chenodeoxycholic acid a drug used in the treatment of cholesterol gallstones, which it gradually dissolves over a period of up to 18 months. It is administered by mouth. A common side-effect is diarrhoea. Trade names: **Chendol**, **Chenofalk**, **Chenocedon**.

cherry angioma *see* ANGIOMA.

chest *n. see* THORAX.

Cheyne-Stokes respiration a striking form of breathing in which there is a cyclical variation in the rate, which becomes slower until breathing stops for several seconds before speeding up to a peak and then slowing again. It occurs when the sensitivity of the respiratory centres in the brain is impaired, particularly in states of coma. [J. Cheyne (1777–1836), Scottish physician; W. Stokes (1804–78), Irish physician]

chiasma *n.* (*pl.* **chiasmata**) **1.** (in genetics) the point at which homologous chromosomes remain in contact after they have started to separate in the first division of *meiosis. Chiasmata occur from the end of prophase to anaphase and represent the point at which mutual exchange of genetic material takes place (*see* CROSSING OVER). **2.** *see* OPTIC CHIASMA.

chickenpox *n.* a highly infectious disease caused by a *herpesvirus (the varicella-zoster virus) that is transmitted by airborne droplets. After an incubation period of 11–18 days a mild fever develops, followed after about 24 hours by an itchy rash of red pimples that soon change to vesicles. These usually start on the trunk or scalp and spread to the face and limbs; they crust over and resolve after about 12 days. Treatment is aimed at reducing the fever and controlling the itching (e.g. by the application of calamine lotion); scarring is unusual. Complications are rare but include secondary infection and occasionally *encephalitis. The patient is infectious from the onset of symptoms until all the spots have gone. One attack usually confers life-long immunity, although the virus may reactivate at a later date and cause shingles (*see* HERPES). In adult patients who are particularly vulnerable, e.g. those with AIDS or who are otherwise immunosuppressed, chickenpox can be a serious disease, which may be treated with *acyclovir or famciclovir. Medical name: **varicella**.

chiclero's ulcer a form of *leishmaniasis of the skin caused by the parasite *Leishmania tropica mexicana*. The disease, occurring in Panama, Honduras, and the Amazon, primarily affects men who visit the forests to collect chicle (gum) and takes the form of an ulcerating lesion on the ear lobe. The sore usually heals spontaneously within six months.

Chief Administrative Medical Officer a public health physician at area level under the NHS (Scotland) Act and the terms of the NHS Act applicable to Wales. *See* NATIONAL HEALTH SERVICE.

Chief Medical Officer (CMO) the government's most senior medical adviser, who is responsible to the Secretary of State for Health for all of the *Department of Health's medical matters.

Chief Nursing Officer the government's chief nursing adviser, who is responsible for providing an expert professional contribution and advice on nursing, midwifery, and health visiting matters to ministers and senior officials.

chigger *n. see* TROMBICULA.

chigoe *n. see* TUNGA.

Chikungunya fever a disease, occurring in Africa and Asia, caused by an *arbovirus and transmitted to man by mosquitoes of the genus *Aëdes*. The disease is similar to *dengue and symptoms include fever, headache, generalized body pain, and an irritating rash. The patient is given drugs to relieve the pain and reduce the fever.

chilblains (perniosis) *pl. n.* dusky red itchy swellings that develop on the extremities in cold weather. They usually settle in two weeks but treatment with *nifedipine is helpful in severe cases. There may be a genetic predisposition to chilblains.

child abuse the maltreatment of children. It may take the form of **sexual abuse**, when a child is involved in sexual activity by an adult; **physical abuse**, when physical injury is caused by cruelty or undue punishment (*see* NONACCIDENTAL INJURY); **neglect**, when basic physical provision for needs is lacking; and **emotional abuse**, when lack of affection and/or hostility from caregivers damage a child's emotional development (*see* ATTACHMENT DISORDER).

childbirth *n. see* LABOUR.

child health clinic (in Britain) a special clinic for the routine care of infants and preschool children, formerly known as a **child welfare centre**. Sometimes these clinics are staffed by doctors, *health visitors, and clinic nurses employed by community trusts; the children attending them are drawn from the neighbourhood around the clinic. Alternatively general practitioners may run their own child health clinic on a regular basis, with health visitors and other staff in attendance; it is unusual for children not registered with the practice to attend such clinics. The service provides screening tests for such conditions as *congenital dislocation of the hip, suppressed squint (*see* COVER TEST), thyroid insufficiency, and impaired speech and/or hearing. The *Guthrie test may also be performed if this has not been done before the baby leaves hospital. The staff of child health clinics also educate mothers (especially those having their first child) in feeding techniques and hygiene and see that children receive the recommended immunizations against infectious diseases. They also ensure that the families of children with disabilities receive maximum support from health and social services and that such children achieve their maximum potential in the preschool period. *See also* COMMUNITY PAEDIATRICIAN.

Child's table a useful guide to the severity of hepatocellular destruction using five criteria: serum bilirubin level, serum albumin level, ascites, neurological disturbance, and nutritional state.

chir- (chiro-) *prefix denoting* the hand(s). *See also* CHEIR-.

chiropody (podiatry) *n.* the study and care of the foot, including its normal structure, its diseases, and their treatment. —**chiropodist** *n.*

chiropractic *n.* a system of treating diseases by manipulation, mainly of the vertebrae of the backbone. It is based on the theory that nearly all disorders can be traced to the incorrect alignment of bones, with consequent malfunctioning of nerves and muscle throughout the body. Practitioners in the UK will be required to register at the General Chiropractic Council, set up in 1997 to regulate the profession.

Chlamydia *n.* a genus of virus-like bacteria that cause disease in man and birds. *Chlamydia psittaci* causes *psittacosis, and *C. trachomatis* is the causative agent of the eye disease *trachoma. Some strains of *Chlamydia*, especially *C. trachomatis*, are a common cause of sexually transmitted infections, being responsible for nonspecific *urethritis in men, *pelvic inflammatory disease in women, and *inclusion conjunctivitis in the newborn. The organisms are usually regarded as Gram-negative bacteria but are of similar size to viruses and all are obligate parasites. —**chlamydial** *adj.*

chloasma (melasma) *n.* ill-defined symmetrical brown patches on the cheeks or elsewhere on the face. Chloasma is a *photosensitivity reaction in women on combined oral contraceptive pills or who are pregnant; very rarely it occurs in men. It can usually be prevented by the use of sunscreens.

chlor- (chloro-) *prefix denoting* **1.** chlorine or chlorides. **2.** green.

chloracne *n.* an occupational acne-like skin disorder that occurs after regular contact with chlorinated hydrocarbons. These chemicals are derived from oil and tar products; 'cutting oils' used in engineering also cause the disease. The skin develops blackheads, papules, and pustules, mainly on hairy parts (such as the forearm). Warts and skin cancer may develop after many years of exposure to these chemicals.

chloral hydrate a sedative and hypnotic drug used, mainly in children and the elderly, to induce sleep or as a daytime sedative. It is rapidly absorbed from the alimentary canal and is usually given by mouth as a syrup, although it can be administered rectally. Toxic effects are usually only seen with overdosage. Prolonged use may lead to *dependence. Trade names: **Noctec, Welldorm elixir**.
    Chloral betaine, in the form of tablets (**Welldorm tablets**), is broken down in the body to chloral hydrate.

chlorambucil *n.* a drug that destroys cancer cells. It is given by mouth and used mainly in the treatment of chronic leukaemias. Prolonged large doses may cause damage to the bone marrow. Trade name: **Leukeran**.

chloramphenicol *n.* an antibiotic, derived from the bacterium *Streptomyces*

venezuelae and also produced synthetically, that is effective against a wide variety of microorganisms. However, due to its serious side-effects, especially damage to the bone marrow, it is usually reserved for serious infections (such as typhoid fever) when less toxic drugs are ineffective. It is also used, in the form of eye drops or ointment, to treat bacterial conjunctivitis. Trade names: **Chloromycetin, Kemicetine**.

chlorbutol *n.* an antibacterial and antifungal agent used as a preservative in injection solutions, in eye and nose drops, in powder form for topical use in irritational skin conditions, and as a gargle or mouthwash (combined with chlorhexidine in **Eludril**).

chlordiazepoxide *n.* a sedative and tranquillizing drug with *muscle relaxant properties, used to relieve tension, fears and anxiety and in the treatment of alcoholism. It is administered by mouth or injection. Common side-effects are nausea, skin reactions, and muscular incoordination. Trade names: **Librium, Diapox, Elenium**. *See also* TRANQUILLIZER.

chlorhexidine *n.* an antiseptic used as a general disinfectant for skin and mucous membranes or as a preservative (for example, in eye drops). Chlorhexidine is used in solution, creams, gels, and lozenges and in some preparations is combined with *cetrimide. In very dilute solutions it can be used as an effective mouthwash for the control of infections of the mouth. Skin sensitivity to chlorhexidine occurs rarely. Trade name: **Hibitane**.

chlorination *n.* the addition of noninjurious traces of chlorine (often one part per million) to water supplies before human consumption to ensure that disease-causing organisms are destroyed. *See also* FLUORIDATION.

chlorine *n.* an extremely pungent gaseous element with antiseptic and bleaching properties. It is widely used to sterilize drinking water and purify swimming pools. In high concentrations it is toxic; it was used in World War I as a poison gas in the trenches. Symbol: Cl.

chlormethiazole *n.* a *sedative and hypnotic drug used to treat insomnia in the elderly (when associated with confusion, agitation, and restlessness) and drug withdrawal symptoms (especially in alcoholism). It is administered by mouth or injection and the most common side-effects are tingling sensations in the nose and sneezing. Trade name: **Heminevrin**.

chlormezanone n. a tranquillizing drug used in the treatment of mild anxiety and tension, including premenstrual tension. It is also used to relieve pain and muscle spasm. Chlormezanone is administered by mouth; the most common side-effects are drowsiness and dizziness. Trade name: **Trancopal**.

chlorocresol n. an antiseptic derived from phenol, used as a general disinfectant and, at low concentrations, as a preservative in injections, creams, and lotions. Strong solutions applied to the skin may cause sensitivity reactions.

chloroform n. a volatile liquid formerly widely used as a general anaesthetic. Because its use as such causes liver damage and affects heart rhythm, chloroform is now used only in low concentrations as a flavouring agent and preservative, in the treatment of flatulence, and in liniments as a *rubefacient.

chloroma n. a tumour that arises in association with *myeloid leukaemia and consists essentially of a mass of leukaemic cells. A freshly cut specimen of the tumour appears green, but the colour rapidly disappears on exposure to air. It shows red fluorescence with ultraviolet light and responds to specific anti-leukaemic treatment.

chlorophenothane n. see DDT.

chlorophyll n. one of a group of green pigments, found in all green plants and some bacteria, that absorb light to provide energy for the synthesis of carbohydrates from carbon dioxide and water (photosynthesis). The two major chlorophylls, a and b, consist of a porphyrin/magnesium complex.

chloropsia n. green vision: a rare symptom of digitalis poisoning.

chloroquine n. a drug used principally in the treatment and prevention of malaria but also used in rheumatoid arthritis, certain liver infections and skin conditions, and lupus erythematosus. It is administered by mouth or injection; a side-effect of prolonged use in large doses is eye damage. Trade names: **Avloclor**, **Nivaquine**.

chlorothiazide n. a *diuretic used to treat fluid retention (oedema) and high blood pressure (hypertension). It is administered by mouth and may cause skin sensitivity reactions, stomach pains, nausea, and reduced blood potassium levels. Trade name: **Saluric**.

chloroxylenol n. an *antiseptic, derived from *phenol but less toxic and more selective in bactericidal activity, used mainly in solution as a skin disinfectant. Trade name: **Dettol**.

chlorphenesin n. a compound, active against bacteria and fungi, that is applied to the skin as a cream or dusting powder to treat fungal infections, such as athlete's foot. Trade name: **Mycil**.

chlorpheniramine n. a potent *antihistamine used to treat such allergies as hay fever, rhinitis, and urticaria. It is administered by mouth or, to relieve severe conditions, by injection. Trade name: **Piriton**.

chlorpromazine n. a phenothiazine *antipsychotic drug used in the treatment of *schizophrenia and *mania; it is also used to treat severe anxiety and agitation and to control nausea and vomiting. It also enhances the effects of *analgesics and is used in terminal illness and preparation for anaesthesia. Chlorpromazine is administered by mouth or injection or as a rectal suppository; common side-effects are drowsiness and dry mouth. It also causes abnormalities of movement, especially *dystonias, *dyskinesia, and *parkinsonism. Trade name: **Largactil**.

chlorpropamide n. a drug that reduces blood sugar levels and is used to treat noninsulin-dependent diabetes in adults. It is administered by mouth and can cause such side-effects as skin sensitivity reactions and digestive upsets. Trade name: **Diabinese**. See also SULPHONYLUREA.

chlortetracycline n. an *antibiotic active against many bacteria and fungi. It is administered by mouth or injection or as ointment or cream (for skin and eye infections); side-effects are those of the other *tetracyclines. Trade names: **Aureomycin**, **Deteclo**.

chlorthalidone n. a thiazide *diuretic used to treat fluid retention (oedema) and high blood pressure (hypertension). It is administered by mouth and may cause skin sensitivity reactions, stomach pains, nausea, and reduced blood potassium levels. Trade name: **Hygroton**.

choana n. (pl. **choanae**) a funnel-shaped opening, particularly either of the two openings between the nasal cavity and the pharynx.

chokedamp n. see BLACKDAMP.

chol- (chole-, cholo-) prefix denoting bile. Example: **cholemesis** (vomiting of).

cholagogue n. a drug that stimulates the flow of bile from the gall bladder and bile ducts into the duodenum.

cholangiocarcinoma n. a malignant tumour of the bile ducts. It is particularly likely to occur at the junction of the two main bile ducts within the liver, causing obstructive jaundice.

cholangiography n. X-ray examination of the bile ducts, used to demonstrate the site and nature of any obstruction to the ducts or to show the presence of stones within them. A medium that is opaque to X-rays is introduced into the ducts either by injection into the bloodstream (**intravenous cholangiography**); direct injection into the liver (**percutaneous transhepatic cholangiography**); direct injection into the bile ducts at operation (**operative cholangiography**); or by injection into the duodenal opening of the bile ducts through a *duodenoscope (**endoscopic retrograde cholangiopancreatography**; see ERCP). See also PERCUTANEOUS TRANSHEPATIC CHOLANGIOPANCREATOGRAPHY.

cholangiolitis n. inflammation of the smallest bile ducts (**cholangioles**). See CHOLANGITIS.

cholangioma n. a rare tumour originating from the bile duct.

cholangitis n. inflammation of the bile ducts. It usually occurs when the ducts are obstructed, especially by stones, or after operations on the bile ducts.

Symptoms include intermittent fever, usually with *rigors, and intermittent jaundice (a combination known as **Charcot's triad**). Initial treatment is by antibiotics, but removal of the obstruction is essential for permanent cure. Liver abscess is a possible complication, and recurrent episodes of cholangitis lead to secondary biliary *cirrhosis. **Sclerosing cholangitis** is a characteristic but rare complication of ulcerative colitis in which all the bile ducts develop irregularities and narrowing.

cholecalciferol n. see VITAMIN D.

cholecyst- prefix denoting the gall bladder. Example: **cholecystotomy** (incision of).

cholecystectomy n. surgical removal of the gall bladder, usually for *cholecystitis or gallstones. Formerly always performed by *laparotomy, the operation is now often done by *laparoscopy (**percutaneous laparoscopic cholecystectomy**). See also MINIMALLY INVASIVE SURGERY.

cholecystenterostomy n. a surgical procedure in which the gall bladder is joined to the small intestine. It is performed in order to allow bile to pass from the liver to the intestine when the common bile duct is obstructed by an irremovable cause.

cholecystitis n. inflammation of the gall bladder. **Acute cholecystitis** is due to bacterial infection, causing fever and acute pain over the gall bladder. It is usually treated by rest and antibiotics. **Chronic cholecystitis** is often associated with *gallstones and causes recurrent episodes of upper abdominal pain. It is also associated with **cholecystitis glandularis proliferans** – thickening of the gall-bladder wall and epithelial changes (crypt formation, hypertrophy). Recurrent bacterial infection may be the cause of chronic cholecystitis, but the physical processes leading to gallstone formation may also be important. It may require treatment by *cholecystectomy. See also CHOLESTEROSIS, MURPHY'S SIGN.

cholecystoduodenostomy n. a form of *cholecystenterostomy in which the gall bladder is joined to the duodenum.

cholecystogastrostomy n. a form of *cholecystenterostomy in which the gall bladder is joined to the stomach. It is rarely performed.

cholecystography *n.* X-ray examination of the gall bladder. A compound that is opaque to X-rays is taken by mouth, absorbed by the intestine, and excreted by the liver into the bile, which is concentrated in the gall bladder. An X-ray photograph (**cholecystogram**) of the gall bladder indicates whether or not it is functioning, and gallstones may be seen as contrasting (nonopaque) areas within it. A fatty meal is usually also given, to demonstrate the ability of the gall bladder to contract. This technique has largely been replaced by ultrasound scanning.

cholecystokinin *n.* a hormone secreted by the cells of the duodenum in response to the presence of partly digested food in the duodenum. It causes contraction of the gall bladder and expulsion of bile into the intestine and stimulates the production of digestive enzymes by the pancreas (*see also* PANCREATIC JUICE). In the brain cholecystokinin functions as a neurotransmitter, involved in the control of satiety.

cholecystotomy *n.* a surgical operation in which the gall bladder is opened, usually to remove gallstones. It is performed only when *cholecystectomy would be impracticable or dangerous.

choledoch- (choledocho-) *prefix denoting* the common bile duct. Example: **choledochoplasty** (plastic surgery of).

choledocholithiasis *n.* stones within the common bile duct. The stones usually form in the gall bladder and pass into the bile duct, but they may develop within the duct after *cholecystectomy.

choledochotomy *n.* a surgical operation in which the common bile duct is opened, to search for or to remove stones within it. It may be performed at the same time as *cholecystectomy or if stones occur in the bile duct after cholecystectomy.

cholelithiasis *n.* the formation of stones in the gall bladder (*see* GALLSTONE).

cholelithotomy *n.* removal of gallstones by *cholecystotomy.

cholera *n.* an acute infection of the small intestine by the bacterium *Vibrio cholerae*, which causes severe vomiting and diarrhoea (known as **ricewater stools**) leading to dehydration. The disease is contracted from food or drinking water contaminated by faeces from a patient. Cholera often occurs in epidemics; outbreaks are rare in good sanitary conditions. After an incubation period of 1–5 days symptoms commence suddenly; the resulting dehydration and the imbalance in the concentration of body fluids can cause death within 24 hours. Initial treatment involves replacing the fluid loss by *oral rehydration therapy; tetracycline eradicates the bacteria and hastens recovery. The mortality rate in untreated cases is over 50%. Vaccination against cholera is effective for only 6–9 months.

choleresis *n.* the production of bile by the liver.

choleretic *n.* an agent that stimulates the secretion of bile by the liver thereby increasing the flow of bile.

cholestasis *n.* failure of normal amounts of bile to reach the intestine, resulting in obstructive *jaundice. The cause may be a mechanical block in the bile ducts, such as a stone (**extrahepatic biliary obstruction**), or liver disease, such as that caused by the drug *chlorpromazine in some hypersensitive individuals (**intrahepatic cholestasis**); it may also occasionally occur in pregnancy. The symptoms are jaundice with dark urine, pale faeces, and usually itching (pruritus).

cholesteatoma *n.* a skin-lined sac containing debris from dead skin cells that grows from the eardrum into the *mastoid bone, eroding normal structures in its path. Left untreated, it can carry infection to the brain, causing meningitis or a cerebral *abscess. Treatment is by means of *mastoidectomy. Rarely, cholesteatoma can arise congenitally in the *temporal bone or central nervous system.

cholesterol *n.* a fatlike material (a *sterol) present in the blood and most tissues, especially nervous tissue. Cholesterol and its esters are important constituents of cell membranes and are precursors of many steroid hormones and bile salts. Western dietary intake is approximately 500–1000 mg/day. Cholesterol is synthesized in the body from acetate, mainly in the liver, and blood concentration is normally 140–300 mg/100 ml (3.6–7.8 mmol/l).

An elevated concentration of cholesterol in the blood (**hypercholesterolaemia**) is often associated with *atheroma, of which cholesterol is a major component. Hypercholesterolaemia and the resulting atheroma have been linked with a high dietary intake of saturated fats and cholesterol. However, current thinking suggests that the damage to blood vessels is actually caused by high levels (over 4.4 mmol/l) of low-density *lipoprotein (LDL), one of the forms in which cholesterol is transported in the bloodstream, in its oxidized form. Therefore increasing the dietary intake of *antioxidants would appear to protect against atherosclerosis. People with **primary** (or **familial**) **hypercholesterolaemia** have a genetic defect causing a lack of LDL receptors, which remove cholesterol from the bloodstream. Drugs are available that lower serum cholesterol and LDL levels. Cholesterol is also a constituent of *gallstones.

cholesterosis *n.* a form of chronic *cholecystitis in which small crystals of cholesterol are deposited on the internal wall of the gall bladder, like the pips of a strawberry: hence its descriptive term **strawberry gall bladder**. The crystals may enlarge to become *gallstones.

cholestyramine *n.* a drug that binds with bile salts so that they are excreted. It is administered by mouth to relieve conditions due to irritant effects of bile salts – such as the itching that occurs in obstructive jaundice – and also to lower the blood levels of cholesterol and other fats. Common side-effects include constipation, diarrhoea, heartburn, and nausea. Trade name: **Questran**.

cholic acid (cholalic acid) *see* BILE ACIDS.

choline *n.* a basic compound important in the synthesis of phosphatidylcholine (lecithin) and other *phospholipids and of *acetylcholine. It is also involved in the transport of fat in the body. Choline is sometimes classed as a vitamin but, although it is essential for life, it can be synthesized in the body.

cholinergic *adj.* **1.** describing nerve fibres that release *acetylcholine as a neu-

rotransmitter. **2.** describing *receptors at which acetylcholine acts to pass on messages from cholinergic nerve fibres. **3.** describing drugs that mimic the actions of acetylcholine (*see* PARASYMPATHOMIMETIC). *Compare* ADRENERGIC.

cholinesterase *n.* an enzyme that breaks down a choline ester into its choline and acid components. The term usually refers to **acetylcholinesterase**, which breaks down the neurotransmitter *acetylcholine into choline and acetic acid. It is found in all *cholinergic nerve junctions, where it rapidly destroys the acetylcholine released during the transmission of a nerve impulse so that subsequent impulses may pass. Other cholinesterases are found in the blood and other tissues.

choline theophyllinate a drug used to dilate the air passages in asthma and chronic bronchitis. It is administered by mouth and can cause digestive upsets and nausea. Trade name: **Choledyl**.

choluria *n.* bile in the urine, which occurs when the level of bile in the blood is raised, especially in obstructive *jaundice. The urine becomes dark brown or orange, and bile pigments and bile salts may be detected in it.

chondr- (chondro-) *prefix denoting* cartilage. Example: **chondrogenesis** (formation of).

chondrin *n.* a material that resembles gelatin, produced when cartilage is boiled.

chondriosome *n. see* MITOCHONDRION.

chondroblast *n.* a cell that produces the matrix of *cartilage.

chondroblastoma *n.* a tumour derived from *chondroblasts, having the appearance of a mass of well-differentiated cartilage.

chondrocalcinosis *n.* the presence of calcium pyrophosphate crystals in joint cartilage. It is seen in *pseudogout.

chondroclast *n.* a cell that is concerned with the absorption of cartilage.

chondrocranium *n.* the embryonic skull, which is composed entirely of cartilage and is later replaced by bone. *See also* MENINX.

chondrocyte *n.* a *cartilage cell, found embedded in the matrix.

chondrodermatitis nodularis helicis a fairly common painful nodule on the upper part of the ear. It occurs mainly in middle-aged or elderly men and characteristically prevents the sufferer from sleeping on the affected side; it is readily treated by being cut out.

chondrodysplasia (chondro-osteodystrophy, chondrodystrophy) *n.* any of various conditions in which there is abnormal cartilage development. It affects long bones and can cause short-limb dwarfism, overgrowth of the epiphysis, or other deformities. *See also* ACHONDROPLASIA.

chondroitin sulphate a mucopolysaccharide that forms an important constituent of cartilage, bone, and other connective tissues. It is composed of glucuronic acid and N-acetyl-D-galactosamine units.

chondroma *n.* a benign tumour of cartilage-forming cells, which may occur at the growing end of any bone but is found most commonly in the bones of the feet and hands. It may be a chance finding on X-ray, it may expand the bone, or it may be the site of a *pathological fracture.

chondromalacia *n.* softening, inflammation, and degeneration of cartilage at a joint. **Chondromalacia patellae** is the most common kind, affecting the undersurface of the kneecap; it results in pain in the front of the knee and grating, which is made worse by kneeling, squatting, and climbing stairs. Treatment is physiotherapy and avoidance of aggravating factors.

chondrosarcoma *n.* a malignant tumour of cartilage cells, occurring in a bone. Treatment is by surgical removal; such tumours are not usually sensitive to radiotherapy or chemotherapy.

chord- (chordo-) *prefix denoting* **1.** a cord. **2.** the notochord.

chorda *n.* (*pl.* **chordae**) a cord, tendon, or nerve fibre. The **chordae tendineae** are stringlike processes in the heart that attach the margins of the mitral and tricuspid valve leaflets to projections of the wall of the ventricle (**papillary muscles**). Rupture of the chordae, through injury, endocarditis, or degenerative changes, results in *mitral incompetence.

chordee *n.* acute angulation of the penis. In *Peyronie's disease, this is due to a localized fibrous plaque in the penis, which fails to engorge on erection. As a result, the penis angulates at this point making intercourse impossible. In a child, downward chordee is an associated deformity in *hypospadias and the more severe forms are corrected surgically.

chordoma *n.* a rare tumour arising from remnants of the embryologic *notochord. The classical sites are the base of skull and the region of the sacrum.

chorea *n.* a jerky involuntary movement particularly affecting the head, face, or limbs. Each movement is sudden but the resulting posture may be prolonged for a few seconds. The symptoms are usually due to disease of the *basal ganglia but may result from drug therapy for *parkinsonism or on the withdrawal of phenothiazines. Such movements are characteristic of *Huntington's disease, in which they are associated with progressive dementia. **Senile chorea** occurs sporadically in elderly people and there is no dementia. **Sydenham's chorea** affects children and is associated with rheumatic fever.

chorion *n.* the embryonic membrane that totally surrounds the embryo from the time of implantation. It is formed from *trophoblast lined with mesoderm and becomes closely associated with the *allantois. The blood vessels (supplied by the allantois) are concentrated in the region of the chorion that is attached to the wall of the uterus and forms the *placenta. *See also* VILLUS. —**chorionic** *adj.*

chorionepithelioma (choriocarcinoma) *n.* a rare form of cancer originating in the outermost of the membranes (chorion) surrounding the fetus. It is a highly malignant tumour usually following a *hydatidiform mole, although it may follow abortion or even a normal pregnancy. The tumour rapidly spreads to the lungs, but is relatively sensitive to treatment with *cytotoxic drugs.

chorionic villus sampling (CVS) a fetal monitoring technique in which a sample of chorionic *villus is extracted through the cervix or abdomen under ultrasound visualization. The earliest recommended time for sampling is the ninth week of pregnancy. The cells so obtained are subjected to chromosomal and biochemical studies to determine if any abnormalities are present in the fetus. This enables the *prenatal diagnosis of such congenital disorders as Down's syndrome and thalassaemia.

chorioretinopathy n. any eye disease involving both the choroid and the retina. *See* CENTRAL SEROUS CHORIORETINOPATHY.

choristoma n. a tumour or mass of tissue composed of tissue not normally found at the affected site. A *dermoid cyst is an example.

choroid n. the layer of the eyeball between the retina and the sclera (*see also* BRUCH'S MEMBRANE). It contains blood vessels and a pigment that absorbs excess light and so prevents blurring of vision. *See* EYE. —**choroidal** adj.

choroidal detachment the separation of the *choroid from the *sclera of the eye as a result of leakage of fluid from the vessels of the choroid. It occurs when pressure inside the eyeball is very low, usually after trauma or intraocular surgery.

choroiditis n. inflammation of the choroid layer of the eye. It may be inflamed together with the iris and ciliary body, but often is involved alone and in patches (**focal** or **multifocal choroiditis**). Vision becomes blurred but the eye is usually painless. *See* UVEITIS.

choroid plexus a rich network of blood vessels, derived from those of the pia mater, in each of the brain's ventricles. It is responsible for the production of *cerebrospinal fluid.

Christmas disease a disorder that is identical in its effects to *haemophilia, but is due to a deficiency of a different blood coagulation factor, the **Christmas factor** (Factor IX). [S. Christmas (20th century), in whom the factor was first identified]

chrom- (chromo-) *prefix denoting* colour or pigment.

chromaffin n. tissue in the medulla of the *adrenal gland consisting of modified neural cells containing granules that are stained brown by chromates. Adrenaline and noradrenaline are released from the granules when the adrenal gland is stimulated by its sympathetic nerve supply. *See also* NEUROHORMONE.

-chromasia *suffix denoting* staining or pigmentation.

chromat- (chromato-) *prefix denoting* colour or pigmentation.

chromatid n. one of the two threadlike strands formed by longitudinal division of a chromosome during *mitosis and *meiosis. They remain attached at the *centromere. Chromatids can be seen between early prophase and metaphase in mitosis and between diplotene and the second metaphase of meiosis, after which they divide at the centromere to form daughter chromosomes.

chromatin n. the material of a cell nucleus that stains with basic dyes and consists of DNA and protein: the substance of which the chromosomes are made. *See* EUCHROMATIN, HETEROCHROMATIN.

chromatography n. any of several techniques for separating the components of a mixture by selective absorption. Two such techniques are quite widely used in medicine, for example to separate mixtures of amino acids. In one of these, **paper chromatography**, a sample of the mixture is placed at the edge of a sheet of filter paper. As the solvent soaks along the paper, the components are absorbed to different extents and thus move along the paper at different rates. In **column chromatography** the components separate out along a column of a powdered absorbent, such as silica or aluminium oxide.

chromatolysis n. the dispersal or disintegration of the microscopic structures within the nerve cells that normally produce proteins. It is part of the cell's response to injury.

chromatophore n. a cell containing pigment. In man chromatophores containing *melanin are found in the skin, hair, and eyes.

chromatopsia *n.* abnormal coloured vision: a rare symptom of various conditions. Sometimes everything looks reddish to patients after removal of their cataracts; patients suffering from digitalis poisoning may see things in green or yellow. Similar disturbances of colour may be experienced by people recovering from inflammation of the optic nerve.

chromoblastomycosis (chromomycosis) *n.* a chronic fungal infection of the skin usually occurring at the site of an injury; for example, a wound from a wood splinter. It produces pigmented wartlike lumps on exposed areas that sometimes ulcerate. In the immunocompromised it may spread rapidly and even prove fatal.

chromosome *n.* one of the threadlike structures in a cell nucleus that carry the genetic information in the form of *genes. It is composed of a long double filament of *DNA coiled into a helix together with associated proteins, with the genes arranged in a linear manner along its length. It stains deeply with basic dyes during cell division (*see* MEIOSIS, MITOSIS). The nucleus of each human somatic cell contains 46 chromosomes, 23 of which are of maternal and 23 of paternal origin (see illustration). Each chromosome can duplicate an exact copy of itself between each cell division (*see* INTERPHASE) so that each new cell formed receives a full set of chromosomes. *See also* CHROMATID, CENTROMERE, SEX CHROMOSOME. —**chromosomal** *adj.*

chron- (chrono-) *prefix denoting* time. Example: **chronophobia** (abnormal fear of).

chronic *adj.* describing a disease of long duration involving very slow changes. Such disease is often of gradual onset. The term does not imply anything about the severity of a disease. *Compare* ACUTE. —**chronicity** *n.*

chronic fatigue syndrome a condition characterized by extreme disabling fatigue that has lasted for at least six months, is made worse by physical or mental exertion, does not resolve with bed rest, and cannot be attributed to other disorders. The fatigue is accompanied by at least some of the following: muscle pain or weakness, poor coordination, joint pain, sore throat, slight fever, painful lymph nodes in the neck and armpits, depression, inability to concentrate, and general malaise. The condition was formerly known as **myalgic encephalomyelitis** (**ME**) and – because it often occurs as a sequel to such viral infections as glandular fever – is sometimes called **postviral fatigue syndrome**. Since the cause is unknown, treatment is limited to relieving the symptoms.

Human male chromosomes, arranged in numbered pairs according to a standard classification. The female set differs only in the sex chromosomes (XX instead of XY).

Chronic Sick and Disabled Persons Act 1970 (in Britain) an Act providing for the identification and care of those suffering from a chronic or degenerative disease for which there is no cure and which can be only partially alleviated by treatment. Such patients are usually distinguished from the elderly who may also suffer from chronic diseases. It is the responsibility of local authorities to identify those with such problems and to ensure that services are available to meet their needs and that the people concerned are aware of the available services. Identification can be difficult because of the lack of clear and agreed definition of what constitutes a disability of such severity as to warrant inclusion in such a register. As there is no compulsion, many general practitioners and community nurses fail to notify the appropriate local authority for reasons of confidentiality and also because many patients fear the stigma of being included on such a register. *See* HANDICAP.

chrys- (chryso-) *prefix denoting* gold or gold salts.

chrysiasis *n.* the deposition of gold in the eye and other tissues as a result of prolonged or excessive treatment with gold salts.

Chrysops *n.* a genus of bloodsucking flies, commonly called deer flies. Female flies, found in shady wooded areas, bite man during the day. Certain species in Africa may transmit the tropical disease *loiasis to man. In the USA *C. discalis* is a vector of *tularaemia.

chrysotherapy *n.* the treatment of disease by the administration of gold or its compounds. The injection or oral administration of *gold salts is extremely effective in the treatment of arthritis in some patients. However, some patients develop potentially severe side-effects, including blood disorders, dermatitis, and impairment of kidney function.

Churg-Strauss syndrome a clinical syndrome comprising severe asthma associated with an increased *eosinophil count in the peripheral blood and eosinophilic deposits in the small vessels of the lungs. It usually responds to oral corticosteroids. Untreated, it may result in severe and widespread systemic *angiitis. [J. Churg (1910–) and L. Strauss (1913–), US pathologists]

Chvosteck's sign twitching of the facial muscles elicited by stimulation of the facial nerve by tapping. This indicates muscular irritability, usually due to calcium depletion (*see* TETANY). [F. Chvosteck (1835–84), Austrian surgeon]

chyle *n.* an alkaline milky liquid found within the *lacteals after a period of absorption. It consists of lymph with a suspension of minute droplets of digested fats, which have been absorbed from the small intestine. It is transported in the lymphatic system to the *thoracic duct. *See also* ASCITES.

chylomicron *n.* a microscopic particle of fat present in the blood after fat has been digested and absorbed from the small intestine.

chyluria *n.* the presence of *chyle in the urine.

chyme *n.* the semiliquid acid mass that is the form in which food passes from the stomach to the small intestine. It is produced by the action of *gastric juice and the churning movements of the stomach.

chymotrypsin *n.* a protein-digesting enzyme (*see* PEPTIDASE). It is secreted by the pancreas in an inactive form, **chymotrypsinogen**, that is converted into chymotrypsin in the duodenum by the action of *trypsin.

chymotrypsinogen *n. see* CHYMOTRYPSIN.

cicatricial *adj.* associated with scarring. For example, **cicatricial alopecia** is a type of baldness associated with scarring (*see* ALOPECIA).

-cide *suffix denoting* killer or killing. Examples: **bactericide** (of bacteria); **infanticide** (of children).

ciliary body the part of the *eye that connects the choroid with the iris. It consists of three zones: the **ciliary ring**, which adjoins the choroid; the **ciliary processes**, a series of about 70 radial ridges behind the iris to which the suspensory ligament of the lens is attached; and the **ciliary muscle**, contraction of which alters the curvature of the lens (*see* ACCOMMODATION).

cilium *n.* (*pl.* **cilia**) **1.** a hairlike process, large numbers of which are found on certain epithelial cells and on certain (ciliate) protozoa. Cilia are particularly characteristic of the epithelium that lines the upper respiratory tract, where their beating serves to remove particles of dust and other foreign material. **2.** an eyelash or eyelid. —**ciliary** *adj.*

cimetidine *n.* an *antihistamine drug that reduces secretion of acid in the stomach and is used to treat stomach and duodenal ulcers, *gastro-oesophageal reflux disease, and other digestive disorders. It is administered by mouth or injection and the most common side-effects are dizziness, diarrhoea, muscular pains, and rash. Trade names: **Dyspamet, Galenamet, Tagamet.**

Cimex *n.* see BED BUG.

CIN see CERVICAL INTRAEPITHELIAL NEOPLASIA.

cinchocaine *n.* a local anaesthetic used in dental and other operations and to relieve pain. It is applied directly to the skin or mucous membranes or injected at the site where anaesthesia is required or into the spine. Side-effects such as yawning, restlessness, excitement, nausea, vomiting, and allergic reactions can sometimes occur. Trade name: **Nupercainal.**

cinchona *n.* the dried bark of *Cinchona* trees, formerly used in medicine to stimulate the appetite and to prevent haemorrhage and diarrhoea. Taken over prolonged periods, it may cause *cinchonism. Cinchona is the source of *quinine.

cinchonism *n.* poisoning caused by an overdose of cinchona or the alkaloids quinine, quinidine, or cinchonine derived from it. The symptoms are commonly ringing noises in the ears, dizziness, blurring of vision (and sometimes complete blindness), rashes, fever, and low blood pressure. Treatment with *diuretics increases the rate of excretion of the toxic compounds from the body.

cineangiocardiography *n.* a form of *angiocardiography in which the X-ray pictures are recorded on cine film. This allows the dynamic movements of the heart to be studied when the film is projected.

cinefluorography *n.* the technique of taking a rapid succession of photographs of the fluorescent screen of a *fluoro-scope, so that the recorded events may be later analysed.

cineradiography *n.* the technique of taking a rapid succession of X-ray photographs, to capture on film events that occur rapidly during a particular radiographic investigation.

cingulectomy *n.* surgical excision of the *cingulum, the part of the brain concerned with anger and depression. The procedure has occasionally been carried out as *psychosurgery for intractable mental illness.

cingulum *n.* (*pl.* **cingula**) **1.** a curved bundle of nerve fibres in each cerebral hemisphere, nearly encircling its connection with the corpus callosum. See CEREBRUM. **2.** a small protuberance on the lingual surface of the crowns of incisor and canine teeth.

ciprofloxacin *n.* a broad-spectrum *quinolone antibiotic that can be given orally and is particularly useful against Gram-negative bacteria, such as *Pseudomonas*, that are resistant to all other oral antibiotics. Side-effects can include nausea, diarrhoea, abdominal pain, and headache. Trade name: **Ciproxin.**

circle of Willis a circle on the undersurface of the brain formed by linked branches of the arteries that supply the brain (see illustration). Most cerebral *aneurysms occur on or near the circle of Willis. [T. Willis (1621–75), English anatomist]

circulatory system see CARDIOVASCULAR SYSTEM.

circum- *prefix denoting* around; surrounding. Example: **circumanal** (surrounding the anus).

circumcision *n.* surgical removal of the foreskin of the penis. This operation is usually performed for religious and ethnic reasons but is sometimes required for medical conditions, mainly *phimosis and *paraphimosis. **Female circumcision** involves removal of the clitoris, *labia minora, and labia majora. The extent of excision varies from tribe to tribe and from country to country. The simplest and least damaging form is **clitoridectomy** (removal of the clitoris); the next form entails excision of the prepuce, clitoris, and all or part of the labia minora. The most extensive form, **infibulation**, involves excision of clitoris, labia minora, and labia majora. The vulval lips are sutured together and a piece of wood or reed is inserted to preserve a small passage for urine and menstrual fluid. In the majority of women who are circumcised, *episiotomy, often extensive, is required to allow delivery of a child.

circumduction *n.* a circular movement, such as that made by a limb.

circumflex nerve a mixed sensory and motor nerve of the upper arm. It arises from the fifth and sixth cervical segments of the spinal cord and is distributed to the deltoid muscle of the shoulder and the overlying skin.

circumoral *adj.* situated around the mouth.

circumstantiality *n.* a disorder of thought in which thinking and speech proceed slowly and with many unnecessary trivial details. It is sometimes seen in organic *psychosis, in *schizophrenia, and in people of pedantic and obsessional personality.

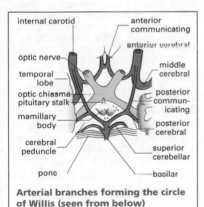

internal carotid

anterior communicating

anterior cerebral

optic nerve

middle cerebral

temporal lobe

optic chiasma
pituitary stalk

posterior communicating

mamillary body

posterior cerebral

cerebral peduncle

superior cerebellar

pons

basilar

Arterial branches forming the circle of Willis (seen from below)

cirrhosis *n.* a condition in which the liver responds to injury or death of some of its cells by producing interlacing strands of fibrous tissue between which are nodules of regenerating cells. The liver becomes tawny and characteristically knobbly (due to the nodules). Causes include *alcoholism (**alcoholic cirrhosis**), viral *hepatitis (**postnecrotic cirrhosis**), chronic obstruction of the common bile duct (**secondary biliary cirrhosis**), autoimmune diseases (**chronic aggressive hepatitis**, **primary biliary cirrhosis**), and chronic heart failure (**cardiac cirrhosis**). In at least half the cases of cirrhosis no cause is found (**cryptogenic cirrhosis**). Complications include *portal hypertension, *ascites, *hepatic encephalopathy, and *hepatoma. Cirrhosis cannot be cured but its progress may be stopped if the cause can be removed. This particularly applies in alcoholism (when all alcohol must be prohibited); in chronic hepatitis (in which corticosteroid treatment may reduce inflammation); in secondary biliary cirrhosis (in which surgery may relieve obstruction); and in cardiac failure that can be treated. —**cirrhotic** *adj.*

cirs- (cirso-) *prefix denoting* a varicose vein. Example: **cirsectomy** (excision of).

cirsoid *adj.* describing the distended knotted appearance of a varicose vein. The term is used for a type of tumour of the scalp (**cirsoid aneurysm**), which is an arteriovenous aneurysm.

CIS *see* CARCINOMA IN SITU.

CISC clean intermittent self-catheterization. *See* INTERMITTENT SELF-CATHETERIZATION.

cisplatin *n.* a heavy-metal compound: a *cytotoxic drug that impedes cell division by damaging DNA. Administered intravenously, it is important in the treatment of testicular and ovarian tumours. It is highly toxic; side-effects include nausea, vomiting, kidney damage, peripheral neuropathy, and hearing loss. Less toxic *analogues of cisplatin are now available (*see* CARBOPLATIN). Trade name: **Neoplatin.**

cisterna *n.* (*pl.* **cisternae**) **1.** one of the enlarged spaces beneath the *arachnoid that act as reservoirs for cerebrospinal fluid. The largest (**cisterna magna**) lies beneath the cerebellum and behind the medulla oblongata. **2.** a dilatation at the lower end of the thoracic duct, into which the great lymph ducts of the lower limbs drain.

cistron *n.* the section of a DNA or RNA

chain that controls the amino-acid sequence of a single polypeptide chain in protein synthesis. A cistron can be regarded as the functional equivalent of a *gene.

citalopram *n.* an antidepressant drug that acts by prolonging the action of the neurotransmitter serotonin (5-hydroxytryptamine) in the brain (*see* SSRI). It is taken by mouth; side-effects may include dizziness, agitation, tremor, nausea, diarrhoea, and drowsiness. Trade name: **Cipramil**.

citric acid an organic acid found naturally in citrus fruits. Citric acid is formed in the first stage of the *Krebs cycle, the important energy-producing cycle in the body.

citric acid cycle *see* KREBS CYCLE.

Citrobacter *n.* a genus of Gram-negative anaerobic rod-shaped bacteria widely distributed in nature. The organisms cause infections of the intestinal and urinary tracts, gall bladder, and the meninges that are usually secondary, occurring in the elderly, newborn, debilitated, and immunocompromised.

citrullinaemia *n.* an inborn lack of one of the enzymes concerned with the chemical breakdown of proteins to urea: in consequence both the amino acid citrulline and ammonia accumulate in the blood. Affected children fail to thrive, and show signs of mental retardation.

citrulline *n.* an *amino acid produced by the liver as a by-product during the conversion of ammonia to *urea.

CJD *see* CREUTZFELDT-JAKOB DISEASE.

clamp *n.* a surgical instrument designed to compress a structure, such as a blood vessel or a cut end of the intestine (see illustration). A variety of clamps have been designed for specific surgical procedures. Blood-vessel clamps are used to stop bleeding from the cut vessels. Intestinal clamps prevent the intestinal contents from leaking into the abdominal cavity during operations on the intestines and are designed either not to damage the intestinal wall (noncrushing clamps) or to close the open end (crushing clamps) prior to suturing.

noncrushing clamp

twin gastrointestinal clamp

Intestinal clamps

Clark's levels the five vertical levels of skin that are successively penetrated by an invading *melanoma. They are: epidermis, papillary dermis, intervening zone, reticular dermis, and subcutaneous tissue. [W. H. Clark (1924–), US dermatologist]

clasp *n.* (in dentistry) the part of a *denture that keeps it in place. It is made of flexible metal.

claudication *n.* limping. **Intermittent claudication** is a cramping pain, induced by exercise and relieved by rest, that is caused by an inadequate supply of blood to the affected muscles. It is most often seen in the calf and leg muscles as a result of *atheroma of the leg arteries. The leg pulses are often absent and the feet may be cold. The treatment is that of atheroma.

claustrophobia *n.* a morbid fear of enclosed places. *Compare* AGORAPHOBIA. *See also* PHOBIA.

claustrum *n.* a thin vertical layer of grey matter in each cerebral hemisphere, between the surface of the *insula and the lenticular nucleus (*see* BASAL GANGLIA).

clavicle *n.* the collar bone: a long slender curved bone, a pair of which form the front part of the shoulder girdle. Each clavicle articulates laterally with the *scapula and medially with the manubrium of the sternum (breastbone). Fracture of the clavicle is a common *sports injury: the majority of cases require no treatment other than supporting the weight of the arm in a sling. —**clavicular** *adj.*

clavulanic acid a drug that interferes with the *penicillinases that inactivate many penicillin-type antibiotics, such as *amoxycillin. Combined with the antibiotic (in **Augmentin** or **Timentin**), clavulanic acid can overcome drug resistance.

clavus n. **1.** see CORN. **2.** a sharp pain in the head, as if a nail were being driven in.

claw-foot n. an excessively arched foot, giving an unnaturally high instep. In most cases the cause is unknown, but the deformity may sometimes be due to an imbalance between the muscles flexing the toes and the shorter muscles that extend them; this type is found in some neuromuscular diseases, such as Friedreich's *ataxia. Surgical treatment is effective in childhood but less so in adult life. Medical name: **pes cavus**.

claw-hand n. flexion and contraction of the fingers with extension at the joints between the fingers and the hand, giving a claw-like appearance. Any kind of damage to the nerves or muscles may lead to clawhand; causes include injuries, *syringomyelia, and leprosy. See also DUPUYTREN'S CONTRACTURE.

clearance (renal clearance) n. a quantitative measure of the rate at which waste products are removed from the blood by the kidneys. It is expressed in terms of the volume of blood that could be completely cleared of a particular substance in one minute.

clearing n. (in microscopy) the process of removing the cloudiness from microscopical specimens after *dehydration by means of a **clearing agent**. This increases the transparency of the specimens. Xylene, cedar oil, methyl benzoate plus benzol, and methyl salicylate plus benzol are commonly used as clearing agents.

cleavage n. (in embryology) the process of repeated cell division of the fertilized egg to form a ball of cells that becomes the *blastocyst. The cells (**blastomeres**) do not grow between divisions and so they decrease in size.

cleft lip (harelip) the congenital deformity of a cleft in the upper lip, on one or both sides of the midline. It occurs when the three blocks of embryonic tissue that go to form the upper lip fail to fuse and

it is often associated with a *cleft palate. Medical name: **cheiloschisis**.

cleft palate a fissure in the midline of the palate due to failure of the two sides to fuse in embryonic development. Only part of the palate may be affected, or the cleft may extend the full length with bilateral clefts at the front of the maxilla; it may be accompanied by a *cleft lip and disturbance of tooth formation. Cleft palates can be corrected by surgery.

cleid- (cleido-, clid-, clido-) prefix denoting the clavicle (collar bone). Example: **cleidocranial** (of the clavicle and cranium).

cleidocranial dysostosis a congenital defect of bone formation in which the skull bones ossify imperfectly and the collar bones (clavicles) are absent.

clemastine n. an antihistamine used for the treatment of symptoms of hay fever, urticaria, and angioneurotic oedema because of its drying effects. It is administered by mouth; commonest side-effects are dizziness, sleepiness, and stomach upset. Trade names: **Aller-eze**, **Tavegil**.

client-centred therapy (Rogerian therapy) a method of psychotherapy in which the therapist refrains from directing his client in what he should do and instead concentrates on communicating understanding and acceptance. Frequently he reflects the client's own words or feelings back to him. The aim is to enable the client to solve his own problems.

climacteric n. **1.** see MENOPAUSE. **2.** (**male climacteric**) declining sexual drive and fertility in men, usually occurring around or after middle age.

clindamycin n. an *antibiotic used to treat serious bacterial infections. It is administered by mouth; possible side-effects are nausea, vomiting, diarrhoea, and occasional hypersensitivity reactions. Trade name: **Dalacin C**.

clinic n. **1.** an establishment or department of a hospital devoted to the treatment of particular diseases or the medical care of out-patients. **2.** a gathering of instructors, students, and patients, usually in a hospital ward, for the examination and treatment of the patients.

clinical audit see MEDICAL AUDIT.

clinical medical officer *see* COMMUNITY HEALTH.

clinical medicine the branch of medicine dealing with the study of actual patients and the diagnosis and treatment of disease at the bedside, as opposed to the study of disease by *pathology or other laboratory work.

clinodactyly *n.* congenital inward bending of a finger, usually the little finger. Clinodactyly may affect both hands and may be found in association with other congenital malformations. No treatment is necessary.

clitoridectomy *n.* the surgical removal of the clitoris (*see* (FEMALE) CIRCUMCISION).

clitoris *n.* the female counterpart of the penis, which contains erectile tissue (*see* CORPUS CAVERNOSUM) but is unconnected with the urethra. Like the penis it becomes erect under conditions of sexual stimulation, to which it is very sensitive.

clivus *n.* (in anatomy) a surface that slopes, such as occurs in part of the sphenoid bone.

CLO columnar-lined oesophagus: *see* BARRETT'S OESOPHAGUS.

cloaca *n.* the most posterior part of the embryonic *hindgut. It becomes divided into the rectum and the urinogenital sinus, which receives the bladder together with the urinary and genital ducts.

clofibrate *n.* a drug that reduces the levels of blood lipids, including cholesterol, and is used to treat atherosclerosis and angina. It is administered by mouth; side-effects can include stomach discomfort, nausea, and diarrhoea. Trade name: **Atromid-S**.

Clomid *n.* *see* CLOMIPHENE.

clomiphene *n.* a synthetic nonsteroidal compound (*see* ANTI-OESTROGEN) that induces ovulation and subsequent menstruation in women who fail to ovulate and is used in the treatment of infertility. It is also used to stimulate ovulation (*see* SUPEROVULATION) for some procedures of assisted conception (e.g. IVF) and to treat some cases of male infertility. Trade name: **Clomid**.

clomipramine *n.* a drug used to treat

various depressive states (*see* ANTIDEPRESSANT). It is administered by mouth or injection; common side-effects are dry mouth and blurred vision. Trade name: **Anafranil**.

clonazepam *n.* a drug with *anticonvulsant properties, used to treat epilepsy and other conditions involving seizures. It is administered by mouth or injection; drowsiness is a common side-effect. Trade name: **Rivotril**.

clone 1. *n.* a group of cells (usually bacteria) descended from a single cell by asexual reproduction and therefore genetically identical to each other and to the parent cell. **2.** *n.* an organism derived from a single cell of its parent and therefore genetically identical to it. The first cloned animal, born in 1997, was produced by fusing a somatic cell of the parent with a denucleated egg cell of a second animal. The resulting 'embryo' was implanted into the uterus of a third animal to complete its development. **3.** *n.* (**gene clone**) a group of identical genes produced by techniques of *genetic engineering. The parent gene is isolated using *restriction enzymes and inserted, via a **cloning vector** (e.g. a bacteriophage), into a bacterium, in which it is replicated. *See also* VECTOR. **4.** *vb.* to form a clone.

clonic *adj.* of, relating to, or resembling clonus. The term is most commonly used to describe the rhythmical limb movements seen as part of a convulsive epileptic seizure (*see* EPILEPSY).

clonidine *n.* a drug used to treat high blood pressure (hypertension) and migraine. It is administered by mouth or injection and commonly causes drowsiness and dry mouth. Trade names: **Catapres**, **Dixarit**.

clonogenic *adj.* describing a cell capable of producing a colony of cells of a predetermined minimum size. Such a cell is known as a **colony forming unit** (**CFU**).

clonorchiasis *n.* a condition caused by the presence of the fluke *Clonorchis sinensis* in the bile ducts. The infection, common in the Far East, is acquired through eating undercooked, salted, or pickled freshwater fish harbouring the larval stage of the parasite. Symptoms include fever, abdominal pain, diarrhoea, liver enlargement, loss of appetite, emaciation and – in advanced cases – cirrhosis and jaundice. Treatment is unsatisfactory although *praziquantel has proved beneficial in some cases.

Clonorchis n. a genus of liver flukes, common parasites of man and other fish-eating mammals in the Far East. The adults of *C. sinensis* cause clonorchiasis. Eggs are passed out in the stools and the larvae undergo their development in two other hosts, a snail and a fish.

clonus n. rhythmical contraction of a muscle in response to a suddenly applied and then sustained stretch stimulus. It is most readily obtained at the ankle when the examiner bends the foot sharply upwards and then maintains an upward pressure on the sole. It is caused by an exaggeration of the stretch reflexes and is usually a sign of disease in the brain or spinal cord.

clopamide n. a *diuretic used to treat fluid retention (oedema) and high blood pressure (hypertension). It is administered by mouth and side-effects are uncommon. Trade name: **Viskaldix**.

clorazepate potassium a tranquillizing drug used to relieve anxiety, tension, and agitation. It is administered by mouth; side-effects can include dizziness, digestive upsets, blurred vision, and, occasionally, drowsiness. Trade name: **Tranxene**.

Clostridium n. a genus of mostly Gram-positive anaerobic spore-forming rodlike bacteria commonly found in soil and in the intestinal tract of man and animals. Many species cause disease in man and animals and produce extremely potent *exotoxins. *C. botulinum* grows freely in badly preserved canned foods, producing a toxin causing serious food poisoning (*botulism); an extremely dilute form of this toxin is now used to treat muscle spasm (*see* BOTULINUM TOXIN). *C. histolyticum, C. oedematiens,* and *C. septicum* all cause *gas gangrene when they infect wounds. *C. tetani* lives as a harmless *commensal in the intestine of animals and man but causes *tetanus on contamination of wounds (with manured soil). The species *C. perfringens* – Welch's bacillus – causes blood poisoning, *food poisoning, and gas

gangrene. Overgrowth of *C. difficile*, a normal inhabitant of the human large intestine, is not uncommon as a complication of some antibiotic therapy and produces a specific condition – **pseudomembranous colitis** – which is life-threatening unless treated promptly.

clotrimazole n. an antifungal drug used to treat all types of fungal skin infections (including ringworm) and vaginal infections. It is applied to the infected part as a cream or solution or as vaginal pessaries and occasionally causes mild burning or irritation. Trade name: **Canesten**.

clotting factors *see* COAGULATION FACTORS.

clotting time *see* COAGULATION TIME.

cloxacillin sodium an antibiotic, derived from penicillin, used to treat many bacterial infections. It is administered by mouth or injection; possible side-effects include diarrhoea and hypersensitivity reactions occur in penicillin-sensitive patients. Trade name: **Orbenin**.

clozapine n. an atypical *antipsychotic drug used in the treatment of schizophrenia and other disorders in patients who are unresponsive to conventional antipsychotics. Administered by mouth, it is notable for the absence of tremors and repetitive movements that are associated with other antipsychotic drugs. Side-effects include dizziness, headache, and increased salivation, and in a few cases the drug may depress levels of white blood cells. Trade name: **Clozaril**.

clubbing n. thickening of the tissues at the bases of the finger and toe nails so that the normal angle between the nail and the digit is filled in. The nail becomes convex in all directions and in extreme cases the digit end becomes bulbous like a club or drumstick. Clubbing is seen in pulmonary tuberculosis, bronchiectasis, empyema, infective endocarditis, cyanotic congenital heart disease, and lung cancer and as a harmless congenital abnormality.

club-foot (talipes) n. a congenital deformity of one or both feet in which the patient cannot stand with the sole of the foot flat on the ground. In the most common variety (**congenital talipes equinovarus**) the foot points downwards, the heel is inverted, and the forefoot twisted. It is diagnosed at birth and may be associated with other congenital abnormalities. Treatment is initially by physiotherapy and strapping or a plaster cast, but if this fails to correct the deformity surgical correction is performed. Other varieties are **talipes varus**, inward deviation of the hind foot; and **talipes valgus**, an outward deviation of the hind foot, which is much less common.

clumping *n.* *see* AGGLUTINATION.

cluttering *n.* an erratic unrhythmical way of speaking in rapid jerky bursts. It can make speech hard to understand, and speech therapy is usually helpful. Unlike *stammering, there are no repetitions or prolonged hesitations of speech.

Clutton's joint a swollen joint in a child, usually the knee, caused by inflammation of the synovial membranes due to congenital syphilis. [H. H. Clutton (1850–1909), British surgeon]

clyster *n.* an old-fashioned term for an *enema.

CMF cyclophosphamide, methotrexate, 5-fluorouracil: the combination used in standard chemotherapy for cancer.

CMO *see* CHIEF MEDICAL OFFICER.

CMV *see* CYTOMEGALOVIRUS.

CNS *see* CENTRAL NERVOUS SYSTEM.

coagulant *n.* any substance capable of converting blood from a liquid to a solid state. *See* BLOOD COAGULATION.

coagulase *n.* an enzyme, formed by disease-producing varieties of certain bacteria of the genus *Staphylococcus*, that causes blood plasma to coagulate. Staphylococci that are positive when tested for coagulase production are classified as belonging to the species *Staphylococcus aureus*.

coagulation *n.* the process by which a colloidal liquid changes to a jelly-like mass. *See* BLOOD COAGULATION.

coagulation factors (clotting factors) a group of substances present in blood plasma that, under certain circumstances, undergo a series of chemical reactions leading to the conversion of blood from a liquid to a solid state (*see* BLOOD CO-

AGULATION). Although they have specific names, most coagulation factors are referred to by an agreed set of Roman numerals (e.g. *Factor VIII, *Factor IX). Lack of any of these factors in the blood results in the inability of the blood to clot. *See also* HAEMOPHILIA.

coagulation time (clotting time) the time taken for blood or blood plasma to coagulate (*see* BLOOD COAGULATION). When measured under controlled conditions and using appropriate techniques, coagulation times may be used to test the function of the various stages of the blood coagulation process.

coagulum *n.* a mass of coagulated matter, such as that formed when blood clots.

coalesce *vb.* to grow together or unite. —**coalescence** *n.*

coal-worker's pneumoconiosis a lung disease caused by coal dust. It affects mainly coal miners but also other exposed workers, such as lightermen, if the lungs' capacity to accommodate and remove the particles is exceeded. *See* PNEUMOCONIOSIS.

coarctation *n.* (of the aorta) a congenital narrowing of a short segment of the aorta. The most common site of coarctation is just beyond the origin of the left subclavian artery from the aorta. This results in high blood pressure (*hypertension) in the upper part of the body and arms and low blood pressure in the legs. The defect is corrected surgically.

Coats' disease a congenital anomaly of the blood vessels of the retina, which are abnormally dilated and leaking. This results in subretinal haemorrhage and massive exudation. [G. Coats (1876–1915), British ophthalmologist]

cobalamin *n.* *see* VITAMIN B_{12}.

cobalt *n.* a metallic element. The artificial radioisotope **cobalt-60**, or **radio-cobalt**, is a powerful emitter of gamma radiation and is used in the radiation treatment of cancer (*see* RADIOTHERAPY, TELECURIETHERAPY). Cobalt itself forms part of the *vitamin B_{12} molecule. Symbol: Co.

cobalt-chromium *n.* a silver-coloured nonprecious alloy of cobalt and chromium used for the metal frame of partial *dentures.

cocaine *n.* an alkaloid that is derived from the leaves of the coca plant (*Erythroxylon coca*) or prepared synthetically and is sometimes used as a local anaesthetic in eye, ear, nose, and throat surgery. It constricts the small blood vessels at the site of application and therefore need not be given with *adrenaline. Since it causes feelings of exhilaration and may lead to psychological *dependence, cocaine has largely been replaced by safer anaesthetics.

cocainism *n.* **1.** the habitual use of, or addiction to, *cocaine in order to experience its intoxicating effects. **2.** the mental and physical deterioration resulting from addiction to cocaine.

cocarcinogen *n.* a substance that enhances the effect of a *carcinogen.

coccidioidomycosis *n.* an infection caused by inhaling the spores of the fungus *Coccidioides immitis*. In 60% of patients infection produces no symptoms at all. In the primary form there is an influenza-like illness that usually resolves within about eight weeks. In a few patients the disease becomes progressive and resembles tuberculosis. Severe or progressive infections are treated with intravenous injections of amphotericin B. The disease is endemic in the desert areas of the Americas, especially the southwestern United States, northern Mexico, and northern Argentina.

coccobacillus *n.* a rod-shaped bacterium (bacillus) that is so small that it resembles a spherical bacterium (coccus). Examples of such bacteria are *Bacteroides* and *Brucella*.

coccus *n.* (*pl.* **cocci**) any spherical bacterium. *See also* GONOCOCCUS, MENINGOCOCCUS, MICROCOCCUS, PNEUMOCOCCUS, STAPHYLOCOCCUS, STREPTOCOCCUS.

cocci- (coccyg-, coccygo-) *prefix denoting* the coccyx. Example: **coccygectomy** (excision of).

coccygodynia (coccydynia) *n.* pain in the lowermost segment of the spine (coccyx) and the neighbouring area.

coccyx *n.* (*pl.* **coccyges** or **coccyxes**) the lowermost element of the *backbone: the vestigial human tail. It consists of four

rudimentary **coccygeal vertebrae** fused to form a triangular bone that articulates with the sacrum. *See also* VERTEBRA. —**coccygeal** *adj.*

cochlea *n.* the spiral organ of the *labyrinth of the ear, which is concerned with the reception and analysis of sound. As vibrations pass from the middle ear through the cochlea, different frequencies cause particular regions of the basilar membrane to vibrate: high notes cause vibration in the region nearest the middle ear; low notes cause vibration in the region nearest the tip of the spiral. The **organ of Corti**, which lies within a central triangular membrane-bound canal (**scala media** or **cochlear duct**), contains sensory hair cells attached to an overlying **tectorial membrane** (see illustration). When the basilar membrane vibrates the sensory cells become distorted and send nerve impulses to the brain via the *cochlear nerve. —**cochlear** *adj.*

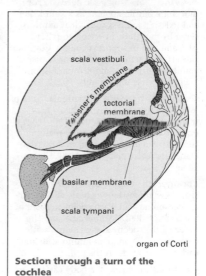

Section through a turn of the cochlea

cochlear duct (scala media) *see* COCHLEA.

cochlear implant a device to improve the hearing of profoundly deaf people who derive no benefit from conventional *hearing aids. It consists of an electrode that is permanently implanted into the inner ear (*cochlea). An external device with a microphone and an electronic processing unit passes information to the electrode using radio-frequency waves. The implant is powered by batteries in the external part of the device.

cochlear nerve the nerve connecting the cochlea to the brain and therefore responsible for the nerve impulses relating to hearing. It forms part of the *vestibulocochlear nerve (cranial nerve VIII).

Cockayne's syndrome a hereditary disorder (inherited as an autosomal *recessive condition) associated with *trisomy of chromosome no. 20. Clinical features include *epidermolysis bullosa, dwarfism, mental retardation, and pigmentary degeneration of the retina. [E. A. Cockayne (1880–1956), British physician]

codeine n. an *analgesic derived from morphine but less potent as a pain killer and sedative and less toxic. It is administered by mouth or injection to relieve pain and also to suppress coughs. Common side-effects include constipation, nausea, vomiting, dizziness, and drowsiness, but *dependence is uncommon.

Codman's triangle a triangular area of new bone seen on X-ray at the edge of a malignant bone tumour resulting from elevation of the *periosteum by malignant tissue. It is most often seen in *osteosarcomas. [E. A. Codman (1869–1940), US surgeon]

codon n. the unit of the *genetic code that determines the synthesis of one particular amino acid. Each codon consists of a section of the DNA molecule, and the order of the codons along the molecule determines the order of amino acids in each protein made in the cell.

-coele *suffix denoting* **1.** a body cavity. Example: **blastocoele** (cavity of blastocyst). **2.** *see* -CELE.

coeli- (coelio-) *prefix denoting* the abdomen or belly. Example: **coeliectasia** (abnormal distension of).

coeliac *adj.* of or relating to the abdominal region. The **coeliac trunk** is a branch of the abdominal *aorta supplying the stomach, spleen, liver, and gall bladder.

coeliac disease a condition in which the small intestine fails to digest and absorb food. Affecting 0.1–0.2% of the population (but much more common in SW Ireland), it is due to a permanent sensitivity of the intestinal lining to the protein gliadin, which is contained in *gluten in the germ of wheat and rye and causes atrophy of the digestive and absorptive cells of the intestine. Symptoms include stunted growth, distended abdomen, and pale frothy foul-smelling stools; the disease can be diagnosed by *biopsy of the jejunum and is treated successfully by a strict and lifelong gluten-free diet. Medical name: **gluten enteropathy**.

coelioscopy n. the technique of introducing an *endoscope through an incision in the abdominal wall to examine the intestines and other organs within the abdominal cavity.

coelom n. the cavity in an embryo between the two layers of mesoderm. It develops into the body cavity.

coenzyme n. a nonprotein organic compound that, in the presence of an *enzyme, plays an essential role in the reaction that is catalysed by the enzyme. Coenzymes, which frequently contain the B vitamins in their molecular structure, include *coenzyme A, *FAD, and *NAD.

coenzyme A a *nucleotide containing pantothenic acid, which is an important coenzyme in the Krebs cycle and in the metabolism of fatty acids.

cofactor n. a nonprotein substance that must be present in suitable amounts before certain *enzymes can act. Cofactors include *coenzymes and metal ions (e.g. sodium and potassium ions).

Cogan's syndrome a disorder in which *keratitis and iridocyclitis (*see* UVEITIS) are associated with tinnitus, vertigo, and bilateral sensorineural deafness. [D. G. Cogan (1908–93), US ophthalmologist]

cognition n. the mental processes by which knowledge is acquired. These include perception, reasoning, acts of creativity, problem-solving, and possibly intuition. *Compare* CONATION.

cognitive psychology the branch of psychology concerned with all human activities relating to knowledge. More specifically, cognitive psychology is concerned with how knowledge is acquired, stored, correlated, and retrieved, by studying the mental processes underlying attention, concept formation, information processing, memory, and speech (**psycholinguistics**). Cognitive psychology views the brain as an information-processing system operating on, and storing, the data acquired by the senses. It investigates this function by experiments designed to measure and analyse human performance in carrying out a wide range of mental tasks. The data obtained allows possible models of the underlying mental processes to be constructed. These models do not purport to represent the actual physiological activity of the brain. Nevertheless, as they are refined by testing and criticism, it is hoped that they may approach close to reality and gradually lead to a clearer understanding of how the brain operates.

cognitive therapy a form of *psychotherapy based on the belief that psychological problems are the products of faulty ways of thinking about the world. For example, a depressed patient may have come to see him- or herself as powerless to change in any way. The therapist assists the patient to identify these false ways of thinking and to avoid them.

cohort study (longitudinal study) a systematic study of a group of people, which may be conducted prospectively or retrospectively. A **prospective cohort study** involves a systematic follow-up for a defined period of time or until the occurrence of a specified event (e.g. onset of illness, retirement, or death) in order to observe their pattern of disease and/or cause of death. For a **retrospective cohort study**, data on the group's exposure and disease experience are already known.

coitus (sexual intercourse, copulation) n. sexual contact between a man and a woman during which the erect penis enters the vagina and is moved within it by pelvic thrusts until *ejaculation occurs. See also ORGASM. —**coital** adj.

coitus interruptus a contraceptive method in which the penis is removed from the vagina before ejaculation of semen (orgasm). The method is unreliable (10–20 pregnancies per 100 woman-years) and it may lead to sexual disharmony and anxiety in one or both partners.

col- (coli-, colo-) *prefix denoting* the colon. Example: **coloptosis** (prolapse of).

colchicine n. a drug obtained from the meadow saffron (*Colchicum autumnale*), used to relieve pain in attacks of gout and in the prevention of attacks of polyserositis. It is administered by mouth; common side-effects are nausea, vomiting, diarrhoea, and stomach pains.

cold (common cold) n. a widespread infectious virus disease causing inflammation of the mucous membranes of the nose, throat, and bronchial tubes. The disease is transmitted by coughing and sneezing. Symptoms commence 1–2 days after infection and include a sore throat, stuffy or runny nose, headache, cough, and general malaise. The disease is mild and lasts only about a week but it can prove serious to young babies and to patients with a pre-existing respiratory complaint.

cold sore *see* HERPES.

colectomy n. surgical removal of the colon. **Total colectomy** is removal of the whole colon, usually for extensive *colitis; **partial colectomy** is removal of a segment of the colon. *See also* HEMICOLECTOMY, PROCTOCOLECTOMY.

colestipol n. a drug used, in conjunction with dietary reduction of cholesterol, to lower *cholesterol levels in the blood in patients with primary hypercholesterolaemia. It binds bile acids, forming a complex that is excreted in the faeces. The reduction in bile acids causes cholesterol to be oxidized to bile acids, decreases low-density *lipoprotein serum levels, and decreases serum cholesterol levels. It is administered by mouth; side-effects include headache, constipation, and abdominal discomfort. Trade name: **Colestid**.

colic n. severe abdominal pain, usually of fluctuating severity, with waves of pain seconds or a few minutes apart. **Infantile colic** is common among babies, due to wind in the intestine associated with feeding difficulties. **Intestinal colic** is due to partial or complete obstruction of the intestine or to constipation. Colic arising from the small intestine is felt in the upper abdomen; colic from the colon is felt in the lower abdomen. Medical names: **enteralgia, tormina**. *See also* BILIARY COLIC.

coliform bacteria a group of Gram-negative rodlike bacteria that are normally found in the gastrointestinal tract and have the ability to ferment the sugar lactose. The group includes the genera *Enterobacter*, **Escherichia*, and **Klebsiella*.

colistin *n.* an **antibiotic administered by mouth to treat gastroenteritis and other bacterial infections. Colistin is a mixture of antimicrobial substances produced by a strain of the bacterium *Bacillus polymyxa*. Trade name: **Colomycin**.

colitis *n.* inflammation of the colon. The usual symptoms are diarrhoea, sometimes with blood and mucus, and lower abdominal pain. It is diagnosed by demonstrating inflammation of the colon's lining (mucosa) by **sigmoidoscopy or barium **enema X-ray. Colitis may be due to infection by **Entamoeba histolytica (**amoebic colitis**) or by bacteria (**infective colitis**); it may also occur in **Crohn's disease (**Crohn's colitis**). Partial or temporary cessation of blood supply to the colon may cause **ischaemic colitis. Ulcerative colitis (idiopathic proctocolitis)** almost always involves the rectum (*see* PROCTITIS) as well as a varying amount of the colon, which become inflamed and ulcerated. Its cause is unknown. It varies in severity from month to month, relapses being treated by drugs, including corticosteroids and drugs containing 5-aminosalicylic acid (sulphasalazine, mesalazine, and olsalazine, as tablets or enemas), and bed rest. Severe, continuous, or extensive colitis may be treated by surgery (*see* COLECTOMY, PROCTOCOLECTOMY). Diarrhoea or pain where inflammation is absent is often due to **mucous colitis** (*see* IRRITABLE BOWEL SYNDROME).

collagen *n.* a protein that is the principal constituent of white fibrous connective tissue (as occurs in tendons). Collagen is also found in skin, bone, cartilage, and ligaments. It is relatively inelastic but has a high tensile strength.

collagen disease an obsolete term for **connective-tissue disease.

collar bone *see* CLAVICLE.

collateral 1. *adj.* accessory or secondary. **2.** *n.* a branch (e.g. of a nerve fibre) that is at right angles to the main part.

collateral circulation 1. an alternative route provided for the blood by secondary vessels when a primary vessel becomes blocked. **2.** the channels of communication between the blood vessels supplying the heart. At the apex of the heart, where the coronary arteries form **anastomoses, these are very complex.

Colles' fracture a fracture of the lower end of the **radius and the tip of the ulna just above the wrist, usually caused by a fall on the outstretched hand. The hand and wrist below the fracture are displaced backwards. The bone is restored to its normal position under anaesthesia, and a plaster cast is applied for about six weeks. Complications are residual deformity and stiffness of the wrist. [A. Colles (1773–1843), Irish surgeon]

colliculus *n.* (*pl.* **colliculi**) a small protuberance or swelling. Two pairs of colliculi, the **superior** and **inferior colliculi**, protrude from the roof of the midbrain (*see* TECTUM).

collimator *n.* a device, used in diagnostic radiology or radiotherapy, to produce a narrow parallel-sided beam of radiation by means of metallic slits that control the size of the beam from a radiation source. The **linear accelerator uses a **multi-leaf collimator**, a specialized form of collimator using electronic fields. Collimators are also used on radiation detectors, in particular in **gamma cameras, for which the exact source of radioactivity needs to be known to produce an accurate image.

collodion *n.* a syrupy solution of nitrocellulose in a mixture of alcohol and ether. When applied to the surface of the body it evaporates to leave a thin clear transparent skin, useful for the protection of minor wounds. Flexible collodion also contains camphor and castor oil, which allow the skin to stretch a little more.

collyrium *n.* a medicated solution used to bathe the eyes.

coloboma *n.* a defect in the development of the eye causing abnormalities ranging in severity from a notch in the lower part of the iris, making the pupil pear-shaped, to defects behind the iris in the *fundus. The enlarged pupil causes dazzle symptoms. A coloboma of the eyelid is a congenital notch in the lid margin.

colon *n.* the main part of the large intestine, which consists of four sections – the **ascending**, **transverse**, **descending**, and **sigmoid colons** (see illustration). The colon has no digestive function but it absorbs large amounts of water and electrolytes from the undigested food passed on from the small intestine. At intervals strong peristaltic movements move the dehydrated contents (faeces) towards the rectum. —**colonic** *adj.*

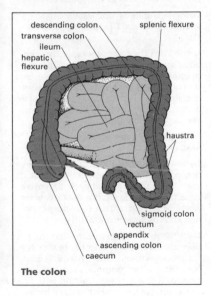

descending colon
transverse colon
ileum
hepatic flexure
splenic flexure
haustra
sigmoid colon
rectum
appendix
ascending colon
caecum

The colon

colonic irrigation washing out the contents of the large bowel by means of copious enemas, using either water, with or without soap, or other medication.

colonoscopy *n.* a procedure for examining the interior of the entire colon and rectum using a flexible illuminated *fibreoptic or video-camera instrument (**colonoscope**) introduced through the anus and guided up the colon by a combination of visual and X-ray control. It is possible to obtain specimens for microscopic examination using flexible forceps passed through the colonoscope and to remove polyps using a *diathermy snare.

colony *n.* a discrete population or mass of microorganisms, usually bacteria, all of which are considered to have developed from a single parent cell. Bacterial colonies that grow on agar plates differ in shape, size, colour, elevation, translucency, and surface texture, depending on the species. This is used as a means of identification. *See also* CULTURE.

colony-stimulating factor (CSF) one of a group of substances (haemopoietic growth factors or hormones) that are produced in the bone marrow and stimulate the production of specific blood cells. Genetically engineered granulocyte colony-stimulating factor (G-CSF) stimulates neutrophil production and also limits bone marrow toxicity from chemotherapy.

colorimeter *n.* an instrument for determining the concentration of a particular compound in a preparation by comparing the intensity of colour in it with that in a standard preparation of known concentration. The instrument is used particularly for measuring the amount of haemoglobin in the blood.

colostomy *n.* a surgical operation in which a part of the colon is brought through the abdominal wall and opened in order to drain or decompress the intestine. The part of the colon chosen depends on the site of obstruction. An **iliac colostomy** opens onto the left lower abdomen; a **transverse colostomy** on the upper abdomen. The colostomy may be temporary, eventually being closed after weeks or months to restore continuity; or permanent, usually when the rectum or lower colon has been removed. An appliance is usually worn over the colostomy opening (*stoma) to prevent soiling the clothes.

colostrum *n.* the first secretion from the breast, occurring shortly after, or sometimes before, birth prior to the secretion of true milk. It is a relatively clear fluid containing serum, white blood cells, and protective antibodies.

colour blindness any of various conditions in which certain colours are confused with one another. True lack of colour appreciation is extremely rare (*see* MONOCHROMAT), but some defect of colour discrimination is present in about 8% of Caucasian males, and 0.4% of Caucasian females. The most common type of colour blindness is **Daltonism (protanopia)** – red-blindness – in which the person cannot distinguish between reds and greens. Occasional cases are due to acquired disease of the retina but in the vast majority it is inherited. The defect is thought to be in the functioning of the light-sensitive cells in the retina responsible for colour perception (*see* CONE). *See also* DEUTERANOPIA, TRICHROMATIC.

colour flow ultrasound imaging *see* DOPPLER ULTRASOUND.

colp- (colpo-) *prefix denoting* the vagina. Example: **colpoplasty** (plastic surgery of).

colpoperineorrhaphy *n.* an operation to repair tears in the vagina and the muscles surrounding its opening, particularly posteriorly.

colporrhaphy *n.* an operation designed to remove lax and redundant vaginal tissue and so reduce the diameter of the vagina in cases of prolapse of the anterior vaginal wall (**anterior colporrhaphy**) or posterior vaginal wall (*see* PROCTOCELE) (**posterior colporrhaphy**).

colposcope (vaginoscope) *n.* an instrument that is inserted into the vagina and permits visual examination of the cervix and the upper part of the vagina (vaginal vault). It is used in the diagnosis of premalignant and early malignant (noninvasive) changes in the cervix. —**colposcopy** *n.*

colposuspension *n.* a surgical operation in which the upper part of the vaginal wall is fixed to the anterior abdominal wall by unabsorbable suture material. Performed through an abdominal incision, this sling operation is used in the surgical treatment of prolapse of the vaginal wall, particularly when stress incontinence exists. *See also* STAMEY PROCEDURE.

colpotomy *n.* an incision made into the wall of the vagina, usually the posterior vaginal wall, close to the cervix (**posterior colpotomy**). This was formerly used to confirm the diagnosis of ectopic pregnancy, but has now been largely superseded by *laparoscopy. Colpotomy is sometimes referred to as **culdocentesis**.

columella *n.* (in anatomy) a part resembling a small column. For example, the **columella cochleae (modiolus)** is the central pillar of the cochlea, around which the spiral cochlear canal winds. The **columella nasi** is the anterior part of the nasal septum.

column *n.* (in anatomy) any pillar-shaped structure, especially any of the tracts of grey matter found in the spinal cord.

coma *n.* a state of unrousable unconsciousness. *See also* GLASGOW SCORING SYSTEM.

combined therapy therapy that combines several types of treatment in order to improve results. It is usually a combination of surgery with radiotherapy and/or chemotherapy for the treatment of malignant tumours (*see* ADJUVANT THERAPY). *See also* SANDWICH THERAPY.

comedo *n.* (*pl.* **comedones**) *see* BLACKHEAD.

commando operation a major operation performed to remove a malignant tumour from the head and neck. Extensive dissection, often involving the face, is followed by reconstruction to restore function and cosmetic acceptability.

commensal *n.* an organism that lives in close association with another of a different species without either harming or benefiting it. For example, some microorganisms living in the gut obtain both food and a suitable habitat but neither harm nor benefit man. *Compare* SYMBIOSIS. —**commensalism** *n.*

comminuted fracture a fracture in which the bone is broken into more than two pieces. A crushing force is usually responsible and there is often extensive injury to surrounding soft tissues.

commissure *n.* **1.** a bundle of nerve fibres that crosses the midline of the central nervous system, often connecting similar structures on each side. **2.** any other tissue connecting two similar structures.

commotio retinae swelling of the retina associated with sudden loss of vision, usually resulting from blunt trauma to the eye.

communicable disease (contagious disease, infectious disease) any disease that can be transmitted from one person to another. This may occur by direct physical contact, by common handling of an object that has picked up infective microorganisms (*see* FOMES), through a disease *carrier, or by spread of infected droplets coughed or exhaled into the air. The most dangerous communicable diseases are on the list of *notifiable diseases.

communicable disease control the control of disease due to infectious agents or their toxic products. *See* CONSULTANT IN COMMUNICABLE DISEASE CONTROL, PUBLIC HEALTH PHYSICIAN.

communicans *adj.* communicating or connecting. The term is applied particularly to blood vessels or nerve fibres connecting two similar structures.

community dentistry the branch of NHS dentistry provided by community trusts. Formerly concerned principally with the treatment of children, it now concentrates on priority groups. Its staff are salaried.

community health preventive services, mainly outside the hospital, involving the surveillance of special groups of the population, such as preschool and school children, women, and the elderly, by means of routine clinical assessment and *screening tests. Routine preventive measures, such as immunization, birth control, and dietary advice, are offered in special clinics staffed by *community nurses, **clinical medical officers**, and **senior clinical medical officers** and sometimes by *community paediatricians. When somebody is identified as having an illness, he (or she) is referred for treatment to a *general practitioner or hospital as appropriate. *See also* CHILD HEALTH CLINIC, COMMUNITY DENTISTRY, SCHOOL HEALTH SERVICE.

Community Health Council (CHC) (in Britain) a group of local residents (usually one per district) appointed to voice the views of patients in relation to the *National Health Service. Serviced by a salaried secretary, these Councils have no executive power but their views must be sought by Health Authorities on all matters that affect the provision of health services in the district. The Health Authority must also receive and consider the annual report of each CHC within its district. Members of a CHC may pay site visits to hospitals or other health service property but not to the private premises of general practitioners or private nursing homes. Patients who are dissatisfied with treatment may be advised by the CHC as to how to submit complaints to the Health Authority or hospital trust.

community hospital *see* HOSPITAL.

community medicine *see* PUBLIC HEALTH MEDICINE.

community midwife (domiciliary midwife) (in Britain) a registered *nurse with special training in midwifery (both hospital and domiciliary practice). The midwife must be registered with the *UKCC in order to practise; this requires regular refresher courses to supplement the basic qualification of **Registered Midwife (RM)**. Community midwives are attached to hospital obstetric units and their work includes **home deliveries** and antenatal and postnatal care in the community.

community nurses (in Britain) a generic term for *health visitors, *community midwives, and *district nurses. *See also* DOMICILIARY SERVICES.

community paediatrician a consultant in paediatrics with special responsibility for the care of children outside the hospital. *See also* COMMUNITY HEALTH.

community physician *see* PUBLIC HEALTH PHYSICIAN.

community services health and social services, including *domiciliary services, that are available in the community but are distinguished from hospital-based services.

community trust an NHS *trust that is concerned with the provision of *community health services and, in some locations, mental health services.

comparative mortality figure *see* OC-CUPATIONAL MORTALITY.

compartment *n.* (in anatomy) any one of the spaces in a limb that are bounded by bone and thick sheets of fascia and enclose the muscles and other tissues of the limb.

compartment syndrome the condition that results from swelling of the muscles in a *compartment of a limb, which raises the pressure within the compartment so that the blood supply to the muscle is cut off, causing *ischaemia and further swelling. If it persists, the muscles and nerves within the compartment die, leading to *Volkmann's contracture. Causes are trauma, damage to blood vessels, and tight casts or bandages. Treatment is to release any tight dressings and to divide the fascia surrounding the compartment to relieve the pressure.

compatibility *n.* the degree to which the body's defence systems will tolerate the presence of intruding foreign material, such as blood when transfused or a kidney when transplanted. Complete compatibility exists between identical twins: a blood transfusion between identical twins will evoke no *antibody formation in the recipient. In severe **incompatibility**, for example between completely unrelated people, there are likely to be swift immune reactions as antibodies attack and destroy any offending antigenic material. *See also* HISTOCOMPATIBILITY, IMMUNITY. —**compatible** *adj.*

compensation *n.* the act of making up for a functional or structural deficiency. For example, compensation for the loss of a diseased kidney is brought about by an increase in size of the remaining kidney, so restoring the urine-producing capacity.

compensation neurosis a fixed preoccupation with real or imaginary disability following an industrial or civil injury, when there is a possibility of financial compensation. The condition tends to deprive the affected person of the motive to overcome the alleged disability and to acknowledge the natural processes of recovery. Uncompensated disability often

persists for many years, but the disorder often clears up soon after a satisfactory settlement.

complement *n.* a substance in the blood, consisting of a group of nine different fractions, that aids the body's defences when antibodies combine with invading antigens. Complement is involved with the breaking up (*lysis), *agglutination, and *opsonization of foreign cells. Following antibody-antigen reaction it may also attract scavenging cells (*phagocytes) to the area of conflict. *See also* IMMUNITY.

complementary medicine *see* ALTERNATIVE MEDICINE.

complement fixation the binding of *complement to the complex that is formed when an antibody reacts with a specific antigen. Because complement is taken up from the serum only when such a reaction has occurred, testing for the presence of complement after mixing a suspension of a known organism with a patient's serum can give confirmation of infection with a suspected organism. The *Wassermann reaction for diagnosing syphilis is a complement-fixation test.

complex *n.* (in psychoanalysis) an emotionally charged and repressed group of ideas and beliefs that is capable of influencing an individual's behaviour. The term in this sense was originally used by Jung, but it is now widely used in a looser sense to denote an unconscious motive.

complication *n.* a disease or condition arising during the course of or as a consequence of another disease.

composite resin a tooth-coloured filling material for teeth. It is composed of two different materials: an inorganic filler chemically held in an organic resin. Composite resins are usually hardened by polymerization initiated by intense light.

compress *n.* a pad of material soaked in hot or cold water and applied to an injured part of the body to relieve the pain of inflammation.

compressed air illness (caisson disease) a syndrome occurring in people working under high pressure in diving bells or at great depths with breathing apparatus. On return to normal atmospheric pressure nitrogen dissolved in the bloodstream expands to form bubbles, causing pain (the **bends**) and blocking the circulation in small blood vessels in the brain and elsewhere (**decompression sickness**). Pain, paralysis, and other features may be eliminated by returning the victim to a higher atmospheric pressure and reducing this gradually, so causing the bubbles to redissolve. Chronic compressed air illness may cause damage to the bones (**avascular necrosis**), heart, and lungs.

compulsion *n.* an *obsession that takes the form of a motor act, such as repetitive washing based on a fear of contamination.

compulsory admission (in Britain) the entry and detention of a person within an institution without his consent, either because of mental illness (*see* MENTAL HEALTH ACT) or severe social deprivation and self-neglect (*see* SECTION 47). *Compare* VOLUNTARY ADMISSION.

computerized tomography (CT) a specialized form of X-ray examination in which the X-ray source and detector (**CT scanner**) rotate around the object to be scanned and the information obtained can be used to produce cross-sectional images by computer (a **CT scan**). A higher radiation dose is received by the patient than with conventional X-rays, but the diagnostic information obtained outweighs the risk. CT scanning can be used for all parts of the body, but is particularly useful in the head, chest, and abdomen. *See also* SPIRAL CT SCANNING.

conation *n.* the group of mental activities (including drives, will, and *instincts) that leads to purposeful action. *Compare* COGNITION.

conception *n.* **1.** (in gynaecology) the start of pregnancy, when a male germ cell (sperm) fertilizes a female germ cell (ovum) in the *Fallopian tube. **2.** (in psychology) an idea or mental impression.

conceptus *n.* the products of conception: the developing fetus and its enclosing membrane at all stages in the uterus.

concha *n.* (*pl.* **conchae**) (in anatomy) any part resembling a shell. For example, the **concha auriculae** is a depression on the outer surface of the pinna (auricle), which

leads to the external auditory meatus of the outer ear. *See also* NASAL CONCHA.

concordance *n.* similarity of any physical characteristic that is found in both of a pair of twins.

concretion *n.* a stony mass formed within such an organ as the kidney, especially the coating of an internal organ (or a foreign body, such as a urinary catheter) with calcium salts. *See also* CALCULUS.

concussion *n.* a condition caused by injury to the head, characterized by headache, confusion, and amnesia. These symptoms may be prolonged and constitute a **post-concussional syndrome**. There may be no recognizable structural damage to the brain, but scans may reveal evidence of *contusion (bruising) within the brain. Repeated concussion eventually causes symptoms suggesting brain damage. *See also* PUNCH DRUNK SYNDROME.

condenser *n.* (in microscopy) an arrangement of lenses beneath the stage of a microscope. It can be adjusted to provide correct focusing of light on the microscope slide.

conditioned reflex a reflex in which the response occurs not to the sensory stimulus that normally causes it but to a separate stimulus, which has been learnt to be associated with it. In Pavlov's classic experiments, dogs learned to associate the sound of a bell with feeding time and would salivate at the bell's sound whether food was then presented to them or not.

conditioning *n.* the establishment of new behaviour by modifying the stimulus/response associations. In **classical conditioning** a stimulus not normally associated with a particular response is presented together with the stimulus that evokes the response automatically. This is repeated until the first stimulus evokes the response by itself (*see* CONDITIONED REFLEX). In **operant conditioning** a response is rewarded (or punished) each time it occurs, so that in time it comes to occur more (or less) frequently (*see* REINFORCEMENT).

condom *n.* a sheath made of latex rubber, plastic, or silk that is fitted over the penis during sexual intercourse. Use of a condom protects both partners against sexually transmitted diseases (including AIDS) and, carefully used, it is a reasonably reliable contraceptive (between 2 and 10 pregnancies per 100 woman-years). A more recent development is the **female condom** (e.g. **Femidom**), which is fitted into the vagina. Manufactured from similar materials as male condoms, they too act as both contraceptives and as barriers to sexually transmitted diseases.

conduct disorder a repetitive and persistent pattern of aggressive or otherwise antisocial behaviour. It is usually recognized in childhood or adolescence and can lead to a *dyssocial or impulsive personality disorder. Treatment is usually with *behaviour therapy or *family therapy.

condylarthrosis (condyloid joint) n. a form of *diarthrosis (freely movable joint) in which an ovoid head fits into an elliptical cavity. Examples are the knee joint and the joint between the mandible (lower jaw) and the temporal bone of the skull.

condyle n. a rounded protuberance that occurs at the ends of some bones, e.g. the *occipital bone, and forms an articulation with another bone.

condyloma n. (pl. **condylomata**) a raised wartlike growth. **Condylomata accuminata** (sing. **condyloma acuminatum**) are warts caused by *human papillomavirus and are found on the vulva, under the foreskin, or on the skin of the anal region. They may be treated with podophyllin or trichloracetic acid; patients should be checked for the presence of other sexually transmitted diseases. **Condylomata lata** (sing. **condyloma latum**) are flat plaques found in the secondary stage of syphilis, occurring in the anogenital region.

cone n. one of the two types of light-sensitive cells in the *retina of the eye (compare ROD). The human retina contains 6–7 million cones; they function best in bright light and are essential for acute vision (receiving a sharp accurate image). The area of the retina called the *fovea contains the greatest concentration of cones. Cones can also distinguish colours. It is thought that there are three types of cone, each sensitive to the wavelength of a different primary colour – red, green, or blue.

Other colours are seen as combinations of these three primary colours.

cone biopsy surgical removal, via a colposcope, of a cone-shaped segment of tissue from the cervix of the uterus. It may be performed if a cervical smear reveals evidence of *cervical intraepithelial neoplasia (CIN): the affected tissue is removed and examined microscopically for confirmation of the diagnosis.

confabulation n. the invention of circumstantial but fictitious detail about events supposed to have occurred in the past. Usually this is to disguise an inability to remember past events. It may be a symptom of any form of loss of memory, but typically occurs in *Korsakoff's syndrome.

confection n. (in pharmacy) a sweet substance that is combined with a medicinal preparation to make it suitable for administration.

conflict n. (in psychology) the state produced when a stimulus produces two opposing reactions. The basic types of conflict situation are **approach–approach**, in which the individual is drawn towards two attractive – but mutually incompatible – goals; **approach–avoidance**, where the stimulus evokes reactions both to approach and to avoid; and **avoidance–avoidance**, in which the avoidance reaction to one stimulus would bring the individual closer to an equally unpleasant stimulus. Conflict has been used to explain the development of neurotic disorders, and the resolution of conflict remains an important part of psychoanalysis. See also CONVERSION.

confluence n. a point of coalescence. The **confluence of the sinuses** is the meeting point of the superior sagittal, transverse, straight, and occipital venous sinuses in the dura mater in the occipital region of the skull.

congenital adj. describing a condition that is recognized at birth or that is believed to have been present since birth. Congenital malformations include all disorders present at birth whether they are inherited or caused by an environmental factor.

congenital dislocation of the hip

(CDH) an abnormality present at birth in which the head of the femur is displaced or easily displaceable from the acetabulum (socket) of the ilium, which is poorly developed; it frequently affects both hip joints. CDH occurs in about 1.5 per 1000 live births, being more common in first-born girls, in breech deliveries, and if there is a family history of the condition. The leg is shortened and has a reduced range of movement, and the skin creases may be asymmetrical. All babies are routinely screened for CDH at birth and at developmental check-ups by gentle manipulation of the hip causing it to be reduced and dislocated with a clunk (see BARLOW'S SIGN, ORTOLANI MANOEUVRE). The diagnosis is confirmed by X-ray or ultrasound scan. Treatment is with a special harness holding the hip reduced. If this is unsuccessful, the hip is reduced under anaesthetic and held with a plaster of Paris cast or the defect is corrected by surgery. Successful treatment of an infant can give a normal hip; if the dislocation is not detected, the hip does not develop normally and osteoarthritis develops at a young age.

congestion *n.* an accumulation of blood within an organ, which is the result of back pressure within its veins (for example congestion of the lungs and of the liver occurs in heart failure). Congestion may be associated with *oedema (accumulation of fluid in the tissues). It is relieved by treatment of the cause.

Congo red a dark-red or reddish-brown pigment that becomes blue in acidic conditions. It is used as a histological *stain. *Amyloidosis is indicated if over 60% of the dye disappears from the blood within one hour of injection.

coniine *n.* an extremely poisonous alkaloid, found in hemlock (*Conium maculatum*), that paralyses the nerves, mainly the motor nerves. Coniine has been included in drug preparations for the treatment of asthma and whooping cough.

coning *n.* prolapse of the brainstem through the *foramen magnum as a result of raised intracranial pressure: it is usually immediately fatal. A similar emergency can occur through the hiatus of the *tentorium.

conization *n.* surgical removal of a cone of tissue. The technique is commonly used in excising a portion of the cervix (neck) of the uterus (see CONE BIOPSY) for the treatment of cervicitis or early cancer (carcinoma in situ).

conjoined twins see SIAMESE TWINS.

conjugate (conjugate diameter, true conjugate) *n.* the distance between the front and rear of the pelvis measured from the most prominent part of the sacrum to the back of the pubic symphysis. Since the true conjugate cannot normally be measured during life it is estimated by subtracting 1.3–1.9 cm from the **diagonal conjugate**, the distance between the lower edge of the symphysis and the sacrum (usually about 12.7 cm). If the true conjugate is less than about 10.2 cm, delivery of an infant through the natural passages may be difficult or impossible, and *Caesarean section may have to be performed.

conjugation *n.* the union of two microorganisms in which genetic material (DNA) passes from one organism to the other. In some bacteria a minute projection on the donor 'male' cell (a **pilus**) forms a bridge with the recipient 'female' cell through which the DNA is transferred. Conjugation is comparable to sexual reproduction in higher organisms.

conjunctiva *n.* the delicate mucous membrane that covers the front of the eye and lines the inside of the eyelids. The conjunctiva lining the eyelids contains many blood vessels but that over the eyeball contains few and is transparent. —**conjunctival** *adj.*

conjunctivitis (pink eye) *n.* inflammation of the conjunctiva, which becomes red and swollen and produces a watery or pus-containing discharge. It causes discomfort rather than pain and does not usually affect vision. Conjunctivitis may be caused by infection by bacteria or viruses (in which case it usually spreads rapidly to the other eye) or physical or chemical irritation. The patient usually recovers with no after-effects in one to three weeks; bacterial infections respond to antibiotic eye drops. **Allergic** (or **vernal**) **conjunctivitis** is acute or chronic inflammation of the cornea usually due to a specific allergen, such as pollen, animal danders, or dust. It is characterized by itching, irritation, redness, watering of the eyes, and light sensitivity. *See also* INCLUSION CONJUNCTIVITIS, TRACHOMA.

connective tissue the tissue that supports, binds, or separates more specialized tissues and organs or functions as a packing tissue of the body. It consists of an amorphous **ground substance** of mucopolysaccharides in which may be embedded white (collagenous), yellow (elastic), and reticular fibres, fat cells, *fibroblasts, *mast cells, and *macrophages (see illustration). Variations in chemical composition of the ground substance and in the proportions and quantities of cells and fibres give rise to tissues of widely differing characteristics, including bone, cartilage, tendons, and ligaments as well as *adipose, *areolar, and *elastic tissues.

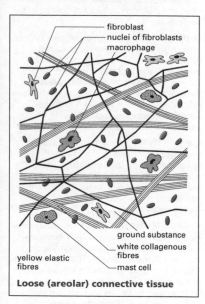

fibroblast
nuclei of fibroblasts
macrophage

ground substance
white collagenous fibres
yellow elastic fibres
mast cell

Loose (areolar) connective tissue

connective-tissue disease any one of a group of diseases that are characterized by inflammatory changes in connective tissue and can affect virtually any body system. Formerly known as **collagen diseases** (connective-tissue disease has been the preferred term since 1978), they include *dermatomyositis, systemic and discoid *lupus erythematosus, *morphoea, *polyarteritis nodosa, and *rheumatoid arthritis.

Conn's syndrome the combination of muscular weakness, abnormally intense thirst (polydipsia), the production of large volumes of urine (polyuria), and hypertension, resulting from excessive production of the hormone aldosterone by the adrenal cortex. 2% of cases of hypertension are due to it. [W. J. Conn (1907–94), US physician]

consanguinity *n.* relationship by blood; the sharing of a common ancestor within a few generations.

conservative treatment treatment aimed at preventing a condition from becoming worse, in the expectation that either natural healing will occur or progress of the disease will be so slow that no drastic treatment will be justified. *Compare* RADICAL TREATMENT.

consolidation *n.* **1.** the state of the lung in which the alveoli (air sacs) are filled with fluid produced by inflamed tissue, as in *pneumonia. It is diagnosed from its dullness to *percussion, bronchial breathing (*see* BREATH SOUNDS) in the patient, and from the distribution of shadows on the chest X-ray. **2.** the stage of repair of a broken bone following *callus formation, during which the callus is transformed by *osteoblasts into mature bone.

constipation *n.* a condition in which bowel evacuations occur infrequently, or in which the faeces are hard and small, or where passage of faeces causes difficulty or pain. The frequency of bowel evacuation varies considerably from person to person and the normal cannot be precisely defined. Constipation developing in a person of previously regular bowel habit may be a symptom of intestinal disease. Recurrent or longstanding constipation is treated by increasing *dietary fibre (roughage), *laxatives, or *enemas. **Faecal impaction**, the end-result of chronic constipation common in senile patients, often requires manual removal of the faecal bolus under an anaesthetic.

constrictor *n.* any muscle that compresses an organ or causes a hollow organ or part to contract.

consultant *n.* a fully trained specialist in a branch of medicine who accepts total responsibility for patient care. In Britain consultants are usually responsible for the care of patients in hospital wards but they are allowed to opt for some sessions in private practice in addition to any National Health Service commitments. After registration, doctors continuing in hospital service are appointed as **senior house officers** and then obtain a **specialist registrar** post (which replaces the old registrar and senior registrar posts) in their chosen specialty. When a specialist registrar has successfully completed a defined college or faculty specialist training programme, he or she is awarded a **Certificate of Completion of Specialist Training** (**CCST**) and is eligible to apply for a consultant post. Doctors who do not complete full specialist training may work in hospitals in subconsultant grades with a variety of titles carrying increasing responsibility, such as **clinical assistant**, **staff grade**, and **associate specialist**. *See also* DOCTOR.

Consultant in Communicable Disease Control (**CCDC**) a consultant within a Health Authority who is responsible for the surveillance, prevention, and control of communicable disease and noncommunicable environmental exposures.

consumption *n.* any disease causing wasting of tissues, especially (formerly) pulmonary tuberculosis. —**consumptive** *adj.*

contact *n.* transmission of an infectious disease by touching or handling an infected person or animal (**direct contact**) or by **indirect contact** with airborne droplets, faeces, etc., containing the infective microorganism.

contact lenses lenses worn directly against the eye, separated from it only by a film of tear fluid. **Corneal microlenses** cover only the cornea, while **haptic lenses** cover some of the surrounding sclera as well. Contact lenses are used mainly in place of glasses to correct long- and shortsightedness and other errors of refraction, but **bandage contact lenses** may be used in a protective capacity to relieve the pain

of a damaged cornea or as part of the treatment of some types of corneal disease. Contact lenses may be made of hard or soft materials, which have very different properties. Hard Perspex lenses have been partly replaced by gas-permeable lenses, which allow oxygen to pass from the atmosphere to the cornea.

contact therapy a form of *radiotherapy in which a radioactive substance is brought into close contact with the part of the body being treated. Needles or capsules of the isotope may be implanted in or around a tumour so that the radiation they emit will destroy it. *Compare* TELECURIETHERAPY.

contagious disease originally, a disease transmitted only by direct physical contact: now usually taken to mean any *communicable disease.

continent diversion *see* URINARY DIVERSION.

contra- *prefix denoting* against or opposite. Example: **contraversion** (turning away from).

contraception *n.* the prevention of unwanted pregnancy, which can be achieved by various means. Hormonal contraceptives (oestrogen and progestogen or progestogen only) act by preventing ovulation. They are usually taken in regular doses in the form of the Pill (*see* ORAL CONTRACEPTIVE), but may also be administered through the skin, by means of an adhesive patch impregnated with the hormones, or by three- or two-monthly injections of a long-acting progestogen. Recently developed methods for continuous administration of the hormones are subcutaneous implants of progestogen, e.g. *levonorgestrel (Norplant); hormonal intrauterine devices (*see* IUS); and vaginal rings containing progestogen, which is released over a period of three months. Methods that aim to prevent fertilization of the ovum include *coitus interruptus, the *condom, the *diaphragm, and surgical intervention (tubal occlusion and vasectomy: *see* STERILIZATION). Methods that aim to prevent implantation of a fertilized ovum in the uterus include the intrauterine contraceptive device (*see* IUCD); these methods can be used after intercourse but before implantation (*see* POST-

COITAL CONTRACEPTION). Couples whose religious beliefs forbid the use of mechanical or hormonal contraceptives may use the *rhythm method, in which intercourse is limited to those days in the menstrual cycle when conception is least likely.

contraction n. the shortening of a muscle in response to a motor nerve impulse. This generates tension in the muscle, usually causing movement.

contracture n. *fibrosis of muscle or connective tissue producing shortening and resulting in deformity of a joint. See also DUPUYTREN'S CONTRACTURE, VOLKMANN'S CONTRACTURE.

contraindication n. any factor in a patient's condition that makes it unwise to pursue a certain line of treatment. For example, an attack of pneumonia in a patient would be a strong contraindication against the use of a general anaesthetic.

contralateral adj. on or affecting the opposite side of the body: applied particularly to paralysis (or other symptoms) occurring on the opposite side of the body from the brain lesion that caused them.

contrast medium any substance that is used to improve the visibility of structures during radiography. Barium, given orally or as an enema to show up the alimentary tract on X-ray, is an example of a contrast medium. Air is occasionally useful as a contrast medium; it may be used to displace the cerebrospinal fluid during X-ray examination of the ventricles of the brain. See also RADIOPAQUE.

contrecoup n. injury of a part resulting from a blow on its opposite side. This may happen, for example, if a blow on the back of the head causes the front of the brain to be pushed against the inner surface of the skull.

controlled drug see MISUSE OF DRUGS ACT 1971.

contusion n. 1. see BRUISE. 2. any of various degrees of bruising of the brain (**cerebral contusion**), resulting from *head injury or surgery. Clinical signs range from *concussion to *coma, reflecting the severity of the trauma.

conus arteriosus the front upper portion of the right ventricle adjoining the pulmonary arteries.

conus medullaris the conical end of the spinal cord, at the level of the lower end of the first lumbar vertebra.

convergence n. 1. (in neurology) the formation of nerve tracts by fibres coming together into one pathway from different regions of the brain. 2. (in ophthalmology) the ability of the eyes to turn inwards and focus on a near point so that a single image is formed on both retinas. The closer the object, the greater the degree of convergence.

conversion n. (in psychiatry) the expression of *conflict as physical symptoms. Psychoanalysts believe that the repressed instinctual drive is manifested as motor or sensory loss, such as paralysis, rather than as speech or action. This is thought to be one of the ways in which *conversion disorder is produced.

conversion disorder a psychological conflict or need that manifests itself as an organic dysfunction or physical symptom. The sufferer may display symptoms of blindness, deafness, loss of sensation, gait abnormalities, or paralysis of various parts of the body. None of these can be accounted for by organic disease. Conversion disorder was formerly known as *hysteria. It is classified with *dissociative disorders (as dissociative (conversion) disorders) in ICD-10 (see INTERNATIONAL CLASSIFICATION OF DISEASES). It is also included under the classification of *somatoform disorders.

convolution n. a folding or twisting, such as one of the many that cause the fissures, sulci, and gyri of the surface of the *cerebrum.

convulsion n. an involuntary contraction of the muscles producing contortion of the body and limbs. Rhythmic convulsions of the limbs are a feature of major *epilepsy. *Febrile convulsions are provoked by fever in otherwise healthy infants and young children.

Cooley's anaemia see THALASSAEMIA. [T. B. Cooley (1871–1945), US paediatrician]

Coombs' test a means of detecting rhesus antibodies on the surface of red blood cells that precipitate proteins (globulins) in the blood serum. The test is used in the diagnosis of haemolytic *anaemia in babies with rhesus incompatibility in whom there is destruction of red blood cells. [R. R. A. Coombs (1921–), British immunologist]

copr- (copro-) *prefix denoting* faeces. Example: **coprophobia** (abnormal fear of).

coprolalia *n.* the repetitive speaking of obscene words. It can be involuntary, as part of the *Gilles de la Tourette syndrome.

coprolith *n.* a mass of hard faeces within the colon or rectum, due to chronic constipation. It may become calcified.

coproporphyrin *n.* a *porphyrin compound formed during the synthesis of protoporphyrin IX, a precursor of *haem. Coproporphyrin is excreted in the faeces in **hereditary coproporphyria.**

co-proxamol *n.* an *analgesic drug consisting of a combination of the drug *paracetamol and the weakly narcotic drug *dextropropoxyphene. It is administered by mouth. Possible side-effects include dizziness, drowsiness, nausea, and vomiting. Trade names: **Distalgesic, Paxalgesic**.

copulation *n. see* COITUS.

cor *n.* the heart.

coracoid process a beaklike process that curves upwards and forwards from the top of the *scapula, over the shoulder joint.

cord *n.* any long flexible structure, which may be solid or tubular. Examples include the spermatic cord, spinal cord, umbilical cord, and vocal cord.

cordectomy *n.* surgical removal of a vocal cord or, more usually, a piece of the vocal cord (**partial cordectomy**).

cordocentesis *n.* the removal of a sample of fetal blood by inserting a hollow needle through the abdominal wall of a pregnant woman, under ultrasound guidance, into the umbilical vein. The blood is subjected to chromosome analysis and biochemical and other tests to determine the presence of abnormalities. *See also* PRENATAL DIAGNOSIS.

cordotomy *n.* a surgical procedure for the relief of severe and persistent pain in the pelvis or lower limbs. The nerve fibres that transmit the sensation of pain to consciousness pass up the spinal cord in special tracts (the **spinothalamic tracts**). In cordotomy the spinothalamic tracts are severed in the cervical (neck) region.

Cordylobia *n. see* TUMBU FLY.

core-and-cluster *n.* a form of housing for handicapped or subnormal people. Institutional organizations are replaced by small self-contained living units associated with a central facility providing more intensive resources.

corectopia *n.* displacement of the pupil towards one side from its normal position in the centre of the iris. When present from birth, the displacement is usually inwards towards the nose. Scarring of the iris from inflammation may also draw the pupil out of position.

corium *n. see* DERMIS.

corn *n.* an area of hard thickened skin on or between the toes: a type of *callosity produced by ill-fitting shoes. The horny skin layers form an inverted pyramid that presses down into the deeper skin layers, causing pain. A corn may be treated by applying salicylic acid or by chiropody. Medical name: **clavus**.

cornea *n.* the transparent circular part of the front of the eyeball. It refracts the light entering the eye onto the lens, which then focuses it onto the retina. The cornea contains no blood vessels and it is extremely sensitive to pain. The innermost layer (**corneal endothelium**) consists of a single layer of cells that cannot regenerate. —**corneal** *adj.*

corneal graft *see* KERATOPLASTY.

corneal ring a ring designed to be inserted into the peripheral tissue of the cornea in order to alter the curvature of the corneal surface. It is undergoing trials to assess its ability to correct errors of refraction. In myopia (short-sightedness), for example, the ring would be required to stretch the corneal tissue peripherally and thus flatten the central corneal curvature in order to correct the myopia.

cornification *n. see* KERATINIZATION.

cornu *n.* (*pl.* **cornua**) (in anatomy) a horn-shaped structure, such as the horn-shaped processes of the hyoid bone and thyroid cartilage. *See also* HORN.

corona *n.* a crown or crownlike structure. The **corona capitis** is the crown of the head.

coronal *adj.* relating to the crown of the head or of a tooth. The **coronal plane** divides the body into dorsal and ventral parts (see illustration).

Coronal plane of section through the body

coronal suture *see* SUTURE.

corona radiata 1. a series of radiating fibres between the cerebral cortex and the internal capsule of the brain. 2. a layer of follicle cells that surrounds a freshly ovulated ovum. The cells are elongated radially to the ovum when seen in section.

coronary angioplasty a procedure, not requiring *thoracotomy, in which a segment of coronary artery narrowed by atheroma is stretched by the inflation of a balloon introduced into it by means of cardiac *catheterization under X-ray screening (*see* ANGIOPLASTY). The site of the obstruction is identified by prior *angio-cardiography. Not all narrowed segments can be improved by angioplasty. *See also* CORONARY BYPASS GRAFT.

coronary arteries the arteries supplying blood to the heart. The **right** and **left coronary arteries** arise from the aorta, just above the aortic valve, and form branches encircling the heart. *See* CORONARY ANGIOPLASTY, CORONARY BYPASS GRAFT.

coronary bypass graft *coronary revascularization in which a segment of a coronary artery narrowed by atheroma is bypassed by an autologous section of healthy saphenous vein or internal mammary artery at *thoracotomy. The improved blood flow resulting from one or more such grafts relieves *angina pectoris and reduces the risk of *myocardial infarction. Recently developed techniques of *minimally invasive surgery have enabled the operation to be performed without the need for thoracotomy.

coronary revascularization a surgical method of improving the blood flow through coronary arteries narrowed by atheroma. *See* CORONARY BYPASS GRAFT.

coronary thrombosis the formation of a blood clot (thrombus) in the coronary artery, which obstructs the flow of blood to the heart. This is usually due to *atheroma and results in the death (infarction) of part of the heart muscle. For symptoms and treatment *see* MYOCARDIAL INFARCTION.

coroner *n.* the official who presides at an *inquest. He must be either a medical practitioner or a lawyer of at least five years' standing.

coronoid process 1. a process on the upper end of the *ulna. It forms part of the notch that articulates with the humerus. 2. the process on the ramus of the *mandible to which the temporalis muscle is attached.

cor pulmonale enlargement of the

right ventricle of the heart that results from diseases of the lungs or the pulmonary arteries. Such diseases include those affecting the structure of the lungs (e.g. emphysema) or their function (e.g. obesity) except when these changes result from congenital heart disease or diseases primarily affecting the left side of the heart.

corpus *n.* (*pl.* **corpora**) any mass of tissue that can be distinguished from its surroundings.

corpus albicans the residual body of scar tissue that remains in the ovary at the point where a *corpus luteum has regressed after its secretory activity has ceased.

corpus callosum the broad band of nervous tissue that connects the two cerebral hemispheres, containing an estimated 300 million fibres. *See* CEREBRUM.

corpus cavernosum either of a pair of cylindrical blood sinuses that form the erectile tissue of the *penis and clitoris. In the penis a third sinus, the corpus spongiosum, encloses the urethra and extends into the glans. All these sinuses have a spongelike structure that allows them to expand when filled with blood.

corpuscle *n.* any small particle, cell, or mass of tissue.

corpus luteum the glandular tissue in the ovary that forms at the site of a ruptured *Graafian follicle after ovulation. It secretes the hormone *progesterone, which prepares the uterus for implantation. If implantation fails the corpus luteum becomes inactive and degenerates. If an embryo becomes implanted the corpus luteum continues to secrete progesterone until the fourth month of pregnancy, by which time the placenta has taken over this function.

corpus spongiosum the blood sinus that surrounds the urethra of the male. Together with the corpora cavernosa, it forms the erectile tissue of the *penis. It is expanded at the base of the penis to form the urethral bulb and at the tip to form the glans penis.

corpus striatum the part of the *basal ganglia in the cerebral hemispheres of the brain consisting of the caudate nucleus and the lentiform nucleus.

correlation *n.* (in statistics) the extent to which one of a pair of characteristics affects the other in a series of individuals. Such pairs of observations can be plotted as a series of points on a graph. If all the points on the resulting **scatter diagram** are in a straight line (which is neither horizontal nor vertical), the **correlation coefficient** may vary within the range of +1, where an increase of one variable is always associated with the corresponding increase in the other, to −1, where an increase of one variable is associated with a constant decrease of the other; a coefficient of 0 indicates no dependence of the one characteristic on the other of a straight line type. The **regression coefficient** is the average extent to which a unit increase of one characteristic influences the increase/decrease of the other. Where several factors appear to correlate with the onset of disease the relative importance of each may be calculated by the statistical technique known as **multivariate analysis**.

Corrigan's pulse (collapsing pulse) a type of pulse that has an exaggerated rise followed by a sudden fall. It is typical of aortic valve incompetence. [Sir D. J. Corrigan (1802–80), Irish physician]

cortex *n.* (*pl.* **cortices**) the outer part of an organ, situated immediately beneath its capsule or outer membrane; for example, the **adrenal cortex** (*see* ADRENAL GLANDS), **renal cortex** (*see* KIDNEY), or *cerebral cortex. —**cortical** *adj.*

corticosteroid (corticoid) *n.* any steroid hormone synthesized by the adrenal cortex. There are two main groups of corticosteroids. The **glucocorticoids** (e.g. *cortisol, *cortisone, and corticosterone) are essential for the utilization of carbohydrate, fat, and protein by the body and for a normal response to stress. Naturally occurring and synthetic glucocorticoids have very powerful anti-inflammatory effects and are used to treat conditions that involve inflammation. The **mineralocorticoids** (e.g. *aldosterone) are necessary for the regulation of salt and water balance.

corticosterone *n.* a steroid hormone (*see*

CORTICOSTEROID) synthesized and released in small amounts by the adrenal cortex.

corticotrophin n. see ACTH.

cortisol n. a steroid hormone: the major glucocorticoid synthesized and released by the human adrenal cortex (see CORTICO-STEROID). It is important for normal carbohydrate metabolism and for the normal response to any stress. See also HYDROCORTI-SONE.

cortisone n. a naturally occurring *corticosteroid that is used mainly to treat deficiency of corticosteroid hormones in *Addison's disease and following surgical removal of the adrenal glands. It is administered by mouth or injection and may cause serious side-effects such as stomach ulcers and bleeding, nervous and hormone disturbances, muscle and bone damage, and eye changes.

cor triloculare a rare congenital condition in which there are three instead of four chambers of the heart due to the presence of a single common ventricle. *Cyanosis (blueness) is common. Most patients die in infancy.

Corynebacterium n. a genus of Gram-positive, mostly aerobic, nonmotile rodlike bacteria that frequently bear club-shaped swellings. Many species cause disease in man, domestic animals, birds, and plants; some are found in dairy products. The species C. diphtheriae (**Klebs-Loeffler bacillus**) is the causative organism of *diphtheria, producing a powerful *exotoxin that is harmful to heart and nerve tissue. It occurs in one of three forms: gravis, intermedius, and mitis.

coryza (cold in the head) n. a catarrhal inflammation of the mucous membrane in the nose due to either a *cold or *hay fever. See also CATARRH.

COSHH (control of substances hazardous to health) (in occupational health) legislation and resulting regulations concerning the duties and responsibilities of employers and employees to ensure that **hazardous substances** used in a workplace (e.g. toxic chemicals in factories, anaesthetic gases in operating theatres, carbonaceous dust arising from photocopying machines in offices) do not affect adversely the operatives themselves or their colleagues.

cost- (costo-) prefix denoting the ribs. Example: **costectomy** (excision of).

costal adj. of or relating to the ribs.

costal cartilage a cartilage that connects a *rib to the breastbone (*sternum). The first seven ribs (true ribs) are directly connected to the sternum by individual costal cartilages. The next three ribs are indirectly connected to the sternum by three costal cartilages, each of which is connected to the one immediately above it.

costalgia n. pain localized to the ribs. This term is now rarely used.

costive adj. constipated.

costochondritis n. see TIETZE'S SYNDROME.

cot death (sudden infant death syndrome, SIDS) the sudden unexpected death of an infant less than two years old (peak occurrence between two and six months) from an unidentifiable cause. There appear to be many factors involved, the most important of which is the position in which the baby is laid to sleep: babies who sleep on their fronts (the prone position) have an increased risk. Other factors increasing the risk include parental smoking, overheating with bedding, prematurity, and a history of cot death within the family. About half the affected infants will have had a viral upper respiratory tract infection within the 48 hours preceding their death, many of these being due to the *respiratory syncytial virus. See also APNOEA MONITOR.

co-trimoxazole n. an antibacterial drug consisting of *sulphamethoxazole and *trimethoprim. Since both these drugs are well absorbed and rapidly excreted – and each potentiates the action of the other – co-trimoxazole is taken by mouth and is particularly useful for treating urinary-tract, respiratory-tract, and gastrointestinal infections. Because of the severity of the side-effects, which are those of the *sulphonamides, co-trimoxazole is now less frequently prescribed than formerly. Trade names: **Bactrim, Septrin**.

cotton-wool spots accumulations of

*axoplasm in the nerve-fibre layer of the retina, which indicate disease (e.g. hypertension, connective-tissue disease, or AIDS).

cotyledon *n.* any of the major convex subdivisions of the mature *placenta. Each cotyledon contains a major branch of the umbilical blood vessels, which branch further into the numerous villi that make up the surface of the cotyledon.

cotyloid cavity *see* ACETABULUM.

couching *n.* an operation for cataract in which the lens is pushed out of the pupil downwards and backwards into the jelly-like vitreous humour by a small knife inserted through the edge of the cornea. It was widely employed in ancient Hindu civilizations and has been practised ever since. Its sole advantage is speed of performance, but modern developments in surgery and anaesthesia leave little place for it today.

coughing *n.* a form of violent exhalation by which irritant particles in the airways can be expelled. Stimulation of the cough reflexes results in the glottis being kept closed until a high expiratory pressure has built up, which is then suddenly released. Medical name: **tussis**.

coulomb *n.* the *SI unit of electric charge, equal to the quantity of electricity transferred by 1 ampere in 1 second. Symbol: C.

coumarin *n.* a drug used to prevent coagulation in the treatment of thrombophlebitis and pulmonary embolism. The main side-effect is haemorrhage.

counselling *n.* **1.** a method of approaching psychological difficulties in adjustment that aims to help the client work out his own problems. The counsellor listens sympathetically, attempting to identify with the client, tries to clarify current problems, and sometimes gives advice. It involves less emphasis on insight and interpretation than does psychotherapy or psychoanalytic therapy. *See also* CLIENT-CENTRED THERAPY. **2.** *see* GENETIC COUNSELLING.

counterextension *n.* *traction on one part of a limb, while the remainder of the limb is held steady: used particularly in the treatment of a fractured femur (thigh bone).

counterirritant *n.* an agent, such as methyl salicylate, that causes irritation when applied to the skin and is used in order to relieve more deep-seated pain or discomfort. —**counterirritation** *n.*

countertraction *n.* the use of an opposing force to balance that being applied during *traction, when a strong continuous pull is applied to a limb so that broken bones can be kept in alignment during healing.

couvade *n.* **1.** a custom in some tribes whereby a father takes to his bed during or after the birth of his child. **2.** a symptom of abdominal pain experienced by a man in relation to his wife's giving birth. It may be due to *conversion disorder, anxiety, or sympathy.

cover-slip *n.* an extremely thin square or circle of glass used to protect the upper surface of a preparation on a microscope slide.

cover test a test used to detect a suppressed *strabismus (squint) in children. The child is asked to look fixedly at an object with one eye while the other is kept open but covered by the hand of the observer. The hand is then withdrawn: if the eye that had been covered is seen to move towards the nose to adjust to the focus of the uncovered eye the child is assumed to have a divergent squint; movement of the eye away from the nose implies a convergent squint.

Cowper's glands (bulbourethral glands) a pair of small glands that open into the urethra at the base of the penis. Their secretion contributes to the seminal fluid, but less than that of the prostate gland or seminal vesicles. [W. Cowper (1660–1709), English surgeon]

cowpox *n.* a virus infection of cows' udders, transmitted to man by direct contact, causing very mild symptoms similar to *smallpox. An attack confers immunity to smallpox. Medical name: **vaccinia**.

cox- (coxo-) *prefix denoting* the hip. Example: **coxalgia** (pain in).

coxa *n.* (*pl.* **coxae**) **1.** the hip bone. **2.** the hip joint.

Coxiella *n.* a genus of rickettsiae that cause disease in animals and man. They are transmitted to man by inhalation and produce disease characterized by inflammation of the lungs, without a rash (*compare* TYPHUS). The single species, *C. burnetii*, causes *Q fever.

Coxsackie virus (echovirus) one of a group of RNA-containing viruses that are able to multiply in the gastrointestinal tract (*see* ENTEROVIRUS). About 30 different types exist. **Type A Coxsackie viruses** generally cause less severe and less well-defined diseases, such as *hand, foot, and mouth disease, although some cause meningitis and severe throat infections (*see* HERPANGINA). **Type B Coxsackie viruses** cause inflammation or degeneration of heart tissue, resulting in pericarditis or myocarditis, or brain tissue, producing meningitis or encephalitis. They can also attack the muscles of the chest wall, the bronchi, pancreas, thyroid, or conjunctiva and recent evidence suggests they may be implicated in diabetes in children and in motor neurone disease. *See also* BORNHOLM DISEASE.

CPA *see* CYPROTERONE.

crab louse *see* PHTHIRUS.

cradle *n.* a framework of metal strips or other material that forms a cage over an injured part of the body of a patient lying in bed, to protect it from the pressure of the bedclothes.

cradle cap a common condition in young babies in which crusty white or yellow scales form a 'cap' on the scalp. It is treated by applying oil or using a special shampoo and usually resolves in the first year of life, although it may represent the start of seborrhoeic *eczema.

cramp *n.* prolonged painful contraction of a muscle. It is sometimes caused by an imbalance of the salts in the body, but is more often a result of fatigue, imperfect posture, or stress. Spasm in the muscles making it impossible to perform a specific task but allowing the use of these muscles for any other movement is called **occupational cramp**. It most often affects the hand muscles for writing (**writer's cramp**).

crani- (cranio-) *prefix denoting* the skull. Example: **cranioplasty** (plastic surgery of).

cranial nerves the 12 pairs of nerves that arise directly from the brain and leave the skull through separate apertures; they are conventionally given Roman numbers, as follows: I *olfactory; II *optic; III *oculomotor; IV *trochlear; V *trigeminal; VI *abducens; VII *facial; VIII *vestibulocochlear; IX *glossopharyngeal; X *vagus; XI *accessory; XII *hypoglossal. *Compare* SPINAL NERVES.

craniometry *n.* the science of measuring the differences in size and shape of skulls.

craniopagus (dicephalus) *n.* *Siamese twins united by their heads.

craniopharyngioma *n.* a brain tumour derived from remnants of **Rathke's pouch**, an embryologic structure from which the pituitary gland is partly formed. The patient may show raised intracranial pressure and *diabetes insipidus due to reduced secretion of the hormone *vasopressin. An X-ray of the skull typically shows calcification within the tumour and loss of the normal skull structure around the pituitary gland.

craniostenosis *n.* premature closing of the *sutures between the cranial bones during development, resulting in the skull remaining abnormally small. *Compare* CRANIOSYNOSTOSIS.

craniosynostosis *n.* premature fusion of some of the cranial bones, usually before birth, so that the skull is unable to expand in certain directions to assume its normal shape under the influence of the growing brain. Depending on which cranial *sutures fuse early, the skull may become elongated from front to back, broad and short, peaked (**oxycephaly** or **turricephaly**), or asymmetrical. *Compare* CRANIOSTENOSIS.

craniotomy *n.* **1.** surgical removal of a portion of the skull, performed to expose the brain and *meninges for inspection or biopsy or to relieve excessive intracranial pressure (as in a subdural *haematoma). **2.** surgical perforation of the skull of a dead fetus during difficult labour, so that delivery may continue.

For both operations the instrument used is called a **craniotome**.

cranium *n.* the part of the skeleton that encloses the brain. It consists of eight bones connected together by immovable joints (*see* SKULL). —**cranial** *adj.*

creatinase (creatine kinase) *n.* an enzyme involved in the metabolic breakdown of creatine to creatinine.

creatine *n.* a product of protein metabolism found in muscle. Its phosphate, **creatine phosphate (phosphocreatine, phosphagen)**, acts as a store of high-energy phosphate in muscle and serves to maintain adequate amounts of *ATP (the source of energy for muscular contraction).

creatinine *n.* a substance derived from creatine and creatine phosphate in muscle. Creatinine is excreted in the urine.

creatinuria *n.* an excess of the nitrogenous compound creatine in the urine.

creatorrhoea *n.* the passage of excessive nitrogen in the faeces due to failure of digestion or absorption in the small intestine. It is found particularly in pancreatic failure. *See* CYSTIC FIBROSIS, PANCREATITIS.

Credé's method a technique for expelling the placenta from the uterus. With the uterus contracted, downward pressure is applied to it through the abdominal wall in the direction of the birth canal. This method has now been largely replaced by the *Brandt Andrews method. [K. S. F. Credé (1819–92), German gynaecologist]

creeping eruption (larva migrans) a skin disease caused either by larvae of certain nematode worms (e.g. *Ancylostoma braziliense*) normally parasitic in dogs and cats or by the maggots of certain flies (*see* HYPODERMA, GASTEROPHILUS). The larvae burrow within the skin tissues, their movements marked by long thin red lines that cause the patient intense irritation. The nematode infections are treated with diethylcarbamazine or thiabendazole; maggots can be surgically removed.

crenation *n.* an abnormal appearance of red blood cells seen under a microscope, in which the normally smooth cell margins appear crinkly or irregular. Crenation may be a feature of certain blood disorders, but most commonly occurs as a result of prolonged storage of a blood specimen prior to preparation of a blood film.

crepitation (rale) *n.* a soft fine crackling sound heard in the lungs through the stethoscope. Crepitations are made either by air passages and alveoli (air sacs) opening up during inspiration or by air bubbling through fluid. They are not normally heard in healthy lungs.

crepitus *n.* **1.** a crackling sound or grating feeling produced by bone rubbing on bone or roughened cartilage, detected on movement of an arthritic joint. Crepitus in the knee joint is a common sign of *chondromalacia patellae in the young and *osteoarthritis in the elderly. **2.** a similar sound heard with a stethoscope over an inflamed lung when the patient breathes in.

cresol *n.* a strong antiseptic effective against many microorganisms and used mostly in soap solutions as a general disinfectant. It is sometimes used in low concentrations as a preservative in injections. Cresol solutions irritate the skin and if taken by mouth are corrosive and cause pain, nausea, and vomiting.

crest *n.* a ridge or linear protuberance, particularly on a bone. Examples include the crest of fibula and the iliac crest (of the ilium).

CREST syndrome a disease characterized by the association of *calcinosis, *Raynaud's phenomenon, (o)esophageal malfunction, sclerodactyly (tapering fingers), and *telangiectasia. It represents a variant of *systemic sclerosis and may be associated with severe pulmonary hypertension.

cretinism *n.* a syndrome of *dwarfism, mental retardation, and coarseness of the skin and facial features due to lack of thyroid hormone from birth (congenital *hypothyroidism).

Creutzfeldt-Jakob disease (CJD) a rapidly progressive rare neurological disease, a form of human *spongiform encephalopathy in which dementia progresses to death after a period of 3–12 months. There is no effective treatment. The causative agent is currently believed to be an abnormal *prion protein that accumulates in the brain and causes widespread destruction of tissue. CJD typically affects middle-aged to elderly people. Some 15% of cases are due to a form of the disease that is inherited as an autosomal *dominant characteristic but most cases are sporadic, susceptibility being genetically determined. A few cases of CJD are acquired: the agent is known to have been transmitted by tissue and organ transplantation and by human growth hormone injections, but the disease may take years to manifest itself. A new variant form of acquired CJD affecting younger people has been linked with the consumption of meat products containing tissue from cattle infected with bovine spongiform encephalopathy (BSE); however, no causative link has yet been established. [H. G. Creutzfeldt (1885–1964) and A. M. Jakob (1884–1931), German psychiatrists]

cribriform plate *see* ETHMOID BONE.

cricoid cartilage the cartilage, shaped like a signet ring, that forms part of the anterior and lateral walls and most of the posterior wall of the *larynx.

cri-du-chat syndrome a congenital condition of severe mental retardation associated with an abnormal facial appearance, spasticity, and a characteristic catlike cry in infancy. It results from a chromosomal abnormality in which there is a loss (*deletion) of part of the short arm of chromosome no. 5.

Crigler-Najjar syndrome a genetic disease in which the liver enzyme glucuronyl transferase, responsible for dealing with bilirubin, is absent. Large amounts of bilirubin accumulate in the blood, and the child becomes progressively more jaundiced. Life expectancy is usually less than two years. [J. F. Crigler (1919–) and V. A. Najjar (1914–), US paediatricians]

Crile's procedure (or **operation**) the standard radical operation for en-bloc removal of malignant lymph nodes of the neck. [G. W. Crile (1864–1943), US surgeon]

crisis *n.* **1.** the turning point of a disease, after which the patient either improves or deteriorates. Since the advent of antibi-

otics, infections seldom reach the point of crisis. **2.** the occurrence of sudden severe pain in certain diseases. *See also* DIETL'S CRISIS.

crista *n.* (*pl.* **cristae**) **1.** the sensory structure within the ampulla of a *semicircular canal within the inner ear (see illustration). The cristae respond to changes in the rate of movement of the head, being activated by pressure from the fluid in the semicircular canals. **2.** one of the infoldings of the inner membrane of a *mitochondrion. **3.** any anatomical structure resembling a crest.

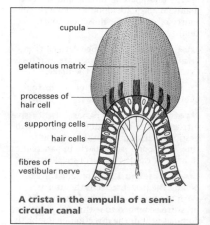

cupula

gelatinous matrix

processes of hair cell

supporting cells

hair cells

fibres of vestibular nerve

A crista in the ampulla of a semicircular canal

Crohn's disease a condition in which segments of the alimentary tract become inflamed, thickened, and ulcerated. It usually affects the terminal part of the ileum; its acute form (**acute ileitis**) may mimic *appendicitis. Chronic disease often causes partial obstruction of the intestine, leading to pain, diarrhoea, and *malabsorption. *Fistulae around the anus, between adjacent loops of intestine, or from intestine to skin, bladder, etc., are characteristic complications. The cause is unknown, but it is thought that an infectious agent might initiate the process (*see* MYCOBACTERIUM). Treatment includes rest, corticosteroids, immunosuppressive drugs, antibiotics, dietary modification, or (in some cases) surgical removal of the affected part of the intestine. Alternative names: **regional enteritis, regional**

ileitis. [B. B. Crohn (1884–1983), US physician]

cromolyn sodium a drug used to prevent and treat asthma and allergic bronchitis. It is administered by inhalation and may cause throat irritation. Trade name: **Intal**.

crossbite n. a condition in which some or all of the lower teeth close outside the upper teeth during normal closure.

cross-dressing n. see TRANSVESTISM.

crossing over (in genetics) the exchange of sections of chromatids that occurs between pairs of homologous chromosomes, which results in the recombination of genetic material. It occurs during *meiosis at a *chiasma.

cross-over trial see INTERVENTION STUDY.

cross-sectional study the collection and analysis of information relating to persons in a population or group at a defined point in time (or within a defined period), with particular reference to their individual characteristics and exposure to factors thought likely to predispose to disease. See also PREVALENCE RATE.

crotamiton n. a drug that destroys mites and is used to treat scabies and similar skin infections and also to relieve itching. It is applied to the skin as a lotion or ointment and sometimes causes reddening and hypersensitivity reactions. Trade name: **Eurax**.

croup n. acute inflammation and obstruction of the respiratory tract, involving the larynx and the main air passages (trachea and bronchi), in young children (usually aged between six months and three years). The usual cause is a virus infection but bacterial secondary infection can occur. The symptoms are those of *laryngitis, accompanied by signs of obstruction – harsh difficult breathing (see STRIDOR), a rising pulse rate, restlessness, and *cyanosis. Treatment by reassurance and humidification of the inspired air usually reverses the alarming symptoms. In severe cases the obstruction may require treatment by *intubation or *tracheostomy. See also EPIGLOTTITIS.

crown n. **1.** the part of a tooth normally visible in the mouth and usually covered by enamel. **2.** a dental *restoration that covers most or all of the natural crown. It may be made of porcelain (sometimes bonded to a metal substructure), gold, a combination of these, or less commonly other materials. Most crowns are like thimbles and are custom made to fit over a trimmed-down tooth. A **post crown** is used to restore a tooth when insufficient of the natural crown remains. A post is inserted into the root and the missing centre of the tooth is built up; over it is fitted a thimble-like crown to restore the natural shape of the tooth. *Root canal treatment is required before a post crown can be made.

crowning n. **1.** the stage of labour when the upper part of the infant's head is encircled by, and just passing through, the vaginal opening. **2.** (in dentistry) the technique of treating and fitting a tooth with an artificial *crown.

cruciate ligaments a pair (anterior and posterior) of ligaments inside each knee joint, which help to prevent excessive anteroposterior glide. Damage to the cruciate ligaments is a common *sports injury, especially in football players.

crude rate the total number of events (e.g. cases of lung cancer) expressed as a percentage (or rate per 1000, etc.) of the whole population. When factors such as age structure or sex of populations may seriously affect their rates (as in *mortality or *morbidity rates) it is more meaningful to compare age/sex specific rates using one or more age groups of a designated sex (e.g. lung cancer in males aged 55–64 years). More complex calculations, which take account of the age bias of a population as a whole, can produce **standardized rates** or – as has been used for deciding resource allocation in the National Health Service – **standardized mortality ratios** (SMR). In these the ratios of subgroups are expressed as percentages of that for a designated or standard population (e.g. England and Wales), particularly applied to the age bracket 15–64 years.

crural adj. **1.** relating to the thigh or leg. **2.** relating to the crura cerebri (see CRUS).

crus n. (pl. **crura**) an elongated process or

part of a structure. The **crus cerebri** is one of two symmetrical nerve tracts situated between the medulla oblongata and the cerebral hemispheres.

crush syndrome kidney failure following massive trauma to, and necrosis of, muscle. It results from acute necrosis of the renal tubules associated with the presence in the blood of *myohaemoglobin, released from the damaged muscle.

cry- (cryo-) *prefix denoting* cold.

cryaesthesia *n.* **1.** exceptional sensitivity to low temperature. **2.** a sensation of coldness.

cryoglobulin *n.* an abnormal protein – an *immunoglobulin (*see* PARAPROTEIN) – that may be present in the blood in certain diseases. Cryoglobulins become insoluble at low temperatures, leading to obstruction of small blood vessels in the fingers and toes in cold weather and producing a characteristic rash. The presence of cryoglobulins (**cryoglobulinaemia**) may be a feature of a variety of diseases, including *macroglobu-linaemia, systemic *lupus erythematosus, and certain infections.

cryoprecipitate *n.* a precipitate produced by freezing and thawing under controlled conditions. An example of a cryoprecipitate is the residue obtained from fresh frozen blood plasma that has been thawed at 4°C. This residue is extremely rich in a clotting factor, Factor VIII (antihaemophilic factor), and is used in the control of bleeding in *haemophilia.

cryopreservation *n.* preservation of tissues by freezing. Cryopreservation of embryos may be employed as part of *in vitro fertilization procedures, for example if there are medical reasons for delaying the pregnancy.

cryoprobe *n.* *see* CRYOSURGERY.

cryoretinopexy *n.* the use of extreme cold to freeze areas of weak or torn retina in order to cause scarring and seal breaks. It is used in *cryosurgery for *retinal detachment.

cryostat *n.* **1.** a chamber in which frozen tissue is sectioned with a *microtome. **2.**

a device for maintaining a specific low temperature.

cryosurgery *n.* the use of extreme cold in a localized part of the body to freeze and destroy unwanted tissues. Cryosurgery is usually undertaken with an instrument called a **cryoprobe**, which has a fine tip cooled by allowing carbon dioxide or nitrous oxide gas to expand within it. Cryosurgery is commonly used for the treatment of retinal detachment (*see* CRYORETINOPEXY), the destruction of certain bone tumours, and the obliteration of skin blemishes.

cryotherapy *n.* the use of cold in the treatment of disorders. *See* CYCLOCRYO-THERAPY, CRYOSURGERY, HYPOTHERMIA. *Compare* THERMOTHERAPY.

crypt *n.* a small sac, follicle, or cavity; for example, the crypts of Lieberkühn (*see* LIEBERKÜHN'S GLANDS), which are intestinal glands.

crypt- (crypto-) *prefix denoting* concealed. Example: **cryptogenic** (of unknown origin).

cryptococcosis (torulosis) *n.* a disease of worldwide distribution, but recognized mainly in the USA, caused by the fungus *Cryptococcus neoformans.* The fungus attacks the lung, resulting in a tumour-like solid mass (**toruloma**), but produces few or no symptoms referable to the lungs. It may spread to the brain, leading to meningitis; this may occur as an opportunistic infection in those suffering from AIDS. The condition responds well to treatment with *amphotericin B.

Cryptococcus *n.* a genus of unicellular yeastlike fungi that cause disease in man. They are found in soil (particularly when enriched with pigeon droppings), and they are common in pigeon roosts and nests. The species *C. neoformans* causes *cryptococcosis.

cryptomenorrhoea *n.* absence of blood flow when the internal symptoms of menstruation are present. The condition may arise because the hymen at the entrance to the vagina lacks an opening (*imperforate hymen) or because of some other obstruction.

cryptophthalmos *n.* apparent absence

of the eyes due to failure of normal eyelid formation during embryonic development, resulting in absence of the opening between the upper and lower eyelids.

cryptorchidism (cryptorchism) *n.* the condition in which the testes fail to descend into the scrotum and are retained within the abdomen or inguinal canal. The operation of *orchidopexy is necessary to bring the testes into the scrotum before puberty in order to allow subsequent normal development; it is thought that the higher temperature in the abdomen interferes with sperm production. —**cryptorchid** *adj., n.*

cryptosporidiosis *n.* an intestinal infection of mammals and birds caused by parasitic protozoa of the genus *Cryptosporidium*, which is usually transmitted to humans via farm animals. Ingestion of water or milk contaminated with infective oocysts results in severe diarrhoea and abdominal cramps, caused by release of a toxin. Most patients recover in 7–14 days, but the disease can persist in the immunocompromised (including AIDS patients), the elderly, and young children.

CSF 1. *see* CEREBROSPINAL FLUID. 2. *see* COLONY-STIMULATING FACTOR.

CS gas a powerful incapacitating gas used in warfare and riot control. The sufferer experiences a burning sensation in the eyes, difficulty in breathing, tightness of the chest, nausea, vomiting, and streaming from the eyes and nose. In confined spaces the gas can prove fatal.

CSOM chronic suppurative otitis media (*see* OTITIS).

CT *see* COMPUTERIZED TOMOGRAPHY.

cubital *adj.* relating to the elbow or forearm; for example the **cubital fossa** is the depression at the front of the elbow.

cuboid bone the outer bone of the *tarsus, which articulates with the fourth and fifth metatarsal bones in front and with the calcaneus (heel bone) behind.

cuirass *n. see* RESPIRATOR.

culdocentesis *n. see* COLPOTOMY.

culdoscope *n.* a tubular instrument with lenses and a light source, used for direct observation of the uterus, ovaries,

and Fallopian tubes (**culdoscopy**). The instrument is passed through the wall of the vagina behind to the neck of the uterus. The culdoscope has now been largely replaced by the *laparoscope.

Culex *n.* a genus of mosquitoes, worldwide in distribution, of which there are some 600 species. Certain species are important as vectors of filariasis (*see also* WUCHERERIA) and viral encephalitis.

culicide *n.* an agent that destroys mosquitoes or gnats.

culmen *n.* an area of the upper surface of the *cerebellum, anterior to the declive and posterior to the central lobule and separated from them by deep fissures.

culture 1. *n.* a population of microorganisms, usually bacteria, grown in a solid or liquid laboratory medium (**culture medium**), which is usually *agar, broth, or *gelatin. A **pure culture** consists of a single bacterial species. A **stab culture** is a bacterial culture growing in a plug of solid medium within a bottle (or tube); the medium is inoculated by 'stabbing' it with a bacteria-coated straight wire. A **stock culture** is a permanent bacterial culture, from which subcultures are made. *See also* TISSUE CULTURE. 2. *vb.* to grow bacteria or other microorganisms in cultures.

cumulative action the toxic effects of a drug produced by repeated administration of small doses at intervals that are not long enough for it to be either broken down or excreted by the body.

cumulus oophoricus a cluster of follicle cells that surround a freshly ovulated ovum. By increasing the effective size of the ovum they may assist its entrance into the end of the Fallopian tube. They are dispersed at fertilization by the contents of the *acrosome.

cuneiform bones three bones in the *tarsus – the **lateral** (external), **intermediate** (middle), and **medial** (internal) cuneiform bones – that articulate respectively with the first, second, and third metatarsal bones in front. All three bones articulate with the navicular bone behind.

cuneus *n.* a wedge-shaped area of *cerebral cortex that forms the inner surface of the occipital lobe.

Cuniculus *n.* a genus of large forest-dwelling rodents, the pacas or spotted cavies, found in South and Central America. In Brazil these animals are a natural reservoir of the parasite *Leishmania braziliensis*, which causes espundia (*see* LEISHMANIASIS).

cupola *n.* **1.** the small dome at the end of the cochlea. **2.** any of several dome-shaped anatomical structures.

cupping *n.* the former practice of applying a heated cup to the skin and allowing it to cool, which causes swelling of the tissues beneath and an increase in the flow of blood in the area. This was thought to draw out harmful excess blood from diseased organs nearby and so promote healing. In **wet cupping** the skin was previously cut, so that blood would actually flow into the cup and could be removed.

cupula *n.* a small dome-shaped structure consisting of sensory hairs embedded in gelatinous material, forming part of a *crista in the ampullae of the semicircular canals of the ear.

curare *n.* an extract from the bark of South American trees (*Strychnos* and *Chondodendron* species) that relaxes and paralyses voluntary muscle. Used for centuries as an arrow poison by South American Indians, curare was formerly employed to control the muscle spasms of tetanus and, more recently, as a muscle relaxant in surgical operations. It has now been replaced in surgery by *tubocurarine.

curettage *n.* the scraping of the skin or the internal surface of an organ or body cavity by means of a spoon-shaped instrument (**curette**), usually to remove diseased tissue or to obtain a specimen for diagnostic purposes (*see also* DILATATION AND CURETTAGE). Curettage of the skin is combined with cauterization; it may be used for the removal of *basal cell carcinoma, seborrhoeic *keratoses, etc., and usually causes little scarring.

curette *n.* a spoon-shaped instrument for scraping tissue from a cavity (*see* CURETTAGE, DILATATION AND CURETTAGE).

curie *n.* a former unit for expressing the activity of a radioactive substance. It has been replaced by the *becquerel. Symbol: Ci.

Curling's ulcers gastric or duodenal ulcers associated with stress from severe injury or major burns. [T. B. Curling (1811–88), British surgeon]

Curschmann's spirals elongated *casts of the smaller bronchi, which are coughed up in bronchial asthma. They unroll to a length of 2 cm or more and have a central core ensheathed in mucus and cell debris. [H. Curschmann (1846–1910), German physician]

Cushing's syndrome the condition resulting from excess amounts of *corticosteroid hormones in the body. Symptoms include weight gain, reddening of the face and neck, excess growth of body and facial hair, raised blood pressure, loss of mineral from the bones (osteoporosis), raised blood glucose levels, and sometimes mental disturbances. The syndrome may be due to overstimulation of the adrenal glands by excessive amounts of the hormone ACTH, secreted either by a tumour of the pituitary gland (**Cushing's disease**) or by a malignant tumour in the lung or elsewhere. Other causes include a benign or malignant tumour of the adrenal gland(s) resulting in excess activity of the gland and prolonged therapy with high doses of corticosteroid drugs (such as prednisone). [H. W. Cushing (1869–1939), US surgeon]

cusp *n.* **1.** any of the cone-shaped prominences on teeth, especially the molars and premolars. **2.** a pocket or fold of the membrane (endocardium) lining the heart or of the layer of the wall of a vein, several of which form a *valve. When the blood flows backwards the cusps fill up and become distended, so closing the valve.

cutaneous *adj.* relating to the skin.

cuticle *n.* **1.** the *epidermis of the skin. **2.** a layer of solid or semisolid material that is secreted by and covers an *epithelium. **3.** a layer of cells, such as the outer layer of cells in a hair.

cutis *n. see* SKIN.

CVP *see* CENTRAL VENOUS PRESSURE.

CVS *see* CHORIONIC VILLUS SAMPLING.

cyan- (cyano-) *prefix denoting* blue.

cyanide *n.* any of the notoriously poisonous salts of hydrocyanic acid. Cyanides combine with and render inactive the enzymes of the tissues responsible for cellular respiration, and therefore they kill extremely quickly; unconsciousness is followed by convulsions and death. Hydrogen cyanide vapour is fatal in less than a minute when inhaled. Sodium or potassium cyanide taken by mouth may also kill within minutes. Prompt treatment with amyl nitrite and sodium thiosulphate or dicobalt *edetate may save life. Cyanides give off a smell of bitter almonds.

cyanocobalamin *n. see* VITAMIN B$_{12}$.

cyanopsia *n.* a condition in which everything looks bluish.

cyanosis *n.* a bluish discoloration of the skin and mucous membranes resulting from an inadequate amount of oxygen in the blood. Cyanosis is associated with heart failure, lung diseases, the breathing of oxygen-deficient atmospheres, and asphyxia. Cyanosis is also seen in *blue babies, because of congenital heart defects. —**cyanotic** *adj.*

cybernetics *n.* the science of communication processes and automatic control systems in both machines and living things; a study linking the working of the brain and nervous system with the functioning of computers and automated feedback devices. *See also* BIONICS.

cycl- (cyclo-) *prefix denoting* **1.** cycle or cyclic. **2.** the ciliary body. Example: **cyclectomy** (excision of).

cyclamate *n.* either of two compounds, sodium or calcium cyclamate, that are thirty times as sweet as sugar and, unlike saccharin, stable to heat. Cyclamates were used as sweetening agents in the food industry until 1969, when their use was banned because they were suspected of causing cancer.

cyclitis *n.* inflammation of the *ciliary body of the eye (*see* UVEITIS). *See also* FUCHS' HETEROCHROMIC CYCLITIS.

cyclizine *n.* a drug with *antihistamine properties, used to prevent and relieve nausea and vomiting in motion sickness, vertigo, disorders of the inner ear, and postoperative sickness. It is administered by mouth; common side-effects are drowsiness and dizziness. Trade name: **Valoid**.

cycloablation *n.* the destruction of part of the *ciliary body of the eye to reduce the production of aqueous humour and hence reduce intraocular pressure. This technique is used in the treatment of advanced glaucoma resistant to other forms of treatment.

cyclocryotherapy *n.* the destruction of part of the *ciliary body (*see* CYCLOABLATION) by freezing. It is used to reduce intraocular pressure in the control of glaucoma.

cyclodialysis *n.* an operation for *glaucoma in which part of the *ciliary body is separated from its attachment to the sclera, producing a cleft between the two. The aqueous humour comes into contact with the exposed surface of the ciliary body and some of it is absorbed from this surface. The pressure within the eye will be reduced if this absorption adds significantly to the drainage of fluid from the eye.

cyclopenthiazide *n.* a *diuretic used to treat fluid retention (oedema), high blood pressure (hypertension), and heart failure. It is administered by mouth and may cause skin sensitivity reactions, nausea, constipation, diarrhoea, and reduced blood potassium levels. Trade name: **Navidrex**.

cyclopentolate *n.* a drug, similar to *atropine, that is used in eye drops to paralyse the ciliary muscles and dilate the pupil for eye examinations and to treat some types of eye inflammation. Trade names: **Minims cyclopentolate, Mydrilate**.

cyclophoria *n.* a type of squint (*see* STRABISMUS) in which the eye, when tested, tends to rotate slightly clockwise or anticlockwise.

cyclophosphamide *n.* a drug used to treat some cancers, often in combination with other *cytotoxic drugs. It also has *immunosuppressive properties and is used in prolonging the survival of tissue transplants and in other conditions requiring a reduced immune response. Cyclophosphamide is administered by mouth or by injection; common side-effects are nausea, vomiting, and – particularly at high doses – hair loss. Trade name: **Endoxana**.

cyclophotoablation n. the use of light or lasers to destroy the *ciliary body of the eye in order to reduce production of aqueous humour and hence reduce intraocular pressure. It is used in the treatment of glaucoma.

cycloplegia n. paralysis of the ciliary muscle of the eye (see CILIARY BODY). This causes inability to alter the focus of the eye and is usually accompanied by paralysis of the muscles of the iris, resulting in fixed dilation of the pupil (**mydriasis**). It is induced by the use of atropine or similar drugs in order to inactivate the muscle in cases of inflammation of the iris and ciliary body. It may also occur after injuries to the eye.

cyclopropane n. a general *anaesthetic, administered by inhalation for all types of surgical operation. It can cause postoperative nausea, vomiting, and headache.

cycloserine n. an *antibiotic, active against a wide range of bacteria, that may be used as supporting treatment in tuberculosis. It is administered by mouth; side-effects, which can be severe, include dizziness, drowsiness, convulsions, and mental confusion.

cyclosporin A a drug that suppresses the immune system and is administered to prevent and treat rejection of a transplanted organ or bone marrow. Trade name: **Sandimmun**.

cyclothymia n. the occurrence of marked swings of mood from cheerfulness to misery. These fluctuations are not as great as those of *manic-depressive psychosis. They usually represent a personality disorder, for which *psychotherapy is sometimes helpful.

cyclotron n. a machine in which charged particles following a spiral path within a magnetic field are accelerated by an alternating electric field. It produces very high-energy electromagnetic radiation, which has been used in the treatment of certain cancers, particularly of the eye. It is little used on account of severe adverse effects on the tissues following treatment.

cyesis n. see PREGNANCY.

cyn- (cyno-) prefix denoting a dog or dogs. Example: **cynophobia** (morbid fear of).

cyproheptadine n. a potent *antihistamine administered by mouth to treat allergies and itching skin conditions; it is also used to stimulate the appetite. Drowsiness is a common side-effect. Trade name: **Periactin**.

cyproterone (cyproterone acetate, CPA) n. a steroid drug that inhibits the effects of male sex hormones (see ANTI-ANDROGEN) and is used to treat various sexual disorders and advanced prostate cancer in men. It is administered by mouth and common side-effects include tiredness, loss of strength, inhibition of sperm formation, infertility, and breast enlargement (gynaecomastia). Trade names: **Androcur**, **Cyprostat**.

cyrtometer n. a device for measuring the shape of the chest and its movements during breathing.

cyst n. **1.** an abnormal sac or closed cavity lined with *epithelium and filled with liquid or semisolid matter. There are many varieties of cysts occurring in different parts of the body. **Retention cysts** arise when the outlet of a glandular duct is blocked, as in *sebaceous cysts. Some cysts are congenital, due to abnormal embryonic development; for example, *dermoid cysts. Others are tumours containing cells that secrete mucus or other substances, and another type of cyst is formed by parasites in the body (see HYDATID CYST). Cysts may occur in the jaws: a **dental cyst** occurs at the apex of a tooth, a **dentigerous cyst** occurs around the crown of an unerupted tooth, and an **eruption cyst** forms over an erupting tooth. See also FIMBRIAL CYST, OVARIAN CYST. **2.** a dormant stage produced during the life cycle of certain protozoan parasites of the alimentary canal, including *Giardia and *Entamoeba. Cysts, passed out in the faeces, have tough outer coats that protect the parasites from unfavourable conditions. The parasites emerge from their cysts when they are eaten by a new host. **3.** a structure formed by and surrounding the larvae of certain parasitic worms.

cyst- (cysto-) *prefix denoting* **1.** a bladder, especially the urinary bladder. Example: **cystoplasty** (plastic surgery of). **2.** a cyst.

cystadenoma *n.* an *adenoma showing a cystic structure.

cystalgia *n.* pain in the urinary bladder. This is common in *cystitis and when there are stones in the bladder and is occasionally present in bladder cancer. Treatment is directed to the underlying cause.

cystectomy *n.* surgical removal of the urinary bladder. This is necessary in the treatment of certain bladder conditions, notably cancer, and necessitates subsequent *urinary diversion. The ureters draining the urine from the kidneys are reimplanted into the colon (*see* URETEROSIGMOIDOSTOMY) or into an isolated segment of intestine (usually the ileum), which is brought to the skin surface as a spout (*see* ILEAL CONDUIT). Alternatively, in **bladder replacement**, a segment of ileum or colon is reconstructed to form a pouch, which is anastomosed to the urethra and acts as a reservoir for the urine. Emptying may be achieved by abdominal straining or *intermittent self-catheterization.

cysteine *n.* a sulphur-containing *amino acid that is an important constituent of many enzymes. The disulphide (S–S) links between adjacent cysteine molecules in polypeptide chains contribute to the three-dimensional molecular structure of proteins.

cystic *adj.* **1.** of, relating to, or characterized by cysts. **2.** of or relating to the gall bladder or urinary bladder.

cystic duct *see* BILE DUCT.

cysticercosis *n.* a disease caused by the presence of tapeworm larvae (*see* CYSTICERCUS) of the species *Taenia solium* in any of the body tissues. Man becomes infected on ingesting tapeworm eggs in contaminated food or drink. The presence of cysticerci in the muscles causes pain and weakness; in the brain the symptoms are more serious, including mental deterioration, paralysis, giddiness, epileptic attacks, and

convulsions, which may be fatal. There is no specific treatment for this cosmopolitan disease although surgical removal of cysticerci may be necessary to relieve pressure on the brain.

cysticercus (bladderworm) *n.* a larval stage of some *tapeworms in which the scolex and neck are invaginated into a large fluid-filled cyst. The cysts develop in the muscles or brain of the host following ingestion of tapeworm eggs. *See* CYSTICERCOSIS.

cystic fibrosis (fibrocystic disease of the pancreas, mucoviscidosis) a hereditary disease affecting cells of the exocrine glands (including mucus-secreting glands, sweat glands, and others). The faulty gene responsible has been identified as lying on chromosome no. 7 and is recessive, i.e. both parents of the patient can be *carriers without being affected by the disease. Affected individuals lack a protein, **cystic fibrosis transmembrane regulator (CFTR)**, that enables the transport of chloride ions across cell membranes: this results in the production of thick mucus, which obstructs the intestinal glands (causing meconium *ileus in newborn babies), pancreas (causing deficiency of pancreatic enzymes resulting in *malabsorption and *failure to thrive), and bronchi (causing *bronchiectasis). Respiratory infections, which may be severe, are a common complication. The sweat contains excessive amounts of sodium and chloride, which is an aid to diagnosis.

Treatment consists of minimizing the effects of the disease by administration of pancreatic enzymes and physiotherapy for the lungs and by preventing and combating secondary infection. *Genetic counselling is essential, as each subsequent child of carrier parents has a one in four chance of being affected (*see also* MOUTHWASH TEST). Some patients are benefiting from revolutionary new treatments, including transplantation of heart and lungs and treatment aimed at altering the genetic content of the faulty cells (*see* GENE THERAPY).

cystine *n.* *see* AMINO ACID.

cystinosis *n.* an inborn defect in the metabolism of amino acids, leading to abnormal accumulation of the amino acid cystine in the blood, kidneys, and lymphatic system. *See also* FANCONI SYNDROME.

cystinuria *n.* an *inborn error of metabolism resulting in excessive excretion of the amino acid cystine in the urine due to a defect of reabsorption by the kidney tubules. It may lead to the formation of cystine stones in the kidney.

cystitis *n.* inflammation of the urinary bladder, often caused by infection (most commonly by the bacterium *Escherichia coli*). It is usually accompanied by the desire to pass urine frequently, with a degree of burning. More severe attacks are often associated with the painful passage of blood in the urine, which is accompanied by a cramplike pain in the lower abdomen persisting after the bladder has been emptied. An acute attack is treated by antibiotic administration and a copious fluid intake. *See also* INTERSTITIAL CYSTITIS.

cystitome *n.* a small knife with a tiny curved or hooked blade, used to cut the lens capsule in the type of operation for cataract in which the capsule is left behind (extracapsular *cataract extraction). *See also* CAPSULOTOMY.

cystocele *n.* prolapse of the base of the bladder in women. It is usually due to weakness of the pelvic floor after childbirth and causes bulging of the anterior wall of the vagina on straining. When accompanied by stress incontinence of urine, surgical repair (anterior *colporrhaphy) is indicated.

cystography *n.* X-ray examination of the urinary bladder after the injection of a contrast medium. The X-ray photographs or films thus obtained are known as **cystograms**. Cystography is most commonly performed to detect reflux of urine from the bladder to the ureters, usually in children (*see* VESICOURETERIC REFLUX). If films are taken during voiding then the urethra can also be observed (*see* URETHROGRAPHY).

cystolithiasis *n.* the presence of stones (calculi) in the urinary bladder. The stones are either formed in the bladder, due to obstruction, urinary retention, and infection (**primary calculi**), or pass to the bladder after being formed in the kidneys

(**secondary calculi**). They cause pain, the passage of bloody urine, and interruption of the urinary stream and should be removed surgically. *See* CALCULUS.

cystometer *n.* an apparatus for measuring the pressure within the bladder. Modern investigations also include measurement of urine flow, and the resultant bladder pressure/flow study (**urodynamic investigation**) provides useful information regarding bladder function.

cystopexy (vesicofixation) *n.* a surgical operation to fix the urinary bladder (or a portion of it) in a different position. It may be performed as part of the repair or correction of a prolapsed bladder.

cystoplasty *n.* the operation of enlarging the capacity of the bladder by incorporating a segment of bowel. In a **clam cystoplasty**, the bladder is cut across longitudinally from one side of the neck to the other side through the dome (fundus) of the bladder and a length of the ileum or colon is inserted as a patch. In the operation of **ileocaecocystoplasty**, the dome is removed by cutting across the bladder transversely above the openings of the ureters; it is replaced by an isolated segment of caecum and terminal ileum. In **ileocystoplasty** the bladder is enlarged by an opened-out portion of small intestine. The bladder may be totally replaced by a reservoir constructed from either small or large intestine (*see* CYSTECTOMY).

cystosarcoma phylloides a malignant tumour of the connective tissue of the breast: it accounts for approximately 1% of all breast cancers. Such tumours may show a wide variation in cell structure. The best treatment for a localized tumour is simple *mastectomy.

cystoscopy *n.* examination of the bladder by means of an instrument (**cystoscope**) inserted via the urethra. The cystoscope consists of a metal sheath surrounding a telescope and light-conducting bundles. Irrigating fluid is conducted via the sheath into the bladder and additional channels are available for the catheters to be inserted into the ureters, diathermy electrodes for removing polyps, etc., or biopsy forceps for taking specimens of tumours or other growths.

cystostomy n. the operation of creating an artificial opening between the bladder and the anterior abdominal wall. This provides a temporary or permanent drainage route for urine.

cystotomy n. surgical incision into the urinary bladder, usually by cutting through the abdominal wall above the pubic symphysis (**suprapubic cystotomy**). This is necessary for such operations as removing stones or tumours from the bladder and for gaining access to the prostate gland in the operation of transvesical *prostatectomy.

cyt- (cyto-) *prefix denoting* 1. cell(s). 2. cytoplasm.

cytarabine n. a *cytotoxic drug used to suppress the symptoms of some types of leukaemia. It is administered by injection and can damage the bone marrow, leading to various blood cell disorders. Other side-effects are nausea, vomiting, mouth ulcers, and diarrhoea. Trade names: **Alexan, Cytosar**.

-cyte *suffix denoting* a cell. Examples: **chondrocyte** (cartilage cell); **osteocyte** (bone cell).

cytidine n. a compound containing cytosine and the sugar ribose. *See also* NUCLEO-SIDE.

cytochemistry n. the study of chemical compounds and their activities in living cells.

cytochrome n. a compound consisting of a protein linked to *haem. Cytochromes act as electron transfer agents in biological oxidation-reduction reactions, particularly those associated with the mitochondria in cellular respiration. *See* ELECTRON TRANSPORT CHAIN.

cytogenetics n. a science that links the study of inheritance (genetics) with that of cells (cytology); it is concerned mainly with the study of the *chromosomes, especially their origin, structure, and functions.

cytokines *pl. n.* protein molecules, released by cells when activated by antigen, that are involved in cell-to-cell communications, acting as enhancing mediators for immune responses through interaction with specific cell-surface receptors on leucocytes. Kinds of cytokines include *interleukins (produced by leucocytes), *lymphokines (produced by lymphocytes), *interferons, and *tumour necrosis factor.

cytokinesis n. division of the cytoplasm of a cell, which occurs at the end of cell division, after division of the nucleus, to form two daughter cells. *Compare* KARYO-KINESIS.

cytology n. the study of the structure and function of cells. The examination of cells under a microscope is used in the diagnosis of various diseases. These cells are obtained by scraping an organ, as in **cervical cytology** (*see* CERVICAL SMEAR), by aspiration (*see* ASPIRATION CYTOLOGY), or they are collected from cells already shed (**exfoliative cytology**). *See also* BIOPSY. —**cytological** *adj*.

cytolysis n. the breakdown of cells, particularly by destruction of their outer membranes.

cytomegalovirus (CMV) n. a member of the herpes group of viruses (*see* HERPESVIRUS). It commonly occurs in humans and normally produces symptoms milder than the common cold. However, in individuals whose immune systems are compromised (e.g. by cancer or AIDS) it can cause more severe effects, and it has been found to be the cause of congenital handicap in infants born to women who have contracted the virus during pregnancy.

cytometer n. an instrument for determining the number of cells in a given quantity of fluid, such as blood, cerebrospinal fluid, or urine. *See* HAEMOCYTOMETER.

cytomorphosis n. the changes undergone by a cell in the course of its life cycle.

cytopenia n. a deficiency of one or more of the various types of blood cells. *See* EOSINOPENIA, ERYTHROPENIA, LYMPHOPENIA, NEUTROPENIA, PANCYTOPENIA, THROMBOCYTOPENIA.

cytophotometry n. the study of chemical compounds in living cells by means of a **cytophotometer**, an instrument that measures light intensity through stained areas of cytoplasm.

cytoplasm n. the jelly-like substance that surrounds the nucleus of a cell. *See* *also* ECTOPLASM, ENDOPLASM, PROTOPLASM. —**cytoplasmic** *adj.*

cytoplasmic inheritance the inheritance of characters controlled by factors present in the cell cytoplasm rather than by genes on the chromosomes in the cell nucleus. Cytoplasmic inheritance is known to occur in lower animals and in plants but has not so far been found in man.

cytosine *n.* one of the nitrogen-containing bases (*see* PYRIMIDINE) that occurs in the nucleic acid DNA.

cytosome *n.* the part of a cell that is outside the nucleus.

cytotoxic drug a drug that damages or destroys cells and is used to treat various types of cancer, either with or without the use of *radiotherapy. Examples are *amsacrine, *cisplatin, *cyclophosphamide, *cytarabine, *mustine, and *anthracycline antibiotics; they offer successful treatment in some conditions and help reduce symptoms and prolong life in others. Cytotoxic drugs destroy cancer cells by inhibiting cell division (i.e. they are **antimitotic**) but they also affect normal cells, particularly in bone marrow, skin, stomach lining, and fetal tissue, and dosage must be carefully controlled. *See also* ANTIMETABOLITE, CHEMOTHERAPY.

cytotrophoblast *n.* the part of a *trophoblast that retains its cellular structure and does not invade the maternal tissues. It forms the outer surface of the *chorion.

dacarbazine (DTIC) *n.* a drug used in the treatment of certain cancers, including *Hodgkin's disease and malignant melanoma. Side-effects include severe vomiting.

dacry- (dacryo-) *prefix denoting* **1.** tears. **2.** the lacrimal apparatus.

dacryoadenitis *n.* inflammation of the tear-producing gland (*see* LACRIMAL APPARATUS).

dacryocystitis *n.* inflammation of the lacrimal sac (in which tears collect), usually occurring when the duct draining the tears into the nose is blocked (*see* LACRIMAL APPARATUS).

dacryocystorhinostomy (DCR) *n.* an operation to relieve blockage of the nasolacrimal duct (which drains tears into the nose), in which a communication is made between the lacrimal sac and the nose by removing the intervening bone. *See* DACRYOCYSTITIS, LACRIMAL APPARATUS.

dacryops *n. Obsolete.* a watering eye.

dactyl- *prefix denoting* the digits (fingers or toes). Examples: **dactylomegaly** (abnormally large size of); **dactylospasm** (painful contraction of).

dactylitis *n.* inflammation of a finger or toe caused by bone infection (as in tuberculous *osteomyelitis) or rheumatic disease or seen in infants with sickle-cell disease.

dactylology *n.* the representation of speech by finger movements: sign language.

Daltonism (protanopia) *n.* red-blindness: a defect in colour vision in which a person cannot distinguish between reds and greens. The term has been used to refer to *colour blindness in general. [J. Dalton (1766–1844), British chemist]

damp *n.* (in mining) any gas encountered underground other than air. *See* BLACKDAMP, FIREDAMP.

danazol *n.* a synthetic *progestogen that

inhibits the secretion by the pituitary gland of gonadotrophins. It is used to treat precocious puberty, breast enlargement in males (gynaecomastia), excessively heavy menstrual periods, and *endometriosis. It is administered by mouth. Possible side-effects include nausea, swelling of the feet and ankles, weight gain, oiliness of the skin, and, in women, excessive growth of facial and body hair. Trade name: **Danol**.

D and C *see* DILATATION AND CURETTAGE.

dandruff *n.* visible scaling from the surface of the scalp. It is extremely common, occurring in about 50% of the population, and is associated with the presence of the yeast *Pityrosporum ovale*. It is the precursor of seborrhoeic *eczema of the scalp, in which there is a degree of inflammation in addition to the greasy scaling. Dandruff can be controlled by shampoos containing tar, selenium sulphide, zinc pyrithione, or imidazole antifungals. Medical name: **pityriasis capitis**.

Dandy-Walker syndrome a form of *cerebral palsy in which the *cerebellum is usually the part of the brain affected. It leads to unsteadiness of balance and an abnormal gait and may be associated with *hydrocephalus. [W. E. Dandy (1886–1946) and A. E. Walker (1907–   ), US surgeons]

dangerous drugs *see* MISUSE OF DRUGS ACT 1971.

danthron *n.* a *laxative administered by mouth; it sometimes colours the urine pink or red. It is usually combined with a faecal softener (e.g. in **Codalax, Normax**).

dantrolene *n.* a *muscle relaxant drug used to relieve muscle spasm in such conditions as cerebral palsy, multiple sclerosis, or spinal cord injury. It is administered by mouth or by injection. Possible side-effects include weakness, dizziness, drowsiness, and vertigo; liver damage sometimes occurs. Trade name: **Dantrium**.

dapsone *n.* a drug (*see* SULPHONE) used to

treat *leprosy and dermatitis herpetiformis. It is administered by mouth or injection; the most common side-effects are allergic skin reactions.

dark adaptation the changes that take place in the retina and pupil of the eye enabling vision in very dim light. Dark adaptation involves activation of the *rods – the cells of the retina that function best in dim light – and the reflex enlargement of the pupil (*see* PUPILLARY REFLEX). *Compare* LIGHT ADAPTATION.

Data Protection Act 1984 (in the UK) legislation by which anyone storing personal information relating to an individual on a computer is responsible for the accuracy of that information and may neither use the information nor pass it on to others without the knowledge and consent of that individual. Users of the information are required to be registered. Individuals about whom information is held can require to see a printout of the information relevant to them and demand to have inaccurate or misleading information amended. Specific exceptions include police, state security, and medical research, but not medical information that may affect employment or promotion.

daunorubicin *n.* an antibiotic that interferes with DNA synthesis and is used in the treatment of acute leukaemia. It is administered by injection. Possible side-effects include loss of hair and damage to bone marrow and heart muscle.

day blindness comparatively good vision in poor light but poor vision in good illumination. The condition is usually congenital and associated with poor *visual acuity and defective colour vision. Acquired cases occur when the *cones (light-sensitive cells) at the back of the retina are selectively destroyed by disease. Medical name: **hemeralopia**. *Compare* NIGHT BLINDNESS.

day-case surgery surgical procedures that can be performed in a single day, without the need to admit the patient for an overnight stay in hospital. Modern techniques of surgery and anaesthesia now enable many surgical cases of minor and intermediate degrees of severity to be treated in this way: examples include many breast lesions, dilatation and curet-

tage, and operations for hernia and varicose veins. Special units are established in many hospitals.

day hospital a hospital in which patients spend a substantial part of the day under medical supervision but do not stay overnight. Day hospitals are mainly used for the treatment of elderly patients and those with mental disorders.

DCR *see* DACRYOCYSTORHINOSTOMY.

DDAVP *see* DESMOPRESSIN.

DDT (chlorophenothane, dicophane) *n.* a powerful insecticide that was formerly widely used against lice, fleas, flies, bed bugs, cockroaches, and other disease-carrying and destructive insects. It is a relatively stable compound that is stored in animal fats, and the quantities now present in the environment – in the form of stores accumulated in animal tissues – have led to its use being restricted. Acute poisoning, from swallowing more than 20 g, produces nervous irritability, muscle twitching, convulsions, and coma, but only a few fatalities have been reported.

de- *prefix denoting* **1.** removal or loss. Examples: **demineralization** (of minerals from bones or teeth); **devascularization** (of blood supply). **2.** reversal.

deafness *n.* partial or total loss of hearing in one or both ears. **Conductive deafness** is due to a defect in the conduction of sound from the external ear to the inner ear. This may be due to perforations of the eardrum, fluid or infection in the middle ear (*see* GLUE EAR, OTITIS MEDIA), or disorders of the small bones in the middle ear (*ossicles). **Sensorineural** (or **perceptive**) **deafness** may be due to a lesion of the *cochlea in the inner ear, the auditory nerve, or the auditory centres in the brain. It may be present from birth (for example if the mother was affected with German measles during pregnancy). In adults it may be brought on by injury, disease (e.g. *Ménière's disease), or prolonged exposure to loud noise; progressive sensorineural deafness (**presbyacusis**) is common with advancing age.

The type of deafness can be diagnosed by various hearing tests (*see* RINNE'S TEST, WEBER'S TEST, AUDIOGRAM), and the treatment depends on the cause. *See also* COCHLEAR IMPLANT, HEARING AID.

deamination *n.* a process, occurring in the liver, that occurs during the metabolism of amino acids. The amino group ($-NH_2$) is removed from an amino acid and converted to ammonia, which is ultimately converted to *urea and excreted.

death *n.* absence of vital functions. Death is diagnosed by permanent cessation of the heartbeat. **Brain death** is defined as permanent functional death of the centres in the brainstem that control breathing, heart rate, and other vital reflexes (including pupillary responses). Usually two independent medical opinions are required before brain death is agreed, but organs such as kidneys may then legally be removed for transplantation surgery before the heart has stopped.

death certificate a medical certificate stating the cause of a person's death, usually also stating the deceased's marital status, occupation, and age. A doctor's diagnosis of the main cause of death, and any contributory causes of death, and his signature are registered in Great Britain at St Catherine's House, London. Death certificates are required by law in the majority of countries throughout the world.

debridement *n.* the process of cleaning an open wound by removal of foreign material and dead tissue, so that healing may occur without hindrance.

debrisoquine *n.* a potent drug used to treat high blood pressure (hypertension). It is administered by mouth; common side-effects are nausea, headache, sweating, and general malaise. Trade name: **Declinax**.

dec- (deca-) *prefix denoting* ten.

Decadron *n. see* DEXAMETHASONE.

decalcification *n.* loss or removal of calcium salts from a bone or tooth.

decapitation *n.* removal of the head, usually the head of a dead fetus to enable delivery to take place. This procedure is very rare nowadays, being undertaken only in dire circumstances when the fetal head is too large to pass through the birth canal, the mother's life is endangered, and Caesarean section impossible.

decapsulation *n. see* DECORTICATION.

decay *n.* (in bacteriology) the decomposition of organic matter due to microbial action.

decerebration *n.* the removal of the higher centres of the brain or cutting across the brain below the cerebrum so that cerebral functions are eliminated. This procedure is carried out on experimental animals, but certain injuries to the brain in man may cause the same severe neurological signs as occur in an animal that has been decerebrated.

deci- *prefix denoting* a tenth.

decibel (dB) *n.* one tenth of a bel: a unit for comparing levels of power (especially sound) on a logarithmic scale. A power source of intensity P has a power level of $10 \log_{10} P/P_0$ decibels, where P_0 is the intensity of a reference source. The decibel is much more widely used than the bel. Silence is 0 dB; a whisper has an intensity of 30 dB, normal speech 60 dB, a shout 90 dB, and a jet aircraft 120 dB.

decidua *n.* the modified mucous membrane that lines the wall of the uterus during pregnancy and is shed with the afterbirth at parturition (*see* ENDOMETRIUM). There are three regions: the **decidua capsularis**, a thin layer that covers the embryo; the **decidua basalis**, where the embryo is attached; and the **decidua parietalis**, which is not in contact with the embryo. —**decidual** *adj.*

deciduoma *n.* a mass of tissue within the uterus derived from remnants of *decidua. *See also* CHORIONEPITHELIOMA (MALIGNANT DECIDUOMA).

deciduous teeth *see* PRIMARY TEETH.

declive *n.* an area of the upper surface of the *cerebellum, posterior to the culmen and anterior to the folium of the middle lobe.

decomposition *n.* the gradual disintegration of dead organic matter, usually foodstuffs or tissues, by the chemical action of bacteria and/or fungi.

decompression *n.* **1.** the reduction of pressure on an organ or part of the body by surgical intervention. Surgical decompression can be effected at many sites: the pressure of tissues on a nerve may be relieved by incision; raised pressure in the fluid of the brain can be lowered by cutting into the *dura mater; and cardiac compression – the abnormal presence of blood or fluid round the heart – can be cured by cutting the sac (pericardium) enclosing the heart. **2.** the gradual reduction of atmospheric pressure for deep-sea divers, who work at artificially high pressures. *See* COMPRESSED AIR ILLNESS.

decompression sickness *see* COMPRESSED AIR ILLNESS.

decongestant *n.* an agent that reduces or relieves nasal congestion. Most nasal decongestants are *sympathomimetic drugs, applied either locally, in the form of nasal sprays or drops, or taken by mouth.

decortication *n.* **1.** the removal of the outside layer (cortex) from an organ or structure, such as the kidney. **2.** an operation for removing the blood clot and scar tissue that forms after bleeding into the chest cavity (haemothorax). **3.** (**decapsulation**) the surgical removal of a *capsule from an organ; for example, the stripping of the membrane that envelops the kidney or of the inflammatory capsule that encloses a chronic abscess, as in the treatment of *empyema.

decubitus *n.* the recumbent position.

decubitus ulcer *see* BEDSORE.

decussation *n.* a point at which two or more structures of the body cross to the opposite side. The term is used particularly for the point at which nerve fibres cross over in the central nervous system.

deep vein thrombosis (DVT) *see* PHLEBOTHROMBOSIS.

deer fly *see* CHRYSOPS.

defecation *n.* a bowel movement in which faeces are evacuated through the rectum and anus. The amount and composition of the food eaten determine to a large degree the bulk of the faeces, and the transit time through the intestinal tract determines the water content. *See* CONSTIPATION, DIARRHOEA.

defence mechanism the means whereby an undesirable impulse can be avoided or controlled. Many defence mech-

anisms have been described, including *repression, *projection, *reaction formation, *sublimation, and *splitting. They may be partly responsible for such problems as tics, stammering, and phobias.

deferent *adj.* **1.** carrying away from or down from. **2.** relating to the vas deferens.

defervescence *n.* the disappearance of a fever, a process that may occur rapidly or take several days, depending upon the cause and treatment given.

defibrillation *n.* administration of a controlled electric shock to restore normal heart rhythm in cases of cardiac arrest due to ventricular *fibrillation. The apparatus (**defibrillator**) administers the shock either through electrodes placed on the chest wall over the heart or directly to the heart after the chest has been opened surgically.

defibrination *n.* the removal of *fibrin, one of the plasma proteins that causes coagulation, from a sample of blood. It is normally done by whisking the blood with a bundle of fine wires, to which the strands of fibrin that form in the blood adhere.

deficiency *n.* (in genetics) *see* DELETION.

deficiency disease any disease caused by the lack of an essential nutrient in the diet. Such nutrients include *vitamins, *essential amino acids, and *essential fatty acids.

degeneration *n.* the deterioration and loss of specialized function of the cells of a tissue or organ. The changes may be caused by a defective blood supply or by disease. Degeneration may involve the deposition of calcium salts, fat (*see* FATTY DEGENERATION), or fibrous tissue in the affected organ or tissue. *See also* INFILTRATION.

deglutition *n.* *see* SWALLOWING.

dehiscence *n.* a splitting open, as of a surgical wound.

dehydration *n.* **1.** loss or deficiency of water in body tissues. The condition may result from inadequate water intake and/or from excessive removal of water from the body; for example, by sweating, vomiting, or diarrhoea. Symptoms include great thirst, nausea, and exhaustion. The condition is treated by drinking plenty of water; severe cases require *oral rehydration therapy or intravenous administration of water and salts (which have been lost with the water). **2.** the removal of water from tissue during its preparation for microscopical study, by placing it successively in stronger solutions of ethyl alcohol. Dehydration follows *fixation and precedes *clearing.

dehydrogenase n. see OXIDOREDUCTASE.

déjà vu a vivid psychic experience in which immediately contemporary events seem to be a repetition of previous happenings. It is a symptom of some forms of *epilepsy. See also JAMAIS VU.

delayed suture a technique used in the closure of contaminated wounds and wounds associated with tissue necrosis, such as are produced by missile injuries. The superficial layers of the wound are left open, to be closed later when the tissues have been cleaned.

deletion (deficiency) n. (in genetics) a type of mutation involving the loss of DNA. The deletion may be small, affecting only a portion of a single gene, or large, resulting in loss of a part of a chromosome and affecting many genes.

Delhi boil see ORIENTAL SORE.

delirium n. an acute disorder of the mental processes accompanying organic brain disease. It may be manifested by delusions, disorientation, hallucinations, or extreme excitement and occurs in metabolic disorders, intoxication, deficiency diseases, and infections.

delirium tremens a psychosis caused by *alcoholism, usually seen as a withdrawal syndrome in chronic alcoholics. Typically it is precipitated by a head injury or an acute infection causing abstinence from alcohol. Features include anxiety, tremor, sweating, and vivid and terrifying visual and sensory hallucinations, often of animals and insects. Severe cases may end fatally.

delivery n. see LABOUR.

delle n. (pl. **dellen**) a localized area of reduced corneal thickness, usually at the

limbus (the junction of the cornea with the sclera), due to local dehydration. It may occur after surgery to correct a squint, due to elevated conjunctiva at the limbus causing poor wetting of the adjacent cornea.

deltoid n. a thick triangular muscle that covers the shoulder joint (see illustration). It is responsible for raising the arm away from the side of the body.

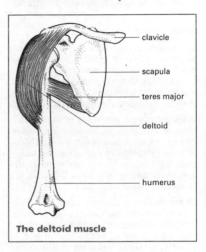

The deltoid muscle

delusion n. an irrationally held belief that cannot be altered by rational argument. In mental illness it is often a false belief that the individual is persecuted by others, is very powerful, is controlled by others, or is a victim of physical disease (see PARANOIA). Delusions may be a symptom of *schizophrenia, *manic-depressive psychosis, or an organic psychosis.

demeclocycline n. an antibiotic that is active against a wide range of bacteria and is used to treat various infections. It is administered by mouth; common side-effects are nausea, diarrhoea, and symptoms resulting from the growth of organisms not sensitive to the drug. Trade name: **Ledermycin**.

dementia n. a chronic or persistent disorder of behaviour and higher intellectual function due to organic brain disease. It is marked by memory disorders, changes in personality, deterioration in personal care, impaired reasoning ability, and disorientation. **Presenile dementia** occurs in young or middle-aged people. Causes of dementia include *Alzheimer's disease and *Pick's disease. A common form, **multi-infarct dementia**, results from the destruction of brain tissue by a series of small strokes. It is important to distinguish these organic conditions from psychological disorders that cause the same symptoms (*see* PSEUDO-DEMENTIA).

demi- *prefix denoting* half.

Demodex *n.* a genus of harmless parasitic mites, the follicle mites, found in the hair follicles and associated sebaceous glands of the face. They resemble tiny worms, about 0.4 mm in length, and their presence may give rise to dermatitis.

demography *n.* the study of populations on a national, regional, or local basis in terms of age, sex, and other *variables, including patterns of migration and survival. It is used in *public health medicine to help identify health needs and *risk factors. *See also* BIOSTATISTICS.

demulcent *n.* a soothing agent that protects the mucous membranes and relieves irritation. Demulcents form a protective film and are used in mouth washes, gargles, etc., to soothe irritation or inflammation in the mouth.

demyelination *n.* damage to the *myelin sheaths surrounding the nerve fibres in the central or peripheral nervous system. This in turn affects the function of the nerve fibres, which the myelin normally supports. Demyelination may be a primary disorder, as in *multiple sclerosis. There may be associated nerve-fibre damage.

denaturation *n.* the changes in the physical and physiological properties of a protein that are brought about by heat, X-rays, or chemicals. These changes include loss of activity (in the case of enzymes) and loss (or alteration) of antigenicity (in the case of *antigens).

dendrite *n.* one of the shorter branching processes of the cell body of a *neurone, which makes contact with other neurones at synapses and carries nerve impulses from them into the cell body.

dendritic cell a type of haemopoietic cell with specialized antigen-presenting functions. *See* APC.

dendritic ulcer a branching ulcer of the surface of the cornea caused by *herpes simplex virus. A similar appearance may be produced by a healing corneal abrasion. Dendritic ulcers tend to recur because the virus lies dormant in the tissues; years may elapse between attacks.

denervation *n.* interruption of the nerve supply to the muscles and skin. The muscle is paralysed and its normal tone (elasticity) is lost. The muscle fibres shrink and are replaced by fat. A denervated area of skin loses all forms of sensation and its subsequent ability to heal and renew its tissues may be impaired.

dengue (breakbone fever) *n.* a disease caused by arboviruses and transmitted to man principally by the mosquito *Aëdes aegypti*. Symptoms, which last for a few days, include severe pains in the joints and muscles, headache, sore throat, fever, running of the eyes, and an irritating rash. These symptoms recur in a usually milder form after an interval of two or three days. Death rarely occurs, but the patient is left debilitated and requires considerable convalescence. A more severe form, **dengue haemorrhagic fever**, characterized by a breakdown of the blood-clotting mechanism with internal bleeding, can affect children. Dengue occurs throughout the tropics and subtropics. Patients are given aspirin and codeine to relieve the pain and calamine lotion is helpful in easing the irritating rash.

dens *n.* a tooth or tooth-shaped structure.

dens invaginatus literally, an infolded tooth: a specific type of tooth malformation that mainly affects upper lateral incisors to varying degrees.

dent- (denti-, dento-) *prefix denoting* the teeth. Example: **dentoalveolar** (relating to the teeth and associated jaw).

dental auxiliary any of several assistants to a dentist. A **dental hygienist** performs scaling and instruction in oral hygiene under the prescription of the dentist. A **dental nurse** helps the dentist at the chairside by preparing materials, passing instruments, and aspirating fluids from the patient's mouth. A **dental technician** constructs dentures, crowns, and orthodontic appliances in the laboratory for the dentist. A **dental therapist** performs treatment on children under the direction of a dentist in the community dental services and in hospitals.

dental caries decay and crumbling of the substance of a tooth. Dental caries is caused by the metabolism of the bacteria in *plaque attached to the surface of the tooth. Acid formed by bacterial breakdown of sugar in the diet causes demineralization of the enamel of the tooth. If no preventive measure or treatment is carried out it spreads into the dentine and progressively destroys the tooth. It is the most common cause of toothache, and once infection has spread to the pulp it may extend through the root canal into the periapical tissues to cause an *apical abscess.

Frequent intake of sugar is a major cause, and the disease is more common in young people and has a predilection for specific sites. Dental caries can be most effectively prevented by restricting the frequency of sugar intake and avoiding sweet food and drinks at bedtime. The resistance of enamel to dental caries can be increased by the application of *fluoride salts to the tooth surface from toothpastes or mouth rinses. *Fluoridation of water also makes teeth resistant to caries during the period of tooth development. Once caries has spread into the dentine, treatment usually consists of removing the decayed part of the tooth using a *drill and replacing it with a *filling.

dental chair the chair on which a patient lies for dental treatment. Electric switches change the position of the patient, and the chair is frequently attached to the *dental unit.

dental floss fine thread, usually of nylon, used to clean some surfaces of teeth.

dental implant *see* IMPLANT.

dental nerve either of two nerves that supply the teeth; they are branches of the trigeminal nerve. The **inferior dental nerve** supplies the lower teeth and for most of its length exists as a single large

bundle; thus anaesthesia of it has a widespread effect (*see* INFERIOR DENTAL BLOCK). The **superior dental nerve**, which supplies the upper teeth, breaks into separate branches at some distance from the teeth and it is possible to anaesthetize these individually with less widespread effect for the patient.

dental nurse *see* DENTAL AUXILIARY.

dental pantomogram (DPT) a special form of tomogram (*see* TOMOGRAPHY) that provides a picture of all the teeth of both jaws on one film.

dental unit a major fixed piece of dental equipment to which are attached the dental drills, aspirator, compressed air syringe, and ultrasonic scaler.

dentate *adj.* **1.** having teeth. **2.** serrated; having toothlike projections.

dentifrice *n.* a paste or powder for cleaning the teeth. Toothpastes contain a fine abrasive; an essential ingredient is suitable flavouring to make their use pleasant. Most toothpastes contain *fluoride salts, which help to prevent dental caries.

dentine *n.* a hard tissue that forms the bulk of a tooth. The dentine of the crown is covered by enamel and that of the root by cementum. The dentine is permeated by fine tubules, which near the centre of the tooth contain cellular processes from the pulp. Exposed dentine is sensitive to touch, heat, and cold.

dentinogenesis *n.* the formation of *dentine by *odontoblasts. Although dentinogenesis continues throughout life, very little dentine is formed later than a few years after tooth eruption unless it is stimulated by caries, abrasion, or trauma. **Dentinogenesis imperfecta** is a hereditary condition in which dentine formation is disturbed; this may result in loss of overlying enamel and excessive wear of the dentine.

dentist *n.* a member of the dental profession, who in the UK must be registered with the General Dental Council unless he holds a medical qualification.

dentistry *n.* the study, management, and treatment of diseases and conditions affecting the mouth, jaws, teeth, and their

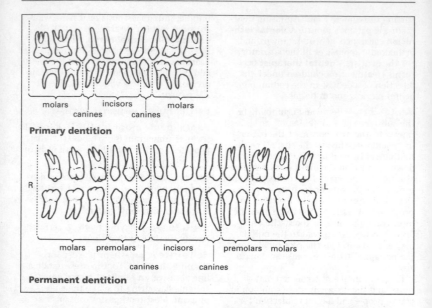

molars · incisors · molars
canines · canines

Primary dentition

R · molars · premolars · incisors · premolars · molars · L
canines · canines

Permanent dentition

supporting tissues. Subdisciplines are: dental public health, *endodontics, oral medicine, oral surgery, *orthodontics, *paediatric dentistry, *periodontology, preventive dentistry, *prosthetic dentistry, and restorative dentistry.

dentition *n.* the arrangement of teeth in the mouth. The **primary dentition** comprises the teeth of young children. It consists of 20 teeth, made up of incisors, canines, and molars only. The lower incisor erupts first at about 6 months of age, and all the primary teeth have usually erupted by the age of 2½ years. The lower incisors are shed first at about 7 years of age, and from this time until about 13 years old both primary and permanent teeth are present; i.e. there is a **mixed dentition**. The **permanent dentition** consists of up to 32 teeth, made up of incisors, canines, premolars, and molars. The first tooth to erupt is the first molar (at the age of 6) and most have appeared by the age of 14 years, although the third molars may not erupt until the age of 18–21 years. See illustrations.

denture *n.* a removable replacement for one or more teeth carried on some type of plate or frame. A **complete denture** replaces all the teeth in one jaw. It is usually made entirely of acrylic resin. A **partial denture** replaces some teeth because others still remain. It is designed to restore function with the least potential damage to the remaining teeth. The framework of the denture base is often made of metal (*cobalt-chromium) because of its strength. (*See also* PROSTHESIS.) **Denture sore mouth** is inflammation of the gum under the denture, caused by a mixed infection of *Candida* and bacteria under a poorly cleaned denture or removable orthodontic appliance. **Denture hyperplasia** is an overgrowth of fibrous tissue covered by mucous membrane, resulting from chronic irritation by a denture.

deodorant *n.* an agent that reduces or removes unpleasant body odours by destroying bacteria that live on the skin and break down sweat. Deodorant preparations often contain an antiseptic.

deontology *n.* the study of ethics and correct behaviour or duty. In medicine this includes consideration of the proper behaviour of a doctor towards his patient, whether a patient should be told if his condition is fatal or not, and similar problems for which there may be no written guidelines. The best-known code of conduct is the *Hippocratic oath.

deoxycholic acid see BILE ACIDS.

deoxycorticosterone n. a hormone, synthesized and released by the adrenal cortex, that regulates salt and water balance. See also CORTICOSTEROID.

deoxyribonuclease n. an enzyme, located in the *lysosomes of cells, that splits DNA at specific places in the molecule.

deoxyribonucleic acid see DNA.

Department of Health (DH) a department of central government that supports the Secretary of State for Health in meeting his or her obligations, which include the *National Health Service, the promotion and protection of the health of the nation, and social care, including the overseeing of personal social services provided by local authorities. The department is staffed by civil servants, including medical and nursing personnel and those from other health professions. The NHS Executive, which is an integral part of the Department, was formally established in 1989 and is responsible for advising government ministers and for formulating and ensuring implementation of policy on health care. It is made up of a headquarters and eight regional offices. Although mainly concerned with the NHS, the DH also oversees private and voluntary provision of health services. Equivalent departments support the ministers responsible for health services in Scotland, Wales, and Northern Ireland. See also DEPARTMENT OF SOCIAL SECURITY.

Department of Social Security a department of central government that supports the Secretary of State for Social Security in meeting his or her obligations, which include the *social services, *National Insurance, and income support and other benefits for those with priority needs.

dependence (drug dependence) n. the physical and/or psychological effects produced by the habitual taking of certain drugs, characterized by a compulsion to continue taking the drug. In **phys-**

ical dependence withdrawal of the drug causes specific symptoms (**withdrawal symptoms**), such as sweating, vomiting, or tremors, that are reversed by further doses. Substances that may induce physical dependence include alcohol and the 'hard' drugs morphine, heroin, and cocaine. Dependence on 'hard' drugs carries a high mortality, partly because overdosage may be fatal and partly because their casual injection intravenously may lead to infections such as *hepatitis and *AIDS. Treatment is difficult and requires specialist skills. Much more common is **psychological dependence**, in which repeated use of a drug induces reliance on it for a state of well-being and contentment, but there are no physical withdrawal symptoms if use of the drug is stopped. Substances that may induce psychological dependence include nicotine in tobacco, cannabis, and many 'soft' drugs, such as barbiturates and amphetamines.

depersonalization n. a state in which a person feels himself becoming unreal or strangely altered, or feels that his mind is becoming separated from his body. Minor degrees of this feeling are common in normal people under stress. Severe feelings of depersonalization occur in anxiety neurosis, in states of *dissociation, in depression and schizophrenia, and in epilepsy (particularly temporal-lobe epilepsy). See also DEREALIZATION, OUT-OF-THE-BODY EXPERIENCE.

depilatory n. an agent applied to the skin to remove hair.

depolarization n. the sudden surge of charged particles across the membrane of a nerve cell or a muscle cell that accompanies a physicochemical change in the membrane and cancels out, or reverses, its resting potential to produce an *action potential. The passage of a *nerve impulse is a rapid wave of depolarization along the membrane of a nerve fibre.

depressant n. an agent that reduces the normal activity of any body system or function. Drugs such as general *anaesthetics, *barbiturates, and opiates are depressants of the central nervous system and respiration. *Cytotoxic drugs, such as azathioprine, are depressants of the levels of white blood cells.

depression *n.* a mental state characterized by excessive sadness. Activity can be agitated and restless or slow and retarded. Behaviour is governed by pessimistic or despairing beliefs, and sleep, appetite, and concentration are disturbed. There are several causes. *Manic-depressive psychosis causes severe depression, a major *affective disorder, in which there may be delusions of being worthless, ill, wicked, or impoverished and hallucinations of accusing voices. Loss and frustration also cause depression, which may be prolonged and disproportionate in **dysthymic disorder** (formerly known as depressive *neurosis). (*See also* PUERPERAL DEPRESSION.) Treatment is with *antidepressant drugs, *cognitive therapy, and/or *psychotherapy. Severe cases may need *electroconvulsive therapy.

depressor *n.* **1.** a muscle that causes lowering of part of the body. The **depressor labii inferioris** is a muscle that draws down and everts the lower lip. **2.** a nerve that lowers blood pressure.

dequalinium *n.* an antiseptic, active against some bacteria and fungi, used as lozenges or paint to treat mouth and throat infections. Trade name: **Labosept.**

derealization *n.* a feeling of unreality in which the environment is experienced as unreal and as flat, dull, or strange. The experience is unwelcome and often frightening. It occurs in association with *depersonalization or with the conditions that cause depersonalization.

dereism *n.* undirected fantasy thinking that fails to respect the realities of life. When this becomes markedly dominant it may be a feature of *schizoid personality or of *schizophrenia.

derm- (derma-, dermo-, dermat(o)-) *prefix denoting* the skin.

-derm *suffix denoting* **1.** the skin. **2.** a germ layer.

Dermacentor *n.* a genus of hard *ticks, worldwide in distribution, the adults of which are parasites of humans and other mammals. The wood tick, *D. andersoni*, transmits Rocky Mountain spotted fever to man in the western USA and the dog tick, *D. variabilis*, is the vector of the milder form of this disease in the east.

dermal *adj.* relating to or affecting the skin, especially the *dermis.

Dermanyssus *n.* a genus of widespread parasitic mites. The red poultry mite, *D. gallinae*, is a common parasite of wild birds in temperate regions but can also infest poultry. It occasionally attacks and takes a blood meal from man, causing itching and mild dermatitis.

dermatitis *n.* an inflammatory condition of the skin caused by outside agents (*compare* ECZEMA, an endogenous disease in which such agents do not play a primary role). **Primary irritant dermatitis** may occur in anyone who has sufficient contact with such irritants as acids, alkalis, solvents, and (especially) detergents. It is the commonest cause of **occupational dermatitis** in hairdressers, nurses, cooks, etc. (*See also* NAPKIN RASH.) In **allergic contact dermatitis** skin changes resembling those of eczema develop as a delayed reaction to contact with a particular allergen, which may be present at low concentrations. The commonest example in women is **nickel dermatitis** from jewellery, jeans studs, etc.; in men **chromium dermatitis** is relatively common. Treatment of dermatitis depends on removing the cause, which is not always possible.

Dermatitis herpetiformis is an uncommon very itchy rash with symmetrical blistering, especially on the knees, elbows, buttocks, and shoulders. It is associated with *gluten sensitivity and responds well to treatment with dapsone.

Dermatobia *n.* a genus of nonbloodsucking flies inhabiting lowland woods and forests of South and Central America. The parasitic maggots of *D. hominis* can cause a serious disease of the skin in humans (*see* MYIASIS). The maggots burrow into the skin, after emerging from eggs transported by bloodsucking insects (e.g. mosquitoes), and produce painful boil-like swellings. Treatment involves surgical removal of the maggots.

dermatochalasis *n.* redundant eyelid skin, which may cause drooping of the upper lid. It occurs as a result of ageing and is therefore seen only in middle-aged and elderly people. *Compare* BLEPHAROCHALASIS.

dermatofibrosarcoma protuberans

a tumour probably derived from *histiocytes that may occur in any part of the body. It is locally invasive but does not *metastasize. It often recurs locally despite excision.

dermatoglyphics n. the study of the patterns of finger, palm, toe, and sole prints. These patterns are formed by skin ridges, the distribution of which is unique to each individual. Abnormalities are found in those with chromosomal aberrations, such as *Down's syndrome. Dermatoglyphics is of value in criminology and is also of interest to anthropologists. See also FINGERPRINT.

dermatology n. the medical specialty concerned with the diagnosis and treatment of skin disorders. **—dermatological** adj. **—dermatologist** n.

dermatome n. **1.** a surgical instrument used for cutting thin slices of skin in some skin grafting operations. **2.** that part of the segmented mesoderm in the early embryo that forms the deeper layers of the skin (dermis) and associated tissues. See SOMITE.

dermatomyositis n. an inflammatory disorder of the skin and underlying tissues, including the muscles. The condition is one of the *connective-tissue diseases. A bluish-red skin eruption occurs on the face, scalp, neck, shoulders, and knuckles and is later accompanied by severe swelling. Dermatomyositis is often associated with internal cancer in adults, though not in children.

Dermatophagoides n. a genus of *mites that have been detected in samples of dust taken from houses in various parts of Europe. The mites may occasionally infest the skin of the scalp and cause dermatitis.

dermatophyte n. a fungus belonging to any one of the three genera (Microsporum, Trichophyton, and Epidermophyton) that can feed on *keratin and cause *ringworm (tinea).

dermatosis n. any disease of skin, particularly one without inflammation. In **juvenile plantar dermatosis**, which affects children up to the age of 14, the skin on the front of the sole becomes red, glazed, and symmetrically cracked. This condition,

which settles spontaneously after a number of years, is believed to be related to the wearing of trainers.

dermis (corium) n. the true *skin: the thick layer of living tissue that lies beneath the epidermis. It consists mainly of loose connective tissue within which are blood capillaries, lymph vessels, sensory nerve endings, sweat glands and their ducts, hair follicles, sebaceous glands, and smooth muscle fibres. **—dermal** adj.

dermographism n. a local reaction caused by pressure on the skin. People with such highly sensitive skin can 'write' on it with a finger or blunt instrument, the pressure producing weals.

dermoid cyst (dermoid) a cyst containing hair, hair follicles, and *sebaceous glands, usually found at sites marking the fusion of developing sections of the body in the embryo. Sometimes a dermoid cyst may develop after an injury. Surgical removal is best undertaken by a plastic surgeon.

descemetocele n. thinning of the *stroma of the cornea to such an extent that *Descemet's membrane is all that is maintaining the integrity of the eyeball. It occurs in severe ulceration of the cornea.

Descemet's membrane the membrane that forms the deepest layer of the *stroma of the cornea of the eye. The endothelium lies between it and the aqueous humour. [J. Descemet (1732–1810), French anatomist]

desensitization n. **1.** (or **hyposensitization**) a method for reducing the effects of a known allergen by injecting, over a period, gradually increasing doses of the allergen, until resistance is built up. See ALLERGY. **2.** a technique used in the *behaviour therapy of phobic states. The thing that is feared is very gradually introduced to the patient, first in imagination and then in reality. At the same time the patient is taught relaxation to inhibit the development of anxiety (see RELAXATION THERAPY). In this way he is able to cope with progressively closer approximations to the feared object or situation.

desferrioxamine n. a drug that combines with iron in body tissues and fluids and is used to treat iron poisoning (including that resulting from prolonged or constant blood transfusion, as for thalassaemia), diseases involving iron storage in parts of the body (*see* HAEMOCHROMATOSIS), and for the diagnosis of such diseases. It is administered by mouth, injection, or as eye drops; reactions and pain sometimes occur on injection. Trade name: **Desferal**.

desipramine *n.* a tricyclic *antidepressant drug administered by mouth or injection; common side-effects are dry mouth, blurred vision, insomnia, and unsteadiness in walking. Trade name: **Pertofran**.

desmoid tumour a dense connective-tissue tumour with a dangerous propensity for repeated local recurrence after treatment. Intra-abdominal desmoids have an association with familial adenomatous *polyposis (FAP).

desmopressin *n.* a synthetic derivative of *vasopressin that causes a decrease in urine output and is used to treat diabetes insipidus. It is also effective in mild haemophilia and von Willebrand's disease. Side-effects include stomach cramps, headache, and flushing of the skin. It is taken intranasally to treat diabetes insipidus and intravenously to treat haemophilia and von Willebrand's disease. Trade name: **DDAVP**.

desmosome *n.* an area of contact between two adjacent cells, occurring particularly in epithelia. The cell membranes at a desmosome are thickened and fine fibres (**tonofibrils**) extend from the desmosome into the cytoplasm.

desogestrel *n.* a *progestogen used in various *oral contraceptives, usually in combination with an oestrogen. Trade names: **Marvelon**, **Mercilon**.

desoximethasone *n.* a corticosteroid applied to the skin as a cream or ointment to reduce inflammation and pruritus. Side-effects include burning, itching, and local skin irritation. Trade name: **Stiedex**.

desquamation *n.* the process in which the outer layer of the *epidermis of the skin is removed by scaling.

detached retina *see* RETINAL DETACHMENT.

detergent *n.* a synthetic cleansing agent that removes all impurities from a surface by reacting with grease and suspended particles, including bacteria and other microorganisms. Some detergents, e.g. *cetrimide, are used solely for cleansing; others may be used as *antiseptics and *disinfectants.

detoxication (detoxification) *n.* **1.** the process whereby toxic substances are removed or toxic effects neutralized. It is one of the functions of the liver. **2.** the 'drying-out' of a patient suffering from *alcoholism.

detrition *n.* the process of wearing away solid bodies (e.g. bones) by friction or use.

detrusor *n.* the muscle of the urinary bladder wall. The functioning of the detrusor and urethral sphincter is assessed by a urodynamic investigation (*see* URODYNAMICS). This is used to diagnose dysfunction, absent and exaggerated reflexes, and instability in the muscle and lack of coordination between the muscle and the sphincter (bladder/sphincter dyssynergia).

Dettol *n.* *see* CHLOROXYLENOL.

detumescence *n.* **1.** the reverse of erection, whereby the erect penis or clitoris becomes flaccid after orgasm. **2.** subsidence of a swelling.

deut- (deuto-, deuter(o)-) *prefix denoting* two, second, or secondary.

deuteranopia *n.* a defect in colour vision in which reds, yellows, and greens are confused. It is thought that the mechanisms for perceiving red light and green light are in some way combined in people with this defect. *Compare* PROTANOPIA, TRITANOPIA. *See also* COLOUR BLINDNESS.

deutoplasm *n.* *see* YOLK.

developmental delay considerable delay in the physical or mental development of children when compared with their peers. There are many causes. **Global delay** describes the state of a child whose overall development is slow in all areas.

developmental disorder any one of a group of conditions in infancy or childhood, that are characterized by delays in biologically determined psychological functions, such as language. They are more common in males than females and tend to follow a course of handicap with gradual improvement. They are classified into **pervasive** conditions, in which many types of development are involved (e.g. *autism), and **specific** disorders, in which the handicap is an isolated problem (such as *dyslexia).

deviance *n.* variation from normal behaviour beyond the limits acceptable to the majority of the conforming peer group; particularly (though not exclusively) applied to sexual habits (*see also* SEXUAL DEVIATION).

deviation *n.* **1.** (in ophthalmology) any abnormal position of one or both eyes. For example, if the eyes are both looking to one side when the head is facing forwards, they are said to be **deviated** to that side. Such deviations of both eyes may occur in brain disease. Deviations of one eye, such as *dissociated vertical deviation, come into the category of squint (*see* STRABISMUS). **2.** *see* SEXUAL DEVIATION.

Devic's disease *see* NEUROMYELITIS OPTICA. [E. Devic (1869–1930), French physician]

devitalization *n.* (in dentistry) removal of a diseased pulp from a tooth. In primary teeth the coronal pulp is removed, followed by fixation of the radicular pulp. For permanent teeth, *see* ROOT CANAL TREATMENT.

dew-point hygrometer *see* HYGROMETER

DEXA (dual-energy X-ray absorptiometry) a method of measuring bone density based on the proportion of a beam of photons that passes through the bone. *See* OSTEOPOROSIS.

dexamethasone *n.* a *corticosteroid drug used principally to treat severe allergies, skin and eye diseases, rheumatic and other inflammatory conditions, and hormone and blood disorders. It is administered by mouth or injection; side-effects include sodium and fluid retention, muscle weakness, convulsions, vertigo, headache, and hormonal disturbances (including menstrual irregularities). Failure of injected (0.5 mg) dexamethasone to inhibit cortisol production (the **dexamethasone suppression test**) is a sensitive test for *phaeochromocytoma. Trade names: **Decadron, Maxidex**.

dexamphetamine *n.* a drug with actions and effects similar to those of *amphetamine. Trade name: **Dexedrine**.

dextr- (dextro-) *prefix denoting* **1.** the right side. Example: **dextroposition** (displacement to the right). **2.** (in chemistry) dextrorotation.

dextran *n.* a carbohydrate, consisting of branched chains of glucose units, that is a storage product of bacteria and yeasts. Preparations of dextran solution are used in transfusions, to increase the volume of plasma.

dextrin *n.* a carbohydrate formed as an intermediate product in the digestion of starch by the enzyme amylase. Dextrin is used in the preparation of pharmaceutical products (as an *excipient) and surgical dressings.

dextrocardia *n.* a congenital defect in which the position of the heart is a mirror image of its normal position, with the apex of the ventricles pointing to the right. It may be associated with other congenital defects and is often combined with **situs invertus**, in which the appendix and liver lie on the left side of the abdomen and the stomach lies on the right side. Isolated dextrocardia produces no adverse effects.

dextromethorphan *n.* a drug used in lozenges, syrups, and linctuses to suppress coughs (*see* ANTITUSSIVE). It sometimes causes drowsiness, dizziness, and digestive upsets. *See also* TRIPROLIDINE.

dextromoramide *n.* an *analgesic used to relieve moderate or severe pain. It is given by mouth, injection, or as suppositories and sometimes causes dizziness, reduced blood pressure, nausea, vomiting, and sleepiness. Dextromoramide is similar to *morphine and can cause morphine-type dependence. Trade name: **Palfium**.

dextropropoxyphene *n.* an *analgesic used to relieve mild or moderate pain. It is administered by mouth, often in combination with other analgesics (*see* CO-PROXAMOL), and sometimes causes dizziness, drowsiness, nausea, and vomiting. Trade name: **Doxolene**.

dextrose *n.* *see* GLUCOSE.

dhobie itch a fungal infection of the

skin that chiefly affects the groin but may spread to the thighs and buttocks. It is caused by *dermatophyte fungi, usually *Trichophyton rubrum*, *T. interdigitale*, and *Epidermophyton floccosum*. Medical name: **tinea cruris**. *See also* RINGWORM.

DI *see* ARTIFICIAL INSEMINATION.

di- *prefix denoting* two or double.

dia- *prefix denoting* **1**. through. **2**. completely or throughout. **3**. apart.

diabetes *n*. any disorder of metabolism causing excessive thirst and the production of large volumes of urine. Used alone, the term most commonly refers to *diabetes mellitus. *See also* DIABETES INSIPIDUS, HAEMOCHROMATOSIS (BRONZE DIABETES). —**diabetic** *adj., n*.

diabetes insipidus a rare metabolic disorder in which the patient produces large quantities of dilute urine and is constantly thirsty. It is due to deficiency of the pituitary hormone *vasopressin, which regulates reabsorption of water in the kidneys, and is treated by administration of the hormone.

diabetes mellitus a disorder of carbohydrate metabolism in which sugars in the body are not oxidized to produce energy due to lack of the pancreatic hormone *insulin. The accumulation of sugar leads to its appearance in the blood (**hyperglycaemia**), then in the urine; symptoms include thirst, loss of weight, and the excessive production of urine. The use of fats as an alternative source of energy leads to disturbances of the *acid-base balance, the accumulation of ketones in the bloodstream (*ketosis), and eventually to **diabetic coma**. There appears to be an inherited tendency to diabetes; the disorder may be triggered by various factors, including physical stress.

Diabetes that starts in childhood or adolescence is usually more severe than that beginning in middle or old age. It is known as **Type I** (or **insulin-dependent**) **diabetes mellitus** as patients have little or no ability to produce the hormone and are entirely dependent on insulin injections for survival. In **Type II** (or **noninsulin-dependent**) **diabetes mellitus**, usually occurring after the age of 40, the pancreas retains some ability to produce

insulin but this is inadequate for the body's needs; patients may require treatment with *oral hypoglycaemic drugs or insulin. In both types of diabetes the diet must be carefully controlled, with adequate carbohydrate for the body's needs. Lack of balance in the diet or in the amount of insulin taken leads to *hypoglycaemia. Long-term complications of diabetes include thickening of the arteries, which can affect the eyes (diabetic *retinopathy).

diabetic retinopathy *see* RETINOPATHY.

diaclast *n*. a surgical instrument used for the destruction of the skull of a fetus. This rare procedure enables a dead fetus to be delivered through the birth canal (*see* DECAPITATION).

diagnosis *n*. the process of determining the nature of a disorder by considering the patient's *signs and *symptoms, medical background, and – when necessary – results of laboratory tests and X-ray examinations. *See also* DIFFERENTIAL DIAGNOSIS, PRENATAL DIAGNOSIS. *Compare* PROGNOSIS. —**diagnostic** *adj*.

diakinesis *n*. the final stage in the first prophase of *meiosis, in which homologous chromosomes, between which crossing over has occurred, are ready to separate.

dialyser *n*. a piece of apparatus for separating components of a liquid mixture by *dialysis, especially an artificial kidney (*see* HAEMODIALYSIS).

dialysis *n*. a method of separating particles of different dimensions in a liquid mixture, using a thin semipermeable membrane whose pores are too small to allow the passage of large particles, such as proteins, but large enough to permit the passage of dissolved crystalline material. A solution of the mixture is separated from distilled water by the membrane; the solutes pass through the membrane into the water while the proteins, etc., are retained. The principle of dialysis is used in the artificial kidney (*see* HAEMODIALYSIS). The peritoneum is used as an autogenous semipermeable membrane in the technique of **peritoneal dialysis**, which is employed when haemodialysis is not appropriate.

diamorphine *n.* *see* HEROIN.

diapedesis *n.* migration of cells through the walls of blood capillaries into the tissue spaces. Diapedesis is an important part of the reaction of tissues to injury (*see* IN-FLAMMATION).

diaphoresis *n.* the process of sweating, especially excessive sweating. *See* SWEAT.

diaphoretic (sudorific) *n.* a drug that causes an increase in sweating, such as *pilocarpine, which stimulates the sweat glands directly. *Antipyretic drugs also have diaphoretic activity, which helps reduce the body temperature in fevers.

diaphragm *n.* **1.** (in anatomy) a thin musculomembranous dome-shaped muscle that separates the thoracic and abdominal cavities. The diaphragm is attached to the lower ribs at each side and to the breastbone and the backbone at the front and back. It bulges upwards against the heart and the lungs, arching over the stomach, liver, and spleen. There are openings in the diaphragm through which the oesophagus, blood vessels, and nerves pass. The diaphragm plays an important role in *breathing. It contracts with each inspiration, becoming flattened downwards and increasing the volume of the thoracic cavity. With each expiration it relaxes and is restored to its dome shape. **2.** a hemispherical rubber cap fitted inside the vagina over the neck (cervix) of the uterus as a contraceptive. When combined with the use of a chemical spermicide the diaphragm provides reliable contraception with a failure rate as low as 2–10 pregnancies per 100 woman-years.

diaphysial aclasis a hereditary abnormality of cartilage and bone growth, resulting in many cartilaginous outgrowths (exostoses) from the long bones. Bone growth may also be retarded, causing stunting and deformity.

diaphysis *n.* the shaft (central part) of a long bone. *Compare* EPIPHYSIS.

diaphysitis *n.* inflammation of the diaphysis (shaft) of a bone, through infection or rheumatic disease. It may result in impaired growth of the bone and consequent deformity.

diarrhoea *n.* frequent bowel evacuation or the passage of abnormally soft or liquid faeces. It may be caused by intestinal infections, other forms of intestinal inflammation (such as *colitis or *Crohn's disease), *malabsorption, anxiety, and the *irritable bowel syndrome. Severe or prolonged diarrhoea may lead to excess losses of fluid, salts, and nutrients in the faeces.

diarthrosis (synovial joint) *n.* a freely movable joint. The ends of the adjoining bones are covered with a thin cartilaginous sheet, and the bones are linked by a ligament (**capsule**) lined with *synovial membrane, which secretes synovial fluid (see illustration). Such joints are classified according to the type of connection between the bones and the type of movement allowed. *See* ARTHRODIC JOINT, CONDYLARTHROSIS, ENARTHROSIS, GINGLYMUS, SADDLE JOINT, TROCHOID JOINT.

synovial membrane

cartilage

synovial cavity

ligament forming capsule

A synovial joint

diaschisis *n.* a temporary loss of reflex activity in the brainstem or spinal cord following destruction of the cerebral cortex. As time passes this state of suppressed reflex activity is replaced by one of unduly exaggerated reflexes and spasticity of the limbs.

diastase *n.* an enzyme that hydrolyses starch in barley grain to produce maltose during the malting process. It has been used to aid the digestion of starch in some digestive disorders.

diastema *n.* a space between two teeth.

diastole *n.* the period between two contractions of the heart, when the muscle of the heart relaxes and allows the chambers to fill with blood. The term usually refers to **ventricular diastole**, which lasts about 0.5 seconds in a normal heart rate of about 70/minute. During exertion this period shortens, so allowing the heart rate to increase. *See also* BLOOD PRESSURE, SYSTOLE. —**diastolic** *adj.*

diastolic pressure *see* BLOOD PRESSURE.

diathermy *n.* the production of heat in a part of the body by means of a high-frequency electric current passed between two electrodes placed on the patient's skin. The heat generated increases blood flow and can be used in the treatment of deep-seated pain in rheumatic and arthritic conditions. *See also* MICROWAVE THERAPY.

The principle of diathermy is also utilized in various surgical instruments: a **diathermy knife**, for example, is used to coagulate tissues. The knife is itself one electrode, the other being a large moistened pad applied to another part of the patient's body. Because blood is coagulated as the knife is used, and small vessels sealed off, virtually bloodless incisions may be made. **Diathermy snares** and **needles** can be used to destroy unwanted tissue and to remove small superficial neoplasms. *See also* ELECTROSURGERY.

diathesis *n.* a higher than average tendency to acquire certain diseases, such as allergies, rheumatic diseases, or gout. Such diseases may run in families, but they are not inherited.

diazepam *n.* a long-acting *benzodiazepine used to treat acute anxiety, delirium tremens, epilepsy, and muscle spasms; it is also used as a *premedication. Diazepam is administered by mouth or injection and can cause addiction; side-effects include drowsiness and lethargy, vertigo, low blood pressure, and skin rashes. Trade names: **Diazemuls**, **Valium**.

diazoxide *n.* a drug used to lower blood pressure in patients with hypertension and also used to treat conditions in which the levels of blood sugar are low (including *insulinoma). It is usually administered (by mouth or (for hypertension) injection) with a diuretic as it causes salt and water retention. Trade name: **Eudemine**.

DIC *see* DISSEMINATED INTRAVASCULAR COAGULATION.

dicephalus *n. see* CRANIOPAGUS.

dichlorphenamide *n.* a *diuretic used to reduce pressure within the eye in the treatment of glaucoma. It is administered by mouth; side-effects include drowsiness, dizziness, digestive upsets, and skin rashes. Trade name: **Daranide**.

dichromatic *adj.* describing the state of colour vision of those who can appreciate only two of the three primary colours. People with such vision match any given colour by a mixture of the two they can distinguish. *Compare* TRICHROMATIC.

DICI (direct intracytoplasmic injection) a former name for *ICSI (intracytoplasmic sperm injection).

Dick test a test for susceptibility to *scarlet fever. If a small quantity of toxin from the bacteria responsible (haemolytic streptococci) is injected under the skin of a person not immune to the disease, a positive reaction results, causing local reddening of the skin. [G. F. Dick (1881–1967) and G. R. H. Dick (1881–1963), US physicians]

diclofenac *n.* an anti-inflammatory drug (*see* NSAID) used to relieve joint pain in osteoarthritis, rheumatoid arthritis, and ankylosing spondylitis. It is administered by mouth; possible side-effects include abdominal pain, nausea, and diarrhoea. Trade names: **Volraman**, **Voltarol**.

dicophane *n. see* DDT.

dicrotism *n.* a condition in which the pulse is felt as a double beat for each contraction of the heart. It may be seen in typhoid fever. —**dicrotic** *adj.*

dictyoma *n.* a tumour of the epithelium lining the *ciliary body of the eye. It may be benign or malignant.

dicyclomine *n.* a drug that reduces spasms of smooth muscle and is used to relieve peptic ulcer, infantile colic, colitis, and related conditions. It is administered by mouth; side-effects include dry mouth, thirst, and dizziness. Trade name: **Merbentyl**.

didanosine (ddI) *n.* an antiviral drug that interferes with the action of the enzyme *reverse transcriptase, by means of which HIV, the cause of AIDS, is able to incorporate itself into the human host cell. The drug is administered by mouth in attempts to prolong the lives of sufferers from AIDS. Possible side-effects include damage to nerves, severe pancreatitis, nausea, vomiting, and headache.

Didronel *n. see* ETIDRONATE.

didym- (didymo-) *prefix denoting* the testis.

dieldrin *n.* an insecticide that attacks the central nervous system of insects and has proved useful in the control of various beetles, flies, and larvae that attack crops. Because of its persistence in and contamination of the environment, its use in the UK is now severely restricted.

diencephalon *n.* an anatomical division of the forebrain, consisting of the epithalamus, thalamus (dorsal thalamus), hypothalamus, and ventral thalamus (subthalamus). *See* BRAIN.

dienoestrol *n.* a synthetic female sex hormone (*see* OESTROGEN) administered topically in the form of a vaginal cream to relieve atrophy, itching, or inflammation of the vagina as part of *hormone replacement therapy. Trade name: **Ortho Dienoestrol**.

diet *n.* the mixture of foods that a person eats. A **balanced diet** contains the correct proportions of all the nutrients, i.e. vitamins, minerals (calcium, phosphorus, potassium, sodium, chlorine, sulphur, magnesium, and the *trace elements), and *dietary fibre, as well as water, carbohydrates and fats (which provide energy), and proteins (required for growth and maintenance).

dietary fibre (roughage) the part of food that cannot be digested and absorbed to produce energy. Dietary fibre falls into four groups: **cellulose**, **hemicelluloses**, **lignins**, and **pectins**. Highly refined foods, such as sucrose, contain no dietary fibre. Foods with a high fibre content include wholemeal cereals and flour, root vegetables, nuts, and fruit. Dietary fibre is considered by some to be helpful in the prevention of many of the diseases of Western civilization, such as *diverticulosis, constipation, appendicitis, obesity, and

diabetes mellitus. Communities consuming high-fibre diets very rarely have any of these diseases.

dietetics *n.* the application of the principles of *nutrition to the selection of food and the feeding of individuals and groups.

diethylcarbamazine *n.* an anthelmintic drug that destroys filariae and is therefore used in the treatment of filariasis, loiasis, and onchocerciasis. It is administered as tablets. Side-effects may include headache, malaise, joint pains, nausea, and vomiting.

diethylpropion *n.* a drug, similar to *amphetamine, that suppresses the appetite and is used in the treatment of obesity. It is administered by mouth and may cause dry mouth, insomnia, depression, headache, constipation, and allergic rashes. Dependence of the amphetamine type can occur. Trade names: **Apesate**, **Tenuate Dospan**.

Dietl's crisis acute obstruction of a kidney causing severe pain in the loins. The obstruction usually occurs at the junction of the renal pelvis and the ureter, causing the kidney to become distended with accumulated urine (*see* HYDRONEPHROSIS). Sometimes the pelvis drains spontaneously, with relief of pain, but acute decompression of the kidney may be required with surgical relief of the obstruction (*pyeloplasty). [J. Dietl (1804–78), Polish physician]

Dieulafoy's lesion an abnormality of small blood vessels in the mucosal lining of the upper stomach that may cause severe spontaneous haemorrhage. The abnormality is difficult to see at *gastroscopy or at surgical exploration and therefore may be overlooked. [G. Dieulafoy (1839–1911), French physician]

differential diagnosis *diagnosis of a condition whose signs and/or symptoms are shared by various other conditions. For example, abdominal pain may be due to any of a large number of different disorders, which must be ruled out in arriving at a correct diagnosis.

differential leucocyte count (differential blood count) a determination of the proportions of the different kinds of white cells (leucocytes) present in a sample of blood. Usually 100 white cells are counted and classified under the microscope or by electronic apparatus, so that the results can readily be expressed as percentages of the total number of leucocytes and the absolute numbers per litre of blood. The information often aids diagnosis of disease.

differentiation *n.* **1.** (in embryology) the process in embryonic development during which unspecialized cells or tissues become specialized for particular functions. **2.** (in oncology) the degree of similarity of tumour cells to the structure of the organ from which the tumour arose. Tumours are classified as well, moderately, or poorly differentiated.

diflunisal *n.* an anti-inflammatory drug (*see* NSAID) derived from salicylic acid and used to control symptoms in osteoarthritis and other painful conditions. It is administered by mouth. Possible side-effects include dyspepsia, diarrhoea, headache, dizziness, tinnitus, and skin rashes. Trade name: **Dolobid**.

di George syndrome a hereditary condition resulting in an inability to fight infections (immunodeficiency) associated with absence of the parathyroid and thymus glands, abnormalities of the heart, and low calcium levels. Affected children are prone to *Candida* infections and often present with *failure to thrive. [A. M. di George (1921–), US paediatrician]

digestion *n.* the process in which ingested food is broken down in the alimentary canal into a form that can be absorbed and assimilated by the tissues of the body. Digestion includes mechanical processes, such as chewing, churning, and grinding food, as well as the chemical action of digestive enzymes and other substances (bile, acid, etc.). Chemical digestion begins in the mouth with the action of *saliva on food, but most of it takes place in the stomach and small intestine, where the food is subjected to *gastric juice, *pancreatic juice, and *succus entericus.

digit *n.* any one of the terminal divisions of a limb: a finger or toe.

digital *adj.* **1.** (in anatomy) relating to a digit. **2.** (in radiology) relating to or utilizing *digitization.

digitalis *n.* an extract from the dried leaves of foxgloves (*Digitalis* species), which contains various substances, including *digitoxin and *digoxin, that stimulate heart muscle. Used to treat heart failure, it is administered by mouth or, in emergency, by injection. High doses can cause nausea, vomiting, loss of appetite, diarrhoea, abdominal pain, and abnormal heart activity. *See also* DIGITALIZATION.

digitalization *n.* the administration of the drug digitalis or one of its purified derivatives to a patient with heart failure until the optimum level has been reached in the heart tissues. At this stage the control of heart failure should be adequate and there should be few side-effects. The process of digitalization may take several days.

digital radiography the application of *digitization to conventional radiography, allowing the storage of images on hard disk and their subsequent retrieval and interpretation using TV monitors rather than photographic film.

digital spot imaging (DSI) X-ray screening in which the images produced can be stored digitally (*see* DIGITIZATION) and either transferred to photographic film or viewed on a TV monitor.

digital subtraction angiography a sophisticated radiological technique in which *digitization allows X-ray examination of blood vessels (*see* ANGIOGRAPHY) to be performed using smaller volumes of contrast material. A digitized image is taken before the contrast medium is added, and this is subtracted by computer from the contrast image. The technique enables blood vessel anatomy and blood supply to an organ to be demonstrated.

digitization *n.* (in radiology) the assignment of a numerical value to each *pixel of a *grey-scale image to allow storage, electronic manipulation, and transfer via computer links of images produced by such devices as X-ray machines, CT scanners, MRI scanners, or ultrasound probes.

digitoxin *n.* a drug that increases heart muscle contraction and is used in heart failure. It is slow-acting but the effects are prolonged. Digitoxin is administered by mouth or injection; possible side-effects are those of *digitalis.

digoxin *n.* a drug that increases heart muscle contraction and is used in heart failure. It is rapidly effective and the effects are short-lived. Digoxin is administered by mouth or injection; side-effects are those of *digitalis. Trade name: **Lanoxin**.

dihydrocodeine *n.* a drug used to relieve pain and suppress coughs (*see* ANALGESIC, ANTITUSSIVE). It is administered by mouth or injection and sometimes causes nausea, dizziness, and constipation. Dependence of the *morphine type can also occur, but this is rare. Trade name: **DHC Continus**.

dihydroergotamine *n.* a derivative of *ergotamine used to prevent and relieve migraine attacks. It is administered by mouth or injection; side-effects are rare but nausea sometimes occurs. Trade name: **Dihydergot**.

dihydrofolate reductase inhibitor any of various drugs that interfere with the conversion of folic acid to its active form in the body. They include *pyrimethamine, *trimethoprim, *triamterene, and *methotrexate. When such drugs are necessary, folate deficiency is treated with *folinic acid rather than folic acid.

diiodohydroxyquinoline *n.* an antiseptic used to treat bowel infections and dysentery caused by amoebae. It is administered by mouth or as pessaries and occasionally causes irritation of the digestive system, headache, itching, and boils.

diiodotyrosine *n.* an iodine-containing substance produced in the thyroid gland from which the *thyroid hormones are derived.

dilaceration *n.* a condition affecting some teeth after traumatic injury, in which the incomplete root continues to form at an abnormal angle to the part already formed. In severe cases it may be necessary to remove the tooth.

dilatation *n.* the enlargement or expansion of a hollow organ (such as a blood vessel) or cavity.

dilatation and curettage (D and C) an operation in which the cervix (neck) of the uterus is dilated, using an instrument called a *dilator, and the lining (endometrium) of the uterus is lightly scraped off with a curette (*see* CURETTAGE). It is performed for a variety of reasons, including the removal of any material remaining after abortion, removal of small tumours, and obtaining a sample of endometrium for histological examination in the diagnosis of gynaecological disorders. Special types of curette to which suction is applied (vabra or suction curettes) may be used to obtain a specimen of endometrium (**vabra curettage**) or to remove the products of conception in abortion (**suction curettage**).

dilator *n.* **1.** an instrument used to enlarge a body opening or cavity. For example, the male urethra may become narrowed by disease and it can sometimes be restored to its original size by inserting a dilator. Dilators (such as **Hegar's dilator**) are also used to enlarge the canal in the cervix of the uterus in the procedure of *dilatation and curettage. **2.** a drug, applied either locally or systemically, that causes expansion of a structure, such as the pupil of the eye or a blood vessel. *See also* VASODILATOR. **3.** a muscle that, by its action, opens an aperture or orifice in the body.

diltiazem *n.* a *calcium antagonist used in the treatment of effort-associated angina and high blood pressure (hypertension). It acts as a vasodilator and is administered by mouth; side-effects include oedema, headache, nausea, dizziness, and skin rash. Trade names: **Britiazem**, **Tildiem**.

dimenhydrinate *n.* an *antihistamine used to prevent and treat motion sickness, nausea and vomiting due to other causes, vertigo, and inner ear disturbances. It is administered by mouth or injection and commonly causes drowsiness, dizziness, digestive upsets, dry mouth, and headache. Trade name: **Dramamine**.

dimercaprol *n.* a drug that combines with metals in the body and is used to treat poisoning by antimony, arsenic, bismuth, gold, mercury, and thallium and in Wilson's disease. It is administered by injection and commonly causes nausea, vomiting, and watering of the eyes. Trade name: **British Anti-Lewisite** (**BAL**).

dimethicone *n.* a silicone preparation used externally to prevent undue drying of the skin and to protect it against irritating external agents. It is commonly used to prevent napkin rash in babies. Trade names: **Conotrane**, **Siopel.**

dimethindine maleate an *antihistamine drug used to treat hay fever, urticaria, and other allergic conditions. It is administered by mouth. Possible side-effects include drowsiness and slowed reactions. Trade names: **Fenostil Retard**, **Vibrocil.**

dimethyl sulphoxide (DMSO) a chemical used in an ointment to treat skin inflammations or in combination with other topically applied drugs to improve their absorption. It may cause skin irritation.

dinoprost *n.* a *prostaglandin drug used to terminate pregnancy or to expel a fetus that has died. It is administered by mouth or as a vaginal tablet or gel. Trade name: **Prostin F2 alpha**.

dioctyl sodium sulphosuccinate a softening agent that is given by mouth or in suppositories, often together with a laxative, to relieve constipation. It is also used in solution to soften ear wax.

diode laser a portable laser used for treating diseases of the retina of the eye by producing small burns in the retina (*see* PHOTOCOAGULATION).

dioptre *n.* the unit of measurement of the power of *refraction of a lens. One dioptre is the power of a lens that brings parallel light rays to a focus at a point one metre from the lens, after passing through it. A stronger lens brings light rays to a focus at a point closer to it than a weaker lens and has a higher dioptric power.

dipeptidase *n.* an enzyme, found in digestive juices, that splits certain products of protein digestion (dipeptides) into their constituent amino acids. The latter are then absorbed by the body.

dipeptide *n.* a compound consisting of two amino acids joined together by a peptide bond (e.g. glycylalanine, a combination of the amino acids glycine and alanine). *See* DIPEPTIDASE.

diphenhydramine *n.* an *antihistamine with sedative properties used to treat allergic conditions, such as hay fever and rhinitis, and – in combination with other drugs – in cough mixtures (e.g. **Benylin**). It is administered by mouth or injection; side-effects include drowsiness, dry mouth, dizziness, and nausea.

diphenoxylate *n.* a drug used, often in combination with *atropine (in **Lomotil**), to treat diarrhoea. It is also used after *colostomy or ileostomy to reduce the frequency and fluidity of the stools. It is administered by mouth; side-effects can include nausea, drowsiness, dizziness, skin reactions, and restlessness.

diphosphonate *n.* any of a class of compounds that bind strongly to bone. This property makes them useful in imaging the skeleton and treating certain bone disorders, such as *Paget's disease of bone.

diphtheria *n.* an acute highly contagious infection, caused by the bacterium *Corynebacterium diphtheriae*, generally affecting the throat but occasionally other mucous membranes and the skin. The disease is spread by direct contact with a patient or carrier or by contaminated milk. After an incubation period of 2–6 days a sore throat, weakness, and mild fever develop. Later, a soft grey membrane forms across the throat, constricting the air passages and causing difficulty in breathing and swallowing; a *tracheostomy may be necessary. Bacteria multiply at the site of infection and release a toxin into the bloodstream, which damages heart and nerves. Death from heart failure or general collapse can follow within four days but prompt administration of antitoxin and penicillin arrests the disease. An effective immunization programme has now made diphtheria rare in most Western countries (*see also* SCHICK TEST).

diphtheroid *adj.* resembling diphtheria (especially the membrane formed in diphtheria) or the bacteria that cause it.

diphyllobothriasis *n.* an infestation of the intestine with the broad tapeworm, *Diphyllobothrium latum*, which sometimes causes nausea, malnutrition, diarrhoea, and anaemia resulting from impaired absorption of vitamin B_{12} through the gut. The infestation, common in Baltic countries, is contracted following ingestion of uncooked fish infected with the larval stage of the tapeworm. The tapeworm can be expelled from the gut with the anthelmintic *mepacrine.

Diphyllobothrium *n.* a genus of large tapeworms that can grow to a length of 3–10 m. The adult of *D. latum*, the broad (or fish) tapeworm, infects fish-eating mammals including man, in whom it may cause serious anaemia (*see* DIPHYLLOBOTHRIASIS). The parasite has two intermediate hosts: a freshwater crustacean and a fish (*see also* PLEROCERCOID).

dipipanone *n.* a potent *analgesic drug used to relieve severe pain. It is administered by mouth or injection and may cause nausea, vomiting, dizziness, and drowsiness. Trade name: **Diconal**.

dipl- (diplo-) *prefix denoting* double.

diplacusis *n.* perception of a single sound as double owing to a defect of the *cochlea in the inner ear.

diplegia *n.* paralysis involving both sides of the body and affecting the legs more severely than the arms. **Cerebral diplegia** is a form of *cerebral palsy in which there is widespread damage, in both cerebral hemispheres, of the brain cells that control the movements of the limbs. —**diplegic** *adj.*

diplococcus *n.* any of a group of nonmotile parasitic spherical bacteria that occur in pairs. The group includes the *pneumococcus.

diploë *n.* the lattice-like tissue that lies between the inner and outer layers of the *skull.

diploid *adj.* describing cells, nuclei, or organisms in which each chromosome except the Y sex chromosome is represented twice. *Compare* HAPLOID, TRIPLOID. —**diploid** *n.*

diplopia *n.* double vision: the simultaneous awareness of two images of the one object. It is usually due to limitation of movement of one eye so that the two eyes cannot simultaneously look at the same object. This may be caused by a defect of the nerves or muscles controlling eye movement or a mechanical restriction of eyeball movement in the orbit. Double vi-

sion that does not disappear on covering one eye can be caused by early cataract (*see also* POLYOPIA).

diplotene *n.* the fourth stage in the first prophase of *meiosis, in which *crossing over occurs between the paired chromatids of homologous chromosomes, which then begin to separate.

diprosopus *n.* a fetal monster with a single trunk and normal limbs but with some degree of duplication of the face.

dipsomania *n.* morbid and insatiable craving for alcohol, occurring in paroxysms. Only a small proportion of alcoholics show this symptom. *See* ALCOHOLISM.

Diptera *n.* a large group of insects, including *mosquitoes, gnats, midges, house flies and *tsetse flies, that possess a single pair of wings. The mouthparts of many species, e.g. mosquitoes and tsetse flies, are specialized for sucking blood; these forms are important in the transmission of disease (*see* VECTOR). *See also* FLY.

Dipylidium *n.* a genus of tapeworms. *D. caninum*, a common parasite of the small intestine of dogs and cats, occasionally infects man but usually produces no obvious symptoms. Fleas are the intermediate hosts, and children in close contact with pets become infected on ingesting fleas harbouring the parasite.

dipyridamole *n.* a drug that dilates the blood vessels of the heart and reduces platelet aggregation. It is given by mouth or injection to prevent thrombosis around prosthetic heart valves. It may cause headache, stomach upsets, and dizziness. Trade name: **Persantin**.

direct intracytoplasmic injection (DICI) a former name for intracytoplasmic sperm injection (*see* ICSI).

director *n.* an instrument used to guide the extent and direction of a surgical incision.

Director of Public Health (DPH) a senior public health doctor of a Health Authority or an NHS Executive regional office. *See also* PUBLIC HEALTH PHYSICIAN.

dis- *prefix denoting* separation.

disability *n.* a loss or restriction of functional ability or activity as a result of im-

pairment of the body or mind. *See also*
HANDICAP.

disability living allowance a state
benefit payable to those under 65 who
have had a disability requiring help for at
least three months and are likely to need
such help for at least a further six
months. It has two components: a care
component, payable at three rates to those
needing help with personal care; and a
mobility component, payable at two rates
to those aged five or over who need help
with walking. The rates depend on the
level of help required.

disability working allowance an income-related benefit payable to those aged
16 or over who are working 16 or more
hours a week and who have a disability
that puts them at a disadvantage in obtaining employment. It is only payable to
those already receiving a 'qualifying
benefit', such as *disability living allowance.

Disabled Living Foundation (in
Britain) a voluntary agency interested in
all aspects of the care of those with disabilities and in improving their quality of
life. It is particularly concerned with aids
to daily living, some of which can be inspected by clients, doctors, and others at a
permanent exhibition at the headquarters
of the Foundation.

disablement *n. see* HANDICAP.

disaccharide *n.* a carbohydrate consisting of two linked *monosaccharide units.
The most common disaccharides are *maltose, *lactose, and *sucrose.

disarticulation *n.* separation of two
bones at a joint. This may be the result of
an injury or it may be done by the surgeon at operation in the course of amputation; for example of a limb, finger, or
toe.

disc *n.* (in anatomy) a rounded flattened
structure, such as an *intervertebral disc
or the *optic disc.

disc cupping an abnormal enlargement
of the central depression of the *optic
disc due to loss of nerve fibres, as occurs
in glaucoma as a result of raised intraocular pressure.

discharge rate the number of cases of

a specified disease or condition discharged
from hospitals related to the population
of the *catchment area: usually expressed
regionally per 10,000.

discission *n.* an obsolete operation for
cataract in which the lens capsule was
ruptured by a fine knife or needle to
allow the substance of the lens to be absorbed naturally into the surrounding
fluid of the eye.

discoid lupus erythematosus (DLE)
see LUPUS ERYTHEMATOSUS.

disease *n.* a disorder with a specific
cause and recognizable signs and symptoms; any bodily abnormality or failure to
function properly, except that resulting
directly from physical injury (the latter,
however, may open the way for disease).

disimpaction *n.* the process of separating the broken ends of a bone when they
have been forcibly driven together during
a fracture.

disinfectant *n.* an agent that destroys
or removes bacteria and other microorganisms and is used to cleanse surgical instruments and other objects. Examples are
*cresol, *hexachlorophane, and *phenol.
Dilute solutions of some disinfectants may
be used as *antiseptics or as preservatives
in solutions of eye drops or injections.

disinfection *n.* the process of eliminating infective microorganisms from contaminated instruments, clothing, or
surroundings by using physical means or
chemicals (*disinfectants).

disinfestation *n.* the destruction of insect pests and other animal parasites. This
generally involves the use of insecticides
applied either topically, as in delousing, or
as a spray for eliminating an infestation
of fleas or bed bugs in the home.

disintegrative psychosis **1.** *see*
HELLER'S SYNDROME. **2.** a pervasive *developmental disorder, often with features of
*autism, occurring as a result of a brain
disease, such as encephalitis, in childhood.

disjunction *n.* the separation of pairs of
homologous chromosomes during meiosis
or of the chromatids of a chromosome
during *anaphase of mitosis or meiosis.
Compare NONDISJUNCTION.

dislocation (luxation) *n.* displacement from their normal position of bones meeting at a joint such that there is complete loss of contact of the joint surfaces. It usually results from trauma (dislocation of the shoulder is common in sports injuries) but may be congenital, in which case it usually affects the hip (*see* CONGENITAL DISLOCATION OF THE HIP). In a traumatic dislocation the bones are restored to their normal positions by manipulation under local or general anaesthesia (*see* REDUCTION). *Compare* SUBLUXATION.

dismemberment *n.* the separating of body parts or the amputation of a leg, arm, or part of a limb.

disoma *n.* a double-bodied fetal monster with a single head.

disopyramide *n.* a *parasympatholytic drug used to treat various heart conditions involving abnormal heart rates. It is administered by mouth; side-effects such as dry mouth, blurred vision, difficulty in urination, and digestive upsets may occur. Trade names: **Dirythmin SA, Rythmodan**.

disorientation *n.* the state produced by loss of awareness of space, time, or personality. It can be the result of drugs, anxiety, or organic disease (such as dementia or *Korsakoff's syndrome).

dispensary *n.* a place where medicines are made up by a pharmacist according to the doctor's prescription and dispensed to patients. A dispensary is often part of an out-patient department in a hospital.

dispensing practice (in Britain) a general practice (usually in a remote area) in which doctors receive special allowances under the terms of the *National Health Service for dispensing the medications they prescribe for their patients. *See also* GENERAL PRACTITIONER.

displacement *n.* (in psychology) the substitution of one type of behaviour for another, usually the substitution of a relatively harmless activity for a harmful one; for example, kicking the cat instead of one's boss.

dissection *n.* the cutting apart and separation of the body tissues along the natural divisions of the organs and different tissues in the course of an operation.

Dissection of corpses is carried out for the study of anatomy.

disseminated *adj.* widely distributed in an organ (or organs) or in the whole body. The term may refer to disease organisms or to pathological changes.

disseminated intravascular coagulation (DIC) a condition resulting from overstimulation of the blood-clotting mechanisms in response to disease or injury, such as severe infection, asphyxia, hypothermia, abruptio placentae, or intrauterine fetal death. The overstimulation results in generalized blood coagulation and excessive consumption of coagulation factors. The resulting deficiency of these may lead to spontaneous bleeding. Transfusions of plasma are given to replace the depleted clotting factors, and treatment of the underlying cause is essential.

disseminated sclerosis *see* MULTIPLE SCLEROSIS.

dissociated vertical deviation (DVD) a condition in which one eye looks upwards when the amount of light entering it is reduced, e.g. when it is covered. The eye returns to its original position when the cover is removed. DVD is an acquired condition chiefly associated with infantile esotropia (convergent *strabismus).

dissociation *n.* (in psychiatry) the process whereby thoughts and ideas can be split off from consciousness and may function independently, thus (for example) allowing conflicting opinions to be held at the same time about the same object. Dissociation may be the main factor in cases of dissociative *fugue and multiple personalities.

dissociative disorder any one of a group of extreme *defence mechanisms that include loss of memory for important personal details (*see* AMNESIA); wandering away from home and the assumption of a new identity (*see* FUGUE); splitting of the personality into two or more distinct personalities (*see* MULTIPLE PERSONALITY DISORDER); and trancelike states with severely reduced response to external stimuli. *Conversion disorder is classified with dissociative disorders (as dissociative (conversion) disorders) in ICD-10 (*see* INTERNATIONAL CLASSIFICATION OF DISEASES).

distal *adj.* **1.** (in anatomy) situated away from the origin or point of attachment or from the median line of the body. For example, the term is applied to a part of a limb that is furthest from the body; to a blood vessel that is far from the heart; and to a nerve fibre that is far from the central nervous system. *Compare* PROXIMAL. **2.** (in dentistry) describing the surface of a tooth away from the midline of the jaw.

Distalgesic *n.* *see* CO-PROXAMOL.

distichiasis *n.* a very rare condition in which there is an extra row of eyelashes behind the normal row. They may rub on the cornea.

distigmine *n.* an *anticholinesterase drug used to treat myasthenia gravis. It is administered by mouth. Possible side-effects include nausea, vomiting, diarrhoea, and excessive salivation. Trade name: **Ubretid**.

distraction *n.* (in orthopaedics) increasing the distance between two points. In *limb lengthening procedures callus can be stretched longitudinally by increasing the distance between pins attached to the bone (*see* CALLOTASIS).

District Health Authority *see* NATIONAL HEALTH SERVICE.

district nurse (home nurse) a trained nurse with special training in *domiciliary services, usually employed by a community trust. District nurses may also be allocated to a designated general practice, an arrangement known as *attachment.

District Planning Team a multidisciplinary team established in a health district to identify gaps in the services and to suggest how they can be improved.

disulfiram *n.* a drug used in the treatment of chronic alcoholism. It acts as a deterrent by producing unpleasant effects when taken with alcohol, including flushing, breathing difficulties, headache, palpitations, nausea, and vomiting. It is administered by mouth; common side-effects are fatigue, nausea, and constipation. Trade name: **Antabuse**.

dithranol *n.* a drug applied to the skin as an ointment or paste to treat *psoriasis. It may irritate the skin on application. Trade names: **Alphodith, Dithrolan**.

diuresis *n.* increased secretion of urine by the kidneys. This normally follows the drinking of more fluid than the body requires, but it can be stimulated by the administration of a *diuretic.

diuretic *n.* a drug that increases the volume of urine produced by promoting the excretion of salts and water from the kidney. The main classes of diuretics act by inhibiting the reabsorption of salts and water from the kidney tubules into the bloodstream. **Thiazide diuretics** (e.g. *bendrofluazide, *chlorthalidone) act at the distal convoluted tubules (*see* NEPHRON), preventing the reabsorption of sodium and potassium. **Potassium-sparing diuretics** (e.g. *amiloride, *spironolactone, *triamterene) prevent excessive loss of potassium at the distal convoluted tubules, and **loop diuretics** (e.g. *frusemide) prevent reabsorption of sodium and potassium in *Henle's loop. Diuretics are used to reduce the oedema due to salt and water retention in disorders of the heart, kidneys, liver, or lungs. Some mild diuretics, including *acetazolamide, are used to reduce the pressure within the eyeball in glaucoma. Thiazides and potassium-sparing diuretics are also used – in conjunction with other drugs – in the treatment of high blood pressure. Treatment with thiazide and loop diuretics often results in potassium deficiency; this is corrected by simultaneous administration of potassium salts or a potassium-sparing diuretic.

divagation *n.* rambling discursive thought and speech. It is not specific to any one psychiatric condition.

divarication *n.* the separation or stretching of bodily structures. **Rectus divarication** is stretching of the *rectus abdominis muscle, a common condition associated with pregnancy or obesity.

divaricator *n.* **1.** a scissor-like surgical instrument used to divide portions of tissue into two separate parts during an operation. **2.** a form of retractor used to open out the sides of an abdominal incision and facilitate access.

divergence n. (in ophthalmology) abduction of the eyes. **Divergence excess** is a type of squint (divergent *strabismus) in which the eyes are deviated outwards more when looking in the distance than for near vision. **Divergence insufficiency** is a type of squint (convergent *strabismus) in which the eyes are deviated slightly inwards only when looking in the distance.

diverticular disease a condition in which there are diverticula (see DIVERTICULUM) in the colon associated with lower abdominal pain and disturbed bowel habit. The pain is due to spasm of the muscle of the intestine and not to inflammation of the diverticula (compare DIVERTICULITIS).

diverticulitis n. inflammation of a *diverticulum, most commonly of one or more colonic diverticula. This type of diverticulitis is caused by infection and causes lower abdominal pain with diarrhoea or constipation; it may lead to abscess formation, which often requires surgical drainage. A Meckel's diverticulum sometimes becomes inflamed due to infection, causing symptoms similar to *appendicitis. Diverticula elsewhere in the alimentary tract are not subject to diverticulitis. Compare DIVERTICULAR DISEASE.

diverticulosis n. a condition in which diverticula exist in a segment of the intestine without evidence of inflammation (compare DIVERTICULITIS).

diverticulum n. (pl. **diverticula**) a sac or pouch formed at weak points in the walls of the alimentary tract. They may be caused by increased pressure from within (**pulsion diverticula**) or by pulling from without (**traction diverticula**). A **pharyngeal diverticulum** occurs in the pharynx and may cause difficulty in swallowing. **Oesophageal diverticula** occur in the middle or lower oesophagus (gullet); they may be associated with muscular disorders of the oesophagus but rarely cause symptoms. **Gastric diverticula** affect the stomach (usually the upper part) and cause no symptoms. **Duodenal diverticula** occur on the concave surface of the duodenal loop; they may be associated with *dyspepsia and an increased risk of choledocholithiasis, but usually cause few symptoms. **Jejunal diverticula** affect the small intestine, are often multiple, and may give rise to abdominal discomfort and *malabsorption due to growth of bacteria within them. **Meckel's diverticulum** occurs in the ileum, about 35 cm from its termination, as a congenital abnormality. It may become inflamed, mimicking *appendicitis; if it contains embryonic remnants of stomach mucosa it may form a *peptic ulcer, causing pain, bleeding, or perforation. **Colonic diverticula**, affecting the colon (particularly the lowest portion), become commoner with increasing age and often cause no symptoms. However they are sometimes associated with abdominal pain or altered bowel habit (see DIVERTICULAR DISEASE) or they may become inflamed (see DIVERTICULITIS).

division n. **1.** the separation of an organ or tissue into parts by surgery. **2.** see CELL DIVISION.

dizygotic twins see TWINS.

DLE discoid lupus erythematosus. See LUPUS ERYTHEMATOSUS.

DMD (Duchenne muscular dystrophy) see MUSCULAR DYSTROPHY.

DMSA dimercaptosuccinic acid labelled with *technetium-99, used as a tracer to obtain *scintigrams of the kidney, by means of a *gamma camera, particularly to show scarring resulting from infection and to assess the relative function of each kidney.

DNA (deoxyribonucleic acid) the genetic material of nearly all living organisms, which controls heredity and is located in the cell nucleus (see CHROMOSOME, GENE). DNA is a *nucleic acid composed of two strands made up of units called *nucleotides (see illustration). The two strands are wound around each other into a double helix and linked together by hydrogen bonds between the bases of the nucleotides (see BASE PAIRING). The genetic information of the DNA is contained in the sequence of bases along the molecule (see GENETIC CODE); changes in the DNA cause *mutations. The DNA molecule can make exact copies of itself by the process of *replication, thereby passing on the genetic information to the daughter cells when the cell divides.

DNA repair a variety of mechanisms

that help to ensure that the genetic sequence, as expressed in the DNA, is maintained and that errors that occur during DNA replication, by mutation, are not allowed to accumulate. An error in the genetic sequence could cause cell death by interfering with the replication process. DNA repair involves the action of enzymes, which detect damage to DNA and effect the repair. Some genetic diseases, including *ataxia telangiectasia and *xeroderma pigmentosum, are due to deficiencies in these enzymes.

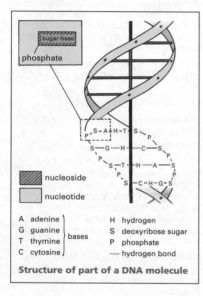

nucleoside

nucleotide

A adenine ⎞
G guanine ⎟ bases
T thymine ⎟
C cytosine ⎠

H hydrogen
S deoxyribose sugar
P phosphate
---- hydrogen bond

Structure of part of a DNA molecule

dobutamine n. a *sympathomimetic drug used to assist in the management of heart failure. It increases the force of contraction of the ventricles and improves the heart output and it may be given by continuous intravenous drip.

Doctor n. **1.** the title given to a recipient of a higher university degree than a Master's degree. The degree *Medicinae Doctor* (MD) is awarded by some British universities as a research degree. In the US the degree is awarded on qualification. **2.** a courtesy title given to a qualified medical practitioner, i.e. one who has been registered by the General Medical Council

(GMC). Most doctors in the UK obtain bachelors' degrees in medicine and surgery (MB, BS) or the diplomas of the conjoint boards of the Royal Colleges of Physicians and Surgeons of England and Scotland or the Society of Apothecaries (e.g. LRCP, MRCS, LMSSA): these degrees or diplomas and one year's hospital experience are required by the GMC before they will register a person as a doctor. Normally it is compulsory to hold two full-time **preregistration appointments** in general subjects at hospitals recognized for this purpose. The doctor has the title **house physician** (or **surgeon**), **resident**, or **intern** and is debarred from independent practice. Surgeons in the UK do not use the title Doctor and are referred to, as a mark of distinction, as Mr. Qualified dentists also use the courtesy title Doctor. *See also* CONSULTANT.

dolich- (dolicho-) *prefix denoting* long. Example: **dolichocolon** (abnormally long colon).

dolichocephaly n. the condition of having a relatively long skull, with a *cephalic index of 75 or less. —**dolichocephalic** adj.

dolor n. pain: one of the classical signs of inflammation in a tissue, the other three being *calor (heat), *rubor (redness), and *tumor (swelling). The pain in inflammation is thought to be due to the release of chemicals from damaged cells.

dolorimetry n. the measurement of pain. *See* ALGESIMETER.

domiciliary consultation **1.** a house call by a *general practitioner made at the request of a patient. **2.** (in Britain) an arrangement in the *National Health Service whereby a hospital specialist, at the request of a general practitioner, visits to advise on the diagnosis or treatment of a patient who, on medical grounds, is unable to attend hospital. The specialist receives special remuneration for this service.

domiciliary midwife *see* COMMUNITY MIDWIFE.

domiciliary services (in Britain) health and social services that are available in the home and are distinguished from hospital-based services. They include the services of such personnel as community nurses employed by community trusts (*see* DISTRICT NURSE, COMMUNITY MIDWIFE, HEALTH VISITOR) and social workers and care assistants employed by social service departments of local authorities. The term **community services** is applied to these services.

dominant *adj.* (in genetics) describing a gene (or its corresponding characteristic) whose effect is shown in the individual whether its *allele is the same or different. If the allele is different it is described as *recessive and its effect is masked. In genetic diseases showing **autosomal dominant** inheritance, the defective gene is dominant and will therefore be inherited by 50% of the offspring (of either sex) of a person with the disease. It will always be expressed in these offspring (since the normal allele inherited from the unaffected parent is recessive). —**dominant** *n.*

domiphen *n.* an *antiseptic administered in the form of lozenges to treat bacterial and fungal infections of the mouth and throat. It is also used in solution for cleansing wounds and burns, for treating fungal infections of the skin, and for general disinfection of skin and mucous membranes. Trade name: **Bradosol**.

domperidone *n.* an antiemetic drug used especially to reduce the nausea and vomiting caused by other drugs (e.g. anticancer drugs). It inhibits the effects of *dopamine, acting to close the sphincter muscle at the upper opening of the stomach (the cardia) and to relax the sphincter at the lower opening (the pylorus). It is administered by mouth or suppository; possible side-effects include breast enlargement and milk secretion. Trade names: **Evoxin**, **Motilium**.

Donald-Fothergill operation (Manchester operation) a surgical operation consisting of anterior *colporrhaphy, amputation of the cervix, and *colpoperineorrhaphy. It is performed for genital prolapse. [A. Donald (1860–1933) and W. E. Fothergill (1865–1926), British gynaecologists]

donor *n.* a person who makes his own tissues or organs available for use by someone else. For example, a donor may provide blood for transfusion (*see* BLOOD DONOR), a kidney for transplantation, or sex cells for *artificial insemination or *oocyte donation.

donor insemination *see* ARTIFICIAL INSEMINATION.

dopa *n.* dihydroxyphenylalanine: a physiologically important compound that forms an intermediate stage in the synthesis of catecholamines (dopamine, adrenaline, and noradrenaline) from the essential amino acid tyrosine. It also plays a role itself in the functioning of certain parts of the brain. The laevorotatory form, *levodopa, is administered for the treatment of *parkinsonism, in which there is a deficiency of the neurotransmitter *dopamine in the brain.

dopamine *n.* a *catecholamine derived from dopa that functions as a *neurotransmitter, acting on specific dopamine receptors and also on adrenergic receptors throughout the body, especially in the *limbic system and *extrapyramidal system of the brain and in the arteries and the heart. It also stimulates the release of noradrenaline from nerve endings. The effects vary with the concentration. Dopamine is used as a drug to increase the strength of contraction of the heart in heart failure, shock, severe trauma, and septicaemia. It is administered by injection in carefully controlled dosage. Possible side-effects include unduly rapid or irregular heartbeat, nausea, vomiting, breathlessness, angina pectoris, and kidney damage.

Certain drugs (**dopamine receptor agonists**) have an effect on the body similar to that of dopamine. They include *amantadine, *bromocriptine, *pergolide, and cabergoline and are used to treat *parkinsonism. Drugs that compete with dopamine to occupy and block the dopamine receptor sites in the body are known as **dopamine receptor antagonists**. They include some *antipsychotic drugs (e.g. the phenothiazines and *butyrophenones) and certain drugs (e.g. *domperidone and *metoclopramide) used to treat nausea and vomiting.

dopamine hypothesis the theory that schizophrenia is caused in part by abnormalities in the metabolism of *dopamine and can be treated in part by drugs (such as *chlorpromazine) that antagonize its action as a neurotransmitter.

Doppler ultrasound a diagnostic technique that utilizes the fact that the frequency of *ultrasound waves changes when they are reflected from a moving surface. It can be used to study the flow in blood vessels and the movement of such structures as heart valves. The frequency detector is contained within the ultrasound probe, which displays the anatomy on a TV screen. Simultaneously the Doppler signal can be displayed next to the anatomical position using a split screen (**duplex scan**). Using electronic techniques, flow, direction, and velocity can each be allocated to different colours and displayed on a colour monitor (**colour flow ultrasound imaging**). [C. J. Doppler (1803–53), Austrian physicist]

dors- (dorsi-, dorso-) *prefix denoting* **1.** the back. Example: **dorsalgia** (pain in). **2.** dorsal.

dorsal *adj.* relating to or situated at or close to the back of the body or to the posterior part of an organ.

dorsiflexion *n.* backward flexion of the foot or hand or their digits; i.e. bending towards the upper surface.

dorsoventral *adj.* (in anatomy) extending from the back (dorsal) surface to the front (ventral) surface.

dorsum *n.* **1.** the back. **2.** the upper or posterior surface of a part of the body; for example, of the hand. *See also* DORSAL.

dose *n.* a carefully measured quantity of a drug that is prescribed by a doctor to be given to a patient at any one time. The **median effective dose (ED$_{50}$)** is the dose of a drug that produces desired effects in 50% of individuals tested. *See also* LD$_{50}$.

dosimeter *n.* **1.** a device used to measure the intensity of a radiation source. **2.** a device to record the amount of radiation received by workers exposed to X-rays or other radiation. Formerly, it consisted of a small piece of photographic film in a holder attached to the clothing, but this film badge has now been replaced by *thermoluminescent dosimeters.

dosimetry *n.* the calculation of appropriate doses for given conditions, usually the calculation of correct amounts of radiation for the treatment of cancer in different parts of the body. *See* RADIOTHERAPY.

double-bind *n.* a disordered pattern of family relationships in which one family member gives contradictory instructions to another (as when a mother asks her child verbally for affection but simultaneously, by her gestures, indicates that the child should remain distant). The result is that any action the child makes will be wrong, and furthermore he cannot escape from the situation. This has been supposed, but not proved, to be a factor in causing schizophrenia.

double-blind trial *see* INTERVENTION STUDY.

double J stents *see* STENT.

double uterus *see* UTERUS DIDELPHYS.

double vision *see* DIPLOPIA.

douche *n.* a forceful jet of water used for cleaning any part of the body, most commonly the vagina. A vaginal douche is extremely unreliable as a method of contraception.

Down's syndrome a condition resulting from a genetic abnormality in which an extra chromosome is present (there are three no. 21 chromosomes instead of the usual two), giving a total of 47 chromosomes rather than the normal 46. The chances of having a Down's child are higher with increasing maternal age. Affected individuals share certain clinical features, including a characteristic flat facial appearance with slanting eyes (as in Mongolian races, which gave the former name, **mongolism**, to the condition), broad hands with short fingers and a single crease across the palm, malformed ears, eyes with a speckled iris (**Brushfield's spots**), short stature, and *hypotonia. Many individuals also have a degree of mental handicap, although the range of ability is wide and some individuals are of normal intelligence. Associated abnormalities, including heart defects (which affect about 40% of Down's children), intestinal malformation, deafness, and squints, may also be present.

*Prenatal diagnosis of Down's syndrome can be obtained by *amniocentesis, *chorionic villus sampling, the *triple marker test, and *nuchal thickness scanning; the condition can be confirmed by chromosomal analysis. Down's syndrome can also occur as a result of chromosomal re-arrangement (*translocation) and as part of a *mosaicism. Medical name: **trisomy 21**. [J. L. H. Down (1828–96), British physician]

doxapram n. a drug that stimulates breathing and has similar effects and uses to those of *nikethamide. Trade name: **Dopram**.

doxazosin n. an *alpha blocker drug used to treat high blood pressure. It is administered by mouth. Possible side-effects include faintness on standing up, weakness, dizziness, and headache. Trade name: **Cardura**.

doxepin n. a drug used to relieve depression, especially when associated with anxiety (see ANTIDEPRESSANT, TRANQUILLIZER). It is administered by mouth; side-effects can include drowsiness, dry mouth, blurred vision, and digestive upsets. Trade name: **Sinequan.**

doxorubicin n. an *anthracycline antibiotic isolated from Streptomyces peucetius caesius and used mainly in the treatment of leukaemia and various other forms of cancer. Doxorubicin acts by interfering with the production of DNA and RNA (see also CYTOTOXIC DRUG). It is administered by injection or infusion; side-effects include bone marrow depression, baldness, gastrointestinal disturbances, and heart damage.

doxycycline n. an *antibiotic used to treat infections caused by a wide range of bacteria and other microorganisms. It is administered by mouth and side-effects are those of the other *tetracyclines. Trade names: **Nordox, Vibramycin**.

DPT see DENTAL PANTOMOGRAM.

DPT vaccine a combined *vaccine against diphtheria, whooping cough (pertussis), and tetanus organisms, prepared from their *toxoids and other antigens. It is given as a course of three doses in the first year of life, at two, three, and four months of age (currently recommended ages). The diphtheria and tetanus components require further boosters.

drachm n. **1.** a unit of weight used in pharmacy. 1 drachm = 3.883 g (60 grains). **2.** a unit of volume used in pharmacy. 1 fluid drachm = 3.696 ml (1/8 fluid ounce).

dracontiasis n. a tropical disease caused by the parasitic nematode Dracunculus medinensis (see GUINEA WORM) in the tissues beneath the skin. The disease is transmitted to man via contaminated drinking water. The initial symptoms, which appear a year after infection, result from the migration of the worm to the skin surface and include itching, giddiness, difficulty in breathing, vomiting, and diarrhoea. Later a large blister forms on the skin, usually on the legs or arms, which eventually bursts and may ulcerate and become infected. Dracontiasis is common in India and West Africa but also occurs in Arabia, Iran, East Africa, and Afghanistan. Treatment involves extracting the worm or administering *thiabendazole, *metronidazole, or *niridazole.

Dracunculus n. see GUINEA WORM.

dragee n. a *pill that has been coated with sugar.

drain **1.** n. a device, usually a tube or wick, used to draw fluid from an internal body cavity to the surface. A drain is sometimes inserted during an operation to ensure that any fluid formed immediately passes to the surface, so preventing an accumulation that may become infected or cause pressure in the operation site. Negative pressure (suction) can be applied through a tube drain to increase its effectiveness. **2.** vb. see DRAINAGE.

drainage n. the drawing off of fluid from a cavity in the body, usually fluid that has accumulated abnormally. For example, serous fluid may be drained from a swollen joint, pus removed from an internal abscess, or urine from an overdistended bladder. See also DRAIN.

drastic n. any agent causing a major change in a body system or function, e.g. strong laxatives.

draw-sheet n. a sheet placed beneath a patient in bed that, when one portion has been soiled or becomes uncomfortably wrinkled, may be pulled under the patient so that another portion may be used. The bed does not have to be remade, and the patient does not have to leave bed.

drepanocyte (sickle cell) n. see SICKLE-CELL DISEASE.

drepanocytosis n. see SICKLE-CELL DISEASE.

dressing n. material applied to a wound or diseased part of the body, with or without medication, to give protection and assist healing.

drill n. (in dentistry) a rotary instrument used to remove tooth substance, particularly in the treatment of caries. It consists of a handpiece that takes variously shaped *burs. Most drilling is done with an air-driven turbine handpiece, but some is performed with a much slower mechanically driven handpiece. Drills usually have a waterspray coolant and may have a fibreoptic light.

drip (intravenous drip) n. apparatus for the continuous injection (*transfusion) of blood, plasma, saline, glucose solution, or other fluid into a vein. The fluid flows under gravity from a suspended bottle through a tube ending in a hollow needle inserted into the patient's vein. The rate of flow can be adjusted according to the rate of drips seen in a transparent section of the tube, but many infusions are now controlled by electronically regulated infusion pumps.

drom- (dromo-) prefix denoting movement or speed.

dromomania n. a pathologically strong impulse to travel, which is said to be present in some vagabonds.

droperidol n. a *butyrophenone antipsychotic drug that produces a state of emotional quietness and mental detachment. It is sometimes used as a premedication before surgery. Trade name: **Droleptan**.

dropsy n. see OEDEMA.

Drosophila n. a genus of very small flies, commonly called fruit flies, that breed in decaying fruit and vegetables. D. melanogaster has been extensively used in genetic research as it has only four pairs of chromosomes and those in its salivary glands are easily recognizable. Adult D. repleta sometimes feed on faecal matter and may transmit disease organisms.

drug n. any substance that affects the structure or functioning of a living organism. Drugs are widely used for the prevention, diagnosis, and treatment of disease and for the relief of symptoms. The term 'medicine' is sometimes preferred for therapeutic drugs in order to distinguish them from narcotics and other addictive drugs that are used illegally.

drug dependence see DEPENDENCE.

drusen pl. n. **1. (macular drusen)** white or yellow deposits of *hyalin in *Bruch's membrane of the choroid. They are often associated with *macular degeneration. **2. (disc drusen)** glistening nodules seen on an irregularly raised *optic disc. Consisting of excess *glia (produced congenitally) that has undergone degeneration and calcification, they can be confused with *papilloedema.

dry mouth a condition that occurs as a result of reduced salivary flow from a variety of causes, including *Sjögren's syndrome, connective tissue diseases, diabetes, excision or absence of a major salivary gland, or radiotherapy to the head that destroys the salivary glands. It causes swallowing and speech difficulties, inflamed gums and teeth, an increased incidence of dental caries, and loss of denture stability in people who have lost their teeth. Patients with their own teeth should be given sugar-free nonacidic saliva substitutes, strict dietary advice, and chlorhexidine mouthwashes; they require special monitoring by their dentist. Medical name: **xerostomia**.

dry socket a painful condition in which the normal healing of a tooth socket has been disturbed. Instead of being filled with a blood clot the socket is empty as a result of a nonspecific infection; treatment is palliative and the condition resolves in 10–14 days.

DSI see DIGITAL SPOT IMAGING.

DSM Diagnostic and Statistical Manual: an influential publication of the American Psychiatric Association in which psychiatric disorders are classified and defined. **DSM-IV** is the current (1994) version.

DTIC n. see DACARBAZINE.

DTPA diethylenetriaminepentaacetic acid

labelled with *technetium-99, used as a tracer to obtain *scintigrams of the kidney over a period of time, by means of a *gamma camera, to show function and reflux.

Duane's syndrome an abnormality of the eye muscles leading most commonly to restricted abduction (outward movement of the eye away from the midline) of one eye. On attempted adduction (inward movement of the eye towards the midline) of that same eye there is retraction of the eye into the orbit and narrowing of the opening between the eyelids. [A. Duane (1858–1926), US ophthalmologist]

Duchenne muscular dystrophy see MUSCULAR DYSTROPHY. [G. B. A. Duchenne (1806–75), French neurologist]

duct n. a tubelike structure or channel, especially one for carrying glandular secretions.

ductless gland see ENDOCRINE GLAND.

ductule n. a small duct or channel.

ductus n. a duct. The **ductus deferens** is the *vas deferens.

ductus arteriosus a blood vessel in the fetus connecting the pulmonary artery directly to the ascending aorta, so bypassing the pulmonary circulation. It normally closes after birth. Failure of the ductus to close (**patent ductus arteriosus**) produces a continuous *murmur, and the consequences are similar to those of a *septal defect. It may close spontaneously in childhood but often requires surgical closure.

Dukes staging a system that compares the extent of tumours of the colon and rectum with their cure rates. It formed the basis for many later systems of cancer staging and is still used. [Sir C. Dukes (1890–1977), British pathologist]

dumbness n. see MUTISM.

Dumdum fever see KALA-AZAR.

dumping syndrome a group of symptoms that sometimes occur after operations on the stomach, particularly *gastrectomy (**postgastrectomy syndrome**). After a meal, especially one rich in carbohydrate, the patient feels faint, weak, and nauseous, has a rapid pulse, and may sweat and become pale. The attack lasts 30 minutes to two hours and is caused by rapid stomach emptying, leading to falls in blood sugar and the drawing of fluid from the blood into the intestine. Avoidance of carbohydrate meals may relieve the syndrome but further surgery is sometimes required.

duo- prefix denoting two.

duoden- (duodeno-) prefix denoting the duodenum. Example: **duodenectomy** (excision of).

duodenal atresia a condition in which the duodenum is narrowed, causing complete obstruction. It presents at birth with vomiting, which is usually bile-stained, and is associated with other congenital abnormalities, particularly *Down's syndrome. Treatment is correction of any fluid imbalance and surgery.

duodenal ulcer an ulcer in the duodenum, caused by the action of acid and pepsin on the duodenal lining (mucosa) of a susceptible individual. It is usually associated with an increased output of stomach acid. Infection of the *antrum of the stomach with *Helicobacter pylori is almost always present. Symptoms include pain in the upper abdomen, especially when the stomach is empty, which often disappears completely for weeks or months; vomiting may occur. Complications include bleeding (see HAEMATEMESIS), perforation, and obstruction due to scarring (see PYLORIC STENOSIS). Symptoms are relieved by antacid medicines; most ulcers heal if treated by an *antisecretory drug, or if H. pylori is eradicated by a combination of a bismuth compound or a *proton-pump inhibitor and antibiotics. Surgery (see GASTRECTOMY, VAGOTOMY) is now rarely required.

duodenoscope n. a fibreoptic or video instrument for examining the interior of the duodenum. An end-viewing instrument is used for most examinations, but a side-viewing instrument is used for *ERCP. The end-viewing instrument is also used for examination of the stomach (it is also known as a **gastroduodenoscope**) and it is usual to combine the two examinations (**gastroduodenoscopy**).

duodenostomy n. an operation in

which the duodenum is brought through the abdominal wall and opened, usually in order to introduce food. *See also* GASTRODUODENOSTOMY.

duodenum *n.* the first of the three parts of the small *intestine. It extends from the pylorus of the stomach to the jejunum. The duodenum receives bile from the gall bladder (via the common bile duct) and pancreatic juice from the pancreas. Its wall contains various glands (including *Brunner's glands) that secrete an alkaline juice, rich in mucus, that protects the duodenum from the effects of the acidic *chyme passing from the stomach. —**duodenal** *adj.*

duplex imaging a method for measuring blood flow using an ultrasound source and a coupled Doppler probe (*see* DOPPLER ULTRASOUND). It is especially useful for estimating venous blood flow.

Dupuytren's contracture forward curvature of the fingers (usually the ring and little fingers) caused by *contracture of the *fascia in the palm and fingers. The condition is treated by surgical excision of the contracted and thickened tissue. [Baron G. Dupuytren (1777–1835), French surgeon]

dura (dura mater, pachymeninx) *n.* the thickest and outermost of the three *meninges surrounding the brain and spinal cord. It consists of two closely adherent layers, the outer of which is identical with the periosteum of the skull. The inner dura extends downwards between the cerebral hemispheres to form the **falx cerebri** and forwards between the cerebrum and cerebellum to form the **tentorium**. A thin film of fluid (not cerebrospinal fluid) separates the inner dura from the arachnoid.

dural *adj.* of, relating to, or affecting the *dura.

DVD *see* DISSOCIATED VERTICAL DEVIATION.

DVT (deep vein thrombosis) *see* PHLEBOTHROMBOSIS.

dwarfism *n.* abnormally short stature from any cause. The most common type of dwarf is the **achondroplastic dwarf** (*see* ACHONDROPLASIA). **Pituitary dwarfs** have a deficiency of *growth hormone

due to a defect in the pituitary gland; they are well proportioned and show no mental retardation, but may be sexually underdeveloped. **Primordial dwarfs** have a genetic defect in their response to growth hormone. Dwarfism is also associated with thyroid deficiency (*see* CRETINISM), in which both physical and mental development is retarded; chronic diseases such as rickets; renal failure; and intestinal malabsorption.

dydrogesterone *n.* a synthetic female sex hormone (*see* PROGESTOGEN) used to treat menstrual abnormalities (such as dysmenorrhoea) and infertility and to prevent miscarriage. It is administered by mouth and may cause mild nausea and breakthrough bleeding. Trade name: **Duphaston**.

dynamic splintage a technique that retains the essentials of splinting but allows some movement of the restrained body part.

dynamometer *n.* a device for recording the force of a muscular contraction. A small hand-held dynamometer may be used to record the strength of a patient's grip. A special optical dynamometer measures the action of the muscles controlling the shape of the lens of the eye.

dyne *n.* a unit of force equal to the force required to impart to a mass of 1 gram an acceleration of 1 centimetre per second per second. 1 dyne = 10^{-5} newton.

-dynia *suffix denoting* pain. Example: **proctodynia** (in the rectum).

dys- *prefix denoting* difficult, abnormal, or impaired. Examples: **dysbasia** (difficulty in walking); **dysgeusia** (impairment of taste).

dysaesthesiae *pl. n.* the abnormal and sometimes unpleasant sensations felt by a patient with partial damage to sensory nerve fibres when his skin is stimulated. *Compare* PARAESTHESIAE.

dysarthria *n.* a speech disorder in which the pronunciation is unclear although the linguistic content and meaning are normal.

dysbarism *n.* any clinical syndrome due to a difference between the atmospheric pressure outside the body and the pressure of air or gas within a body cavity (such as the paranasal sinuses or the middle ear). *See* COMPRESSED AIR ILLNESS.

dysbulia *n.* any disturbance of the will or of the mental processes that lead to purposeful action.

dyschezia *n.* a form of constipation resulting from a long period of voluntary suppression of the urge to defecate. The rectum becomes distended with faeces and bowel movements are difficult or painful.

dyschondroplasia (Ollier's disease) *n.* a condition due to faulty ossification of cartilage, resulting in development of many benign cartilaginous tumours (*see* CHONDROMA). The bones involved may become stunted and deformed. There is an increased risk of developing malignant tumours.

dyschromatopsia *n.* any defect of colour vision.

dyscoria *n.* any abnormality in the shape of the pupil.

dyscrasia *n.* an abnormal state of the body or part of the body, especially one due to abnormal development or metabolism. In classical medicine the term was used for the imbalance of the four *humours, which was believed to be the basic cause of all diseases.

dysdiadochokinesis (adiadochokinesis) *n.* clumsiness in performing rapidly alternating movements. It is often recognized by asking the patient to tap with his fingers on the back of his other hand. It is a sign of disease of the cerebellum or its intracerebral connections.

dysentery *n.* an infection of the intestinal tract causing severe diarrhoea with blood and mucus. **Amoebic dysentery (amoebiasis)** is caused by the protozoan *Entamoeba histolytica* and results in ulceration of the intestines and occasionally in the formation of abscesses in the liver (**amoebic** or **tropical abscesses**), lungs, testes, or brain. The parasite is spread by food or water contaminated by infected faeces. Symptoms appear days or even years after infection and include diarrhoea, indigestion, loss of weight, and anaemia. Prolonged treatment with drugs,

including metronidazole and tetracyclines, is usually effective in treating the condition. Amoebic dysentery is mainly confined to tropical and subtropical countries.

Bacillary dysentery is caused by bacteria of the genus *Shigella* and is spread by contact with a patient or carrier or through food or water contaminated by their faeces. Epidemics are common in overcrowded insanitary conditions. Symptoms, which develop 1–6 days after infection, include diarrhoea, nausea, cramp, and fever and they persist for about a week. An attack may vary from mild diarrhoea to an acute infection causing serious dehydration and bleeding from the gut. In most cases, provided fluid losses are replaced, recovery occurs within 7–10 days; antibiotics may be given to eliminate the bacteria. *Compare* CHOLERA.

dysfunctional uterine bleeding *see* MENORRHAGIA.

dysgenesis *n.* faulty development. **Gonadal dysgenesis** is failure of the ovaries or testes to develop (*see* TURNER'S SYNDROME).

dysgerminoma (germinoma, gonocytoma) *n.* a malignant tumour of the ovary, thought to arise from primitive germ cells; it is homologous to the *seminoma of the testis. About 15% of such tumours affect both ovaries; outside the ovary they have been recorded in the anterior mediastinum and in the pineal gland. Dysgerminomas may occur from infancy to old age, but the average age of patients is about 20 years. They are very sensitive to *radiotherapy.

Dysgerminomas are also known as **large cell carcinomas** or **alveolar sarcomas of the ovary**.

dysgraphia *n. see* AGRAPHIA.

dyskariosis *n.* the abnormal condition of a cell that has a nucleus showing the features characteristic of the earliest stage of malignancy, while retaining relatively normal cytoplasm. It may be seen, for example, in the squamous and columnar epithelial cells of a *cervical smear.

dyskinesia *n.* a group of involuntary movements that appear to be a fragmentation of the normal smoothly controlled limb and facial movements. They include *chorea, *dystonia, and those involuntary movements occurring as side-effects to the use of levodopa and the phenothiazines.

dyslalia *n.* a speech disorder in which the patient uses a vocabulary or range of sounds that is peculiar to him. It is a feature of the defective speech acquired by children who have been aphasic from birth (*see* APHASIA).

dyslexia *n.* a developmental disorder selectively affecting a child's ability to learn to read and write. The condition affects boys more often than girls and can create serious educational problems. It is sometimes called **specific dyslexia**, **developmental reading disorder**, or **developmental word blindness** to distinguish it from acquired difficulties with reading and writing. *Compare* ALEXIA. —**dyslexic** *adj.*

dyslogia *n.* disturbed and incoherent speech. This may be due to *dementia, *aphasia, *mental retardation, or mental illness.

dysmenorrhoea *n.* painful menstruation, of which there are two main forms. **Primary** (**spasmodic**) **dysmenorrhoea** usually begins with the first period and is heralded by cramping lower abdominal pains starting just before or with the menstrual flow and continuing during menstruation. It is often associated with nausea, vomiting, headache, faintness, and symptoms of peripheral vasodilatation. The cause is thought to be related to excessive *prostaglandin production. **Secondary** (**congestive**) **dysmenorrhoea** usually affects older women who complain of a congested ache with lower abdominal cramps, which usually start from a few days to two weeks before menstruation. Causes include *pelvic inflammatory disease, *endometriosis, fibroids, and the presence of an IUCD.

dysmnesic syndrome a disorder of memory in which new information is not learned but old material is well remembered. *See* KORSAKOFF'S SYNDROME.

dysmorphophobia *n.* a fixed distressing belief that one's body is deformed and repulsive, or an excessive fear that it might become so.

dysostosis *n.* the abnormal formation of bone or the formation of bone in abnormal places, such as a replacement of cartilage by bone.

dyspareunia *n.* painful or difficult sexual intercourse experienced by a woman. Psychological or physical factors may be responsible (*see* VAGINISMUS).

dyspepsia (**indigestion**) *n.* disordered digestion: usually applied to pain or discomfort in the lower chest or abdomen after eating and sometimes accompanied by nausea or vomiting. —**dyspeptic** *adj.*

dysphagia *n.* a condition in which the action of swallowing is either difficult to perform, painful (*see* ODYNOPHAGIA), or in which swallowed material seems to be held up in its passage to the stomach. It is caused by painful conditions of the mouth and throat, obstruction of the pharynx or oesophagus by diseases of the wall or pressure from outside, or by abnormalities of muscular activity of the pharynx or oesophagus.

dysphasia *n. see* APHASIA.

dysphemia *n. see* STAMMERING.

dysphonia *n.* difficulty in voice production. This may be due to a disorder of the larynx, pharynx, tongue, or mouth, or it may be *psychogenic. *Compare* DYSARTHRIA, APHASIA.

dysplasia (**alloplasia**, **heteroplasia**) *n.* abnormal development of skin, bone, or other tissues. *See also* BRONCHOPULMONARY DYSPLASIA, FIBROUS DYSPLASIA. —**dysplastic** *adj.*

dyspnoea *n.* laboured or difficult breathing. (The term is often used for a sign of laboured breathing apparent to the doctor, **breathlessness** being used for the subjective feeling of laboured breathing.) Dyspnoea can be due to obstruction to the flow of air into and out of the lungs (as in bronchitis and asthma), various diseases affecting the tissue of the lung (including pneumoconiosis, emphysema, tuberculosis, and cancer), and heart disease.

dyspraxia *n. see* APRAXIA.

dyssocial *adj.* describing a personality disorder characterized by callous unconcern for others, irresponsibility, violence, disregard for social rules, and an incapacity to maintain enduring relationships.

dyssynergia (asynergia) *n.* lack of coordination, especially clumsily uncoordinated movements found in patients with disease of the cerebellum. They include **dysmetria** (the application of inappropriate force for a movement), intention *tremor, *dysdiadochokinesis, and a staggering wide-based gait.

dysthymic disorder *see* DEPRESSION, NEUROSIS.

dystocia *n.* difficult birth, caused by abnormalities in the fetus or the mother. The most common causes of **fetal dystocia** are excessive size or *malpresentation of the baby. **Maternal dystocia** may result if the pelvis is abnormally small, the uterine muscles fail to contract, or the neck of the uterus fails to expand. If the cause of dystocia cannot be eliminated, it may be necessary to deliver the baby by Caesarean section or to operate in such a way that it can be removed with the minimum possible risk to the mother.

dystonia *n.* a postural disorder often associated with disease of the *basal ganglia in the brain. There may be spasm in the muscles of the face, shoulders, neck, trunk, and limbs. The arm is often held in a rotated position and the head may be drawn back and to one side. Dystonic conditions, including *blepharospasm, may be helped by the injection of *botulinum toxin. —**dystonic** *adj.*

dystrophia myotonica (myotonic dystrophy) a type of *muscular dystrophy in which the muscle weakness and wasting is accompanied by an unnatural prolongation of the muscular contraction after any voluntary effort (*see* MYOTONIA). The muscles of the face, temples, and neck are especially wasted. Baldness, endocrine malfunction, and cataracts also occur. The disease can affect both sexes (it is inherited as an autosomal *dominant character).

dystrophy (dystrophia) *n.* a disorder of an organ or tissue, usually muscle, due to impaired nourishment of the affected part. The term is applied to several unrelated conditions; for example, *muscular dystrophy, *Fuch's endothelial dystrophy, and **dystrophia adiposogenitalis** (*see* FRÖHLICH'S SYNDROME).

dysuria *n.* difficult or painful urination. This is usually associated with urgency and frequency of urination if due to *cystitis or *urethritis. The pain is burning in nature and is relieved by curing the underlying cause. A high fluid intake usually helps

E

Eales' disease inflammation of the blood vessels of the retina occurring in young adults. It is characterized by leakage from abnormal growths of new vessels as well as recurrent haemorrhages into the vitreous humour. [H. Eales (1852–1913), British physician]

ear *n.* the sense organ concerned with hearing and balance (see illustration). Sound waves, transmitted from the outside into the external auditory meatus, cause the eardrum (tympanic membrane) to vibrate. The small bones (ossicles) of the middle ear – the malleus, incus, and stapes – transmit the sound vibrations to the fenestra ovalis, which leads to the inner ear (*see* LABYRINTH). Inside the *cochlea the sound vibrations are converted into nerve impulses. Vibrations emerging from the cochlea could cause pressure to build up inside the ear, but this is released through the *Eustachian tube. The *semicircular canals, *saccule, and *utricle – also in the inner ear – are all concerned with balance.

earache *n. see* OTITIS, OTALGIA.

eardrum *n. see* TYMPANIC MEMBRANE.

earwax *n. see* CERUMEN.

Ebola virus a virus responsible for an acute infection in humans with features similar to those of *Marburg disease. Transmission is by contact with infected blood and other body fluids and the incubation period is 2–21 days (7 days on average). The mortality rate is 53–88%, but intensive treatment (including rehydration) in the early stages of the disease can halt its rapid and usually irreversible progression to haemorrhaging of internal organs. Sporadic but short-lived outbreaks have occurred in Africa since 1976, when the virus was first identified during an outbreak in the region of the Ebola river, in Zaïre (now Democratic Republic of Congo). An unknown species of animal is assumed to act as a reservoir for the virus between outbreaks of the disease in humans.

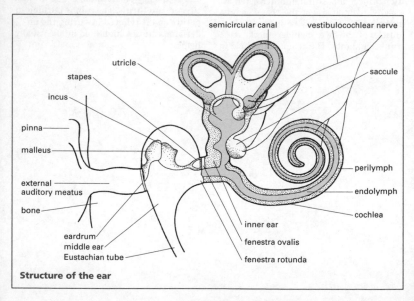

Structure of the ear

Ebstein's anomaly a form of congenital heart disease affecting the right side of the heart: the muscle is unusually thin and the heart valves are abnormal. It causes breathlessness and sometimes cyanosis. If mild, life expectancy is normal. If severe, corrective surgery may be necessary. [W. Ebstein (1836–1912), German physician]

eburnation *n.* the wearing down of the cartilage at the articulating surface of a bone, exposing the underlying bone. This is an end result of *osteoarthritis.

EB virus (EBV) *see* EPSTEIN-BARR VIRUS.

ec- *prefix denoting* out of or outside.

ecbolic *n.* an agent, such as *oxytocin, that induces childbirth by stimulating contractions of the uterus.

ecchondroma *n.* (*pl.* **ecchondromata**) a benign cartilaginous tumour (*see* CHONDROMA) that protrudes beyond the margins of a bone. *Compare* ENCHONDROMA.

ecchymosis *n.* a bruise: an initially bluish-black mark on the skin, resulting from the release of blood into the tissues either through injury or through the spontaneous leaking of blood from the vessels (as in some blood diseases).

eccrine *adj.* **1.** describing sweat glands that are distributed all over the body. Their ducts open directly onto the surface of the skin and they are densest on the soles of the feet and the palms of the hands. *Compare* APOCRINE. **2.** *see* MEROCRINE.

ecdemic *adj.* not occurring normally in the population of a country: applied sometimes to unusual diseases brought in from abroad by immigrants or travellers. *Compare* ENDEMIC.

ecdysis *n.* the act of shedding skin; *desquamation.

ECG *n.* *see* ELECTROCARDIOGRAM.

echinococciasis (echinococcosis) *n.* *see* HYDATID DISEASE.

Echinococcus *n.* a genus of small parasitic tapeworms that reach a maximum length of only 8 mm. Adults are found in the intestines of dogs, wolves, or jackals. If the eggs are swallowed by man, who can act as a secondary host, the resulting lar-

vae penetrate the intestine and settle in the lungs, liver, or brain to form large cysts, usually 5–10 cm in diameter (*see* HYDATID DISEASE). Two species causing this condition are *E. granulosus* and *E. multilocularis*.

echoacousia *n.* a false sensation of echoing after normally heard sound owing to a defect of the cochlea in the inner ear.

echocardiography *n.* the use of *ultrasound waves to investigate and display the action of the heart as it beats. Used in the diagnosis and assessment of congenital and acquired heart diseases, it is safe, painless, and reliable and reduces the need for cardiac *catheterization. **M-mode echocardiography** uses a single beam of ultrasound. The image produced is not anatomical but permits precise measurement of cardiac dimensions and the diagnosis of valvular, myocardial, and pericardial disease. **Real-time echocardiography** uses a pulsed array of ultrasound beams to build up a moving image on a TV monitor of the chambers and valves of the heart. In **Doppler echocardiography** ultrasound reflected from moving red blood cells is subject to the Doppler effect (change of pitch with velocity relative to the observer), which can be used to calculate blood flow and pressure within the heart and great vessels. It is useful in the diagnosis and assessment of valve disease and intracardial shunts.

echoencephalography *n.* investigation of structures within the skull by detecting the echoes of ultrasonic pulses. The chief value of the method was in detecting those disorders causing a displacement of the midline structures of the brain. The technique has largely been superseded by *computerized tomography (CT) and *magnetic resonance imaging (MRI).

echography *n.* an obsolete term for ultrasound imaging. *See* ULTRASONOGRAPHY.

echokinesis *n.* *see* ECHOPRAXIA.

echolalia *n.* pathological repetition of the words spoken by another person. It may be a symptom of language disorders, *autism, *catatonia, or *Gilles de la Tourette syndrome.

echo planar imaging (EPI) an imaging technique, based on *nuclear magnetic resonance (NMR), that provides a real-time snapshot with, apparently, the same image quality as NMR. This method, which is still in the early stages of development, may provide new insights into fetal pathology.

echopraxia (echokinesis) *n.* pathological imitation of the actions of another person. It may be a symptom of *catatonia or of *latah.

echovirus *n.* one of a group of about 30 RNA-containing viruses, originally isolated from the human intestinal tract, that were found to produce pathological changes in cells grown in culture, although they were not clearly associated with any specific disease. These viruses – which were accordingly termed *enteric cytopathic human orphan* viruses – are now more commonly known as *Coxsackie viruses. *Compare* REOVIRUS.

eclabium *n.* the turning outward of a lip.

eclampsia *n.* the occurrence of one or more convulsions not caused by other conditions, such as epilepsy or cerebral haemorrhage, in a woman with *pre-eclampsia. The onset of convulsions may be preceded by a sudden rise in blood pressure and/or a sudden increase in *oedema and development of *oliguria. The convulsions are usually followed by coma. Eclampsia is a threat to both mother and baby and must be treated immediately.

ECMO *see* EXTRACORPOREAL MEMBRANE OXYGENATION.

ECoG *see* ELECTROCOCHLEOGRAPHY.

ecology (bionomics) *n.* the study of the relationships between man, plants and animals, and the environment, including the way in which human activities may affect other animal populations and alter natural surroundings. —**ecological** *adj.* —**ecologist** *n.*

econazole *n.* an antifungal drug used to treat ringworm and candidosis. It is administered as a cream, lotion, spray powder, or vaginal pessary. Possible side-effects may include local irritation and burning. Trade names: **Ecostatin**, **Pevaryl**.

ecraseur *n.* a surgical device, resembling

a *snare, that is used to sever the base of a tumour during its surgical removal.

ecstasy *n.* a sense of extreme well-being and bliss. The word applies particularly to *trance states dominated by religious thinking. While not necessarily pathological, it can be caused by epilepsy (especially of the temporal lobe) or by schizophrenia.

Ecstasy *n.* the street name for methylenedioxymethamphetamine (MDMA), a mildly hallucinogenic drug that generates feelings of euphoria in those who take it. Its most common side-effect is hyperthermia; drinking large quantities of water to combat the intense thirst produced by taking the drug may result in fatal damage to the body's fluid balance. Its manufacture, sale, use, and possession are illegal.

ECT *see* ELECTROCONVULSIVE THERAPY.

ect- (ecto-) *prefix denoting* outer or external.

ectasia (ectasis) *n.* the dilatation of a tube, duct, or hollow organ.

ecthyma *n.* an infection of the skin caused by both *Streptococcus pyogenes* and *Staphylococcus aureus*. The full thickness of the epidermis is involved (*compare* IMPETIGO, which is a superficial infection). Ecthyma heals slowly and causes scarring. It may be associated with poor hygiene or depressed immunity.

ectoderm *n.* the outer of the three *germ layers of the early embryo. It gives rise to the nervous system and sense organs, the teeth and lining of the mouth, and to the *epidermis and its associated structures (hair, nails, etc.). —**ectodermal** *adj.*

ectomorphic *adj.* describing a *body type that is relatively thin, with a large skin surface in comparison to weight. —**ectomorph** *n.* —**ectomorphy** *n.*

-ectomy *suffix denoting* surgical removal of a segment or all of an organ or part. Examples: **appendicectomy** (of the appendix); **prostatectomy** (of the prostate gland).

ectoparasite *n.* a parasite that lives on the outer surface of its host. Some ectoparasites, such as bed bugs, maintain only periodic contact with their hosts, whereas others, such as the crab louse, have a permanent association. *Compare* ENDOPARASITE.

ectopia *n.* **1.** the misplacement, due either to a congenital defect or injury, of a bodily part. **2.** the occurrence of something in an unnatural location (*see also* EC-TOPIC BEAT, ECTOPIC PREGNANCY). —**ectopic** *adj.*

ectopic beat (extrasystole) a heartbeat due to an impulse generated somewhere in the heart outside the sinoatrial node. Ectopic beats are generally premature in timing; they are classified as **supraventricular** if they originate in the atria and **ventricular** if they arise from a focus in the ventricles. They may be produced by any heart disease, by nicotine from smoking, or by caffeine from excessive tea or coffee consumption; they are common in normal individuals. The patient may be unaware of their presence or may feel that his heart has 'missed a beat'. Ectopic beats may be suppressed by drugs such as quinidine, propranolol, and lignocaine; avoidance of smoking and reduction in excessive tea or coffee intake may help. *See* ARRHYTHMIA.

ectopic hormone a hormone produced by cells that do not usually produce it. Some tumour cells secrete hormones; for example, lung cancer cells secrete vasopressin.

ectopic pregnancy (extrauterine pregnancy) the development of a fetus at a site other than in the uterus. This may happen if the fertilized egg cell remains in the ovary or in the tube leading from near the ovary to the uterus (the Fallopian tube) or if it lodges in the free abdominal cavity. The most common type of ectopic pregnancy is a **tubal** (or **oviducal**) **pregnancy**, which occurs in Fallopian tubes that become blocked or inflamed. The growth of the fetus may cause the tube to rupture and bleed. In many cases the fetus dies within three months of conception and the products are absorbed into the maternal circulation. Rarely, the pregnancy may continue until a live baby can be delivered by Caesarean section. The condition may be diagnosed by ultrasound and the products of conception may be re-

moved by laparoscopy before damage is done to the Fallopian tube.

ectoplasm *n.* the outer layer of cytoplasm in cells, which is denser than the inner cytoplasm (*endoplasm) and concerned with activities such as cell movement. —**ectoplasmic** *adj.*

ectro- *prefix denoting* congenital absence.

ectrodactyly *n.* congenital absence of all or part of one or more fingers.

ectromelia *n.* congenital absence or gross shortening (aplasia) of the long bones of one or more limbs. *See also* AMELIA, HEMIMELIA, PHOCOMELIA.

ectropion *n.* turning out of the eyelid, away from the eyeball. The commonest type is **senile ectropion**, in which the lower eyelid droops because of laxity of the eyelid in old age. If the muscle that closes the eye (orbicularis oculi) is paralysed the lower lid also droops. Ectropion may also occur if scarring causes contraction of the surrounding facial skin.

eczema *n.* a common itchy skin disease characterized by reddening (*erythema) and vesicle formation, which may lead to weeping and crusting. It is endogenous, or constitutional, i.e. outside agents do not play a primary role (*compare* DERMATITIS), but in some contexts the terms 'dermatitis' and 'eczema' are used interchangeably. There are five main types: (1) **atopic eczema**, which affects up to 20% of the population and is associated with asthma and hay fever; (2) **seborrhoeic eczema** (or **dermatitis**), which involves the scalp, eyelids, nose, and lips, is associated with the presence of *Pityrosporum* yeasts, and is common in patients with AIDS; (3) **discoid** (or **nummular**) **eczema**, which is characterized by coin-shaped lesions and occurs only in adults; (4) *pompholyx, affecting the hands and feet; (5) **gravitational** (or **stasis**) **eczema**, associated with poor venous circulation and incorrectly known as **varicose eczema**.

Treatment of eczema is with topical or systemic corticosteroids but emollients are very important, especially in treating mild cases. Newer treatments include *PUVA or cyclosporin A. —**eczematous** *adj.*

edentulous *adj.* lacking teeth: usually

applied to people who have lost some or all of their teeth.

edetate *n.* a salt of **ethylenediamine-tetraacetic acid (EDTA)**, which is used as a *chelating agent in the treatment of poisoning. **Dicobalt edetate** is an antidote to cyanide, administered by intravenous injection as soon as possible after poisoning. **Calcium disodium edetate** is used to treat poisoning by heavy metals, such as lead and strontium.

edrophonium *n.* a drug that stimulates skeletal muscles (*see* PARASYMPATHOMIMETIC). It is administered by injection in a test for diagnosis of *myasthenia gravis. Side-effects can include nausea and vomiting, increased saliva flow, diarrhoea, and stomach pains. Trade name: **Tensilon**.

EDTA (ethylenediaminetetraacetic acid) *see* EDETATE.

Edwards' syndrome a condition resulting from a genetic abnormality in which an extra chromosome is present – there are three no. 18 chromosomes instead of the usual two. Affected babies, who rarely survive, have a characteristic abnormally shaped head, low birth weight, prominent heels ('rocker-bottom feet'), heart abnormalities, and severe mental retardation. [J. H. Edwards (1928–   ), British geneticist]

EEG (electroencephalogram) *see* ELECTROENCEPHALOGRAPHY.

effector *n.* any structure or agent that brings about activity in a muscle or gland, such as a motor nerve that causes muscular contraction or glandular secretion. The term is also used for the muscle or gland itself.

efferent *adj.* **1.** designating nerves or neurones that convey impulses from the brain or spinal cord to muscles, glands, and other effectors; i.e. any motor nerve or neurone. **2.** designating vessels or ducts that drain fluid (such as lymph) from an organ or part. *Compare* AFFERENT.

effleurage *n.* a form of *massage in which the hands are passed continuously and rhythmically over a patient's skin in one direction only, with the aim of increasing blood flow in that direction and aiding the dispersal of any swelling due to *oedema.

effort syndrome a condition of marked anxiety about the condition of one's heart and circulatory system. This is accompanied by a heightened consciousness of heartbeat and respiration, which in turn is worsened by the anxiety it induces. Treatment is commonly with reassurance and *tranquillizers; the use of psychotherapy is only occasionally necessary.

effusion *n.* **1.** the escape of pus, serum, blood, lymph, or other fluid into a body cavity as a result of inflammation or the presence of excess blood or tissue fluid in an organ or tissue. **2.** fluid that has escaped into a body cavity.

eflornithine *n.* a drug recently approved by the World Health Organization for the treatment of *sleeping sickness. It is administered by mouth and intravenous injection. Possible side-effects include diarrhoea, hair loss, convulsions, and damage to bone marrow. Trade name: **DMFO**.

egg cell *see* OVUM.

ego *n.* (in psychoanalysis) the part of the mind that develops from a person's experience of the outside world and is most in touch with external realities. In Freudian terms the ego is said to reconcile the demands of the *id (the instinctive unconscious mind), the *superego (moral conscience), and reality.

eidetic *adj.* *see* IMAGERY.

eikonometer *n.* an instrument for measuring the size of images on the retina of the eye.

Eisenmenger reaction a condition in which *pulmonary hypertension is associated with a *septal defect, so that blood flows from the right to the left side of the heart or from the pulmonary artery to the aorta. This allows blue blood, poor in oxygen, to bypass the lungs and enter the general circulation. This reduces the oxygen content of the arterial blood in the aorta and its branches, resulting in a patient with a dusky blue appearance (*cyanosis) and an increased number of red blood cells (*polycythaemia). There is no curative treatment at this stage, but the patient may be helped by the control of heart failure and polycythaemia. The condition may be prevented by appropriate treatment of the septal defect before irreversible pulmonary hypertension develops. [V. Eisenmenger (1864–1932), German physician]

ejaculation *n.* the discharge of semen from the erect penis at the moment of sexual climax (orgasm) in the male. The constituents of semen are not released simultaneously, but in the following sequence: the secretion of *Cowper's glands followed by that of the *prostate gland and the spermatozoa and finally the secretion of the *seminal vesicles. *See also* PREMATURE EJACULATION.

elastic cartilage a type of *cartilage in which elastic fibres are distributed in the matrix. It is yellowish in colour and is found in the external ear.

elastic tissue strong extensible flexible *connective tissue rich in yellow **elastic fibres**. These fibres are long, thin, and branching and are composed primarily of an albumin-like protein, **elastin**. Elastic tissue is found in the dermis of the skin, in arterial walls, and in the walls of the alveoli of the lungs.

elastin *n.* protein forming the major constituent of *elastic tissue fibres.

elastography *n.* an ultrasonic imaging technique that displays the elasticity of soft tissues. It has been found useful in demonstrating abnormalities of both muscle and breast tissue.

elastosis *n.* degeneration of the yellow fibres in connective tissues and skin (*see* ELASTIC TISSUE).

elation (exaltation) *n.* a state of cheerful excitement and enthusiasm. Marked elation of mood is a characteristic of *mania or *hypomania.

elbow *n.* the hinge joint (*see* GINGLYMUS) between the bones of the upper arm (humerus) and the forearm (radius and ulna). It is a common site of fractures and dislocation.

electrocardiogram (ECG) *n.* a recording of the electrical activity of the heart on a moving paper strip (see illustration). The ECG tracing is recorded by means of

an apparatus called an **electrocardiograph** (*see* ELECTROCARDIOGRAPHY). It aids in the diagnosis of heart disease, which may produce characteristic changes in the ECG.

P wave due to atrial contraction
Q, R, S, and T waves due to ventricular activity

Typical electrocardiograms

electrocardiography *n.* a technique for recording the electrical activity of the heart. Electrodes connected to the recording apparatus (**electrocardiograph**) are placed on the skin of the four limbs and chest wall; the record itself is called an *electrocardiogram (ECG). In conventional **scalar electrocardiography** 12 leads (*see* LEAD[2]) are recorded, but more may be employed in special circumstances (for example, an oesophageal lead, from an electrode within the gullet, may be used in the analysis of arrhythmias).

Vectorcardiography is less commonly used in Britain, but may be employed to obtain a three-dimensional impression of electrical activity of the heart.

electrocardiophonography *n.* a technique for recording heart sounds and murmurs simultaneously with the ECG, which is used as a reference tracing. The sound is picked up by a microphone placed over the heart. The tracing is a **phonocardiogram**. It provides a permanent record of heart sounds and murmurs and is useful in their analysis.

electrocautery *n.* the destruction of diseased or unwanted tissue by means of a needle or snare that is electrically heated.

Warts, polyps, and other growths can be burned away by this method.

electrocoagulation *n.* the coagulation of body tissues by means of a high-frequency electric current concentrated at one point as it passes through them. Electrocoagulation, using a *diathermy knife, permits bloodless incisions to be made during operation.

electrocochleography (ECoG) *n.* a test to measure electrical activity produced within the *cochlea in response to a sound stimulus. It is used in the diagnosis of Ménière's disease and other forms of sensorineural *deafness.

electroconvulsive therapy (ECT) a treatment for severe depression and occasionally for schizophrenia and mania. A convulsion is produced by passing an electric current through the brain. The convulsion is modified by giving a *muscle relaxant drug and an *anaesthetic, so that in fact only a few muscle twitches are produced. The means by which ECT acts is not yet known. The procedure can also produce confusion, loss of memory, and headache, which almost always pass off within a few hours. These side-effects are reduced by unilateral treatment, in which the current is passed only through the nondominant hemisphere of the brain.

electrodesiccation *n.* *see* FULGURATION.

electroencephalogram (EEG) *n.* *see* ELECTROENCEPHALOGRAPHY.

electroencephalography *n.* the technique for recording the electrical activity from different parts of the brain and converting it into a tracing called an **electroencephalogram (EEG)**. The machine that records this activity is known as an **encephalograph**. The pattern of the EEG reflects the state of the patient's brain and his level of consciousness in a characteristic manner. Electroencephalography is mostly used in the diagnosis and management of epilepsy.

electroglottography *n.* a method of assessing laryngeal function using external recording electrodes.

electrokymography *n.* the technique of recording the movements of an organ, especially the heart, by means of a *fluoroscope and a photoelectric recording system.

electrolyte *n.* a solution that produces ions (an ion is an atom or group of atoms that conduct electricity); for example, sodium chloride solution consists of free sodium and free chloride ions. In medical usage electrolyte usually means the ion itself; thus the term **serum electrolyte level** means the concentration of separate ions (sodium, potassium, chloride, bicarbonate, etc.) in the circulating blood. Concentrations of various electrolyte levels can be altered by many diseases, in which electrolytes are lost from the body (as in vomiting or diarrhoea) or are not excreted and accumulate (as in renal failure). When electrolyte concentrations are severely diminished they can be corrected by administering the appropriate substance by mouth or by intravenous drip. When excess of an electrolyte exists it may be removed by *dialysis or by special resins in the intestine, taken by mouth or by enema. *See also* ANION.

electromyography *n.* continuous recording of the electrical activity of a muscle by means of electrodes inserted into the muscle fibres. The tracing is displayed on an oscilloscope. The technique is used for diagnosing various nerve and muscle disorders and assessing progress in recovery from some forms of paralysis.

electronarcosis *n.* the induction of sleep by passing weak electrical currents through the brain. It is seldom used in Western psychiatry.

electron microscope a microscope that uses a beam of electrons as a radiation source for viewing the specimen. The resolving power (ability to register fine detail) is a thousand times greater than that of an ordinary light microscope. The specimen must be examined in a vacuum, which necessitates special techniques for preparing it, and the electrons are usually focused onto a fluorescent screen (for direct viewing) or onto a photographic plate (for a photograph, or **electron micrograph**). A **transmission electron microscope** is used to examine thin sections at high magnification. A **scanning electron microscope** reveals the surfaces of objects at various magnifications; its great depth of focus is advantageous.

electron transport chain a series of enzymes and proteins in living cells through which electrons are transferred, via a series of oxidation-reduction reactions. This ultimately leads to the conversion of chemical energy into a readily usable and storable form. The most important electron transport chain is the **respiratory chain**, present in mitochondria and functioning in cellular respiration.

electrooculography *n.* an electrical method of recording eye movements. Tiny electrodes are attached to the skin at the inner and outer corners of the eye, and as the eye moves an alteration in the potential between these electrodes is recorded. The size of this potential at rest also gives an indication of the health of the retina. The recording itself is called an **electrooculogram (EOG)**.

electrophoresis *n.* the technique of separating electrically charged particles, particularly proteins, in a solution by passing an electric current through the solution. The rate of movement of the different components depends upon their charge, so that they gradually separate into bands. Electrophoresis is widely used in the investigation of body chemicals, such as the analysis of the different proteins in blood serum.

electroretinography *n.* a method of recording changes in the electrical potential of the retina when it is stimulated by light; the recording itself is called an **electroretinogram (ERG)**. One electrode is placed on the eye in a contact lens and the other is usually attached to the back of the head. In retinal disease the pattern of electrical change is altered. The technique is useful in diagnosing retinal diseases when opacities, such as cataract, make it difficult to view the retina or when the disease produces little visible change in the retina.

electrosurgery *n.* the use of a high-frequency electric current from a fine wire electrode (a *diathermy knife) to cut tissue. The ground electrode is a large metal plate. When used correctly, little heat spreads to the surrounding tissues, in contrast to *electrocautery.

electrotherapy *n.* the passage of electric currents through the body's tissues to stimulate the functioning of nerves and the muscles that they supply. The technique is used to treat the muscles of patients with various forms of paralysis due to nerve disease or muscle disorder. *See also* FARADISM, GALVANISM.

electuary *n.* a pharmaceutical preparation in which the drug is made up into a paste with syrup or honey.

elephantiasis *n.* gross enlargement of the skin and underlying connective tissues caused by obstruction of the lymph vessels, which prevents drainage of lymph from the surrounding tissues. Inflammation and thickening of the walls of the vessels and their eventual blocking is commonly caused by the parasitic filarial worms *Wuchereria bancrofti* and *Brugia malayi*. The parts most commonly affected are the legs but the scrotum, breasts, and vulva may also be involved. Elastic bandaging is applied to the affected parts and the limbs are elevated and rested. Larval forms in the blood are killed with diethylcarbamazine. *See also* FILARIASIS.

elevator *n.* **1.** an instrument that is used to raise a depressed broken bone, for example in the skull or cheek. A specialized **periosteal elevator** is used in orthopaedics to strip the fibrous tissue (periosteum) covering bone. **2.** a lever-like instrument used to ease a tooth or root out of its socket during extraction.

elimination *n.* (in physiology) the entire process of excretion of metabolic waste products from the blood by the kidneys and urinary tract.

ELISA *see* ENZYME-LINKED IMMUNOSORBENT ASSAY.

elixir *n.* a preparation containing alcohol (ethanol) or glycerine, which is used as the vehicle for bitter or nauseous drugs.

elliptocytosis *n.* the presence of significant numbers of abnormal elliptical red cells (**elliptocytes**) in the blood. Elliptocytosis may occur as a hereditary disorder or be a feature of certain blood diseases, such as *myelofibrosis or iron-deficiency *anaemia.

Elschnig pearls round or oval transparent cystic structures seen through the pupil of the eye, due to proliferation of lens epithelial cells following extracapsular *cataract extraction. They can grow to occlude the pupil and hence cause reduction in vision. [A. Elschnig (1863–1939), German ophthalmologist]

elutriation *n.* the separation of a fine powder from a coarser powder by mixing them with water and decanting the upper layer while it still contains the finer particles. The heavier coarse particles sink to the bottom more rapidly.

em- *prefix. see* EN-.

emaciation *n.* wasting of the body, caused by such conditions as malnutrition, tuberculosis, cancer, or parasitic worms.

emasculation *n.* strictly, surgical removal of the penis. The term is often used to mean loss of male physical and emotional characteristics, either as a result of removal of the testes (castration) or of emotional stress.

embalming *n.* the preservation of a dead body by the introduction of chemical compounds that delay putrefaction. Embalming is employed mainly so that a body can be transported long distances and funeral rites can be conducted without undue haste. In the USA it is a routine hygienic measure.

embedding *n.* (in microscopy) the fixing of a specimen within a mass of firm material in order to facilitate the cutting of thin sections for microscopical study. The embedding medium, e.g. paraffin wax for light microscopy or Araldite for electron microscopy, helps to keep the specimen intact.

embolectomy *n.* surgical removal of an *embolus in order to relieve arterial obstruction. The embolus may be removed by cutting directly into the affected artery (**arteriotomy**). In some instances it is removed by a balloon *catheter, which is manipulated beyond the embolus from a small arteriotomy in an accessible artery. The catheter is then withdrawn carrying the embolus with it. In some cases of pulmonary embolism, embolectomy may be life saving. It may also prevent gangrene in cases of a limb artery embolus.

embolism *n.* the condition in which an embolus becomes lodged in an artery and obstructs its blood flow. The most common form of embolism is *pulmonary embolism, in which a blood clot is carried in the circulation to lodge in the pulmonary artery. An embolus in any other artery constitutes a **systemic embolism**. In this case a common source of the embolus is a blood clot within the heart in mitral valve disease or following *myocardial infarction. The clinical features depend upon the site at which an embolus lodges (for example, a stroke may result from a cerebral embolism and gangrene caused by a limb embolism). Treatment is by *anticoagulant therapy with heparin and warfarin. Major embolism is treated by *embolectomy or *streptokinase to remove or dissolve the embolus. *See also* AIR EMBOLISM.

embolization (therapeutic embolization) *n.* the introduction of embolic material to reduce or completely obstruct bloodflow in such conditions as congenital arteriovenous malformations (*see* ANGIOMA), angiodysplasia, malignant tumours, or arterial rupture. Under X-ray screening control, a cannula is inserted into the artery supplying the affected area and occluding material, such as microspheres, metallic coils, or PVA (polyvinyl alcohol) foam, is injected. The procedure simplifies subsequent surgery or replaces it.

embolus *n.* (*pl.* **emboli**) material, such as a blood clot, fat, air, amniotic fluid, or a foreign body, that is carried by the blood from one point in the circulation to lodge at another point (*see* EMBOLISM).

embrasure *n.* the space formed between adjacent teeth.

embrocation *n.* a lotion rubbed onto the body to treat sprains and strains.

embryo *n.* an animal at an early stage of development, before birth. In man the term refers to the products of conception within the uterus up to the eighth week of development, during which time all the main organs are formed (see illustration). *Compare* FETUS. **—embryonic** *adj.*

embryology *n.* the study of growth and development of the embryo and fetus

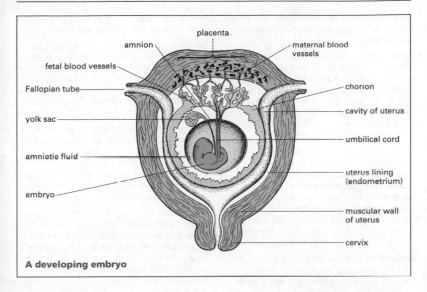

A developing embryo

from fertilization of the ovum until birth.
—**embryological** *adj.*

embryonic disc the early embryo before the formation of *somites. It is a flat disc of tissue bounded dorsally by the amniotic cavity and ventrally by the yolk sac. The formation of the *primitive streak and *archenteron in the embryonic disc determines the orientation of the embryo, which then becomes progressively elongated.

embryoscopy *n.* examination of an embryo or fetus during the first 12 weeks of pregnancy by means of a fibreoptic *endoscope inserted through the cervix; it can be performed as early as five weeks gestation. Access to the fetal circulation may be obtained through the instrument and direct visualization of the embryo permits the diagnosis of malformations.

embryo transfer the transfer of an embryo from an in vitro culture into the uterus. *See also* IN VITRO FERTILIZATION.

emesis *n. see* VOMITING.

emetic *n.* an agent that causes vomiting. Strong emetics, such as *apomorphine, are used to induce vomiting following drug overdose. Substances such as common salt, which irritate the stomach nerves if taken in sufficient quantities, also cause vomiting. Some emetics, e.g. *ipecacuanha, are *expectorants at low doses.

eminence *n.* a projection, often rounded, on an organ or tissue, particularly on a bone. An example is the **iliopubic eminence** on the hip bone.

Emiscan *n.* trade name for *computerized tomography.

emissary veins a group of veins within the skull that drain blood from the venous sinuses of the dura mater to veins outside the skull.

emission *n.* the flow of semen from the erect penis, usually occurring while the subject is asleep (**nocturnal emission**).

EMLA cream a cream containing a eutectic mixture of local anaesthetics (hence the name). Applied to the skin as a thick coating, it gives a helpful degree of local anaesthesia, allowing blood samples to be taken and facilitating biopsy procedures in young children.

emmetropia *n.* the state of refraction of the normal eye, in which parallel light rays are brought to a focus on the retina with the accommodation relaxed. Distant objects are seen clearly without any effort to focus. *Compare* AMETROPIA, HYPERMETRO-PIA, MYOPIA.

emollient *n.* an agent that soothes and softens the skin. Emollients are fats and oils, such as lanolin and liquid paraffin; they are used alone as moisturizers to lessen the need for active drug therapy (such as corticosteroids for eczema) and in skin preparations as a base for a more active drug, such as an antibiotic.

emotion *n.* a state of arousal that can be experienced as pleasant or unpleasant. Emotions can have three components: **subjective**, **physiological**, and **behavioural**. For example, fear can involve an unpleasant subjective experience, an increase in physiological measures such as heart rate, sweating, etc., and a tendency to flee from the fear-provoking situation.

empathy *n.* the ability to understand the thoughts and emotions of another person. In a psychotherapist empathy is often considered to be one of the necessary qualities enabling successful treatment. *See* ALEXITHYMIA.

emphysema *n.* air in the tissues. In **pulmonary emphysema** the air sacs (*alveoli) of the lungs are enlarged and damaged, which reduces the surface area for the exchange of oxygen and carbon dioxide. Severe emphysema causes breathlessness, which is made worse by infections. There is no specific treatment, and the patient may become dependent on oxygen. The mechanism by which emphysema develops is not understood, although it is known to be particularly common in men in Britain and is associated with chronic bronchitis, smoking, and advancing age.

In **surgical emphysema** air may escape into the tissues of the chest and neck from leaks in the lungs or oesophagus; occasionally air escapes into other tissues during surgery, and bacteria may form gas in soft tissues. The presence of gas or air gives the affected tissues a characteristic crackling feeling to the touch, and it may be visible on X-rays. It is easily absorbed once the leak or production is stopped.

empirical *adj.* describing a system of treatment based on experience or observation, rather than of logic or reason.

Employment Service (in Britain) an executive agency within the Department of Employment for running public employment services. It has special responsibility to find employment for and if necessary train (or retrain) those who are handicapped from any cause.

empyema (pyothorax) *n.* pus in the *pleural cavity, usually secondary to infection in the lung or in the space below the diaphragm. Empyema is a life-threatening condition, which can be relieved by aspiration or drainage of the pus or by decapsulation (*see* DECORTICATION).

emulsion *n.* a preparation in which fine droplets of one liquid (such as oil) are dispersed in another liquid (such as water). In pharmacy medicines are prepared in the form of emulsions to disguise the taste of an oil, which is dispersed in a flavoured liquid.

en- (em-) *prefix denoting* in; inside.

enalapril *n.* a drug used in the treatment of high blood pressure (hypertension) and heart failure. It inhibits the action of angiotensin (*see* ACE INHIBITOR), which results in decreased vasopressor (blood-vessel constricting) activity and decreased aldosterone secretion. It is administered by mouth; side-effects include headache, dizziness, fatigue, and diarrhoea. Trade name: **Innovace**.

enamel *n.* the extremely hard outer covering of the crown of a *tooth. It is formed before tooth eruption by *ameloblasts and consists of crystalline *hydroxyapatite.

enarthrosis *n.* a ball-and-socket joint: a type of *diarthrosis (freely movable joint), e.g. the shoulder joint and the hip joint. Such a joint always involves a long bone, which is thus allowed to move in all planes.

encapsulated *adj.* (of an organ, tumour, bacterium, etc.) enclosed in a *capsule.

encephal- (encephalo-) *prefix denoting* the brain.

encephalin (enkephalin) *n.* a peptide occurring naturally in the brain and having effects resembling those of morphine or other opiates. *See also* ENDORPHIN.

encephalitis *n.* inflammation of the brain. It may be caused by a viral or bacterial infection or it may be part of an allergic response to a systemic viral illness or vaccination (*see* ENCEPHALOMYELITIS). **Viral encephalitis** is endemic in some parts of the world; it may also occur epidemically or sporadically. One form – **encephalitis lethargica** – reached epidemic proportions shortly after World War I and was marked by headache and drowsiness, progressing to coma (hence its popular name – **sleepy sickness**). Encephalitis can cause postencephalitic *parkinsonism. Another type of encephalitis that occurs sporadically is due to herpes simplex.

encephalocele *n. see* NEURAL TUBE DEFECTS.

encephalography *n.* any of various techniques for recording the structure of the brain or the activity of the brain cells. Examples are *echoencephalography, *electroencephalography, and *pneumoencephalography.

encephaloid *adj.* having the appearance of brain tissue: applied to certain tumours, for example **encephaloid carcinoma of the breast**.

encephalomyelitis *n.* an acute inflammatory disease affecting the brain and spinal cord. It is sometimes part of an overwhelming virus infection but **acute disseminated encephalomyelitis** is a form of delayed tissue hypersensitivity provoked by a mild infection or vaccination 7–10 days earlier. Survival through the acute phase of the illness is often followed by a remarkably complete recovery.

encephalomyelopathy *n.* any condition in which there is widespread disease of the brain and spinal cord. **Necrotizing encephalomyelopathy of childhood** is a progressive illness with extensive destruction of nerve cells throughout the central nervous system. It is thought to be caused by a disorder of metabolism.

encephalon *n. see* BRAIN.

encephalopathy *n.* any of various diseases that affect the functioning of the brain. *See* HEPATIC ENCEPHALOPATHY, SPONGIFORM ENCEPHALOPATHY, WERNICKE'S ENCEPHALOPATHY.

enchondroma *n.* (*pl.* **enchondromata**) a benign cartilaginous tumour (*see* CHONDROMA) occurring in the growing zone (metaphysis) of a bone and not protruding beyond its margins. Such tumours are often solitary; when multiple tumours occur the condition is known as **enchondromatosis**. *Compare* ECCHONDROMA.

encopresis *n.* incontinence of faeces. The term is used for faecal soiling in a child who has gained bowel control but passes formed stools in unacceptable places. The underlying problem is behavioural and treatment is often difficult. Encopresis must be distinguished from chronic constipation with overflow.

encounter group a form of group psychotherapy. The emphasis is on encouraging close relationships between group members and on the expression of feelings. To this end, physical contact and confrontations between group members are arranged by the group leader. The stress of the experience can be damaging to maladjusted people.

encysted *adj.* enclosed in a cyst.

end- (endo-) *prefix denoting* within or inner. Example: **endonasal** (within the nose).

endarterectomy *n.* a surgical 're-bore' of an artery that has become obstructed by *atheroma with or without a blood clot (thrombus): the former operation is known as **thromboendarterectomy**. The inner part of the wall is removed together with any clot that is present. This restores patency and arterial blood flow to the tissues beyond the obstruction. The technique is most often applied to obstruction of the carotid arteries (**carotid endarterectomy**) or of the arteries that supply the legs.

endarteritis *n.* chronic inflammation of the inner (intimal) portion of the wall of an artery, which most often results from late syphilis. Thickening of the wall produces progressive arterial obstruction and symptoms from inadequate blood supply to the affected part (*ischaemia). The arteries to the brain are often involved, giving rise to meningovascular syphilis.

Endarteritis of the aorta may obstruct the mouths of the coronary arteries, supplying the heart. Endarteritis of the arteries to the wall of the aorta (the vasa vasorum) contributes to *aneurysm formation. The syphilitic infection may be eradicated with penicillin.

end artery the terminal branch of an artery, which does not communicate with other branches. The tissue it supplies is therefore probably completely dependent on it for its blood supply.

endemic *adj.* occurring frequently in a particular region or population: applied to diseases that are generally or constantly found among people in a particular area. *Compare* ECDEMIC, EPIDEMIC, PANDEMIC.

endemic syphilis *see* BEJEL.

endocarditis *n.* inflammation of the lining of the heart cavity (endocardium) and valves. It is most often due to rheumatic fever or results from bacterial infection (**bacterial endocarditis**). Temporary or permanent damage to the heart valves may result. The main features are fever, changing heart murmurs, heart failure, and embolism. Treatment consists of rest and antibiotics; surgery may be required to repair damaged heart valves.

endocardium *n.* a delicate membrane, formed of flat endothelial cells, that lines the heart and is continuous with the lining of arteries and veins. At the openings of the heart cavities it is folded back on itself to form the cusps of the valves. It presents a smooth slippery surface, which does not impede blood flow. —**endocardial** *adj.*

endocervicitis *n.* inflammation of the membrane that lines the cervix (neck) of the uterus, usually caused by infection. Surface cells (epithelium) may die, resulting in a new growth of healthy epithelium over the affected area. The condition is accompanied by a thick mucoid discharge.

endocervix *n.* the mucous membrane (*endometrium) lining the cervix (neck) of the uterus.

endochondral *adj.* within the material of a cartilage.

endocrine gland (ductless gland) a gland that manufactures one or more *hormones and secretes them directly into the bloodstream (and not through a duct to the exterior). Endocrine glands include the pituitary, thyroid, parathyroid, and adrenal glands, the ovary and testis, the placenta, and part of the pancreas.

endocrinology *n.* the study of the *endocrine glands and the substances they secrete (*hormones). —**endocrinologist** *n.*

endoderm *n.* the inner of the three *germ layers of the early embryo, which gives rise to the lining of most of the alimentary canal and its associated glands, the liver, gall bladder, and pancreas. It also forms the lining of the bronchi and alveoli of the lung and most of the urinary tract. —**endodermal** *adj.*

endodermal sinus tumour a rare tumour of fetal remnants of the ovaries or testes.

endodontics *n.* the study, treatment, and prevention of diseases of the pulp of teeth and their sequelae. A major part of treatment is *root canal treatment.

endogenous *adj.* arising within or derived from the body. *Compare* EXOGENOUS.

endolymph *n.* the fluid that fills the membranous *labyrinth of the ear.

endolymphatic duct a blind-ended duct that leads from the sacculus and joins a duct from the utriculus of the membranous *labyrinth of the ear.

endolymphatic sac a dilatation at the end of the *endolymphatic duct that removes waste products from the inner ear.

endometrial ablation the removal of the entire endometrium by means of a technique (**laser ablation**) in which a special type of laser, known as a **Nd:YAG laser** (neodymium:yttrium–aluminium–garnet laser), is used to destroy the endometrium in situ. The operation is usually performed under local anaesthetic by using a *hysteroscope. The same effect may be achieved by *electrocoagulation (*see also* TRANSCERVICAL RESECTION OF THE ENDOMETRIUM). Ablation may be used as an alternative to hysterectomy or hormone therapy in the treatment of abnormally heavy menstrual bleeding (*see* MENORRHAGIA) or *endometrial hyperplasia.

endometrial hyperplasia an increase in the thickness of the cells of the *endometrium, usually due to prolonged exposure to unopposed oestrogen, which can be endogenous, as in *anovulatory menstrual cycles; or exogenous, deriving, for example, from *hormone replacement therapy or an oestrogen-secreting tumour. Atypical cells may or may not be present. The presence of atypical cells may lead to endometrial carcinoma. Treatment can include progestogen therapy or surgery (*see* ENDOMETRIAL ABLATION).

endometriosis *n.* the presence of tissue similar to the lining of the uterus (*see* ENDOMETRIUM) at other sites in the pelvis; it is thought to be caused by retrograde *menstruation. When the tissue has infiltrated the wall of the uterus (myometrium) the condition is known as **adenomyosis**. The tissue may also be found in the ovary, Fallopian tubes, pelvic ligaments, on the pelvic peritoneum, and even in the cervix and the vagina. This tissue undergoes the periodic changes similar to those of the endometrium and causes pelvic pain and severe *dysmenorrhoea. The pain continues throughout and after menstruation. Symptoms disappear if pregnancy occurs and after the menopause. Treatment during the reproductive years is largely confined to the use of drugs (e.g. *danazol), although restricted surgical treatment may also be necessary. The formation of pelvic *adhesions is a common sequel to endometriosis. In such circumstances the uterus, Fallopian tubes, and ovaries may need to be surgically removed in order to alleviate the symptoms.

endometritis *n.* inflammation of the *endometrium due to acute or chronic infection. It may be caused by foreign bodies, bacteria, viruses, or parasites. In the acute phase it may occur in the period immediately after childbirth (puerperium) but the chronic phase may not be associated with pregnancy (as in tuberculous endometritis). Chronic endometritis in women with IUDs may be responsible for the contraceptive action.

endometrium *n.* the mucous membrane lining the uterus, which becomes progressively thicker and more glandular and has an increased blood supply in the latter part of the menstrual cycle. This prepares the endometrium for implantation of the embryo, but if this does not occur much of the endometrium breaks down and is lost in menstruation. If pregnancy is established the endometrium becomes the *decidua, which is shed after birth. —**endometrial** *adj.*

endomorphic *adj.* describing a *body type that is relatively fat, with highly developed viscera and weak muscular and skeletal development. —**endomorph** *n.* —**endomorphy** *n.*

endomorphin *n. see* ENDORPHIN.

endomyocarditis *n.* an acute or chronic inflammatory disorder of the muscle and lining membrane of the heart. When the membrane surrounding the heart (pericardium) is also involved the condition is termed **pancarditis**. The principal causes are rheumatic fever and virus infections. There is enlargement of the heart, murmurs, embolism, and frequently arrhythmias. The treatment is that of the cause and complications. *See also* ENDOCARDITIS.

A chronic condition, **endomyocardial fibrosis**, is seen in Black Africans: the cause is unknown.

endomysium *n.* the fine connective tissue sheath that surrounds a single *muscle fibre.

endoneurium *n.* the layer of fibrous tissue that separates individual fibres within a *nerve.

endoparasite *n.* a parasite that lives inside its host, for example in the liver, lungs, gut, or other tissues of the body. *Compare* ECTOPARASITE.

endopeptidase *n.* a digestive enzyme (e.g. *pepsin) that splits a whole protein into small peptide fractions by splitting the linkages between peptides in the interior of the molecule. *Compare* EXOPEPTIDASE. *See also* PEPTIDASE.

endophthalmitis *n.* inflammation, usually due to infection, within the eye.

endoplasm *n.* the inner cytoplasm of cells, which is less dense than the *ectoplasm and contains most of the cell's structures. —**endoplasmic** *adj.*

endoplasmic reticulum (ER) a system

of membranes present in the cytoplasm of cells. ER is described as **rough** when it has *ribosomes attached to its surface and **smooth** when ribosomes are absent. It is the site of manufacture of proteins and lipids and is concerned with the transport of these products within the cell (*see also* GOLGI APPARATUS).

end organ a specialized structure at the end of a peripheral nerve, acting as a receptor for a particular sensation. Taste buds, in the tongue, are end organs subserving the sense of taste.

endorphin (endomorphin) *n.* one of a group of chemical compounds, similar to the *encephalins, that occur naturally in the brain and have pain-relieving properties similar to those of the opiates. They are also responsible for sensations of pleasure. The endorphins are derived from a substance found in the pituitary gland known as **beta-lipotrophin**; they are thought to be concerned with controlling the activity of the endocrine glands.

endoscope *n.* any instrument used to obtain a view of the interior of the body. Examples of endoscopes include the *auriscope and the *gastroscope. Essentially, most endoscopes consist of a tube with a light at the end and an optical system or a miniature video camera for transmitting an image to the examiner's eye. *See also* FIBRESCOPE. —**endoscopic** *adj.* —**endoscopy** *n.*

endoscopic retrograde cholangio-pancreatography *see* ERCP.

endospore *n.* the resting stage of certain bacteria, particularly species of the genera *Bacillus* and *Clostridium*. In adverse conditions the bacterium can become enclosed within a tough protective coat, allowing the cell to survive. On return of favourable conditions the spore changes back to the vegetative form.

endostapler *n.* a stapling instrument (*see* STAPLE) used endoscopically for fixing tissues or joining them together.

endosteum *n.* the membrane that lines the marrow cavity of a bone.

endothelioma *n.* any tumour arising from or resembling endothelium. It may arise from the linings of blood or lymph vessels (**haemangioendothelioma** and **lymphangioendothelioma** respectively); from the linings of the pleural cavity or the peritoneal cavity (*see* MESOTHELIOMA); or from the meninges (*see* MENINGIOMA).

endothelium *n.* the single layer of cells that lines the heart, blood vessels, and lymphatic vessels. It is derived from embryonic mesoderm. The **corneal endothelium** is the innermost layer of the *cornea. *Compare* EPITHELIUM.

endothermic *adj.* describing a chemical reaction associated with the absorption of heat. *Compare* EXOTHERMIC.

endotoxin *n.* a poison generally harmful to all body tissues, contained within certain Gram-negative bacteria and released only when the bacterial cell is broken down or dies and disintegrates. *Compare* EXOTOXIN.

endotracheal *adj.* within or through the trachea (windpipe). *See* INTUBATION.

end-plate *n.* the area of muscle cell membrane immediately beneath the motor nerve ending at a *neuromuscular junction. Special receptors in this area trigger muscular contraction when the nerve ending releases its *neurotransmitter.

end-stage renal failure (ESRF) the most advanced stage of kidney failure, which is reached when the *glomerular filtration rate (GFR) falls to 5 ml/min (normal GFR = 120 ml/min).

enema *n.* (*pl.* **enemata** or **enemas**) a quantity of fluid infused into the rectum through a tube passed into the anus. An **evacuant enema** (soap or olive oil) is used to remove faeces. A **barium enema** using barium sulphate, which is opaque to X-rays, is given to demonstrate the colon by X-ray. The large bowel is best investigated by a **double-contrast barium enema**, which uses air *insufflation to distend the bowel. A **therapeutic enema** is used to insert drugs into the rectum, usually corticosteroids in the treatment of *procto-colitis.

enervation *n.* **1.** weakness; loss of strength. **2.** the surgical removal of a nerve.

enflurane *n.* a volatile drug used to induce and maintain general anaesthesia. It is administered by inhalation. Possible side-effects include seizures, hepatitis, and kidney damage.

engagement n. (in obstetrics) the stage of pregnancy that occurs when the presenting part of the fetus has descended into the mother's pelvis. Engagement of the fetal head occurs when the widest part has passed through the pelvic inlet.

engram n. the supposed physical basis of an individual memory.

enkephalin n. see ENCEPHALIN.

enophthalmos n. a condition in which the eye is abnormally sunken into the socket. It may follow fractures of the floor of the orbit that allow the eye to sink downwards and backwards.

enoxacin n. see QUINOLONE.

enoxaparin n. see LOW-MOLECULAR-WEIGHT HEPARIN.

enoximone n. an *inotropic drug used in heart failure to increase the force and output of the heart. It is administered by injection. Trade name: **Perfan**.

ensiform cartilage see XIPHOID PROCESS.

ENT see OTORHINOLARYNGOLOGY.

Entamoeba n. a genus of widely distributed amoebae, of which some species are parasites of the digestive tract of man. *E. histolytica* invades and destroys the tissues of the intestinal wall, causing amoebic *dysentery and ulceration of the gut wall (see also AMOEBOMA); infection of the liver with this species (amoebic hepatitis) is common in tropical countries. *E. coli* is a harmless intestinal parasite; *E. gingivalis*, found within the spaces between the teeth, is associated with periodontal disease and gingivitis.

enter- (entero-) prefix denoting the intestine. Example: **enterolith** (calculus in).

enteral adj. of or relating to the intestinal tract.

enteral feeding see NUTRITION.

enteralgia n. see COLIC.

enterectomy n. surgical removal of part of the intestine.

enteric adj. relating to or affecting the intestine.

enteric-coated adj. describing tablets that are coated with a substance that enables them to pass through the stomach and into the intestine unchanged. Enteric-coated tablets contain drugs that are destroyed by the acid contents of the stomach.

enteric fever see PARATYPHOID FEVER, TYPHOID FEVER.

enteritis n. inflammation of the small intestine, usually causing diarrhoea. **Infective enteritis** is caused by viruses or bacteria; **radiation enteritis** is caused by X-rays or radioactive isotopes. See also CROHN'S DISEASE (REGIONAL ENTERITIS), GASTROENTERITIS.

enterobiasis (oxyuriasis) n. a disease, common in children throughout the world, caused by the parasitic nematode *Enterobius vermicularis* (see THREADWORM) in the large intestine. The worms do not cause any serious lesions of the gut wall although, rarely, they may provoke appendicitis. The emergence of the female from the anus at night irritates and inflames the surrounding skin, causing the patient to scratch and thereby contaminate fingers and nails with infective eggs. The eggs may reinfect the same child or be spread to other children. Worms may occasionally enter the vulva and cause a discharge from the vagina. Enterobiasis responds well to treatment with *piperazine compounds.

Enterobius (Oxyuris) n. see THREADWORM.

enterocele n. a hernia of the *pouch of Douglas (between the rectum and uterus) into the upper part of the posterior vaginal wall. It may contain loops of small bowel.

enterocentesis n. a surgical procedure in which a hollow needle is pushed through the wall of the stomach or intestines to release an abnormal accumulation of gas or fluid or to introduce a catheter for feeding (see GASTROSTOMY, ENTEROSTOMY).

enterocolitis n. inflammation of the

colon and small intestine. *See also* COLITIS, ENTERITIS, NECROTIZING ENTEROCOLITIS.

enterogastrone *n.* a hormone from the small intestine (duodenum) that inhibits the secretion of gastric juice by the stomach. It is released when the stomach contents pass into the small intestine.

enterogenous *adj.* borne by or carried in the intestine.

enterokinase *n.* the former name for *enteropeptidase.

enterolith *n.* a stone within the intestine. It usually builds up around a gallstone or a swallowed fruit stone.

enteromegaly *n. Rare.* enlargement (usually increased diameter) of the intestine.

enteropathy *n.* disease of the small intestine. *See also* COELIAC DISEASE (GLUTEN-INDUCED ENTEROPATHY).

enteropeptidase *n.* an enzyme secreted by the glands of the small intestine that acts on trypsinogen to produce *trypsin.

enteropexy *n.* a surgical operation in which part of the intestine is fixed to the abdominal wall. This was formerly performed for visceroptosis (a condition in which the abdominal organs were thought to have descended to a lower than normal position), but it is no longer carried out.

enteroptosis *n.* a condition in which loops of intestine (especially transverse *colon) are in a low anatomical position. At one time this was thought to cause various abdominal symptoms, and operations were devised to correct it. It is now known that no symptoms result from simple anatomical variations of this sort.

enterorrhaphy *n.* the surgical procedure of stitching an intestine that has either perforated or been divided during an operation.

enteroscope *n.* an illuminated optical instrument used to inspect the interior of the small intestine. The image is transmitted through a fibreoptic bundle or by a tiny video-camera. The **push** type, about 280 cm long and of variable stiffness, is introduced by guidance under direct vision. The **sonde** type, about 280 cm long, has an inflatable balloon that pulls the instrument through the length of the intestine by peristalsis. The enteroscope is useful in diagnosing the cause of haemorrhage of the small intestine or of *strictures. —**enteroscopy** *n.*

enterostomy *n.* an operation in which the small intestine is brought through the abdominal wall and opened (*see* DUODENOSTOMY, JEJUNOSTOMY, ILEOSTOMY) or is joined to the stomach (**gastroenterostomy**) or to another loop of small intestine (**entero-enterostomy**).

enterotomy *n.* surgical incision into the intestine.

enterotoxin *n.* a poisonous substance that has a particularly marked effect upon the gastrointestinal tract, causing vomiting, diarrhoea, and abdominal pain.

enterovirus *n.* any virus that enters the body through the gastrointestinal tract, multiplies there, and then (generally) invades the central nervous system. Enteroviruses include *Coxsackie viruses and *polioviruses.

enterozoon *n.* any animal species inhabiting or infecting the gut of another. *See also* ENDOPARASITE.

enthesis *n.* the junction of tendon and bone.

enthesopathy *n.* any rheumatic disease resulting in inflammation of *entheses. Ankylosing *spondylitis, *psoriatic arthritis, and *Reiter's disease are examples.

entoptic phenomena visual sensations caused by changes within the eye itself, rather than by the normal light stimulation process. The commonest are tiny floating spots (**floaters**) that most people can see occasionally, especially when gazing at a brightly illuminated background (such as a blue sky).

entrapment neuropathy pain, muscle wasting, and paralysis resulting from pressure on a nerve in conditions in which it is subjected to compression by surrounding structures. *See* CARPAL TUNNEL SYNDROME.

entropion *n.* inturning of the eyelid towards the eyeball. The lashes may rub against the eye and cause irritation (*see* TRICHIASIS). The commonest type is **spastic**

entropion of the lower eyelid, due to spasm of the muscle that closes the eye (orbicularis oculi). Entropion may also be caused by scarring of the lining membrane (conjunctiva) of the lid.

enucleation *n.* a surgical operation in which an organ, tumour, or cyst is completely removed. In ophthalmology it is an operation in which the eyeball is removed but the other structures in the socket (e.g. eye muscles) are left in place. Commonly a plastic ball is temporarily buried in the socket to give a better cosmetic result prior to fitting an artificial eye.

enuresis *n.* the involuntary passing of urine. The most common form is bedwetting (**nocturnal enuresis**) by children (the majority of children are dry during the day by the age of three years and at night by four). Nocturnal enuresis is occasionally caused by underlying disorders of the urinary tract, particularly infection, but in the majority of children the problem is behavioural; there is often a family history. The condition usually settles spontaneously as the child grows older, but it may persist into teenage – and rarely adult – life. It can be treated by behavioural techniques, such as the use of a nocturnal alarm (*see* BELL AND PAD) or *reinforcement of periods of continence with a reward system, or by drug treatment. Enuresis that starts in adulthood is usually associated with a disorder of the bladder or a neurological disease, such as multiple sclerosis. *See also* INCONTINENCE. —**enuretic** *adj.*

environment *n.* any or all aspects of the surroundings of an organism, both internal and external, which influence its growth, development, and behaviour.

Environmental Health Officer (EHO) a person, employed by a local authority, with special training in such aspects of environmental health and pollution as housing, sanitation, food, clean air, noise, and water supplies (formerly known as a **Public Health Inspector**). Though not a registered medical practitioner, the EHO is responsible for the organization of the environmental health department. If medical (epidemiological) advice is required, the appropriate *public health physician (proper officer) acts in an advisory or consultant capacity.

enzyme *n.* a protein that, in small amounts, speeds up the rate of a biological reaction without itself being used up in the reaction (i.e. it acts as a catalyst). An enzyme acts by binding with the substance involved in the reaction (the **substrate**) and converting it into another substance (the **product** of the reaction). An enzyme is relatively specific in the type of reaction it catalyses; hence there are many different enzymes for the various biochemical reactions. Each enzyme requires certain conditions for optimum activity, particularly correct temperature and pH, the presence of *coenzymes, and the absence of specific inhibitors. Enzymes are unstable and are easily inactivated by heat or certain chemicals. They are produced within living cells and may act either within the cell (as in cellular respiration) or outside it (as in digestion). The names of enzymes usually end in '-ase'; enzymes are named according to the substrate upon which they act (as in lactase), or the type of reaction they catalyse (as in hydrolase).
     Enzymes are essential for the normal functioning and development of the body. Failure in the production or activity of a single enzyme may result in metabolic disorders; such disorders are often inherited and some have serious effects. —**enzymatic** *adj.*

enzyme-linked immunosorbent assay (ELISA) a sensitive technique for measuring the amount of a substance. An antibody that will bind to the substance is produced; the amount of an easily measured enzyme that then binds to the antibody complex enables accurate measurement.

EOG *see* ELECTROOCULOGRAPHY.

eonism *n.* the adoption of female manners and dress by a man. *See* TRANSSEXUALISM, TRANSVESTITISM.

eosin *n.* a red acidic dye, produced by the reaction of bromine and fluorescein, used to stain biological specimens for microscopical examination. Eosin may be used in conjunction with a contrasting blue alkaline dye taken up by different parts of the same specimen.

eosinopenia *n.* a decrease in the number of eosinophils in the blood.

eosinophil *n.* a variety of white blood cell distinguished by the presence in its cytoplasm of coarse granules that stain orange-red with *Romanowsky stains. The function of the eosinophil is poorly understood, but it is capable of ingesting foreign particles, is present in large numbers in lining or covering surfaces within the body, and is involved in allergic responses. There are normally $40–400 \times 10^6$ eosinophils per litre of blood.

eosinophilia *n.* an increase in the number of eosinophils in the blood. Eosinophilia occurs in response to certain drugs and in a variety of diseases, including allergies, parasitic infestations, and certain forms of leukaemia.

eparterial *adj.* situated on or above an artery.

ependyma *n.* the extremely thin membrane, composed of cells of the *glia (**ependymal cells**), that lines the ventricles of the brain and the choroid plexuses. It is responsible for helping to form cerebrospinal fluid. —**ependymal** *adj.*

ependymoma *n.* a cerebral tumour derived from the glial (non-nervous) cells lining the cavities of the ventricles of the brain (*see* EPENDYMA). It may obstruct the flow of cerebrospinal fluid, causing a *hydrocephalus.

ephebiatrics *n.* the branch of medicine concerned with the common disorders of children and adolescents. *Compare* PAEDIATRICS.

ephedrine *n.* a drug that causes constriction of blood vessels and widening of the bronchial passages (*see* SYMPATHOMIMETIC). It is used mainly in the treatment of asthma and other allergic conditions and chronic bronchitis. It is administered by mouth or by inhalation and may cause nausea, vomiting, insomnia, headache, and nervousness.

EPI *see* ECHO PLANAR IMAGING.

epi- *prefix denoting* above or upon.

epiblepharon *n.* an abnormal fold of skin, present from birth, stretching across the eye just above the lashes of the upper eyelid or in front of them in the lower lid. It may cause the lower lashes to turn upwards or inwards against the eye. It usually disappears within the first year of life.

epicanthus (epicanthic fold) *n.* a vertical fold of skin from the upper eyelid that covers the inner corner of the eye. It is normal in Mongolian races and occurs abnormally in certain congenital conditions, e.g. *Down's syndrome. —**epicanthal**, **epicanthic** *adj.*

epicardia *n.* the part of the *oesophagus, about 2 cm long, that extends from the level of the diaphragm to the stomach.

epicardium *n.* the outermost layer of the heart wall, enveloping the myocardium. It is a serous membrane that forms the inner layer of the serous *pericardium. —**epicardial** *adj.*

epicondyle *n.* the protuberance above a *condyle at the end of an articulating bone.

epicranium *n.* the structures that cover the cranium, i.e. all layers of the scalp.

epicranius *n.* the muscle of the scalp. The **frontal** portion, at the forehead, is responsible for raising the eyebrows and wrinkling the forehead; the **occipital** portion, at the base of the skull, draws the scalp backwards.

epicritic *adj.* describing or relating to sensory nerve fibres responsible for the fine degrees of sensation, as of temperature and touch. *Compare* PROTOPATHIC.

epidemic *n.* a sudden outbreak of infectious disease that spreads rapidly through the population, affecting a large proportion of people. The commonest epidemics today are of influenza. *Compare* ENDEMIC, PANDEMIC. —**epidemic** *adj.*

epidemiology *n.* the study of the occurrence, distribution, and control of infectious and noninfectious diseases in populations, which is a basic part of *public health medicine. Originally restricted to the study of epidemic infectious diseases, such as smallpox and cholera, it now covers all forms of disease that relate to the environment and ways of life. It thus includes the study of the links between smoking and cancer, and diet and coro-

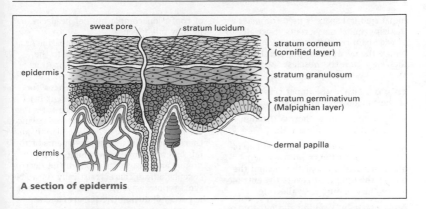

A section of epidermis

nary disease, as well as *communicable diseases.

epidermis *n.* the outer layer of the *skin, which is divided into four layers (see illustration). The innermost **Malpighian** or **germinative layer (stratum germinativum)** consists of continuously dividing cells. The other three layers are continually renewed as cells from the germinative layer are gradually pushed outwards and become progressively impregnated with keratin (see KERATINIZATION). The outermost layer (**stratum corneum**) consists of dead cells whose cytoplasm has been entirely replaced by keratin. It is thickest on the soles of the feet and palms of the hands. —**epidermal** *adj.*

epidermoid *adj.* having the appearance of epidermis (the outer layer of the skin): used to describe certain tumours of tissues other than the skin.

epidermoid cyst *see* SEBACEOUS CYST.

epidermolysis bullosa any one of a group of genetically determined disorders characterized by blistering of skin and mucous membranes. In the simple forms the blistering is induced by injury. In the more serious (dystrophic) forms the blistering may occur spontaneously; some of the dystrophic forms of the disease are fatal.

Epidermophyton *n.* a genus of fungi that grow on the skin, causing *ringworm. *See also* DERMATOPHYTE.

epidiascope *n.* an apparatus for projecting a greatly magnified image of an object, such as a specimen on a microscope slide, on to a screen.

epididymectomy *n.* the surgical removal or excision of the epididymis.

epididymis *n.* (*pl.* **epididymides**) a highly convoluted tube, about seven metres long, that connects the *testis to the vas deferens. The spermatozoa are moved passively along the tube over a period of several days, during which time they mature and become capable of fertilization. They are concentrated and stored in the lower part of the epididymis until ejaculation. —**epididymal** *adj.*

epididymitis *n.* inflammation of the epididymis. The usual cause is infection spreading down the vas deferens from the bladder or urethra, resulting in pain, swelling, and redness of the affected half of the scrotum. The inflammation may spread to the testicle (**epididymo-orchitis**). Treatment is by administration of antibiotics and analgesics.

epididymovasostomy *n.* the operation of connecting the vas deferens to the epididymis to bypass obstruction of the latter. It is performed in an attempt to cure *azoospermia caused by this blockage.

epidural (extradural) *adj.* on or over the dura mater (the outermost of the three membranes covering the brain and spinal cord). The **epidural space** is the space between the dura mater of the spinal cord and the vertebral canal. The spinal epidural space is used for anaesthetizing spinal nerve roots, especially to provide pain relief during childbirth or to reduce the need for deep general anaesthesia (e.g. to relax muscles). *See also* SPINAL ANAESTHESIA.

epigastrium *n.* the upper central region of the *abdomen. —**epigastric** *adj.*

epigastrocele *n.* a *hernia through the upper central abdominal wall.

epiglottis *n.* a thin leaf-shaped flap of cartilage, covered with mucous membrane, situated immediately behind the root of the tongue. It covers the entrance to the *larynx during swallowing.

epiglottitis *n.* swelling and inflammation of the epiglottis and other parts of the *supraglottis, obstructing air flow to the lungs. It is usually caused by the bacterium *Haemophilus influenzae*. Treatment is by administration of antibiotics, careful observation, and possible *intubation or *tracheostomy.

epikeratophakia *n.* eye surgery to correct errors of *refraction in which the curvature of the cornea is altered using donor corneal tissue, which has been frozen and shaped using a lathe to produce a tissue lens that is then sutured onto the cornea.

epilation *n.* the removal of a hair by its roots. This can be done mechanically (by plucking or using wax) or by electrolysis; lasers for epilation are now available.

epilepsy *n.* a disorder of brain function characterized by recurrent seizures that have a sudden onset. The term **idiopathic** is used to describe epilepsy that is not associated with structural damage to the brain. Seizures may be generalized or partial. **Generalized epilepsy** may take the form of **major**, or **tonic-clonic**, seizures (formerly called **grand mal**), in which, at the onset, the patient falls to the ground unconscious with his muscles in a state of spasm. The lack of any respiratory movement may result in a bluish discoloration of the skin and lips (cyanosis). This – the tonic phase – is replaced by convulsive movements (the clonic phase) when the tongue may be bitten and urinary incontinence may occur. Movements gradually cease and the patient may rouse in a state

of confusion, complaining of headache, or he may fall asleep.

Partial epilepsy may be idiopathic or a symptom of structural damage to the brain. In one type of partial idiopathic epilepsy, often affecting children, the seizures take the form of **absences** (formerly called **petit mal** in children): brief spells of unconsciousness lasting for a few seconds, during which posture and balance are maintained. The eyes stare blankly and there may be fluttering movements of the lids and momentary twitching of the fingers and mouth. In children the electroencephalogram characteristically shows bisynchronous wave and spike discharges (3 per second) during the seizures and at other times. Attacks are sometimes provoked by overbreathing or intermittent photic stimulation. As the stream of thought is completely interrupted, children with frequent seizures may have learning difficulties. This form of epilepsy seldom appears before the age of three or after adolescence. It often subsides spontaneously in adult life, but it may be followed by the onset of major or partial epilepsy.

In partial epilepsy due to brain damage, called **focal epilepsy**, the nature of the seizure depends upon the location of the damage in the brain. In a **Jacksonian** motor seizure the convulsive movements might spread from the thumb to the hand, arm, and face (this spread of symptoms is called the **march**). **Temporal lobe** (or **psychomotor**) **epilepsy** is caused by disease in the cortex of the temporal lobe or the adjacent parietal lobe of the brain. Its symptoms may include *hallucinations of smell, taste, sight, and hearing, paroxysmal disorders of memory, and *automatism. Throughout an attack the patient is in a state of clouded awareness and afterwards he may have no recollection of the event (*see also* DÉJÀ VU, JAMAIS VU).

The different forms of epilepsy can be controlled by the use of antiepileptic drugs (*see* ANTICONVULSANT). Surgical resection of focal epileptogenic lesions in the brain is appropriate in a strictly limited number of cases. —**epileptic** *adj., n.*

epileptogenic *adj.* having the capacity to provoke epileptic seizures.

epiloia *n. see* TUBEROUS SCLEROSIS.

epimenorrhagia n. see MENORRHAGIA.

epimenorrhoea n. menstruation at shorter intervals than is normal.

epimysium n. the fibrous elastic tissue that surrounds a *muscle.

epinephrine n. see ADRENALINE.

epineural adj. derived from or situated on the neural arch of a vertebra.

epineurium n. the outer sheath of connective tissue that encloses the bundles (fascicles) of fibres that make up a *nerve.

epiphenomenon n. an unusual symptom or event that may occur simultaneously with a disease but is not necessarily directly related to it. Compare COMPLICATION.

epiphora n. watering of the eye, in which tears flow onto the cheek. It is due to some abnormality of the tear drainage system (see LACRIMAL APPARATUS).

epiphysis n. 1. the end of a long bone, which is initially separated by cartilage from the shaft (diaphysis) of the bone and develops separately. It eventually fuses with the diaphysis to form a complete bone. Injuries of the epiphysis are defined in the **Salter and Harris classification**. 2. see PINEAL GLAND. —**epiphyseal** adj.

epiphysitis n. inflammation of the end (epiphysis) of a long bone. It may result in retardation of growth and deformity of the affected bone.

epiplo- prefix denoting the omentum. Example: **epiplocele** (hernia containing omentum).

epiploon n. see OMENTUM.

epiretinal membrane (cellophane maculopathy) a transparent membrane that forms on the retina, over the *macula. Contraction of this causes wrinkling of the retina (**macular pucker**) and hence distorted vision.

episclera n. the outermost covering of the *sclera of the eye, which provides nutritional support to the sclera.

episcleritis n. inflammation of the *episclera, resulting in a red painful eye that is sensitive to light. It is usually a be-

nign condition, which will settle without treatment.

episio- prefix denoting the vulva. Example: **episioplasty** (plastic surgery of).

episiotomy n. an incision into the tissues surrounding the opening of the vagina (perineum) during a difficult birth, at the stage when the infant's head has partly emerged through the opening of the birth passage. The aim is to enlarge the opening in a controlled manner so as to make delivery easier and to avoid extensive tearing of adjacent tissues.

epispadias n. a congenital abnormality in which the opening of the *urethra is on the dorsal (upper) surface of the penis. Surgical correction is carried out in infancy.

epistasis n. 1. the stopping of a flow or discharge, as of blood. 2. a type of gene action in which one gene can suppress the action of another (nonallelic) gene. The term is sometimes used for any interaction between nonallelic genes. —**epistatic** adj.

epistaxis n. see NOSEBLEED.

epithalamus n. part of the forebrain, consisting of a narrow band of nerve tissue in the roof of the third ventricle (including the region where the choroid plexus is attached) and the *pineal gland. See also BRAIN.

epithalaxia n. loss of layers of epithelial cells from the lining of the intestine.

epithelioma n. a tumour of *epithelium, the covering of internal and external surfaces of the body: a former term for *carcinoma.

epithelium n. the tissue that covers the external surface of the body and lines hollow structures (except blood and lymphatic vessels). It is derived from embryonic ectoderm and endoderm. Epithelial cells may be flat and scalelike (**squamous**), **cuboidal**, or **columnar**. The latter may bear cilia or brush borders or secrete mucus or other substances (see GOBLET CELL). The cells rest on a common **basement membrane**, which separates epithelium from underlying *connective tissue. Epithelium may be either **simple**, consisting of a single layer of cells; **stratified**, consisting of several layers; or **pseudostratified**, in which the cells appear to be arranged in layers but in fact share a common basement membrane (see illustration). *See also* ENDOTHELIUM, MESOTHELIUM. —**epithelial** *adj.*

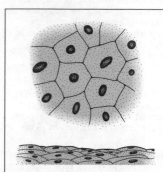

Stratified squamous epithelium, surface view above and sectional view below

basement membrane

Simple cuboidal epithelium

goblet cell

Ciliated columnar epithelium

basement membrane

Pseudostratified ciliated epithelium

Types of epithelium

epitrichium (periderm) *n.* the most superficial layer of the skin, one cell in thickness, that is only present early in embryonic development. It protects the underlying *epidermis until it is fully formed.

eponychium *n.* see NAIL.

eponym *n.* a disease, structure, or species named after a particular person, usually the person who first discovered or described it. Eponyms are widespread in medicine, but they are being replaced as more descriptive terms become necessary. Thus the eponyms islets of Langerhans, aqueduct of Sylvius, and Hashimoto's disease are more likely to be designated in text books as pancreatic islands, cerebral aqueduct, and autoimmune thyroiditis, respectively. —**eponymous** *adj.*

epoophoron *n.* see PAROOPHORON.

epoprostenol *n.* a *prostaglandin drug used immediately before and during renal dialysis to prevent clotting of blood in the shunt. It is administered by intravenous injection.

Epstein-Barr virus (EB virus, EBV) the virus, belonging to the *herpesvirus group, that is the causative agent of *glandular fever. It attacks B-*lymphocytes; an imbalance in the immune response to this gives rise to the clinical features of the disease. EB virus is also implicated in hepatitis and in certain cancers (e.g. *Burkitt's lymphoma and *Hodgkin's disease). [Sir M. A. Epstein (1921–) and Y. M. Barr (1932–), British pathologists]

epulis *n.* a swelling on the gum. Most such swellings are due to fibrous hyperplasia, but an epulis may be the opening of a *sinus tract.

equi- *prefix denoting* equality.

equinia *n.* see GLANDERS.

Erb's palsy weakness or paralysis of the shoulder and arm caused by injury to the upper roots of a baby's *brachial plexus during birth. This may happen if, during a difficult delivery, excess traction applied to the head damages the fifth cervical root of the spinal cord. The muscles of the shoulder and the flexors of the elbow are paralysed and the arm hangs at the side internally rotated at the shoulder.

Recovery may be spontaneous, but in some cases nerve grafts or muscle transfers are required. [W. H. Erb (1840–1921), German neurologist]

ERCP (endoscopic retrograde cholangiopancreatography) the technique in which a catheter is passed through a *duodenoscope into the *ampulla of Vater of the common bile duct and injected with a radiopaque medium to outline the pancreatic duct and bile ducts radiologically. It is widely used in the diagnosis of obstructive jaundice and pancreatic disease. See also PAPILLOTOMY.

erectile adj. capable of causing erection or becoming erect. The penis is composed largely of erectile tissue.

erection n. the sexually active state of the penis, which becomes enlarged and rigid (due to the erectile tissue being swollen with blood) and capable of penetrating the vagina. The term is also applied to the clitoris in a state of sexual arousal.

erepsin n. a mixture of protein-digesting enzymes (see PEPTIDASE) secreted by the intestinal glands. It is part of the *succus entericus.

erethism n. **1.** a state of abnormal mental excitement or irritability. **2.** rapid response to a stimulus.

erg n. a unit of work or energy equal to the work done when the point of application of a force of 1 dyne is displaced through a distance of 1 centimetre in the direction of the force. 1 erg = 10^{-7} joule.

ERG see ELECTRORETINOGRAPHY.

erg- (ergo-) prefix denoting work or activity.

ergocalciferol n. see VITAMIN D.

ergograph n. an apparatus for recording the work performed by the muscles of the body when undergoing activity. Ergographs are useful for assessment of the capabilities of athletes undergoing training.

ergometrine n. a drug that stimulates contractions of the uterus. It is administered by injection to assist labour and to control bleeding following delivery. Trade name: **Syntometrine**.

ergonomics n. the study of man in relation to his work and working surroundings. This broad science involves the application of psychological as well as physiological principles to the design of buildings, machinery, vehicles, packaging, implements, and anything else with which man comes into contact.

ergosterol n. a plant sterol that, when irradiated with ultraviolet light, is converted to ergocalciferol (vitamin D_2). See VITAMIN D.

ergot n. a fungus (*Claviceps purpurea*) that grows on rye. It produces several important alkaloids, chemically related to LSD, including *ergotamine and *ergometrine, which are used in medicine in the treatment of migraine and in childbirth. Eating bread made with rye infected with the fungus has led to sporadic outbreaks of *ergotism over the centuries.

ergotamine n. a drug that causes constriction of blood vessels and is used to relieve migraine. It is administered by mouth, injection, inhalation, or in suppositories. Common side-effects are nausea and vomiting, and ergotism may develop as a result of high doses. Trade names: **Lingraine**, **Migril**.

ergotism n. poisoning caused by eating rye infected with the fungus *ergot. The chief symptom is gangrene of the fingers and toes, with diarrhoea and vomiting, nausea, and headache. In the Middle Ages the disease was known as **St Anthony's fire**, because of the inflamed appearance of the tissues afflicted with gangrene and the belief that a pilgrimage to St Anthony's tomb would result in cure.

erogenous adj. describing certain parts of the body, the physical stimulation of which leads to sexual arousal.

erosion n. **1.** an eating away of surface tissue by physical or chemical processes, including those associated with inflammation. A **cervical erosion** is an abnormal area of epithelium that may develop at the neck of the uterus due to tissue damage caused at childbirth or by attempts at abortion. In the skin an erosion represents a superficial type of ulceration and therefore heals quite readily. **2.** (in dentistry) loss of surface tooth substance, usually caused by repeated application of acid, which softens the enamel surface. It may result from excessive intake of citrus drinks, citrus fruits, or carbonated drinks or by regurgitation of acid from the stomach, as in bulimia nervosa, hiatus hernia, alcoholism, or stress. The teeth become very sensitive. The cause should be corrected; severe cases may require extensive dental restorations.

erot- (eroto-) *prefix denoting* sexual desire or love. Example: **erotophobia** (morbid dread of).

eroticism *n.* **1.** those elements in thought, imagination, pictorial imagery, literature, or the arts that tend to arouse sexual excitement or desire. **2.** actual sexual arousal. **3.** a greater than average disposition for sex and all its manifestations. **4.** sexual interest or excitement prompted by contemplation or stimulation of areas of the body not normally associated with sexuality. The terms **anal eroticism** and **oral eroticism** are used both in a theoretical Freudian sense and in reference to adult physical sexual activity.

erotomania *n.* a delusion that the individual is loved by some person, often a person of importance. Sometimes, but not always, this progresses to schizophrenia.

eructation *n.* belching: the sudden raising of gas from the stomach.

eruption *n.* **1.** the outbreak of a rash. A **bullous eruption** is an outbreak of blisters. **2.** (in dentistry) the emergence of a growing tooth from the gum into the mouth.

erysipelas *n.* a streptococcal infection of the skin, especially the face, characterized by redness and swelling; it usually has a sharply-defined margin, which can differentiate erysipelas from the otherwise similar *cellulitis. The patient is ill, with a high temperature. *Penicillin V is the treatment of choice.

erysipeloid *n.* an infection of the skin and underlying tissues with *Erysipelothrix insidiosa, developing usually in people handling fish, poultry, or meat. Infection enters through scratches or cuts on the hands, and is normally confined to a finger or hand, which becomes reddened;

sometimes systemic illness develops. Treatment is with penicillin.

Erysipelothrix *n.* a genus of Gram-positive nonmotile rod-shaped bacteria with a tendency to form filaments. They are parasites of mammals, birds, and fish. *E. insidiosa* (formerly *E. rhusiopathiae*) is a widely distributed species causing the disease *erysipeloid.

erythema *n.* flushing of the skin due to dilatation of the blood capillaries in the dermis. It may be physiological or a sign of inflammation or infection. **Erythema nodosum** is characterized by tender bruiselike swellings on the shins and is often associated with streptococcal infection. In **erythema multiforme** the eruption, which can take various forms, is characterized by so-called target lesions that may be recurrent and follow herpes simplex infection. **Erythema ab igne** is a reticular pigmented rash on the lower legs or elsewhere caused by persistent exposure to radiant heat.

erythr- (erythro-) *prefix denoting* **1.** redness. Example: **erythuria** (excretion of red urine). **2.** erythrocytes.

erythraemia *n. see* POLYCYTHAEMIA VERA.

erythrasma *n.* a chronic skin infection due to the bacterium *Corynebacterium minutissimum*, occurring in such areas as the armpits, groin, and toes, where skin surfaces are in contact. It fluoresces coralpink under *Wood's light and can be treated with antifungal creams or with antibiotics.

erythroblast *n.* any of a series of nucleated cells (*see* NORMOBLAST, PROERYTHROBLAST) that pass through a succession of stages of maturation to form red blood cells (*erythrocytes). Erythroblasts are normally present in the blood-forming tissue of the bone marrow, but they may appear in the circulation in a variety of diseases, (*see* ERYTHROBLASTOSIS). *See also* ERYTHROPOIESIS.

erythroblastosis *n.* the presence in the blood of the nucleated precursors of the red blood cells (*erythroblasts). This may occur when there is an increase in the rate of red cell production, as in haemorrhagic or haemolytic *anaemia, or in infiltrations of the bone marrow by tumours, etc.

erythroblastosis foetalis a severe but rare haemolytic *anaemia affecting new-born infants due to destruction of the infant's red blood cells by factors present in the mother's serum. It is usually caused by incompatibility of the rhesus blood groups between mother and infant (*see* RHESUS FACTOR).

erythrocyanosis *n.* mottled purplish discoloration on the legs and thighs, usually of adolescent girls or fat boys before puberty. The disorder sometimes occurs in older women and is worse in cold weather. Weight loss is the best treatment because it reduces the insulating effect of a thick layer of fat.

erythrocyte (red blood cell) *n.* a *blood cell containing the red pigment *haemoglobin, the principal function of which is the transport of oxygen. A mature erythrocyte has no nucleus and its shape is that of a biconcave disc, approximately 7 μm in diameter. There are normally about 5×10^{12} erythrocytes per litre of blood. *See also* ERYTHROPOIESIS.

erythrocyte sedimentation rate *see* ESR.

erythrocytic *adj.* describing those stages in the life cycle of the malarial parasite (*see* PLASMODIUM) that develop inside the red blood cells (*see* TROPHOZOITE). *Compare* EXOERYTHROCYTIC.

erythroderma (exfoliative dermatitis) *n.* abnormal reddening, flaking, and thickening of the skin affecting a wide area of the body. Commoner after the age of 50, erythroderma affects men three times as often as women; it may result from pre-existing skin disease, such as eczema or psoriasis, or be caused by drugs or lymphoma.

erythroedema *n.* *see* PINK DISEASE.

erythrogenesis *n.* *see* ERYTHROPOIESIS.

erythromelalgia *n.* painful paroxysmal dilation of the blood vessels of the skin, usually affecting the extremities; the skin feels hot. Some patients may respond to aspirin.

erythromycin *n.* an *antibiotic used to

treat infections caused by a wide range of bacteria and other microorganisms. It is administered by mouth or injection. Side-effects are rare and mild, though nausea, vomiting, and diarrhoea occur occasionally. Trade names: **Erymax**, **Erythrocin**.

erythron *n.* that part of the blood-forming system of the body that is directed towards the production of red blood cells. The erythron is not a single organ but is dispersed throughout the blood-forming tissue of the *bone marrow. *See also* ERYTHROPOIESIS.

erythropenia *n.* a reduction in the number of red blood cells (*erythrocytes) in the blood. This usually, but not invariably, occurs in *anaemia.

erythroplasia *n.* an abnormal red patch of skin that occurs in the mouth or on the genitalia and is precancerous.

erythropoiesis (erythrogenesis) *n.* the process of red blood cell (*erythrocyte) production, which normally occurs in the blood-forming tissue of the *bone marrow. The ultimate precursor of the red cell is the *haemopoietic stem cell, but the earliest precursor that can be identified microscopically is the *proerythroblast. This divides and passes through a series of stages of maturation termed respectively early, intermediate, and late *normoblasts, the latter finally losing its nucleus to become a mature red cell. *See also* HAEMOPOIESIS.

erythropoietin *n.* a hormone secreted by certain cells in the kidney in response to a reduction in the amount of oxygen reaching the tissues. Erythropoietin increases the rate of red cell production (*erythropoiesis) and is the mechanism by which the rate of erythropoiesis is controlled.

erythropsia *n.* red vision: a symptom sometimes experienced after removal of a cataract and also in snow blindness.

eschar *n.* a scab or slough, as produced by the action of heat or a corrosive substance on living tissue.

Escherichia *n.* a genus of Gram-negative, generally motile, rodlike bacteria that have the ability to ferment carbohydrates, usually with production of gas, and are found in the intestines of man and many animals. *E. coli* – a lactose-fermenting species – is usually not harmful but some strains cause gastrointestinal infections. Ingestion of the pathogenic serotype *E. coli 0157*, derived from infected meat, causes colitis with bloody diarrhoea, which may give rise to the complications of *haemolytic uraemic syndrome or thrombocytopenic *purpura (*see also* FOOD POISONING). *E. coli* is widely used in laboratory experiments for bacteriological and genetic studies.

eserine *n. see* PHYSOSTIGMINE.

esophoria *n.* a tendency to squint in which the eye, when covered, tends to turn inwards towards the nose. *See also* HETEROPHORIA.

esotropia *n.* convergent *strabismus: a type of squint.

espundia (mucocutaneous leishmaniasis) *n.* a disease of the skin and mucous membranes caused by the parasitic protozoan *Leishmania braziliensis* (*see* LEISHMANIASIS). Occurring in South and Central America, espundia takes the form of ulcerating lesions on the arms and legs; the infection may also spread to the mucous membranes of the nose and mouth, causing serious destruction of the tissues.

ESR (erythrocyte sedimentation rate) the rate at which red blood cells (erythrocytes) settle out of suspension in blood plasma, measured under standardized conditions. The ESR increases if the level of certain proteins in the plasma rises, as in rheumatic diseases, chronic infections, and malignant disease, and thus provides a simple but valuable screening test for these conditions.

essence *n.* a solution consisting of an essential oil dissolved in alcohol.

essential *adj.* describing a disorder that is not apparently attributable to an outside cause; for example, essential *hypertension.

essential amino acid an *amino acid that is essential for normal growth and development but cannot be synthesized by the body. Essential amino acids are normally obtained from protein-rich foods in the diet, such as liver, eggs, and dairy

products. There are nine essential amino acids: tryptophan, lysine, phenylalanine, histidine, threonine, valine, methionine, leucine, and isoleucine.

essential fatty acid one of a group of unsaturated fatty acids that are essential for growth but cannot be synthesized by the body. These essential fatty acids are **linoleic, linolenic,** and **arachidonic acids**; of these, only linoleic acid need be included in the diet as the other two can be synthesized from it in the body. Large amounts of linoleic acid occur in maize (corn) oil and soya bean oil; smaller amounts in pork fat.

essential oil a volatile oil derived from an aromatic plant. Essential oils are used in various pharmaceutical preparations.

esterase *n.* an enzyme that catalyses the hydrolysis of esters into their constituent acids and alcohols. For example, fatty-acid esters are broken down to form fatty acids plus alcohol.

ESWL extracorporeal shock-wave lithotripsy. *See* LITHOTRIPSY.

ethacrynic acid a *diuretic used to treat fluid retention (oedema), such as that associated with heart failure and kidney and liver disorders. It is administered by mouth or injection. Common side-effects are loss of appetite, difficulty in swallowing, nausea, vomiting, and diarrhoea. Trade name: **Edecrin**.

ethambutol *n.* a drug used in the treatment of tuberculosis, in conjunction with other drugs. It is administered by mouth and occasionally causes visual disturbances, which cease when the drug is withdrawn. Allergic rashes and digestive upsets may also occur. Trade name: **Myambutol**.

ethanol (ethyl alcohol) *n. see* ALCOHOL.

ether *n.* a volatile liquid formerly used as an anaesthetic administered by inhalation, though now largely replaced by safer and more efficient drugs. It also has laxative action when administered by mouth. Ether irritates the respiratory tract and affects the circulation.

ethical committee (in Britain) a group including lay people, medical practitioners, and other experts set up (especially in a hospital) to monitor investigations, concerned with teaching or research, that involve the use of human subjects. It is responsible for ensuring that patients are adequately informed of the procedures involved in a research project (including the use of dummy or placebo treatments as controls), that the tests and/or therapies are safe, and that no-one is pressurized into participating.

ethinyloestradiol *n.* a synthetic female sex hormone (*see* OESTROGEN) administered by mouth to treat symptoms of the menopause and menstrual disorders and to suppress lactation in mothers not breast-feeding. It is mainly used, however, in combination with a progestogen, in *oral contraceptives (e.g. **Conova 30**, **Femodene**).

ethionamide *n.* a drug used to treat tuberculosis, usually in conjunction with other drugs. It is administered by mouth or in suppositories. Loss of appetite, nausea, and vomiting are common side-effects. Trade name: **Trescatyl**.

ethisterone *n.* a synthetic female sex hormone (*see* PROGESTOGEN) used, often in combination with an *oestrogen, to treat menstrual disorders, particularly amenorrhoea. It was formerly used in hormone pregnancy tests. It is administered by mouth.

ethmoid bone a bone in the floor of the cranium that contributes to the nasal cavity and orbits. The part of the ethmoid forming the roof of the nasal cavity – the **cribriform plate** – is pierced with many small holes through which the olfactory nerves pass. *See also* NASAL CONCHA, SKULL.

ethnology *n.* the study of the different races of mankind and their variations: a branch of anthropology that deals mainly with cultural and social differences between groups and the problems, medical and otherwise, that arise from their particular ways of life. —**ethnic** *adj.*

ethosuximide *n.* an *anticonvulsant drug used to control epileptic seizures. It is administered by mouth; side-effects such as drowsiness, depression, and digestive disturbances may occur but are usually temporary. Trade names: **Emeside**, **Zarontin**.

ethylene *n.* an inflammable gas sometimes used as an anaesthetic administered by inhalation. There are usually no toxic effects, but nausea and vomiting commonly occur after its use.

ethyloestrenol *n.* a steroid drug with *anabolic properties, used to treat conditions involving wasting of protein and bone, such as osteoporosis. It is administered by mouth and sometimes causes nausea, water retention, and menstrual disturbances at high doses. Trade name: **Orabolin**.

ethynodiol *n.* a synthetic female sex hormone (*see* PROGESTOGEN) that is used to treat menstrual disorders and in *oral contraceptives. It is administered by mouth, usually in combination with an *oestrogen. Side-effects can include nausea, vomiting, headache, breast swelling, weight gain, fluid retention, and breakthrough bleeding. Trade name: **Femulen**.

etidronate *n.* a *biphosphonate drug that is administered orally or by intravenous infusion to treat various disorders of bone metabolism, including Paget's disease, hypercalcaemia caused by malignant tumours, and (in combination with calcium carbonate) osteoporosis of the vertebrae. Side-effects include diarrhoea and nausea. Trade names: **Didronel**, **Didronel IV**, **Didronel PMO**.

etiology *n. see* AETIOLOGY.

etoposide (VP16-213) *n.* a *cytotoxic drug derived from an extract of the mandrake plant. It is administered intravenously or by mouth, primarily in the treatment of bronchial carcinoma, lymphomas, and testicular tumours. Side-effects include alopecia, nausea, and marrow suppression. Trade name: **Vepesid**.

eu- *prefix denoting* **1.** good, well, or easy. **2.** normal.

eubacteria *pl. n.* a very large group of bacteria with rigid cell walls and – typically – flagella for movement. The group comprises the so-called 'true' bacteria, excluding those, such as spirochaetes and mycoplasmas, with flexible cell walls.

eucalyptol *n.* a volatile oil that has a mild irritant effect on the mucous membranes of the mouth and digestive system.

It is taken as pastilles or inhaled as vapour to relieve catarrh. Large doses may cause nausea, vomiting, and diarrhoea.

euchromatin *n.* chromosome material (*see* CHROMATIN) that stains most deeply during mitosis and represents the major genes. *Compare* HETEROCHROMATIN.

eugenics *n.* the science that is concerned with the improvement of the human race by means of the principles of genetics. It is mainly concerned with the detection and, where possible, the elimination of genetic disease in man.

eumenorrhoea *n.* regular menstruation. This does not necessarily indicate regular ovulation.

eupepsia *n.* the state of normal or good digestion: freedom from digestive symptoms.

euphoria *n.* a state of optimism, cheerfulness, and well-being. A morbid degree of euphoria is characteristic of *mania and *hypomania. *See also* ECSTASY, ELATION.

euplastic *adj.* describing a tissue that heals quickly after injury.

euploidy *n.* the condition of cells, tissues, or organisms in which there is one complete set of chromosomes or a whole multiple of this set in each cell. *Compare* ANEUPLOIDY. —**euploid** *adj., n.*

Eustachian tube the tube that connects the middle *ear to the pharynx. It allows the pressure on the inner side of the eardrum to remain equal to the external pressure. [B. Eustachio (1520–74), Italian anatomist]

euthanasia *n.* the act of taking life to relieve suffering. In **voluntary euthanasia** the sufferer asks for measures to be taken to end his life. This may be accomplished by active steps, usually the administration of a drug, or by **passive euthanasia** – the deliberate withholding of treatment. In **compulsory euthanasia** society or a person acting on authority gives instructions to terminate the life of a person, such as an infant, who cannot express his wishes. In no country is compulsory euthanasia legal, but many societies exist to promote the cause of voluntary euthanasia.

euthyroid *adj.* having a thyroid gland that functions normally. *Compare* HYPERTHYROIDISM, HYPOTHYROIDISM. —**euthyroidism** *n.*

evacuator *n.* a device for sucking fluid out of a cavity. In its simplest form it consists of a hollow rubber bulb that is attached, via a valve system, to a tube inserted into the cavity. Another valve leads to a discharge tube. Evacuators may be used to empty the bladder of unwanted material during such operations as the removal of a calculus or transurethral *prostatectomy.

evagination *n.* the protrusion of a part or organ from a sheathlike covering or by eversion of its inner surface.

eventration *n.* **1.** protrusion of the intestines through the abdominal wall. **2.** (of the diaphragm) abnormal elevation of part of the diaphragm due to a congenital weakness (but without true herniation), as observed by X-ray.

event sampling (in psychology) a way of recording behaviour in which the presence of a particular kind of behaviour is noted whenever it occurs. It is used for precise descriptions of behaviour and for following the course of *behaviour modification. *See also* TIME SAMPLING.

eversion *n.* a turning outward; in **eversion of the cervix** the edges of the cervix (neck) of the uterus turn outward after having been torn during childbirth.

evisceration *n.* **1.** (in surgery) **a.** the removal of part of the viscera. **b.** the protrusion of an organ through a surgical incision. **2.** (in ophthalmology) an operation in which the contents of the eyeball are removed, the empty outer envelope (sclera) being left behind. *Compare* ENUCLEATION.

Ewing's sarcoma a malignant tumour of bone occurring in children and young adults. Distinguished from *osteosarcoma by J. Ewing in 1921, it commonly arises in the femur but is liable to spread to other bones and to the lung. It usually presents with pain, often associated with fever and *leucocytosis. The tumour is sensitive to radiotherapy, and systemic therapy with *cytotoxic drugs has improved its prognosis. [J. Ewing (1866–1943), US pathologist]

ex- (exo-) *prefix denoting* outside or outer.

exaltation *n.* *see* ELATION.

exanthem *n.* a rash or eruption, such as that occurring in measles. **Exanthem subitum** is another name for *roseola (infantum). —**exanthematous** *adj.*

excavator *n.* **1.** a spoon-shaped surgical instrument that is used to scrape out diseased tissue, usually for laboratory examination. **2.** a type of hand instrument with spoon ends used for removing decayed dentine from teeth. It may also be used as a *curette.

exchange transfusion a technique for treating *haemolytic disease in newborn infants. Using a syringe with a three-way tap, blood is withdrawn from the baby (via the umbilical vein), ejected, and replaced by an equal amount of donor blood compatible with the mother's blood, without detaching the syringe. By many repetitions of this exchange, red blood cells liable to be destroyed and bilirubin released from those already destroyed are removed, while keeping the baby's blood volume and number of red cells constant. Exchange transfusion can also be used in *sickle-cell disease, as a temporary treatment during a crisis.

excimer laser a laser that can remove very thin sheets of tissue from the surface of the cornea of the eye. This can be done to alter the curvature of the corneal surface, for example to treat myopia (**photorefractive keratectomy**; *see* LASIK), or to remove diseased (e.g. calcified) tissue from the corneal surface (**photothera-peutic keratectomy**).

excipient *n.* a substance that is combined with a drug in order to render it suitable for administration; for example in the form of pills. Excipients should have no pharmacological action themselves.

excise *vb.* to cut out tissue, an organ, or a tumour from the body. —**excision** *n.*

excitation *n.* (in neurophysiology) the triggering of a conducted impulse in the membrane of a muscle cell or nerve fibre. During excitation a polarized membrane becomes momentarily depolarized and an *action potential is set up.

excoriation *n.* the destruction and removal of the surface of the skin or the covering of an organ by scraping, the application of a chemical, or other means.

excrescence *n.* an abnormal outgrowth on the surface of the body, such as a wart.

excreta *n.* any waste material discharged from the body, especially faeces.

excretion *n.* the removal of the waste products of metabolism from the body, mainly through the action of the *kidneys. Excretion also includes the loss of water, salts, and some urea through the sweat glands and carbon dioxide and water vapour from the lungs, and the term is also used to include the egestion of faeces.

exenteration *n.* (in ophthalmology) an operation in which all the contents of the eye socket (orbit) are removed, leaving only the bony walls intact. The bone is covered by a skin graft. This operation is sometimes necessary when there is a malignant tumour in the orbit.

exercise *n.* any activity resulting in physical exertion that is intended to maintain physical fitness, to condition the body, or to correct a physical deformity. Exercises may be done actively by the person or passively by a therapist. **Aerobic exercises** are intended to increase oxygen consumption (as in running) and to benefit the lungs and cardiovascular system, in contrast to *isometric exercises. In **isotonic exercises**, the muscles contract and there is movement, but the force remains the same; this improves joint mobility and muscle strength.

exflagellation *n.* the formation and release of mature flagellated male sex cells (*see* MICROGAMETE) by the *microgameto-cytes of the malarial parasite (*see* PLASMODIUM). The process, which is completed in 10–15 minutes, occurs after the microgametocytes have been transferred from man to the stomach of a mosquito.

exfoliation *n.* **1.** flaking off of the upper layers of the skin. **2.** separation of a surface epithelium from the underlying tissue. **3.** the natural shedding of primary teeth. —**exfoliative** *adj.*

exhalation (expiration) *n.* the act of

breathing air from the lungs out through the mouth and nose. *See* BREATHING.

exhibitionism *n.* exposure of the genitals to another person, as a sexually deviant act. The word is often broadened to mean public flaunting of any quality of the individual.

exo- *prefix.* *see* EX-.

exocoelom *n.* *see* EXTRAEMBRYONIC COELOM.

exocrine gland a gland that discharges its secretion by means of a duct, which opens onto an epithelial surface. An exocrine gland may be **simple**, with a single unbranched duct, or **compound**, with branched ducts and multiple secretory sacs. The illustration shows some different types of these glands. Examples of exocrine glands are the sebaceous and sweat glands. *See also* SECRETION.

simple tubular   simple alveolar

compound   compound   compound
tubular   alveolar   tubulo-alveolar

Types of exocrine glands

exoenzyme *n.* an *enzyme that acts outside the cell that produced it. Examples of exoenzymes are the digestive enzymes.

exoerythrocytic *adj.* describing those stages in the life cycle of the malarial parasite (*see* PLASMODIUM) that develop in the cells of the liver. Each parasite (*sporozoite) divides repeatedly to produce a schizont containing many merozoites.

exogenous *adj.* originating outside the body or part of the body: applied particularly to substances in the body that are derived from the diet rather than built up by the body's own processes of metabolism. *Compare* ENDOGENOUS.

exomphalos *n.* an umbilical *hernia.

exopeptidase *n.* an enzyme (e.g. *trypsin) that takes part in the digestion of proteins by splitting off the terminal amino acids of a polypeptide chain. *Compare* ENDOPEPTIDASE. *See also* PEPTIDASE.

exophoria *n.* a tendency to squint in which the eye, when covered, tends to turn outwards. *See also* HETEROPHORIA.

exophthalmic goitre (Graves's disease) *see* THYROTOXICOSIS.

exophthalmometer (proptometer) *n.* an instrument for measuring the degree of protrusion of the eyeball. The distance measured is that from the rim of bone at the outer edge of the eye, forwards to the surface of the front of the cornea.

exophthalmos *n.* protrusion of the eyeballs in their sockets. This can result from injury or disease of the eyeball or socket but is most commonly associated with overactivity of the thyroid gland (*see* THYROTOXICOSIS).

exosmosis *n.* outward osmotic flow. *See also* OSMOSIS.

exostosis *n.* a benign outgrowth of bone with a cap of cartilage, arising from the surface of a bone. *See* OSTEOMA.

exothermic *adj.* describing a chemical reaction in which energy is released in the form of heat. *Compare* ENDOTHERMIC.

exotic *adj.* describing a disease occurring in a region of the world far from where it might be expected. Thus malaria and leishmaniasis are regarded as exotic when they are diagnosed in patients in Britain.

exotoxin *n.* a highly potent poison, often harmful to only a limited range of tissues, that is produced by a bacterial cell and secreted into its surrounding medium. It is generally unstable, being rendered inactive by heat, light, and chemicals. Exotoxins are produced by such bacteria as those causing *botulism, *diphtheria, and *tetanus. *Compare* ENDO-TOXIN.

exotropia *n.* divergent *strabismus: a type of squint.

expectorant *n.* a drug that enhances the secretion of sputum by the air passages so that it is easier to cough up. Expectorants are used in cough mixtures; they act by increasing the bronchial secretion or make it less viscous (*see* MUCOLYTIC). Drugs such as *ipecacuanha are **stimulant expectorants** in small quantities: they irritate the lining of the stomach, which provides a stimulus for the reflex production of sputum by the glands in the bronchial mucous membrane. At higher doses they produce vomiting.

expectoration *n.* the act of spitting out material brought into the mouth by coughing.

expiration *n.* **1.** the act of breathing out air from the lungs: exhalation. **2.** dying.

explant 1. *n.* live tissue transferred from the body (or any organism) to a suitable artificial medium for culture. The tissue grows in the artificial medium and can be studied for diagnostic or experimental purposes. Tumour growths are sometimes examined in this way. **2.** *n.* silicone rubber material sutured to the outside of the eyeball over a retinal tear or hole (*see* PLOMBAGE). The resulting indent allows the retina to reattach. **3.** *vb.* to transfer live tissue for culture outside the body. —**explantation** *n.*

exploration *n.* (in surgery) an investigative operation on a wound, tissue, or cavity. It may be undertaken to determine the cause of symptoms. —**exploratory** *adj.*

exposure *n.* (in behaviour therapy) a method of treating fears and phobias that involves confronting the individual with the situation he has been avoiding, so allowing the fears to wane by *habituation. It can be achieved gradually by *desensitization or *graded self-exposure or suddenly by *flooding.

expressed emotion a measure of the degree of warmth or hostility in a relationship between two people, assessed when one person is talking about the other. High levels of criticism and hostility from family members can worsen the prognosis of mentally ill patients.

exsanguination *n.* **1.** depriving the body of blood; for example, as a result of an accident causing severe bleeding or – very rarely – through uncontrollable bleeding during a surgical operation. **2.** a technique for providing a bloodless field to facilitate delicate or haemorrhagic operative procedures. —**exsanguinate** *vb.*

exsiccation *n.* drying up, as may occur in tissues deprived of an adequate supply of water during dehydration or starvation.

exstrophy *n.* a severe congenital abnormality in which the bladder fails to close during development: the baby is born with an absent lower abdominal wall and the internal surface of the posterior bladder wall is exposed. It is associated with *epispadias, total urinary incontinence, and undescended testes.

exsufflation *n.* the forcible removal of secretions from the air passages by some form of suction apparatus.

extension *n.* **1.** the act of extending or stretching, especially the muscular movement by which a limb is straightened. **2.** the application of *traction to a fractured or dislocated limb in order to restore it to its normal position.

extensor *n.* any muscle that causes the straightening of a limb or other part.

exteriorization *n.* a surgical procedure in which an organ is brought from its normal site to the surface of the body. This may be done as a temporary or permanent measure; for example, the intestine may be brought to the surface of the abdomen (*see* COLOSTOMY). The process is also sometimes used in physiological experiments on animals.

external fixator an apparatus consisting of a rigid frame that connects pins passed through the skin into the bone above and below a fracture. This immobilizes the fracture, and is used particularly to treat some compound fractures. An external fixator is also used for *limb lengthening.

exteroceptor *n.* a sensory nerve, ending in the skin or a mucous membrane, that is responsive to stimuli from outside the body. *See also* CHEMORECEPTOR, RECEPTOR.

extinction *n.* (in psychology) the weakening of a conditioned reflex that takes place if it is not maintained by *reinforcement. This is used as a method of treatment when undesirable behaviour (e.g. destructiveness) is reduced simply by withdrawing whatever rewards it (e.g. the fuss made by other people).

extirpation *n.* the complete surgical removal of tissue, an organ, or a growth.

extra- *prefix denoting* outside or beyond.

extracellular *adj.* situated or occurring outside cells; for example, **extracellular fluid** is the fluid surrounding cells.

extracorporeal *adj.* situated or occurring outside the body. **Extracorporeal circulation** is the circulation of the blood outside the body, as through a *heart-lung machine or an artificial kidney (*see* HAEMODIALYSIS).

extracorporeal membrane oxygenation (ECMO) a new technique that is accepted as a rescue treatment for otherwise fatal respiratory failure in newborn babies or infants due to prematurity or overwhelming septicaemia (e.g. meningitis). It involves modified prolonged *cardiopulmonary bypass to support gas exchange, which allows the lungs to rest and recover. ECMO is only available in selected high-technology centres.

extract *n.* a preparation containing the pharmacologically active principles of a drug, made by evaporating a solution of the drug in water, alcohol, or ether.

extraction *n.* **1.** the surgical removal of a part of the body. Extraction of teeth is usually achieved by applying extraction *forceps to the crown or root of the tooth to dislocate it from its socket. When this is not possible, for example because the tooth or root is deeply buried within the bone, extraction is performed surgically by removing bone and, where necessary, dividing the tooth. **2.** the act of pulling

out a baby from the body of its mother during childbirth.

extractor *n.* an instrument used to pull out a natural part of the body, to remove a foreign object, or to assist delivery of a baby (*see* VACUUM EXTRACTOR).

extradural *adj.* *see* EPIDURAL.

extraembryonic coelom (exocoelom) the cavity, lined with mesoderm, that surrounds the embryo from the earliest stages of development. It communicates temporarily with the coelomic cavity within the embryo (peritoneal cavity). Late in pregnancy it becomes almost entirely obliterated by the growth of the *amnion, which fuses with the *chorion.

extraembryonic membranes the membranous structures that surround the embryo and contribute to the placenta and umbilical cord. They include the *amnion, *chorion, *allantois, and *yolk sac. In man the allantois is always very small and by the end of pregnancy the amnion and chorion have fused into a single membrane and the yolk sac has disappeared.

extrapleural *adj.* relating to the tissues of the chest wall outside the parietal *pleura.

extrapyramidal system the system of nerve tracts and pathways connecting the cerebral cortex, basal ganglia, thalamus, cerebellum, reticular formation, and spinal neurones in complex circuits not included in the *pyramidal system. The extrapyramidal system is mainly concerned with the regulation of stereotyped reflex muscular movements.

extrasensory perception (ESP) a supposed way of perceiving that involves none of the known senses. **Clairvoyance** is the extrasensory perception of current events; **precognition** is extrasensory perception of future events; **telepathy** is the extrasensory perception of the thoughts of others.

extrasystole *n.* *see* ECTOPIC BEAT.

extrauterine *adj.* outside the uterus.

extravasation *n.* the leakage and spread of blood or fluid from vessels into the surrounding tissues, which follows injury, burns, inflammation, and allergy.

conjunctiva — — sclera

eyelash — — choroid

iris —

lens — vitreous humour

aqueous humour —

cornea — — blind spot

— optic nerve

suspensory
ligament — — retina

ciliary body — — extrinsic muscle

The eye (sagittal section)

extraversion *n.* *see* EXTROVERSION.

extrinsic muscle a muscle, such as any of those controlling movements of the eyeball, that has its origin some distance from the part it acts on. *See also* EYE.

extroversion *n.* **1.** (or **extraversion**) an enduring personality trait characterized by interest in the outside world rather than the self. People high in extroversion (**extroverts**), as measured by questionnaires and tests, are gregarious and outgoing, prefer to change activities frequently, and are not susceptible to permanent *conditioning. Extroversion was first described by Carl Jung as a tendency to action rather than thought, to scientific rather than philosophical interests, and to emotional rather than intellectual reactions. *Compare* INTROVERSION. **2.** a turning inside out of a hollow organ, such as the uterus (which sometimes occurs after childbirth).

extrovert *n.* *see* EXTROVERSION.

extrusion *n.* (in dentistry) **1.** the forced eruption of a tooth by means of an orthodontic appliance; for example, to realign a tooth that has been accidentally forced into the jaw. **2.** the partial lifting of a tooth from its socket as a result of traumatic injury.

exudation *n.* the slow escape of liquid (called the **exudate**) containing proteins and white cells through the walls of intact blood vessels, usually as a result of inflammation. Exudation is a normal part of the body's defence mechanisms.

eye *n.* the organ of sight: a three-layered roughly spherical structure specialized for receiving and responding to light. The outer fibrous coat consists of the sclera and the transparent cornea; the middle vascular layer comprises the choroid, ciliary body, and iris; and the inner sensory layer is the retina (see illustration).

Light enters the eye through the cornea, which refracts the light through the aqueous humour onto the lens. By adjustment of the shape of the lens (*see* ACCOMMODATION) light is focused through the vitreous humour onto the retina. In the retina light-sensitive cells (*see* CONE, ROD) send nerve impulses to the brain via the optic nerve. The arrangement of the two eyes at the front of the head provides *binocular vision. Each eye is contained in an *orbit, and movement of the eye within the orbit is controlled by extrinsic eye muscles (see illustration).

eyeball *n.* the body of the *eye, which is roughly spherical, is bounded by the *sclera, and lies in the *orbit. It is closely associated with accessory structures – the eyelids, conjunctiva, and lacrimal (tear-producing) apparatus – and its movements are controlled by three pairs of extrinsic eye muscles (see illustration).

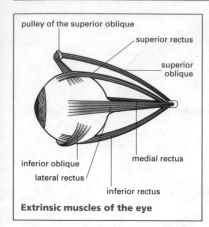

pulley of the superior oblique

superior rectus

superior oblique

medial rectus

inferior oblique

lateral rectus

inferior rectus

Extrinsic muscles of the eye

eyebrow *n.* the small fringe of hair on the bony ridge just above the eye. It helps to prevent moisture from running into the eye. Anatomical name: **supercilium**.

eyeground *n.* the inside of the eye as seen through an ophthalmoscope; the ocular fundus.

eyelash *n.* one of the long stiff hairs that form a row projecting outwards from the front edge of the upper and lower eyelids. The eyelashes help keep dust away from the eye. Anatomical name: **cilium**.

eyelid *n.* the protective covering of the eye. Each eye has two eyelids consisting of skin, muscle, connective tissue (**tarsus**), and sebaceous glands (**meibomian** or **tarsal glands**). Each eyelid is lined with membrane (*conjunctiva) and fringed with eyelashes. Stimulation of the pain receptors in the cornea causes the eyelids to close in a reflex action. Inflammation of a meibomian gland can result in a *chalazion. Anatomical names: **blepharon**, **palpebra**.

eyepiece *n.* the lens or system of lenses of an optical instrument, such as a microscope, that is nearest to the eye of the examiner. It usually produces a magnified image of the previous image formed by the instrument. *Compare* OBJECTIVE.

eyespot *n.* a small light-sensitive area of pigment found in some protozoans and other lower organisms.

eyestrain *n.* a sense of fatigue brought on by use of the eyes for prolonged close work or in persons who have an uncorrected error of *refraction or an imbalance of the muscles that move the eyes. Symptoms are usually aching or burning of the eyes, accompanied by headache and even general fatigue if the eyes are not rested. Medical name: **asthenopia**.

Fabry's disease *see* ANGIOKERATOMA. [J. Fabry (1860–1930), German dermatologist]

face-bow *n.* (in dentistry) an instrument for transferring the jaw relationship of a patient to an *articulator to allow reproduction of the lateral and protrusive movements of the lower jaw.

face-lift *n.* plastic surgery designed to correct sagging facial tissues. Eyelid drooping can be corrected at the same procedure.

facet *n.* a small flat surface on a bone or tooth, especially a surface of articulation.

facial nerve the seventh *cranial nerve (VII): a mixed sensory and motor nerve that supplies the muscles of facial expression, the taste buds of the front part of the tongue, the sublingual salivary glands, and the lacrimal glands. A small branch to the middle ear regulates the tension on the ear ossicles.

facial paralysis paralysis of the facial nerve, causing weakness and loss of function of the muscles it serves. It occurs in *Bell's palsy.

-facient *suffix denoting* causing or making. Example: **abortifacient** (causing abortion).

facies *n.* **1.** facial expression, often a guide to a patient's state of health as well as his emotions. The typical facies seen in adenoids is the vacant look, with the mouth drooping open. A **Hippocratic facies** is the sallow face, sagging and with listless staring eyes, that some read as the expression of approaching death. **2.** (in anatomy) a specified surface of a bone or other body part.

facilitation *n.* (in neurology) the phenomenon that occurs when a neurone receives, through a number of different synapses, impulses that are not powerful enough individually to start an *action potential but whose combined activity brings about some *depolarization of the membrane. In this facilitated state any small additional depolarization will suffice to trigger off an impulse in the cell.

facio- *prefix denoting* the face. Examples: **faciobrachial** (relating to the face and arm); **faciolingual** (relating to the face and tongue); **facioplegia** (paralysis of).

factitious *adj.* produced artificially, either deliberately or by accident, and therefore not to be taken into account when the results of an experiment are considered or a diagnosis is being made.

factor *n.* (in biochemistry) a substance that is essential to a physiological process, often a substance the nature of which is unknown. *See also* COAGULATION FACTORS, GROWTH FACTOR.

Factor VIII (antihaemophilic factor) a *coagulation factor normally present in blood. Deficiency of the factor, which is inherited by males from their mothers, results in classic *haemophilia. *See also* VON WILLEBRAND'S DISEASE.

Factor IX (Christmas factor) a *coagulation factor normally present in blood. Deficiency of the factor results in *haemophilia.

Factor XI a *coagulation factor normally present in blood. Deficiency of the factor is inherited, but rarely causes spontaneous bleeding. However, bleeding does occur after surgery or trauma to the blood vessels.

Factory Inspectorate the largest and oldest of the statutory bodies responsible for monitoring the health and safety of factory workers. It is administered by the Department of Employment through the Health and Safety Executive under the terms of the Health and Safety at Work Act. Requirements include a routine examination of young persons and those exposed to toxic hazards (e.g. lead) and the adequate guarding of machinery. Ensuring that the atmosphere inside the factory is free from poisonous fumes and chemicals may cause some conflict with local authorities, whose *Environmental Health

Officers have responsibility to prevent atmospheric pollution.

facultative *adj.* describing an organism that is not restricted to one way of life. A **facultative parasite** can live either as a parasite or, in different conditions, as a nonparasite able to survive without a host. *Compare* OBLIGATE.

FAD (flavin adenine dinucleotide) a *coenzyme, derived from riboflavin, that takes part in many important oxidation-reduction reactions. It consists of two phosphate groups, adenine, and ribose.

fading *n.* (in behaviour modification) *see* PROMPTING.

faecal impaction *see* CONSTIPATION, IMPACTED.

faecalith *n.* a small hard mass of faeces, found particularly in the vermiform appendix: a cause of inflammation.

faeces *n.* the waste material that is eliminated through the anus. It is formed in the *colon and consists of a solid or semisolid mass of undigested food remains (chiefly cellulose) mixed with *bile pigments (which are responsible for the colour), bacteria, various secretions (e.g. mucus), and some water. —**faecal** *adj.*

Fahrenheit temperature temperature expressed on a scale in which the melting point of ice is assigned a temperature of 32° and the boiling point of water a temperature of 212°. For most medical purposes the Celsius (centigrade) scale has replaced the Fahrenheit scale. The formula for converting from Fahrenheit (F) to Celsius (C) is: $C = 5/9(F - 32)$. *See also* CELSIUS TEMPERATURE. [G. D. Fahrenheit (1686–1736), German physicist]

failure to thrive (FTT) failure of an infant to grow satisfactorily compared with the average for that community. It is detected by regular measurements and plotting on *centile charts. It can be the first indication of a serious underlying condition, such as kidney or heart disease or malabsorption, or it may result from problems at home, particularly *nonaccidental injury.

fainting *n.* *see* SYNCOPE.

falciform ligament a fold of peritoneum separating the right and left lobes of the liver and attaching it to the diaphragm and the anterior abdominal wall as far as the umbilicus.

Fallopian tube (oviduct, uterine tube) either of a pair of tubes that conduct ova (egg cells) from the ovary to the uterus (*see* REPRODUCTIVE SYSTEM). The ovarian end opens into the abdominal cavity via a funnel-shaped structure with fingerlike projections (**fimbriae**) surrounding the opening. Movements of the fimbriae at ovulation assist in directing the ovum to the Fallopian tube. The ovum is fertilized near the ovarian end of the tube. [G. Fallopius (1523–63), Italian anatomist]

falloposcope *n.* a narrow flexible fibreoptic *endoscope used to view the inner lining of the Fallopian tubes (*see* FALLOPOSCOPY).

falloposcopy *n.* observation of the interior of a Fallopian tube using a *falloposcope introduced via a *hysteroscope.

Fallot's tetralogy *see* TETRALOGY OF FALLOT.

false pregnancy *see* PSEUDOCYESIS.

false rib *see* RIB.

falx (falx cerebri) *n.* (*pl.* **falces**) a sickle-shaped fold of the *dura mater that dips inwards from the skull in the midline, between the cerebral hemispheres.

familial *adj.* describing a condition or character that is found in some families but not in others. It is often inherited.

familial adenomatous polyposis (FAP) *see* POLYPOSIS.

family doctor *see* GENERAL PRACTITIONER.

Family Health Services Authority (FHSA) (in Britain) a former authority responsible for running general medical services (general practitioners and also dentists, pharmacists, and opticians working outside hospitals) for a given population. In 1996 FHSAs merged with District Health Authorities to form new Health Authorities. *See* NATIONAL HEALTH SERVICE.

family planning 1. the use of *contraception to limit or space out the numbers of children born to a couple. 2. provision of contraceptive methods within a com-

munity or nation. *See also* GENETIC COUN-
SELLING.

family practitioner *see* GENERAL PRACTI-
TIONER.

family therapy a form of *psychotherapy based on the belief that psychological problems are the products of
abnormalities in communication between
family members. All family members are
therefore seen together, when possible, in
order to clarify and modify the ways they
relate together (*see* GENOGRAM, PARADOX,
SCULPTING).

famotidine *n.* a drug used for the treatment of duodenal ulcers and conditions of
excessive gastric acid secretion, such as
the Zollinger-Ellison syndrome. It is administered by mouth and intravenously;
side-effects are headache, diarrhoea, and
dizziness. Trade name: **Pepcid**.

Fanconi syndrome a disorder of the
proximal kidney tubules, which may be
inherited or acquired and is most common
in children. It is characterized by the urinary excretion of large amounts of amino
acids, glucose, and phosphates (though
blood levels of these substances are normal). Symptoms may include osteomalacia,
rickets, muscle weakness, and *cystinosis.
Treatment is directed to the cause. [G.
Fanconi (1892–1979), Swiss paediatrician]

fantasy *n.* a complex sequence of imagination in which several imaginary elements are woven together into a story.
An excessive preoccupation with one's
own imaginings may be symptomatic
of a difficulty in coping with reality. In
psychoanalytic psychology, **unconscious
fantasies** are supposed to control behaviour, so that psychological symptoms can
be symbols of or defences against such
fantasies (*see* SYMBOLISM).

farad *n.* the *SI unit of capacitance,
equal to the capacitance of a capacitor between the plates of which a potential difference of 1 volt appears when it is
charged with 1 coulomb of electricity.
Symbol: F.

faradism *n.* the use of induced rapidly
alternating electric currents to stimulate
nerve and muscle activity. *See also* ELEC-
TROTHERAPY.

farcy *n.* *see* GLANDERS.

farmer's lung an occupational lung disease caused by allergy to fungal spores
that grow in inadequately dried stored
hay, straw, or grain, which then becomes
mouldy. It is an allergic *alveolitis, such as
also results from sensitivity to many
other allergens. An acute reversible form
can develop a few hours after exposure; a
chronic form, with the gradual development of irreversible breathlessness, occurs
with or without preceding acute attacks.
Avoidance of the allergen is the main
principle of treatment, but most farmers
are able to continue to farm by taking appropriate precautions.

fascia *n.* (*pl.* **fasciae**) connective tissue
forming membranous layers of variable
thickness in all regions of the body. Fascia
surrounds the softer or more delicate organs and is divided into **superficial fascia**
(found immediately beneath the skin) and
deep fascia (which forms sheaths for
muscles).

fasciculation *n.* brief spontaneous contraction of a few muscle fibres, which is
seen as a flicker of movement under the
skin. It is most often associated with disease of the lower motor neurones (e.g.
*motor neurone disease). Fasciculation
may be seen in the calf muscles of normal
individuals.

fasciculus (fascicle) *n.* a bundle, e.g. of
nerve or muscle fibres.

fasciitis *n.* inflammation of *fascia. It
may result from bacterial infection or
from a rheumatic disease, such as
*Reiter's syndrome or ankylosing
spondylitis. *See also* NECROTIZING FASCIITIS,
PLANTAR FASCIITIS.

Fasciola *n.* a genus of *flukes. *F. hepatica*,
the liver fluke, normally lives as a parasite
of sheep and other herbivorous animals
but sometimes infects man (*see* FASCIOLIA-
SIS).

fascioliasis *n.* an infestation of the bile
ducts and liver with the liver fluke,
Fasciola hepatica. Man acquires the infection through eating wild watercress on
which the larval stages of the parasite are
present. The symptoms include fever, dyspepsia, vomiting, loss of appetite, abdominal pain, and coughing; the liver may also

be extensively damaged (causing **liver rot**). Anthelmintics are used in the treatment of fascioliasis.

fasciolopsiasis *n.* a disease, common in the Far East, caused by the fluke *Fasciolopsis buski* in the small intestine. At the site of attachment of the adult flukes in the intestine there may be inflammation with some ulceration and bleeding. Symptoms include diarrhoea, and in heavy infections the patient may experience loss of appetite, vomiting, and (later) swelling of the face, abdomen, and legs. Death may follow in cases of severe ill health and malnutrition. The flukes can be removed with an anthelmintic (such as praziquantel).

Fasciolopsis *n.* a genus of large parasitic flukes widely distributed throughout eastern Asia and especially common in China. The adults of *F. buski*, the giant intestinal fluke, live in the human small intestine. Man becomes infected with the fluke on eating uncooked water chestnuts contaminated with fluke larvae and the resulting symptoms can be serious (*see* FASCIOLOPSIASIS).

fastigium *n.* the highest point of a fever.

fat *n.* a substance that contains one or more fatty acids (in the form of *triglycerides) and is the principal form in which energy is stored by the body (in *adipose tissue). It also serves as an insulating material beneath the skin (in the subcutaneous tissue) and around certain organs (including the kidneys). Fat is one of the three main constituents of food (*see also* CARBOHYDRATE, PROTEIN); it is necessary in the diet to provide an adequate supply of *essential fatty acids and for the efficient absorption of fat-soluble vitamins from the intestine. Excessive deposition of fat in the body leads to *obesity. *See also* BROWN FAT, LIPID.

fatigue *n.* **1.** mental or physical tiredness, following prolonged or intense activity. Muscle fatigue may be due to the waste products of metabolism accumulating in the muscles faster than they can be removed by the venous blood. Incorrect or inadequate food intake or disease may predispose a person to fatigue. **2.** the inability of an organism, an organ, or a tissue to give a normal response to a stimulus until a certain recovery period has elapsed.

fatty acid an organic acid with a long straight hydrocarbon chain and an even number of carbon atoms. Fatty acids are the fundamental constituents of many important lipids, including *triglycerides. Some fatty acids can be synthesized by the body; others, the *essential fatty acids, must be obtained from the diet. Examples of fatty acids are **palmitic acid**, **oleic acid**, and **stearic acid**. *See also* FAT.

fatty degeneration deterioration in the health of a tissue due to the deposition of abnormally large amounts of fat in its cells. The accumulation of fat in the liver and heart may seriously impair their functioning. The deposition of fat may be linked with incorrect diet, excessive alcohol consumption, or a shortage of oxygen in the tissues caused by poor circulation or a deficiency of haemoglobin.

fauces *n.* the opening leading from the mouth into the pharynx. It is surrounded by the **glossopalatine arch** (which forms the anterior pillars of the fauces) and the **pharyngopalatine arch** (the posterior pillars).

favism *n.* an inherited defect in the enzyme glucose-6-phosphate dehydrogenase causing the red blood cells to become sensitive to a chemical in broad beans. It results in destruction of red blood cells (haemolysis), which may lead to severe anaemia, requiring blood transfusion. Favism occurs in parts of the Mediterranean and Iran. *See also* GLUCOSE-6-PHOSPHATE DEHYDROGENASE DEFICIENCY.

favus *n.* a type of *ringworm of the scalp that is caused by the fungus *Trichophyton schoenleinii*. Favus, which is rare in Europe, is typified by yellow crusts made up of the threads of fungus and skin debris, which form honeycomb-like masses.

fear *n.* an emotional state evoked by the threat of danger and usually characterized by unpleasant subjective experiences as well as physiological and behavioural changes. Fear is often distinguished from *anxiety in having a specific object. Associated physiological changes can include increases in heart rate, blood pressure, sweating, etc. Behavioural changes can include an avoidance of fear-producing objects or situations and may be extremely disabling; for example, fear of open spaces. These specific disabling fears are known as *phobias. *Beta blockers relieve the physiological manifestations of fear and are useful in the treatment of short-term fears, such as the fear of hearing the results of an examination. Tranquillizers, such as diazepam, carry a risk of developing dependence, and *behaviour therapy or *cognitive therapy are preferred for disabling and persistent fears.

febricula *n.* a fever of low intensity or short duration.

febrifuge *n.* a treatment or drug that reduces or prevents fever. *See* ANTIPYRETIC.

febrile *adj.* relating to or affected with fever.

febrile convulsion (febrile seizure) an epileptic-type seizure associated with a fever. Such seizures affect up to 4% of children, usually aged between six months and six years, and generally last less than 10 minutes. Seizures do not lead to mental retardation or cerebral palsy, although the risk of developing *epilepsy is around 2%, especially when other risk factors, such as family history, are present. Seizures may be recurrent, but the risk of this can be minimized by attempts to reduce the fever. The underlying infection is usually viral, but more serious conditions, such as meningitis, should be excluded.

feedback *n.* the coupling of the output of a process to the input. Feedback mechanisms are important in regulating many physiological processes; for example, hormone output and enzyme-mediated reactions. In **negative feedback**, a rise in the output of a substance (e.g. a hormone) will inhibit a further increase in its production, either directly or indirectly. In **positive feedback**, a rise in the output of a substance is associated with an increase in the output of another substance, either directly or indirectly.

Fehling's test a test for detecting the presence of sugar in urine; it has now been replaced by better and easier methods. It uses **Fehling's solution**, of which

there are two components: Fehling's I (a copper sulphate solution) and Fehling's II (a solution of potassium sodium tartrate and sodium hydroxide). Boiling Fehling's solution is added to an equal volume of boiling urine; a yellowish or brownish coloration indicates the presence of sugar. [H. von Fehling (1812–85), German chemist]

Feingold diet a diet that purports to treat many illnesses by the elimination of artificial food colourings, preservatives, and salicylates from the diet. It has been recommended for the treatment of *attention deficit disorder, but is of unproved value.

feminization *n.* the development of female secondary sexual characteristics (enlargement of the breasts, loss of facial hair, and fat beneath the skin) in the male, either as a result of an endocrine disorder or of hormone therapy.

femoral *adj.* of or relating to the thigh or to the femur.

femoral artery an artery arising from the external iliac artery at the inguinal ligament. It is situated superficially, running down the front medial aspect of the thigh. Two-thirds of the way down it passes into the back of the thigh, continuing downward behind the knee as the **popliteal artery**.

femoral epiphysis *see* FEMUR.

femoral nerve the nerve that supplies the quadriceps muscle at the front of the thigh and receives sensation from the front and inner sides of the thigh. It arises from the second, third, and fourth lumbar nerves.

femoral triangle (Scarpa's triangle) a triangular depression on the inner side of the thigh bounded by the sartorius and adductor longus muscles and the inguinal ligament. The pulse can be felt here as the femoral artery lies over the depression.

femur (thigh bone) *n.* a long bone between the hip and the knee (see illustration). The head of the femur articulates with the acetabulum of the *hip bone. The **greater** and **lesser trochanters** are protuberances on which the gluteus and psoas major muscles, respectively, are inserted. The **lateral** and **medial condyles**

articulate with the *tibia and the concave grooved **patellar surface** accommodates the kneecap (patella).

The narrowed end of the femur (**femoral neck**), which carries the head, is the commonest site of fracture of the leg in elderly women. Partial dislocation of the **femoral epiphysis**, the growth area of the upper end of the bone, leads to deformity of the head of the femur and premature degeneration of the hip joint.

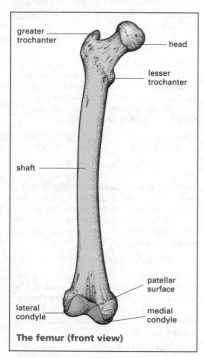

greater trochanter
head
lesser trochanter
shaft
patellar surface
lateral condyle
medial condyle

The femur (front view)

fenbufen *n.* an anti-inflammatory drug (*see* NSAID) used to relieve inflammation and the resulting pain and stiffness. It is administered by mouth. Possible side-effects include nausea, vomiting, and skin rashes. Trade name: **Lederfen**.

fenestra *n.* (in anatomy) an opening resembling a window. The **fenestra ovalis** (**fenestra vestibuli**) – the oval window – is the opening between the middle *ear and the vestibule of the inner ear. It is

closed by a membrane to which the stapes is attached. The **fenestra rotunda** (**fenestra cochleae**) – the round window – is the opening between the scala tympani of the cochlea and the middle ear. Sound vibrations leave the cochlea through the fenestra rotunda which, like the fenestra ovalis, is closed by a membrane.

fenestration *n.* a surgical operation in which a new opening is formed in the bony *labyrinth of the inner ear as part of the treatment of deafness due to *otosclerosis. It is rarely performed today, having been superseded by *stapedectomy.

fenoprofen *n.* an *analgesic drug that also reduces inflammation (*see* NSAID) and is used to treat arthritic conditions. It is administered by mouth and may cause digestive upsets, drowsiness, dizziness, sweating, and headache. Trade names: **Fenopron, Progesic**.

fermentation *n.* the biochemical process by which organic substances, particularly carbohydrate compounds, are decomposed by the action of enzymes to provide chemical energy. An example is **alcoholic fermentation**, in which enzymes in yeast decompose sugar to form ethyl alcohol and carbon dioxide.

ferning *n.* a test to determine if the amniotic membrane surrounding the fetus has ruptured in late pregnancy. A typical pattern of amniotic fluid crystallization occurs when the amniotic fluid dries.

ferri- (ferro-) *prefix denoting* iron.

ferritin *n.* an iron-protein complex that is one of the forms in which iron is stored in the tissues.

ferrous sulphate an *iron salt administered by mouth to treat or prevent iron-deficiency anaemia. There are few serious side-effects; stomach upsets and diarrhoea may be prevented by taking the drug with meals. Similar preparations used to treat anaemia include ferrous fumarate and ferrous succinate.

fertility rate the number of live births occurring in a year per 1000 women of child-bearing age (usually 15 to 44 years). A less reliable measure of fertility can be obtained from the **live birth rate** (the number of live births per 1000 of the population) or the **natural increase** (the excess of live births over deaths). More rarely quoted are the **gross reproduction rate** (the rate at which the child-bearing female population is reproducing itself) and the **net reproduction rate**, which takes into account female mortality before the age of reproduction.

fertilization n. the fusion of a spermatozoon and an ovum. Rapid changes in the membrane of the ovum prevent other spermatozoa from penetrating. Penetration stimulates the completion of meiosis and the formation of the second polar body. Once the male and female pronuclei have fused the zygote starts to divide by cleavage.

FESS see FUNCTIONAL ENDOSCOPIC SINUS SURGERY.

festination n. the short tottering steps that characterize the gait of a patient with *parkinsonism.

fetal alcohol syndrome a condition of newborn babies that results from the toxic effects on the fetus of maternal alcohol abuse. Babies have a low birth weight and growth is retarded; there may be head and facial abnormalities and possibly mental retardation. The greater the alcohol abuse, the more severe the fetal manifestations.

fetal blood sampling a technique, usually carried out during labour, in which a sample of blood is withdrawn from a vein in the scalp of the fetus. From this is determined the degree of fetal *acidosis. The normal pH of fetal blood is 7.35 (range 7.45–7.25). The lower the level, the more likely is the fetus to be suffering from *hypoxia, indicating an urgent need to terminate the labour; if the pH is allowed to fall below a level of 7.10, the life of the fetus is endangered.

fetal implant (fetal graft) the introduction of an ovum, fertilized in vitro and developed to the *blastocyst stage, into the uterus of a postmenopausal woman in order that she may become pregnant. Before this procedure, the woman's uterus must be prepared, by hormone therapy, to receive and nurture the blastocyst. Hormone treatment is continued throughout the pregnancy.

fetal transplant specific cells taken from a healthy newly aborted fetus and transplanted into a person suffering from a specific disease. These fetal cells take over the function of the specific diseased or damaged cells of the host. Examples are fetal brain cells transplanted into the affected part of the brain in a patient suffering from Parkinson's disease, and fetal pancreatic cells transplanted into the pancreas of a juvenile diabetic. Other diseases are being investigated experimentally with a view to using fetal transplants. Potentially, such procedures involve ethical considerations.

feticide n. the destruction of a fetus in the uterus; for example by injection of a lethal substance into the fetal heart to achieve a late-stage termination of pregnancy.

fetishism n. sexual attraction to an inappropriate object (known as a **fetish**). This may be a part of the body (e.g. the foot or the hair), clothing (e.g. underwear or shoes), or other objects (e.g. leather handbags or rubber sheets). In all these cases the fetish has replaced the normal object of sexual love, in some cases to the point at which sexual relationships with another person are impossible or are possible only if the fetish is either present or fantasized. Treatment can involve *psychotherapy or behaviour therapy using *aversion therapy and masturbatory conditioning of desirable sexual behaviour. See also SEXUAL DEVIATION.

feto- prefix denoting a fetus.

fetor (foetor) n. an unpleasant smell. **Fetor oris** is bad breath (*halitosis).

fetoscopy n. the inspection of a fetus before birth by passing a special fibreoptic instrument known as a **fetoscope** through the abdomen of a pregnant woman into her uterus. Fetoscopy, usually performed in the 18th–20th week of gestation, allows the inspection of the fetus for visible abnormalities and blood sampling by inserting a hollow needle under direct vision into a placental blood vessel. The blood can then be examined for abnormalities and hence the *prenatal diagnosis of blood disorders (such as thalassaemia, haemophilia, and sickle-cell disease) and Duchenne muscular dystrophy.

fetus (foetus) *n.* a mammalian *embryo during the later stages of development within the uterus. In human reproduction it refers to an unborn child from its eighth week of development. —**fetal** *adj.*

fetus papyraceous a twin fetus that has died in the uterus and become flattened and mummified.

Feulgen reaction a method of demonstrating the presence of DNA in cell nuclei. The tissue section under investigation is first hydrolysed with dilute hydrochloric acid and then treated with *Schiff's reagent. A purple coloration develops in the presence of DNA. [R. Feulgen (1884–1955), German chemist]

FEV *see* FORCED EXPIRATORY VOLUME.

fever (pyrexia) *n.* a rise in body temperature above the normal, i.e. above an oral temperature of 98.6°F (37°C) or a rectal temperature of 99°F (37.2°C). Fever is generally accompanied by shivering, headache, nausea, constipation, or diarrhoea. A rise in temperature above 105°F (40.5°C) may cause delirium and, in young children, *convulsions too. Fevers are usually caused by bacterial or viral infections and can accompany any infectious illness, from the common cold to *malaria. An **intermittent fever** is a periodic rise and fall in body temperature, often returning to normal during the day and reaching its peak at night, as in malaria. A **remittent fever** is one in which body temperature fluctuates but does not return to normal. *See also* RELAPSING FEVER.

FHSA *see* FAMILY HEALTH SERVICES AUTHORITY.

fibr- (fibro-) *prefix denoting* fibres or fibrous tissue.

fibre *n.* **1.** (in anatomy) a threadlike structure, such as a muscle cell, a nerve fibre, or a collagen fibre. **2.** (in dietetics) *see* DIETARY FIBRE. —**fibrous** *adj.*

fibre optics the use of fibres for the transmission of light images. Synthetic fibres with special optical properties can be used in instruments to relay pictures of the inside of the body for direct observation or photography. *See* FIBRESCOPE. —**fibreoptic** *adj.*

fibrescope *n.* an *endoscope that uses *fibre optics for the transmission of images from the interior of the body. Fibrescopes have a great advantage over the older endoscopes as they are flexible and can be introduced into relatively inaccessible cavities of the body.

fibril *n.* a very small fibre or a constituent thread of a fibre (for example, a *myofibril of a muscle fibre). —**fibrillar**, **fibrillary** *adj.*

fibrillation *n.* a rapid and chaotic beating of the many individual muscle fibres of the heart, which is consequently unable to maintain effective synchronous contraction. The affected part of the heart then ceases to pump blood.

Fibrillation may affect the atria or ventricles independently. **Atrial fibrillation**, a common type of *arrhythmia, results in rapid and irregular heart and pulse rates. The main causes are atherosclerosis, chronic rheumatic heart disease, and hypertensive heart disease. It may also complicate various other conditions, including chest infections and thyroid overactivity. The heart rate is controlled by the administration of *digoxin; in some cases the heart rhythm can be restored to normal by *cardioversion. Anticoagulant therapy with *warfarin reduces the risk of blood-clot formation, which could cause a stroke.

When **ventricular fibrillation** occurs the heart stops beating (*see* CARDIAC ARREST). It is most commonly the result of *myocardial infarction.

fibrin *n.* the final product of the process of *blood coagulation, produced by the action of the enzyme thrombin on a soluble precursor fibrinogen. The product thus formed (**fibrin monomer**) links up (polymerizes) with similar molecules to give a fibrous meshwork that forms the basis of a blood clot, which seals off the damaged blood vessel.

fibrinogen *n.* a substance (*coagulation factor), present in blood plasma, that is acted upon by the enzyme thrombin to produce the insoluble protein fibrin in the final stage of *blood coagulation. The normal level of fibrinogen in plasma is 2–4 g/1 (4–6 g/l during pregnancy).

fibrinogenopenia *n. see* HYPOFIBRINO-GENAEMIA.

fibrinoid *adj.* resembling the protein fibrin.

fibrinokinase *n.* one of a group of substances (activators) that convert the inactive substance plasminogen to the active enzyme *plasmin, which digests blood clots (*see* FIBRINOLYSIS). Fibrinokinase is insoluble in water and can be extracted from animal tissue.

fibrinolysin *n. see* PLASMIN.

fibrinolysis *n.* the process by which blood clots are removed from the circulation, involving digestion of the insoluble protein *fibrin by the enzyme *plasmin. The latter exists in the plasma as an inactive precursor (plasminogen), which is activated in parallel with the *blood coagulation process. Normally a balance is maintained between the processes of coagulation and fibrinolysis in the body; an abnormal increase in fibrinolysis leads to excessive bleeding.

fibrinolytic *adj.* describing a group of drugs that are capable of breaking down the protein fibrin, which is the main constituent of blood clots, and are therefore used to disperse blood clots (thrombi) that have formed within the circulation. They include *streptokinase, *alteplase, *anistreplase, and *urokinase. Possible side-effects include bleeding at needle puncture sites, headache, backache, blood spots in the skin, and allergic reactions.

fibroadenoma *n. see* ADENOMA.

fibroblast *n.* a widely distributed cell in *connective tissue that is responsible for the production of both the ground substance and of the precursors of collagen, elastic fibres, and reticular fibres.

fibrocartilage *n.* a tough kind of *cartilage in which there are dense bundles of fibres in the matrix. It is found in the intervertebral discs and pubic symphysis.

fibrocyst *n.* a benign tumour of fibrous connective tissue containing cystic spaces. **—fibrocystic** *adj.*

fibrocystic disease of the pancreas *see* CYSTIC FIBROSIS.

fibrocyte *n.* an inactive cell present in fully differentiated *connective tissue. It is derived from a *fibroblast.

fibrodysplasia *n.* abnormal development affecting connective tissue.

fibroelastosis *n.* overgrowth or disturbed growth of the yellow (elastic) fibres in *connective tissue, especially **endocardial fibroelastosis**, overgrowth and thickening of the wall of the heart's left ventricle.

fibroepithelial polyp a fibrous overgrowth covered by epithelium, often occurring inside the mouth in response to chronic irritation. It is sometimes called an *epulis.

fibroid 1. *n.* (**fibromyoma, uterine fibroid**) a benign tumour of fibrous and muscular tissue, one or more of which may develop in the muscular wall of the uterus. Fibroids often cause pain and excessive menstrual bleeding and they may become extremely large. They do not threaten life, but render pregnancy unlikely. It is usually women over 30 years of age who are affected. Some fibroids can be removed surgically; in other cases removal of the uterus (hysterectomy) may be necessary. If, as frequently happens, discomfort and other symptoms are absent, surgery is not required. **2.** *adj.* resembling or containing fibres.

fibroma *n.* (*pl* **fibromas** or **fibromata**) a nonmalignant tumour of connective tissue.

fibromyoma *n.* a tumour of muscular and fibrous material, usually occurring in the uterus (*see* FIBROID).

fibronectin *n.* a large glycoprotein that acts as a host defence mechanism. In the plasma it induces phagocytosis and on the cell surface it induces protein linkage which is important in the formation of new epithelium in wound healing. It is also involved in platelet aggregation. It is concentrated in connective tissue and the endothelium of the capillaries.

fibroplasia *n.* the production of fibrous tissue, occurring normally during the healing of wounds. **Retrolental fibropla-**

sia is the abnormal proliferation of fibrous tissue immediately behind the lens of the eye, leading to blindness. It is most commonly seen in newborn preterm infants, in whom it is associated with high concentrations of inhaled oxygen.

fibrosarcoma n. a malignant tumour of connective tissue, derived from *fibroblasts. Fibrosarcomas may arise in soft tissue or bone; they can affect any organ but are most common in the limbs, particularly the leg. They occur in people of all ages and may be congenital. The cells of these tumours show varying degrees of differentiation; the less well differentiated tumours containing elements of histiocytes have been recently reclassified as **malignant fibrous histiocytomas**.

fibrosis n. thickening and scarring of connective tissue, most often a consequence of inflammation or injury. **Pulmonary interstitial fibrosis** is thickening and stiffening of the lining of the air sacs (alveoli) of the lungs, causing progressive breathlessness. See also CYSTIC FIBROSIS, RETROPERITONEAL FIBROSIS.

fibrositis n. inflammation of fibrous connective tissue, especially an acute inflammation of back muscles and their sheaths, causing pain and stiffness. See also MUSCULAR RHEUMATISM.

fibrous dysplasia a developmental abnormality in which changes occur in bony tissue. Trabecular bone is replaced by fibrous tissue, resulting in aching and a tendency to pathological fracture. In **monostotic fibrous dysplasia** one bone is affected; **polyostotic fibrous dysplasia** involves many bones.

fibula n. the long thin outer bone of the lower leg. The head of the fibula articulates with the *tibia just below the knee; the lower end projects laterally as the **lateral malleolus**, which articulates with one side of the *talus.

field n. (in radiotherapy) an area of the body selected for treatment with radiotherapy. For example, a **mantle field** comprises the neck, armpits, and central chest, for the radiotherapy of Hodgkin's disease. Radiation is administered to the defined area by focusing the beam of particles emitted by the radiotherapy machine and shielding the surrounding area of the body.

field of vision see VISUAL FIELD.

figlu test a test for folic acid or vitamin B_{12} deficiency. A dose of the amino acid histidine, which requires the presence of folic acid or vitamin B_{12} for its complete breakdown, is given by mouth. In the absence of these vitamins, *formiminoglutamic acid* (figlu) – an intermediate product in histidine metabolism – accumulates and can be detected in the urine.

FIGO staging a classification drawn up by the International Federation of Gynaecology and Obstetrics to define the extent of the spread of cancers of the ovary, uterus, and cervix.

filament n. a very fine threadlike structure, such as a chain of bacterial cells. —**filamentous** adj.

filaria n. (pl. **filariae**) any of the long threadlike nematode worms that, as adults, are parasites of the connective and lymphatic tissues of man capable of causing disease. They include the genera *Brugia, *Loa, *Onchocerca, and *Wuchereria. Filariae differ from the intestinal nematodes (see HOOKWORM) in that they undergo part of their development in the body of a bloodsucking insect, e.g. a mosquito, on which they subsequently depend for their transmission to another human host. See also MICROFILARIA. —**filarial** adj.

filariasis n. a disease, common in the tropics and subtropics, caused by the presence in the lymph vessels of the parasitic nematode worms *Wuchereria bancrofti* and *Brugia malayi* (see FILARIA). The worms, which are transmitted to man by various mosquitoes (including *Aëdes, Culex, Anopheles*, and *Mansonia*), bring about inflammation and eventual blocking of lymph vessels, which causes the surrounding tissues to swell (see ELEPHANTIASIS). The rupture of urinary lymphatics may lead to the presence of *chyle in the urine. Filariasis is treated with the drug *diethylcarbamazine.

filiform adj. shaped like a thread; for example, the threadlike **filiform papillae** of the *tongue.

filling *n.* (in dentistry) the operation of inserting a specially prepared substance into a cavity drilled in a tooth, often in the treatment of dental caries. The filling may be **temporary** or **permanent**, and various materials may be used (*see* AMALGAM, CEMENT, COMPOSITE RESIN, GOLD).

filum *n.* a threadlike structure. The **filum terminale** is the slender tapering terminal section of the spinal cord.

fimbria *n.* (*pl.* **fimbriae**) a fringe or fringelike process, such as any of the finger-like projections that surround the opening of the ovarian end of the *Fallopian tube. —**fimbrial** *adj.*

fimbrial cyst a simple cyst of the *fimbria of the Fallopian tube.

finasteride *n.* a drug that causes shrinkage of the prostate gland and is administered by mouth for relieving the symptoms caused by an enlarged gland obstructing the outflow of urine from the bladder. The drug acts by reducing androgenic stimulation of the prostate, inhibiting the enzyme responsible for converting testosterone to its more active metabolite, 5-dehydroxytestosterone (5-DHT), within the gland. Trade name: **Proscar.**

fine-needle aspiration cytology (FNAC) a technique that uses samples obtained by fine-needle aspiration to provide information on the cells of tumours or cysts. It is useful for excluding the presence of malignant cells in cysts of the breast and thyroid. *See also* ASPIRATION CYTOLOGY.

fingerprint *n.* the distinctive pattern of minute ridges in the outer horny layer of the skin. Every individual has a unique pattern of loops (70%), whorls (25%), or arches (5%) (see illustration). Fingerprint patterns can show the presence of inherited disorders. *See also* DERMATOGLYPHICS.

firedamp *n.* (in mining) an explosive mixture of gases, usually containing a high proportion of methane, occasionally encountered in pockets underground. It can be distinguished from *blackdamp (chokedamp), which does not ignite.

first aid procedures used in an emergency to help a wounded or ill patient before the arrival of a doctor or admission to hospital.

first intention *see* INTENTION.

fission *n.* a method of asexual reproduction in which the body of a protozoan or bacterium splits into two equal parts (**binary fission**), as in the *amoebae, or more than two equal parts (**multiple fission**), for example sporozoite formation in the malarial parasite (*see* PLASMODIUM). The resulting products of fission eventually grow into complete organisms.

double loop   tented loop   radial loop

arch   whorl   ulnar loop

Ridges on the hand, with details of the most common fingerprints

fissure *n.* **1.** (in anatomy) a groove or cleft; *e.g.* the **fissure of Sylvius** is the groove that separates the temporal lobe of the brain from the frontal and parietal lobes. **2.** (in pathology) a cleftlike defect in the skin or mucous membrane caused by some disease process. *See* ANAL FISSURE. **3.** (in dentistry) a naturally occurring groove in the enamel on the surface of a tooth, especially a molar. It is a common site of dental caries.

fissure sealant (in dentistry) a material that is bonded to the enamel surface of teeth to seal the fissures, in order to prevent dental caries. Composite resins, unfilled resins, and glass ionomer cements have been used as fissure sealants.

fistula *n.* (*pl.* **fistulae**) an abnormal communication between two hollow organs or between a hollow organ and the exterior. Many fistulae are caused by infection or injury. For example, an **anal fistula** may develop after an abscess in the rectum has burst (*see* ISCHIORECTAL ABSCESS), creating an opening between the anal canal and the surface of the skin. (*See also* VESICO-VAGINAL FISTULA.) *Crohn's disease has a particular tendency to cause fistulae to form between adjacent loops of bowel or from bowel to bladder, vagina, or skin. Some fistulae result from malignant growths or ulceration: a carcinoma of the colon may invade and ulcerate the adjacent wall of the stomach, causing a **gastrocolic fistula**. Other fistulae develop as complications of surgery: after gall-bladder surgery, for example, bile may continually escape to the surface through the wound producing a **biliary fistula**. Fistulae may also be a form of congenital abnormality; examples include a **tracheo-oesophageal fistula** (between the windpipe and gullet) and a **rectovaginal fistula** (between the rectum and vagina).

fit *n.* a sudden attack. The term is commonly used specifically for the seizures of *epilepsy but it is also used more generally, e.g. a fit of coughing.

fixation *n.* **1.** (in psychoanalysis) a failure of psychological development, in which traumatic events prevent a child from progressing to the next developmental stage. This is said to be a cause of mental illness and of personality disorder. *See also* PSYCHOSEXUAL DEVELOPMENT. **2.** a procedure for the hardening and preservation of tissues or microorganisms to be examined under a microscope. Fixation kills the tissues and ensures that their original shape

and structure are retained as closely as possible. It also prepares them for sectioning and staining. The specimens can be immersed in a chemical *fixative or subjected to *freeze-drying.

fixative (fixing agent) *n.* a chemical agent, e.g. alcohol or osmium tetroxide, used for the preservation and hardening of tissues for microscopical study. *See* FIXATION.

FK506 *see* TACROLIMUS.

flaccid *adj.* **1.** flabby and lacking in firmness. **2.** characterized by a decrease in muscle tone (e.g. flaccid *paralysis). —**flaccidity** *n.*

flagellate *n.* a type of *protozoan with one or more fine whiplike threads (*see* FLAGELLUM) projecting from its body surface, by means of which it is able to swim. Some flagellates are parasites of humans and are therefore of medical importance. *See* TRYPANOSOMA, LEISHMANIA, GIARDIA, TRICHOMONAS.

flagellation *n.* the act of whipping oneself or others as a means of obtaining sexual pleasure (*see* MASOCHISM, SADISM). A person displaying this sexual deviation is called a **flagellant** or **flagellomane**.

flagellum *n.* (*pl.* **flagella**) a fine long whiplike thread attached to certain types of cell (e.g. spermatozoa and some unicellular organisms). Flagella are responsible for the movement of the organisms to which they are attached.

flail chest a condition of the chest associated with an unstable ribcage following multiple fractures of the ribs and sternum. It leads to asphyxia unless corrected promptly.

flap *n.* **1.** (in surgery) a strip of tissue dissected away from the underlying structures but left attached at one end so that it retains its blood and nerve supply in a *pedicle. The flap is then used to repair a defect in another part of the body. The free end of the flap is sewn into the area to be repaired and after about three weeks, when the flap has 'healed into' its new site, the other end is detached and the remainder of the flap is sewn in. Flaps are commonly used by plastic surgeons in treating patients who have suffered severe skin and tissue loss after mutilating operations (e.g. *mastectomy) or after burns or injuries not amenable to repair by split skin grafting (*see* SKIN GRAFT). Skin flaps may also be used to cover the end of a bone in an amputated limb. In neurosurgery combined skin and bone (**osteoplastic**) flaps are commonly raised to provide access to the cranium. **2.** (in dentistry) a piece of mucous membrane and periosteum attached by a broad base. It is lifted back to expose the underlying bone and enable a procedure such as surgical *extraction to be performed. It is subsequently replaced.

flare *n.* **1.** reddening of the skin that spreads outwards from a focus of infection or irritation in the skin. **2.** the red area surrounding an urticarial weal. **3.** (**aqueous flare**) the visible passage of a beam of light through the aqueous humour, which is a sign of inflammation of the anterior segment of the eye. The light is scattered by proteins in the aqueous humour that have exuded from blood vessels (*see* EXUDATION).

flashback *n.* vivid involuntary reliving of the perceptual abnormalities experienced during a previous episode of drug intoxication, including *hallucinations and *derealization.

flat-foot *n.* absence of the arching of the foot, so that the sole lies flat upon the ground. It may be present in infancy or be acquired in adult life, usually either from prolonged standing or from excessive weight. Flat feet need treatment (exercises) only if they cause pain. Medical name: **pes planus**.

flatulence *n.* **1.** the expulsion of gas or air from the stomach through the mouth; belching. **2.** a sensation of abdominal distension. —**flatulent** *adj.*

flatus *n.* intestinal gas, composed partly of swallowed air and partly of gas produced by bacterial fermentation of intestinal contents. It consists mainly of hydrogen, carbon dioxide, and methane in varying proportions. Indigestible nonabsorbable carbohydrates in some foods (e.g. beans) cause increased volumes of flatus.

flatworm (platyhelminth) *n.* any of the flat-bodied worms, including the

*flukes and *tapeworms. Both these groups contain many parasites of medical importance.

flav- (flavo-) *prefix denoting* yellow.

flavin adenine dinucleotide *see* FAD.

flavin mononucleotide *see* FMN.

flavoprotein *n.* a compound consisting of a protein bound to either *FAD or *FMN (called **flavins**). Flavoproteins are constituents of several enzyme systems involved in intermediary metabolism.

flea *n.* a small wingless bloodsucking insect with a laterally compressed body and long legs adapted for jumping. Adult fleas are temporary parasites on birds and mammals and those species that attack man (*Pulex*, *Xenopsylla*, and *Nosopsyllus*) may be important in the transmission of various diseases. Their bites are not only a nuisance but may become a focus of infection. Appropriate insecticide powders are used to destroy fleas in the home.

flecainide *n.* a drug used to control irregular heart rhythms. It is administered by mouth. Possible side-effects include nausea, vomiting, dizziness, vertigo, jaundice, visual disturbances, and some nerve damage. Trade name: **Tambocor**.

Fleischer ring a deposit of iron in the form of a ring in the epithelium of the cornea, which is seen, for example, around the base of the 'cone' of the cornea in *keratoconus. It is best visualized using cobalt blue light. [B. Fleischer (1848–1904), German physician]

flexibilitas cerea *see* CATATONIA.

flexion *n.* the bending of a joint so that the bones forming it are brought towards each other. **Plantar flexion** is the bending of the toes (or fingers) downwards, towards the sole (or palm). *See also* DORSIFLEXION.

flexor *n.* any muscle that causes bending of a limb or other part.

flexure *n.* a bend in an organ or part, such as the **hepatic** and **splenic flexures** of the *colon.

floaters *pl. n.* opacities in the vitreous humour of the eye, which cast a shadow on the retina and are therefore seen as dark shapes against a bright background in good illumination. They are a form of *entopic phenomenon.

floccillation n. see CARPHOLOGY.

flocculation n. a reaction in which normally invisible material leaves solution to form a coarse suspension or precipitate as a result of a change in physical or chemical conditions. Flocculation tests using serum and special reagents are useful in diagnosing liver abnormalities. See also AGGLUTINATION.

flocculus n. a small ovoid lobe of the *cerebellum, overhung by the posterior lobe and connected centrally with the nodulus in the midline.

flooding n. **1.** excessive bleeding from the uterus, as in *menorrhagia or miscarriage. **2.** (in psychology) (also called **implosion**) a method of treating *phobias in which the patient is exposed intensively and at length to the feared object, either in reality or fantasy. Although it is distressing and needs good motivation if treatment is to be completed, it is an effective and rapid form of therapy.

floppy baby syndrome see AMYOTONIA CONGENITA.

flosequinan n. a drug that acts on the smooth muscle of arteries and veins to cause these to relax and widen. This greatly reduces the load on the heart in patients with heart failure without affecting the blood supply to the various parts of the body. The drug is still being evaluated; side-effects include headache, dizziness, and palpitations.

flow cytometry a technique in which cells are tagged with a fluorescent dye and then directed single file through a laser beam. The intensity of *fluorescence induced by the laser beam is proportional to the amount of DNA in the cells.

flowmeter n. an instrument for measuring the flow of a liquid or gas. Anaesthetic equipment has to be fitted with flowmeters so that the administration of anaesthetic gases in different proportions can be controlled. Flowmeters are widely used by asthma sufferers to measure their ability to expire air.

flucloxacillin n. a semisynthetic *peni-

cillin, readily absorbed when taken by mouth and effective against bacteria that produce *penicillinase. A possible side-effect is an allergic reaction to penicillin. Trade names: **Floxapen, Magnapen**.

fluconazole n. an antifungal drug used to treat candidosis in any part of the body, externally or internally. It is administered by mouth. Possible side-effects include nausea and vomiting. Trade name: **Diflucan**.

fluctuation n. the characteristic feeling of a wave motion produced in a fluid-filled part of the body by an examiner's fingers. If fluctuation is present when a swelling is examined, this is an indication that there is fluid within it and that the swelling is not due to a solid growth.

flucytosine n. an antifungal drug that is effective against systemic infections, including cryptococcosis and candidosis. It can be administered by mouth; side-effects may include nausea and vomiting, diarrhoea, rashes, and blood disorders.

fludrocortisone n. a synthetic *corticosteroid used to treat disorders of the adrenal glands. It is administered by mouth and side-effects include muscle weakness, bone disorders, digestive and skin disorders, and fluid retention. Trade name: **Florinef**.

fluke n. any of the parasitic flatworms belonging to the group Trematoda. Adult flukes, which have suckers for attachment to their host, are parasites of man, occurring in the liver (**liver flukes**; see FASCIOLA), lungs (see PARAGONIMUS), gut (see HETEROPHYES), and blood vessels (**blood flukes**; see SCHISTOSOMA) and often cause serious disease. Eggs, passed out with the stools, hatch into larvae called *miracidia, which penetrate an intermediate snail host. Miracidia give rise asexually to *redia larvae and finally *cercariae in the snail's tissues. The released cercariae may enter a second intermediate host (such as a fish or crustacean); form a cyst (*metacercaria) on vegetation; or directly penetrate the human skin.

flumazenil n. a *benzodiazepine antagonist drug, used in anaesthesia to reverse the effects of benzodiazepines on the nervous system. It is administered by injection. Trade name: **Anexate**.

flunisolide *n.* an anti-inflammatory corticosteroid drug used in the long-term treatment of bronchial asthma and rhinitis. It is administered as an inhalation or a spray; the most common side-effects are nausea and vomiting, headache, upper respiratory-tract infections, and local irritation. Trade name: **Syntaris**.

flunitrazepam *n.* a *benzodiazepine drug used for the short-term treatment of insomnia. It is administered by mouth. Trade name: **Rohypnol**.

fluocinonide *n.* a synthetic corticosteroid used topically to reduce inflammation. It is applied to the skin as a cream, gel, ointment, or solution. Side-effects include burning, itching, and local eruptions. Trade name: **Metosyn**.

fluorescein sodium a water-soluble orange dye that glows with a brilliant green colour when blue light is shone on it. A dilute solution is used to detect defects in the surface of the cornea, since it stains areas where the *epithelium is not intact. In retinal *angiography it is injected into a vein and its circulation through the blood vessels of the retina is viewed and photographed by a special camera.

fluorescence *n.* the emission of light by a material as it absorbs radiation from outside. The radiation absorbed may be visible or invisible (e.g. ultraviolet rays or X-rays). *See* FLUOROSCOPE. —**fluorescent** *adj.*

fluoridation *n.* the addition of *fluoride to drinking water in order to reduce *dental caries. Drinking water with a fluoride ion content of one part per million is effective in reducing caries throughout life when given during the years of tooth development. *See also* FLUOROSIS.

fluoride *n.* a compound of fluorine. The incorporation of fluoride ions in the enamel of teeth makes them more resistant to *dental caries. The ions enter enamel during its formation, and after tooth eruption by surface absorption. The addition of fluoride to public water supplies is called *fluoridation. Fluoride may also be applied topically in toothpaste or by a dentist. If the water supply contains

too little fluoride, fluoride salts may be given to children in the form of mouthwashes, drops, or tablets.

fluoroscope *n.* an instrument on which X-ray images may be viewed directly, without taking and developing X-ray photographs. For diagnostic purposes it has been replaced by *image intensifiers and TV monitors (*see* X-RAY SCREENING).

fluorosis *n.* the effects of high *fluoride intake. Dental fluorosis is characterized by mottled enamel, which is opaque and may be stained. Its incidence increases when the level of fluoride in the water supply is above 2 parts per million. The mottled enamel is resistant to dental caries. When the level is over 8 parts per million systemic fluorosis may occur, with calcification of ligaments.

fluorouracil *n.* a drug that prevents cell growth (*see* ANTIMETABOLITE) and is used in the treatment of cancers of the digestive system and breast. It can be administered by mouth or by injection. Side-effects, which may be severe, include digestive and skin disorders, mouth ulcers, hair loss, nail changes, and blood disorders. Fluorouracil is also applied as a cream to treat certain skin conditions, including skin cancer.

fluoxetine *n.* an *antidepressant drug that acts by prolonging the action of the neurotransmitter serotonin (5 hydroxytryptamine) in the brain (*see* SSRI). It is administered by mouth. Possible side-effects include nausea, vomiting, diarrhoea, insomnia, anxiety, fever, skin rash, and convulsions. Trade name: **Prozac**.

flupenthixol *n.* a thioxanthene *antipsychotic drug used to treat schizophrenia and other psychoses. It is administered by mouth and by injection. Possible side-effects include sedation and involuntary movements. Trade names: **Depixol**, **Fluanxol**.

fluphenazine *n.* a phenothiazine *antipsychotic drug used for the treatment of schizophrenia and other psychotic disorders. It is administered by mouth or injection. Side-effects include abnormal muscular movements. Trade names: **Modecate**, **Moditen**.

flurazepam *n.* a benzodiazepine drug

used to treat insomnia and sleep disturbances (see HYPNOTIC). It is administered by mouth and sometimes causes morning drowsiness, dizziness, and muscle incoordination. Trade name: **Dalmane**.

flurbiprofen n. an analgesic that relieves inflammation (see NSAID), used in the treatment of rheumatoid arthritis and osteoarthritis and to prevent contraction of the pupil during eye surgery. Side-effects may include gastrointestinal upset, diarrhoea, and nausea. Trade names: **Froben, Ocufen**.

flush n. reddening of the face and/or neck. **Hectic flush** occurs in such wasting diseases as pulmonary tuberculosis. A **hot flush**, accompanied by a feeling of heat, occurs in some emotional disorders and during the menopause (see VASOMOTOR SYMPTOMS).

fluspirilene n. an *antipsychotic drug used to treat schizophrenia. It is administered by injection; side-effects can include fatigue, digestive upsets, and drowsiness. Trade name: **Redeptin**.

flutter n. a disturbance of normal heart rhythm that – like *fibrillation – may affect the atria or ventricles. However, the arrhythmia is less rapid and less chaotic. The causes and treatment are similar to those of fibrillation. See also CARDIAC ARREST, DEFIBRILLATION.

fluvoxamine n. an *antidepressant drug that acts by prolonging the action of the neurotransmitter serotonin (5-hydroxytryptamine) in the brain (see SSRI). It is taken by mouth; side-effects may include sleepiness, agitation, tremor, vomiting, and diarrhoea. Trade name: **Faverin**.

flux n. an abnormally copious flow from an organ or cavity. **Alvine flux** is *diarrhoea.

fly n. a two-winged insect belonging to a large group called the Diptera. The mouthparts of flies are adapted for sucking and sometimes also for piercing and biting. Fly larvae (maggots) may infest human tissues and cause disease (see MYIASIS).

FMN (flavin mononucleotide) a derivative of riboflavin (vitamin B_2) that is the immediate precursor of *FAD and functions as a *coenzyme in various oxidation-reduction reactions.

FNAC see FINE-NEEDLE ASPIRATION CYTOLOGY.

focal distance (of the eye) the distance between the lens and the point behind the lens at which light from a distant object is focused. In a normally sighted person the point of focus is on the retina, but in *myopia (short-sightedness) the focus is in front of the retina and in *hypermetropia (long-sightedness) the point of focus is beyond the retina.

focus **1.** n. the point at which rays of light converge after passing through a lens. **2.** n. the principal site of an infection or other disease. **3.** vb. (in ophthalmology) to accommodate (see also ACCOMMODATION).

foetus n. see FETUS.

fold n. (in anatomy and embryology) the infolding of two surfaces or membranes.

folic acid (pteroylglutamic acid) a B vitamin that is important in the synthesis of nucleic acids. The metabolic role of folic acid is interdependent with that of *vitamin B_{12} (both are required by rapidly dividing cells) and a deficiency of one may lead to deficiency of the other. A deficiency of folic acid results in the condition of megaloblastic anaemia. Good sources of folic acid are liver, yeast extract, and green leafy vegetables. The actual daily requirement of folate is not known but the suggested daily intake is 200 µg/day for an adult, which should be doubled shortly before conception and during the first three months of pregnancy to prevent neural tube defects (e.g. spina bifida) and other congenital malformations (e.g. cleft lip and cleft palate) in the fetus.

folie à deux (communicated insanity) a condition in which two people who are closely involved with each other share a system of *delusions. Sometimes one member of the pair has developed a *psychosis and has imposed it on the other by a process of suggestion; sometimes both members are schizophrenic and elaborate their delusions or hallucinations together. More than two people may be involved (**folie à trois, folie à quatre**, etc.). Treatment usually involves separation of the affected people and management according to their individual requirements.

folinic acid a derivative of folic acid involved in purine synthesis. Administered by mouth or by injection, it is used to reverse the biological effects of methotrexate and other *dihydrofolate reductase inhibitors and so to prevent excessive toxicity. This action is termed **folinic acid rescue**. Trade name: **Leucovorin**.

folium n. (pl. **folia**) a thin leaflike structure, such as any of the folds on the surface of the cerebellum.

follicle n. **1.** (in anatomy) a small secretory cavity, sac, or gland, such as any of the cavities in the *ovary in which the ova are formed. See also GRAAFIAN FOLLICLE, HAIR FOLLICLE. **2.** (in ophthalmology) any of the smooth translucent elevations of the conjunctiva produced by an immune response. They are usually associated with viral inflammation. —**follicular** adj.

follicle-stimulating hormone (FSH) a hormone (see GONADOTROPHIN) synthesized and released by the anterior pituitary gland. FSH stimulates ripening of the follicles in the ovary and formation of sperm in the testes. It is administered by injection to treat sterility due to lack of ovulation, amenorrhoea, and decreased sperm production. Stimulation of ovulation by FSH may, in some cases, lead to multiple pregnancy.

folliculitis n. inflammation of hair follicles in the skin, commonly caused by infection. Folliculitis caused by *Pityrosporum* yeasts may be a marker for the diagnosis of AIDS.

fomentation n. see POULTICE.

fomes n. (pl. **fomites**) any object that is used or handled by a person with a *communicable disease and may therefore become contaminated with the infective organisms and transmit the disease to a subsequent user. Common fomites are towels, bed-clothes, cups, and money.

fontanelle n. an opening in the skull of a fetus or young infant due to incomplete *ossification of the cranial bones and the resulting incomplete closure of the *sutures. The **anterior fontanelle** occurs where the coronal, frontal, and sagittal sutures meet; the **posterior fontanelle** occurs where the sagittal and lambdoidal sutures meet (see illustration).

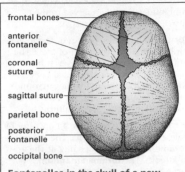

frontal bones
anterior fontanelle
coronal suture
sagittal suture
parietal bone
posterior fontanelle
occipital bone

Fontanelles in the skull of a newborn infant (from above)

food handler a person engaged in the preparation, storage, cooking, and serving of food. Such people should be free from infectious conditions, either in the form of overt disease or as carriers. They may be subject to inspection to prove freedom from infection, particularly those who handle food that is either to be eaten raw or has previously been subjected to cooking (e.g. meat pies, paté).

food poisoning an illness affecting the digestive system that results from eating food that is contaminated either by bacteria or bacterial toxins or, less commonly, by residues of insecticides (on fruit and vegetables) or poisonous chemicals such as lead or mercury. It can also be caused by eating poisonous fungi, berries, etc. Symptoms commence 1–24 hours after ingestion and include vomiting, diarrhoea, abdominal pain, and nausea. Food-borne infections are caused by bacteria of the genera *Salmonella, *Campylobacter, and *Listeria in foods of animal origin. The disease is transmitted by human carriers who handle the food, by shellfish growing in sewage-polluted waters, or by vegetables fertilized by manure. Toxin-producing bacteria causing food poisoning include those of the genus *Staphylococcus*, which rapidly multiply in warm foods; pathogenic *Escherichia coli*; and the species *Clostridium perfringens*, which multiplies in reheated cooked meals. A rare form of food poisoning – *botulism – is caused by toxins produced by the bacterium *Clostridium botulinum*, which may contaminate badly preserved canned foods. *See also* GASTROENTERITIS.

foot *n.* the terminal organ of the lower limb. From a surgical point of view, the human foot comprises the seven bones of the *tarsus, the five metatarsal bones, and the phalangeal bones plus the surrounding tissues; anatomically, the bones and tissues of the ankle are excluded.

foramen *n. (pl.* **foramina**) an opening or hole, particularly in a bone. The **apical foramen** is the small opening at the apex of a tooth. The **foramen magnum** is a large hole in the occipital bone through which the spinal cord passes. The **foramen ovale** is the opening between the two atria of the fetal heart, which allows blood to flow from the right to the left side of the heart by displacing a membranous valve.

forced expiratory volume (FEV) the volume of air exhaled in a given period (usually limited to 1 second in tests of vital capacity). FEV is reduced in patients with obstructive airways disease and diminished lung volume.

forced preferential looking test (FPL test) a test used to evaluate the *visual acuity of infants and young children by observing whether the child looks at a blank screen or one with stripes, the spatial frequency of which can be changed.

forceps *n.* a pincer-like instrument designed to grasp an object so that it can be held firm or pulled. Specially designed forceps – of which there are many varieties – are used by surgeons and dentists in operations (see illustration). The forceps used in childbirth are so designed as to fit firmly round the baby's head without damaging it. Dental **extraction forceps** are specially designed to fit the various shapes of teeth. By having long handles and short beaks they provide considerable leverage.

forebrain *n.* the furthest forward division of the *brain, consisting of the *dien-cephalon and the two cerebral hemispheres.

foregut *n.* the front part of the embryonic gut, which gives rise to the oesophagus (gullet), stomach, and part of the small intestine (from which the liver and pancreas develop).

bone-holding forceps

volsella

sinus forceps

dissecting forceps

dressing forceps

obstetrical forceps

dental extraction forceps

Types of forceps

forensic medicine the branch of medicine concerned with the scientific investigation of the causes of injury and death in unexplained circumstances, particularly when criminal activity is suspected. Such investigations are carried out chiefly by pathologists at the request of a *coroner, in conjunction with other experts and police investigators.

forequarter amputation an operation involving removal of an entire arm, including the scapula and clavicle. It is usually performed for soft tissue or bone sarcomas arising from the upper arm or shoulder. *Compare* HINDQUARTER AMPUTATION.

foreskin *n. see* PREPUCE.

forewaters *n.* the *amniotic fluid that escapes from the uterus through the vagina when that part of the amnion lying in front of the presenting part of the fetus ruptures, either spontaneously or by *amniotomy. Spontaneous rupture is usual in labour but rupture may occur before labour starts (premature rupture of membranes).

formaldehyde *n.* the aldehyde derivative of formic acid, formerly used as a vapour to sterilize and disinfect rooms and such items as mattresses and blankets. The toxic vapour is produced by boiling *formalin in an open container or using it in a sealed autoclave.

formalin *n.* a solution containing 40% formaldehyde in water, used as a sterilizing agent and, in pathology, as a fixative. It is lethal to bacteria, viruses, fungi, and spores and is used to treat wools and hides to kill anthrax spores. Heating the solution produces the irritating vapour of *formaldehyde, which is also used for disinfection.

forme fruste an atypical form of a disease in which the usual symptoms fail to appear and its progress is stopped at an earlier stage than would ordinarily be expected.

formication *n.* a prickling sensation said to resemble the feeling of ants crawling over the skin. It is sometimes a symptom of drug intoxication and has also been reported by patients with Parkinson's disease.

formulary *n.* a compendium of formulae used in the preparation of medicinal drugs.

fornix *n.* (*pl.* **fornices**) an arched or vault-like structure, especially the **fornix cerebri**, a triangular structure of white matter in the brain, situated between the hippocampus and hypothalamus. The **fornix of the vagina** is any of three vaulted spaces at the top of the vagina, around the cervix of the uterus.

Forrest screening a national breast screening programme, introduced in 1988, in which regular *mammography is available for all women between the ages of 50 and 64. It enables the early diagnosis of breast cancer in order to improve treatment and reduce mortality. [Sir P. Forrest (1923–), Scottish surgeon]

foscarnet *n.* an antiviral drug used in the treatment of infections caused by herpesviruses, including *cytomegaloviruses, that are resistant to *acyclovir, especially in patients with AIDS. It is administered by intravenous injection. Possible side-effects include thirst and increased urine output, nausea and vomiting, fatigue, headache, and kidney damage. Trade name: **Foscavir**.

fossa *n.* (*pl.* **fossae**) a depression or hollow. The **cubital fossa** is the triangular hollow at the front of the elbow joint; the **iliac fossa** is the depression in the inner surface of the ilium; the **pituitary fossa** is the hollow in the sphenoid bone in which the pituitary gland is situated; a **tooth fossa** is a pit in the enamel on the surface of a tooth.

fovea *n.* (in anatomy) a small depression, especially the shallow pit in the retina at the back of the eye. It contains a large number of *cones and is therefore the area of greatest acuity of vision: when the eye is directed at an object, the part of the image that is focused on the fovea is the part that is most accurately registered by the brain. *See also* MACULA (LUTEA).

foveola *n.* (in anatomy) a small depression.

FPL test *see* FORCED PREFERENTIAL LOOKING TEST.

fracture *n.* breakage of a bone, either complete or incomplete. A **simple fracture** involves a clean break with little damage to surrounding tissues and no break in the overlying skin. If a bone end pierces the overlying skin the fracture is **compound** or **open**, and there is a risk of infection (*see* OSTEOMYELITIS). Treatment of a simple fracture includes realignment of the bone ends where there is displacement, immobilization by external splints or internal fixation, followed by *rehabilitation. *See also* COLLES' FRACTURE, COMMINUTED FRACTURE, GREENSTICK FRACTURE, PATHOLOGICAL FRACTURE, SCAPHOID FRACTURE, SMITH'S FRACTURE.

fraenectomy *n.* an operation to remove the fraenum, including the underlying fibrous tissue.

fraenum (frenum, frenulum) *n.* **1.** any of the folds of mucous membrane under the tongue or between the gums and the upper or lower lips. **2.** any of several other structures of similar appearance.

fragile-X syndrome a major genetic disorder caused by a constriction near the end of the long arm of an *X chromosome. The fragile-X syndrome is second only to *Down's syndrome as a cause of mental retardation. Affected males have unusually high foreheads, unbalanced faces, large jaws, long protruding ears, and large testicles. They have an IQ below 50 and are prone to violent outbursts. Folic acid helps to control their behaviour. About one-third of the females with this mutation on one of their two X chromosomes are also mentally retarded. Screening for the characteristic chromosome can be done by *amniocentesis or *chorionic villus sampling.

fragilitas *n.* abnormal brittleness or fragility, for example of the hair (**fragilitas crinium**) or the bones (**fragilitas ossium**; *see* OSTEOGENESIS IMPERFECTA).

framboesia *n.* *see* YAWS.

framycetin *n.* an *antibiotic used mainly in the form of an ointment, cream, or eye or ear drops to treat skin, eye, and ear infections. Skin sensitivity sometimes occurs. Trade names: **Sofradex**, **Soframycin**.

fraternal twins *see* TWINS.

freckle *n.* a small brown spot on the skin commonly found on the arms and face of red-haired or blond people. Freckles,

which are harmless, appear where there is excessive production of the pigment melanin without any increase in numbers of melanocytes after exposure to sunlight. *Compare* LENTIGO.

free association (in *psychoanalysis) a technique in which the patient is encouraged to pursue a particular train of ideas as they enter consciousness. *See also* ASSOCIATION OF IDEAS.

free-floating anxiety an all-pervasive unfocused fear that is not produced by any appropriate cause or attached to any particular idea. Such anxiety is a feature of the *generalized anxiety disorder.

freeze drying a method for the *fixation of histological specimens, involving a minimum of chemical and physical change. Specimens are immersed in isopentane cooled to −190°C in liquid air. This fixes the tissue instantly, without the formation of large ice crystals (which would cause structural changes). The tissue is then dehydrated in a vacuum for about 72 hours at −32.5°C.

freeze etching a technique for preparing specimens for electron microscopy. The unfixed tissue is frozen and then split with a knife and a layer of ice is sublimed from the exposed surface. The resultant image is thus not distorted by chemical fixatives.

Frei test a rarely used diagnostic test for the sexually transmitted disease *lymphogranuloma venereum. A small quantity of the virus, inactivated by heat, is injected into the patient's skin. If the disease is present a small red swelling appears at the site of injection within 48 hours. [W. S. Frei (1885–1943), German dermatologist]

fremitus *n.* vibrations or tremors in a part of the body, detected by feeling with the fingers or hand (*palpation) or by listening (*auscultation). The term is most commonly applied to vibrations perceived through the chest when a patient breathes, speaks (**vocal fremitus**), or coughs. The nature of the fremitus gives an indication as to whether the chest is affected by disease. For example, loss of vocal fremitus suggests the presence of fluid in the pleural cavity; its increase suggests consolidation of the underlying lung.

frenulum *n. see* FRAENUM.

frenum *n. see* FRAENUM.

frequency *n.* (of urine) the frequent passage of urine, which usually indicates genitourinary disorders and diseases but also accompanies *polyuria.

frequency distribution (in statistics) presentation of the characteristics (*variables) of a series of individuals (e.g. their heights, weights, or blood pressures) in tabular form or as a histogram (bar chart) so as to indicate the proportion of the series that have different measurements. In a **normal** or **Gaussian distribution** the number of readings and their range on either side of the *mean value is symmetrical; in a **skewed distribution** (e.g. **Poisson**) the measurements are bunched on one side of the mean and spread out over a wider range on the other.

Fresnel prism a flexible plastic prism that can be stuck to spectacle lenses to provide a prism to correct double vision (*diplopia). [A. J. Fresnel (1788–1827), French physicist]

Freudian *adj.* relating to or describing the work and ideas of Sigmund Freud (1856–1939): applied particularly to the school of psychiatry based on his teachings (*see* PSYCHOANALYSIS).

friction murmur (friction rub) a scratching sound, heard over the heart with the aid of the stethoscope, in patients who have *pericarditis. It results from the two inflamed layers of the pericardium rubbing together during activity of the heart.

Friedman's test an obsolete pregnancy test based on the ability of urine of pregnant women (containing human chorionic gonadotrophin) to induce the development of corpora lutea in a female rabbit. [M. Friedman (1903–), US physiologist]

Friedreich's ataxia *see* ATAXIA. [N. Friedreich (1825–82), German neurologist]

frigidity *n.* lack of sexual desire or inability to achieve orgasm. The phenomenon may affect either sex, but the term is almost always applied to women only.

In some cases the woman feels revulsion towards sexual activity.

fringe medicine *see* ALTERNATIVE MEDICINE.

Fröhlich's syndrome a disorder of the *hypothalamus (part of the brain) affecting males: the boy is overweight with sexual development absent and disturbances of sleep and appetite. Medical name: **dystrophia adiposogenitalis**. [A. Fröhlich (1871–1953), Austrian neurologist]

Froin's syndrome a condition in which the cerebrospinal fluid (CSF) displays a combination of yellow colour and high protein content. It is characteristic of a block to the spinal circulation of CSF caused by a tumour. [G. Froin (1874–1932), French physician]

frontal *adj.* **1.** of or relating to the forehead (*see* FRONTAL BONE). **2.** denoting the *anterior part of a body or organ.

frontal bone the bone forming the forehead and the upper parts of the orbits; it contains several air spaces (**frontal sinuses**: *see* PARANASAL SINUSES). At birth it consists of right and left halves, joined by a suture that usually closes during infancy. *See* SKULL.

frontal lobe the anterior part of each cerebral hemisphere (*see* CEREBRUM), extending as far back as the deep central sulcus (cleft) of its upper and outer surface. Immediately anterior to the central sulcus lies the motor cortex, responsible for the control of voluntary movement; the area further forward – the *prefrontal lobe – is concerned with behaviour, learning, judgment, and personality.

frontal sinus *see* PARANASAL SINUSES.

frostbite *n.* damage to the tissues caused by freezing. The affected parts, usually the nose, fingers, or toes, become pale and numb. Ice forms in the tissues, which may thus be destroyed, and amputation may become necessary. Frostbitten parts should not be rubbed, since there is no blood circulation in the tissues, but they may be gently warmed in tepid water. Precautions must be taken against bacterial infection, to which frostbitten skin is highly susceptible.

frottage *n.* rubbing up against somebody (usually in a crowd) as a means of obtaining sexual pleasure. A person displaying this sexual deviation is called a **frotteur**; frotteurs are almost exclusively males.

frozen shoulder chronic painful stiffness of the shoulder joint. This may follow injury, a stroke, or *myocardial infarction or may gradually develop for no apparent reason. Treatment is by gentle stretching and exercises, sometimes combined with *corticosteroid injection into the joint. *See also* CAPSULITIS.

frozen watchfulness the state of a child who is unresponsive to its surroundings but is clearly aware of them. The child is usually expressionless and difficult to engage but of normal intelligence. Frozen watchfulness is usually a marker of *child abuse.

fructose *n.* a simple sugar found in honey and in such fruit as figs. Fructose is one of the two sugars in *sucrose. Fructose from the diet can be used to produce energy by the process known as *glycolysis, which takes place in the liver. Fructose is important in the diet of diabetics since, unlike glucose, fructose metabolism is not dependent on insulin.

fructosuria (levulosuria) *n.* the presence of fructose (levulose) in the urine.

frusemide *n.* a loop *diuretic used to treat fluid retention (oedema) associated with heart, liver, or kidney disease and also high blood pressure. It is administered by mouth or injection; common side-effects are nausea and vomiting. Trade name: **Lasix**.

FSH *see* FOLLICLE-STIMULATING HORMONE.

FTT *see* FAILURE TO THRIVE.

Fuchs' endothelial dystrophy a hereditary condition in which the endothelium of the cornea fails to function with age; small whitish deposits of hyalin are seen on the inner surface of the cornea (**cornea guttata**). It results in thickening and swelling of the cornea (*bullous keratopathy) and hence reduced vision. Treatment is corneal transplantation (*see* KERATOPLASTY), which both improves vision and reduces pain. [E. Fuchs (1851–1913), German ophthalmologist]

Fuchs' heterochromic cyclitis a condition characterized by chronic low-grade inflammation of the ciliary body and iris (anterior *uveitis) affecting one eye and depigmentation of the affected iris (*heterochromia). Glaucoma and cataract can develop in the affected eye.

fuchsin (magenta) *n.* any one of a group of reddish to purplish dyes used in staining bacteria for microscopic observation and capable of killing various disease-causing microorganisms. **Acid fuchsin (acid magenta)** is a mixture of sulphonated fuchsins; **basic fuchsin (basic magenta)** and **new (trimethyl) fuchsin** are basic histological dyes (basic fuchsin is also an antifungal agent).

Fuchs' spots pigmented lesions in the macular area of the retina that are seen in severely myopic (short-sighted) individuals. They are breaks in *Bruch's membrane allowing choroidal *neovascularization and can result in reduced vision. [E. Fuchs]

-fuge *suffix denoting* an agent that drives away, repels, or eliminates. Example: **febrifuge** (a drug that reduces fever).

fugue *n.* a period of memory loss during which the patient leaves his usual surroundings and wanders aimlessly or starts a new life elsewhere. It is often preceded by psychological conflict and depression (*see* DISSOCIATIVE DISORDER) or it may be associated with organic mental disease.

fulguration (electrodesiccation) *n.* the destruction with a *diathermy instrument of warts, growths, or unwanted areas of tissue, particularly inside the bladder. This latter operation is performed via the urethra and viewed through a cystoscope.

fulminating (fulminant, fulgurant) *adj.* describing a condition or symptom that is of very sudden onset, severe, and of short duration.

fumigation *n.* the use of gases or vapours to bring about *disinfestation of clothing, buildings, etc. Sulphur dioxide, formaldehyde, and chlorine are common fumigating agents.

functional disorder a condition in which a patient complains of symptoms for which no physical cause can be found.

Such a condition is frequently an indication of a psychiatric disorder. *Compare* ORGANIC DISORDER.

functional endoscopic sinus surgery (FESS) surgery of the *paranasal sinuses using *endoscopes. Routes of sinus drainage and aeration that are blocked by disease are cleared and enlarged, allowing the rest of the sinuses to return to normal.

functional independence measure a table recommended by the WHO for assessing the degree of whole-person disability, being particularly useful for judging the extent of recovery from serious injury. It has five grades, ranging from 0 (fully independent) to 4 (completely dependent).

Functional Recovery Index an international index, published by the World Health Organization, that grades the degree of recovery after serious injury.

fundholder *n.* (in the NHS) *see* GENERAL PRACTITIONER.

fundoplication *n.* a surgical operation for *gastro-oesophageal reflux disease in which the upper part of the stomach is wrapped around the lower oesophagus. The commonest technique is named after Rudolf Nissen, a Swiss surgeon.

fundoscopy (ophthalmoscopy) *n.* examination of the interior of the eye by means of an *ophthalmoscope.

fundus *n.* **1.** the base of a hollow organ: the part farthest from the opening; e.g. the fundus of the stomach, bladder, or uterus. **2.** the interior concavity forming the back of the eyeball, opposite the pupil. **Fundus flavimaculatus** is a hereditary disease of the retina in which white material is deposited in the fundus at the level of the retinal pigment epithelium (*see* RETINA). It usually causes loss of central vision, but good vision may persist into adulthood. **Fundus albipúnctatus** is a hereditary disease in which the fundus shows widespread distribution of uniform-sized white dots, resulting in poor *dark adaptation.

fungicide *n.* an agent that kills fungi. *See also* ANTIFUNGAL.

fungoid **1.** *adj.* resembling a fungus. **2.** *n.* a fungus-like growth.

fungus *n.* (*pl.* **fungi**) a simple organism (formerly regarded as a plant) that lacks the green pigment chlorophyll. Fungi include the *yeasts, rusts, moulds, and mushrooms. They live either as *saprophytes or as *parasites of plants and animals; some species infect and cause disease in man. Some yeasts are a good source of vitamin B and many antibiotics are obtained from the moulds (*see* PENICILLIN). —**fungal** *adj.*

funiculitis *n.* inflammation of the spermatic cord. This usually arises in association with *epididymitis and causes pain and swelling of the involved cord. Treatment is by administration of antibiotics and analgesics.

funiculus *n.* **1.** any of the three main columns of white matter found in each lateral half of the spinal cord. **2.** a bundle of nerve fibres enclosed in a sheath; a fasciculus. **3.** (formerly) the spermatic cord or umbilical cord.

funis *n.* (in anatomy) any cordlike structure, especially the umbilical cord.

funnel chest depression of the breastbone and inward curving of the costal cartilages articulating with it, resulting in deformity of the chest. It may displace the heart to the left and can cause slight breathlessness. Medical name. **pectus excavatum.**

furcation *n.* the place where the roots fork on a multirooted tooth.

furor *n.* indiscriminate violence and destructiveness, occurring especially during a period of mental confusion due to *epilepsy.

furuncle *n.* *see* BOIL.

furunculosis *n.* the occurrence of several *boils (furuncles) at the same time, usually caused by *Staphylococcus aureus* infection. Treatment includes thorough daily disinfection of the skin and incision (lancing), which may be more effective than antibiotic therapy.

fusidic acid a steroid antibiotic used in the form of its salt, sodium fusidate, against penicillin-resistant staphylococci.

It has no value against streptococci and is usually prescribed in conjunction with another antibiotic, such as *flucloxacillin. It is administered by mouth. Possible side-effects include nausea, vomiting, and skin rashes. Trade name: **Fucidin**.

fusiform *adj.* spindle-shaped; tapering at both ends.

fusion *n.* the joining together of two structures. For example, the surgical fusion of two or more vertebra is performed to stabilize an unstable spine. Fusion of the *epiphyses during growth is the cause of arrested growth of stature.

Fusobacterium *n.* a genus of Gram-negative rodlike bacteria with tapering ends. Most species are normal inhabitants of the mouth of animals and man and produce no harmful effects, but anaerobic *Fusobacterium* species are associated with *ulcerative gingivitis.

G

GABA *see* GAMMA-AMINOBUTYRIC ACID.

gabapentin *n. see* ANTICONVULSANT.

Gaffkya *n.* a genus of bacteria now classified as *Micrococcus*.

gag *n.* (in medicine) an instrument that is placed between a patient's teeth to keep his mouth open.

galact- (galacto-) *prefix denoting* **1.** milk. Example: **galactosis** (formation of). **2.** galactose.

galactagogue *n.* an agent that stimulates the secretion of milk or increases milk flow.

galactocele *n.* **1.** a breast cyst containing milk, caused by closure of a milk duct. **2.** an accumulation of milky liquid in the sac surrounding the testis (*see* HYDROCELE).

galactorrhoea *n.* **1.** abnormally copious milk secretion. **2.** secretion of milk after breast feeding has been stopped.

galactosaemia *n.* an inborn inability to utilize the sugar galactose, which in consequence accumulates in the blood. Untreated, affected infants fail to thrive and become mentally retarded, but if galactose is eliminated from the diet growth and development may be normal.

galactose *n.* a simple sugar and a constituent of the milk sugar *lactose. Galactose is converted to glucose in the liver. The enzyme necessary for this conversion is missing in infants with a rare inherited metabolic disease called *galactosaemia.

galea *n.* **1.** a helmet-shaped part, especially the **galea aponeurotica**, a flat sheet of fibrous tissue (*see* APONEUROSIS) that caps the skull and links the two parts of the *epicranius muscle. **2.** a type of head bandage.

galenical *n.* a pharmaceutical preparation of a drug of animal or plant origin.

gallamine *n.* a drug administered by injection to produce muscle relaxation during anaesthesia (*see* MUSCLE RELAXANT). It is also used in a diagnostic test for *myasthenia gravis. Trade name: **Flaxedil**.

gall bladder a pear-shaped sac (7–10 cm long), lying underneath the right lobe of the liver, in which *bile is stored (see illustration). Bile passes (via the hepatic duct) to the gall bladder from the liver, where it is formed, and is released into the duodenum (through the common bile duct) under the influence of the hormone *cholecystokinin, which is secreted when food is present in the duodenum. The gall bladder is a common site of stone formation (*see* GALLSTONE).

The gall bladder and pancreas and their associated ducts

gallium *n.* a silvery metallic element. A radioisotope of gallium is used for the detection of lymphomas and areas of infection (such as an abscess) following intravenous injection.

gallstone *n.* a hard mass composed of bile pigments, cholesterol, and calcium salts, in varying proportions, that can form in the gall bladder. The formation of gallstones (**cholelithiasis**) occurs when the physical characteristics of bile alter so that cholesterol is less soluble, though chronic inflammation of the gall bladder (see CHOLECYSTITIS) or diminished contractility may also be a contributory factor. Gallstones may exist for many years without causing symptoms. However, they may cause severe pain (see BILIARY COLIC) or they may pass into the common bile duct and cause obstructive *jaundice or *cholangitis. Gallstones are usually diagnosed by ultrasonography, but those containing calcium may be seen on a plain X-ray (opaque stones). Cholelithiasis is usually treated by surgical removal of the gall bladder (see CHOLECYSTECTOMY) or by removing the stones themselves, which can be either dissolved using bile salts given by mouth or shattered by ultrasound waves. There is no need for treatment if the stones are causing no symptoms.

galvanism n. (formerly) any form of medical treatment using electricity. **Interrupted galvanism** is a form of *electrotherapy in which direct current, in impulses lasting for 30 to 100 milliseconds, is used to stimulate the activity of nerves or the muscles they supply. See also FARADISM.

Gam-Anon n. see GAMBLERS ANONYMOUS.

Gamblers Anonymous (GA) an organization, founded in the United States in 1957 and established in the UK in 1964, that seeks to assist compulsive gamblers. The despair, humiliation, and loneliness of compulsive gamblers is neither widely known nor understood. Invariably their addiction leads to bankruptcy, loss of jobs, rejection by family and friends, and ultimately to criminal means of obtaining money with which to gamble. GA offers a form of group therapy similar to that provided by *Alcoholics Anonymous. Senior members help the new members to face their creditors and to work out repayment budgets that will eventually free them from their obligations. The sister organization, **Gam-Anon**, provides advice and encouragement for the families of compulsive gamblers.

gamete n. a mature sex cell: the *ovum of the female or the *spermatozoon of the male. Gametes are haploid, containing half the normal number of chromosomes.

gamete intrafallopian transfer

(GIFT) a procedure for assisting conception, suitable only for women with healthy Fallopian tubes. In over 50% of women in whom infertility is diagnosed, the tubes are normal but some other factor, such as endometriosis, prevents conception. Using needle *aspiration, under laparoscopic or ultrasonic guidance, ova are removed from the ovary. After being mixed with the partner's spermatozoa, they are introduced into a Fallopian tube, where fertilization takes place. The fertilized ovum can subsequently become implanted in the uterus.

gametocide n. a drug that kills *gametocytes. Drugs such as *primaquine destroy gametocytes of the malaria parasite (see PLASMODIUM), so interrupting the life cycle and preventing infection of the mosquito.

gametocyte n. any of the cells that are in the process of developing into gametes by undergoing *gametogenesis. See also OOCYTE, SPERMATOCYTE.

gametogenesis n. the process by which spermatozoa and ova are formed. In both sexes the precursor cells undergo *meiosis, which halves the number of chromosomes. However, the timing of events and the size and number of gametes produced are very different in the male and female. See OOGENESIS, SPERMATOGENESIS.

gamma aminobutyric acid (GABA) an amino acid found in the central nervous system, predominantly in the brain, where it acts as an inhibitory *neurotransmitter.

gamma benzene hexachloride an insecticide used in creams, lotions, solutions, or shampoos to treat infestations caused by scabies, mites, and lice (including head lice). Mild skin reactions occasionally occur.

gamma camera a piece of apparatus that detects radioactivity in the form of gamma rays emitted by radioactive isotopes that have been introduced into the body as *tracers. It contains an activated sodium iodide crystal (see SCINTILLATOR) and a large array of photomultiplier tubes. Using lead *collimators, the position of the source of the radioactivity can be plotted and displayed on a TV monitor or photographic film (*see* SCINTIGRAM).

gammaglobulin any of a class of proteins, present in the blood *plasma, identified by their characteristic rate of movement in an electric field (*see* ELECTROPHORESIS). Almost all gammaglobulins are *immunoglobulins. Injection of gammaglobulin provides temporary protection against *hepatitis A and has recently been shown to reduce the incidence of coronary artery involvement in *Kawasaki disease. *See also* GLOBULIN.

gamma rays electromagnetic radiation of wavelengths shorter than X-rays, given off by certain radioactive substances. Gamma rays have greater penetration than X-rays; they are harmful to living tissues and can be used to sterilize certain materials and to kill bacteria as a means of food preservation. Controlled doses are used in *radiotherapy.

gamo- *prefix denoting* marriage.

ganciclovir *n.* an antiviral drug used to treat severe *cytomegalovirus infections, mainly in patients with AIDS. It is administered by injection. Possible side-effects include nausea, vomiting, diarrhoea, infertility, confusion, seizures, and disturbance of bone marrow blood-cell production. Trade name: **Cymevene**.

gangli- (ganglio-) *prefix denoting* a ganglion.

ganglion *n.* (*pl.* **ganglia**) **1.** (in neurology) any structure containing a collection of nerve cell bodies and often also numbers of synapses. In the *sympathetic nervous system chains of ganglia are found on each side of the spinal cord, while in the *parasympathetic system ganglia are situated in or nearer to the organs innervated. Swellings in the posterior sensory *roots of the spinal nerves are termed ganglia; these contain cell bodies but no synapses. Within the central nervous system certain well-defined masses of nerve cells are called ganglia (or **nuclei**); for example, the *basal ganglia. **2.** an abnormal but harmless swelling (cyst) that sometimes forms in tendon sheaths, especially at the wrist.

ganglioside *n.* one of a group of *glycolipids found in the brain, liver, spleen, and red blood cells (they are particularly abundant in nerve cell membranes). Gangliosides are chemically similar to *cerebrosides but contain additional carbohydrate groups.

gangosa *n.* a lesion that occasionally appears in the final stage of *yaws, involving considerable destruction of the tissues of both the hard palate and the nose.

gangrene *n.* death and decay of part of the body due to deficiency or cessation of blood supply. The causes include disease, injury, or *atheroma in major blood vessels, frostbite or severe burns, and diseases such as *diabetes mellitus and *Raynaud's disease. **Dry gangrene** is death and withering of tissues caused simply by a cessation of local blood circulation. **Moist gangrene** is death and putrefactive decay of tissue caused by bacterial infection. *See also* GAS GANGRENE.

Ganser state (pseudodementia) a syndrome characterized by approximate answers, i.e. the patient gives grossly and absurdly false replies to questions, but the reply shows that the question has been understood. For example, the question "What colour is snow?" may elicit the reply "Green". This can be accompanied by odd behaviour or episodes of *stupor. The condition is due to *conversion disorder or to conscious malingering. [S. J. M. Ganser (1853–1931), German psychiatrist]

Gardnerella *n.* a genus of anaerobic bacteria. *G. vaginalis* is a cause of vaginitis and, in pregnant women, of late miscarriage.

Gardner's syndrome a variant form of familial adenomatous *polyposis in which polyps in the colon are associated with fibromas and *osteomas (benign tumours), especially of the skull and jaw, and multiple *sebaceous cysts. [E. J. Gardner (1909–), US physician]

gargoylism *n. see* HUNTER'S SYNDROME, HURLER'S SYNDROME.

gas gangrene death and decay of wound tissue infected by the soil bacterium *Clostridium perfringens*. Toxins produced by the bacterium cause putrefactive decay of connective tissue with the generation of gas. Treatment is usually by surgery.

Gasterophilus n. a genus of widely distributed non-bloodsucking beelike flies. The parasitic maggots normally live in the alimentary canal of horses but, rarely, can also infect man and cause an inflamed itching eruption of the skin (see CREEPING ERUPTION).

gastr- (gastro-) prefix denoting the stomach. Examples: **gastralgia** (pain in); **gastrocolic** (relating to the stomach and colon).

gastrectasia n. dilatation of the stomach. This may be caused by *pyloric stenosis or it may occur as a complication of some abdominal operations or trauma.

gastrectomy n. a surgical operation in which the whole or a part of the stomach is removed. **Total gastrectomy**, in which the oesophagus is joined to the duodenum, is usually performed for stomach cancer but occasionally for the *Zollinger-Ellison syndrome. In **partial** (or **subtotal**) **gastrectomy** the upper third or half of the stomach is joined to the duodenum or small intestine (**gastroenterostomy**); this operation was used in severe cases of *peptic ulcers before the advent of effective drug treatment. After gastrectomy capacity for food is reduced, sometimes leading to weight loss. Other complications of gastrectomy include *dumping syndrome, anaemia, and *malabsorption.

gastric adj. relating to or affecting the stomach.

gastric glands tubular glands that lie in the mucous membrane of the stomach wall. There are three varieties: the **cardiac**, **fundic** (**oxyntic**), and **pyloric glands**, and they secrete *gastric juice.

gastric juice the liquid secreted by the *gastric glands of the stomach. Its main digestive constituents are hydrochloric acid, mucin, *rennin, and pepsinogen. The acid acts on pepsinogen to produce *pepsin, which functions best in an acid medium. The acidity of the stomach contents also kills unwanted bacteria and other organisms that have been ingested with the food. Gastric juice also contains *intrinsic factor, which is necessary for the absorption of vitamin B_{12}.

gastric ulcer an ulcer in the stomach, caused by the action of acid, pepsin, and bile on the stomach lining (mucosa). The output of stomach acid is not usually increased. Taking *NSAIDs (nonsteroidal anti-inflammatory drugs) or *corticosteroids are predisposing factors. *Helicobacter pylori is often present. Symptoms include vomiting and pain in the upper abdomen soon after eating, and such complications as bleeding (see also HAEMATEMESIS), *perforation, and obstruction due to scarring may occur. Symptoms are relieved by antacid medicines, but most ulcers heal if treated by an *antisecretory drug. Surgery may be required if the ulcer fails to heal. Since stomach cancer may mimic a gastric ulcer, all gastric ulcers should be examined by a *gastroscope to aid in their differentiation.

gastrin n. a hormone produced in the mucous membrane of the pyloric region of the stomach (see G-CELL). Its secretion is stimulated by the presence of food. It is circulated in the blood to the rest of the stomach, where it stimulates the production of *gastric juice.

gastrinoma n. a rare tumour that secretes excess amounts of the hormone gastrin, causing the *Zollinger-Ellison syndrome. Such tumours most frequently occur in the pancreas; about half of them are malignant.

gastritis n. inflammation of the lining (mucosa) of the stomach. **Acute gastritis** is caused by ingesting excess alcohol or other irritating or corrosive substances, resulting in vomiting. **Chronic gastritis** is associated with smoking and chronic alcoholism and may be caused by bile entering the stomach from the duodenum, but most cases are caused by the bacterium *Helicobacter pylori. It has no definite symptoms, but the patient is liable to develop gastric ulcers or gastric cancer. **Atrophic gastritis**, in which the stomach lining is atrophied, may succeed chronic gastritis but may occur spontaneously as an *autoimmune disease.

gastrocele n. a *hernia of the stomach.

gastrocnemius n. a muscle that forms the greater part of the calf of the leg (see illustration). It flexes the knee and foot (so that the toes point downwards).

gastrocolic reflex a wave of peristalsis

produced in the colon by introducing food into a fasting stomach.

gastroduodenoscope *n. see* DUODENO-SCOPE, GASTROSCOPE.

gastroduodenoscopy *n.* the technique of viewing the inside of the stomach and duodenum with an endoscope. *See also* DUODENOSCOPE.

gastroduodenostomy *n.* a surgical operation in which the *duodenum (usually the third or fourth part) is joined to an opening made in the stomach in order to bypass an obstruction (such as *pyloric stenosis) or to facilitate the exit of food from the stomach after vagotomy. *See also* DUODENOSTOMY.

gastroenteritis *n.* inflammation of the stomach and intestine. It is usually due to acute infection by viruses or bacteria or to food-poisoning toxins and causes vomiting and diarrhoea. The illness usually lasts 3–5 days. Fluid loss is sometimes severe, especially in infants, and intravenous fluid replacement may be necessary.

femur

fibula

tibia

gastrocnemius

soleus

Achilles tendon

Gastrocnemius and soleus muscles

gastroenterology *n.* the study of gastrointestinal disease, which includes disease of any part of the digestive tract and also of the liver, biliary tract, and pancreas.

gastroenterostomy *n.* a surgical operation in which the small intestine is joined to an opening made in the stomach. The usual technique is *gastroduodenostomy.

Gastrografin *n.* trade name for meglumine diatrizoate, a water-soluble contrast medium used in angiography and urography.

gastroileac reflex the relaxation of the *ileocaecal valve caused by the presence of food in the stomach.

gastrojejunostomy *n.* a surgical operation in which the *jejunum is joined to an opening made in the stomach. This is done in preference to *gastroduodenostomy if the latter operation is technically difficult or in special operations to avoid a backflow of bile into the stomach.

gastrolith *n.* a stone in the stomach, which usually builds up around a *bezoar.

gastro-oesophageal reflux a condition in which the stomach contents reflux into the oesophagus because of permanent or intermittent impairment of the usual mechanisms preventing this. It may give rise to *oesophagitis.

gastro-oesophageal reflux disease (GORD) the syndrome caused by abnormal *gastro-oesophageal reflux, which includes symptoms of *heartburn, regurgitation, and *odynophagia, in which *oesophagitis may be present.

gastro-oesophagostomy *n.* a surgical operation in which the *oesophagus (gullet) is joined to the stomach, bypassing the natural junction when this is obstructed by *achalasia, *stricture (narrowing) of the oesophagus, or cancer. This operation is rarely performed, because gastric juices entering the oesophagus through the artificial junction cause inflammation and stricture.

gastropexy *n.* surgical attachment of the stomach to the abdominal wall.

gastroplasty *n.* surgical alteration of the shape of the stomach without removal of any part. The term was originally used for correction of an acquired deformity, e.g. narrowing due to a peptic ulcer, but has more recently been applied to techniques for reducing the size of the stomach in the treatment of morbid obesity, e.g. vertical banded gastroplasty.

gastroptosis *n.* a condition in which the stomach hangs low in the abdomen. Although the diagnosis was once used to explain various abdominal complaints, it is now known that the stomach may assume various anatomical positions without causing any symptoms.

gastroschisis *n.* a congenital defect in the abdominal wall, which fails to close to the right of a normal umbilical cord. Gut prolapses through the defect and has no covering. Treatment is surgical.

gastroscope *n.* an illuminated optical instrument used to inspect the interior of the stomach. For many years these were rigid or semirigid instruments affording only limited views, but modern fully flexible instruments, which transmit the image through a fibreoptic bundle or by a tiny video camera, allow all areas of the stomach to be seen and photographed and specimens taken for microscopic examination. Therapeutic procedures (e.g. to arrest haemorrhage, remove a polyp, or produce a *gastrostomy) may be performed. As the same instruments can usually be introduced into the duodenum they are also known as **gastroduodenoscopes** or **oesophagogastroduodenoscopes**. —**gastroscopy** *n.*

gastrostaxis *n.* an obsolete term for *haematemesis (bleeding from the stomach).

gastrostomy *n.* a surgical procedure in which an opening is made into the stomach from the outside. It is usually performed to allow food and fluid to be poured directly into the stomach when swallowing is impossible because of disease or obstruction of the oesophagus. Sometimes it is used temporarily after operations on the oesophagus, until healing has occurred. Formerly a gastrostomy was always performed surgically, but it can now be done using an *endoscope (**percutaneous endoscopic gastrostomy**) or by direct puncture under radiological guidance.

gastrotomy *n.* a procedure during abdominal surgery in which the stomach is opened, usually to allow inspection of the interior (e.g. to find a point of bleeding), to remove a foreign body, or to allow the oesophagus to be approached from below (e.g. to pull down a tube through a constricting growth).

gastrula *n.* an early stage in the development of many animal embryos. It consists of a double-layered ball of cells formed by invagination and movement of cells in the preceding single-layered stage (blastula) in the process of **gastrulation**. It contains a central cavity, the *archenteron, which opens through the **blastopore** to the outside. True gastrulation only occurs in the embryos of amphibians and certain fish, but a similar process occurs in the embryonic disc in other vertebrates, including man.

Gaucher's disease a genetically determined (autosomal *recessive) disease resulting from the deposition of glucocerebrosides (*see* CEREBROSIDE) in the brain and other tissues (especially bone). It causes mental retardation, abnormal limb posture and spasticity, and difficulty with swallowing. Carrier detection and *prenatal diagnosis are possible; enzyme replacement therapy is used in treatment. [P. C. E. Gaucher (1854–1918), French physician]

gauss *n.* a unit of magnetic flux density equal to 1 maxwell per square centimetre. 1 gauss = 10^{-4} tesla.

Gaussian distribution *see* FREQUENCY DISTRIBUTION, SIGNIFICANCE. [K. F. Gauss (1777–1855), German mathematician]

gauze *n.* thin open-woven material used in several layers for the preparation of dressings and swabs.

gavage *n.* forced feeding: any means used to get an unwilling or incapacitated patient to take in food by mouth, especially via a stomach tube.

G-cell *n.* any of the cells of the mucous membrane of the stomach that are responsible for the production of *gastrin. They occur mainly in the gastric *antrum. Increased production of G-cells is associated with duodenal ulcer and the *Zollinger-Ellison syndrome: gastrin acts to increase the production of acid by the oxyntic (parietal) cells of the gastric glands.

gel *n.* a colloidal suspension that has set to form a jelly. Some insoluble drugs are administered in the form of gels.

gelatin *n.* a jelly-like substance formed when tendons, ligaments, etc. containing *collagen (a protein) are boiled in water. Gelatin has been used in medicine as a source of protein in the treatment of malnutrition, in pharmacy for the manufacture of capsules and suppositories, and in bacteriology for preparing culture media.

gemeprost *n.* a *prostaglandin drug, administered as a vaginal pessary to terminate pregnancy. It causes powerful contractions of the uterus at any stage of pregnancy. Trade name: **Cervagem**.

gemfibrozil *n.* a drug used to lower very low-density *lipoproteins in patients with high *triglyceride serum levels who have not responded to diet, weight reduction, or exercise. It is administered by mouth; side-effects include diarrhoea, abdominal pain, and nausea and vomiting. Trade name: **Lopid**.

gemmule *n.* one of the minute spines or surface extensions of a *dendrite, through which contact is made with another neurone at a *synapse.

gene *n.* the basic unit of genetic material, which is carried at a particular place on a *chromosome. Originally it was regarded as the unit of inheritance and mutation but is now usually defined as a sequence of *DNA or *RNA that acts as the unit controlling the formation of a single polypeptide chain (see CISTRON). In diploid organisms, including man, genes occur as pairs of *alleles. Various kinds of gene have been discovered: **structural genes** determine the biochemical makeup of the proteins; **regulator genes** control the rate of protein production (see OPERON). **Architectural genes** are responsible for the integration of the protein into the structure of the cell, and **temporal genes** control the time and place of action of the other genes and largely control the *differentiation of the cells and tissues of the body.

gene clone *see* CLONE.

General Dental Council a statutory body that controls the practice of dentistry in the UK.

general dental services a part of the NHS dental service. Dentists are included on the dental list of the appropriate Health Authority and are independent contractors. They are paid partly by capitation (per head) and partly by item of service. They are entirely responsible for the financial management of their own practices.

generalized anxiety disorder a state of inappropriate and sometimes severe anxiety, without adequate cause, that lasts for at least six months. It affects about 2% of the population, women twice as often as men, and often develops in early adult life. It can, however, start at any age. There is a hereditary tendency to develop the disorder and about 25% of immediate relatives of sufferers are also affected. The disorder is thought to be caused by a disturbance of the functions of neurotransmitters, such as adrenaline or GABA, in the frontal lobes or the *limbic system of the brain. Symptoms include shakiness, *bruxism, restlessness, fatigability, breathlessness, palpitations, sweating, clammy hands, dry mouth, lightheadedness, diarrhoea, flushing, and *globus hystericus. Treatment is with beta blockers, antihistamines, and antidepressants.

general paralysis of the insane (GPI) a late consequence of syphilitic infection. The symptoms are those of a *dementia and spastic weakness of the limbs. Deafness, epilepsy, and *dysarthria may occur. The infecting organism can be detected in the brain cells and tests for syphilis in blood and cerebrospinal fluid are usually positive. When the symptoms are combined with those of *tabes dorsalis, the resulting condition is called **tabo-paresis**. Vigorous treatment with procaine penicillin is required, but recovery is likely to be limited.

general practitioner (GP) a doctor (also known as a **family doctor** or **family practitioner**) who is the main agent of *primary health care, through whom patients make first contact with health services for a new episode of illness or fresh developments of chronic diseases. Advice and treatment are provided for those who do not require the expertise of a *consultant or other specialist services of hospitals (see SECONDARY HEALTH CARE). In the British *National Health Service patients on the practice list of a GP receive care without payment on an open-access basis.

A practitioner may have private patients in addition to NHS patients; a few have exclusively private practices. No NHS patient may be charged for a NHS prescription by the GP (except in a *dispensing practice, where a statutory charge is made for the medication); similarly a medical certificate on which to base a claim for *social security payment must be given without charge. Conversely, no private patient may receive a NHS prescription. Two or more practitioners may form a partnership sharing fees and work loads, including cross-cover for each other's NHS patients. When they share premises, administrative and nursing staff, and other resources this constitutes a **group practice**; the premises from which they operate may be privately owned or may be a publicly owned *health centre. Remuneration of GPs is based on a quarterly capitation fee for each registered patient (higher for those over 65 years of age) regardless of the number of consultations; however, additional claims can be made for some services (e.g. antenatal care and household calls made outside normal working hours). A practice with at least 5000 patients may apply to become a **fundholder**, with responsibility for managing its own NHS budget, including the power to purchase the services it requires for its own patients from whichever hospital or other health-care provider gives the best service. *See also* INDEPENDENT CONTRACT.

generic *adj.* **1.** denoting a drug name that is not protected by a trademark. **2.** of or relating to a *genus.

-genesis *suffix denoting* origin or development. Example: **spermatogenesis** (development of spermatozoa).

gene therapy treatment directed to curing genetic disease by introducing normal genes into patients to overcome the effects of defective genes, using techniques of *genetic engineering. The most radical approach would be to do this at a very early stage in the embryo, so that the new gene would be incorporated into the germ cells (ova and sperm) and would therefore be inheritable. However, this approach is not considered to be either safe or ethical, because the consequences would affect all descendants of the patient, and it is not being pursued. In **somatic cell gene therapy** the healthy gene is inserted into *somatic cells (such as the *stem cells of the bone marrow) that give rise to other cells. All the surviving descendants of these modified cells will then be normal and, if present in sufficient numbers, the condition will be cured (the defective gene will, however, still be present in the germ cells).

At present, gene therapy is most feasible for treating disorders caused by a defect in a single recessive gene, so that the deficiency can be overcome by the introduction of a normal allele (therapy for disorders caused by dominant genes (e.g. Huntington's disease) would require the modification or replacement of the defective allele as its effect is expressed in the presence of a normal allele). Examples of such recessive disorders include *adenosine deaminase (ADA) deficiency and *cystic fibrosis. Gene therapy trials for the former condition have already begun: lymphocyte stem cells are isolated from the patient, using *monoclonal antibodies, and incubated with *retroviruses that have been genetically engineered to contain the normal ADA gene (*see* VECTOR). This gene thus becomes integrated into the stem cells, which – when returned to the patient's bone marrow – can then produce normal lymphocytes.

Clinical trials for the gene therapy of cystic fibrosis involve using *liposomes to introduce the normal gene into the lungs of sufferers via an inhaler.

Gene therapy for certain types of cancer is also undergoing clinical trials. Here the approach is aimed at introducing into the cancer cells tumour-suppressing genes, such as *$p53$ (which prevents uncontrolled cell division), or genes that direct the production of substances (such as *interleukin 2) that stimulate the immune system to destroy the tumour cells.

genetic code the information carried by *DNA and *messenger RNA that determines the sequence of amino acids in every protein and thereby controls the nature of all proteins made by the cell. The genetic code is expressed by the sequence of *nucleotide bases in the nucleic acid molecule, a unit of three consecutive bases (a **codon**) coding for each amino acid. The code is translated into protein at the ribosomes (see TRANSCRIPTION, TRANSLATION). Any changes in the genetic code result in the insertion of incorrect amino acids in a protein chain, giving a *mutation.

genetic counselling the procedure by which patients and their families are given advice about the nature and consequences of inherited disorders, the possibility of becoming affected or having affected children, and the various options that are available to them for the prevention, diagnosis, and management of such conditions. Genetic counselling should be available at prenatal and postnatal clinics, and also through family planning clinics.

genetic drift the tendency for variations to occur in the genetic composition of small isolated inbreeding populations by chance. Such populations become genetically rather different from the original population from which they were derived.

genetic engineering (recombinant DNA technology) the techniques involved in altering the characteristics of an organism by inserting genes from another organism into its DNA. This altered DNA (known as **recombinant DNA**) is usually produced by isolating foreign genes, often by the use of *restriction enzymes, and inserting them into bacterial DNA, often using viruses as *vectors. Once inserted, the foreign gene may use the cell machinery of its host to synthesize the protein that it originally coded for in the organism it was derived from. For example, the human genes for *insulin, *interferon, and *growth hormone production have been incorporated into bacterial DNA and such genetically engineered bacteria are used in the commercial production of these substances. Some other applications of genetic engineering include DNA analysis, the production of *monoclonal antibodies, and – more recently – *gene therapy.

genetics n. the science of inheritance. It attempts to explain the differences and similarities between related organisms and the ways in which characters are passed from parents to their offspring. **Human** and **medical genetics** are concerned with the study of inherited diseases. See also CYTOGENETICS, MENDEL'S LAWS.

genetic screening *screening tests to discover individuals whose *genotypes are associated with specific diseases (see also MOUTHWASH TEST). Such individuals may later develop the disease itself or pass it on to their children (see CARRIER). The recent use of genetic screening to diagnose the sex of the fetus so that the parents may 'choose' the sex of their children has caused considerable controversy.

geni- (genio-) prefix denoting the chin.

-genic suffix denoting 1. producing. 2. produced by.

genicular adj. relating to the knee joint: applied to arteries that supply the knee.

geniculum n. a sharp bend in an anatomical structure, such as the bend in the facial nerve in the medial wall of the middle ear.

genion n. (in *craniometry) the tip of the protuberance of the chin.

genioplasty n. an operation performed in plastic surgery to alter the size and shape of the chin. This can be built up with grafted bone, cartilage, or artificial material.

genital adj. relating to the reproductive organs or to reproduction.

genital herpes see HERPES.

genitalia pl. n. the reproductive organs of either the male or the female. However, the term is usually used in reference to the external parts of the reproductive system. See also VULVA.

genito- prefix denoting the reproductive organs. Examples: **genitoplasty** (plastic surgery of); **genitourinary** (relating to the reproductive and excretory systems).

genitourinary medicine the medical specialty concerned with the study and treatment of *sexually transmitted diseases.

genodermatosis n. any genetically determined skin disorder, such as *ichthyosis, *neurofibromatosis, or *xeroderma pigmentosum.

genogram n. a technique of family *psychotherapy, in which a family tree and a family history of a particular psychological disorder are constructed in view of the whole family to help them understand each other better.

genome n. the total genetic material of an organism, comprising the genes contained in its chromosomes; sometimes the term is used for the basic *haploid set of chromosomes of an organism. The human genome comprises 23 pairs of chromosomes (see HUMAN GENOME PROJECT).

genotype n. **1.** the genetic constitution of an individual or group, as determined by the particular set of genes it possesses. **2.** the genetic information carried by a pair of alleles, which determines a particular characteristic. **3.** a gene or pattern of genes the precise details of which are defined. *Compare* PHENOTYPE.

gentamicin n. an *aminoglycoside antibiotic used to treat infections caused by a wide range of bacteria. It can be administered by injection or applied in a cream to the skin or in drops to the ears and eyes. Kidney and ear damage may occur at high doses. Trade names: **Cidomycin, Garamycin, Genticin.**

gentian violet **1.** a dye used for staining tissues and microorganisms for microscopical study. **2.** *see* METHYL VIOLET.

genu n. **1.** the knee. **2.** any bent anatomical structure resembling the knee. —**genual** *adj.*

genus n. (*pl.* **genera**) a category used in the classification of animals and plants. A genus consists of several closely related and similar species; for example the genus *Canis* includes the dog, wolf, and jackal.

genu valgum abnormal in-curving of the legs, resulting in excessive separation of the feet when the knees are in contact. *See* KNOCK-KNEE.

genu varum abnormal outward curving of the legs, resulting in separation of the knees. *See* BOW-LEGS.

geo- *prefix denoting* the earth or soil.

geophagia n. the eating of dirt. *See* PICA.

ger- (gero-, geront(o)-) *prefix denoting* old age.

geriatrics n. the branch of medicine concerned with the diagnosis and treatment of disorders that occur in old age and with the care of the aged. *See also* GERONTOLOGY.

germ n. any microorganism, especially one that causes disease. *See also* INFECTION.

German measles a mild highly contagious virus infection, mainly of childhood, causing enlargement of lymph nodes in the neck and a widespread pink rash. The disease is spread by close contact with a patient. After an incubation period of 2–3 weeks a headache, sore throat, and slight fever develop, followed by swelling and soreness of the neck and the eruption of a rash of minute pink spots, spreading from the face and neck to the rest of the body. The spots disappear within seven days but the patient remains infectious for a further 3–4 days. An infection usually confers immunity. As German measles can cause fetal malformations during early pregnancy, girls should be immunized against the disease before puberty. Most children now receive immunization via the *MMR vaccine in their second year. Medical name: **rubella**. *Compare* SCARLET FEVER.

germ cell (gonocyte) any of the embryonic cells that have the potential to develop into spermatozoa or ova. The term is also applied to any of the cells undergoing gametogenesis and to the gametes themselves.

germicide n. an agent that destroys microorganisms, particularly those causing disease. *See* ANTIBIOTIC, ANTIFUNGAL, ANTISEPTIC, DISINFECTANT.

germinal *adj.* **1.** relating to the early developmental stages of an embryo or tissue. **2.** relating to a germ.

germinal epithelium the epithelial covering of the ovary, which was formerly thought to be the site of formation of *oogonia. It is now thought that the oogonia persist in a dormant state from the prenatal period until required in reproductive life.

germinal vesicle the nucleus of a mature *oocyte, prior to fertilization. It is considerably larger than the nucleus of other cells.

germ layer any of the three distinct types of tissue found in the very early stages of embryonic development (*see* EC-TODERM, ENDODERM, MESODERM). The germ layers can be traced throughout embryonic development as they differentiate to form the entire range of body tissues.

germ plasm the substance postulated by 19th century biologists (notably Weismann) to be transmitted via the gametes from one generation to the next and to give rise to the body cells.

gerontology *n.* the study of the changes in the mind and body that accompany ageing and the problems associated with them.

Gerota's nodes pararectal lymph nodes, i.e. lymph nodes situated beside the rectum. [D. Gerota (1867–1939), Hungarian anatomist]

Gerstmann's syndrome a group of symptoms that represent a partial disintegration of the patient's recognition of his *body image. It consists of an inability to name the individual fingers, misidentification of the right and left sides of the body, and inability to write or make mathematical calculations (*see* ACALCULIA, AGRAPHIA). It is caused by disease in the association area of the left parietal lobe of the brain. [J. G. Gerstmann (1888–1969), US neurologist]

gestaltism *n.* a school of psychology that regards mental processes as wholes (**gestalts**) that cannot be broken down into constituent parts. From this was developed **gestalt therapy**, which aims at achieving a suitable gestalt within the patient that includes all facets of functioning.

gestation *n.* the period during which a fertilized egg cell develops into a baby that is ready to be delivered. Gestation averages 266 days in humans (or 280 days from the first day of the last menstrual period). *See also* PREGNANCY.

gestodene *n.* a *progestogen used in oral contraceptives in combination with an oestrogen. Trade names: **Femodene**, **Minulet**.

GFR *see* GLOMERULAR FILTRATION RATE.

Ghon's focus the lesion produced in the lung of a previously uninfected person by tubercle bacilli. It is a small focus of granulomatous inflammation, which may become visible on a chest X-ray if it grows large enough or if it calcifies. A Ghon focus usually heals without further trouble, but in some patients tuberculosis spreads from it via the lymphatics, the air spaces, or the bloodstream. [A. Ghon (1866–1936), Czech pathologist]

ghost vessels empty transparent blood vessels that persist in the cornea after regression of the inflammatory process that stimulated their development.

giant cell any large cell, such as a *megakaryocyte. Giant cells may have one or many nuclei.

giant-cell arteritis *see* ARTERITIS.

Giardia *n.* a genus of parasitic pear-shaped protozoa inhabiting the small intestine of man. They have four pairs of *flagella, two nuclei, and two sucking discs used for attachment to the intestinal wall. *Giardia* is usually harmless but may occasionally cause diarrhoea (*see* GIARDIASIS).

giardiasis (lambliasis) *n.* a disease caused by the parasitic protozoan *Giardia lamblia* in the small intestine. Man becomes infected by eating food contaminated with cysts containing the parasite. Symptoms include diarrhoea, nausea, bellyache, and flatulence, as well as the passage of pale fatty stools (steatorrhoea). Large numbers of the parasite may interfere with the absorption of food through the gut wall. The disease occurs throughout the world and is particularly common in children; it responds well to oral doses of quinacrine and *metronidazole.

gibbus (gibbosity) *n.* a sharply angled curvature of the backbone, resulting from collapse of a vertebra. Infection with tuberculosis was a common cause.

Giemsa's stain a mixture of *methylene blue and *eosin, used for distinguishing different types of white blood cell and for detecting parasitic microorganisms in blood smears. It is one of the *Romanowsky stains. [G. Giemsa (1867–1948), German chemist]

GIFT *see* GAMETE INTRAFALLOPIAN TRANSFER.

gigantism *n.* abnormal growth causing excessive height, most commonly due to oversecretion during childhood of *growth hormone (somatotrophin) by the pituitary gland. In **eunuchoid gigantism** the tall stature is due to delayed puberty, which results in continued growth of the long bones before their growing ends (epiphyses) fuse. *See also* ACROMEGALY.

Gilbert's syndrome familial unconjugated hyperbilirubinaemia: a condition due to an inherited congenital deficiency of the enzyme UDP glucuronyl transferase in the liver cells. Patients become mildly jaundiced, especially if they fast or have some minor infection. Occasionally they have mild abdominal discomfort. The jaundice can be diminished by small doses of phenobarbitone, which stimulates enzyme activity. The condition is harmless. [N. A. Gilbert (1858–1927), French physician]

Gilles de la Tourette syndrome (Tourette's syndrome) a condition of severe and multiple *tics, including vocal tics, grunts, and involuntary obscene speech (*coprolalia). The patient may also involuntarily repeat the words or imitate the actions of others (*see* PALILALIA). The condition usually starts in childhood and becomes chronic; the causes are unknown. Drug treatment (for example, with *pimozide) is sometimes successful. [G. Gilles de la Tourette (1857–1904), French neurologist]

Gimbernat's ligament a portion of the medial end of the *inguinal ligament that is reflected along the upper part of the pubic bone. It is used to hold stitches during repairs of a femoral *hernia. [A. de Gimbernat (1734–1816), Spanish surgeon and anatomist]

gingiv- (gingivo-) *prefix denoting* the gums. Example: **gingivoplasty** (plastic surgery of).

gingiva *n.* (*pl.* **gingivae**) the gum: the layer of dense connective tissue and overlying mucous membrane that covers the alveolar bone and necks of the teeth. —**gingival** *adj.*

gingivectomy *n.* the surgical removal of excess gum tissue. It is a specific procedure of periodontal surgery.

gingivitis *n.* inflammation of the gums (*see* GINGIVA) caused by *plaque on the surfaces of the teeth at their necks. The gums are swollen and bleed easily. **Chronic gingivitis** is an early stage of *periodontal disease but is reversible with good oral hygiene. *Ulcerative gingivitis is painful and destructive. Gingival overgrowth may be caused by drug therapy, e.g. phenytoin.

ginglymus (hinge joint) *n.* a form of *diarthrosis (freely movable joint) that allows angular movement in one plane only, increasing or decreasing the angle between the bones. Examples are the knee joint and the elbow joint.

girdle *n.* (in anatomy) an encircling or arching arrangement of bones. *See also* PELVIC GIRDLE, SHOULDER GIRDLE.

glabella *n.* the smooth rounded surface of the *frontal bone in the middle of the forehead, between the two eyebrows.

gladiolus *n.* the middle and largest segment of the *sternum.

gland *n.* an organ or group of cells that is specialized for synthesizing and secreting certain fluids, either for use in the body or for excretion. There are two main groups of glands: the *exocrine glands, which discharge their secretions by means of ducts, and the *endocrine glands, which secrete their products – hormones – directly into the bloodstream. *See also* SECRETION.

glanders (equinia) *n.* an infectious disease of horses, donkeys, and mules that is caused by the bacterium *Pseudomonas mallei* and can be transmitted to man. Symptoms include fever and inflammation (with possible ulceration) of the lymph nodes (a form of the disease known as **farcy**), skin, and nasal mucous membranes. In the untreated acute form death may follow in 2–20 days. In the more common chronic form, many patients survive without treatment. Administration of sulphonamides or streptomycin is usually effective.

glandular fever an infectious disease, caused by the Epstein-Barr virus, that affects the lymph nodes in the neck, armpits, and groin; it mainly affects adolescents and young adults. After an incubation period of 5–7 days, symptoms commence with swelling and tenderness of the lymph nodes, fever, headache, a sore throat, lethargy, and loss of appetite. In some cases the liver is affected, causing *hepatitis, or the spleen is enlarged. Glandular fever is diagnosed by the presence of large numbers of *monocytes in the blood. Complications are rare but symptoms may persist for weeks before recovery. Medical name: **infectious mononucleosis**.

glans (glans penis) *n.* the acorn-shaped end part of the *penis, formed by the expanded end of the corpus spongiosum (erectile tissue). It is covered by the prepuce (foreskin), unless this has been removed by circumcision. The term glans is also applied to the end of the *clitoris.

glare *n.* the undesirable effects of scattered stray light on the retina, causing reduced contrast and visual performance as well as annoyance and discomfort.

Glasgow scoring system (Glasgow coma scale) a numerical system used to estimate a patient's level of consciousness after head injury. Each of the following are numerically graded: eye opening (4), motor response (6), and verbal response (5). The higher the score, the greater the level of consciousness: a score of 7 indicates a coma.

glaucoma *n.* a condition in which loss of vision occurs because of an abnormally high pressure in the eye. In most cases there is no other ocular disease. This is known as **primary glaucoma** and there are two pathologically distinct types: acute and chronic simple. In **acute** (or **angle-closure**) **glaucoma**, there is an abrupt rise in pressure due to sudden closure of the angle between the cornea and iris where aqueous humour usually drains from the eye. This is accompanied by pain and marked blurring of vision associated with inflammation of the anterior segment. In the more common **chronic simple** (or **open-angle**) **glaucoma**, the pressure increases gradually, usually without producing pain, and the visual loss is insidious. The same type of visual loss may rarely occur in eyes with a normal pressure: this is called **low-tension glaucoma**. Primary glaucoma occurs increasingly with age and is an important cause of blindness. **Secondary glaucoma** may occur when other ocular disease impairs

the normal circulation of the aqueous humour and causes the intraocular pressure to rise.

In all types of glaucoma the eventual problem is to reduce the intraocular pressure. Drops are inserted into the eye at regular intervals to improve the outflow of aqueous humour from the eye, and drops and tablets (such as *acetazolamide) are used to reduce the production of aqueous humour. If this treatment is ineffective, surgery may be performed to make a new channel through which the aqueous humour may drain from the eye in sufficient quantities to allow the pressure to return to normal. Such operations are known as **drainage** or **filtering operations**.

gleet *n.* a discharge of purulent mucus from the penis or vagina resulting from chronic *gonorrhoea.

glenohumeral *adj.* relating to the glenoid cavity and the humerus: the region of the shoulder joint.

glenoid cavity (glenoid fossa) the socket of the shoulder joint: the pear-shaped cavity at the top of the *scapula into which the head of the humerus fits.

gli- (glio-) *prefix denoting* **1.** glia. **2.** a glutinous substance.

glia (neuroglia) *n.* the special connective tissue of the central nervous system, composed of different cells, including the *oligodendrocytes, *astrocytes, ependymal cells (see EPENDYMA), and *microglia, with various supportive and nutritive functions (see illustration). Glial cells outnumber the neurones by between five and ten to one, and make up some 40% of the total volume of the brain and spinal cord. —**glial** *adj.*

gliadin *n.* a protein, soluble in alcohol, that is obtained from wheat. It is one of the constituents of *gluten.

glibenclamide *n.* a drug that reduces the level of sugar in the blood and is used to treat noninsulin-dependent diabetes (see SULPHONYLUREA). It is administered by mouth. Side-effects include mild digestive upsets and skin reactions. Trade names: **Daonil, Euglucon**.

gliclazide *n.* a *sulphonylurea oral hypoglycaemic drug used in the treatment of noninsulin-dependent (Type II) *diabetes. Trade name: **Diamicron**.

Ependymal cells

Protoplasmic astrocyte

Fibrous astrocyte

Microglia

Oligodendroglia

Types of glia

gliding joint *see* ARTHRODIC JOINT.

glioblastoma (spongioblastoma) *n.* the most aggressive type of brain tumour derived from non-nervous (glial) tissue (*see* ASTROCYTOMA). Its rapid enlargement destroys normal brain cells, with a progressive loss of function, and raises the intracranial pressure, causing headache, vomiting, and drowsiness. Treatment is rarely curative and the prognosis is poor.

glioma *n.* any tumour of non-nervous cells (*glia) in the nervous system. The term is sometimes also used for all tumours that arise in the central nervous system, including *astrocytomas, *oligodendrogliomas, medulloblastomas, and ependymomas. Tumours of low-grade ma-

lignancy produce symptoms by pressure on surrounding structures; those of high-grade malignancy may be invasive.

gliosome *n.* a *lysosome in an *astrocyte.

glipizide *n.* a drug used to control high blood-glucose levels (hyperglycaemia) in patients with noninsulin-dependent diabetes after diet control has failed (*see* SULPHONYLUREA). It is administered by mouth; side-effects are hypoglycaemia, nausea and vomiting, and skin rash. Trade names: **Glibenese**, **Minodiab**.

globin *n.* a protein, found in the body, that can combine with iron-containing groups to form *haemoglobin (which is found in red blood cells) and *myohaemoglobin (found in muscle).

globulin *n.* one of a group of simple proteins that are soluble in dilute salt solutions and can be coagulated by heat. A range of different globulins is present in the blood (the **serum globulins**, including alpha (α), beta (β), and *gamma (γ) globulins). Some globulins have important functions as antibodies (*see* IMMUNOGLOBULIN); others are responsible for the transport of lipids, iron, or copper in the blood.

globulinuria *n.* the presence in the urine of globulins.

globus *n.* a spherical or globe-shaped structure; for example the **globus pallidus**, part of the lenticular nucleus in the brain (*see* BASAL GANGLIA).

globus hystericus the sense of having a 'lump in the throat' that can neither be swallowed nor brought up. This feeling often accompanies acute anxiety, sadness, or mental conflict and is due to a constriction of the circularly placed muscles around the lower part of the pharynx.

glomangioma (glomus tumour) *n. see* GLOMUS.

glomerular filtration rate (GFR) the rate at which substances are filtered from the blood of the glomeruli into the Bowman's capsules of the *nephrons. It is calculated by measuring the *clearance of specific substances (e.g. creatinine) and is an index of renal function.

glomerulitis *n.* any one of a variety of

lesions of the glomeruli (*see* GLOMERULUS) associated with acute or chronic kidney disease. Such lesions are recognized by electron microscopic examination, using immunofluorescent staining techniques, of kidney biopsy specimens taken during the course of the disease.

glomerulonephritis (glomerular nephritis) *n.* any of a group of kidney diseases involving the glomeruli (*see* GLOMERULUS), usually thought to be the result of antibody-antigen reactions that localize in the kidneys because of their filtering function. **Acute nephritis** is marked by blood in the urine and fluid and urea retention. It may be related to a recent streptococcal throat infection and usually settles completely, with rapid return of normal kidney function. Other forms of nephritis present with chronic *haematuria or with the *nephrotic syndrome; children often eventually recover completely, but adults are more likely to progress to **chronic nephritis** and eventual kidney failure.

glomerulus *n.* (*pl.* **glomeruli**) **1.** the network of blood capillaries contained within the cuplike end (**Bowman's capsule**) of a *nephron. It is the site of primary filtration of waste products from the blood into the kidney tubule. **2.** any other small rounded mass

glomus *n.* (*pl.* **glomera**) a small communication between a tiny artery and vein in the skin of the limbs. It is concerned with the regulation of temperature. Occasionally its malformation and overgrowth produces a harmless but often painful tumour (**glomus tumour** or **glomangioma**), usually occurring in the skin at the ends of the fingers or toes. It may be cauterized or removed surgically.

glomus jugulare a collection of chemoreceptors within a dilatation of the internal jugular vein at its origin at the base of the skull. It is a site of origin for *chemodectomas.

gloss- (glosso-) *prefix denoting* the tongue. Examples: **glossopharyngeal** (relating to the tongue and pharynx); **glossoplasty** (plastic surgery of).

glossa *n. see* TONGUE.

glossectomy *n.* surgical removal of the

tongue, an operation usually carried out for cancer in this structure.

Glossina *n. see* TSETSE.

glossitis *n.* inflammation of the tongue. Causes include anaemia, candidosis, and vitamin deficiency. 'Geographical tongue' is a benign glossitis in which areas of *erythema change from day to day.

glossolalia *n.* nonsense speech that mimics normal speech in that it is appropriately formed into an imitation of syllables, words, and sentences. It can be uttered in *trance states and during sleep.

glossopharyngeal nerve the ninth *cranial nerve (IX), which supplies motor fibres to part of the pharynx and to the parotid salivary glands and sensory fibres to the posterior third of the tongue and the soft palate.

glossoplegia *n.* paralysis of the tongue.

glottis *n.* the space between the two *vocal folds. The term is often applied to the vocal folds themselves or to that part of the larynx associated with the production of sound.

gluc- (gluco-) *prefix denoting* glucose. Example: **glucosuria** (urinary excretion of).

glucagon *n.* a hormone, produced by the pancreas, that causes an increase in the blood sugar level and thus has an effect opposite to that of *insulin. Glucagon is administered by injection to counteract diabetic *hypoglycaemia.

glucagonoma *n.* a pancreatic tumour that secretes glucagon and produces attacks of *hypoglycaemia.

glucocorticoid *n. see* CORTICOSTEROID.

glucokinase *n.* an enzyme (a *hexokinase), found in the liver, that catalyses the conversion of glucose to glucose-6-phosphate. This is the first stage of *glycolysis.

gluconeogenesis *n.* the biochemical process in which glucose, an important source of energy, is synthesized from noncarbohydrate sources, such as amino acids. Gluconeogenesis occurs mainly in the liver and kidney and meets the needs of the body for glucose when carbohydrate is not available in sufficient amounts in the diet.

glucosamine *n.* the amino sugar of glucose, i.e. glucose in which the hydroxyl group is replaced by an amino group. Glucosamine is a component of *mucopolysaccharides and *glycoproteins: for example, *hyaluronic acid, found in synovial fluid, and *heparin.

glucose (dextrose) *n.* a simple sugar containing six carbon atoms (a hexose). Glucose is an important source of energy in the body and the sole source of energy for the brain. Free glucose is not found in many foods (grapes are an exception); however, glucose is one of the constituents of both sucrose and starch, both of which yield glucose after digestion. Glucose is stored in the body in the form of *glycogen. The concentration of glucose in the blood is maintained at around 5 mmol/l by a variety of hormones, principally *insulin and *glucagon. If the blood-glucose concentration falls below this level neurological and other symptoms may result (*see* HYPOGLYCAEMIA). Conversely, if the blood-glucose level is raised above its normal level, to 10 mmol/l, the condition of *hyperglycaemia develops. This is a symptom of *diabetes mellitus.

glucose-6-phosphate dehydrogenase deficiency a hereditary (X-linked) condition in which the absence of the enzyme glucose-6-phosphate dehydrogenase (G6PD), which functions in carbohydrate metabolism, results in the breakdown of the red blood cells (*haemolysis), usually after exposure to *oxidants, such as drugs, or infections. The breakdown causes acute attacks that are characterized by pallor, loin pain, and rigors. There are several varieties of G6PD deficiency: African (which is sensitive to some antimalarial drugs), European (including *favism), and oriental. Treatment involves identifying and avoiding agents that trigger the haemolysis and treating acute attacks symptomatically.

glucose tolerance test a test used in the diagnosis of *diabetes mellitus. A quantity of glucose is given to the patient by mouth, after 10–16 hours of fasting, and the concentration of sugar in the blood and urine is determined at 30-minute intervals during the next two hours. These readings indicate the ability of the patient's body to utilize glucose.

glucoside *n. see* GLYCOSIDE.

glucuronic acid a sugar acid derived from glucose. Glucuronic acid is an important constituent of *chondroitin sulphate (found in cartilage) and *hyaluronic acid (found in synovial fluid).

glue ear a common condition in which viscous fluid accumulates in the middle ear, causing *deafness. It is most frequently seen in children and is due to malfunction of the *Eustachian tube. Many cases resolve spontaneously; treatment, if required, consists of surgical incision of the eardrum (*myringotomy), drainage of the fluid, and the insertion of a *grommet. Medical name: **secretory otitis media**.

glutamate dehydrogenase (glutamic acid dehydrogenase) an important enzyme involved in the *deamination of amino acids.

glutamic acid (glutamate) *see* AMINO ACID, NEUROTRANSMITTER.

glutamic oxaloacetic transaminase (GOT) an enzyme involved in the *transamination of amino acids. This enzyme is present in blood serum (**serum GOT, SGOT**); measurement of SGOT may be used in the diagnosis of acute *myocardial infarction and acute liver disease. This enzyme has been renamed **aspartate aminotransferase (AST)**, but the old abbreviation is still widely used.

glutamic pyruvic transaminase (GPT) an enzyme involved in the *transamination of amino acids. High levels of this enzyme are found in the liver, and measurement of GPT in the serum (**serum GPT, SGPT**) is of use in the diagnosis and study of acute liver disease. This enzyme has been renamed **alanine aminotransferase (ALT)**, but the old abbreviation is still widely used.

glutaminase *n.* an enzyme, found in the kidney, that catalyses the breakdown of the amino acid glutamine to ammonia and glutamic acid: a stage in the production of urea.

glutamine *n. see* AMINO ACID.

glutathione *n.* a peptide containing the amino acids glutamic acid, cysteine, and glycine. It functions as a *coenzyme in several oxidation-reduction reactions. Glutathione serves as an *antioxidant: it reacts with potentially harmful oxidizing agents and is itself oxidized (*see also* SELENIUM). This is important in ensuring the proper functioning of proteins, haemoglobin, membrane lipids, etc. High levels of glutathione in the blood are associated with longevity.

glutelin *n.* one of a group of simple proteins found in plants and soluble only in dilute acids and bases. An example is **glutenin**, found in wheat (*see* GLUTEN).

gluten *n.* a mixture of the two proteins **gliadin** and **glutenin**. Gluten is present in wheat and rye and is important for its baking properties: when mixed with water it becomes sticky and enables air to be trapped and dough to be formed. Sensitivity to gluten leads to *coeliac disease in children.

gluteus *n.* one of three paired muscles of the buttocks (**gluteus maximus, gluteus medius** and **gluteus minimus**). They are responsible for movements of the thigh. —**gluteal** *adj.*

glyc- (glyco-) *prefix denoting* sugar.

glyceride *n.* a *lipid consisting of glycerol (an alcohol) combined with one or more fatty acids. See also* TRIGLYCERIDE.

glycerin (glycerol) *n.* a clear viscous liquid obtained by hydrolysis of fats and mixed oils and produced as a by-product in the manufacture of soap. It is used as an *emollient in many skin preparations, as a laxative (particularly in the form of *suppositories), and as a sweetening agent in the pharmaceutical industry.

glyceryl trinitrate (nitroglycerin) a drug that dilates blood vessels and is used to prevent and treat angina (*see* VASODILATOR). It is administered by mouth (tablets or sprays), skin patches, or injection; large doses may cause flushing, headache, and fainting. Trade names: **Glytrin Spray, Nitrolingual Pumpspray, Sustac, Transiderm-Nitro.**

glycine *n. see* AMINO ACID.

glycobiology *n.* the study of the chemistry, biochemistry, and other aspects of carbohydrates and carbohydrate complexes, especially *glycoproteins. Elucidation of the structure and role of the sugar molecules of glycoproteins has important medical implications and has led to the development of new drugs, such as *tissue plasminogen activators, drugs that affect the immune system, and antiviral drugs.

glycocholic acid *see* BILE ACIDS.

glycogen *n.* a carbohydrate consisting of branched chains of glucose units. Glycogen is the principal form in which carbohydrate is stored in the body: it is the counterpart of starch in plants. Glycogen is stored in the liver and muscles and may be readily broken down to glucose.

glycogenesis *n.* the biochemical process, occurring chiefly in the liver and in muscle, by which glucose is converted into glycogen.

glycogenolysis *n.* a biochemical process, occurring chiefly in the liver and in muscle, by which glycogen is broken down into glucose.

glycolipid *n.* a *lipid containing a sugar molecule (usually galactose or glucose). The *cerebrosides are examples of glycolipids.

glycolysis *n.* the conversion of glucose, by a series of ten enzyme-catalysed reactions, to lactic acid. Glycolysis takes place in the cytoplasm of cells and the first nine reactions (converting glucose to pyruvate) form the first stage of cellular *respiration. The process involves the production of a small amount of energy (in the form of ATP), which is used for biochemical work. The final reaction of glycolysis (converting pyruvate to lactic acid) provides energy for short periods of time when oxygen consumption exceeds demand; for example, during bursts of intense muscular activity. *See also* LACTIC ACID.

glycoprotein *n.* one of a group of compounds consisting of a protein combined with a carbohydrate (such as galactose or mannose). Examples of glycoproteins are certain enzymes, hormones, and antigens.

glycoside *n.* a compound formed by replacing the hydroxyl (–OH) group of a sugar by another group. (If the sugar is glucose the compound is known as a **glucoside**.) Glycosides found in plants include some pharmacologically important products (such as *digitalis). Other plant glycosides are natural food toxins, present in cassava, almonds, and other plant products, and may yield hydrogen cyanide if the plant is not prepared properly before eating.

glycosuria *n.* the presence of glucose in the urine in abnormally large amounts. Only very minute quantities of this sugar may be found normally in the urine. Higher levels may be associated with diabetes mellitus, kidney disease, and some other conditions.

gnath- (gnatho-) *prefix denoting* the jaw. Example: **gnathoplasty** (plastic surgery of).

gnathion *n.* the lowest point of the midline of the lower jaw (mandible).

Gnathostoma *n.* a genus of parasitic nematodes. Adult worms are commonly found in the intestines of tigers, leopards, and dogs. The presence of the larval stage of *G. spinigerum* in man, who is not the normal host, causes a skin condition called *creeping eruption.

gnotobiotic *adj.* describing germ-free conditions or a germ-free animal that has been inoculated with known microorganisms.

GnRH *see* GONADOTROPHIN-RELEASING HORMONE.

GnRH analogue *see* GONADOTROPHIN-RELEASING HORMONE, LHRH ANALOGUE.

goblet cell a column-shaped secretory cell found in the *epithelium of the respiratory and intestinal tracts. Goblet cells secrete the principal constituents of mucus.

goitre *n.* a swelling of the neck due to enlargement of the thyroid gland. This may be due to lack of dietary iodine, which is necessary for the production of thyroid hormone: the gland enlarges in an attempt to increase the output of hormone. This was the cause of **endemic goitre**, formerly common in regions where the diet lacked iodine. **Sporadic goitre** may be due to simple overgrowth (hyperplasia) of the gland or to a tumour.

In **exophthalmic goitre (Graves's disease)** the swelling is associated with overactivity of the gland and is accompanied by other symptoms (*see* THYROTOXICOSIS). Autoimmune thyroiditis can be associated with goitre (*see* HASHIMOTO'S DISEASE).

gold *n.* **1.** a bright yellow metal that is very malleable. In dentistry pure gold is occasionally used as a filling. Alloys are used for *crowns, *inlays, and *bridges, either alone or veneered with a tooth-coloured material. Gold alloys are now only rarely used as the metal framework for partial dentures, *cobalt-chromium alloys being used instead. **2.** (in pharmacology) any of several compounds of the metal gold, used in the treatment of rheumatoid arthritis. **Sodium aurothiomalate (Myocrisin)** is administered by intramuscular injection. Common side-effects include mouth ulcers, itching, blood disorders, skin reactions, and inflammation of the colon and kidneys. *Auranofin is a gold compound administered orally.

golfer's elbow inflammation of the origin of the muscle on the inside of the elbow caused by overuse. Treatment is by rest, anti-inflammatory medication, or steroid injection. *Compare* TENNIS ELBOW.

Golgi apparatus a collection of vesicles and folded membranes in a cell, usually connected to the *endoplasmic reticulum. It stores and later transports the proteins manufactured in the endoplasmic reticulum. The Golgi apparatus is well developed in cells that produce secretions, e.g. pancreatic cells producing digestive enzymes. [C. Golgi (1844–1926), Italian histologist]

Golgi cells types of *neurones (nerve cells) within the central nervous system. **Golgi type I neurones** have very long axons that connect different parts of the system; **Golgi type II neurones**, also known as **microneurones**, have only short axons or sometimes none.

Golgi tendon organ *see* TENDON ORGAN.

Gomori's method a method of staining for the demonstration of enzymes, especially phosphatases and lipases, in histological specimens. [G. Gomori (1904–57), Hungarian histochemist]

gomphosis *n.* a form of *synarthrosis

(immovable joint) in which a conical process fits into a socket. An example is the joint between the root of a tooth and the socket in the jawbone.

gonad *n.* a male or female reproductive organ that produces the gametes. *See* OVARY, TESTIS.

gonadorelin *n.* a synthetic analogue of gonadotrophin-releasing hormone (*see* LHRH ANALOGUE), administered by intravenous injection to stimulate the production of pituitary gonadotrophins. It is used in the treatment of *amenorrhoea and certain types of infertility.

gonadotrophin (gonadotrophic hormone) *n.* any of several hormones synthesized and released by the pituitary gland that act on the testes or ovaries (gonads) to promote production of sex hormones and either sperm or ova. Their production is controlled by *gonadotrophin-releasing hormone. The main gonadotrophins are *follicle-stimulating hormone and *luteinizing hormone. They may be given by injection to treat infertility. *See also* HUMAN CHORIONIC GONADOTROPHIN.

gonadotrophin-releasing hormone (GnRH) a peptide hormone produced in the hypothalamus and transported via the bloodstream to the pituitary gland, where it controls the synthesis and release of pituitary *gonadotrophins. **GnRH analogues**, which are also known as *LHRH analogues, are used to treat endometriosis, fibroids, some types of infertility, and prostate cancer.

gonagra *n.* gout in the knee.

goni- (gonio-) *prefix denoting* an anatomical angle or corner.

goniometer *n.* an instrument for measuring angles, such as those made in joint movements.

gonion *n.* the point of the angle of the lower jawbone (mandible).

goniopuncture *n.* a rarely performed operation for congenital glaucoma (*see* BUPHTHALMOS) to enable fluid to be drawn from the eye. Using a fine knife, an incision is made from within the eye into Schlemm's canal, at the junction of the cornea and sclera, and continued outwards until the knife appears beneath the conjunctiva. This creates a pathway for fluid to drain from the anterior chamber of the eye to the subconjunctival tissue. The tip of the knife within the eye is observed through a special contact lens.

gonioscope *n.* a special lens used for viewing the structures around the edge of the anterior chamber of the eye (in front of the iris). These structures are hidden behind the sclera at the periphery of the cornea and are not accessible to direct viewing.

goniotomy (trabeculotomy) *n.* an operation for congenital glaucoma (*see* BUPHTHALMOS). A fine knife is used to make an incision into Schlemm's canal from within the eye. It is the first stage of *goniopuncture.

gonococcus *n.* (*pl.* **gonococci**) the causative agent of gonorrhoea: the bacterium *Neisseria gonorrhoeae. —**gonococcal** *adj.*

gonocyte *n.* *see* GERM CELL.

gonorrhoea *n.* a sexually transmitted disease, caused by the bacterium *Neisseria gonorrhoeae*, that affects the genital mucous membranes of either sex. Symptoms develop about a week after infection and include pain on passing urine and discharge of pus (known as **gleet**) from the penis (in men) or vagina (in women); some infected women, however, experience no symptoms. If a pregnant woman has gonorrhoea, her baby's eyes may become infected during passage through the birth canal (*see* OPHTHALMIA NEONATORUM). In untreated cases, the infection may spread throughout the reproductive system, causing sterility; severe inflammation of the urethra in men can prevent passage of urine (a condition known as *stricture). Later complications include arthritis, inflammation of the heart valves (*endocarditis), and infection of the eyes, causing conjunctivitis. Treatment with sulphonamides, penicillin, or tetracycline in the early stages of the disease is usually effective.

good neighbour scheme (in Britain) a voluntary experimental scheme organized by social service departments of local authorities to bridge the gap in the care of the elderly between total independence and the provision of a care assistant. *See also* SOCIAL SERVICES.

goose flesh the reaction of the skin to cold or fear. The blood vessels contract and the small muscle attached to the base of each hair follicle also contracts, causing the hairs to stand up: this gives the skin an appearance of plucked goose skin.

GORD *see* GASTRO-OESOPHAGEAL REFLUX DISEASE.

gorget *n.* an instrument used in the operation for removal of stones from the bladder. It is a *director or guide with a wide groove.

goserelin *n. see* LHRH ANALOGUE.

Gott shunt a heparin-bonded shunt used to bypass sections of aorta that are being operated on. It is one of several shunts used in operations on the heart and arteries.

A gouge

gouge *n.* a curved chisel used in orthopaedic operations to cut and remove bone (see illustration).

goundou (anákhré) *n.* a condition following an infection with *yaws in which the nasal processes of the upper jaw bone thicken (*see* HYPEROSTOSIS) to form two large bony swellings, about 7 cm in diameter, on either side of the nose. The swellings not only obstruct the nostrils but also interfere with the field of vision. Initial symptoms include persistent headache and a bloody purulent discharge from the nose. Early cases can be treated with injections of penicillin; otherwise surgical removal of the growths is necessary. Goundou occurs in central Africa and South America.

gout *n.* a disease in which a defect in uric acid metabolism causes an excess of the acid and its salts (urates) to accumulate in the bloodstream and the joints respectively. It results in attacks of acute gouty arthritis and chronic destruction of the joints and deposits of urates (**tophi**) in the skin and cartilage, especially of the ears. The excess of urates also damages the kidneys, in which stones may form. Treatment with drugs that increase the excretion of urates (*uricosuric drugs) or with *allopurinol, which slows their formation, can control the disease. Acute attacks of gout are treated with anti-inflammatory analgesics. *See also* PODAGRA.

Graafian follicle a mature follicle in the ovary prior to ovulation, containing a large fluid-filled cavity that distends the surface of the ovary. The *oocyte develops inside the follicle, attached to one side. [R. de Graaf (1641–73), Dutch physician and anatomist]

graded self-exposure a technique used in the *behaviour therapy of phobias. A hierarchy of fears (increasingly fearful stimuli) is set up and the patients expose themselves to each level of the hierarchy in turn. Exposure continues until *habituation occurs before proceeding to the next highest level of the hierarchy. The patient is then ultimately able to cope with the feared object or situation.

graft **1.** *n.* any organ, tissue, or object used for *transplantation to replace a faulty part of the body. A *skin graft is a piece of skin cut from a healthy part of the body and used to heal a damaged area of skin. A **bone graft** is healthy bone collected from the patient or from another person and used to fill a defect in a bone or as a stimulus to fracture healing. A healthy kidney removed from one person and transplanted to another individual is described as a **kidney** (or **renal**) **graft**. Corneal grafts are taken from a recently dead individual to repair corneal opacity (*see* KERATOPLASTY). Diseased coronary arteries may be replaced by a *coronary bypass graft. Artificial tubes and valves are used to replace diseased peripheral arteries and heart valves, respectively. **2.** *vb.* to transplant an organ or tissue. *See also* HETEROGRAFT, HOMOGRAFT.

graft-versus-host disease (GVHD) a condition that occurs following bone marrow transplantation and sometimes blood transfusion, in which lymphocytes from the graft attack specific tissues in the host. The skin, gut, and liver are the most severely affected. Drugs that suppress the immune reaction, such as steroids and *cyclosporin A, reduce the severity of the rejection.

grain *n.* a unit of mass equal to 1/7000 of a pound (avoirdupois). 1 grain = 0.0648 gram.

gram *n.* a unit of mass equal to one thousandth of a kilogram. Symbol: g.

-gram *suffix denoting* a record; tracing. Example: **electrocardiogram** (record of an electrocardiograph).

gramicidin *n.* an *antibiotic that acts against a wide range of bacteria. It is used alone or in combination with other antibiotics or antiseptics in ointments, solutions, or sprays for the treatment of infected ulcers, wounds, and burns.

Gram's stain a method of staining bacterial cells, used as a primary means of identification. A film of bacteria spread onto a glass slide is dried and heat-fixed, stained with a violet dye, treated with decolourizer (e.g. alcohol), and then counterstained with red dye. **Gram-negative** bacteria lose the initial stain but take up the counterstain, so that they appear red microscopically. **Gram-positive** bacteria retain the initial stain, appearing violet microscopically. These staining differences are based on variations in the structure of the cell wall in the two groups. [H. C. J. Gram (1853–1938), Danish physician]

grand mal (major epilepsy) *see* EPILEPSY.

grand multiparity the condition of a woman who has had six or more previous pregnancies. Such women are more prone to the accidents of labour and to some of the diseases of pregnancy.

granular cast a cellular *cast derived from a kidney tubule. In certain kidney diseases, notably acute *glomerulonephritis, abnormal collections of renal tubular cells are shed from the kidney, often as a cast of the tubule. The casts can be observed on microscopic examination of the centrifuged deposit of a specimen of urine. Their presence in the urine indicates continued activity of the disease.

granulation *n.* the growth of small rounded outgrowths, made up of small blood vessels and connective tissue, on the healing surface of a wound (when the edges do not fit closely together) or an ulcer. Granulation is a normal stage in the healing process.

granulocyte *n.* any of a group of white blood cells that, when stained with *Romanowsky stains, are seen to contain granules in their cytoplasm. They can be subclassified on the basis of the colour of the stained granules into *neutrophils, *eosinophils, and *basophils.

granulocytopenia *n.* a reduction in the number of *granulocytes (a type of white cell) in the blood. *See* NEUTROPENIA.

granuloma *n.* (*pl.* **granulomata** or **granulomas**) a mass of *granulation tissue produced in response to chronic infection, inflammation, a foreign body, or to unknown causes. Infections giving rise to granulomata include tuberculosis, syphilis, *granuloma inguinale, leprosy, and some fungal diseases, such as coccidioidomycosis. Granulomata may occur as reactions to such foreign bodies as starch and talc following surgical procedures or to some metals, such as beryllium and zirconium. Sarcoidosis and Crohn's disease are granulomatous diseases of which the causes are not known. A granuloma may also occur around the apex of a tooth root as a result of inflammation or infection of its pulp. —**granulomatous** *adj.*

granuloma annulare a chronic skin condition of unknown cause. In the common localized type there is a ring or rings of closely set papules, 1–5 cm in diameter, found principally on the hands and arms.

granuloma inguinale an infectious disease caused by *Calymmatobacterium granulomatis*, which is known to be transmitted during sexual intercourse. It is marked by a pimply rash on and around the genital organs, which develops into a granulomatous ulcer. The disease responds to treatment with tetracyclines and streptomycin.

granulomatosis *n.* any condition marked by multiple widespread *granulomata. *See also* WEGENER'S GRANULOMATOSIS.

granulopoiesis *n.* the process of production of *granulocytes, which normally occurs in the blood-forming tissue of the graph- 282

*bone marrow. Granulocytes are ultimately derived from a *haemopoietic stem cell, but the earliest precursor that can be identified microscopically is the *myeloblast. This divides and passes through a series of stages of maturation termed respectively *promyelocyte, *myelocyte, and *metamyelocyte, before becoming a mature granulocyte. *See also* HAEMOPOIESIS.

graph- (grapho-) *prefix denoting* handwriting.

-graph *suffix denoting* an instrument that records. Example: **electrocardiograph** (instrument recording heart activity).

graphology *n.* the study of the characteristics of handwriting to obtain indications about a person's psychological make-up or state of health. It is possible to detect certain signs of physical disease, such as fine nervous tremors or irregularity of the pulse.

grattage *n.* the process of brushing or scraping the surface of a slowly healing ulcer or wound to remove *granulation tissue, which – though a stage in the healing process – sometimes overgrows or becomes infected and therefore delays healing. Grattage is used in the treatment of *trachoma.

gravel *n.* small stones formed in the urinary tract. The stones usually consist of calcareous debris or aggregations of other crystalline material. The passage of gravel from the kidneys is usually associated with severe pain (**ureteric colic**) and may cause blood in the urine. *See also* CALCULUS.

Graves's disease (exophthalmic goitre) *see* THYROTOXICOSIS. [R. J. Graves (1797–1853), Irish physician]

gravid *adj.* pregnant.

Grawitz tumour *see* HYPERNEPHROMA. [P. A. Grawitz (1850–1932), German pathologist]

gray *n.* the *SI unit of absorbed dose of ionizing radiation, being the absorbed dose when the energy per unit mass imparted to matter by ionizing radiation is 1 joule per kilogram. It has replaced the rad. Symbol: Gy.

green monkey disease *see* MARBURG DISEASE.

greenstick fracture an incomplete break in a bone in which part of the outer shell (cortex) remains intact. It occurs in children, who have more flexible bones. *See also* FRACTURE.

grey matter the darker coloured tissues of the central nervous system, composed mainly of the cell bodies of neurones, branching dendrites, and glial cells (*compare* WHITE MATTER). In the brain grey matter forms the *cerebral cortex and the outer layer of the cerebellum; in the spinal cord the grey matter lies centrally and is surrounded by white matter.

grey scale (in radiology) a scale representing the gradation of densities in a black-and-white image. Contrast between structures can be altered by increasing or decreasing the number of divisions.

gripe *n.* severe abdominal pain (*see* COLIC).

griseofulvin *n.* an *antibiotic administered by mouth to treat fungal infections of the hair, skin, and nails, such as ringworm. Mild and temporary side-effects such as headache, skin rashes, and digestive upsets may occur. Trade names: **Fulcin, Grisovin**.

groin *n.* the external depression on the front of the body that marks the junction of the abdomen with either of the thighs. *See also* INGUINAL.

grommet *n.* a flanged metal or plastic tube that is inserted in the eardrum in cases of *glue ear. It allows air to enter the middle ear, bypassing the patient's own nonfunctioning *Eustachian tube.

ground substance the matrix of *connective tissue, in which various cells and fibres are embedded.

group practice *see* GENERAL PRACTITIONER.

group therapy 1. (group psychotherapy) *psychotherapy involving at least two patients and a therapist. The patients are encouraged to understand and to analyse their own and one another's problems. *See also* ENCOUNTER GROUP, PSYCHODRAMA. **2.** therapy in which people with the same problem, such as *alcoholism, meet and discuss together their difficulties and possible ways of overcoming them.

growth factor any of various chemicals, particularly polypeptides, that have a variety of important roles in the stimulation of new cell growth and cell maintenance. They bind to the cell surface on receptors. Specific growth factors can cause new cell proliferation (**epidermal growth factor, haemopoietic growth factor**) and the migration of cells (**fibroblast growth factor**) and play a role in wound healing (**platelet-derived growth factor; PDGF**). Some growth factors act in the embryonic stage of development; for example, *nerve growth factor. It is thought that some growth factors that induce cell proliferation are involved in the abnormal regulation of growth seen in cancer when produced in excessive amounts (e.g. **insulin-like growth factor, IGF-I**). Growth factors produced locally around a carcinoma (e.g. **vascular endothelial growth factor**) are important in the encouragement of invasion by the tumour; other factors (e.g. autocrine motility factor, migration-stimulating factor) are also significant. *See also* BONE GROWTH FACTOR.

growth hormone (GH, somatotrophin) a hormone, synthesized and stored in the anterior pituitary gland, that promotes growth of the long bones in the limbs and increases protein synthesis (via *somatomedin). Its release is controlled by the opposing actions of **growth-hormone releasing hormone** and *somatostatin. Excessive production of growth hormone results in *gigantism before puberty and *acromegaly in adults. Lack of growth hormone in children causes *dwarfism.

grumous *adj.* coarse; lumpy; clotted; often used to describe the appearance of the centre of wounds or diseased cells or the surface of a bacterial culture.

GSI genuine stress incontinence. *See* INCONTINENCE.

guaiphenesin *n.* an *expectorant used in cough mixtures and tablets.

guanethidine *n.* a drug that is used to reduce high blood pressure (*see* SYMPATHOLYTIC). It is administered by mouth;

common side-effects are diarrhoea, faintness, and dizziness. Trade name: **Ismelin**.

guanine *n.* one of the nitrogen-containing bases (*see* PURINE) that occurs in the nucleic acids DNA and RNA.

guanosine *n.* a compound containing guanine and the sugar ribose. *See also* NUCLEOTIDE.

gubernaculum *n.* (*pl.* **gubernacula**) either of a pair of fibrous strands of tissue that connect the gonads to the inguinal region in the fetus. In the male they guide and possibly move the testes into the scrotum before birth. In the female the ovaries descend only slightly within the abdominal cavity and the gubernacula persist as the round ligaments connecting the ovaries and uterus to the abdominal wall.

Guillain-Barré syndrome (postinfective polyneuropathy) a disease of the peripheral nerves in which there is numbness and weakness in the limbs. It usually develops 10–20 days after a respiratory or gastrointestinal infection (commonly with *Campylobacter*) that provokes an allergic response in the peripheral nerves. A rapidly progressive form of the disease is called **Landry's paralysis**: paralysis starts in the hands and feet and ascends to the neck; involvement of the respiratory muscles may require mechanical ventilation. Recovery is usually excellent although often prolonged. Treatment with immunoglobulins may speed recovery and reduce long-term disability. *See* POLYRADICULITIS. [G. Guillain (1876–1961) and A. Barré (1880–1967), French neurologists]

A tonsil guillotine

guillotine *n.* (in surgery) **1.** an instrument used for removing the tonsils. It is loop-shaped and contains a sliding knife blade (see illustration). **2.** an encircling suture to control the escape of fluid or blood from an orifice or to close a gap.

guinea worm a nematode worm, *Dracunculus medinensis*, that is a parasite of man. The white threadlike adult female, 60–120 cm long, lives in the connective tissues beneath the skin. It releases its larvae into a large blister on the legs or arms; when the limbs are immersed in water the larvae escape and are subsequently eaten by tiny water fleas (*Cyclops*), inside which their development continues. The disease *dracontiasis results from drinking water contaminated with *Cyclops*.

Gulf War syndrome a variety of symptoms, mainly neurological (including chronic fatigue, dizziness, amnesia, digestive upsets, and muscle wasting), that have been attributed to exposure of armed forces personnel to chemicals (e.g. insecticides) used during the Gulf War (1991) or possibly to the effects of vaccines and tablets given to protect personnel against the anticipated threat of chemical and biological warfare during the conflict. Medical research into the syndrome is continuing.

gullet *n. see* OESOPHAGUS.

gum *n.* (in anatomy) *see* GINGIVA.

gumboil *n.* the opening on the surface of the gum of a *sinus tract from a chronic abscess associated with the roots of a tooth. It may be accompanied by varying degrees of swelling, pain, and discharge.

gumma *n.* a small soft tumour, characteristic of the tertiary stage of *syphilis, that occurs in connective tissue, the liver, brain, testes, heart, or bone.

gumshield *n.* a soft flexible cover that fits over the teeth for protection in contact sports. The best type is specially made to fit the individual.

gunshot wound a common cause of both military and civil injuries. Gunshot wounds are usually produced by high-velocity missiles: deep-seated tissue destruction of thermal origin is a major complication.

gustation *n.* the sense of taste or the act of tasting.

gustatory *adj.* relating to the sense of taste or to the organs of taste.

gut *n.* **1.** *see* INTESTINE. **2.** *see* CATGUT.

Guthrie test examination of a drop of blood to exclude the presence of *phenylketonuria. This rare metabolic disorder (with an estimated incidence of 1/20,000) has severe consequences in terms of mental handicap unless the child receives a special diet from an early age. It is performed once milk feeding has been established, on the sixth or seventh day of life. [R. Guthrie (1916–   ), US paediatrician]

gutta *n.* (*pl.* **guttae**) (in pharmacy) a drop. Drops are the form in which medicines are applied to the eyes and ears.

gutta-percha *n.* the juice of an evergreen Malaysian tree, which is hard at room temperature but becomes soft and elastic when heated in hot water. On cooling, gutta-percha will retain any deformity imparted to it when hot; thus it was used in dentistry as an impression material and as a temporary filling material. It has been superseded for these purposes by better materials, but is still used in the form of gutta-percha points as the principal core of *root fillings.

guttate *adj.* describing lesions in the skin that are shaped like drops.

GVHD *see* GRAFT-VERSUS-HOST DISEASE.

gyn- (gyno-, gynaec(o)-) *prefix denoting* women or the female reproductive organs.

gynaecology *n.* the study of diseases of women and girls, particularly those affecting the female reproductive system. *Compare* OBSTETRICS. **—gynaecological** *adj.* **—gynaecologist** *n.*

gynaecomastia *n.* enlargement of the breasts in the male, due either to hormone imbalance or to hormone therapy.

gypsum *n. see* PLASTER OF PARIS.

gyr- (gyro-) *prefix denoting* **1.** a gyrus. **2.** a ring or circle.

gyrus *n.* (*pl.* **gyri**) a raised convolution of the *cerebral cortex, between two sulci (clefts).

Haab's striae splits or tears in *Descemet's membrane occurring during infancy, commonly as a result of childhood glaucoma. [O. Haab (1850–1931), German ophthalmologist]

habit *n.* a sequence of learned behaviour occurring in a particular context or as a response to particular events. Habits organize life, often in minute detail. They are often the result of *conditioning, are performed automatically and unconsciously, and reduce decision-making. Habits, once established, often persist after the original causal factors no longer operate. Behavioural psychology is based on the premise that one form of conditioning can be replaced by another.

habitual abortion *see* ABORTION.

habituation *n.* **1.** (in psychology) a simple type of learning consisting of a gradual waning response by the subject to a continuous or repeated stimulus that is not associated with *reinforcement. **2.** (in pharmacology) the condition of being psychologically dependent on a drug, following repeated consumption, marked by reduced sensitivity to its effects and a craving for the drug if it is withdrawn. *See also* DEPENDENCE.

habitus *n.* an individual's general physical appearance, especially when this is associated with a constitutional tendency to a particular disease.

haem *n.* an iron-containing compound (a *porphyrin) that combines with the protein globin to form *haemoglobin, found in the red blood cells.

haem- (haema-, haemo-, haemat(o)-) *prefix denoting* blood. Examples: **haematogenesis** (formation of); **haemophobia** (fear of).

haemagglutination *n.* the clumping of red blood cells (*see* AGGLUTINATION). It is caused by an antibody–antigen reaction or some viruses and other substances.

haemangioblastoma (Lindau's tumour) *n.* a tumour of the brain or spinal cord arising in the blood vessels of the meninges or brain. It is often associated with *phaeochromocytoma and *syringomyelia. *See also* VON HIPPEL-LINDAU DISEASE.

haemangioma *n.* a benign tumour of blood vessels. It often appears on the skin as a type of birthmark; the strawberry *naevus is an example. *See also* ANGIOMA.

Haemaphysalis *n.* a genus of hard *ticks. Certain species transmit tick *typhus in the Old World; *H. spinigera* transmits the virus causing *Kyasanur Forest disease in India.

haemarthrosis *n.* joint pain and swelling caused by bleeding into a joint. This may follow injury or may occur spontaneously in a disease of the blood, such as *haemophilia. Treatment is by immobilization, cold compresses, and correction of the blood disorder (if present). Removal of blood from the joint may relieve the pain.

haematemesis *n.* the act of vomiting blood. The blood may have been swallowed (e.g. following nosebleed or tonsillectomy) but more often arises from bleeding in the oesophagus, stomach, or duodenum. Common causes are gastric and duodenal ulcers, and varicose veins in the oesophagus. If much blood is lost, it is usually replaced by blood transfusion. If bleeding does not stop spontaneously it may be arrested by coagulation of the bleeding point using either a *laser or a *heater-probe, or by the injection of *adrenaline or a sclerosing material: all these techniques are applied through an *endoscope. *See also* MELAENA.

haemathidrosis (haematidrosis) *n.* *see* HAEMATOHIDROSIS.

haematin *n.* a chemical derivative of *haemoglobin formed by removal of the protein part of the molecule and oxidation of the iron atom from the ferrous to the ferric form.

haematinic *n.* a drug that increases the

amount of *haemoglobin in the blood, e.g. *ferrous sulphate and other iron-containing compounds. Haematinics are used, often in combination with vitamins and *folic acid, to prevent and treat anaemia due t to iron deficiency. They are used particularly to prevent anaemia during pregnancy. Digestive disturbances sometimes occur with haematinics.

haematocoele n. a swelling caused by leakage of blood into a cavity, especially that of the tunica vaginalis, the membrane overlying the front and sides of the *testis. A **parametric (pelvic) haematocoele** is a swelling near the uterus formed by the escape of blood, usually from a Fallopian tube in ectopic pregnancy.

haematocolpos n. the accumulation of menstrual blood in the vagina because the hymen at the entrance to the vagina lacks an opening. See CRYPTOMENORRHOEA.

haematocrit n. see PACKED CELL VOLUME.

haematocyst n. a cyst that contains blood.

haematogenous (haematogenic) adj. **1.** relating to the production of blood or its constituents; haematopoietic. **2.** produced by, originating in, or carried by the blood.

haematohidrosis (haemathidrosis, haematidrosis) n. the secretion of sweat containing blood.

haematology n. the study of blood and blood-forming tissues and the disorders associated with them. —**haematological** adj. —**haematologist** n.

haematoma n. an accumulation of blood within the tissues that clots to form a solid swelling. Injury, disease of the blood vessels, or a clotting disorder of the blood are the usual causative factors. An **intracranial haematoma** causes symptoms by compressing the brain and by raising the pressure within the skull. A blunt injury to the head, especially the temple, may tear the middle meningeal artery, giving rise to a rapidly accumulating **extradural haematoma** requiring urgent surgical treatment. In elderly people a relatively slight head injury may tear the veins where they cross the space beneath the dura, giving rise to a **subdural haematoma**. Excellent results are obtained by surgical treatment. An **intracerebral haematoma** may be a consequence of severe head injury but is more often due to atheromatous disease of the cerebral arteries and high blood pressure resulting in bleeding into the brain. See also PERIANAL HAEMATOMA.

haematometra n. **1.** accumulation of menstrual blood in the uterus. **2.** any abnormally copious bleeding in the uterus.

haematomyelia n. bleeding into the tissue of the spinal cord. This may result in acutely developing symptoms that mimic *syringomyelia.

haematopoiesis n. see HAEMOPOIESIS.

haematoporphyrin n. a type of *porphyrin produced during the metabolism of haemoglobin.

haematosalpinx (haemosalpinx) n. the accumulation of menstrual blood in the *Fallopian tubes.

haematoxylin n. a colourless crystalline compound extracted from logwood (*Haematoxylon campechianum*) and used in various histological stains. When oxidized haematoxylin is converted to **haematein**, which imparts a blue colour to certain parts of cells, especially cell nuclei. **Heidenhain's iron haematoxylin** is used to stain sections that are to be photographed, since it gives great clarity at high magnification.

haematuria n. the presence of blood in the urine. The blood may come from the kidneys, one or both ureters, the bladder, or the urethra, as a result of injury or disease.

haemin n. a chemical derivative of haemoglobin formed by removal of the protein part of the molecule, oxidation of the iron atom, and combination with an acid to form a salt (*compare* HAEMATIN). **Chlorohaemin** forms characteristic crystals, the identification of which provides the basis of a chemical test for blood stains.

haemo- *prefix. see* HAEM-.

Haemobartonella n. see BARTONELLA.

haemochromatosis (bronze dia-

betes, iron-storage disease) *n.* a hereditary disorder in which there is excessive absorption and storage of iron. This leads to damage and functional impairment of many organs, including the liver, pancreas, and endocrine glands. The main features are a bronze colour of the skin, diabetes, and liver failure. Iron may be removed from the body by blood letting or an iron *chelating agent may be administered. *Compare* HAEMOSIDEROSIS.

haemoconcentration *n.* an increase in the proportion of red blood cells relative to the plasma, brought about by a decrease in the volume of plasma. Haemoconcentration may occur in any condition in which there is a severe loss of water from the body. *Compare* HAEMODILUTION.

haemocytometer *n.* a special glass chamber of known volume into which diluted blood is introduced. The numbers of the various blood cells present are then counted visually, through a microscope. Haemocytometers have been largely replaced by electronic cell counters.

haemodialysis *n.* a technique of removing waste materials or poisons from the blood using the principle of *dialysis. Haemodialysis is performed on patients whose kidneys have ceased to function; the process takes place in an **artificial kidney**, or **dialyser**. The stream of blood taken from an artery is circulated through the dialyser on one side of a semipermeable membrane, while a solution of similar electrolytic composition to the patient's blood circulates on the other side. Water and waste products from the patient's blood filter through the membrane, whose pores are too small to allow passage of blood cells and proteins. The purified blood is then returned to the patient's body through a vein.

haemodilution *n.* a decrease in the proportion of red blood cells relative to the plasma, brought about by an increase in the total volume of plasma. This may occur in a variety of conditions, including pregnancy and enlargement of the spleen (*see* HYPERSPLENISM). *Compare* HAEMOCONCENTRATION.

haemoglobin *n.* a substance contained within the red blood cells (*erythrocytes)

and responsible for their colour, composed of the pigment **haem** (an iron-containing *porphyrin) linked to the protein **globin**. Haemoglobin has the unique property of combining reversibly with oxygen and is the medium by which oxygen is transported within the body. It takes up oxygen as blood passes through the lungs and releases it as blood passes through the tissues. Blood normally contains 12–18 g/dl of haemoglobin. *See also* MYOHAEMOGLOBIN, OXYHAEMOGLOBIN.

haemoglobinometer *n.* an instrument for determining the concentration of *haemoglobin in a sample of blood, which is a measure of its ability to carry oxygen.

haemoglobinopathy *n.* any of a group of inherited diseases, such as *thalassaemia and *sickle-cell disease, in which there is an abnormality in the production of haemoglobin.

haemoglobinuria *n.* the presence in the urine of free haemoglobin. The condition occurs if haemoglobin, released from disintegrating red blood cells, cannot be taken up rapidly enough by blood proteins. The condition sometimes follows strenuous exercise. It is also associated with certain infectious diseases (such as blackwater fever), ingestion of certain chemicals (such as arsenic), and injury.

haemogram *n.* the results of a routine blood test, including an estimate of the blood haemoglobin level, the *packed cell volume, and the numbers of red and white blood cells (*see* BLOOD COUNT). Any abnormalities seen in microscopic examination of the blood are also noted.

haemolysin *n.* a substance capable of bringing about destruction of red blood cells (*haemolysis). It may be an antibody or a bacterial toxin.

haemolysis *n.* the destruction of red blood cells (*erythrocytes). Within the body, haemolysis may result from defects within the red cells or from poisoning, infection, or the action of antibodies; it may occur in mismatched blood transfusions. It usually leads to anaemia. Haemolysis of blood specimens may result from unsatisfactory collection or storage or be brought about intentionally as part of an analytical procedure (*see* LAKING).

haemolytic *adj.* causing, associated with, or resulting from destruction of red blood cells (*erythrocytes). For example, a **haemolytic antibody** is one that causes destruction of red cells; a **haemolytic anaemia** is due to red-cell destruction (*see* ANAEMIA).

haemolytic disease of the newborn the condition resulting from destruction (haemolysis) of the red blood cells of the fetus by antibodies in the mother's blood passing through the placenta. This most commonly happens when the red blood cells of the fetus are Rh positive (i.e. they have the *rhesus factor) but the mother's red cells are Rh negative. The fetal cells are therefore incompatible in her circulation and evoke the production of antibodies. This may result in very severe anaemia of the fetus, leading to heart failure with oedema (*hydrops fetalis) or stillbirth. When the anaemia is less severe the fetus may reach term in good condition, but the accumulation of the bile pigment bilirubin from the destroyed cells causes severe jaundice after birth, which may require *exchange transfusion. If untreated it may cause serious brain damage (*see* KERNICTERUS).

A blood test early in pregnancy enables the detection of antibodies in the mother's blood and the adoption of various precautions for the infant's safety. Some cases of predictably very severe haemolytic disease have been successfully treated by intrauterine transfusion. The incidence of the disease has been greatly reduced by preventing the formation of antibodies in a Rh negative mother. If at birth or after an abortion the baby's blood is found to be incompatible with the mother's (i.e. Rh positive) she is given an injection of Rh antibody (anti-D immunoglobulin). This rapidly destroys any Rh positive fetal cells so that they do not remain long enough to stimulate antibody production in her blood (which could affect her next pregnancy).

haemolytic uraemic syndrome a condition in which sudden rapid destruction of red blood cells (*see* HAEMOLYSIS) causes acute renal failure due partly to obstruction of small arteries in the kidneys. The haemolysis also causes a reduction in the number of platelets, which can lead to severe haemorrhage. The syndrome may occur as a result of septicaemia following a respiratory or gastrointestinal infection (especially by pathogenic *Escherichia coli), eclamptic fits in pregnancy (*see* ECLAMPSIA), or as a reaction to certain drugs. There may also be small sporadic outbreaks of the condition without any obvious cause.

haemopericardium *n.* the presence of blood within the membranous sac (pericardium) surrounding the heart, which may result from injury, tumours, rupture of the heart (e.g. following myocardial infarction), or a leaking aneurysm. The heart is compressed (**cardiac tamponade**) and the circulation impaired; a large fall in blood pressure and cardiac arrest may result. Surgical drainage of the blood may be life saving.

haemoperitoneum *n.* the presence of blood in the peritoneal cavity, between the lining of the abdomen or pelvis and the membrane covering the organs within.

haemophilia *n.* a hereditary disorder in which the blood clots very slowly, due to a deficiency of either of two *coagulation factors: Factor VIII (antihaemophilic factor) or Factor IX (Christmas factor). The patient may experience prolonged bleeding following any injury or wound, and in severe cases there is spontaneous bleeding into muscles and joints. Bleeding in haemophilia may be treated by transfusions of plasma (which contains the missing factor). Alternatively concentrated preparations of Factor VIII or Factor IX, obtained by freezing fresh plasma, may be administered (*see* CRYOPRECIPITATE). Haemophilia is controlled by a *sex-linked gene, which means that it is almost exclusively restricted to males: women can carry the disease – and pass it on to their sons – without being affected themselves. —**haemophiliac** *n.*

Haemophilus *n.* a genus of Gram-negative aerobic nonmotile parasitic rodlike bacteria frequently found in the respiratory tract. They can grow only in the presence of certain factors in the blood and/or certain coenzymes: they are cultured on fresh blood *agar. Most species are pathogenic: *H. aegyptius* causes conjunctivitis, and *H. ducreyi* soft sore (chancroid). *H. influenzae* is associated with acute and chronic respiratory infections (*see also* EPIGLOTTITIS) and is a common secondary cause of *influenza infections; *H. influenzae* type B is an important cause of bacterial *meningitis in young children (*see* HIB VACCINE).

haemophthalmia *n.* bleeding into the *vitreous humour of the eye: vitreous haemorrhage.

haemopneumothorax *n.* the presence of both blood and air in the pleural cavity, usually as a result of injury. Both must be drained out to allow the lung to expand normally. *See also* HAEMOTHORAX.

haemopoiesis *n.* the process of production of blood cells and platelets which continues throughout life, replacing aged cells (which are removed from the circulation). In healthy adults, haemopoiesis is confined to the *bone marrow, but in embryonic life and in early infancy, as well as in certain diseases, it may occur in other sites (**extramedullary haemopoiesis**). *See also* ERYTHROPOIESIS, LEUCOPOIESIS, THROMBOPOIESIS. —**haemopoietic** *adj.*

haemopoietic stem cell the cell from which all classes of blood cells are derived. It cannot be identified microscopically, although some workers believe that it is identical in appearance with a *lymphocyte. It can be demonstrated by *tissue culture of the blood-forming tissue of the bone marrow, as well as in certain other sites. *See also* HAEMOPOIESIS.

haemoptysis *n.* the coughing up of blood. This symptom should always be taken seriously, however small the amount. In some patients the cause is not serious; in others it is never found. But it should always be reported to a doctor.

haemorrhage (bleeding) *n.* the escape of blood from a ruptured blood vessel, externally or internally. Arterial blood is bright red and emerges in spurts, venous blood is dark red and flows steadily, while damage to minor vessels may produce only an oozing. Rupture of a major blood vessel such as the femoral artery can lead to the loss of several litres of blood in a few minutes, resulting in *shock, collapse,

and death, if untreated. *See also* HAEMATEMESIS, HAEMATURIA, HAEMOPTYSIS.

haemorrhagic *adj.* associated with or resulting from blood loss (*see* HAEMORRHAGE). For example, **haemorrhagic anaemia** is due to blood loss (*see* ANAEMIA).

haemorrhagic disease of the newborn a temporary disturbance in blood clotting caused by *vitamin K deficiency and affecting infants on the second to fourth day of life. It varies in severity from mild gastrointestinal bleeding to profuse bleeding into many organs, including the brain. It is more common in breast-fed and *preterm infants. The condition can be prevented by giving all babies vitamin K, either by injection or orally, shortly after birth. Medical name: **melaena neonatorum**.

haemorrhoidectomy *n.* the surgical operation for removing *haemorrhoids, which are tied and then excised. Possible complications are bleeding or, later, anal stricture (narrowing). The operation is usually performed only for second- or third-degree haemorrhoids that have not responded to simple measures.

haemorrhoids (piles) *pl. n.* enlargement of the normal spongy blood-filled cushions in the wall of the anus (**internal haemorrhoids**), usually a consequence of prolonged constipation or, occasionally, diarrhoea. They most commonly occur at three main points equidistant around the circumference of the anus. Uncomplicated haemorrhoids are seldom painful; any pain is usually caused by a *fissure. The main symptom is bleeding, and in **first-degree haemorrhoids**, which never appear at the anus, bleeding at the end of defaecation is the only symptom. **Second-degree haemorrhoids** protrude beyond the anus as an uncomfortable swelling but return spontaneously; **third-degree haemorrhoids** remain outside the anus and need to be returned by pressure.

First- and second-degree haemorrhoids may respond to bowel regulation using a high-fibre diet with faecal softening agents. If bleeding persists, an irritant fluid (a sclerosing agent) may be injected around the swollen cushions to make them shrivel up. Other effective treatments are infrared coagulation and the application of elastic bands. Third-degree haemorrhoids often require surgery (see HAEMORRHOIDECTOMY), especially if they become *strangulated (producing severe pain and further enlargement).

External haemorrhoids are either prolapsed internal haemorrhoids or – more often – *perianal haematomas or the residual skin tags remaining after a perianal haematoma has healed.

haemosalpinx n. see HAEMATOSALPINX.

haemosiderin n. a substance composed of a protein shell containing iron salts which may be present inside certain cells, being one of the forms in which iron is stored within the body. It is insoluble and may be demonstrated microscopically in suitably stained tissue preparations.

haemosiderosis n. a disorder caused by excessive deposition of iron, which in turn results from excessive intake or administration of iron, usually in the form of blood transfusions. It results in damage to various organs, including the heart and liver. Compare HAEMOCHROMATOSIS.

haemostasis n. the arrest of bleeding, involving the physiological processes of *blood coagulation and the contraction of damaged blood vessels. The term is also applied to various surgical procedures (for example the application of *ligatures or *diathermy to cut vessels) used to stop bleeding.

haemostatic (styptic) n. an agent that stops or prevents haemorrhage; for example, *phytomenadione and *thromboplastin. Haemostatics are used to control bleeding due to various causes and may be used in treating bleeding disorders, such as haemophilia.

haemothorax n. blood in the pleural cavity, usually due to injury. If the blood is not drained dense fibrous *adhesions occur between the pleural surfaces, which can impair the normal movement of the lung. The blood may also become infected (see EMPYEMA).

haemozoin n. an iron-containing pigment present in the organisms that cause malaria (*Plasmodium species).

hair n. a threadlike keratinized outgrowth of the epidermis of the *skin. It develops inside a tubular **hair follicle**. The part above the skin consists of three layers: an outer **cuticle**; a **cortex**, forming the bulk of the hair and containing the pigment that gives the hair its colour; and a central core (**medulla**), which may be hollow. The **root** of the hair, beneath the surface of the skin, is expanded at its base to form the **bulb**, which contains a matrix of dividing cells. As new cells are formed the older ones are pushed upwards and become keratinized to form the root and shaft. A hair may be raised by a small erector muscle in the dermis, attached to the hair follicle.

hairball n. see TRICHOBEZOAR.

hair follicle a sheath of epidermal cells and connective tissue that surrounds the root of a *hair.

hair papilla a projection of the dermis that is surrounded by the base of the hair bulb. It contains the capillaries that supply blood to the growing *hair.

hairy cell an abnormal white blood cell that has the appearance of an immature lymphocyte with fine hairlike cytoplasmic projections around the perimeter of the cell. It is found in a rare form of leukaemia (**hairy-cell leukaemia**) most commonly occurring in young men.

halfway house a residential home for a group of people where some professional supervision is available. It is used as a stage in the rehabilitation of the mentally ill, usually when they have just been discharged from hospital and are able to work but are not yet ready for independent life.

halitosis n. bad breath. Causes of temporary halitosis include recently eaten strongly flavoured food, such as garlic or onions, and drugs such as paraldehyde. Other causes include mouth breathing, *periodontal disease, and infective conditions of the nose, throat, and lungs (especially *bronchiectasis). Constipation, indigestion, and some liver diseases may also cause the condition.

hallucination n. a false perception of something that is not really there. Hallucinations may be visual, auditory, tactile, gustatory (of taste), or olfactory (of smell). They may be provoked by psychological illness (such as *schizophrenia) or physical disorders in the brain (such as temporal lobe *epilepsy or stroke) or they may be caused by drugs or sensory deprivation. Hallucinations should be distinguished from dreams and from *illusions (since they occur at the same time as real perceptions and are not based upon real stimuli).

hallucinogen n. a drug that produces hallucinations, e.g. *cannabis and *lysergic acid diethylamide. Hallucinogens were formerly used to treat certain types of mental illness. —**hallucinogenic** adj.

hallux n. (pl. **halluces**) the big toe.

hallux rigidus painful stiffness of the joint between the big toe and the first metatarsal bone, usually resulting from osteoarthritis. Conservative treatment is often successful, but in some cases *arthrodesis or *arthroplasty is required.

hallux valgus displacement of the big toe towards the others. It is often associated with a *bunion.

hallux varus displacement of the big toe away from the others.

haloperidol n. a *butyrophenone antipsychotic drug used to relieve anxiety and tension in the treatment of schizophrenia and other psychiatric disorders. It is administered by mouth or injection; muscular incoordination and restlessness are common side-effects. Trade names: **Haldol**, **Serenace**.

halophilic adj. requiring solutions of high salt concentration for healthy growth. Certain bacteria are halophilic. —**halophile** n.

halos pl. n. coloured rings seen around lights by people with acute congestive glaucoma and sometimes by people with cataract.

halothane n. a potent general *anaesthetic administered by inhalation, used for inducing and maintaining anaesthesia in all types of surgical operations. Reduced blood pressure and irregular heartbeat may occur during halothane anaesthesia. Trade name: **Fluothane**.

hamartoma n. an overgrowth of mature tissue in which the elements show disordered arrangement and proportion in comparison to normal. The overgrowth is benign but malignancy may occur in any of the constituent tissue elements.

hamate bone (unciform bone) a hook-shaped bone of the wrist (see CARPUS). It articulates with the capitate and triquetral bones at the sides, with the lunate bone behind, and with the fourth and fifth metacarpal bones in front.

hammer n. (in anatomy) see MALLEUS.

hammer toe a deformity of a toe, most often the second, caused by fixed flexion of the first joint. A corn often forms over the deformity, which may be painful. If severe pain does not respond to strapping or corrective footwear, it may be necessary to perform *arthrodesis at the affected joint.

hamstring n. any of the tendons at the back of the knee. They attach the **hamstring muscles** (the biceps femoris, semitendinosus, and semimembranosus) to their insertions in the tibia and fibula.

hamulus n. (pl. **hamuli**) any hooklike process, such as occurs on the hamate, lacrimal, and sphenoid bones and on the cochlea.

hand n. the terminal organ of the upper limb. From a surgical point of view, the human hand comprises the eight bones of the *carpus (wrist), the five metacarpal bones, and the phalangeal bones plus the surrounding tissues; anatomically, the bones and tissues of the wrist are excluded. The hand is a common site of infections and injuries, many of which are of industrial origin for which compensation may be claimed.

handedness n. the preferential use of one hand, rather than the other, in voluntary actions. Ambidexterity – the ability to use either hand with equal skill – is very rare. About 90% of people are right-handed and this correlates with the half of the brain that is dominant for speech: some 97% of right-handed people have left-hemisphere dominance for speech, whereas only 60% of left-handed people are right-hemisphere dominant for speech.

hand, foot, and mouth disease a

self-limiting disease, mainly affecting young children, caused by *Coxsackie virus A16. A feeling of mild illness is accompanied by mouth ulcers and painful blisters on the hands and feet.

handicap *n.* **1.** partial or total inability to perform a social, occupational, or other activity that the affected person wants to do. It reflects the extent to which an individual is disadvantaged by some partial or total *disability when compared with those in a peer group who have no such disability. A handicap is usually related to an identifiable structural **impairment**. It may also reflect functional impairment, which may be unsuspected by the individual and discovered by clinical observation or testing. The alternative terms **abnormality**, **defect**, or **malformation** (for impairment) and **malfunction** (for disability) are used by many authorities, which may sometimes cause confusion; in an attempt to resolve this, a working group of the *World Health Organization has suggested using the generic term **disablement**, but this has gained only limited acceptance. *See also* INTERNATIONAL CLASSIFICATION OF DISEASES. **2.** *see* MENTAL HANDICAP.

Hand-Schüller-Christian disease *see* RETICULOENDOTHELIOSIS. [A. Hand (1868–1949), US paediatrician; A. Schüller (1874–1958), Austrian neurologist; H. A. Christian (1876–1951), US physician]

Hansen's bacillus *see* MYCOBACTERIUM. [G. H. A. Hansen (1841–1912), Norwegian physician]

Hansen's disease *see* LEPROSY.

hantavirus *n.* one of a genus of viruses that infect rats, mice, and voles and cause disease in humans when the secretions or excreta of these rodents are inhaled or ingested. The disease was first reported from the area of the Hantaan river, which separates North from South Korea, but hantavirus infections also occur in Japan, China, Russia, Europe, and the USA: in Britain it can affect farm, nature conservancy, and sewage workers and those engaged in water sports. The symptoms vary according to the strain of the infecting virus. Many patients have a mild influenza-like illness, but severe cases are characterized by high fever, headache, shock, nausea and vomiting, and *petechiae in the skin; there may be kidney pain and rapidly progressive kidney damage leading to kidney failure. A particularly virulent strain in the USA attacks the lungs, leading to rapid respiratory failure. The mortality rate in these severe cases is high.

haploid (monoploid) *adj.* describing cells, nuclei, or organisms that have a single set of unpaired chromosomes. In man the gametes are haploid following *meiosis. *Compare* DIPLOID, TRIPLOID. —**haploid** *n.*

haplotype *n.* a complete set of *HLA antigens inherited from either parent.

hapt- (hapto-) *prefix denoting* touch.

hapten *n. see* ANTIGEN.

haptoglobin *n.* a protein present in blood plasma that binds with free haemoglobin to form a complex that is rapidly removed from the circulation by the liver. Depletion of plasma haptoglobin is a feature of anaemias in which red blood cells are destroyed inside the circulation with the release of haemoglobin into the plasma and its loss in the urine.

harara *n.* a severe and itchy inflammation of the skin occurring in people continuously subjected to the bites of the *sandfly *Phlebotomus papatasii*. The incidence of this allergic skin reaction, prevalent in the Middle East, may be checked by controlling the numbers of sandflies.

harelip *n. see* CLEFT LIP.

Harrison's sulcus a depression on both sides of the chest wall of a child between the pectoral muscles and the lower margin of the ribcage. It is caused by exaggerated suction of the diaphragm when breathing in and develops in conditions in which the airways are partially obstructed or when the lungs are abnormally congested due to some congenital abnormality of the heart. [E. Harrison (1789–1838), British physician]

Hartmann's operation a method of reconstruction after surgical removal of distal colon and proximal rectum, in which the rectal stump is closed off and the divided end of the colon is brought out as a *colostomy. The technique allows for a second-stage joining up of the bowel ends with no colostomy. [H. Hartmann (1860–1952), French surgeon]

Hartmann's pouch a saclike dilatation of the gall-bladder wall near its outlet; it is a common site for finding *gallstones.

Hartmann's solution a *physiological solution used for infusion into the circulation. In addition to essential ions, it also contains glucose. [A. F. Hartmann (1898–1964), US paediatrician]

Hartnup disease a rare hereditary defect in the absorption of the amino acid tryptophan, leading to mental retardation, thickening and roughening of the skin on exposure to light, and lack of muscular coordination. The condition is similar to *pellagra. Treatment with nicotinamide is usually effective. [Hartnup, the family in whom it was first reported]

harvest mite *see* TROMBICULA.

Hashimoto's disease chronic inflammation of the thyroid gland (**thyroiditis**) due to the formation of antibodies against normal thyroid tissue (autoantibodies; *see* THYROID ANTIBODIES). Its features include a firm swelling of the thyroid and partial or total failure of secretion of thyroid hormones; often there are autoantibodies to other organs, such as the stomach. Women are more often affected than men and the condition often occurs in families. [H. Hashimoto (1881–1934), Japanese surgeon]

hashish *n.* *see* CANNABIS.

haustrum *n.* one of the pouches on the external surface of the *colon.

Haversian canal one of the small canals (diameter about 50 μm) that ramify throughout compact *bone. *See also* HAVERSIAN SYSTEM. [C. Havers (1650–1702), English anatomist]

Haversian system one of the cylindrical units of which compact *bone is made. A **Haversian canal** forms a central tube, around which are alternate layers of bone matrix (**lamellae**) and **lacunae** containing bone cells. The lacunae are linked by minute channels (**canaliculi**).

hay fever a form of *allergy due to the pollen of grasses, trees, and other plants, characterized by inflammation of the membrane lining the nose and sometimes

of the conjunctiva (*see* (ALLERGIC) CONJUNCTIVITIS). The symptoms of sneezing, running or blocked nose, and watering eyes are due to histamine release and often respond to treatment with *antihistamines. If the allergen is identified, it may be possible to undertake *desensitization. Medical name: **allergic rhinitis**.

hazardous substance (in occupational health) *see* COSHH.

HCG *see* HUMAN CHORIONIC GONADOTROPHIN.

head *n.* **1.** the part of the body that contains the brain and the organs of sight, hearing, smell, and taste. **2.** the rounded portion of a bone, which fits into a groove of another to form a joint; for example, the head of the humerus or femur.

headache *n.* pain felt deep within the skull. Most headaches are caused by emotional stress or fatigue but some are symptoms of serious intracranial disease. *See also* MIGRAINE.

headgear *n.* (in dentistry) a strap that is fixed round the back of the head and/or the neck and attached to an *orthodontic appliance to aid tooth movement. It is normally worn at night and for part of the day.

head injury an injury usually resulting from a blow to the head and often associated with brain injury. It may result in *contusion or – if the blood vessels in the head are torn – to a *haematoma. The level of consciousness of a patient following a head injury can be assessed using the *Glasgow scoring system. Head injuries are an important cause of death due to accidents: legislation to impose protective headgear at industrial sites and on construction workers and motorcyclists has reduced their incidence.

Heaf test a skin test to determine whether or not an individual is immune to tuberculosis. A spring-loaded gun mounted with very short needles produces a circle of six punctures in the forearm through which *tuberculin is introduced. If the test is positive a reaction causes the skin to become red and raised, indicating that the individual is immune. If the test is negative a vaccine (*BCG) can be given. [F. R. G. Heaf (20th century), British physician]

Health and Safety Executive (HSE) (in Britain) a statutory body responsible for the health and safety of workers (including factory, office, and agricultural workers). *See also* COSHH.

Health Authority *see* NATIONAL HEALTH SERVICE.

Health Board a Health Authority in Scotland and Northern Ireland. *See* NATIONAL HEALTH SERVICE.

health care *see* PRIMARY HEALTH CARE, SECONDARY HEALTH CARE, TERTIARY HEALTH CARE.

health centre (in Britain) a building, owned or leased by a community trust or a Health Authority, that houses personnel and/or services from one or several sections of the National Health Service (e.g. *general practitioners, *district nurses, dentists, *child health clinics, and facilities for X-rays, laboratory tests, and electrocardiography). Services provided by local authorities, such as social services, chiropody, and child psychology, may also operate from such a centre.

health education persuasive methods used to encourage people (either individually or collectively) to adopt lifestyles that the educators believe will improve health and to reject habits regarded as harmful to health or likely to shorten life expectancy. The term is also used in a broader sense to include instruction about bodily function, etc., so that the public is better informed about health issues. *See also* HEALTH PROMOTION.

health promotion a programme of surveillance planned on a community basis to maintain the best possible health and quality of life of the members of that community, both collectively and individually. Programmes include a blend of such personal services as *health education, immunization, and *screening tests, with environmental monitoring of the atmosphere, housing, and water and food supplies, as well as occupational hazards (*see* OCCUPATIONAL HEALTH SERVICE).

Health Service Commissioner (Health Service Ombudsman) an official responsible to Parliament and appointed to protect the interests of patients in relation to administration of and provision of health care by the *National Health Service. He can investigate complaints and allegations of maladministration by a Health Authority or trust and also complaints about GPs, dentists, pharmacists, and opticians (including actions arising from clinical judgment of practitioners).

health service manager an administrator with special training and skills in management who is concerned with running hospitals and other health services. Generally, the basic training for managers is in disciplines other than health; however, doctors, nurses, and others may fill such posts, sometimes combining them with professional appointments. *See also* NATIONAL HEALTH SERVICE.

health service planning balancing the needs of a community, assessed by such indices as mortality, morbidity, and disability, with the resources available to meet these needs in terms of medical manpower (ensuring the numbers in training grades meet but do not exceed future requirements for career grades) and technical resources, such as hospitals (capital planning), equipment, and medicines. *See also* MEDICAL AUDIT.

health visitor (public health nurse) a trained nurse with specialist qualifications in *health promotion and public health. Most of the work of health visitors is focused on families with children but can be extended to other targeted groups in the population (e.g. the elderly) to meet health needs in the wider community. Health visitors do not carry out practical nursing care but seek to educate, in particular by drawing attention to unmet needs in terms of health care and those of the social services likely to improve health.

hearing aid an electronic device to enable a deaf person to hear, consisting of a miniature sound receiver, an amplifier, and either an earpiece or a vibrator to transfer the amplified sound to the ear. The earpiece fits into the ear; the vibrator (used in cases of conductive *deafness) fits behind the ear and transmits through the bone directly to the inner ear. The aid is powered by a battery, and the whole unit is usually small enough to fit behind or within the ear inconspicuously. *See also*

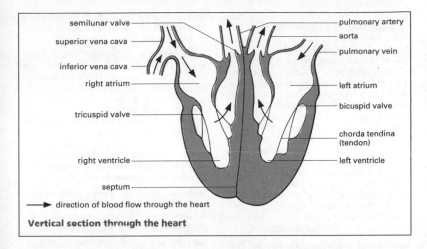

semilunar valve
superior vena cava
inferior vena cava
right atrium
tricuspid valve
right ventricle
septum
pulmonary artery
aorta
pulmonary vein
left atrium
bicuspid valve
chorda tendina (tendon)
left ventricle

→ direction of blood flow through the heart

Vertical section through the heart

BONE-ANCHORED HEARING AID, COCHLEAR IMPLANT.

heart *n.* a hollow muscular cone-shaped organ, lying between the lungs, with the pointed end (**apex**) directed downwards, forwards, and to the left. The heart is about the size of a closed fist. Its wall consists largely of *cardiac muscle (myocardium), lined and surrounded by membranes (see ENDOCARDIUM, PERICARDIUM). It is divided by a **septum** into separate right and left halves, each of which is divided into an upper *atrium and a lower *ventricle (see illustration). Deoxygenated blood from the *venae cavae passes through the right atrium to the right ventricle. This contracts and pumps blood to the lungs via the *pulmonary artery. The newly oxygenated blood returns to the left atrium via the pulmonary veins and passes through to the left ventricle. This forcefully contracts, pumping blood out to the body via the *aorta. The direction of blood flow within the heart is controlled by *valves.

heart attack *see* MYOCARDIAL INFARCTION.

heart block a condition in which conduction of the electrical impulses generated by the natural pacemaker of the heart (the *sinoatrial node) is impaired, so that the pumping action of the heart is slowed down. In **partial** or **incomplete heart block** conduction between atria and

ventricles is delayed (**first degree heart block**) or not all the impulses are conducted from the atria to the ventricles (**second degree heart block**). In **third degree** or **complete heart block** no impulses are conducted and the ventricles beat at their own slow intrinsic rate (20–40 per minute).

Heart block may be congenital or it may be due to heart disease, including myocardial infarction, myocarditis, cardiomyopathy, and disease of the valves. It is most frequently seen in the elderly as the result of chronic degenerative scarring around the conducting tissue. There may be no symptoms, but when very slow heart and pulse rates occur the patient may develop heart failure or *Stokes-Adams syndrome. Symptoms may be abolished by the use of an artificial *pacemaker.

heartburn (pyrosis) *n.* discomfort or pain, usually burning in character, that is felt behind the breastbone and often appears to rise from the abdomen towards or into the throat. It may be accompanied by the appearance of acid or bitter fluid in the mouth and is usually caused by regurgitation of stomach contents into the gullet or by *oesophagitis.

heart failure a condition in which the pumping action of the ventricle of the heart is inadequate. This results in back pressure of blood, with congestion of the lungs and liver. The veins in the neck becomed engorged and fluid accumulates in the tissues (see OEDEMA). There is a reduced flow of arterial blood from the heart, which in extreme cases results in peripheral circulatory failure (cardiogenic shock). Heart failure may result from any condition that overloads, damages, or reduces the efficiency of the heart muscle. Common causes are coronary thrombosis, hypertension, chronic disease of the valves, and arrhythmias. The patient experiences breathlessness, even when lying flat, and oedema of the legs.

Treatment consists of rest, a low salt diet, diuretic drugs (e.g. frusemide), and digitalis derivatives (e.g. digoxin). Structural abnormalities, such as defective valves, may be corrected surgically.

heart-lung machine an apparatus for taking over temporarily the functions of both the heart and the lungs during heart surgery. It incorporates a pump, to maintain the circulation, and equipment to oxygenate the blood. Blood is taken from the body by tubes inserted into the superior and inferior venae cavae, and the oxygenated blood is returned under pressure into a large artery, such as the femoral artery. The surgeon is therefore able to undertake the repair or replacement of heart valves or perform other surgical operations involving the heart and great blood vessels.

heater-probe n. a device that can be passed through an endoscope to apply controlled heat in order to coagulate a bleeding peptic ulcer.

heat exhaustion fatigue and collapse due to the low blood pressure and blood volume that result from loss of body fluids and salts after prolonged or unaccustomed exposure to heat. It is most common in new arrivals in a hot climate and is treated by giving drinks or intravenous injections of salted water.

heatstroke (sunstroke) n. raised body temperature (pyrexia), absence of sweating, and eventual loss of consciousness due to failure or exhaustion of the temperature-regulating mechanism of the body. It is potentially fatal unless treated immediately: the body should be cooled by applying damp cloths and body fluids restored by giving drinks or intravenous injections of salted water.

hebephrenia n. a form of *schizophrenia. It is typically a chronic condition, and the most prominent features are disordered thinking; inappropriate emotions with thoughtless cheerfulness, apathy, or querulousness; and silly behaviour. It typically starts in adolescence or young adulthood. Social and occupational rehabilitation are the most important therapies for most patients; drugs such as the *phenothiazines or butyrophenones can also help. —**hebephrenic** adj.

Heberden's node a bony thickening arising at the terminal joint of a finger in *osteoarthritis. It is often inherited. [W. Heberden (1710–1801), British physician]

hebetude n. apathy and emotional dullness. This is not a symptom specific to any one condition; extreme degrees are found in *schizophrenia and *dementia.

hectic adj. occurring regularly. A **hectic fever** is a fever that typically develops in the afternoons, in cases of pulmonary tuberculosis.

hecto- prefix denoting a hundred.

heel n. the part of the foot that extends behind the ankle joint, formed by the **heel bone** (see CALCANEUS).

Hegar's sign an indication of pregnancy detectable between the 6th and 12th weeks: used before modern urine tests for pregnancy were available. If the fingers of one hand are inserted into the vagina and those of the other are placed over the pelvic cavity, the lower part of the uterus feels very soft compared with the body of the uterus above and the cervix below. [A. Hegar (1830–1914), German gynaecologist]

helc- (helco-) prefix denoting an ulcer.

Helicobacter n. a genus of spiral flagellated Gram-negative bacteria. The species H. pylori (formerly classified as Campylobacter pylori) is found in the stomach within the mucous layer. It occurs in the majority of middle-aged people and causes progressive gastritis. It is almost invariably present in duodenal ulceration and usually in gastric ulceration. Eradication of the organism (using various combinations of bismuth, antibiotics, and *antisecretory drugs) leads to healing of the ulcer. *H. pylori* has also been implicated in some forms of stomach cancer and in heart disease.

helicopter-based emergency medical services *see* HEMS.

helicotrema *n.* the narrow opening between the scala vestibuli and the scala tympani at the tip of the *cochlea in the ear.

helio- *prefix denoting* the sun.

heliotherapy *n.* the use of sunlight to promote healing; sunbathing.

helix *n.* the outer curved fleshy ridge of the *pinna of the outer ear.

Heller's operation *see* ACHALASIA. [E. Heller (1877–1964), Austrian pathologist]

Heller's syndrome (disintegrative psychosis) a rare mental illness of childhood. Abnormalities of behaviour may be the only sign at first but the condition progresses to psychotic manifestations, such as *stereotypies and hallucinations, and ultimately to dementia. Nearly always a physical cause can be found. The illness progresses to severe incapacity or death. [T. Heller (20th century)]

Heller's test a test for the presence of protein (albumin) in the urine. A quantity of urine is carefully poured onto the same quantity of pure nitric acid in a test tube. A white ring forms at the junction of the liquids if albumin is present. However, a similar result may be obtained if the urine contains certain drugs or is very concentrated. A dark brown ring indicates the presence of an abnormally high level of potassium indoxyl sulphate in the urine (*see* INDICANURIA). [J. F. Heller (1813–71), Austrian pathologist]

HELLP syndrome a form of severe *pre-eclampsia affecting many body systems and characterized by haemolysis, elevated liver enzymes, and a low platelet count (hence the name). It constitutes an emergency requiring prompt termination of the pregnancy.

Helly's fluid a mixture of potassium dichromate, sodium sulphate, mercuric chloride, formaldehyde, and distilled

water, used in the preservation of bone marrow. [K. Helly (20th century), Swiss pathologist]

helminth *n.* any of the various parasitic worms, including the *flukes, *tapeworms, and *nematodes.

helminthiasis *n.* the diseased condition resulting from an infestation with parasitic worms (helminths).

helminthology *n.* the study of parasitic worms.

helper T-cell a type of T-*lymphocyte that plays a key role in cell-mediated immunity by recognizing foreign antigen on the surface of target cells when this is associated with the individual's *MHC antigens, having been processed by antigen-presenting cells. Helper T-cells stimulate the production of cytotoxic T-cells (*see* KILLER CELL), which destroy the target cells.

hemeralopia *n.* *see* DAY BLINDNESS.

hemi- *prefix denoting* (in medicine) the right or left half of the body. Example: **hemianaesthesia** (anaesthesia of one side of the body).

hemiachromatopsia *n.* loss of colour appreciation in one half of the visual field.

hemianopia *n.* absence of half of the normal field of vision. The commonest type is **homonymous hemianopia**, in which the same half (right or left) is lost in both eyes. Sometimes the inner halves of the visual field are lost in both eyes, producing a **binasal hemianopia**, while in others the outer halves are lost, producing a **bitemporal hemianopia**. Very rarely both upper halves or both lower halves are lost, producing an **altitudinal hemianopia**.

hemiarthroplasty *n.* replacement of the end of a bone on one side of a joint with a prosthesis (*see* ARTHROPLASTY). It is the treatment for some fractures of the hip and shoulder.

hemiballismus *n.* a violent involuntary movement usually restricted to one arm and primarily involving the proximal muscles. It is a symptom of disease of the *basal ganglia.

hemicolectomy *n.* surgical removal of about half the *colon (large intestine), usually the right section (**right hemi-colectomy**) with subsequent joining of the *ileum to the transverse colon. This is performed for disease of the terminal part of the ileum (such as *Crohn's disease) or of the caecum or ascending colon (such as cancer or Crohn's disease).

hemicrania n. **1.** a headache affecting only one side of the head, usually *migraine. **2.** absence of half of the skull in a developing fetus.

hemihypertrophy n. a condition in which one side of the body is larger than the other. It is often benign but can be associated with *nephroblastoma.

hemimelia n. congenital absence or gross shortening (aplasia) of the distal portion of the arms or legs. Sometimes only one of the two bones of the distal arm (radius and ulna) or leg (tibia and fibula) may be affected. See also ECTROMELIA.

hemiparesis n. see HEMIPLEGIA.

hemiplegia (hemiparesis) n. paralysis of one side of the body. Movements of the face and arm are often more severely affected than those of the leg. It is caused by disease affecting the opposite (contralateral) hemisphere of the brain.

hemisacralization n. fusion of the fifth lumbar vertebra to one side only of the sacrum. See SACRALIZATION.

hemisphere n. one of the two halves of the *cerebrum, not in fact hemispherical but more nearly quarter-spherical.

hemizygous adj. describing genes that are carried on an unpaired chromosome, for example the genes on the X chromosome in man. —**hemizygote** n.

hemlock n. the plant Conium maculatum, found in Britain and central Europe. It is a source of the poisonous alkaloid *coniine.

hemp n. see CANNABIS.

HEMS helicopter-based emergency medical services: a fast method for the provision of first aid and the rapid transport of the seriously injured (primary use) or the critically ill (secondary use) to a hospital.

Henle's loop the part of a kidney tubule that forms a loop extending towards the centre of the kidney. It is surrounded by blood capillaries, which absorb water and selected soluble substances back into the bloodstream. [F. G. J. Henle (1809–85), German anatomist]

Henoch-Schönlein purpura (Schönlein-Henoch purpura, anaphylactoid purpura) a common, and frequently recurrent, form of *purpura found especially (but not exclusively) in young children. It is characterized by red weals and a purple rash on the buttocks and lower legs due to bleeding into the skin from inflamed capillaries, together with arthritis, gastrointestinal symptoms, and (in some cases) nephritis. There is no specific treatment. [E. H. Henoch (1820–1910), German paediatrician; J. L. Schönlein (1793–1864), German physician]

henry n. the *SI unit of inductance, equal to the inductance of a closed circuit with a magnetic flux of 1 weber per ampere of current. Symbol: H.

Hensen's node (primitive knot) the rounded front end of the embryonic *primitive streak. [V. Hensen (1835–1924), German pathologist]

heparin n. an *anticoagulant produced in liver cells, some white blood cells, and certain other sites, which acts by inhibiting the action of the enzyme *thrombin in the final stage of *blood coagulation. An extracted purified form of heparin is widely used for the prevention of blood coagulation both in patients with thrombosis and similar conditions and in blood collected for examination. The drug is usually administered by injection and the most important side-effect is bleeding. See also LOW-MOLECULAR-WEIGHT HEPARIN.

hepat- (hepato-) prefix denoting the liver. Examples: **hepatopexy** (surgical fixation of); **hepatorenal** (relating to the liver and kidney).

hepatalgia n. pain in or over the liver. It is caused by liver inflammation (especially an abscess) or swelling (as in cardiac failure or *steatosis).

hepatectomy n. the operation of removing the liver. **Partial hepatectomy** is the removal of one or more lobes of the liver; it may be carried out after severe injury or to remove a tumour localized in one part of the liver.

hepatic *adj.* relating to the liver.

hepatic duct *see* BILE DUCT.

hepatic encephalopathy (portosystemic encephalopathy) a condition in which brain function is impaired by the presence of toxic substances, absorbed from the colon, which are normally removed or detoxified by the liver. It occurs when the liver is severely damaged (as in cirrhosis) or bypassed. Symptoms include drowsiness, confusion, difficulty in performing tasks (e.g. writing), and coma. Treatment consists of stopping protein intake and administering antibiotics (to prevent bacterial production of toxins) and enemas and cathartics (to remove colonic toxins).

hepatic flexure the bend in the *colon, just underneath the liver, where the ascending colon joins the transverse colon.

hepaticostomy *n.* a surgical operation in which a temporary or permanent opening is made into the main duct carrying bile from the liver.

hepatic vein one of several short veins originating within the lobes of the liver as small branches, which unite to form the hepatic veins. These lead directly to the inferior vena cava, draining blood from the liver.

hepatitis *n.* inflammation of the liver caused by viruses, toxic substances, or immunological abnormalities. **Infectious hepatitis** is caused by viruses, several types of which have been isolated as specific causes of the disease and can be detected by blood tests, including hepatitis A, hepatitis B, hepatitis C, hepatitis D, and hepatitis E. Other viral causes of hepatitis include the *Epstein-Barr virus. *See also* ENTAMOEBA.

Hepatitis A (epidemic hepatitis) is transmitted by food or drink contaminated by a carrier or patient and commonly occurs where sanitation is poor. After an incubation period of 15–40 days, the patient develops fever and sickness. Yellow discoloration of the skin (*see* JAUNDICE) appears about a week later and persists for up to three weeks. The patient may be infectious throughout this period. Serious complications are unusual and an attack often confers immunity. Injection

of *gammaglobulin provides temporary protection, but active immunization is preferable.

Hepatitis B (formerly known as **serum hepatitis**) is transmitted by infected blood or blood products contaminating hypodermic needles, blood transfusions, or tattooing needles, by sexual contact, or by contact with any other body fluid (e.g. milk, sweat); it often occurs in drug addicts. Symptoms, which develop suddenly after an incubation period of 1–6 months, include headache, fever, chills, general weakness, and jaundice. Most patients make a gradual recovery but the mortality rate is 5–20%. A vaccine is available.

Hepatitis C (formerly known as **non-A, non-B hepatitis**) has a mode of transmission similar to that of hepatitis B; symptoms include fatigue, sore bones, and dryness of the eyes. **Hepatitis D** is a defective virus and occurs only with or after infection with hepatitis B. Patients with D virus usually have severe chronic hepatitis. **Hepatitis E** is transmitted by infected food or drink and can cause acute hepatitis.

Chronic hepatitis continues for months or years, eventually leading to *cirrhosis (*see also* HEPATOMA). It may be caused by persistent infection with a hepatitis virus (usually hepatitis B, C, or D), which may respond to treatment with *interferon, or by *autoimmune disease, treated by *corticosteroids or *immunosuppressive therapy.

hepatization *n.* the conversion of lung tissue, which normally holds air, into a solid liver-like mass during the course of acute lobar *pneumonia.

hepato- *prefix.* *see* HEPAT-.

hepatoblastoma *n.* a malignant tumour of the liver occurring in children, made up of embryonic liver cells. It is often confined to one lobe of the liver; such cases may be treated by a partial *hepatectomy.

hepatocellular *adj.* relating to or affecting the cells of the liver.

hepatocyte *n.* the principal cell type in the *liver: a large cell with many metabolic functions, including synthesis, storage, detoxification, and bile production.

hepatoma n. a malignant tumour of the liver, originating in mature liver cells. In Western countries it is rare in normal livers, but often develops in patients with cirrhosis, particularly after hepatitis B or C infection. In Africa and other tropical countries it is frequent, possible causes including fungi (see AFLATOXIN) and other ingested toxins. Hepatomas often synthesize *alpha-fetoprotein, which circulates in the blood and is a useful indicator of these tumours.

The term hepatoma is often, though incorrectly, used to include malignant tumours arising in the bile duct (see CHOLANGIOCARCINOMA).

hepatomegaly n. enlargement of the liver to such an extent that it can be felt below the rib margin. This may be due to congestion (as in heart failure), inflammation, infiltration (e.g. by fat), or tumour.

hepatotoxic adj. damaging or destroying liver cells. Certain drugs, such as *paracetamol, can cause liver damage at high doses or with prolonged use.

hept- (hepta-) prefix denoting seven.

hereditary adj. transmitted from parents to their offspring; inherited.

heredity n. the process that causes the biological similarity between parents and their offspring. *Genetics is the study of heredity.

heredo- prefix denoting heredity.

hermaphrodite n. an individual in which both male and female sex organs are present or in which the sex organs contain both ovarian and testicular cells. Human hermaphrodites are very rare. —**hermaphroditism** n.

hernia n. the protrusion of an organ or tissue out of the body cavity in which it normally lies. An **inguinal hernia** (or **rupture**) occurs in the lower abdomen; a sac of peritoneum, containing fat or part of the bowel, bulges through a weak part (**inguinal canal**) of the abdominal wall. It may result from physical straining or coughing. A **scrotal hernia** is an inguinal hernia so large that it passes into the scrotum; a **femoral hernia** is similar to an inguinal hernia but protrudes at the top of the thigh, through the point at which the

femoral artery passes from the abdomen to the thigh. A **diaphragmatic hernia** is the protrusion of an abdominal organ through the diaphragm into the chest cavity; the most common type is the **hiatus hernia,** in which the stomach passes partly or completely into the chest cavity through the hole (**hiatus**) for the oesophagus (gullet). This may be associated with *gastro-oesophageal reflux. An **umbilical hernia** (or **exomphalos**) is the protrusion of abdominal organs into the umbilical cord, due to a fault in embryonic development. It is present at birth and can be treated surgically.

Hernias may be complicated by becoming impossible to return to their normal site (**irreducible**); swollen and fixed within their sac (**incarcerated**); or cut off from their blood supply, becoming painful and eventually gangrenous (**strangulated**). The best treatment for hernias, especially if they are painful, is surgical repair (see HERNIOPLASTY).

hernia-en-glissade an inguinal *hernia that has an element of descent ('slide') of related structures alongside the sac.

hernio- prefix denoting a hernia.

hernioplasty n. the surgical operation to repair a hernia, in which the abnormal opening is sewn up and/or the weakness strengthened with suture material. The recommended techniques for repair include a layered suture repair (**Shouldice operation**) or the insertion of a mesh of polypropylene (**Lichtenstein operation**).

herniorrhaphy n. surgical repair of a hernia. It can be performed through a *laparoscope. See also HERNIOTOMY.

herniotomy n. excision of a hernial sac: the first stage of the surgical repair of a hernia. In infants and young muscular subjects it is all that is needed to cure the hernia.

heroin n. a white crystalline powder derived from *morphine but with a shorter duration of action. Like morphine it is a powerful narcotic analgesic whose continued use leads to *dependence. It is used medicinally (as **diamorphine**) for the relief of severe pain.

herpangina n. an acute viral infection, occurring predominantly in children, that causes a fever of sudden onset associated with malaise and acute ulceration of the soft palate and tonsillar area. It usually lasts 2–5 days.

herpes *n.* inflammation of the skin or mucous membranes that is caused by *herpesviruses and characterized by collections of small blisters. There are two types of **herpes simplex virus (HSV)**: type I causes the common **cold sore**, usually present on or around the lips; type II is mainly associated with **genital herpes** and is sexually transmitted. However, types I and II can both cause either genital herpes or cold sores, depending on the site of initial infection. HSV blisters are contagious through skin-to-skin contact and are recurrent in some people. HSV can also affect the conjunctiva (*see also* DENDRITIC ULCER).
Herpes zoster (shingles) is caused by the varicella-zoster virus, which also causes chickenpox. Following an attack of chickenpox, the virus lays dormant in the dorsal root ganglia of the spinal cord. Later, under one of a number of influences, the virus migrates down the sensory nerve to affect one or more *dermatomes on the skin in a band, causing the characteristic shingles rash. One side of the face or an eye (**ophthalmic zoster**) may be involved. Shingles may be chronically painful (**post-herpetic neuralgia**), especially in the elderly. *See also* RAMSAY HUNT SYNDROME.
Treatment of all forms of herpes is with an appropriate preparation of *acyclovir or related drugs; shingles may require potent analgesics.

herpesvirus *n.* one of a group of DNA-containing viruses causing latent infections in both man and animals. The herpesviruses are the causative agents of *herpes and chickenpox. The group also includes the *cytomegalovirus and *Epstein-Barr virus. **Herpesvirus simiae (virus B)** causes an infection in monkeys similar to herpes simplex, but when transmitted to man it can produce fatal encephalitis.

hertz *n.* the *SI unit of frequency, equal to one cycle per second. Symbol: Hz.

Herxheimer reaction *see* JARISCH-HERXHEIMER REACTION.

heter- (hetero-) *prefix denoting* difference; dissimilarity.

heterochromatin *n.* chromosome material (*see* CHROMATIN) that stains most deeply when the cell is not dividing. It is thought not to represent major genes but may be involved in controlling these genes, and also in controlling mitosis and development. *Compare* EUCHROMATIN.

heterochromia *n.* colour difference in the iris of the eye, which is usually congenital but is occasionally secondary to inflammation of the iris (as in *Fuchs' heterochromic cyclitis). In **heterochromia iridis** one iris differs in colour from the other; in **heterochromia iridum** one part of the iris differs in colour from the rest. —**heterochromic** *adj.*

heterogametic *adj.* describing the sex that produces two different kinds of gamete, which carry different *sex chromosomes, and that therefore determines the sex of the offspring. In humans men are the heterogametic sex: the sperm cells carry either an X or a Y chromosome. *Compare* HOMOGAMETIC.

heterogeneity *n.* (in oncology) variability or differences in the properties of cells within a tumour.

heterograft (xenograft) *n.* a living tissue graft that is made from an animal of one species to another of a different species. For example, attempts have been made to graft animal organs into humans. *Bioengineering techniques are now available to produce animals whose *MHC is compatible with that of another species. *See also* XENOTRANSPLANTATION.

heterophoria *n.* a tendency to squint. Under normal circumstances both the eyes work together and look at the same point simultaneously, but if one eye is covered it will move out of alignment with the object the other eye is still viewing. When the cover is removed the eye immediately returns to its normal position. Most people have some small degree of the type of heterophoria known as **exophoria**, in which the covered eye turns outwards, away from the nose (*compare* ESOPHORIA). Heterophoria often produces eyestrain because of the unconscious effort required to keep the two eyes aligned. *See also* STRABISMUS.

Heterophyes *n.* a genus of small parasitic *flukes occurring in Egypt and the Far East. Adult flukes of the species *H. heterophyes* live in the small intestine of man and other fish-eating animals; in man the flukes can produce serious symptoms (*see* HETEROPHYIASIS). The fluke has two intermediate hosts, a snail and a mullet fish.

heterophyiasis *n.* an infestation of the small intestine with the parasitic fluke *Heterophyes heterophyes*. Man becomes infected on eating raw or salted fish that contains the larval stage of the fluke. The presence of adult flukes may provoke symptoms of abdominal pain and diarrhoea; if the eggs reach the brain, spinal cord, and heart (via the bloodstream) they produce serious lesions.
Tetrachloroethylene may be used in treatment of the infection.

heteroplasty *n.* the grafting of tissue from an animal of one species to another of a different species.

heteropsia *n.* different vision in each eye.

heterosexuality *n.* the pattern of sexuality in which sexual behaviour and thinking are directed towards people of the opposite sex. It includes both normal and deviant forms of sexual activity. —**heterosexual** *adj., n.*

heterosis *n.* hybrid vigour: the increased sturdiness, resistance to disease, etc., of individuals whose parents are of different races or species compared both with their parents and with the offspring of genetically similar parents.

heterotopia (heterotopy) *n.* the displacement of an organ or part of the body from its normal position.

heterotrophic (organotrophic) *adj.* describing organisms (known as heterotrophs) that use complex organic compounds to synthesize their own organic materials. Most heterotrophs are **chemoheterotrophic**, i.e. they use the organic compounds as an energy source. This group includes the majority of bacteria and all animals and fungi. *Compare* AUTOTROPHIC.

heterotropia *n. see* STRABISMUS.

heterozygous *adj.* describing an individual in whom the members of a pair of genes determining a particular characteristic are dissimilar. *See* ALLELE. *Compare* HOMOZYGOUS. —**heterozygote** *n.*

hex- (hexa-) *prefix denoting* six.

hexacanth *n. see* ONCOSPHERE.

hexachlorophane *n.* a disinfectant similar to *phenol, formerly used in soaps and creams to treat skin disorders. Its use in medicinal products was limited by law in 1973 because of the toxic effects it might produce when absorbed into the body. Trade names: **Dermalex**, **Ster-Zac D.C.**

hexachromia *n.* the ability to distinguish only six of the seven colours of the spectrum, the exception being indigo. Most people cannot distinguish indigo from blue or violet.

hexamine (methenamine) *n.* an *antiseptic with a wide range of antibacterial activity, used to treat infections and inflammation of the urinary tract, such as cystitis. High doses may cause irritation of the stomach or bladder. Trade name: **Hiprex**.

hexokinase *n.* an enzyme that catalyses the conversion of glucose to glucose-6-phosphate. This is the first stage of *glycolysis.

hexosamine *n.* the amino derivative of a *hexose sugar. The two most important hexosamines are *glucosamine and galactosamine.

hexose *n.* a simple sugar with six carbon atoms. Hexose sugars are the sugars most frequently found in food. The most important hexose is *glucose.

hiatus *n.* an opening or aperture. For example, the diaphragm contains hiatuses for the oesophagus and aorta.

hiatus hernia *see* HERNIA.

Hib vaccine a vaccine that gives protection against the bacterium *Haemophilus influenzae* type B (Hib). Before the introduction of the vaccine in the UK in 1992, Hib was the commonest cause of meningitis in children under the age of two. The vaccine, which has an excellent safety record, is currently given with the triple DPT vaccine at two, three and four months of age.

hiccup *n.* abrupt involuntary lowering of the diaphragm and closure of the sound-producing folds at the upper end of the trachea, producing a characteristic sound as the breath is drawn in. Hiccups, which usually occur repeatedly, may be caused by indigestion or more serious disorders, such as alcoholism. Medical name: **singultus**.

Hickman catheter a fine plastic cannula inserted into a vein in the neck to allow administration of drugs and repeated blood samples. The catheter is tunnelled for several centimetres beneath the skin to prevent infection entering the bloodstream. It is used most frequently in patients receiving long-term chemotherapy.

hidr- (hidro-) *prefix denoting* sweat. Example: **hidropoiesis** (formation of).

hidradenitis suppurativa an inflammatory condition of the *apocrine sweat glands, which first become active at adolescence; it occurs in the armpits and groin. In women the condition responds to *anti-androgen therapy. Antibiotics and antiseptics are also used.

hidrosis *n.* **1.** the excretion of sweat. **2.** excessive sweating.

hidrotic *n.* an agent that causes sweating. *Parasympathomimetic drugs are hidrotics.

hilum *n.* (*pl.* **hila**) a hollow situated on the surface of an organ, such as the kidney or spleen, at which structures such as blood vessels, nerve fibres, and ducts enter or leave it.

hindbrain *n.* the part of the *brain comprising the cerebellum, pons, and medulla oblongata. The pons and medulla contain the nuclei of many of the cranial nerves, which issue from their surfaces, and the reticular formation in the midline is the fourth *ventricle.

hindgut *n.* the back part of the embryonic gut, which gives rise to part of the large intestine, the rectum, bladder, and urinary ducts. *See also* CLOACA.

hindquarter amputation an operation involving removal of an entire leg and part or all of the pelvis associated with it. It is usually performed for soft tissue or bone sarcomas arising from the upper thigh, hip, or buttock. *Compare* FOREQUARTER AMPUTATION.

hinge joint *see* GINGLYMUS.

hip *n.* the region of the body where the thigh bone (femur) articulates with the *pelvis: the region on each side of the pelvis.

hip bone (innominate bone) a bone formed by the fusion of the ilium, ischium, and pubis. It articulates with the femur by the **acetabulum** of the ilium, a deep socket into which the head of the femur fits (*see* HIP JOINT). Between the pubis and ischium, below and slightly in front of the acetabulum, is a large opening – the **obturator foramen**. The right and left hip bones form part of the *pelvis.

hip girdle *see* PELVIC GIRDLE.

hip joint the ball-and-socket joint (*see* ENARTHROSIS) between the head of the femur and the acetabulum (socket) of the ilium (*see* HIP BONE). It is a common site of osteoarthritis and rheumatoid arthritis, which is often treated surgically (by *hip replacement). *See also* CONGENITAL DISLOCATION OF THE HIP.

Hippelates *n.* a genus of small flies. The adults of *H. pallipes* are suspected of transmitting *yaws in the West Indies. Other species of *Hippelates* may be involved in the transmission of conjunctivitis.

hippocampal formation a curved band of cortex lying within each cerebral hemisphere: in evolutionary terms one of the brain's most primitive parts. It forms a portion of the *limbic system and is involved in the complex physical aspects of behaviour governed by emotion and instinct.

hippocampus *n.* a swelling in the floor of the lateral *ventricle of the brain. It contains complex foldings of cortical tissue and is involved, with other connections of the *hippocampal formation, in the workings of the *limbic system.
—**hippocampal** *adj.*

Hippocratic oath the oath taken by a doctor that binds him to observe the code of behaviour and practice followed by the Greek physician Hippocrates (460–370 BC), called the 'Father of Medicine', and the students of the medical school in Cos where he taught.

Hippuran n. trade name for sodium iodohippurate, used as a contrast medium in radiology of the urinary tract. Labelled with iodine-131, it can be used to measure renal function.

hippus n. abnormal rhythmical variations in the size of the pupils, independent of the intensity of the light falling on the eyes. It is occasionally seen in various diseases of the nervous system.

hip replacement a surgical procedure developed for replacing a diseased hip joint with a prosthesis. A plastic cup forms the socket, and the head of the femur is replaced by a metal ball on a stem placed inside the femur. There are many types of prosthesis, which can be fixed to the bone with or without cement. *See also* ARTHROPLASTY.

Hirschsprung's disease a congenital condition in which the rectum and sometimes part of the lower colon have failed to develop a normal nerve network. The affected portion does not expand or conduct the contents of the bowel, which accumulate in and distend the upper colon. Symptoms, which are usually apparent in the first weeks of life, are abdominal pain and swelling and severe or complete constipation. Diagnosis is by X-ray and by microscopic examination of samples of the bowel wall, which shows the absence of nerve cells. Treatment is by surgery to remove the affected segment and join the remaining (normal) colon to the anus. *See also* MEGACOLON. [H. Hirschsprung (1830–1916), Danish physician]

hirsutism n. the presence of coarse pigmented hair on the face, chest, upper back, or abdomen in a female as a result of *hyperandrogenism (excessive production of androgen). *See also* VIRILIZATION.

hirudin n. an *anticoagulant present in the salivary glands of *leeches and in certain snake venoms, that prevents *blood coagulation by inhibiting the action of the enzyme *thrombin.

hist- (histio-, histo-) *prefix denoting* tissue.

histaminase n. an enzyme, widely distributed in the body, that is responsible for the inactivation of histamine.

histamine n. a compound derived from the amino acid histidine. It is found in nearly all tissues of the body, associated mainly with the *mast cells. Histamine has pronounced pharmacological activity, causing dilation of blood vessels and contraction of smooth muscle (for example, in the lungs). It is an important mediator of inflammation and is released in large amounts after skin damage (such as that due to animal venoms and toxins), producing a characteristic skin reaction (consisting of flushing, a flare, and a weal). Histamine is also released in anaphylactic reactions and allergic conditions, including asthma, and gives rise to some of the symptoms of these conditions. *See also* ANAPHYLAXIS, ANTIHISTAMINE.

histamine acid phosphate a derivative of *histamine that was formerly used to test for acid secretion in the stomach in conditions involving abnormal gastric secretion, such as *Zollinger-Ellison syndrome.

histidine n. an *amino acid from which *histamine is derived.

histiocyte n. a fixed *macrophage, i.e. one that is stationary within connective tissue.

histiocytoma n. a tumour that contains *macrophages or *histiocytes, large cells with the ability to engulf foreign matter and bacteria. *See also* FIBROSARCOMA (MALIGNANT FIBROUS HISTIOCYTOMA).

histiocytosis n. any of a group of diseases in which there are abnormalities in certain large phagocytic cells (*histiocytes), leading to biochemical defects, such as abnormal storage of fats (as in *Gaucher's disease), and other poorly understood conditions, such as Hand-Schüller-Christian disease and Letterer-Siwe disease (*see* RETICULOENDOTHELIOSIS).

histochemistry n. the study of the identification and distribution of chemical compounds within and between cells, by means of stains, indicators, and light and electron microscopy. —**histochemical** adj.

histocompatibility n. the form of *compatibility that depends upon tissue components, mainly specific glycoprotein antigens in cell membranes. A high degree of histocompatibility is necessary for a tissue graft or organ transplant to be successful. —**histocompatible** adj.

histogenesis n. the formation of tissues.

histogram n. a form of statistical graph in which values are plotted in the form of rectangles on a chart; a bar-chart.

histoid adj. 1. resembling normal tissue. 2. composed of one type of tissue.

histological grade the degree of *differentiation of a tumour; for example, of a breast tumour.

histology n. the study of the structure of tissues by means of special staining techniques combined with light and electron microscopy. —**histological** adj.

histone n. a simple protein that combines with a nucleic acid to form a *nucleoprotein.

Histoplasma n. a genus of parasitic yeastlike fungi. The species *H. capsulatum* causes the respiratory infection *histoplasmosis.

histoplasmin n. a preparation of antigenic material from a culture of the fungus *Histoplasma capsulatum*, used to test for the presence of the disease *histoplasmosis by subcutaneous injection.

histoplasmosis n. an infection caused by inhaling spores of the fungus *Histoplasma capsulatum*. The primary pulmonary form usually produces no symptoms or harmful effects and is recognized retrospectively by X-rays and positive *histoplasmin skin testing. Occasionally, progressive histoplasmosis, which resembles tuberculosis, develops. The fungus may spread via the bloodstream to attack other organs, such as the liver, spleen, lymph nodes, or intestine. Symptomatic disease is treated with intravenous amphotericin-B. The spores are found in soil contaminated by faeces, especially from chickens and bats. The disease is endemic in the northern and central USA, Argentina, Brazil, Venezuela, and parts of Africa.

histotoxic adj. poisonous to tissues: applied to certain substances and conditions.

HIV (human immunodeficiency virus) a *retrovirus responsible for *AIDS. There are two varieties, HIV-1 and HIV-2; the latter is most common in Africa. See also HTLV.

hives n. see URTICARIA.

HLA system human leucocyte antigen system: a series of four gene families (termed A, B, C, and D) that code for polymorphic proteins expressed on the surface of most nucleated cells. Individuals inherit from each parent one gene (or set of genes) for each subdivision of the HLA system. If two individuals have identical HLA types, they are said to be histocompatible. Successful tissue transplantation requires a minimum number of HLA differences between donor and recipient tissues.

hobnail liver the liver of a patient with cirrhosis, which has a knobbly appearance caused by regenerating nodules separated by bands of fibrous tissue.

Hodgkin's disease a malignant disease of lymphatic tissues – a form of *lymphoma – usually characterized by painless enlargement of one or more groups of lymph nodes in the neck, armpits, groin, chest, or abdomen; the spleen, liver, bone marrow, and bones may also be involved. Apart from the enlarging nodes, there may also be weight loss, fever, profuse sweating at night, and itching (known as **B symptoms**). Hodgkin's disease is distinguished from other forms of lymphoma by the presence of large binucleate cells (**Sternberg-Reed cells**) in the cancerous lymph nodes. Treatment depends on the extent of disease and may include surgery, radiotherapy, drug therapy, or a combination of these. Drugs used in the treatment of the disease include nitrogen mustard, vincristine, procarbazine, prednisone, chlorambucil, and vinblastine. Many patients can be cured; in the early stages of the disease this may be in the order of 85% or more. [T. Hodgkin (1798–1866), British physician]

hole in the heart *see* SEPTAL DEFECT.

holistic *adj.* describing an approach to patient care in which the physical, mental, and social factors in the patient's condition are taken into account, rather than just the diagnosed disease. The term is applied to a range of orthodox and unorthodox methods of treatment. *See also* ALTERNATIVE MEDICINE.

Hollister ring a watertight adherent ring placed around an intestinal *stoma and incorporating a flange to which a disposable plastic bag could be attached. It was the forerunner of modern disposable stoma bags.

Holmes-Adie syndrome *see* ADIE'S SYNDROME.

holo- *prefix denoting* complete or entire.

holocrine *adj.* describing a gland or type of secretion in which the entire cell disintegrates when the product is released.

home delivery *see* COMMUNITY MIDWIFE.

home help *see* CARE ASSISTANT.

home nurse *see* DISTRICT NURSE.

homeo- (homoeo-) *prefix denoting* similar; like.

homeopathic (homoeopathic) *adj.* **1.** of or relating to *homeopathy. **2.** infinitesimally small, as applied to the dose of a drug.

homeopathy (homoeopathy) *n.* a system of medicine based on the theory that 'like cures like'. The patient is treated with extremely small quantities of drugs that are themselves capable of producing symptoms of his particular disease. The system was founded by Samuel Hahnemann (1755–1843) at the end of the 18th century and is followed by a minority of doctors in the UK. There is a Royal London Homeopathic Hospital. *See also* ALTERNATIVE MEDICINE. **—homeopathist** *n.*

homeostasis *n.* the physiological process by which the internal systems of the body (e.g. blood pressure, body temperature, *acid-base balance) are maintained at equilibrium, despite variations in the external conditions. **—homeostatic** *adj.*

homo- *prefix denoting* the same or common.

homocystinuria *n.* an *inborn error of metabolism caused by an enzyme deficiency resulting in an excess of homocysteine (an intermediate in the synthesis of the amino acid *cysteine) in the blood and the presence of homocystine (an oxidized form of cysteine) in the urine. Clinically affected individuals are mentally retarded, excessively tall with long fingers (due to overgrowth of bones), and have a tendency to form blood clots in the veins and arteries. Treatment is by diet, which may allow for normal development if the disease is recognized early enough.

homoeopathy *n. see* HOMEOPATHY.

homogametic *adj.* describing the sex that produces only one kind of gamete, which carries the same *sex chromosome, and that therefore does not determine the sex of the offspring. In humans women are the homogametic sex: each egg cell carries an X chromosome. *Compare* HETEROGAMETIC.

homogenize *vb.* to reduce material to a uniform consistency, e.g. by crushing and mixing. Organs and tissues are homogenized to determine their overall content of a particular enzyme or other substance. **—homogenization** *n.*

homogentisic acid a product formed during the metabolism of the amino acids phenylalanine and tyrosine. In normal individuals homogentisic acid is oxidized by the enzyme **homogentisic acid oxidase**. In rare cases this enzyme is lacking and a condition known as *alcaptonuria, in which large amounts of homogentisic acid are excreted in the urine, results.

homograft (allograft) *n.* a living tissue or organ graft between two members of the same species; for example, a heart transplant from one person to another. Such grafts will not survive unless the recipient is treated to suppress his body's automatic rejection of the foreign tissue or the grafted organ is from an identical twin. *See also* TRANSPLANTATION.

homoiothermic *adj.* warm-blooded: able to maintain a constant body temperature independently of, and despite variations in, the temperature of the surroundings.

Mammals (including humans) and birds are homoiothermic. *Compare* POIKILOTHER-MIC. —**homoiothermy** *n.*

homolateral *adj. see* IPSILATERAL.

homologous *adj.* **1.** (in anatomy) describing organs or parts that have the same basic structure and evolutionary origin, but not necessarily the same function or superficial structure. *Compare* ANALO-GOUS. **2.** (in genetics) describing a pair of chromosomes of similar shape and size and having identical gene loci. One member of the pair is derived from the mother; the other from the father.

homonymous *adj.* describing a visual defect in which the visual field to one side of the body is restricted in both eyes (*see* HEMIANOPIA).

homoplasty *n.* surgical repair of defective or damaged tissues or organs with a *homograft.

homosexuality *n.* the condition of being sexually attracted, covertly or overtly, by members of one's own sex: it can affect either sex (*see also* LESBIANISM). The cause of homosexuality remains unclear, although there is some evidence of a genetic basis. Homosexuality is no longer regarded as a psychological disorder, but help is sometimes offered to individuals wishing to change their sexual orientation. There are no drugs available for changing sexual orientation, although it is possible to depress the sexual drive. Persons seeking help for their homosexuality are more likely to benefit from *counselling to reduce any anxiety and guilt that may be associated with the condition, rather than trying to change their sexual behaviour. —**homosexual** *adj., n.*

homozygous *adj.* describing an individual in whom the members of a pair of genes determining a particular characteristic are identical. *See* ALLELE. *Compare* HETEROZYGOUS. —**homozygote** *n.*

homunculus *n.* **1.** (or **manikin**) a dwarf with no deformity or abnormality other than small size. **2.** (or **manikin**) a small jointed anatomical model of a man. **3.** (in early biological theory) a miniature human being thought to be contained within each of the reproductive cells.

hook *n.* a surgical instrument with a bent or curved tip, used to hold, lift, or retract tissue at operation.

hookworm *n.* either of two nematode worms, *Necator americanus* or *Ancylostoma duodenale*, which live as parasites in the intestine of man. Both species, also known as the New and Old World hookworms respectively, are of great medical importance (*see* HOOKWORM DISEASE).

hookworm disease a condition resulting from an infestation of the small intestine by hookworms. Hookworm larvae live in the soil and infect man by penetrating the skin. The worms travel to the lungs in the bloodstream and from there pass via the windpipe and gullet to the small intestine. Heavy hookworm infections may cause considerable damage to the wall of the intestine, leading to a serious loss of blood; this, in conjunction with malnutrition, can provoke severe anaemia. Symptoms include abdominal pain, diarrhoea, debility, and mental inertia. The disease occurs throughout the tropics and subtropics and is prevalent in areas of poor personal hygiene and sanitation. *Bephenium hydroxynaphthoate, reliable and easy to administer, is used in treatment.

hordeolum *n. see* STYE.

hormone *n* a substance that is produced in one part of the body (by an *endocrine gland, such as the thyroid, adrenal, or pituitary), passes into the bloodstream and is carried to other (distant) organs or tissues, where it acts to modify their structure or function. Examples of hormones are corticosteroids (from the adrenal cortex), growth hormone (from the pituitary gland), and androgens (from the testes).

hormone replacement therapy (HRT) the use of female hormones for the relief of symptoms resulting from cessation of ovarian function, either at the time of the natural *menopause or following surgical removal of the ovaries. Oestrogenic hormones may be prescribed orally, transdermally (as skin patches or gel), or by subcutaneous implant. The combination of progestogen with oestrogen is preferred if the woman has retained her uterus, since administration of oestrogen alone might cause overstimulation of the endometrium or even cancer; overstimulation may result in uterine bleeding. HRT is effective against *vasomotor symptoms (e.g. hot flushes), genitourinary atrophy (causing vaginal dryness) and in preventing *osteoporosis; there is usually also an improvement in psychological well-being, and HRT is claimed to prevent coronary heart disease. It is most efficacious in preventing the above conditions if prescribed as soon as the earliest symptoms of the menopause are detected.

horn *n.* (in anatomy) a process, outgrowth, or extension of an organ or other structure. It is often paired. In the spinal cord crescent-shaped areas of grey matter (seen in cross section) are known as the dorsal and ventral horns.

Horner's syndrome a syndrome consisting of a constricted pupil, drooping of the upper eyelid (*ptosis), and an absence of sweating over the affected side of the face. The symptoms are due to a disorder of the sympathetic nerves in the brainstem or cervical (neck) region. [J. F. Horner (1831–86), Swiss ophthalmologist]

horseshoe kidney an anatomical variation in kidney development whereby the lower poles of both kidneys are joined together. This usually causes no trouble but it may be associated with impaired drainage of urine from the kidney by the ureters, which cross in front of the united lower segment.

hospice *n.* an institution that specializes in the care of terminally ill patients with special concern for death with dignity: narcotic drugs are used in carefully controlled doses for the relief of pain.

hospital *n.* an institution providing medical or psychiatric care and treatment of patients. Such care may be residential (in-patient), including the care of patients for a whole day and their return home at night (day stay). Out-patient services include consultation with specialists by prior appointment, X-rays, laboratory tests, physiotherapy, and accident and emergency services for those requiring urgent care. Most health districts have a **district general hospital (DGH)**, which provides sufficient basic services for the population of the district. Some larger hospitals have resources that are more highly specialized, to meet the needs of a wider population, providing so-called **regional** or **supraregional (national)** services. Such hospitals often provide training for medical students (**teaching** or **university hospitals**) and for postgraduate education. Some smaller hospitals – known as **community hospitals** – may be staffed by general practitioners and are intended for people for whom home care is not practicable on social grounds. Since 1991 hospitals have become self-governing NHS *trusts, independent of Health Authority control, their income deriving chiefly from contracts to provide services to Health Authorities and fundholding general practitioners. *See also* INDEPENDENT CONTRACT.

Hospital Activity Analysis *see* HOSPITAL IN-PATIENT ENQUIRY.

hospital fatality ratio *see* CASE FATALITY RATIO.

hospital infection *see* NOSOCOMIAL INFECTION.

Hospital In-patient Enquiry (in Britain) a statistical review, organized jointly by the *Department of Health and the *Office for National Statistics, providing information about in-patients treated in National Health Service hospitals. The data, based on a sample of episodes of illness (as distinct from individual patients), include diagnosis on discharge or death, duration on the waiting list, and length of stay. More detailed information, including aspects of therapy while in the hospital, are included in **Hospital Activity Analysis**. *Compare* RECORD LINKAGE.

host *n.* an animal or plant in or upon which a *parasite lives. An **intermediate host** is one in which the parasite passes its larval or asexual stages; a **definitive host** is one in which the parasite develops to its sexual stage.

Hounsfield unit the numerical unit assigned electronically to each *pixel in a *computerized tomography (CT) image according to its X-ray density. The scale runs from −1000 (air) to +1000 (compact bone), with 0 indicating water density. The unit was named after Sir Godfrey Hounsfield (1919–), who developed CT scanning in the 1950s. Symbol: H.

hourglass stomach a deformity of the stomach in which the 'waist' is constricted by fibrosis caused by a chronic peptic ulcer, producing an upper and a lower cavity separated by a narrow channel. **Teapot** and **handbag** are other stomach shapes associated with a chronic peptic ulcer.

housemaid's knee (prepatellar bursitis) a fluid-filled swelling of the bursa in front of the kneecap, often resulting from frequent kneeling. Treatment – and prevention – is by avoidance of kneeling. *See also* BURSITIS.

house physician/surgeon *see* DOCTOR.

HPV *see* HUMAN PAPILLOMAVIRUS.

H₂-receptor antagonist *see* ANTIHISTAMINE.

H₂ receptors *see* ANTIHISTAMINE.

HRT *see* HORMONE REPLACEMENT THERAPY.

HSE *see* HEALTH AND SAFETY EXECUTIVE.

5-HT 5-hydroxytryptamine (*see* SEROTONIN).

HTLV (human T-cell leukaemia/lymphoma virus or **lymphocytotrophic virus)** a family of viruses that includes the AIDS virus, HTLV-III (or *HIV). HTLV-I causes lymphoma.

Hudson-Stähli line a linear horizontal yellowish line seen in the deep epithelium of ageing corneas. [A. C. Hudson (1875–1962), British ophthalmologist; J. Stähli (20th century), Swiss ophthalmologist]

human chorionic gonadotrophin (HCG) a hormone, similar to the pituitary *gonadotrophins that is produced by the placenta during pregnancy. Large amounts are excreted in the urine, and this is used as the basis for most *pregnancy tests. The level of HCG in the serum is one of the indicators used in the *triple marker test for Down's syndrome. HCG maintains the secretion of *progesterone by the corpus luteum of the ovary, the secretion of pituitary gonadotrophins being blocked during pregnancy. HCG is given by injection to treat delayed puberty, undescended testes, premenstrual tension, and (with *follicle-stimulating hormone) sterility due to lack of ovulation.

Human Fertilization and Embryology Act 1990 an Act of Parliament that makes provisions for human embryos and children produced as a result of artificial insemination, in vitro fertilization, or any other method of assisted conception. The increasing use of such methods means that it is no longer possible to define legal parentage solely on a genetic basis. Under the Act, a person must give written informed consent before tissue is removed for use in assisted conception. The legal mother is defined as the woman who has given birth to the child, regardless of genetic parentage, unless the child is subsequently adopted or (in the case of children born to *surrogate mothers) a *section 30 order is made. The legal father is generally the genetic father except when the latter is a licensed sperm donor or when the donor's sperm is used after his death. When a wife conceives as a result of assisted conception, her spouse may be regarded as the child's legal father, even if he is not the genetic father, as long as he consented to her treatment.

The Act also established a **Human Fertilization and Embryology Authority**, which controls and reviews research involving the use of embryos and issues licences for this research and for treatment in assisted conception. It also maintains a register of persons whose gametes are used for assisted conception and of children born as a result. Children over the age of 18 can apply to the Authority for information concerning their ethnic and genetic background.

Human Genome Project a massive international research project to elucidate the entire sequence of genes on all the human chromosomes. The human genome comprises some 3000 million nucleotide base pairs (*see* DNA) forming about 100,000 genes, distributed between 23 pairs of chromosomes. The sequence of these bases, along the length of each chromosome, is currently being determined in several centres in different parts of the world. The Human Genome Project is by far the most ambitious biological research programme of all time. Beginning in 1988, it was scheduled to last for 15 years, but recent advances in methods of automating gene sequencing, made in a French laboratory, suggest that the project will be completed sooner than this. Knowledge of the entire human genome will be of incalculable value to medicine and human biology. It has already resulted in the identification of the genes associated with many hereditary disorders and revealed the existence of a genetic basis or component for many other diseases not previously known to have one. Theoretically, this would enable the development of drugs to alleviate conditions caused by deficiency of specific proteins and the large-scale genetic screening of populations known to be susceptible to particular disorders.

human immunodeficiency virus see HIV.

human leucocyte antigen system see HLA SYSTEM.

human papillomavirus (HPV) a virus – a member of the *papovavirus group – that causes warts, including genital warts. There are over 50 strains of HPV: certain strains are considered to be causative factors in the development of anal and genital cancers, especially cervical cancer, but additional factors are necessary before the cells become malignant. HPV is one of the most common sexually transmitted infections. In women the presence of HPV may be detected on colposcopic examination, although techniques using DNA amplification (see POLYMERASE CHAIN REACTION) give more accurate results and suggest that up to 40% of a normal, apparently healthy, female population may harbour these viruses. In women with an abnormal cervical smear, the DNA test is found to be positive in a much higher percentage and is therefore a useful indicator of a high risk of developing cancer of the cervix.

humectant 1. *n.* a substance that is used for moistening. 2. *adj.* causing moistening.

humerus *n.* the bone of the upper arm. The **head** of the humerus articulates with the *scapula at the shoulder joint. At the lower end of the shaft the **trochlea** articulates with the *ulna and part of the radius. The radius also articulates with a rounded protuberance (the **capitulum**) close to the trochlea. Depressions (**fossae**) at the front and back of the humerus accommodate the ulna and radius, respec-

tively, when the arm is flexed or straightened.

humoral *adj.* circulating in the bloodstream; humoral *immunity requires circulating antibodies.

humour *n.* a body fluid. See AQUEOUS HUMOUR, VITREOUS HUMOUR.

Hunner's ulcer see INTERSTITIAL CYSTITIS. [G. L. Hunner (1868–1957), US urologist]

Hunter's syndrome a hereditary disorder caused by deficiency of an enzyme that results in the accumulation of protein–carbohydrate complexes and fats in the cells of the body (see MUCOPOLYSACCHARIDOSIS). This leads to mental retardation, enlargement of the liver and spleen, and prominent coarse facial features (**gargoylism**). The disease is *sex-linked, being restricted to males, although females can be *carriers. Medical name: **mucopolysaccharidosis type II**. [C. H. Hunter (1872–1955), US physician]

Huntington's disease (Huntington's chorea) a hereditary disease caused by a defect in a single gene that is inherited as an autosomal *dominant characteristic, tending to appear in half of the children of the parents with this condition. Symptoms, which begin to appear in early middle age, include unsteady gait and jerky involuntary movements (see CHOREA), accompanied later by behavioural changes, and progressive dementia. The defective gene, which is located on chromosome no. 4, has now been identified, and *genetic screening is possible for those at risk. [G. Huntington (1850–1916), US physician]

Hurler's syndrome a hereditary disorder caused by deficiency of an enzyme that results in the accumulation of protein–carbohydrate complexes and fats in the cells of the body (see MUCOPOLYSACCHARIDOSIS). This leads to severe mental retardation, enlargement of the liver and spleen, heart defects, deformities of the bones, and coarsening and thickening of facial features (**gargoylism**). A bone marrow transplant offers the only hope of treatment. Medical name: **mucopolysaccharidosis type I**. [G. Hurler (1889–1965), Austrian paediatrician]

Hürthle cell tumour a malignant tumour of the thyroid gland that arises from **Hürthle cells**, large eosinophilic cells occasionally occurring in the gland. This carcinoma is not as common as **papillary**, **follicular**, or **anaplastic** thyroid carcinomas. [K. W. Hürthle (1860–1945), German histologist]

Hutchinson's teeth narrowed and notched permanent incisor teeth: a sign of congenital *syphilis. [J. Hutchinson (1828–1913), British surgeon]

hyal- (hyalo-) *prefix denoting* **1.** glassy; transparent. **2.** hyalin. **3.** the vitreous humour of the eye.

hyalin *n.* a clear glassy material produced as the result of degeneration in certain tissues, particularly connective tissue and epithelial cells.

hyaline cartilage the most common type of *cartilage: a bluish-white elastic material with a matrix of chondroitin sulphate in which fine collagen fibrils are embedded.

hyaline membrane disease *see* RESPIRATORY DISTRESS SYNDROME.

hyalitis *n.* inflammation of the *vitreous body of the eye. *See also* ASTEROID HYALOSIS.

hyaloid artery a fetal artery lying in the *hyaloid canal of the eye and supplying the lens.

hyaloid canal a channel within the vitreous humour of the *eye. It extends from the centre of the optic disc, where it communicates with the lymph spaces of the optic nerve, to the posterior wall of the lens.

hyaloid membrane the transparent membrane that surrounds the *vitreous humour of the eye, separating it from the retina.

hyaluronic acid an acid *mucopolysaccharide that acts as the binding and protective agent of the ground substance of connective tissue. It is also present in the synovial fluid around joints and in the vitreous and aqueous humours of the eye.

hyaluronidase *n.* an enzyme that depolymerizes *hyaluronic acid and therefore increases the permeability of connective tissue. Hyaluronidase is found in the testes, in semen, and in other tissues.

hybrid *n.* the offspring of a cross between two genetically unlike individuals. A hybrid, whose parents are usually of different species or varieties, is often sterile.

HYCOSY (hysterosalpingo-contrast sonography) an out-patient technique that tests for blocked Fallopian tubes. Using *transvaginal ultrasonography and an echo contrast medium, flow along the tubes can be reliably visualized. *See also* DOPPLER ULTRASOUND.

hydatid *n.* a bladder-like cyst formed in various human tissues following the growth of the larval stage of an *Echinococcus tapeworm. E. granulosus produces a single large fluid-filled cyst, called **unilocular hydatid**, which gives rise internally to smaller daughter cysts. The entire hydatid is bound by a fibrous capsule. E. multilocularis forms aggregates of many smaller cysts with a jelly-like matrix, called an **alveolar hydatid**, and enlarges by budding off external daughter cysts. Alveolar hydatids are not delimited by fibrous capsules and produce malignant tumours, which invade and destroy human tissues. *See also* HYDATID DISEASE.

hydatid disease (hydatidosis, echinococciasis, echinococcosis) a condition resulting from the presence in the liver, lungs, or brain of *hydatid cysts. The cysts of *Echinococcus multilocularis* form malignant tumours; those of *E. granulosus* exert pressure as they grow and thereby damage surrounding tissues. The presence of hydatids in the brain may result in blindness and epilepsy, and the rupture of any cyst can cause severe allergic reactions including fever and *urticaria. Treatment may necessitate surgical removal of the cysts. Spread of hydatid disease, particularly common in sheep-raising countries, can be prevented by the deworming of dogs.

hydatidiform mole (hydatid mole, vesicular mole) a collection of fluid-filled sacs that develop when the membrane (chorion) surrounding the embryo degenerates in early pregnancy. These sacs give the placenta the appearance of a bunch of grapes. The embryo dies, the uterus enlarges, and there is a discharge of pinkish liquid and cysts from the vagina. A malignant condition may subsequently develop (*see* CHORIONEPITHELIOMA).

hydatidosis *n.* *see* HYDATID DISEASE.

hydr- (hydro-) *prefix denoting* water or a watery fluid.

hydraemia *n.* the presence in the blood of more than the normal proportion of water.

hydralazine *n.* a drug that lowers blood pressure and is used, usually in conjunction with *diuretics, to treat hypertension. It is given by mouth or by injection; side-effects, including rapid heart rate, headache, faintness, and digestive upsets, can occur, especially at high doses. Trade name: **Apresoline**.

hydramnios (hydramnion) *n.* the presence of an abnormally large amount of *amniotic fluid surrounding the fetus from about the 20th week of pregnancy. The uterus becomes swollen, which causes breathlessness, there is excess fluid in the body tissues, and there may be a difficult birth. Hydramnios is often associated with twin pregnancies or with fetal abnormalities, e.g. *anencephaly. The diagnosis is confirmed by ultrasound scan.

hydrargyria *n.* *see* MERCURIALISM.

hydrarthrosis *n.* swelling at a joint caused by excessive synovial fluid. The condition usually involves the knees and may be recurrent. Often no cause is apparent; in some cases rheumatoid arthritis develops later.

hydrocalycosis *n.* *see* CALIECTASIS.

hydrocele *n.* the accumulation of watery liquid in a sac, usually the sac surrounding the testes. This condition is characterized by painless enlargement of the scrotum; it is treated surgically, by drainage of the fluid or removal of the sac.

hydrocephalus *n.* an abnormal increase in the amount of cerebrospinal fluid within the ventricles of the brain. In childhood, before the sutures of the skull have fused, hydrocephalus makes the head enlarge. In adults, because of the unyielding nature of the skull, hydrocephalus raises the intracranial pressure with consequent drowsiness and vomiting.

Hydrocephalus may be caused by obstruction to the outflow of cerebrospinal fluid from the ventricles or a failure of its reabsorption into the cerebral sinuses. *Spina bifida may be associated with hydrocephalus in childhood. Treatment is to divert the excess cerebrospinal fluid into the abdominal cavity, where it is absorbed. This is achieved by tunnelling a thin tube from the ventricles to the abdomen (**ventriculo-peritoneal shunt**) or atrium (**ventriculo-atrial shunt**).

hydrochloric acid a strong acid present, in a very dilute form, in gastric juice. The secretion of excess hydrochloric acid by the stomach results in the condition *hyperchlorhydria.

hydrochlorothiazide *n.* a *diuretic used to treat fluid retention (oedema) and high blood pressure. It is administered by mouth, and side-effects can include digestive upsets, skin reactions, and dizziness. Trade names: **Esidrex**, **Hydrosaluric**.

hydrocortisone *n.* a pharmaceutical preparation of the steroid hormone *cortisol. Hydrocortisone is used in the treatment of adrenal failure (*Addison's disease) and inflammatory, allergic, and rheumatic conditions (including rheumatoid arthritis, colitis, and eczema). It may be given by mouth, by injection, or in the form of a cream or ointment. Possible side-effects of hydrocortisone therapy include peptic ulcers, bone and muscle damage, suppression of growth in children, and the signs of *Cushing's syndrome.

hydrocyanic acid (prussic acid) an intensely poisonous volatile acid that can cause death within a minute if inhaled. It has a smell of bitter almonds. *See* CYANIDE.

hydrogenase *n.* an enzyme that catalyses the addition of hydrogen to a compound in reduction reactions.

hydrogen bond a weak electrostatic bond formed by linking a hydrogen atom between two electronegative atoms (e.g. nitrogen or oxygen). The large number of hydrogen bonds in proteins and nucleic acids are responsible for maintaining the stable molecular structure of these compounds.

hydrogen peroxide a colourless liquid used as a disinfectant for cleansing wounds and, diluted, as a deodorant mouthwash or as ear drops for removing wax. Strong solutions irritate the skin.

hydrolase *n.* an enzyme that catalyses the hydrolysis of compounds. Examples are the *peptidases.

hydroma *n. see* HYGROMA.

hydronephrosis *n.* distension and dilatation of the pelvis of the kidney. This is due to an obstruction to the free flow of urine from the kidney. An obstruction at or below the neck of the bladder will result in hydronephrosis of both kidneys. The term **primary pelvic hydronephrosis** is used when the obstruction, usually functional, is at the junction of the renal pelvis and ureter. Surgical relief by *pyeloplasty is advisable to avoid the back pressure atrophy of the kidney and the complications of infection and stone formation. —**hydronephrotic** *adj.*

hydropericarditis *n. see* HYDROPERI-CARDIUM.

hydropericardium *n.* accumulation of a clear serous fluid within the membranous sac surrounding the heart. It occurs in many cases of *pericarditis (**hydropericarditis**). If the heart is compressed the fluid is withdrawn (aspirated) via a needle inserted into the pericardial sac through the chest wall (**pericardiocentesis**). *See also* HYDROPNEUMOPERICARDIUM.

hydroperitoneum *n. see* ASCITES.

hydrophobia *n. see* RABIES.

hydrophthalmos *n. see* BUPHTHALMOS.

hydropneumopericardium *n.* the presence of air and clear fluid within the pericardial sac around the heart, which is most commonly due to entry of air during pericardiocentesis (*see* HYDROPERI-CARDIUM). The presence of air does not affect the management of the patient.

hydropneumoperitoneum *n.* the presence of fluid and gas in the peritoneal cavity. This may be due either to the introduction of air through an instrument being used to remove the fluid; because a perforation in the digestive tract has allowed the escape of fluid and gas; or because gas-forming bacteria are growing in the peritoneal fluid.

hydropneumothorax *n.* the presence of air and fluid in the pleural cavity. If the patient is shaken the fluid makes a splashing sound (called a **succussion splash**). An *effusion of serous fluid commonly complicates a *pneumothorax, and must be drained.

hydrops *n.* an abnormal accumulation of fluid in body tissues or cavities. For example, **corneal hydrops** is the sudden painful accumulation of fluid in the cornea seen in *keratoconus. It results in a sudden reduction of vision. *See also* HY-DROPS FETALIS, MÉNIÈRE'S DISEASE (ENDOLYM-PHATIC HYDROPS).

hydrops fetalis severe oedema that develops before birth. The excess fluid collects in the body cavities, particularly in the peritoneal cavity (*see* ASCITES) and the pleural cavity. There are several causes for this, but the most common is severe anaemia associated with *haemolytic disease of the newborn. Other causes are congenital heart disease, kidney disease, and lung disease. Treatment can be undertaken before birth with intrauterine blood transfusions to the fetus; without treatment the mortality is high. Antenatal ultrasound scanning enables early recognition of hydrops fetalis.

hydrosalpinx *n.* the accumulation of watery fluid in one of the *Fallopian tubes, which becomes swollen.

hydrostatic accouchement the management of normal labour with the mother partially immersed in a water bath.

hydrotherapy *n.* the use of water in the treatment of disorders: today restricted in orthodox medicine to exercises done in remedial swimming pools for the *rehabilitation of arthritic or partially paralysed patients.

hydrothorax *n.* fluid in the pleural cavity. *See also* HYDROPNEUMOTHORAX.

hydrotubation *n.* the introduction of a fluid (usually a dye) through the cervix (neck) of the uterus under pressure to allow visualization, by *laparoscopy, of the passage of the dye through the Fallopian tubes. It is used to test whether or not the tubes are blocked in the investigation of infertility.

hydroureter *n.* an accumulation of urine in one of the tubes (ureters) leading from the kidneys to the bladder. The ureter becomes swollen and the condition usually results from obstruction of the ureter by a stone or a misplaced artery.

hydroxocobalamin *n.* a cobalt-containing drug administered by injection to treat conditions involving vitamin B$_{12}$ deficiency, such as pernicious anaemia. Trade names: **Cobalin-H**, **Neo-Cytamen**.

hydroxyapatite *n.* **1.** the crystalline component of bones and teeth, consisting of a complex form of calcium phosphate. **2.** a biocompatible ceramic material that is a synthetic form of natural hydroxyapatite. Some joint replacement prostheses are coated with synthetic hydroxyapatite, which encourages bone to grow on to the implant. The material is also used in some forms of middle-ear surgery.

hydroxychloroquine *n.* a drug similar to *chloroquine, used mainly to treat lupus erythematosus and rheumatoid arthritis. Side-effects such as skin reactions, hair loss, and digestive upsets may occur and prolonged use can lead to eye damage. Trade name: **Plaquenil**.

hydroxyprogesterone *n.* a synthetic female sex hormone (*see* PROGESTOGEN) administered by injection to prevent miscarriage and to treat menstrual disorders. There may be pain at the injection site, and progestogens taken by mouth are often preferred. Trade name: **Proluton**.

hydroxyproline *n.* a compound, similar in structure to the *amino acids, found only in *collagen.

5-hydroxytryptamine *n.* *see* SEROTONIN.

hydroxyurea *n.* a drug that prevents cell growth and is used to treat some types of leukaemia. It is administered by mouth. Hydroxyurea may lower the white cell content of the blood due to its effects on the bone marrow. Trade name: **Hydrea**.

hydroxyzine *n.* an *antihistamine drug with sedative properties, used to relieve anxiety, tension, and agitation and to treat nausea and vomiting. It is administered by mouth and may cause drowsiness, headache, dry mouth, and itching. Trade name: **Atarax**.

hygiene *n.* the science of health and the study of ways of preserving it, particularly by promoting cleanliness.

hygr- (hygro-) *prefix denoting* moisture.

hygroma (hydroma) *n.* a type of cyst. It may develop from a *lymphangioma (**cystic hygroma**) or from the liquified remains of a subdural *haematoma (**subdural hygroma**).

hygrometer *n.* an instrument for measuring the relative humidity of the atmosphere, i.e. the ratio of the moisture in the air to the moisture it would contain if it were saturated at the same temperature and pressure. In the **dew-point hygrometer** a polished surface is reduced in temperature until the water vapour from the atmosphere forms on it. The temperature of this dew point enables the relative humidity of the atmosphere to be calculated. In the **wet-and-dry bulb hygrometer**, there are two thermometers mounted side by side, the bulb of one being surrounded by moistened muslin. The thermometer with the wet bulb will register a lower temperature than that with the dry bulb owing to the cooling effect of the evaporating water. The temperature difference enables the relative humidity to be calculated.

hymen *n.* the membrane that covers the opening of the vagina at birth but usually perforates spontaneously before puberty. If the initial opening is small it may tear, with slight loss of blood, at the first occasion of sexual intercourse.

Hymenolepis *n.* a genus of small widely distributed parasitic tapeworms. The dwarf tapeworm, *H. nana*, only 40 mm in length, lives in the human intestine. Fleas can be important vectors of this species, and children in close contact with flea-infested dogs are particularly prone to infection. *H. diminuta* is a common parasite of rodents; man occasionally becomes infected on swallowing stored cereals contaminated with insect pests – the intermediate hosts for this parasite. Symptoms of abdominal pain, diarrhoea, loss of appetite, and headache are obvious only in heavy infections of either species. Treatment involves a course of *anthelmintics.

hymenotomy n. incision of the hymen at the entrance to the vagina. This operation may be performed on a young girl if the membrane completely closes the vagina and thus impedes the flow of menstrual blood. It is also carried out to alleviate dyspareunia (painful intercourse).

hyo- *prefix denoting* the hyoid bone. Example: **hyoglossal** (relating to the hyoid bone and tongue).

hyoglossus n. a muscle that serves to depress the tongue. It has its origin in the hyoid bone.

hyoid bone a small isolated U-shaped bone in the neck, below and supporting the tongue. It is held in position by muscles and ligaments between it and the styloid process of the temporal bone.

hyoscine (scopolamine) n. a drug that prevents muscle spasm (see PARASYMPATHO-LYTIC). It is used in the treatment of gastric or duodenal ulcers, spasm in the digestive system, and difficult or painful menstruation and also to relax the uterus in labour. It can also be used to calm excitement in some psychiatric conditions, for preoperative medication, for motion sickness, and to dilate the pupil and paralyse the muscles of the eye for examination. It is administered by mouth or injection. Side-effects are rare but can include dry mouth, blurred vision, difficulty in urination, and increased heart rate. Trade names: **Buscopan**, **Scopoderm**.

hyp- (hypo-) *prefix denoting* **1.** deficiency, lack, or small size. Example: **hypognathous** (having a small lower jaw). **2.** (in anatomy) below; beneath. Example: **hypoglossal** (under the tongue).

hypalgesia n. an abnormally low sensitivity to pain.

Hypaque n. trade name for diatrizoate sodium, used as a water-soluble contrast medium in radiology of the urinary tract.

hyper- *prefix denoting* **1.** excessive; abnormally increased. **2.** (in anatomy) above.

hyperacusis n. abnormally acute hearing or painful sensitivity to sounds.

hyperadrenalism n. overactivity of the adrenal glands. See CUSHING'S SYNDROME.

hyperaemia n. the presence of excess blood in the vessels supplying a part of the body. In **active hyperaemia** (**arterial hyperaemia**) the arterioles are relaxed and there is an increased blood flow. In **passive hyperaemia** the blood flow from the affected part is obstructed.

hyperaesthesia n. excessive sensibility, especially of the skin.

hyperalgesia n. an abnormal state of increased sensitivity to painful stimuli.

hyperandrogenism n. excessive secretion of androgen in women. It is associated with *hirsutism, acne, sparse or infrequent menstruation (oligomenorrhoea), *metrorrhagia, absent or infrequent ovulation, infertility, endometrial *hyperplasia, *hyperlipidaemia, *hyperglycaemia, and hypertension; all these conditions may be the result of mutations in specific genes. See also VIRILIZATION.

hyperbaric *adj.* at a pressure greater than atmospheric pressure.

hyperbaric oxygenation a technique for exposing a patient to oxygen at high pressure. It is used to treat carbon monoxide poisoning, gas gangrene, compressed air illness, and acute breathing difficulties. It is also used in some cases during heart surgery.

hypercalcaemia n. the presence in the blood of an abnormally high concentration of calcium. **Idiopathic hypercalcaemia** is a congenital condition associated with mental retardation and heart defects. Hypercalcaemia can also be caused by excessive ingestion of vitamin D. *Compare* HYPOCALCAEMIA.

hypercalcinuria (hypercalcuria) n. the presence in the urine of an abnormally high concentration of calcium.

hypercapnia (hypercarbia) n. the presence in the blood of an abnormally high concentration of carbon dioxide.

hyperchloraemia n. the presence in the blood of an abnormally high concentration of chloride.

hyperchlorhydria n. a greater than normal secretion of hydrochloric acid by the stomach, usually associated with a *duodenal ulcer. Extremely high levels of acid secretion are found in the *Zollinger-Ellison syndrome.

hypercholesterolaemia *n. see* CHOLESTEROL.

hyperchromatism *n.* the property of the nuclei of certain cells (for example, those of tumours) to stain more deeply than normal. —**hyperchromatic** *adj.*

hyperdactylism (polydactylism) *n.* the condition of having more than the normal number of fingers or toes. The extra digits are commonly undersized (rudimentary) and are usually removed surgically shortly after birth.

hyperdynamia *n.* excessive activity of muscles.

hyperemesis gravidarum severe vomiting during pregnancy. It starts in early pregnancy and may continue to produce marked dehydration and subsequent liver damage. Rarely, the condition worsens in spite of active treatment; under such circumstances it may be necessary to terminate the pregnancy.

hyperextension *n.* extension of a joint or limb beyond its normal limit.

hyperglycaemia *n.* an excess of glucose in the bloodstream. It may occur in a variety of diseases, most notably in *diabetes mellitus, due to insufficient insulin in the blood and excessive intake of carbohydrates. Untreated it may progress to diabetic coma.

hypergraphia *n.* a style of writing characterized by excessive verbosity, pedantic insistence on much nonessential detail, and obsessive inclusiveness that is a feature of the type of personality disturbance frequently associated with severe epilepsy. People manifesting hypergraphia will seldom accept that they have a communication problem.

hyperidrosis (hyperhidrosis) *n.* excessive sweating, which may occur in certain diseases, such as thyrotoxicosis or fevers, or following the use of certain drugs.

hyperinsulinism *n.* **1.** excessive secretion o of the hormone insulin by the islet cells of the pancreas. **2.** metabolic disturbance due to administration of too much insulin.

hyperkalaemia *n.* the presence in the blood of an abnormally high concentration of *potassium, usually due to failure of the kidneys to excrete it. *See also* ELECTROLYTE.

hyperkeratosis *n.* thickening of the outer horny layeof the skin. It may occur as an inherited disorder, affecting the palms and soles.

hyperkinesia *n.* a state of overactive restlessness in children. —**hyperkinetic** *adj.*

hyperkinetic disorder *see* ATTENTION DEFICIT DISORDER.

hyperlipidaemia (hyperlipaemia) *n.* the presence in the blood of an abnormally high concentration of fats.

hyperlipoproteinaemia *n.* the presence in the blood of abnormally high concentrations of *lipoproteins.

hypermetropia (long-sightedness) *n.* the condition in which parallel light rays are brought to a focus behind the retina when the *accommodation is relaxed (see illustration). Moderate degrees of hypermetropia may not cause blurred vision in children and young adults because of their ability to accommodate, but for older people and those with greater degrees of hypermetropia near vision is more blurred than distance vision. Normal vision can be restored by wearing spectacles with convex lenses. *Compare* EMMETROPIA, MYOPIA.

hypermotility *n.* excessive movement or activity, especially of the stomach or intestine.

hypernatraemia *n.* the presence in the blood of an abnormally high concentration of *sodium. *See also* ELECTROLYTE.

hypernephroma (Grawitz tumour, renal cell carcinoma) *n.* a malignant tumour of kidney cells, so called because it is said to resemble part of the adrenal gland and at one time was thought to originate from this site. It may be present for some years before giving rise to symptoms, which include fever, loin pain and swelling, and blood in the urine. Treatment is by surgery but tumours are apt to recur locally. The tumour spreads via the bloodstream and can often be seen growing along the renal vein. Secondary growths from a renal cell carcinoma in the lung have a characteristic 'cannon-ball' appearance. These tumours are relatively insensitive to radiotherapy and cytotoxic drugs but some respond to such hormones as progestogens and testosterone.

hyperopia *n.* the usual US term for *hypermetropia.

hyperosmia *n.* an abnormally acute sense of smell.

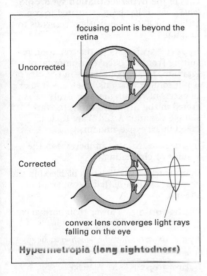

focusing point is beyond the retina

Uncorrected

Corrected

convex lens converges light rays falling on the eye

Hypermetropia (long sightedness)

hyperostosis *n.* excessive enlargement of the outer layer of a bone. The condition is harmless and is usually recognized as an incidental finding on X-ray. It commonly affects the frontal bone of the skull (**hyperostosis frontalis**). **Infantile cortical hyperostosis** (or **Caffey's disease**) affects infants under six months. There is swelling of the long bones, jaw, and shoulder blade, with pain and a fever. The condition settles spontaneously.

hyperparathyroidism *n.* overactivity of the parathyroid glands. *See also* VON RECKLINGHAUSEN'S DISEASE.

hyperpiesia *n. see* HYPERTENSION.

hyperplasia *n.* the increased production and growth of normal cells in a tissue or organ. The affected part becomes larger but retains its normal form. During pregnancy the breasts grow in this manner. *See also* ENDOMETRIAL HYPERPLASIA. *Compare* HYPERTROPHY, NEOPLASM.

hyperpnoea *n.* an increase in the rate of breathing that is proportional to an increase in metabolism; for example, on exercise. *Compare* HYPERVENTILATION.

hyperpraxia *n.* excessive motor activity, such as is seen in *mania and *attention deficit disorder.

hyperpyrexia *n.* a rise in body temperature above 106°F (41.1°C). *See* FEVER.

hypersensitive *adj.* prone to respond abnormally to the presence of a particular antigen, which may cause a variety of tissue reactions ranging from *serum sickness to an allergy (such as hay fever) or, at the severest, to anaphylactic shock (*see* ANAPHYLAXIS). It is thought that when the normal antigen-antibody defence reaction is followed by tissue damage this may be due to an abnormality in the working of the *complement system. *See also* ALLERGY, IMMUNITY. —**hypersensitivity** *n.*

hypersomnia *n.* sleep lasting for exceptionally long periods, as occurs in some cases of brain inflammation.

hypersplenism *n.* a decrease in the numbers of red cells, white cells, and platelets in the blood resulting from destruction or pooling of these cells by an enlarged spleen. Hypersplenism may occur in any condition in which there is enlargement of the spleen (*see* SPLENOMEGALY).

hypersthenia *n.* an abnormally high degree of strength or physical tension in all or part of the body.

hypertension *n.* high *blood pressure, i.e. elevation of the arterial blood pressure above the normal range expected in a particular age group. Hypertension may be of unknown cause (**essential hypertension** or **hyperpiesia**). It may also result from kidney disease, including narrowing (stenosis) of the renal artery (**renal hypertension**), endocrine diseases (such as Cushing's disease or phaeochromocytoma) or disease of the arteries (such as coarctation of the aorta), when it is known as

secondary or **symptomatic hypertension.**

Complications that may arise from hypertension include atherosclerosis, heart failure, cerebral haemorrhage, and kidney failure, but treatment may prevent their development. Hypertension is symptomless until the symptoms of its complications develop. Some cases of hypertension may be cured by eradicating the cause. Most cases, however, depend upon long-term drug therapy to lower the blood pressure and maintain it within the normal range. The drugs used include thiazide *diuretics, *beta blockers, *methyldopa, *guanethidine, and many others. Combinations of drugs may be needed to obtain optimum control. *See also* PORTAL HYPERTENSION, PULMONARY HYPERTENSION.

hyperthermia (hyperthermy) *n.* **1.** exceptionally high body temperature (about 41°C or above). *See* FEVER. **2.** treatment of disease by inducing fever. *Compare* HYPOTHERMIA.

hyperthyroidism *n.* overactivity of the thyroid gland, either due to a tumour, overgrowth of the gland, or Graves's disease. *See* THYROTOXICOSIS.

hypertonia (hypertonicity) *n.* exceptionally high tension in muscles.

hypertonic *adj.* **1.** describing a solution that has a greater osmotic pressure than another solution. *See* OSMOSIS. **2.** describing muscles that demonstrate an abnormal increase in *tonicity.

hypertrichosis *n.* excessive growth of hair (*see* HIRSUTISM).

hypertrophy (hypertrophia) *n.* increase in the size of a tissue or organ brought about by the enlargement of its cells rather than by cell multiplication (as during normal growth and tumour formation). Muscles undergo this change in response to increased work. *Compare* HYPERPLASIA.

hypertropia *n. see* STRABISMUS.

hyperuricaemia (lithaemia) *n.* the presence in the blood of an abnormally high concentration of uric acid. *See* GOUT.

hyperuricuria (lithuria) *n.* the presence in the urine of an abnormally high concentration of uric acid.

hyperventilation *n.* breathing at an abnormally rapid rate at rest. This causes a reduction of the carbon dioxide concentration of arterial blood, leading to dizziness, tingling (paraesthesiae) in the lips and limbs, tetanic cramps in the hands, and tightness across the chest. If continued, hyperventilation may cause loss of consciousness. This sequence of events occurs in the **hyperventilation syndrome** (**HVS**), which has been estimated to contribute to 10% of out-patient referrals to hospital.

hypervitaminosis *n.* the condition resulting from excessive consumption of vitamins. This is not serious in the case of water-soluble vitamins, when any intake in excess of requirements is easily excreted in the urine. However, the fat-soluble vitamins A and D are toxic if taken in excessive amounts.

hypervolaemia *n.* an increase in the volume of circulating blood.

hyphaema *n.* a collection of blood in the chamber of the eye that lies in front of the iris.

hyphedonia *n.* a lower than normal capacity for achieving enjoyment.

hypn- (hypno-) *prefix denoting* **1.** sleep. **2.** hypnosis.

hypnagogic *adj. see* IMAGERY.

hypnopompic *adj. see* IMAGERY.

hypnosis *n.* a sleeplike state, artificially induced in a person by a **hypnotist**, in which the mind is more than usually receptive to suggestion and memories of past events – apparently forgotten – may be elicited by questioning. Hypnotic suggestion has been used for a variety of purposes in medicine, for example as a cure for addiction and in other forms of *psychotherapy.

hypnotherapy *n.* any form of psychotherapy that utilizes hypnosis.

hypnotic (soporific) *n.* a drug that produces sleep by depressing brain function. Hypnotics include benzodiazepines (such as *nitrazepam and *temazepam), *chloral hydrate, and some sedative *antihistamines (e.g. *promethazine). Hypnotics are used for insomnia and sleep disturbances, especially in mental illnesses and in the elderly. They often cause hangover effects in the morning.

hypnotism *n.* the induction of *hypnosis.

hypo- *prefix. see* HYP-.

hypoaesthesia *n.* a condition in which the sense of touch is diminished; uncommonly this may be extended to include other forms of sensation.

hypobaric *adj.* at a pressure lower than that of the atmosphere.

hypobulia *n.* mild deficiency of will power. *See* ABULIA.

hypocalcaemia *n.* the presence in the blood of an abnormally low concentration of calcium. *See* TETANY. *Compare* HYPERCALCAEMIA.

hypocapnia *n. see* ACAPNIA.

hypochloraemia *n.* the presence in the blood of an abnormally low concentration of chloride.

hypochlorhydria *n.* reduced secretion of hydrochloric acid by the stomach. *See* ACHLORHYDRIA.

hypochondria *n.* preoccupation with the physical functioning of the body and with fancied ill health. It may amount to a handicapping neurosis and dominate a person's life. In the most severe form there are delusions of ill health, usually due to underlying *depression. When symptoms reach the level sufficient to be classified as a disorder, it is called **hypochondriasis** (in *DSM-IV) or **hypochondriacal disorder** (in ICD-10). Treatment with reassurance, *antidepressant drugs, and/or psychotherapy is usual, but the condition is often chronic. —**hypochondriac** *adj., n.*

hypochondrium *n.* the upper lateral portion of the *abdomen, situated beneath the lower ribs. —**hypochondriac** *adj.*

Hypoderma *n.* a genus of non-blood-sucking beelike insects – the warble flies – widely distributed in Europe, North America, and Asia. Cattle are the usual

hosts for the parasitic maggots, but rare and accidental infections of man have occurred (*see* MYIASIS), especially in farm workers. The maggots migrate beneath the skin surface, producing an inflamed linear lesion similar to that of *creeping eruption.

hypodermic *adj.* beneath the skin: usually applied to subcutaneous *injections. The term is also applied to the syringe used for such injections, and sometimes – loosely – to any injection.

hypodontia *n.* a reduction in the normal number of teeth through congenital absence.

hypofibrinogenaemia (fibrinogeno-penia) *n.* a deficiency of the clotting factor *fibrinogen in the blood, which results in an increased tendency to bleed. It may occur as an inherited disorder in which either production of fibrinogen is impaired or the fibrinogen produced does not function in the normal way (**dysfibrinogenaemia**). Alternatively, it may be acquired. For example, it is the commonest cause of blood coagulation failure during pregnancy, when the blood fibrinogen level falls below the normal pregnancy level of 4–6 g/l. This usually occurs as a complication of severe *abruptio placentae, prolonged retention of a dead fetus, or amniotic fluid embolism.

hypogammaglobulinaemia *n.* a deficiency of the protein *gammaglobulin in the blood. It may occur in a variety of inherited disorders or as an acquired defect, as in certain *lymphomas. Since gammaglobulin consists mainly of antibodies (*immunoglobulins), hypogammaglobulinaemia results in an increased susceptibility to infections.

hypogastrium *n.* that part of the central *abdomen situated below the region of the stomach. —**hypogastric** *adj.*

hypogeusia *n.* a condition in which the sense of taste is abnormally weak. *See also* HYPOAESTHESIA.

hypoglossal nerve the twelfth *cranial nerve (XII), which supplies the muscles of the tongue and is therefore responsible for the movements of talking and swallowing.

hypoglycaemia *n.* a deficiency of glucose in the bloodstream, causing muscular weakness and incoordination, mental confusion, and sweating. If severe it may lead to **hypoglycaemic coma**. Hypoglycaemia most commonly occurs in *diabetes mellitus, as a result of insulin overdosage and insufficient intake of carbohydrates. It is treated by administration of glucose: by injection if the patient is in a coma, by mouth otherwise. **—hypoglycaemic** *adj.*

hypogonadism *n.* impaired function of the testes or ovaries, causing absence or impairment of the *secondary sexual characteristics.

hypohidrosis *n. see* ANHIDROSIS.

hypoinsulinism *n.* a deficiency of insulin due either to inadequate secretion of the hormone by the pancreas or to inadequate treatment of diabetes mellitus.

hypokalaemia *n.* the presence of abnormally low levels of potassium in the blood: occurs in dehydration. *See* ELECTROLYTE.

hypomania *n.* a mild degree of *mania. Elated mood leads to faulty judgment; behaviour lacks the usual social restraints and the sexual drive is increased; speech is rapid and animated; the individual is energetic but not persistent and tends to be irritable. The abnormality is not so great as in mania and the patient may appear normal and 'a bit of a character' to those who do not know him (*see* ELATION, EUPHORIA). Treatment follows the same principles as for mania, and it may be difficult to prevent an individual from damaging his own interests with extravagant behaviour. **—hypomanic** *adj., n.*

hypomenorrhoea *n.* the release of an abnormally small quantity of blood at menstruation. The duration of bleeding may be normal or less than normal.

hyponatraemia *n.* the presence in the blood of an abnormally low concentration of *sodium: occurs in dehydration. *See* ELECTROLYTE.

hypoparathyroidism *n.* subnormal activity of the parathyroid glands, causing a fall in the blood concentration of calcium and muscular spasms (*see* TETANY).

hypopharynx *n. see* LARYNGOPHARYNX.

hypophysectomy *n.* the surgical removal or destruction of the pituitary gland (hypophysis) in the brain. The operation may be conducted by opening the skull or by the insertion of special needles that produce a very low temperature (*see* CRYOSURGERY). Radiotherapy (e.g. by insertion of needles of radioactive *yttrium) can also be used to destroy parts of the pituitary.

hypophysis *n. see* PITUITARY GLAND.

hypopiesis *n.* abnormally reduced blood pressure in the absence of organic disease (*see* HYPOTENSION).

hypopituitarism *n.* subnormal activity of the pituitary gland, causing *dwarfism in childhood and a syndrome of impaired sexual function, pallor, and premature ageing in adult life (*see* SIMMOND'S DISEASE).

hypoplasia *n.* underdevelopment of an organ or tissue. **Dental hypoplasia** is the defective formation of parts of a tooth due to illnesses such as measles or starvation while the tooth is being formed. It is marked by transverse lines of brown defective enamel, which define the date of the illness.

hypoplastic left heart a congenital heart disorder in which the left side of the heart, particularly the left ventricle, is underdeveloped. The first part of the aorta may also be abnormal. Affected babies usually develop severe heart failure within the first few days of life. Diagnosis can be confirmed on *echocardiography. Prognosis is generally very poor – most babies die within the first few weeks – but milder cases may be amenable to surgery. It is the commonest cause of death in the neonatal period due to heart disease.

hypopraxia *n.* **1.** a condition of diminished and enfeebled activity. **2.** a lack of interest in, or a disinclination for, activity; listlessness.

hypoproteinaemia *n.* a decrease in the quantity of protein in the blood. It may result from malnutrition, impaired protein production (as in liver disease), or increased loss of protein from the body (as in the *nephrotic syndrome). It results in swelling (*oedema), because of the accumulation of fluid in the tissues, and increased susceptibility to infections. *See also* HYPOGAMMAGLOBULINAEMIA.

hypoprothrombinaemia *n.* a deficiency of the clotting factor *prothrombin in the blood, which results in an increased tendency to bleed. It may occur as an inherited defect, as the result of liver disease, vitamin K deficiency, or anticoagulant treatment.

hypopyon *n.* pus in the chamber of the eye that lies in front of the iris.

hyposensitive *adj.* less than normally responsive to the presence of antigenic material. *Compare* HYPERSENSITIVE. —**hyposensitivity** *n.*

hyposensitization *n.* *see* DESENSITIZATION.

hyposmia *n.* a condition in which the sense of smell is exceptionally weak. *See also* HYPOAESTHESIA.

hypospadias *n.* a congenital abnormality in which the opening of the *urethra is on the underside of the penis: either on the glans penis (**glandular hypospadias**), at the junction of the glans with the shaft (**coronal hypospadias**), or on the shaft itself (**penile hypospadias**). All varieties can be treated surgically, and neither micturition nor sexual function need be impaired. *See* MAGPI OPERATION.

hypostasis *n.* accumulation of fluid or blood in a dependent part of the body, under the influence of gravity, in cases of poor circulation. Hypostatic congestion of the lung bases may be seen in debilitated patients who are confined to bed. It predisposes to pneumonia (hypostatic pneumonia) but it may be prevented by careful nursing and physiotherapy. A similar condition affects the dependent parts of the body after death. —**hypostatic** *adj.*

hyposthenia *n.* a state of physical weakness or abnormally low muscular tension.

hyposthenuria *n.* the secretion of urine of low specific gravity. The inability to concentrate the urine occurs in patients at the final stage of chronic renal failure.

hypotension *n.* a condition in which the arterial *blood pressure is abnormally low. It occurs after excessive fluid loss (e.g. through diarrhoea, burns, or vomiting) or

following severe blood loss (haemorrhage) from any cause. Other causes include myocardial infarction, pulmonary embolism, severe infections, allergic reactions, arrhythmias, acute abdominal conditions (e.g. pancreatitis), Addison's disease, and drugs (e.g. an overdose of the drugs used to treat hypertension).

Some people experience a temporary fall in blood pressure when rising from a horizontal position (**orthostatic hypotension**). Temporary hypotension may result in a simple faint (syncope). The patient becomes light-headed, sweats, and may develop impaired consciousness. In severe cases peripheral circulatory failure (cardiogenic shock) develops, with unrecordable blood pressure, weak pulses, and suppression of urine production. The patient is placed flat, with legs elevated, and given oxygen. Fluid and blood are replaced by an intravenous infusion as required. Specific treatment of the cause is provided (e.g. corticosteroids in Addison's disease).

hypothalamus *n.* the region of the forebrain in the floor of the third ventricle, linked with the thalamus above and the *pituitary gland below (*see* BRAIN). It contains several important centres controlling body temperature, thirst, hunger, and eating, water balance, and sexual function. It is also closely connected with emotional activity and sleep and functions as a centre for the integration of hormonal and autonomic nervous activity through its control of the pituitary secretions (*see* NEUROENDOCRINE SYSTEM, PITUITARY GLAND). —**hypothalamic** *adj.*

hypothenar *adj.* describing or relating to the fleshy prominent part of the palm of the hand below the little finger. *Compare* THENAR.

hypothermia *n.* **1.** accidental reduction of body temperature below the normal range in the absence of protective reflex actions, such as shivering. Often insidious in onset, it is particularly liable to occur in babies and the elderly if they are living in poorly heated homes and have inadequate clothing. **2.** deliberate lowering of body temperature for therapeutic purposes. This may be done during surgery, in order to reduce the patient's requirement for oxygen.

hypothymia *n.* a diminished intensity of emotional response. It is a feature of *asthenic personalities, and of some chronic schizophrenics and some depressives.

hypothyroidism *n.* subnormal activity of the thyroid gland. If present at birth and untreated it leads to *cretinism. In adult life it causes mental and physical slowing, undue sensitivity to cold, slowing of the pulse, weight gain, and coarsening of the skin (**myxoedema**). The condition can be treated by administration of thyroxine.

hypotonia *n.* a state of reduced tension in muscle.

hypotonic *adj.* **1.** describing a solution that has a lower osmotic pressure than another solution. *See* OSMOSIS. **2.** describing muscles that demonstrate diminished *tonicity.

hypotrichosis *n.* a condition in which less hair develops than normal.

hypotropia *n.* *see* STRABISMUS.

hypoventilation *n.* breathing at an abnormally shallow and slow rate, which results in an increased concentration of carbon dioxide in the blood. **Alveolar hypoventilation** may be primary, which is very rare, or secondary, which can be due to destructive lesions of the brain or to an acquired blunting of respiratory drive arising from failure of the respiratory pump.

hypovitaminosis *n.* a deficiency of a vitamin caused either through lack of the vitamin in the diet or from an inability to absorb or utilize it.

hypovolaemia (oligaemia) *n.* a decrease in the volume of circulating blood. *See* SHOCK.

hypoxaemia *n.* reduction of the oxygen concentration in the arterial blood, recognized clinically by the presence of central and peripheral *cyanosis. When the partial pressure of oxygen (pO_2) falls below 8.0 kPa (60 mmHg), the condition is defined as respiratory failure.

hypoxia *n.* a deficiency of oxygen in the tissues. *See also* ANOXIA, HYPOXAEMIA.

hypsarrhythmia *n.* a severe abnormality on an EEG (*see* ENCEPHALOGRAPHY) that demonstrates a chaotic pattern of brain activity. It is usually characteristic of *infantile spasms.

hyster- (hystero-) *prefix denoting* **1.** the uterus. **2.** hysteria.

hysterectomy *n.* the surgical removal of the uterus, either through an incision in the abdominal wall (**abdominal hysterectomy**) or through the vagina (**vaginal hysterectomy**). **Subtotal hysterectomy** (rarely performed now) involves removing the body of the uterus but leaving the neck (cervix); in **total hysterectomy** the entire uterus is removed. The operation is performed for cancerous conditions affecting the uterus and for nonmalignant conditions (e.g. fibroids) in which there is excessive menstrual bleeding. Although pregnancy is no longer possible, hysterectomy does not affect sexual desire or activity.

hysteria *n.* **1.** formerly, a neurosis characterized by emotional instability, repression, dissociation, some physical symptoms (*see* HYSTERICAL), and vulnerability to suggestion. Two types were recognized: **conversion hysteria**, now known as *conversion disorder; and **dissociative hysteria**, comprising a group of conditions now generally regarded as *dissociative disorders. *See also* NEUROSIS. **2.** a state of great emotional excitement.

hysterical *adj.* **1.** formerly, describing a symptom that is not due to organic disease, is produced unconsciously, and from which the individual derives some gain. What were known as hysterical symptoms are characteristic of *conversion disorder. **2.** describing a kind of *personality disorder characterized by instability and shallowness of feelings and by superficiality and a tendency to manipulate in personal relationships.

hysterosalpingography *n.* *see* UTEROSALPINGOGRAPHY.

hysterosalpingosonography *n.* visualization of the Fallopian tubes by means of an ultrasound beam, usually directed via a vaginal probe, after a contrast medium has been passed through them via the cervix. *See also* TRANSVAGINAL ULTRA-SONOGRAPHY.

hysteroscope (uteroscope) *n.* a tubular instrument with a light source for observing the interior of the uterus. *See also* ENDOSCOPE.

hysterotomy *n.* an operation for removal of the fetus by incision of the uterus through the abdomen before the 24th week of gestation; after this time the operation is called *Caesarean section. Hysterotomy is now rarely performed owing to improvements in the efficiency of drugs now available for inducing abortion, e.g. *mifepristone.

-iasis *suffix denoting* a diseased condition. Example: **leishmaniasis** (disease caused by *Leishmania* species).

iatro- *prefix denoting* **1.** medicine. **2.** doctors.

iatrogenic *adj.* describing a condition that has resulted from treatment, as either an unforeseen or inevitable side-effect.

IBD *see* INFLAMMATORY BOWEL DISEASE.

IBS *see* IRRITABLE BOWEL SYNDROME.

ibuprofen *n.* an anti-inflammatory drug (*see* NSAID), used in the treatment of arthritic conditions. It is administered by mouth and sometimes causes skin rashes and digestive upsets. Trade names: **Brufen, Junifen.**

ICD *see* INTERNATIONAL CLASSIFICATION OF DISEASES. The latest version is **ICD-10**.

ICG angiography indocyanine green *angiography.

ichor *n.* a watery material oozing from wounds or ulcers.

ichthyosis *n.* a genetically determined skin disorder (*see* GENODERMATOSIS) in which there is abnormal scaling of the skin (the scaly condition of the skin is reflected in the name of this disorder, which is derived from the Greek word for fish). Ichthyosis may be caused by a variety of genetic defects in skin shedding; the pattern of scaling varies according to the underlying defect. The commonest form, **ichthyosis vulgaris**, is inherited as an autosomal *dominant and occurs in 1 in 300 of the population. Treatment of ichthyosis is mainly by the regular use of emollients. *See also* XERODERMA.

ICIDH *see* INTERNATIONAL CLASSIFICATION OF DISEASES.

ICSH (interstitial-cell-stimulating hormone) *see* LUTEINIZING HORMONE.

ICSI (intracytoplasmic sperm injection) a technique of assisted conception in cases of male infertility caused by inability of the spermatozoa to penetrate the barriers surrounding the ovum, in which a single spermatozoon is injected into the cytoplasm of an ovum in vitro. The fertilized ovum is then implanted into the uterus.

icterus *n. see* JAUNDICE.

ictus *n.* a stroke or any sudden attack. The term is often used for an epileptic seizure, stressing the suddenness of its onset.

id *n.* (in psychoanalysis) a part of the unconscious mind governed by the instinctive forces of *libido and the death wish. These violent forces seek immediate release in action or in symbolic form. The id is therefore said to be governed by the pleasure principle and not by the demands of reality or of logic. In the course of individual development some of the functions of the id are taken over by the *ego.

-id *suffix denoting* relationship or resemblance to. Example: **spermatid** (a stage of sperm formation).

ideation *n.* the process of thinking or of having *imagery or ideas.

identical twins *see* TWINS.

identification *n.* (in psychological development) the process of adopting other people's characteristics more or less permanently. Identification with a parent is important in personality formation, and has been especially implicated in the development of a moral sense and of an appropriate sex role.

ideo- *prefix denoting* **1.** the mind or mental activity. **2.** ideas.

ideomotor *adj.* describing or relating to a motor action that is evoked by an idea. **Ideomotor apraxia** is the inability to translate the idea of a complex behaviour into action.

idio- *prefix denoting* peculiarity to the individual.

idiopathic *adj.* denoting a disease or condition the cause of which is not known or that arises spontaneously. —**idiopathy** *n.*

idiopathic thrombocytopenic purpura (ITP) an *autoimmune disease in which platelets are destroyed, leading to spontaneous bruising (*see* PURPURA). Acute ITP is a relatively mild disease of children, who usually recover without treatment. A chronic form of the disease, typically affecting adults, is more serious, requiring treatment with corticosteroids or, if there is no response, with splenectomy. If both fail, immunosuppressive drugs may be effective. Platelet concentrates are used for life-threatening bleeding.

idiosyncrasy *n.* an unusual and unexpected sensitivity exhibited by an individual to a particular drug or food. —**idiosyncratic** *adj.*

idiot savant an individual whose overall functioning is at the level of mental retardation but who has one or more special intellectual abilities that are advanced to a high level. Musical ability, calculating ability, and rote memory are examples of abilities that may be highly developed. Many such individuals suffer from *autism.

idioventricular *adj.* affecting or peculiar to the ventricles of the heart. The term is most often used to describe the very slow beat of the heart's ventricles under the influence of their own natural subsidiary pacemaker (**idioventricular rhythm**).

idoxuridine *n.* an iodine-containing antiviral drug that inhibits the growth of viruses and is used to treat herpes infections of the eye. It is administered in eye drops or ointment and may cause irritation and stinging on application. Trade names: **Herpid**, **Idoxene**.

ifosfamide *n.* a *cytotoxic drug used in the treatment of malignant disease, particularly sarcomas, testicular tumours, and lymphomas. It is administered intravenously by injection or infusion. Side-effects include nausea, vomiting, alopecia, and haemorrhagic cystitis; concomitant administration of *mesna is recommended to prevent cystitis. Trade name: **Mitoxana.**

IGF insulin-like growth factor, which includes IGF-I and IGF-II. *See* GROWTH FACTOR, SOMATOMEDIN.

IL-2 *n. see* INTERLEUKIN.

ile- (ileo-) *prefix denoting* the ileum. Examples: **ileocaecal** (relating to the ileum and caecum); **ileocolic** (relating to the ileum and colon).

ileal conduit a segment of small intestine (ileum) used to convey urine from the ureters to the exterior into an appliance (*see also* URINARY DIVERSION). The ureters are implanted into an isolated segment of bowel, usually ileum but sometimes sigmoid colon, one end of which is brought through the abdominal wall to the skin surface. This end forms a spout, or **stoma**, which projects into a suitable urinary appliance. The ureters themselves cannot be used for this purpose as they tend to narrow and retract if brought through the skin. The operation is performed if the bladder has to be removed or bypassed; for example, because of cancer.

ileal pouch (perineal pouch) a reservoir made from loops of ileum to replace a surgically removed rectum, avoiding the need for a permanent *ileostomy.

ileectomy *n.* surgical removal of the ileum (small intestine) or part of the ileum.

ileitis *n.* inflammation of the ileum (small intestine). It may be caused by *Crohn's disease, tuberculosis, the bacterium *Yersinia enterocolitica*, or typhoid or it may occur in association with ulcerative *colitis (when it is known as **backwash ileitis**).

ileocaecal valve a valve at the junction of the small and large intestines consisting of two membranous folds that close to prevent the backflow of food from the colon and caecum to the ileum.

ileocolitis *n.* inflammation of the ileum and the colon (small and large intestines). The commonest causes are *Crohn's disease and tuberculosis.

ileocolostomy *n.* a surgical operation in which the ileum is joined to some part of the colon. It is usually performed when the right side of the colon has been removed or if it is desired to bypass either the terminal part of the ileum or right side of the colon.

ileocystoplasty *n. see* CYSTOPLASTY.

ileorectal anastomosis (ileoproctostomy) a surgical operation in which the ileum is joined to the rectum, usually after surgical removal of the colon (*see* COLECTOMY).

ileostomy *n.* a surgical operation in which the ileum is brought through the abdominal wall to create an artificial opening (**stoma**) through which the intestinal contents can discharge, thus bypassing the colon. Various types of bag may be worn to collect the effluent. The operation is usually performed in association with *colectomy; or to allow the colon to rest and heal in cases of colitis; or following injury or surgery to the colon. It can be used as an alternative to a *colostomy.

ileum *n.* the lowest of the three portions of the small *intestine. It runs from the jejunum to the *ileocaecal valve. —**ileal**, **ileac** *adj.*

ileus *n.* intestinal obstruction, usually obstruction of the small intestine (ileum). **Paralytic** or **adynamic ileus** is functional obstruction of the ileum due to loss of intestinal movement (peristalsis), which may be caused by abdominal surgery (*see* LAPAROTOMY), spinal injuries, deficiency of potassium in the blood (hypokalaemia), or peritonitis. Treatment consists of intravenous administration of fluid and nutrients and removal of excess stomach secretions by tube until peristalsis returns. If possible, the underlying condition is treated. Mechanical obstruction of the ileum may be caused by a gallstone entering the bowel through a fistula or widened bile duct (**gallstone ileus**); thickened *meconium in newborn babies with *cystic fibrosis (**meconium ileus**); or intestinal worms, usually the threadworm *Enterobius vermicularis* (**verminous ileus**).

ili- (ilio-) *prefix denoting* the ilium.

iliac arteries the arteries that supply most of the blood to the lower limbs and pelvic region. The right and left **common iliac arteries** form the terminal branches of the abdominal aorta. Each branches

into the **external iliac artery** and the smaller **internal iliac artery**.

iliacus *n.* a flat triangular muscle situated in the area of the groin. This muscle acts in conjunction with the *psoas muscle to flex the thigh.

iliac veins the veins draining most of the blood from the lower limbs and pelvic region. The right and left **common iliac veins** unite to form the inferior vena cava. They are each formed by the union of the **internal** and **external iliac veins**.

iliopsoas *n.* a composite muscle made up of the *iliacus and *psoas muscles, which have a common tendon.

ilium *n.* the haunch bone: a wide bone forming the upper part of each side of the *hip bone (*see also* PELVIS). There is a concave depression (**iliac fossa**) on the inside of the pelvis; the right iliac fossa provides space for the vermiform appendix. —**iliac** *adj.*

illusion *n.* a false perception due to misinterpretation of the stimuli arising from an object. For example, a patient may misinterpret the conversation of others as the voices of enemies conspiring to destroy him. Illusions can occur in quite normal people, when they are usually spontaneously corrected. They may also occur in almost any psychiatric syndrome, especially *depression. *Compare* HALLUCINATION.

Optical illusions are perceptions that do not agree with the actual object in the external world. They are produced by deceptive qualities of the stimulus and are in no way pathological.

image intensifier an electronic device that provides a TV image from an X-ray source using *photomultiplier tubes in place of conventional photographic film.

imagery *n.* the production of vivid mental representations by the normal processes of thought. **Hypnagogic imagery** occurs just before falling asleep, and the images are often very distinct. **Hypnopompic imagery** occurs in the state between sleep and full wakefulness. Like hypnagogic imagery, the experiences may be very vivid. **Eidetic imagery**, commoner in children than adults, is the production of images of exceptional clarity, which may be recalled long after being first experienced.

imaging *n.* the production of images of organs or tissues using radiological procedures, particularly by using scanning techniques. *See also* COMPUTERIZED TOMOGRAPHY, MAGNETIC RESONANCE IMAGING, ULTRASONOGRAPHY.

imago *n.* (in psychoanalysis) the internal unconscious representation of an important person in the individual's life, particularly a parent.

imidazole *n.* one of a group of chemically related antifungal drugs that are also effective against a wide range of bacteria; some (e.g. *thiabendazole and *mebendazole) are also used as anthelmintics. The group includes *econazole, *clotrimazole, *ketoconazole, and *miconazole. They are administered by mouth or externally as creams.

imipramine *n.* a drug administered by mouth or injection to treat depression (*see* ANTIDEPRESSANT). Its effects may be slow to develop; common side-effects include dry mouth, blurred vision, constipation, sweating, and rapid heartbeat. Trade name: **Tofranil**.

imitation *n.* acting in the same way as another person, either temporarily or permanently. This is one of the mechanisms of *identification. It can be used in therapy (*see* MODELLING).

immersion foot *see* TRENCH FOOT.

immobilization *n.* the procedure of making a normally movable part of the body, such as a joint, immovable. This helps an infected, diseased, or injured tissue (bone, joint, or muscle) to heal. Immobilization may be temporary (for example, by means of a plaster of Paris cast on a limb) or it may be permanent. Permanent immobilization of a joint is achieved by means of the operation of *arthrodesis.

immune *adj.* protected against a particular infection by the presence of specific antibodies against the organisms concerned. *See* IMMUNITY.

immune response the response of the *immune system to antigens. There are two types of immune response produced

by two populations of *lymphocytes. B-lymphocytes (or B-cells) are responsible for **humoral immunity**, producing free antibodies that circulate in the bloodstream; and T-lymphocytes (or T-cells) are responsible for **cell-mediated immunity** (*see* HELPER T-CELL, KILLER CELL, SUPPRESSOR T-CELL).

immune system the organs responsible for *immunity. The primary *lymphoid organs are the thymus and the bone marrow; the secondary lymphoid organs are the lymph nodes and lymphoid aggregates (spleen, tonsils, gastrointestinal lymph tissue, and Peyer's patches).

immunity *n.* the body's ability to resist infection, afforded by the presence of circulating *antibodies and white blood cells. Antibodies are manufactured specifically to deal with the antigens associated with different diseases as they are encountered. **Active immunity** arises when the body's own cells produce, and remain able to produce, appropriate antibodies following an attack of a disease or deliberate stimulation (*see* IMMUNIZATION). **Passive immunity**, which is only short-lived, is provided by injecting ready-made antibodies in *antiserum taken from another person or an animal already immune. Babies have passive immunity, conferred by antibodies from the maternal blood and *colostrum, to common diseases for several weeks after birth. *See also* IMMUNE RESPONSE.

immunization *n.* the production of *immunity by artificial means. Passive immunity, which is temporary, may be conferred by the injection of an *antiserum, but the production of active immunity calls for the use of treated antigens, to stimulate the body to produce its own antibodies: this is the procedure of *vaccination (also called **inoculation**). The material used for immunization (the *vaccine) may consist of live bacteria or viruses so treated that they are harmless while remaining antigenic or completely dead organisms or their products (e.g. toxins) chemically or physically altered to produce the same effect.

immuno- *prefix denoting* immunity or immunological response.

immunoassay *n.* any of various techniques for determining the levels of anti-

gen and antibody in a tissue. *See* IMMUNO-
ELECTROPHORESIS, IMMUNOFLUORESCENCE,
RADIOIMMUNOASSAY.

immunocompromised *adj.* describing
patients in whom the immune response is
reduced or defective due to *immunosuppression. Such patients are vulnerable to
opportunistic infections.

immunodeficiency *n.* deficiency in the
*immune response. This can be acquired,
as in *AIDS, but there are many varieties
of primary immunodeficiency occurring
as inherited disorders characterized by
*hypogammaglobulinaemia.

immunoelectrophoresis *n.* a technique for identifying antigenic fractions
in a serum. The components of the serum
are separated by *electrophoresis and allowed to diffuse through agar gel towards
a particular antiserum. Where the antibody meets its antigen, a band of precipi-
tation occurs. *See also* PRECIPITIN.

immunofluorescence *n.* a technique
for observing the amount and/or distribution of antibody or antigen in a tissue section. The antibodies are labelled (directly
or indirectly) with a fluorescent dye (e.g.
fluorescein) and applied to the tissue,
which is observed through an ultraviolet
microscope. In **direct immunofluorescence** the antibody is labelled before
being applied to the tissue. In **indirect
immunofluorescence** the antibody is labelled after it has bound to the antigen,
by means of fluorescein-labelled anti-
immunoglobulin serum. —**immunofluorescent** *adj.*

immunogenicity *n.* the property that
enables a substance to provoke an immune response, including foreignness (*see*
ANTIGEN), size, route of entry into the
body, dose, number and length of exposures to the antigen, and host genetic
make-up.

immunoglobulin (Ig) *n.* one of a group
of structurally related proteins (gamma
*globulins) that act as antibodies. Several
classes of Ig with different functions are
distinguished – IgA, IgD, IgE, IgG, and
IgM. They can be separated by *immunoelectrophoresis. *See* ANTIBODY.

immunological tolerance a failure of
the body to distinguish between materials

that are 'self', and therefore to be tolerated, and those that are 'not self', against
which antibodies are produced. For example, the body fails to produce antibodies
against foreign materials if an antigen has
previously been introduced into the body
before the antibody-producing system is
mature; apparently the presence of antigen within the growing cells inhibits antibody formation.

immunology *n.* the study of *immunity
and all of the phenomena connected with
the defence mechanisms of the body.
—**immunological** *adj.*

immunophoresis *n.* a technique, relying upon the *precipitin reaction, for
identifying an unknown antigen or testing for an antibody in a serum. Antibody
and antigen are allowed to diffuse towards each other in agar gel.

immunosuppression *n.* suppression of
the *immune response, usually by disease
(e.g. AIDS) or by drugs (e.g. steroids, azathioprine, cyclosporin A).

immunosuppressive *n.* a drug, such as
*azathioprine or *cyclophosphamide, that
reduces the body's resistance to infection
and other foreign bodies by suppressing
the immune system. Immunosuppressives
are used to maintain the survival of organ
and tissue transplants and to treat various
*autoimmune diseases, including rheuma-
toid arthritis. *Cyclosporin A is the immunosuppressive usually used in organ
transplant recipients. Because immunity is
lowered during treatment with immunosuppressives, there is an increased susceptibility to infection and certain types of
cancer.

immunotherapy *n.* the prevention or
treatment of disease using agents that
may modify the immune response. It is a
largely experimental approach, studied
most widely in the treatment of cancer.
See BIOLOGICAL RESPONSE MODIFIER.

immunotoxin *n.* one of a new class of
drugs undergoing clinical trials for the
treatment of leukaemia. Immunotoxins
combine *monoclonal antibodies, which
can specifically target cancerous cells, with
a highly toxic compound (such as *ricin)
that inactivates the cells' *ribosomes and
thus inhibits protein synthesis. Because

the toxin does not attack the whole cell only tiny amounts are required.

immunotransfusion *n.* the transfusion of an *antiserum to treat or give temporary protection against a disease.

impacted *adj.* firmly wedged. An **impacted tooth** (usually a wisdom tooth) is one that cannot erupt into a normal position because it is obstructed by other tissues. **Impacted faeces** are so hard and dry that they cannot pass through the anus without special measures being taken (*see* CONSTIPATION). An **impacted fracture** is one in which the bone ends are driven into each other. —**impaction** *n.*

impairment *n. see* HANDICAP.

impalpable *adj.* describing a structure within the body that cannot be detected (or that can be detected only with difficulty) by feeling with the hand.

imperforate *adj.* lacking an opening. Occasionally girls at puberty are found to have an **imperforate hymen** (a fold of membrane close to the vaginal orifice), which impedes the flow of menstrual blood.

imperforate anus (proctatresia) partial or complete obstruction of the anus: a condition, discovered at birth, due to failure of the anus to develop normally in the embryo. There are several different types of imperforate anus; these include **developmental anal stenosis**, **persistent anal membrane**, and **covered anus** (due to fused genital folds). If the anal canal fails to develop, the rectum ends blindly above the muscles of the perineum. Most mild cases of imperforate anus can be treated by a simple operation. If the defect is extensive a temporary opening is made in the colon (*see* COLOSTOMY), with later surgical reconstruction of the rectum and anus.

impetigo *n.* a superficial bacterial infection of the skin. **Nonbullous impetigo** is caused by *Staphylococcus aureus*, *Streptococcus* species, or both organisms; it mainly affects young children and is highly contagious, with yellowish-brown crusting. **Bullous impetigo** is caused by *Staph. aureus*; it is characterized by blisters, is less contagious than the nonbullous form, and occurs at any age. Treatment of impetigo is with topical

antibiotics; systemic antibiotics may occasionally be needed.

implant *n.* **1.** a drug (such as a subcutaneous hormone implant), a prosthesis (such as an artificial hip, an **intraocular lens implant** (*see* CATARACT), a *breast implant, a *cochlear implant, or a *artificial heart implant), or a radioactive source (such as radium needles) that is put into the body. **2.** (in dentistry) a rigid structure that is embedded in bone or under its periosteum to provide support for replacement teeth on a *denture or a *bridge. Recent types (**osseointegrated implants**) consist of a number of special titanium alloy inserts, placed in the jawbone, onto which abutments are fitted after the bone has healed. Later an artificial-tooth superstructure is bolted onto the abutments. Osseointegrated implants are also used to retain facial *prostheses. *See also* OSSEOINTEGRATION.

implantation *n.* **1.** (or **nidation**) the attachment of the early embryo to the lining of the uterus, which occurs at the *blastocyst stage of development, six to eight days after ovulation. The site of implantation determines the position of the placenta. **2.** the placing of a substance (e.g. a drug) or an object (e.g. an artificial pacemaker) within a tissue. **3.** the surgical replacement of damaged tissue with healthy tissue (*see* TRANSPLANTATION).

implosion *n. see* FLOODING.

impotence *n.* inability in a man to have sexual intercourse. Impotence may be **erectile**, in which the penis does not become firm enough to enter the vagina, or **ejaculatory**, in which penetration occurs but there is no ejaculation of semen (orgasm). Either of these kinds of impotence may be due to a physical disease, such as diabetes (**organic**), or to a psychological or emotional problem (**psychogenic**). Treatment is by means of a penile *prosthesis or injection into the corpora cavernosa of the penis (e.g. *alprostadil). *Sildenafil is an orally administered drug that improves blood flow to the penis.

impression *n.* (in dentistry) a mould made of the teeth and surrounding soft tissues or of a toothless jaw. A soft impression material (e.g. silicone or alginate) is placed over the teeth or jaw and sets within several minutes, producing an elastic mould. Impressions may also be taken with hard-setting materials (e.g. plaster or zinc oxide–eugenol cement). After removal from the mouth a plaster model is made; on this are constructed *restorations of teeth, *dentures, or *orthodontic appliances.

imprinting n. (in animal behaviour) a rapid and irreversible form of learning that takes place in some animals during the first hours of life. Animals attach themselves in this way to members of their own species, but if they are exposed to creatures of a different species during this short period, they become attached to this species instead.

impulse n. (in neurology) see NERVE IMPULSE.

in- (im-) prefix denoting **1.** not. **2.** in; within; into.

inanition n. a condition of exhaustion caused by lack of nutrients in the blood. This may arise through starvation, malnutrition, or intestinal disease.

inappetence n. lack of desire, usually for food.

in articulo mortis Latin: at the moment of death.

inborn error of metabolism any one of a group of inherited conditions in which there is a disturbance in either the structure, synthesis, function, or transport of protein molecules. There are over 1500 inborn errors of metabolism; examples are *phenylketonuria, *homocystinuria, and *hypogammaglobulinaemia.

inbreeding n. the production of offspring by parents who are closely related; for example, who are first cousins or siblings. The amount of inbreeding in a population is largely controlled by culture and tradition. Compare OUTBREEDING.

incapacity benefit a state benefit payable to those under the state retirement age who are incapable of work because of an illness or disability but who do not qualify for statutory sick pay; it replaced invalidity benefit and sickness benefit in 1995. Entitlement depends on an adequate record of National Insurance contributions. It is paid at three basic

rates. Short-term incapacity benefit is payable at the lower rate for the first 28 weeks of incapacity and at the higher rate for the 29th–52nd weeks. Long-term benefit is payable, at the highest rate, after 52 weeks. For the first 28 weeks of incapacity claims are made by an 'own occupation' test, based on the production of a *medical certificate. After 28 weeks claimants must undergo a medical test to assess their capacity for work-related activities (an 'all work' test) as well as completing a questionnaire. Doctors must certify in all cases the material supplied. Compare SEVERE DISABLEMENT ALLOWANCE.

incarcerated adj. confined or constricted so as to be immovable: applied particularly to a type of *hernia.

incidence rate a measure of morbidity based on the number of new episodes of illness arising in a population over a period of time. It can be expressed in terms of sick persons or episodes per 1000 individuals at risk. Compare PREVALENCE RATE.

incision n. **1.** the surgical cutting of soft tissues, such as skin or muscle, with a knife or scalpel. **2.** the cut so made.

incisor n. any of the four front teeth in each jaw, two on each side of the midline. See also DENTITION.

incisure n. (in anatomy) a notch, small hollow, or depression.

inclusion bodies particles occurring in the nucleus and cytoplasm of cells usually as a result of virus infection. Their presence can sometimes be used to diagnose such an infection.

inclusion conjunctivitis a sexually transmitted disease caused by Chlamydia trachomatis. It can be transmitted to infants at birth, with the disease clinically apparent 5–13 days after birth. Diagnosis is by cell culture. Treatment in the newborn is with topical erythromycin; adults require oral tetracycline or doxycycline for three weeks.

income support An income-related benefit payable to those whose income does not exceed a specified minimum. It replaced supplementary benefit in 1988.

incompatibility n. see COMPATIBILITY.

incompetence *n.* impaired function of the valves of the heart or veins, which allows backward leakage of blood. *See* AORTIC REGURGITATION, MITRAL INCOMPETENCE, VARICOSE VEINS.

incontinence *n.* **1.** the inappropriate involuntary passage of urine, resulting in wetting. **Stress incontinence** is the leak of urine on coughing and straining. It is common in women in whom the muscles of the pelvic floor are weakened after childbirth. **Genuine stress incontinence (GSI)** is incontinence in women for which a physical (as opposed to a psychological) cause can be identified. **Overflow incontinence** is leakage from a full bladder, which occurs most commonly in elderly men with bladder outflow obstruction or in patients with neurological conditions affecting bladder control. **Urge incontinence** is leakage of urine that accompanies an intense desire to pass water with failure of restraint. *See also* ENURESIS. **2.** inability to control bowel movements (**faecal incontinence**).

incoordination *n.* (in neurology) an impairment in the performance of precise movements. These are dependent upon the normal function of the whole nervous system, and incoordination may result from a disorder in any part of it. *See* APRAXIA, ATAXIA, DYSSYNERGIA.

incubation *n.* **1.** the process of develop ment of an egg or a culture of bacteria. **2.** the care of a premature baby in an *incubator.

incubation period (latent period) **1.** the interval between exposure to an infection and the appearance of the first symptoms. **2.** (in bacteriology) the period of development of a bacterial culture.

incubator *n.* a transparent container for keeping premature babies in controlled conditions and protecting them from infection. Other forms of incubator are used for cultivating bacteria in Petri dishes and for hatching eggs.

incus *n.* a small anvil-shaped bone in the middle *ear that articulates with the malleus and the stapes. *See* OSSICLE.

independent contract (in Britain) a special arrangement whereby *hospitals or *general practitioners working in the *National Health Service receive budgeted funds to provide services of their own selection, without direction from Health Authorities. However, basic services must be provided for the population of the Health Authority in which the service is located at an agreed rate.

Inderal *n.* *see* PROPRANOLOL.

indican *n.* a compound excreted in the urine as a detoxification product of *indoxyl. Indican is formed by the conjugation of indoxyl with sulphuric acid and potassium on the decomposition of tryptophan.

indicanuria *n.* the presence in the urine of an abnormally high concentration of *indican. This may be a sign that the intestine is obstructed.

indication *n.* (in medicine) a strong reason for believing that a particular course of action is desirable. In a wounded patient, the loss of blood, which would lead to circulatory collapse, is an indication for blood transfusion. *Compare* CONTRAINDICATION.

indigestion *n.* *see* DYSPEPSIA.

indocyanine green angiography *see* ANGIOGRAPHY.

indole *n.* a derivative of the amino acid tryptophan, excreted in the urine and faeces. Abnormal patterns of urinary indole excretion are found in some mentally retarded patients.

indolent *adj.* describing a disease process that is failing to heal or has persisted. The term is applied particularly to ulcers of skin or mucous membrane.

indomethacin *n.* an anti-inflammatory drug (*see* NSAID), used in the treatment of arthritic conditions. It is administered either by mouth or in suppositories; common side effects are headache, dizziness, and digestive upsets. Trade names: **Indocid, Indomod**.

indoramin *n.* an *alpha blocker drug used to treat high blood pressure. It is administered by mouth. Possible side-effects can include drowsiness, nasal congestion, dry mouth, and failure of ejaculation. Trade names: **Baratol, Doralese**.

indoxyl *n.* an alcohol derived from *indole by bacterial action. It is excreted in the urine as *indican.

induction *n.* **1.** (in obstetrics) the starting of labour by artificial means. **Medical induction** is carried out using such drugs as *prostaglandins or *oxytocin, which stimulate uterine contractions. **Surgical induction** is performed by *amniotomy (artificial rupture of membranes), usually supplemented by oxytocic drugs. Induction of labour is carried out if the wellbeing or life of mother or child is threatened by continuance of the pregnancy **2.** (in anaesthesia) initiation of *anaesthesia. General anaesthesia is usually induced by the intravenous injection of rapid short-acting narcotic drugs, e.g. thiopentone.

induration *n.* abnormal hardening of a tissue or organ. *See also* SCLEROSIS.

indusium *n.* a thin layer of grey matter covering the upper surface of the *corpus callosum between the two cerebral hemispheres.

industrial disease *see* OCCUPATIONAL DISEASE.

industrial injuries disablement benefit a state benefit payable to a person disabled by injury or a prescribed industrial disease sustained or contracted in the course of employment (*see* OCCUPATIONAL DISEASE). The benefit is payable as a weekly amount. The amount of the benefit depends on the degree of disablement, which is assessed by a specialist or a board of two doctors. To be entitled to benefit, the disablement must be assessed as being at least 14% of total disability (1% in the case of pneumoconiosis, byssinosis, and diffuse mesothelioma). The benefit is payable if the claimant is still suffering disability 15 weeks or more after the date of the accident or onset of the disease. It is payable for a period assessed as the time for which the claimant is likely to suffer the disability. The assessment can be reviewed if the claimant's condition deteriorates or if he or she is still disabled at the end of the period of assessment.

inertia *n.* (in physiology) sluggishness or absence of activity in certain smooth muscles. In **uterine inertia** the muscular wall of the uterus fails to contract adequately

during labour, making the process excessively long. This inertia may be present from the start of labour or it may develop because of exhaustion following strong contractions.

in extremis Latin: at the point of death.

infant *n.* a child incapable of any form of independence from its mother: the term is usually used to refer to a child under one year of age, especially a premature or newborn child. In legal use the term denotes a child up to the age of seven years.

infanticide *n.* (in Britain) under the terms of the Infanticide Act 1938, the felony of child destruction by the natural mother within 12 months of birth when the balance of her mind is disturbed because she has not fully recovered from childbirth and/or lactation. Under such circumstances a charge that would have been one of murder is reduced to manslaughter.

infantile *adj.* **1.** denoting conditions occurring in adults that are recognizable in childhood, e.g. poliomyelitis (**infantile paralysis**) and **infantile scurvy**. **2.** of, relating to, or affecting infants.

infantile spasms (salaam attacks) a rare but serious form of epilepsy that usually begins between three and eight months of age. The spasms are involuntary flexing movements of the arms, legs, neck, and trunk; each spasm lasts 1–3 seconds and is associated with flushing of the face, and runs of spasms occur over a period of several minutes. They may occur many times in one day. The baby fails to respond to human contact and development is usually profoundly slowed. An EEG pattern of *hypsarrhythmia is usual and diagnostic. Diagnosis may be delayed as spasms are sometimes confused with colic. Immediate recognition and treatment with corticosteroids or ACTH offers a chance of arresting the disease, but outcome depends primarily on the nature of the underlying brain abnormality.

infantilism *n.* persistence of childlike physical or psychological characteristics into adult life.

infant mortality rate (IMR) the number of deaths of infants under one year of age per 1000 live births in a given year. Included in the IMR are the **neonatal mortality rate** (calculated from deaths occurring in the first four weeks of life) and **postneonatal mortality rate** (from deaths in the remainder of the first year). Neonatal deaths are further subdivided into **early** (first week) and **late** (second, third, and fourth weeks). In prosperous countries neonatal deaths account for about two-thirds of infant mortalities, the majority being in the first week (in the UK the major cause is prematurity and related problems). The IMR is usually regarded more as a measure of social affluence than a measure of the quality of antenatal and/or obstetric care; the latter is more truly reflected in the **perinatal mortality rate** (the number of deaths after 24 weeks of gestation, including stillbirths, and during the first week of life per 1000 total births). *See also* STILL-BIRTH RATE.

infarct *n. see* INFARCTION.

infarction *n.* the death of part or the whole of an organ that occurs when the artery carrying its blood supply is obstructed by a blood clot (thrombus) or an *embolus. For example, *myocardial infarction, affecting the muscle of the heart, follows coronary thrombosis. A small localized area of dead tissue produced as a result of an inadequate blood supply is known as an **infarct**.

infection *n.* invasion of the body by harmful organisms (pathogens), such as bacteria, fungi, protozoa, rickettsiae, or viruses. The infective agent may be transmitted by a patient or *carrier in airborne droplets expelled during coughing and sneezing or by direct contact, such as kissing or sexual intercourse (*see* SEXUALLY TRANSMITTED DISEASE); by animal or insect *vectors; by ingestion of contaminated food or drink; or from an infected mother to the fetus during pregnancy or birth. Pathogenic organisms present in soil, organisms from animal intermediate hosts, or those living as *commensals on the body can also cause infections. Organisms may invade via a wound or bite or through mucous membranes. After an *incubation period symptoms appear, usually consisting of either localized inflammation and pain or more remote effects.

Treatment with drugs is usually effective against most infections but there is no specific treatment for many of the common viral infections, including the common cold and influenza.

infectious disease *see* COMMUNICABLE DISEASE.

infectious mononucleosis *see* GLANDULAR FEVER.

inferior *adj.* (in anatomy) lower in the body in relation to another structure or surface.

inferior dental block a type of injection to anaesthetize the inferior *dental nerve. Inferior dental block is routinely performed to allow dental procedures to be carried out on the lower teeth on one side of the mouth.

inferior dental canal a bony canal in the *mandible on each side. It carries the inferior *dental nerve and vessels and for part of its length its outline is visible on a radiograph.

inferiority complex **1.** an unconscious and extreme exaggeration of feelings of insignificance or inferiority, which is shown by behaviour that is defensive or compensatory (such as aggression). **2.** (in psychoanalysis) a *complex said to result from the conflict between Oedipal wishes (*see* OEDIPUS COMPLEX) and the reality of the child's lack of power. This gives rise to repressed feelings of personal inferiority.

infertility *n.* inability in a woman to conceive or in a man to induce conception. Female infertility may be due to failure to ovulate, to obstruction of the *Fallopian tubes, or to disease of the lining of the uterus (endometrium). Possible treatments (depending on the cause) include administration of drugs (such as *clomiphene or *LHRH analogues), surgery (*see* SALPINGOGRAPHY, SALPINGOSTOMY, SALPINGOLYSIS) to restore patency of the Fallopian tubes, *gamete intrafallopian transfer (GIFT), and *in vitro fertilization. Causes of male infertility include decreased numbers or motility of spermatozoa (*see* OLIGOSPERMIA) and total absence of sperm (*see* AZOOSPERMIA). *See also* ANDROLOGY, STERILITY.

infestation *n.* the presence of animal parasites either on the skin (for example ticks) or inside the body (for example tapeworms).

infibulation *n.* *see* (FEMALE) CIRCUMCISION.

infiltration *n.* **1.** the abnormal entry of a substance (**infiltrate**) into a cell, tissue, or organ. Examples of infiltrates are blood cells, cancer cells, fat, starch, or calcium and magnesium salts. **2.** the injection of a local anaesthetic solution into the tissues to cause local *anaesthesia. Infiltration anaesthesia is routinely used to anaesthetize upper teeth to allow dental procedures to be carried out.

inflammation *n.* the body's response to injury, which may be acute or chronic. **Acute inflammation** is the immediate defensive reaction of tissue to any injury, which may be caused by infection, chemicals, or physical agents. It involves pain, heat, redness, swelling, and loss of function of the affected part. Blood vessels near the site of injury are dilated, so that blood flow is locally increased. White blood cells enter the tissue and begin to engulf bacteria and other foreign particles. Similar cells from the tissues (*see* MACROPHAGE) remove and consume the dead cells, sometimes with the production of pus, enabling the process of healing to commence. In certain circumstances healing does not occur and **chronic inflammation** ensues.

inflammatory bowel disease (IBD) any of a group of inflammatory conditions of the intestine that include (among others) *ulcerative colitis and *Crohn's disease.

influenza *n.* a highly contagious virus infection that affects the respiratory system. The viruses are transmitted by coughing and sneezing. Symptoms commence after an incubation period of 1–4 days and include headache, fever, loss of appetite, weakness, and general aches and pains. They may continue for about a week. With bed rest and aspirin most patients recover, but a few may go on to develop pneumonia, either a primary influenzal viral pneumonia or a secondary bacterial pneumonia. Either of these may lead to death from haemorrhage within the lungs. The main bacterial organisms responsible for secondary infection are *Streptococcus pneumoniae, Haemophilus influenzae,* and *Staphylococcus aureus,* against which appropriate antibiotic therapy must be given. An influenzal infection provides later protection only against the specific strain of virus concerned; the same holds true for immunization.

informed consent a legal requirement that physicians or researchers inform a patient undergoing surgery or invasive tests or a subject involved in a clinical trial of the nature, risks, and probable outcome of the treatment or research. The patient signs an agreement stating that he or she has been informed and accepts the treatment, surgery, or research protocol. Without informed consent, the physician or researcher is violating the patient's rights, regardless of whether the treatment is appropriate and successful.

infra- *prefix denoting* below.

infrared radiation the band of electromagnetic radiation that is longer in wavelength than the red of the visible spectrum. Infrared radiation is responsible for the transmission of radiant heat. It may be used in physiotherapy to warm tissues, reduce pain, and improve circulation, but is not as effective as *diathermy for deep structures. Special photographic film, which is sensitive to infrared radiation, is used in *thermography.

infundibulum *n.* any funnel-shaped channel or passage, particularly the hollow conical stalk that extends downwards from the hypothalamus and is continuous with the posterior lobe of the pituitary gland.

infusion *n.* **1.** the slow injection of a substance, usually into a vein (**intravenous infusion**). This is a common method for replacing water, electrolytes, and blood products and is also used for the continuous administration of drugs (e.g. antibiotics, painkillers) or *nutrition. *See also* DRIP. **2.** the process whereby the active principles are extracted from plant material by steeping it in water that has been heated to boiling point (as in the making of tea). **3.** the solution produced by this process.

ingesta *pl. n.* food and drink that is introduced into the alimentary canal through the mouth.

ingestion *n.* **1.** the process by which food is taken into the alimentary canal. It involves chewing and swallowing. **2.** the process by which a phagocytic cell takes in solid material, such as bacteria.

ingravescent *adj.* gradually increasing in severity.

ingrowing toenail downward curving of the sides of a toenail, which causes chafing of the skin alongside the nail resulting in inflammation around the base of the nail.

inguinal *adj.* relating to or affecting the region of the groin (inguen).

inguinal canal either of a pair of openings that connect the abdominal cavity with the scrotum in the male fetus. The inguinal canals provide a route for the descent of the testes into the scrotum, after which they normally become obliterated.

inguinal hernia *see* HERNIA.

inguinal ligament (Poupart's ligament) a ligament in the groin that extends from the anterior superior iliac spine to the pubic tubercle. It is part of the *aponeurosis of the external oblique muscle of the abdomen.

INH *see* ISONIAZID.

inhalation *n.* **1.** (or **inspiration**) the act of breathing air into the lungs through the mouth and nose. *See* BREATHING. **2.** a gas, vapour, or aerosol breathed in for the treatment of conditions of the respiratory tract. —**inhaler** *n.*

inhibition *n.* **1.** (in physiology) the prevention or reduction of the functioning of an organ, muscle, etc., by the action of certain nerve impulses. **2.** (in psychoanalysis) an inner command that prevents one from doing something forbidden. Some inhibitions are essential for social adjustment, but excessive inhibitions can severely restrict one's life. **3.** (in psychology) a tendency not to carry out a specific action, produced each time the action is carried out.

inhibitor *n.* a substance that prevents the occurrence of a given process or reaction. *See also* MAO INHIBITOR.

inion *n.* the projection of the occipital bone that can be felt at the base of the skull.

initiation *n.* (in oncology) the first step in the development of cancer (*see* CARCINO-GENESIS).

initiator (in oncogenesis) *n.* a substance that induces an irreversible change in a cell's DNA that can result in a cancer. An example is dimethylbenzanthracene. *Compare* PROMOTER.

injection *n.* introduction into the body of drugs or other fluids by means of a syringe, usually drugs that would be destroyed by the digestive processes if taken by mouth. Common routes for injection are into the skin (**intracutaneous** or **intradermal**); below the skin (**subcutaneous**), e.g. for insulin; into a muscle (**intramuscular**), for drugs that are slowly absorbed; and into a vein (**intravenous**), for drugs to be rapidly absorbed. *Enemas are also regarded as injections.

injury scoring system (injury severity scale, ISS) a system used, particularly in *triage, for grading the severity of an injury. *See also* ABBREVIATED INJURY SCALE.

inlay *n.* **1.** a substance or piece of tissue inserted to replace a defect in a tissue. For example, a bone graft may be inlaid into an area of missing or damaged bone. **2.** (in dentistry) a rigid restoration inserted into a tapered cavity in a tooth. It is held in place with a cement *lute. While cast gold has been the most widely used material, porcelain and composite resin are also used.

inlet *n.* an aperture providing the entrance to a cavity, such as that of the pelvis.

innate *adj.* describing a condition or characteristic that is present in an individual at birth and is inherited from his parents. *See also* CONGENITAL.

inner ear *see* LABYRINTH.

innervation *n.* the nerve supply to an area or organ of the body, which can carry either motor impulses to the structure or sensory impulses away from it towards the brain.

innocent *adj.* (of a tumour) benign; not malignant.

innominate artery (brachiocephalic artery) a short artery originating as the first large branch of the *aortic arch, passing upwards to the right, and ending at the lower neck near the right sternoclavicular joint. Here it divides into the right common carotid and the right subclavian arteries.

innominate bone *see* HIP BONE.

innominate vein (brachiocephalic vein) either of two veins, one on each side of the neck, formed by the junction of the external jugular and subclavian veins. The two veins join to form the superior vena cava.

ino- *prefix denoting* **1.** fibrous tissue. **2.** muscle.

inoculation *n.* the introduction of a small quantity of material, such as a vaccine, in the process of *immunization: a more general name for *vaccination.

inoculum *n.* any material that is used for inoculation.

inosine pranobex a drug that increases the efficiency of the immune system by increasing the number of T-lymphocytes and enhancing the activity of natural killer cells. Some early trials in HIV-positive people suggest that the drug could delay progression to AIDS. Trade name: **Imunovir**.

inositol *n.* a compound, similar to a hexose sugar, that is a constituent of some cell phospholipids. Inositol is present in many foods, in particular in the bran of cereal grain. It is sometimes classified as a vitamin but it can be synthesized by most animals and there is no evidence that it is an essential nutrient in humans.

inositol triphosphate (IP₃) a short-lived biochemical *second messenger formed from *phospholipid in the cell membrane when a chemical messenger (e.g. a hormone or serotonin) binds to receptors on the cell surface. Inositol triphosphate triggers the rapid release of calcium into the cell fluid, which initiates various cellular processes, such as smooth muscle contraction and the release of glucose, histamine, etc. Inositol triphosphate exists for only a few seconds before being converted to inositol by the action of a sequence of enzymes.

inotropic *adj.* affecting the contraction of heart muscle. Drugs such as *digitalis, *dobutamine, and *enoximone have positive inotropic action, stimulating heart muscle contractions and causing the heart rate to increase. *Beta-blocker drugs, such as *propranolol, have negative inotropic action, reducing heart muscle contractions and causing the heart rate to decrease.

INOVE balloon *see* VALVOTOMY.

in-patient *n.* a patient who is admitted to a bed in a hospital ward and remains there for a period of time for treatment, examination, or observation. *Compare* OUTPATIENT.

inquest *n.* an official judicial enquiry into the cause of a person's death: carried out when the death is sudden or takes place under suspicious circumstances. The results of medical and legal investigations that have been carried out are considered by a *coroner, sitting with or without a jury, and made publicly known. *See also* AUTOPSY.

insanity *n.* a degree of mental illness such that the affected individual is not responsible for his actions or is not capable of entering into a legal contract. The term is a legal rather than a medical one.

insect *n.* a member of a large group of mainly land-dwelling *arthropods. The body of the adult is divided into a head, thorax, and abdomen. The head bears a single pair of sensory antennae; the thorax bears three pairs of legs and, in most insects, wings (these are absent in some parasitic groups, such as lice and fleas). Some insects are of medical importance. Various bloodsucking insects transmit tropical diseases, for example the female *Anopheles* mosquito transmits malaria and the tsetse fly transmits sleeping sickness. The bites of lice can cause intense irritation and, secondarily, bacterial infection. The organisms causing diarrhoea and dysentery can be conveyed to food on the bodies of flies. *See also* MYIASIS.

insecticide *n.* a preparation used to kill destructive or disease-carrying insects. Ideally, an insecticide should have no toxic effects when ingested by human beings or animals, but modern powerful compounds have inherent dangers and have caused fatalities. Some insect powders contain organic phosphorus compounds and fluorides; when ingested accidentally they may cause damage to the nervous system. The use of such compounds is generally under strict control. *See also* DDT, DIELDRIN.

insemination *n.* introduction of semen into the vagina. *See also* ARTIFICIAL INSEMINATION, INTRAUTERINE INSEMINATION.

insertion *n.* (in anatomy) the point of attachment of a muscle (e.g. to a bone) that is relatively movable when the muscle contracts. *Compare* ORIGIN.

insight *n.* (in psychology) knowledge of oneself. The term is applied particularly to a patient's recognition that he has psychological problems; in this sense absence of insight is a feature of psychosis. The term is also applied to the patient's accuracy of understanding the development of his personality and his problems; in this sense insight is enhanced by psychotherapy.

insolation *n.* exposure to the sun's rays. *See also* HEATSTROKE.

insomnia *n.* inability to fall asleep or to remain asleep for an adequate length of time, so that tiredness is virtually permanent. Insomnia may be associated with disease, particularly if there are painful symptoms, but is more often caused by worry.

inspiration *n. see* INHALATION.

inspissated *adj.* (of secretions, etc.) thickened or dried by evaporation or dehydration.

instillation *n.* **1.** the application of liquid medication drop by drop, as into the eye. **2.** the medication, such as eye drops, applied in this way.

instinct *n.* **1.** a complex pattern of behaviour innately determined, which is characteristic of all individuals of the same species. The behaviour is released and modified by environmental stimuli, but its pattern is relatively uniform and predetermined. **2.** an innate drive that urges the individual towards a particular

goal (for example, *libido in psychoanalytic psychology).

institutionalization *n.* a condition produced by long-term residence in an unstimulating impersonal institution (such as some residential care homes and orphanages). The individual adapts to the behaviour characteristic of the institution to such an extent that he is handicapped in other environments. The features often include apathy, dependence, and a lack of personal responsibility. Some symptoms, such as *stereotypy, are commoner in the institutionalized.

insufficiency *n.* inability of an organ or part, such as the heart or kidney, to carry out its normal function.

insufflation *n.* the act of blowing gas or a powder, such as a medication, into a body cavity.

insula *n.* an area of the *cerebral cortex that is overlapped by the sides of the deep lateral sulcus (cleft) in each hemisphere.

insulin *n.* a protein hormone, produced in the pancreas by the beta cells of the *islets of Langerhans, that is important for regulating the amount of sugar (glucose) in the blood. Insulin secretion is stimulated by a high concentration of blood sugar. Lack of this hormone gives rise to *diabetes mellitus, in which large amounts of sugar are present in the blood and urine. This condition may be treated successfully by insulin injections.

insulinase *n.* an enzyme found in such tissues as the liver and kidney, that is responsible for the normal breakdown of insulin in the body.

insulinoma *n.* an insulin-producing tumour of the beta cells in the *islets of Langerhans of the pancreas. Symptoms can include sweating, faintness, episodic loss of consciousness, and other features of *hypoglycaemia (*see* WHIPPLE'S TRIAD). Single tumours can be removed surgically. Multiple very small tumours scattered throughout the pancreas cannot be treated by surgery but do respond to drugs that poison the beta cells, including *diazoxide.

insulin shock a condition in which excess insulin in the body decreases the amount of glucose in the blood (*see* HYPO-GLYCAEMIA). If not treated with glucose or glucagon, coma and death can occur.

insult *n.* an injury or physical trauma.

Intal *n.* *see* CROMOLYN SODIUM.

integration *n.* the blending together of the *nerve impulses that arrive through the thousands of synapses at a nerve cell body. Impulses from some synapses cause *excitation, and from others *inhibition; the overall pattern decides whether an individual nerve cell is activated to transmit a message or not.

integument *n.* **1.** the skin. **2.** a membrane or layer of tissue covering any organ of the body.

intelligence quotient (IQ) an index of intellectual development. In childhood and adult life it represents intellectual ability relative to the rest of the population; in children it can also represent rate of development (*mental age as a percentage of chronological age). Most *intelligence tests are constructed so that the resulting intelligence quotients in the general population have a *mean of about 100 and a *standard deviation of about 15.

intelligence test a standardized assessment procedure for the determination of intellectual ability. The score produced is usually expressed as an *intelligence quotient. Most tests present a series of different kinds of problems to be solved. The best known are the Wechsler Adult Intelligence Scale (WAIS), the Wechsler Intelligence Scale for Children (WISC), and the Stanford Binet Intelligence Scale. Scores on intelligence tests are used for such purposes as the diagnosis of *mental retardation and the assessment of intellectual deterioration.

intensive therapy unit (ITU) a hospital unit designed to give intensive care, provided by specialist multidisciplinary staff, to a selected group of seriously ill patients or to those in need of special postoperative techniques (e.g. heart or chest patients).

intention *n.* a process of healing. Healing by **first intention** is the natural healing of a wound or surgical incision when the edges are brought together under aseptic conditions and *granulation tissue forms. In healing by **second intention** the wound edges are separated and the cavity is filled with granulation tissue over which epithelial tissue grows from the wound edges. In healing by **third intention** the wound ulcerates, granulations are slow to form, and a scar forms at the wound site.

intention tremor *see* TREMOR.

inter- *prefix denoting* between. Examples: **intercostal** (between the ribs); **intertrochanteric** (between the trochanters).

intercalated *adj.* describing structures, tissues, etc., that are inserted or situated between other structures.

intercellular *adj.* situated or occurring between cells.

intercostal muscles muscles that occupy the spaces between the ribs and are responsible for controlling some of the movements of the ribs. The superficial **external intercostals** lift the ribs during inspiration; the deep **internal intercostals** draw the ribs together during expiration.

intercurrent *adj.* going on at the same time: applied to an infection contracted by a patient who is already suffering from an infection or other disease.

interferon *n.* a substance that is produced by cells infected with a virus and has the ability to inhibit viral growth (*see* CYTOKINES). Interferon is active against many different viruses, but particular interferons are effective only in the species that produces them. There are three types of human interferon: **alpha** (from white blood cells), **beta** (from fibroblasts), and **gamma** (from lymphocytes).

Human interferon can now be produced in bacterial host cells by *genetic engineering for clinical use in treating hepatitis B and C, hairy-cell leukaemia, Kaposi's sarcoma, and multiple sclerosis. Side-effects, including flulike symptoms, lethargy, and depression, may be severe. Trade names: **Immukin, Intron A, Roferon-A, Viraferon, Wellferon**.

interkinesis *n.* **1.** the resting stage between the two divisions of *meiosis. **2.** see INTERPHASE.

interleukin n. any of a family of proteins that control some aspects of haemopoiesis and the immune response (see CYTOKINES). Many interleukins are currently characterized; **interleukin 2 (IL-2)** stimulates T-lymphocytes and is being investigated for the treatment of cancer (see ALDESLEUKIN).

intermittent claudication see CLAUDICATION.

intermittent fever a fever that rises, subsides, then returns again. See MALARIA.

intermittent self-catheterization (clean intermittent self-catheterization, ISC, CISC) a procedure in which the patient periodically passes a disposable catheter through the urethra into the bladder for the purpose of emptying it of urine. It is increasingly used in the management of patients of both sexes (including children) with chronic *retention and large residual urine volumes, often due to *neuropathic bladder. ISC may prevent back pressure and dilatation of the upper urinary tract with consequent infection and incontinence.

intern n. see DOCTOR.

International Classification of Diseases (ICD) a list of all known diseases and syndromes, including mental and behavioural disorders, published by the *World Health Organization every ten years (approximately). Over the years the classification has moved from being disease-orientated to include a wider framework of illness and other health problems. The latest version, **ICD-10**, was published in 1992 and employs alphanumeric coding. It is used in many countries as the principal means of classifying both mortality and morbidity experience and allows comparison of morbidity and mortality rates nationally and internationally. A parallel list, the **International Classification of Impairments, Disabilities and Handicaps (ICIDH)**, has also been compiled and is being used experimentally. See also HANDICAP.

interneurone n. a neurone in the central nervous system that acts as a link between the different neurones in a *reflex

arc. It usually possesses numerous branching processes (dendrites) that make possible extensive and complex circuits and pathways within the brain and spinal cord.

internode n. the length of *axon covered with a myelin sheath. Internodes are separated by nodes of Ranvier, where the sheath is absent.

interobserver error (in statistical surveys) see VALIDITY.

interoceptor n. any *receptor organ composed of sensory nerve cells that respond to and monitor changes within the body, such as the stretching of muscles or the acidity of the blood.

interparietal bone (inca bone, incarial bone) the bone lying between the *parietal bones, at the back of the skull.

interpeduncular adj. situated between the peduncles of the cerebrum or cerebellum.

interphase (interkinesis) n. the period when a cell is not undergoing division (mitosis), during which activities such as DNA synthesis occur.

intersex n. an individual who shows anatomical characteristics of both sexes. See HERMAPHRODITE, PSEUDOHERMAPHRODITISM. —**intersexuality** n.

interstice n. a small space in a tissue or between parts of the body. —**interstitial** adj.

interstitial cells (Leydig cells) the cells interspersed between the seminiferous tubules of the *testis. They secrete *androgens in response to stimulation by *luteinizing hormone from the anterior pituitary gland.

interstitial-cell-stimulating hormone see LUTEINIZING HORMONE.

interstitial cystitis a chronic nonbacterial inflammation of the bladder accompanied by an urgent desire to pass urine frequently and bladder pain; it is usually associated with an ulcer in the bladder wall (**Hunner's ulcer**). The cause is unknown and *contracture of the bladder eventually occurs. Treatment is by *balloon distension of the bladder under spinal or epidural anaesthetic, instillation of anti-inflammatory solutions into the bladder, and administration of steroids or *NSAIDs. Bladder enhancement or augmentation (see CYSTOPLASTY) may be required for a contracted bladder.

intertrigo *n.* superficial inflammation of two skin surfaces that are in contact, such as between the thighs or under the breasts, particularly in obese people. It is caused by friction and sweat and is often aggravated by infection, especially with *Candida*.

interventional radiology an application of radiology whereby therapeutic or diagnostic procedures can be performed under direct radiological vision. It is used in many forms of *minimally invasive surgery, including *angioplasty, visualization of obstructions in the bile ducts (see (PERCUTANEOUS) CHOLANGIOGRAPHY), and the removal of kidney stones (see PERCUTANEOUS NEPHROLITHOTOMY). See also MAGNETIC RESONANCE IMAGING.

intervention study a comparison of the outcome between two or more groups of patients that are deliberately subjected to different regimes (usually of treatment but sometimes of a preventive measure, such as vaccination). Wherever possible those entering the trial should be allocated to their respective groups by means of random numbers, and one such group (**controls**) should have no active treatment (**randomized controlled trial**). Ideally neither the patient nor the person assessing the outcome should be aware of which therapy is allocated to which patient (**blind trial**), nor should the doctor responsible for treatment (**double-blind trial**), and the groups should exchange treatment after a prearranged period (**crossover trial**).

intervertebral disc the flexible plate of fibrocartilage that connects any two adjacent vertebrae in the backbone. At birth the central part of the disc – the **nucleus pulposus** – consists of a gelatinous substance, which becomes replaced by cartilage with age. The intervertebral discs account for one quarter of the total length of the backbone; they act as shock absorbers, protecting the brain and spinal cord from the impact produced by run-

ning and other movements. *See also* PROLAPSED INTERVERTEBRAL DISC.

intestinal flora bacteria normally present in the intestinal tract. Some are responsible for the synthesis of *vitamin K. By producing a highly acidic environment in the intestine they may also prevent infection by pathogenic bacteria that cannot tolerate such conditions.

intestinal juice *see* SUCCUS ENTERICUS.

intestinal obstruction blockage of the intestines producing symptoms of vomiting, distension, and abdominal pain; failure to pass flatus or faeces (complete constipation) is usual. The causes may be acute (e.g. hernia) or chronic (e.g. tumours, Crohn's disease). Conservative management is by nasogastric suction ('suck') and replacement of water and electrolytes ('drip'), but most cases require surgical cure by removing the underlying cause.

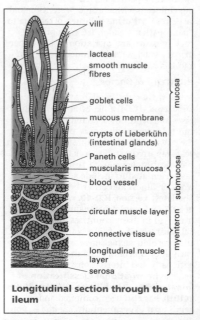

villi

lacteal

smooth muscle fibres

goblet cells

mucous membrane

crypts of Lieberkühn (intestinal glands)

Paneth cells

muscularis mucosa

blood vessel

circular muscle layer

connective tissue

longitudinal muscle layer

serosa

mucosa

submucosa

myenteron

Longitudinal section through the ileum

intestine (bowel, gut) *n.* the part of the *alimentary canal that extends from the stomach to the anus. It is divided into two main parts – the small intestine and the large intestine. The **small intestine** is divided into the *duodenum, *jejunum, and *ileum. It is here that most of the processes of digestion and absorption of food take place. The surface area of the inside of the small intestine is increased by the presence of finger-like projections called **villi** (see illustration). Glands in the mucous layer of the intestine secrete digestive enzymes and mucus. The **large intestine** consists of the *caecum, vermiform *appendix, *colon, and *rectum. It is largely concerned with the absorption of water from the material passed from the small intestine. The contents of the intestines are propelled forwards by means of rhythmic muscular contractions (see PERISTALSIS). —**intestinal** adj.

intima (tunica intima) n. **1**. the inner layer of the wall of an *artery or *vein. It is composed of a lining of endothelial cells and an elastic membrane. **2**. the inner layer of various other organs or parts.

intolerance n. the inability of a patient to tolerate a particular drug, manifested by various adverse reactions.

intoxication n. the symptoms of poisoning due to ingestion of any toxic material, including alcohol and heavy metals.

intra- prefix denoting inside; within. Examples: **intralobular** (within a lobule); **intrauterine** (within the uterus).

intracellular adj. situated or occurring inside a cell or cells.

intracranial adj. within the skull.

intracytoplasmic sperm injection see ICSI.

intradermal adj. within the skin. An **intradermal injection** is made into the skin.

intramuscular adj. within a muscle. An **intramuscular injection** is made into a muscle.

intraobserver error (in statistical surveys) see VALIDITY.

intraocular adj. of or relating to the area within the eyeball. An **intraocular lens implant** is a plastic lens placed inside the eye after *cataract extraction to replace the natural lens.

intrastromal keratomileusis an operation to correct severe degrees of myopia (short-sightedness). A disc of corneal tissue (from the *stroma of the cornea) is removed, frozen, and remodelled on a lathe, then replaced into the cornea to alter its curvature and thus reduce the myopia. *Excimer laser treatment, which is easier to perform, is also now being used for treating severe myopia (see LASIK).

intrathecal adj. **1**. within the *meninges of the spinal cord. An **intrathecal injection** is made into the meninges. **2**. within a sheath, e.g. a nerve sheath.

intrauterine contraceptive device see IUCD.

intrauterine growth retardation (IUGR) the condition resulting in the birth of a baby whose birth weight is abnormally low in relation to its gestational age (i.e. **small for dates**; **SFD**). Causes include maternal disease (e.g. infection, malnutrition, high blood pressure, smoking, and alcoholism), poor socioeconomic conditions, multiple pregnancy (e.g. twins), and fetal disease. It may be associated with *preterm birth.

intrauterine insemination (IUI) a procedure for assisting conception in cases of male infertility caused by inability of the spermatozoa to penetrate the cervical mucus or the barriers surrounding the ovum. The spermatozoa, which may be chemically treated in vitro to improve their motility and *acrosome reaction, are injected into the uterus through the vagina.

intravenous adj. into or within a vein. See INFUSION, INJECTION.

intravenous feeding see NUTRITION.

intravenous pyelogram (IVP) a succession of X-ray films of the urinary tract following the injection into a vein of a *contrast medium. This material is concentrated and excreted by the kidneys, and the IVP reveals details of the kidneys, the ureters, and subsequently the bladder. An IVP tests kidney function and reveals the presence of stones, tumours, or obstruction in the urinary tract. See also PYELOGRAPHY.

intraversion n. see INTROVERSION.

intra vitam Latin: during life.

intravitreal *adj.* within the vitreous humour of the eye.

intrinsic factor a glycoprotein secreted in the stomach. The secretion of intrinsic factor is necessary for the absorption of *vitamin B$_{12}$; a failure of secretion of intrinsic factor leads to a deficiency of the vitamin and the condition of *pernicious anaemia.

intrinsic muscle a muscle that is contained entirely within the organ or part it acts on. For example, there are intrinsic muscles of the tongue, whose contractions change the shape of the tongue.

intro- *prefix denoting* in; into.

introitus *n.* (in anatomy) an entrance into a hollow organ or cavity.

introjection *n.* (in psychoanalysis) the process of adopting, or of believing that one possesses, the qualities of another person. This can be a form of *defence mechanism. *See also* IDENTIFICATION.

intromission *n.* the introduction of one organ or part into another, e.g. the penis into the vagina.

introversion *n.* **1.** (or **intraversion**) an enduring personality trait characterized by interest in the self rather than the outside world. People high in introversion (**introverts**), as measured by questionnaires and psychological tests, tend to have a small circle of friends, like to persist in activities once they have started, and are highly susceptible to permanent *conditioning. Introversion was first described by Carl Jung as a tendency to distancing oneself from others, to philosophical interests, and to reserved defensive reactions. *Compare* EXTROVERSION. **2.** a turning inwards of a hollow organ (such as the uterus) on itself.

introvert *n.* *see* INTROVERSION.

intubation *n.* the introduction of a tube into part of the body for the purpose of diagnosis or treatment. Thus **gastric intubation** may be performed to remove a sample of the stomach contents for analysis or to administer drugs directly into the stomach. In **endotracheal intubation** a tube is inserted through the nose or mouth into the trachea to maintain an airway or to facilitate administration of general anaesthetics or oxygen.

intumescence *n.* a swelling or an increase in the volume of an organ.

intussusception *n.* the telescoping (**invagination**) of one part of the bowel into another: most common in young children under the age of four. As the contents of the intestine are pushed onwards by muscular contraction more and more intestine is dragged into the invaginating portion, resulting in obstruction. Symptoms include intermittent colic or pain, vomiting, and the passing of red jelly with the stools; if the condition does not receive prompt surgical treatment, shock from gangrene of the bowel may result. A barium or Gastrografin enema may confirm the diagnosis and in many cases may relieve the intussusception.

inulin *n.* a carbohydrate with a high molecular weight, used in a test of kidney function called **inulin clearance**. Inulin is filtered from the bloodstream by the kidneys. By injecting it into the blood and measuring the amount that appears in the urine over a given period, it is possible to calculate how much filtrate the kidneys are producing in a given time.

inunction *n.* the rubbing in with the fingers of an ointment or liniment.

invagination *n.* **1.** the infolding of the wall of a solid structure to form a cavity. This occurs in some stages of the development of embryos. **2.** *see* INTUSSUSCEPTION.

invalidity benefit a former benefit under the Social Security Acts that replaced sickness benefit after 28 six-day weeks. Both sickness and invalidity benefits were replaced by *incapacity benefit in 1995.

invasion *n.* the spread of *cancer into neighbouring normal structures; it is one of the cardinal features of malignancy.

inversion *n.* **1.** the turning inwards or inside-out of a part or organ: commonly applied to the state of the uterus after childbirth when its upper part is pulled through the cervical canal. **2.** a chromosome mutation in which a block of genes within a chromosome are in reverse order, due to that section of the chromosome becoming inverted. The centromere may be included in the inverted segment (**pericentric inversion**) or not (**paracentric inversion**).

invertebrate 1. *n.* an animal without a backbone. The following are invertebrate groups of medical importance: *insects, *ticks, *nematodes, *flukes, and *tapeworms. 2. *adj.* not possessing a backbone.

in vitro Latin: describing biological phenomena that are made to occur outside the living body (traditionally in a test-tube).

in vitro fertilization (IVF) fertilization of an ovum outside the body, the resultant *zygote being incubated to the *blastocyst stage and then implanted in the uterus. The technique, pioneered in Britain, resulted in 1978 in the birth of the first **test-tube baby**. IVF is employed when a woman has blocked Fallopian tubes or some other impediment to the union of sperm and ovum in the reproductive tract. The mother-to-be is given hormone therapy causing a number of ova to mature at the same time (*see* SUPEROVULATION). Several of them are then removed from the ovary through a laparoscope. The ova are mixed with spermatozoa from her partner and incubated in a culture medium until the blastocyst is formed. The blastocyst is then implanted in the mother's uterus and the pregnancy allowed to continue normally.

in vivo Latin: describing biological phenomena that occur or are observed occurring within the bodies of living organisms.

involucrum *n.* a growth of new bone, formed from the *periosteum, that sometimes surrounds a mass of infected and dead bone in osteomyelitis.

involuntary muscle muscle that is not under conscious control, such as the muscle of the gut, stomach, blood vessels, and heart. *See also* CARDIAC MUSCLE, SMOOTH MUSCLE.

involution *n.* 1. the shrinking of the womb to its normal size after childbirth. 2. atrophy of an organ in old age.

involutional melancholia a severe

*depression, usually psychotic, appearing for the first time in the involutional period of middle life (approximately 40–55 for women, 50–65 for men). Such an illness classically has characteristic features, including agitation; delusions of ill-health, poverty, sin, and sometimes of the nonexistence of the world; and preoccupations with death and loss. However, the features are not always classical, and many authorities do not regard the condition as a clinical entity separate from depressive psychosis. *See* MANIC-DEPRESSIVE PSYCHOSIS.

iodine *n.* an element required in small amounts for healthy growth and development. An adult body contains about 30 mg of iodine, mostly concentrated in the thyroid gland: this gland requires iodine to synthesize *thyroid hormones. A deficiency of iodine leads to *goitre. The daily requirement of iodine in an adult is thought to be about 140 μg per day; dietary sources of iodine are sea food and vegetables grown in soil containing iodide and also iodized table salt. Radioactive isotopes of iodine (usually iodine-131) are used in the diagnosis and treatment of diseases of the thyroid gland. Water-soluble contrast agents used in X-ray examinations are organic chemicals containing iodine. Iodine is also used as an antiseptic. Symbol: I.

iodism *n.* iodine poisoning. The main features are a characteristic staining of the mouth and odour on the breath. Vomited material may be yellowish or bluish. There is pain and burning in the throat, intense thirst, and diarrhoea, with dizziness, weakness, and convulsions. Emergency treatment includes administration of starch or flour in water and lavage with sodium thiosulphate solution.

IOL intraocular lens implant. *See* CATARACT.

ion *n.* an atom or group of atoms that has lost one or more electrons, making it electrically charged and therefore more chemically active. *See* ANION, CATION, ELECTROLYTE, IONIZATION.

ionization *n.* the process of producing *ions. Some molecules ionize in solution (*see* ELECTROLYTE). Ions can also be produced when ionizing radiation dislodges one or more electrons from an atom or molecule.

iontophoresis *n.* the technique of introducing through the skin, by means of an electric current, charged particles of a drug, so that it reaches a deep site. The method has been used to transfer salicylate ions through the skin in the treatment of deep rheumatic pain. *See also* CATAPHORESIS.

iopanoic acid *n.* a *radiopaque iodine-containing compound used in *cholecystography to outline the gall bladder.

IOUS intraoperative ultrasound examination (*see* ULTRASONOGRAPHY).

ipecacuanha *n.* a plant extract used in small doses, usually in the form of tinctures and syrups, as an *expectorant to relieve coughing and to induce vomiting. Ipecacuanha irritates the digestive system, and high doses may cause severe digestive upsets.

ipratropium *n.* a bronchodilator drug used in the treatment of chronic reversible airways obstruction (*see* BRONCHOSPASM). Ipratropium is administered by inhalation; side-effects include nausea, palpitations, and headache. Trade name: **Atrovent**.

iprindole *n.* a drug administered by mouth for the treatment of depression (*see* ANTIDEPRESSANT). Response may take place gradually, and side-effects, such as dry mouth, blurred vision, constipation, and sweating, may occur. Trade name: **Prondol**.

ipsilateral (ipselateral, homolateral) *adj.* on or affecting the same side of the body: applied particularly to paralysis (or other symptoms) occurring on the same side of the body as the brain lesion that caused them. *Compare* CONTRALATERAL.

IQ *see* INTELLIGENCE QUOTIENT.

irid- (irido-) *prefix denoting* the iris.

iridectomy *n.* an operation on the eye in which a part of the iris is removed.

iridencleisis *n.* an operation for *glaucoma in which a small incision is made into the eye, beneath the *conjunctiva and close to the cornea, and part of the iris is drawn into it. The iris acts like a wick and keeps the incision open for the drainage of fluid from the front chamber of the eye to the tissue beneath the conjunctiva.

iridocyclitis *n.* inflammation of the iris and ciliary body of the eye. *See* UVEITIS.

iridodialysis *n.* a tear, caused by injury to the eye, in the attachment of the iris to the ciliary body. Usually a dark crescentic gap is seen at the edge of the iris where the tear has occurred, and the pupil pulls away from the site of the tear.

iridodonesis *n.* tremulousness of the iris when the eye is moved. It is due to absence of support from the lens, against which the iris normally lies, and occurs when the lens is absent or dislocated from its normal position.

iridoplegia *n.* paralysis of the iris, which is usually associated with *cycloplegia and results from injury, inflammation, or the use of pupil-dilating eye drops. In the case of injury, the pupil is usually larger than normal and moves little, if at all, in response to light and drugs.

iridotomy *n.* an operation on the eye in which an incision is made in the iris using a knife or a *YAG laser.

iris *n.* the part of the eye that regulates the amount of light that enters. It forms a coloured muscular diaphragm across the front of the lens; light enters through a central opening, the **pupil**. A ring of muscle round the margin contracts in bright light, causing the pupil to become smaller (*see* PUPILLARY REFLEX). In dim light a set of radiating muscles contract and the constricting muscles relax, increasing the size of the pupil. The outer margin of the iris is attached to the *ciliary body.

iris bombé an abnormal condition of the eye in which the iris bulges forward towards the cornea. It is due to pressure from the aqueous humour behind the iris when its passage through the pupil to the anterior chamber of the eye is blocked (**pupil-block glaucoma**).

iritis *n.* inflammation of the iris. *See* UVEITIS.

iron *n.* an element essential to life. The body of an adult contains on average 4 g of iron, over half of which is contained in *haemoglobin in the red blood cells, the rest being distributed between *myohaemoglobin in muscles, *cytochromes, and iron stores in the form of *ferritin and *haemosiderin. Iron is an essential component in the transfer of oxygen in the body. The absorption and loss of iron is very finely controlled. A good dietary source is meat, particularly liver. The recommended daily intake of iron is 10 mg per day for men and 12 mg per day for women during their reproductive life. A deficiency of iron may lead to *anaemia. Symbol: Fe.

Many preparations of iron are used to treat iron-deficiency anaemia. These include preparations taken by mouth, such as *ferrous sulphate, and those administered by injection, such as *iron dextran.

iron dextran a drug containing *iron and *dextran, administered by intramuscular or intravenous injection to treat iron-deficiency anaemia. Side-effects can include pain at the site of injection, rapid beating of the heart, and allergic reactions. Trade name: **Imferon.**

iron lung *see* RESPIRATOR.

iron-storage disease *see* HAEMOCHROMATOSIS.

irradiation *n.* **1.** exposure of the body's tissues to ionizing radiation. The source may be background radiation, diagnostic X-rays, radiotherapy, or nuclear accidents. **2.** exposure of a substance or object to ionizing radiation. Irradiation of food with gamma rays, which kill bacteria, is a technique used in food preservation.

irreducible *adj.* unable to be replaced in a normal position: applied particularly to a type of *hernia.

irrigation *n.* the process of washing out a wound or hollow organ with a continuous flow of water or medicated solution. Techniques are available for washing out the entire intestinal tract (**whole-gut irrigation**) as a prelude to surgery on the lower intestine.

irritability *n.* (in physiology) the property of certain kinds of tissue that enables them to respond in a specific way to outside stimuli. Irritability is shown by nerve cells, which can generate and transmit electrical impulses when stimulated appropriately, and by muscle cells, which

contract when stimulated by nerve impulses.

irritable bowel syndrome (IBS, spastic colon, mucous colitis) a common condition in which recurrent abdominal pain with constipation and/or diarrhoea continues for years without any general deterioration in physical health. There is no detectable structural disease; the symptoms are caused by abnormal muscular contractions in the intestine and heightened sensitivity to such stimuli as stretching or distension. The cause is unknown, but the condition is often associated with stress or anxiety and may follow severe infection of the intestine. Tests may be needed to rule out organic disease. Treatment is based on removing anxiety (psychotherapy), dietary adjustment and faecal softening agents, and drugs to reduce spasm or diminish pain sensitivity.

irritant *n.* any material that causes irritation of a tissue, ranging from nettles (causing pain and swelling) to tear gas (causing watering of the eyes). Chronic irritation by various chemicals can give rise to *dermatitis.

isch- (ischo-) *prefix denoting* suppression or deficiency.

ischaemia *n.* an inadequate flow of blood to a part of the body, caused by constriction or blockage of the blood vessels supplying it. Ischaemia of heart muscle produces *angina pectoris. Ischaemia of the calf muscles of the legs on exercise (causing intermittent *claudication) or at rest (producing *rest pain) is common in elderly subjects with atherosclerosis of the vessels at or distal to the point where the aorta divides into the iliac arteries. —**ischaemic** *adj.*

ischi- (ischio-) *prefix denoting* the ischium.

ischiorectal abscess an abscess in the space between the sheet of muscle that assists in control of the rectum (levator ani) and the pelvic bone. It may occur spontaneously, but is often secondary to an anal fissure, thrombosed *haemorrhoids, or other disease of the anus. Symptoms are severe throbbing pain near the anus with swelling and fever; it may cause an anal *fistula. Pus is drained from the abscess by surgical incision.

ischium *n.* a bone forming the lower part of each side of the *hip bone (*see also* PELVIS). —**ischiac, ischial** *adj.*

ischuria *n.* retention or suppression of the urine. *See* ANURIA, RETENTION.

island *n.* (in anatomy) an area of tissue or group of cells clearly differentiated from surrounding tissues.

islet *n.* (in anatomy) a small group of cells that is structurally distinct from the cells surrounding it.

islets of Langerhans small groups of cells, scattered through the material of the *pancreas, that secrete the hormones *insulin and *glucagon. There are three main histological types of cells: alpha (α), beta (β), and delta cells; these cells produce glucagon, insulin, and *somatostatin, respectively.

iso- *prefix denoting* equality, uniformity, or similarity.

isoagglutinin (isohaemagglutinin) *n.* one of the antibodies occurring naturally in the plasma that cause *agglutination of red blood cells of a different group.

isoagglutinogen *n.* one of the *antigens naturally occurring on the surface of red blood cells that is attacked by an isoagglutinin in blood plasma of a different group, so causing *agglutination.

isoantibody *n.* an *antibody that occurs naturally against the components of foreign tissues from an individual of the same species.

isoantigen *n.* an antigen that forms a natural component of an individual's tissues. Thus the antigens of the *HLA system are isoantigens, as are the agglutinogens of the different *blood groups.

isodactylism *n.* a congenital defect in which all the fingers are the same length.

isoenzyme (isozyme) *n.* a physically distinct form of a given enzyme. Isoenzymes catalyse the same type of reaction but have slight physical and immunological differences. Isoenzymes of

dehydrogenases, oxidases, transaminases, phosphatases, and proteolytic enzymes are known to exist.

isohaemagglutinin *n. see* ISOAGGLUTININ.

isoimmunization *n.* the development of antibodies (**isoantibodies**) within an individual against antigens from another individual of the same species.

isolation *n.* **1.** the separation of a person with an infectious disease from noninfected people. *See also* QUARANTINE. **2.** (in surgery) the separation of a structure from surrounding structures by the use of instruments.

isoleucine *n.* an *essential amino acid. *See also* AMINO ACID.

isomerase *n.* any one of a group of enzymes that catalyse the conversion of one isomer of a compound into another.

isometheptene *n.* a *sympathomimetic drug used in the treatment of migraine, either alone or in combination with paracetamol (as **Midrid**). It is administered by mouth. Possible side-effects include dizziness.

isometric exercises (isometrics) a system of exercises based on the principle of **isometric contraction** of muscles. This occurs when the fibres are called upon to contract and do work, but despite an increase in tension do not shorten in length. It can be induced in muscles that are used when a limb is made to pull or push against something that does not move. The exercises increase fitness and build muscle.

isometropia *n.* an equal power of *refraction in both eyes.

isomorphism *n.* the condition of two or more objects being alike in shape or structure. It can exist at any structural level, from molecules to whole organisms. —**isomorphic, isomorphous** *adj.*

isoniazid (isonicotinic acid hydrazide, INH) *n.* a drug used in the treatment of *tuberculosis, usually taken by mouth. Because tuberculosis bacteria soon become resistant to isoniazid, it is usually given in conjunction with streptomycin and other antibiotics. Occasional side-effects include digestive disturbances and dry mouth; high doses or prolonged treatment may cause inflammation of the nerves, which can be countered by including pyridoxine (vitamin B_6) in the preparation.

isoprenaline n. a *sympathomimetic drug used to dilate the air passages in asthma and other bronchial conditions. It also stimulates the heart and is used to treat some heart conditions involving reduced heart activity. It is administered by inhalation, by mouth, by injection, or in suppositories. Side-effects such as increased heart rate, palpitations, chest pain, dizziness, and fainting may occur. Trade names: **Medihaler-Iso, Saventrine**.

isosorbide dinitrate a drug used for the treatment of angina in patients unable to take glyceryl trinitrate. It acts by relaxing the smooth muscle of both arteries and veins, thus causing dilation. It is administered by mouth; side-effects are rare, but include headache, hypotension, nausea and vomiting, and skin rash. Trade names: **Cedocard, Isoket, Isordil, Sorbitrate**.

isosthenuria n. inability of the kidneys to produce either a concentrated or a dilute urine. This occurs in the final stages of renal failure.

isotonic adj. **1.** describing solutions that have the same osmotic pressure. See OSMOSIS. **2.** describing muscles that have equal *tonicity.

isotonic exercises see EXERCISE.

isotope n. any one of the different forms of an element, possessing the same number of protons (positively charged particles) in the nucleus, and thus the same atomic number, but different numbers of neutrons. Isotopes therefore have different atomic weights. Radioactive isotopes decay into other isotopes or elements, emitting alpha, beta, or gamma radiation. Some radioactive isotopes may be produced artificially by bombarding elements with neutrons. These are known as **nuclides** and are used extensively in *radiotherapy for the treatment of cancer.

isotretinoin n. a drug related to vitamin A (see RETINOID) and used in the treatment of severe acne that has failed to respond

to other treatment. It is administered by mouth. Possible side-effects include dry skin, nose bleeds, eyelid and lip inflammation, muscle, joint, and abdominal pains, diarrhoea, and some disturbances of vision. Trade name: **Roaccutane**.

isoxsuprine n. a drug that dilates blood vessels and is used to improve blood flow in such conditions as cerebrovascular disease and arteriosclerosis and to inhibit contractions in premature labour. It is administered by mouth or injection and rarely it may cause flushing, increased heart rate, dizziness, and nausea. Trade name: **Duvalidan**.

isozyme n. see ISOENZYME.

ispaghula husk a bulking agent (see LAXATIVE) used to treat constipation, *diverticulitis, and *irritable bowel syndrome. It is administered by mouth. Trade names: **Colven, Fybogel**.

ISS see INJURY SCORING SYSTEM.

isthmus n. a constricted or narrowed part of an organ or tissue, such as the band of thyroid tissue connecting the two lobes of the thyroid gland.

itch n. local discomfort or irritation of the skin, prompting the sufferer to scratch or rub the affected area. It is the main symptom of skin disease. See PRURITUS.

-itis suffix denoting inflammation of an organ, tissue, etc. Examples: **arthritis** (of a joint); **peritonitis** (of the peritoneum).

ITU see INTENSIVE THERAPY UNIT.

IUCD (intrauterine contraceptive device) a plastic or metal coil, spiral, or other shape, about 25 mm long, that is inserted into the cavity of the uterus to prevent conception. Its exact mode of action is unknown but it is thought to interfere with implantation of the embryo. Early IUCDs (such as the **Lippes loop**) were made of plastic; later variants (such as the **Gravigard**) are covered with copper, which slowly dissolves and augments the contraceptive action. Devices such as the **Progestasert** release small amounts of a contraceptive hormone drug. About one-third of women fitted with an IUCD find the side-effects (heavy menstrual bleeding or back pain) unacceptable, but most have no complaints. The unwanted pregnancy rate is about 2 per 100 woman-years. If pregnancy should occur there is normally no need to remove the device (it may, however, be shed spontaneously). *See also* POSTCOITAL CONTRACEPTION.

IUGR *see* INTRAUTERINE GROWTH RETARDATION.

IUI *see* INTRAUTERINE INSEMINATION.

IUS (intrauterine system) a hormonal contraceptive device consisting of a plastic T-shaped frame that is inserted into the uterus. It carries a hormone (progestogen) in a sleeve around its stem and has two fine threads attached to its base, by which it can be removed. It provides a long-term method of contraception that is also reversible. Trade name: **Mirena**.

ivermectin *n.* a drug used in the treatment of *onchocerciasis. It is administered by mouth and acts by killing the immature forms (*microfilariae) of the parasite. Side-effects, which are mild, include itching and swollen lymph nodes.

IVF *see* IN VITRO FERTILIZATION.

IVP *see* INTRAVENOUS PYELOGRAM.

Ixodes *n.* a genus of widely distributed parasitic ticks. Several species are responsible for transmitting *Lyme disease, *tularaemia, Queensland tick typhus, and *Russian spring-summer encephalitis. The bite of a few species can give rise to a serious paralysis, caused by a toxin in the tick's saliva.

ixodiasis *n.* any disease caused by the presence of *ticks.

Ixodidae *n.* a family of *ticks.

J

Jacksonian epilepsy *see* EPILEPSY. [J. H. Jackson (1835–1911), British neurologist]

Jacquemier's sign a bluish or purplish coloration of the vagina: a possible indication of pregnancy. [J. M. Jacquemin (1806–79), French obstetrician]

jactitation *n.* restless tossing and turning of a person suffering from a severe disease, frequently one with a high fever.

jamais vu one of the manifestations of temporal lobe *epilepsy, in which there is a sudden feeling of unfamiliarity with everyday surroundings.

Jarisch-Herxheimer reaction (Herxheimer reaction) exacerbation of the symptoms of syphilis that may occur on starting antibiotic therapy for the disease. The effect is transient and requires no treatment. [A. Jarisch (1850–1902), Austrian dermatologist; K. Herxheimer (1861–1944), German dermatologist]

jaundice *n.* a yellowing of the skin or whites of the eyes, indicating excess bilirubin (a bile pigment) in the blood. Jaundice is classified into three types. **Obstructive jaundice** occurs when bile made in the liver fails to reach the intestine due to obstruction of the *bile ducts (e.g. by gallstones) or to *cholestasis. The urine is dark, the faeces pale, and the patient may itch. **Hepatocellular jaundice** is due to disease of the liver cells, such as *hepatitis, when the liver is unable to utilize the bilirubin, which accumulates in the blood. The urine may be dark but the faeces retain their colour. **Haemolytic jaundice** occurs when there is excessive destruction of red cells in the blood (*see* HAEMOLYSIS). Urine and faeces retain their normal colour. Medical name: **icterus**.

jaw *n.* either the *maxilla (upper jaw) or the *mandible (lower jaw). The jaws form the framework of the mouth and provide attachment for the teeth.

jejun- (jejuno-) *prefix denoting* the jejunum.

jejunal biopsy removal of a piece of the lining (mucosa) of the upper small intestine. This can be done by a surgical operation but is usually performed by a gastroduodenoscope or a special metal capsule, swallowed by the patient. When the capsule is in the *jejunum a small knife within it is triggered by suction on an attached tube, cutting off a small piece of mucosa. The specimen may be examined microscopically to assist in the diagnosis of *coeliac disease, *Whipple's disease, or intestinal infections, or its enzyme content may be measured chemically to detect, for example, *lactase deficiency.

jejunal ulcer *see* PEPTIC ULCER, ZOLLINGER-ELLISON SYNDROME.

jejunectomy *n.* surgical removal of the jejunum or part of the jejunum.

jejunoileostomy *n.* an operation in which the jejunum is joined to the ileum (small intestine), when either the end of the jejunum or the beginning of the ileum has been removed or is to be bypassed. It is usually performed for intestinal disease (e.g. Crohn's disease). It was formerly used for the treatment of obesity but has been abandoned because of serious side-effects.

jejunostomy *n.* a surgical operation in which the jejunum is brought through the abdominal wall and opened. It can enable the insertion of a catheter into the jejunum for short-term infusion of nutrients or other substances.

jejunotomy *n.* a surgical incision into the jejunum in order to inspect the interior or remove something from within it.

jejunum *n.* part of the small *intestine. It comprises about two-fifths of the whole small intestine and connects the duodenum to the ileum. —**jejunal** *adj.*

jerk *n.* the sudden contraction of a muscle in response to a nerve impulse. The **knee jerk** (*see* PATELLAR REFLEX) is the reflex kicking movement produced by contraction of the quadriceps muscle of the thigh after it has been stretched by tapping the tendon below the knee. Eliciting this and other jerks, such as the ankle and elbow jerks, is a means of testing the nerve pathways, via the spinal cord, which are involved in *reflexes.

jigger n. see TUNGA.

joint n. the point at which two or more bones are connected. The opposing surfaces of the two bones are lined with cartilaginous, fibrous, or soft (synovial) tissue. The three main classes of joint are *diarthrosis (freely movable), *amphiarthrosis (slightly movable), and *synarthrosis (immovable).

joule n. the *SI unit of work or energy, equal to the work done when the point of application of a force of 1 newton is displaced through a distance of 1 metre in the direction of the force. In electrical terms the joule is the work done per second when a current of 1 ampere flows through a resistance of 1 ohm. Symbol: J. See also CALORIE.

jugular adj. relating to or supplying the neck or throat.

jugular vein any one of several veins in the neck. The **internal jugular** is a very large paired vein running vertically down the side of the neck and draining blood from the brain, face, and neck. It ends behind the sternoclavicular joint, where it joins the subclavian vein. The **external jugular** is a smaller paired vein running superficially down the neck to the subclavian vein and draining blood from the face, scalp, and neck. Its tributary, the **anterior jugular**, runs down the front of the neck.

jugum n. (in anatomy) a ridge or furrow that connects two parts of a bone.

jumper's knee (patellar tendinitis) a form of *tendinitis that occurs in athletes and dancers. Repeated sudden contracture of the quadriceps muscle at take-off causes inflammation of the attachment of the patellar tendon to the lower end of the patella. Treatment is rest, physiotherapy, and anti-inflammatory medication.

junction n. (in anatomy) the point at which two different tissues or structures are in contact. See also NEUROMUSCULAR JUNCTION.

juvenile polyp see POLYP.

juxta- prefix denoting proximity to. Example: **juxta-articular** (near a joint).

Kahn reaction a test for syphilis, in which antibodies specific to the disease are detected in a sample of the patient's blood by means of a *precipitin reaction. This test is not as reliable as some. [R. L. Kahn (20th century), US bacteriologist]

kala-azar (visceral leishmaniasis, Dumdum fever) *n.* a tropical disease caused by the parasitic protozoan *Leishmania donovani*. The parasite, which is transmitted to man by *sandflies, invades the cells of the lymphatic system, spleen, and bone marrow. Symptoms include enlargement and subsequent lesions of the liver and spleen; anaemia; a low *leucocyte count; weight loss; and irregular fevers. The disease occurs in Asia, South America, the Mediterranean area, and Africa. Drugs containing antimony, with supplementary pentamidine, are used in the treatment of this potentially fatal disease.

kallidin *n.* a naturally occurring polypeptide consisting of ten amino acids. Kallidin is a powerful vasodilator and causes contraction of smooth muscle; it is formed in the blood under certain conditions. *See* KININ.

kallikrein *n.* one of a group of enzymes found in the blood and body fluids that act on certain plasma globulins to produce bradykinin and kallidin. *See* KININ.

kanamycin *n.* an *antibiotic used to treat a wide range of bacterial infections. It is administered mainly by injection but is given by mouth for infections of the intestine and by inhalation for respiratory infections. Mild side-effects sometimes occur; these include skin rashes, fever, headache, nausea, vomiting, and tingling sensations. Trade name: **Kannasyn**.

kaolin *n.* a white clay that contains aluminium and silicon and is purified and powdered for use as an adsorbent. It is taken by mouth to treat the diarrhoea and vomiting due to food poisoning and other digestive disorders. Kaolin is also used in dusting powders and poultices.

Kaposi's sarcoma a malignant tumour arising from blood vessels in the skin and appearing as purple to dark brown plaques or nodules. It is common in Africa but rare in the Western world, except in patients with *AIDS. The tumour evolves slowly; radiotherapy is the treatment of choice but chemotherapy may be of value in metastatic disease. [M. Kaposi (1837–1902), Austrian dermatologist]

Kartagener's syndrome a hereditary condition in which the heart and other internal organs lie on the opposite side of the body to the norm (i.e. the heart lies on the right; *see* DEXTROCARDIA); it is associated with chronic sinusitis and bronchiectasis. [M. Kartagener (1897–1975), German physician]

kary- (karyo-) *prefix denoting* a cell nucleus.

karyokinesis *n.* division of the nucleus of a cell, which occurs during cell division before division of the cytoplasm (**cytokinesis**). *See* MITOSIS.

karyolysis *n.* the breakdown of a cell nucleus, which occurs during cell *necrosis and is preceded by fragmentation of the nucleus (**karyorrhexis**).

karyoplasm *n.* *see* NUCLEOPLASM.

karyosome *n.* the dense mass of *chromatin found in the cell nucleus, which is composed mainly of chromosomes.

karyotype **1.** *n.* the *chromosome set of an individual or species described in terms of both the number and structure of the chromosomes. **2.** *n.* the representation of the chromosome set in a diagram. **3.** *vb.* to determine the karyotype of a cell, as by microscopic examination.

katathermometer *n.* a thermometer used to measure the cooling power of the air surrounding it, having its bulb covered with water-moistened material. The instrument is brought to a steady temperature of 100°F and then exposed to the air. The time taken for the temperature recorded by the thermometer to fall to 95°F gives an index of the air's cooling power.

Kawasaki disease (mucocutaneous lymph node syndrome) a condition of unknown cause affecting young children, usually less than five years old, and characterized by fever, conjunctivitis, a sore throat, and a generalized rash and reddening of the palms and soles. This is followed by peeling of the fingers and toes. The fever usually persists for 1–2 weeks. In approximately one-fifth of children there is involvement of the coronary arteries and heart muscle (myocardium), resulting in *myocarditis and *aneurysms of the coronary arteries. About 2% of cases are fatal. The aneurysms will usually resolve spontaneously but slowly. Treatment involves aspirin therapy, and *gammaglobulin has recently been shown to reduce the risk of coronary artery disease. [T. Kawasaki (20th century), Japanese physician]

Kayser-Fleischer ring a brownish-yellow ring in the outer rim of the cornea of the eye. It is a deposit of copper granules and is diagnostic of *Wilson's disease. When well developed it can be seen by unaided observation, but faint Kayser-Fleischer rings may only be detected by specialized ophthalmological examination. [B. Kayser (1869–1954), German ophthalmologist; B. Fleischer (1848–1904), German physician]

Kehr's sign pain in the left shoulder caused by irritation of the undersurface of the diaphragm by blood leaking from a ruptured spleen. The pain impulses are referred along the *phrenic nerve. [H. Kehr (1862–1913), German surgeon]

Kell antigens a group of antigens that may or may not be present on the surface of red blood cells, forming the basis of a *blood group. This group is important in blood transfusion reactions. [Mrs Kell (20th century), patient in whom they were first demonstrated]

Keller's operation an operation for *hallux valgus (*see also* BUNION) or *hallux rigidus, usually reserved for elderly patients. It involves excision of the base of the first (proximal) phalanx of the big toe; the gap thus created fills with fibrous tis-

sue. The toe will be slightly shorter and floppy. [W. L. Keller (1874–1959), US surgeon]

keloid *n.* an overgrowth of fibrous scar tissue following trauma to the skin. It does not resolve spontaneously but may be flattened by applied pressure or with injections of potent corticosteroids. Keloid formation is particularly common at certain sites, such as the breastbone or ear lobe; surgical excision of benign (nonmalignant) lesions from such sites is therefore best avoided. A **hypertrophic scar** is similar, but resolves over a period of months.

kelvin *n.* the *SI unit of temperature, formally defined as the fraction 1/273.16 of the temperature of the triple point of water. A temperature in kelvins is equal to a Celsius temperature plus 273.15°C. Symbol: K.

Kemp echoes *see* OTOACOUSTIC EMISSIONS.

kerat- (kerato-) *prefix denoting* **1.** the cornea. Example: **keratopathy** (disease of). **2.** horny tissue, especially of the skin.

keratalgia *n.* pain arising from the cornea.

keratectasia *n.* bulging of the cornea at the site of scar tissue (which is thinner than normal corneal tissue).

keratectomy *n.* an operation in which a part of the cornea is removed, usually a superficial layer. This procedure is now frequently done by an *excimer laser, as in **photorefractive keratectomy**, in which the shape of the cornea is altered to correct long- or short-sightedness. *See also* AUTOMATED LAMELLAR KERATECTOMY.

keratin *n.* one of a family of proteins that are the major constituents of the nails, hair, and the outermost layers of the skin. The cytoplasm of epithelial cells, including *keratinocytes, contains a network of keratin filaments.

keratinization (cornification) *n.* the process by which cells become horny due to the deposition of *keratin within them. It occurs in the *epidermis of the skin and associated structures (hair, nails, etc.), where the cells become flattened, lose their nuclei, and are filled with keratin as they approach the surface.

keratinocyte n. a type of cell that makes up 95% of the cells of the epidermis. Keratinocytes migrate from the deeper layers of the epidermis and are finally shed from the surface of the skin.

keratitis n. inflammation of the *cornea of the eye. The eye waters and is very painful and vision is blurred. It may be due to physical or chemical agents (abrasions, exposure to dust, chemicals, ultraviolet light, etc.) or result from infection. In **disciform keratitis** a disc-shaped patch of oedema and inflammation develops in the cornea, usually as an immune response to viral infection, commonly herpes simplex virus. **Filamentary keratitis** is associated with small mucoid deposits of epithelial filaments on the surface of the cornea, which come off to leave small corneal erosions that cause severe pain until they heal. Keratitis not due to infection usually responds to keeping the eyes covered until the corneal surface has healed; infections often require specific drug treatment, e.g. with antibiotics.

keratoacanthoma n. a firm nodule that appears singly on the skin, grows to 1–2 cm across in about six weeks, and usually disappears gradually during the next few months. Men are affected more often than women, commonly between the ages of 50 and 70. Keratoacanthomas occur mainly on the face; the cause is not known. Spontaneous healing may leave an unsightly scar; therefore treatment by curettage and cautery, or excision, may be required.

keratocele (descemetocele) n. outward bulging of the base of a deep ulcer of the cornea. The deep layer of the cornea (Descemet's membrane) is elastic and relatively resistant to perforation; it therefore bulges when the overlying cornea has been destroyed.

keratoconjunctivitis n. combined inflammation of the cornea and conjunctiva of the eye. **Keratoconjunctivitis sicca** is dryness of the cornea and conjunctiva due to deficiency production of tears. It may be associated with systemic disorders, such as *Sjögren's syndrome, systemic lupus, systemic sclerosis, and sarcoidosis.

keratoconus n. conical cornea: an abnormal condition of the eye in which the cornea, instead of having a regular curvature, comes to a rounded apex towards its centre. The 'cone' tends to become sharper over a period of years.

keratoglobus (megalocornea) n. a congenital disorder of the eye in which the whole cornea bulges forward in a regular curve. Compare KERATOCONUS.

keratomalacia n. a progressive nutritional disease of the eye due to vitamin A deficiency. The cornea softens and may become perforated. This condition is very serious and blindness is usually inevitable. See also XEROPHTHALMIA.

keratome n. any instrument designed for cutting the cornea. The simplest type has a flat triangular blade attached at its base to a handle, the other two sides being very sharp and tapering to a point. Power-driven keratomes have oscillating or rotating blades. An automated keratome is used in *automated lamellar keratectomy.

keratometer (ophthalmometer) n. an instrument for measuring the radius of curvature of the cornea. It is used for assessing the degree of abnormal curvature of the cornea in *astigmatism. Usually the vertical and horizontal curvatures are measured. All keratometers work on the principle that the size of the image of an object reflected from a convex mirror (in this case, the cornea) depends on the curvature of the mirror. The steeper the curve, the smaller the image. —**keratometry** n.

keratomileusis n. see INTRASTROMAL KERATOMILEUSIS, LASIK (LASER IN SITU KERATOMILEUSIS).

keratopathy n. any disorder relating to the cornea. See BAND KERATOPATHY, BULLOUS KERATOPATHY.

keratoplasty (corneal graft) n. an eye operation in which any diseased parts of the cornea are replaced by clear corneal tissue from a donor. All layers of the cornea may need to be replaced (**penetrating keratoplasty**) or only the superficial layers, the deeper layer remaining (**lamellar keratoplasty**). In the latter case the thickness of the replacement cornea is correspondingly reduced. Lamellar keratoplasty has the advantage over penetrating keratoplasty of not requiring the eye to be opened, and therefore the risk of infection is greatly reduced.

keratoprosthesis *n.* an optically clear prosthesis that is implanted into the cornea to replace an area that has become opaque. Due to its poor success rate, it is used only as a last resort in an attempt to restore some sight to patients with severe disease and dry eyes when corneal transplantation (*see* KERATOPLASTY) is certain to fail.

keratoscope (Placido's disc) *n.* an instrument for detecting abnormal curvature of the cornea. It consists of a black disc, about 20 cm in diameter, marked with concentric white rings. The examiner looks through a small lens in the centre at the reflection of the rings in the patient's cornea. A normal cornea will reflect regular concentric images of the rings; a cornea that is abnormally curved (for example in *keratoconus) or scarred reflects distorted rings. Modern keratoscopes can print out a contour map of the corneal surface.

keratosis *n.* a horny overgrowth of the skin. **Actinic** (or **solar**) **keratoses** are red spots with a scaly surface, found in older fair-skinned people who have been chronically overexposed to the sun. They may occasionally become malignant. **Seborrhoeic keratoses** (or **basal-cell papillomas**), less correctly known as **seborrhoeic warts**, never become malignant. They are superficial yellowish spots, occurring especially on the trunk in middle age, that slowly darken and become warty over the years.

keratotomy *n.* an incision into the cornea. *See* ACUATE KERATOTOMY, RADIAL KERATOTOMY.

keratouveitis *n.* inflammation involving both the cornea (*see* KERATITIS) and the uvea (*see* UVEITIS).

kerion *n.* an uncommon and severe form of *ringworm of the scalp consisting of a painful inflamed mass. It is caused by a type of ringworm fungus that usually infects animal species.

kernicterus *n.* staining and subsequent damage of the brain by bile pigment (bilirubin), which may occur in severe cases of *haemolytic disease of the new-

born. Immature brain cells in the *basal ganglia are affected, and as brain development proceeds a pattern of *cerebral palsy emerges at about six months, with uncoordinated movements, deafness, disturbed vision, and feeding and speech difficulties.

Kernig's sign a symptom of *meningitis in which the hamstring muscles in the legs are so stiff that the patient is unable to extend his legs at the knee when the thighs are held at a right angle to the body. [V. Kernig (1840–1917), Russian physician]

Kernohan's phenomenon (or **syndrome**) *hemiplegia that is *ipsilateral to the brain lesion that caused it, due to pressure of the lesion (which is often a haematoma) on surrounding structures in the brain. [J. W. K. Kernohan (20th century), US pathologist]

ketamine *n.* a drug used to produce anaesthesia, mainly in children. It is administered by injection. Trade name: **Ketalar**.

ketoacidosis *n.* a condition in which *acidosis is accompanied by *ketosis, such as occurs in diabetes mellitus. Symptoms include nausea and vomiting, abdominal tenderness, confusion or coma, extreme thirst, and weight loss. It is a life-threatening situation.

ketoconazole *n.* an antifungal drug (*see* IMIDAZOLE) used in the treatment of such fungal diseases as *candidosis, *histoplasmosis, and *blastomycosis. It is taken by mouth; side-effects include dizziness, drowsiness, nausea, and vomiting. Trade name: **Nizoral**.

ketogenesis *n.* the production of *ketone bodies. These are normal products of lipid metabolism and can be used to provide energy. The condition of *ketosis can occur when excess ketone bodies are produced.

ketogenic diet a diet that promotes the formation of *ketone bodies in the tissues. A ketogenic diet is one in which the principal energy source is fat rather than carbohydrate.

ketonaemia *n.* the presence in the blood of *ketone bodies.

ketone *n.* any member of a group of organic compounds consisting of a carbonyl group (=CO) flanked by two alkyl groups. The ketones acetoacetic acid, acetone, and β-hydroxybutyrate (known as **ketone** (or **acetone**) **bodies**) are produced during the metabolism of fats. *See also* KETOSIS.

ketonuria (acetonuria) *n.* the presence in the urine of *ketone (acetone) bodies. This may occur in diabetes mellitus, starvation, or after persistent vomiting and results from the partial oxidation of fats. Ketone bodies may be detected by adding a few drops of 5% sodium nitroprusside solution and a solution of ammonia to the urine; the gradual development of a purplish-red colour indicates their presence.

ketoprofen *n.* an anti-inflammatory drug (*see* NSAID), administered by mouth to treat various arthritic and rheumatic diseases. Side-effects are rare, but indigestion sometimes occurs. Trade names: **Orudis, Oruvail**.

ketose *n.* a simple sugar that terminates with a keto group (–C=O); for example, *fructose.

ketosis *n.* raised levels of *ketone bodies in the body tissues. Ketone bodies are normal products of fat metabolism and can be oxidized to produce energy. Elevated levels arise when there is an imbalance in fat metabolism, such as occurs in diabetes mellitus or starvation. Ketosis may result in severe *acidosis. *See also* KETONURIA.

keyhole surgery *see* MINIMALLY INVASIVE SURGERY.

khat (qat, kat) *n.* the leaves of the shrub *Catha edulis*, which contain a stimulant. In the Yemen these leaves are wrapped around betel nuts and chewed: this habit is associated with the development of oral *leucoplakia.

kidney *n.* either of the pair of organs responsible for the excretion of nitrogenous wastes, principally urea, from the blood (see illustration). The kidneys are situated at the back of the abdomen, below the diaphragm, one on each side of the spine; they are supplied with blood by the renal arteries. Each kidney is enclosed in a fibrous capsule and is composed of an outer **cortex** and an inner **medulla**. The active units of the kidney are the *nephrons, within the cortex and medulla, which filter the blood under pressure and then reabsorb water and selected substances back into the blood. The *urine thus formed is conducted from the nephrons via the renal tubules into the **renal pelvis** and from here to the ureter, which leads to the bladder. *See also* HAEMODIALYSIS, HORSESHOE KIDNEY, RENAL FUNCTION TESTS.

Kienböck's disease necrosis of the *lunate bone of the wrist caused by interruption of its blood supply (*see* OSTEOCHONDRITIS). It usually follows chronic stress to the bone or injury (often trivial) and presents with pain and stiffness of the wrist. Treatment is rest, but some cases require surgical shortening of the ulna or *fusion of the wrist. [R. Kienböck (1871–1953), Austrian radiologist]

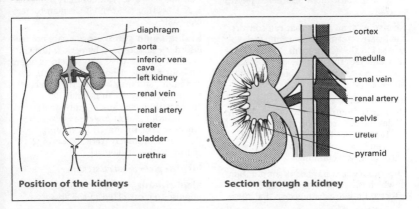

diaphragm
aorta
inferior vena cava
left kidney
renal vein
renal artery
ureter
bladder
urethra

cortex
medulla
renal vein
renal artery
pelvis
ureter
pyramid

Position of the kidneys   **Section through a kidney**

killer cell (cytotoxic T-cell) a type of T-*lymphocyte that destroys cancerous or virus-infected cells. In order to act, they require the presence on the surface of the target cell of foreign antigen that has been 'presented' by macrophages (*see* APC) and recognized by *helper T-cells. *Compare* NATURAL KILLER CELL.

kilo- *prefix denoting* a thousand.

kilocalorie *n.* one thousand calories. *See* CALORIE.

kilogram *n.* the *SI unit of mass equal to 1000 grams and defined in terms of the international prototype (a cylinder of platinum-iridium alloy) kept at Sèvres, near Paris. Symbol: kg.

kin- (kine-) *prefix denoting* movement.

kinaesthesia *n.* the sense that enables the brain to be constantly aware of the position and movement of muscles in different parts of the body. This is achieved by means of *proprioceptors, which send impulses from muscles, joints, and tendons. Without this sense, coordinated movement would be impossible with the eyes closed.

kinaesthesiometer *n.* an instrument for measuring a patient's awareness of the muscular and joint movements of his own body: used during the investigation of nervous and muscular disorders and certain forms of brain damage.

kinanaesthesia *n.* inability to sense the positions and movements of parts of the body, with consequent disordered physical activity.

kinase *n.* **1.** an agent that can convert the inactive form of an enzyme (*see* PROENZYME) to the active form. **2.** an enzyme that catalyses the transfer of phosphate groups. An example is *phosphofructokinase.

kinematics *n.* the study of motion and the forces required to produce it. This includes the different forces at work during the movement of a single part of the body, and more complex movements such as running and climbing.

kineplasty *n.* a method of amputation in which the muscles and tendons of the affected limb are arranged so that they can be integrated with a specially made artificial replacement. This enables direct movement of the artificial hand or limb by the muscles.

-kinesis *suffix denoting* movement.

kinetochore *n.* *see* CENTROMERE.

kinin *n.* one of a group of naturally occurring polypeptides that are powerful *vasodilators, which lower blood pressure, and cause contraction of smooth muscle. The kinins **bradykinin** and **kallidin** are formed in the blood by the action of proteolytic enzymes (**kallikreins**) on certain plasma globulins (**kininogens**). Kinins are not normally present in the blood, but are formed under certain conditions; for example when tissue is damaged or when there are changes in the pH and temperature of the blood. They are thought to play a role in inflammatory response.

kiss of life *see* MOUTH-TO-MOUTH RESPIRATION.

Klebsiella *n.* a genus of Gram-negative rodlike nonmotile bacteria, mostly lactose-fermenting, found in the respiratory, intestinal, and urinogenital tracts of animals and man. The species *K. oxytoca* is associated with human urinary infections; *K. pneumoniae* is associated with pneumonia and other respiratory infections. The species *K. rhinoscleromatis* causes *rhinoscleroma, a chronic infection of the nose and pharynx.

Klebs-Loeffler bacillus *see* CORYNEBACTERIUM. [T. Klebs (1834–1913) and F. A. J. Loeffler (1852–1915), German bacteriologists]

Kleine-Levin syndrome a rare episodic disorder characterized by periods (usually of a few days or weeks) in which sufferers eat enormously, sleep for most of the day and night, and may become more dependent or aggressive than normal. Between episodes they are usually quite unaffected. The disorder almost always resolves spontaneously. [W. Kleine (20th century), German neuropsychiatrist; M. Levin (20th century), US neurologist]

klepto- *prefix denoting* stealing.

kleptomania *n.* a pathologically strong impulse to steal, often in the absence of any desire for the stolen object(s). It is sometimes associated with *depression.

Klinefelter's syndrome a genetic disorder in which there are three sex chromosomes, XXY, rather than the normal XX or XY. Affected individuals are apparently male, but are tall and thin, with small testes, failure of normal sperm production (azoospermia), enlargement of the breasts (gynaecomastia), and absence of facial and body hair. [H. F. Klinefelter (1912–   ), US physician]

Klumpke's paralysis a partial paralysis of the arm caused by injury to a baby's *brachial plexus during birth. This may result from an obstetric manoeuvre in which the arm is raised at the shoulder to an extreme degree, which damages the lower cervical (neck) and upper thoracic (chest) nerve roots of the spinal cord. It results in weakness and wasting of the muscles of the hand. [A. Klumpke (1859–1927), French neurologist]

kneading n. see PETRISSAGE.

knee n. the hinge joint (see GINGLYMUS) between the end of the femur, the top of the tibia, and the back of the *patella (kneecap). It is commonly involved in *sports injuries (such as a torn meniscus or ligament) and is a common site of osteoarthritis and rheumatoid arthritis; it can be replaced by an artificial joint.

knee-elbow position the buttocks-up position commonly assumed by patients undergoing anorectal examinations.

knight's-move thought a form of thought disorder, characteristic of *schizophrenia, in which the *associations of ideas are bizarre and tortuous.

knock-knee n. abnormal in-curving of the legs, resulting in a gap between the feet when the knees are in contact. In severe cases there is stress on the knee, ankle, and foot joints, resulting eventually in degenerative arthritis. The condition may be corrected by *osteotomy. Medical name: **genu valgum**.

Kocher manoeuvre a method for *reduction of a dislocated shoulder by manipulation. [E. T. Kocher (1841–1917), Swiss surgeon]

Koch's bacillus see MYCOBACTERIUM. [R. Koch (1843–1910), German bacteriologist]

Koebner phenomenon (isomorphic response) a phenomenon that occurs in skin diseases, especially psoriasis and lichen planus, in which the characteristic lesions of the disease appear in linear form in response to such trauma as cuts, burns, or scratches. [H. Koebner (1834–1904), German dermatologist]

Köhler's disease necrosis of the *navicular bone of the foot (see OSTEOCHONDRITIS). It occurs in children, causing pain and limping, and is treated by strapping the foot and rest. [A. Köhler (1874–1947), German physician]

koilonychia n. the development of thin (brittle) concave (spoon-shaped) nails, a common disorder that can occur with anaemia due to iron deficiency, though the cause is not known. Any underlying disease should be treated.

Koplik's spots small red spots with bluish-white centres that often appear on the mucous membranes of the mouth in *measles. [H. Koplik (1858–1927), US physician]

koro n. a state of acute anxiety, seen especially in certain cultures (such as that of the Chinese of SE Asia), characterized by a sudden belief that the penis is shrinking into the abdomen and will disappear: the sufferer is convinced that disappearance of the penis means death. Occasionally women have a similar belief that their breasts are disappearing into their body. It is usually treated with tranquillizing drugs and reassurance.

Korsakoff's syndrome (Korsakoff's psychosis) an organic disorder affecting the brain that results in a memory defect in which new information fails to be learnt although events from the past are still recalled; *disorientation for time and place; and a tendency to invent material to fill memory blanks (see CONFABULATION). The commonest cause of the condition is alcoholism, especially when this has led to deficiency of thiamin (vitamin B_1). Large doses of thiamin are given as treatment. The condition often becomes chronic. [S. S. Korsakoff (1854–1900), Russian neurologist]

KPTT kaolin partial thromboplastin time:

a method for estimating the degree of anticoagulation induced by heparin therapy for venous thrombosis.

K-ras n. a gene that mutates to form an important *oncogene for the causation of human lung and colon cancer.

kraurosis n. shrinking of a body part, usually the vulva in elderly women (**kraurosis vulvae**).

Krebs cycle (citric acid cycle) a complex cycle of enzyme-catalysed reactions, occurring within the cells of all living animals, in which acetate, in the presence of oxygen, is broken down to produce energy in the form of *ATP (via the *electron transport chain) and carbon dioxide. The cycle is the final step in the oxidation of carbohydrates, fats, and proteins; some of the intermediary products of the cycle are used in the synthesis of amino acids. [Sir H. A. Krebbs (1900–81), British biochemist]

Krukenberg tumour a rapidly developing malignant growth in one or (more often) both ovaries. The tumour is secondary to a primary growth in the stomach or intestine. [F. E. Krukenberg (1871–1946), German pathologist]

krypton-81m n. a radioactive gas that is the shortest-lived isotope in medical use (half-life 13 seconds). It can be used to investigate the function of the lungs. The patient breathes a small quantity of the gas, the arrival of which in different parts of the lungs is recorded by means of a *gamma camera. *See also* RUBIDIUM-81.

Küntscher nail a metal rod that is inserted down the middle of the femur (thigh bone) to stabilize a transverse fracture of the shaft. [G. Küntscher (1902–72), German orthopaedic surgeon]

Kupffer cells phagocytic cells that line the sinusoids of the *liver (*see* MACROPHAGE). They are particularly concerned with the formation of *bile and are often seen to contain fragments of red blood cells and pigment granules that are derived from the breakdown of haemoglobin. [K. W. von Kupffer (1829–1902), German anatomist]

kuru (trembling disease) n. a disease that affects only members of the Fore tribe of New Guinea. It involves a progressive degeneration of the nerve cells of the central nervous system, particularly in the region of the brain that controls movement. Muscular control becomes defective and shiver-like tremors occur in the trunk, limbs, and head. Kuru affects mainly women and children and usually proves fatal within 9–12 months. It is thought to be caused by a *prion and transmitted by cannibalism. *See also* SPONGIFORM ENCEPHALOPATHY.

Kussmaul breathing the slow deep respiration associated with acidosis. [A. Kussmaul (1822–1902), German physician]

Kveim test a test used for the diagnosis of *sarcoidosis. Tissue from a lymph node of a person suffering from the disease is injected intradermally; the development of a granuloma at the injection site indicates that the subject has sarcoidosis. [M. A. Kveim (20th century), Norwegian physician]

kwashiorkor n. a form of malnutrition due to a diet deficient in protein and energy-producing foods, common among certain African tribes. Kwashiorkor develops when, after prolonged breast feeding, the child is weaned onto an inadequate traditional family diet. The diet is such that it is physically impossible for the child to consume the required quantity in order to obtain sufficient protein and energy. Kwashiorkor is most common in children between the ages of one and three years. The symptoms are *oedema, loss of appetite, diarrhoea, general discomfort, and apathy; the child fails to thrive and there is usually associated gastrointestinal infection.

Kyasanur Forest disease a tropical disease, common in southern India, caused by a virus transmitted to man through the bite of the forest-dwelling tick *Haemaphysalis spinigera.* Symptoms include fever, headache, muscular pains, vomiting, conjunctivitis, exhaustion, bleeding of nose and gums and, subsequently, internal bleeding and the *necrosis of various tissues. General therapy, in the absence of specific treatment, involves relief of dehydration and loss of blood; analgesics are given to alleviate pain.

kymograph n. an instrument for recording the flow and varying pressure

of the blood within the blood vessels.
—**kymography** n.

kypho- prefix denoting a hump.

kyphos n. a sharply localized forward angulation of the spine, resulting in the appearance of a lump (the deformity of the traditional hunchback). The deformity is due to collapse of the anterior part of a vertebra, usually caused by osteoporosis, a secondary malignant deposit, or tuberculosis.

kyphoscoliosis n. abnormal curvature of the spine both forwards and sideways: *kyphosis combined with *scoliosis. The deformity may occur during growth for no apparent reason (**idiopathic kyphoscoliosis**) or may result from any of several diseases involving the vertebrae and spinal muscles. Special braces can reduce the ex-

tent of the deformity if this is mild. Severe deformity requires surgical correction by *fusion of the spine.

kyphosis n. excessive outward curvature of the spine, causing hunching of the back. A **mobile kyphosis** may be caused by bad posture or muscle weakness or may develop to compensate for another condition, such as hip deformity. A **fixed kyphosis** may result from collapse of the vertebrae (as in senile *osteoporosis), from *osteochondritis in the young, or from ankylosing *spondylitis. Lesser degrees of fixed kyphosis may be balanced by *lordosis (inward curvature) in another part of the spine. Treatment depends on the cause, and may include physiotherapy, bracing, and spinal *osteotomy in severe cases. See also KYPHOS, KYPHOSCOLIOSIS.

labelling index the proportion of cells in a sample of tissue that are producing DNA. Cells that are synthesizing DNA take up tritiated thymidine, which shows up on an autoradiograph (*see* AUTORADIOGRAPHY) of the sample.

labetalol *n.* a combined alpha- and beta-blocking drug (*see* SYMPATHOLYTIC), sometimes found to be more effective in the treatment of high blood pressure than beta blockers. It is administered by mouth or intravenous infusion. Possible side-effects include faintness on standing up, scalp tingling, and difficulty with urination and ejaculation. Trade names: **Labrocol**, **Trandate**.

labial *adj.* **1.** relating to the lips or to a labium. **2.** designating the surface of a tooth adjacent to the lips.

labio- *prefix denoting* the lip(s).

labiomancy *n.* lip-reading.

labioplasty (cheiloplasty) *n.* surgical repair of injury or deformity of the lips (*cleft lip).

labium *n.* (*pl.* **labia**) a lip-shaped structure, especially either of the two pairs of skin folds that enclose the *vulva. The larger outer pair are known as the **labia majora** and the smaller inner pair the **labia minora**.

labour *n.* the sequence of actions by which a baby and the afterbirth (placenta) are expelled from the uterus at childbirth. The process usually starts spontaneously about 280 days after conception, but it may be started by artificial means (*see* INDUCTION). In the first stage the muscular wall of the uterus begins contracting while the muscle fibres of the cervix relax so that the cervix expands. A portion of the membranous sac (amnion) surrounding the baby is pushed into the opening and ruptures under the pressure, releasing *amniotic fluid to the exterior. In the second stage the baby's head appears at the cervix and the contractions of the uterus strengthen. The passage of the in-

fant through the vagina is assisted by contractions of the abdominal muscles and conscious pushing by the mother. When the top of the baby's head appears at the vaginal opening the whole infant is eased clear of the vagina, and the umbilical cord is cut. If the emergence of the head is impeded an incision may be made in the surrounding tissue (*see* EPISIOTOMY). In the final stage the placenta and membranes are pushed out by the continuing contraction of the uterus, which eventually returns to its unexpanded state. The average duration of labour is about 12 hours in first pregnancies and about 8 hours in subsequent pregnancies. The pain of labour may be reduced if the mother trains her abdominal muscles during the prenatal period and by the use of drugs (**accelerated labour**). *See also* CAESAREAN SECTION.

labrum *n.* (*pl.* **labra**) a lip or liplike structure; occurring, for example, around the margins of the articulating socket (acetabulum) of the hip bone.

Membranous labyrinth of the right ear

labyrinth (inner ear) *n.* a convoluted system of cavities and ducts comprising the organs of hearing and balance. The **membranous labyrinth** is a series of interconnected membranous canals and chambers consisting of the *semicircular canals, *utricle, and *saccule (concerned with balance) and the central cavity of the *cochlea (concerned with hearing). (See illustration.) It is filled with a fluid, **endolymph**. The **bony labyrinth** is the system of the bony canals and chambers that surround the membranous labyrinth. It is embedded in the petrous part of the *temporal bone and is filled with fluid (**perilymph**).

labyrinthectomy *n.* a surgical procedure to ablate (see ABLATION) the structures of the *labyrinth, usually performed for cases of severe Ménière's disease.

labyrinthitis (otitis interna) *n.* inflammation of the inner ear (labyrinth). See OTITIS.

laceration *n.* a tear in the flesh producing a wound with irregular edges.

lacertus *n.* a band of fibres or a tendon-like structure.

lacrimal apparatus the structures that produce and drain away fluid from the eye (see illustration). The **lacrimal gland** secretes *tears, which drain away through small openings (**puncta**) at the inner corner of the eye into two **lacrimal canaliculi**. From there the tears pass into the nasal cavity via the **lacrimal sac** and the *nasolacrimal duct.

lacrimal gland
lacrimal canaliculus
lacrimal sac
nasal cavity
excretory ducts of lacrimal glands
punctum
nasolacrimal duct

The lacrimal apparatus

lacrimal bone the smallest bone of the face: either of a pair of rectangular bones that contribute to the orbits. See SKULL.

lacrimal nerve a branch of the *ophthalmic nerve that supplies the lacrimal gland (see LACRIMAL APPARATUS) and conjunctiva.

lacrimation *n.* the production of excess tears; crying. See also LACRIMAL APPARATUS.

lacrimator *n.* an agent that irritates the eyes, causing excessive secretion of tears.

lact- (lacti-, lacto-) *prefix denoting* **1.** milk. **2.** lactic acid.

lactalbumin *n.* a milk protein present in milk at a lower concentration than *casein. Unlike casein, it is not precipitated from milk under acid conditions; it is therefore a constituent of cheese made from whey rather than curd.

lactase *n.* an enzyme, secreted by the glands of the small intestine, that converts lactose (milk sugar) into glucose and galactose during digestion.

lactation *n.* the secretion of milk by the *mammary glands of the breasts, which usually begins at the end of pregnancy. A fluid called *colostrum is secreted before the milk is produced; both secretions are released in response to the sucking action of the infant on the nipple. Lactation is controlled by hormones (see PROLACTIN, OXYTOCIN); it stops when the baby is no longer fed at the breast.

lacteal *n.* a blind-ended lymphatic vessel that extends into a villus of the small *intestine. Digested fats are absorbed into the lacteals.

lactic acid a compound that forms in the cells as the end-product of glucose metabolism in the absence of oxygen (see GLYCOLYSIS). During strenuous exercise pyruvic acid is reduced to lactic acid, which may accumulate in the muscles and cause cramp. Lactic acid (owing to its low pH) is an important food preservative. The lactic acid produced by the fermentation of milk is responsible for the preservation and flavour of cheese, yoghurt, and other fermented milk products.

lactiferous *adj.* transporting or secreting milk, as the **lactiferous ducts** of the breast.

lactifuge *n.* a drug that reduces the secretion of milk. Some oestrogenic drugs have this effect and are used to suppress milk production in mothers not breast-feeding.

Lactobacillus *n.* a genus of Gram-positive nonmotile rodlike bacteria capable of growth in acid media and of producing lactic acid from the fermentation of carbohydrates. They are found in fermenting animal and plant products, especially dairy products, and in the alimentary tract and vagina. They are responsible for the souring of milk. The species *L. acidophilus* is found in milk and is associated with dental caries. It occurs in very high numbers in the faeces of breast- or bottle-fed infants.

lactogenic hormone *see* PROLACTIN.

lactose *n.* a sugar, consisting of one molecule of glucose and one of galactose, found only in milk. Lactose is split into its constituent sugars by the enzyme *lactase, which is secreted in the small intestine. This enzyme is missing or is of low activity in certain people of some Eastern and African races. This leads to the inability to absorb lactose, known as **lactose intolerance**.

lactosuria *n.* the presence of milk sugar (*lactose) in the urine. This often occurs during pregnancy and breastfeeding or if the milk flow is suppressed.

lactulose *n.* a disaccharide sugar that acts as a gentle but effective *laxative. It is administered by mouth but is not absorbed or broken down, remaining intact until it reaches the colon. There it is split by bacteria into simpler sugars that help to retain water, thereby softening the stools. Trade names: **Duphalac, Lactulose**.

lacuna *n.* (*pl.* **lacunae**) (in anatomy) a small cavity or depression; for example, one of the spaces in compact bone in which a bone cell lies.

laetrile *n.* a cyanide-containing compound extracted from peach stones. It has been used in *alternative medicine in the treatment of various forms of cancer.

laevo- *prefix. see* LEVO-.

laevocardia *n.* the normal position of the heart, in which its apex is directed towards the left. *Compare* DEXTROCARDIA.

lagaena (lagena) *n.* the closed end of the spiral *cochlea. This term is more commonly used to describe the structure homologous to the cochlea in primitive vertebrates.

lagophthalmos *n.* any condition in which the eye does not close completely. It may lead to corneal damage from undue exposure.

laking *n.* the physical or chemical treatment of blood to abolish the structure of the red cells and thus form a homogeneous solution. Laking is an important preliminary step in the analysis of haemoglobin or enzymes present in red cells.

-lalia *suffix denoting* a condition involving speech.

lallation (lalling) *n.* **1.** unintelligible speech-like babbling, as heard from infants. **2.** the immature substitution of one consonant for another (e.g. 'l' for 'r').

lambda *n.* the point on the skull at which the lambdoidal and sagittal *sutures meet.

lambdoidal suture *see* SUTURE.

lambliasis *n.* *see* GIARDIASIS.

lamella *n.* (*pl.* **lamellae**) **1.** a thin layer, membrane, scale, or plate-like tissue or part. In *bone tissue, lamellae are thin bands of calcified matrix arranged concentrically around a Haversian canal. **2.** a thin gelatinous medicated disc used to apply drugs to the eye. The disc is placed on the eyeball; the gelatinous material dissolves and the drug is absorbed.

lamina *n.* (*pl.* **laminae**) a thin membrane or layer of tissue.

laminectomy (rachiotomy) *n.* surgical cutting into the backbone to obtain access to the spinal cord. The surgeon excises the rear part (the posterior arch) of one or more vertebrae. The operation is performed to remove tumours, to treat injuries to the spine, such as prolapsed intervertebral (slipped) disc (in which the affected disc is removed), or to relieve pressure on the spinal cord or roots.

lamotrigine *n.* an anticonvulsant drug used in the control of epilepsy. It is administered by mouth. Possible side-effects include nausea, headache, double vision, dizziness, *ataxia, and skin rashes. Trade name: **Lamictal**.

lanatoside *n.* a drug similar to *digitalis, used in the treatment of heart failure. It is administered by mouth or injection. High doses may cause loss of appetite, nausea, vomiting, headache, disturbed vision, and abnormal heart activity. Trade name: **Cedilanid**.

Lancefield classification a classification of the *Streptococcus* bacteria based on the presence or absence of antigenic carbohydrate on the cell surface. Species are classified into the groups A–S. Most species causing disease in man belong to groups A, B, and D. [R. C. Lancefield (1895–1981), US bacteriologist]

lancet *n.* a broad two-edged surgical knife with a sharp point.

lancinating *adj.* describing a sharp stabbing or cutting pain.

Landry's paralysis a rapidly progressive form of the *Guillain-Barré syndrome. [J. B. O. Landry (1826–65), French physician]

Lange curve an obsolescent method of detecting excess globulins in the protein of the cerebrospinal fluid. It was useful in the diagnosis of neurosyphilis and multiple sclerosis but has been superseded by more specific tests. [Described in 1912 by F. A. Lange, German physician]

Langer's lines normal permanent skin creases. Incisions parallel to Langer's lines heal well and are less visible. [C. R. von E. Langer (1819–87), Austrian anatomist]

lansoprazole *n. see* PROTON-PUMP INHIBITOR.

lanugo *n.* fine hair covering the body and limbs of the human fetus. It is most profuse at about the 28th week of gestation and is shed around 40 weeks.

laparo- *prefix denoting* the loins or abdomen.

laparoscope (peritoneoscope) *n.* a surgical instrument (a type of *endoscope) comprising an illuminated viewing tube that is inserted through the abdominal wall to enable the surgeon to view the abdominal organs (*see* LAPAROSCOPY). It can be used as a means to allow surgical procedures to be carried out with special instruments without using a surgical incision.

laparoscopy (peritoneoscopy) *n.* examination of the abdominal structures (which are contained within the peritoneum) by means of an illuminated tubular instrument (*laparoscope). This is passed through a small incision in the wall of the abdomen after injecting carbon dioxide into the abdominal cavity (pneumoperitoneum). In addition to being a diagnostic aid, it is used when taking a biopsy, aspirating cysts, and dividing adhesions. Surgery, including *cholecystectomy, *fundoplication, *colectomy, *hemicolectomy, and the occlusion of Fallopian tubes for sterilization, can also be performed through a laparoscope, using either a laser or diathermy to control bleeding (*see also* MINIMALLY INVASIVE SURGERY). The laparoscope is also used for collecting ova for *in vitro fertilization and in performing certain gynaecological operations using a laser (**laser laparoscopy**). —**laparoscopic** *adj.*

laparotomy *n.* a surgical incision into the abdominal cavity. The operation is done to examine the abdominal organs as a help to diagnosis; for example, to establish the spread of a growth (**exploratory laparotomy**) or as a prelude to major surgery.

lardaceous *adj.* resembling lard: often applied to tissue infiltrated with the starchlike substance amyloid (*see* AMYLOIDOSIS).

Lariam *n. see* MEFLOQUINE.

larva *n.* (*pl.* **larvae**) the preadult or immature stage hatching from the egg of some animal groups, e.g. insects and nematodes, which may be markedly different from the sexually mature adult and have a totally different way of life. For example, the larvae of some flies are parasites of animals and cause disease whereas the adults are free-living. —**larval** *adj.*

larva migrans *see* CREEPING ERUPTION.

laryng- (laryngo-) *prefix denoting* the larynx.

laryngeal reflex a cough produced by irritating the larynx.

laryngeal stroboscopy a method of studying the movements of the *vocal folds of the *larynx by using stroboscopic light (controlled intermittent flashes) to slow or freeze the movement.

laryngectomy n. surgical removal of the whole or a part of the larynx, as in the treatment of laryngeal carcinoma. Speech can be restored in many patients using special techniques and appliances.

laryngismus n. closure of the vocal folds by sudden contraction of the laryngeal muscles, followed by a noisy indrawing of breath. It occurs in young children and was in the past associated with low-calcium rickets. Now it occurs when the larynx has been irritated following administration of anaesthetic, when a foreign body has lodged in the larynx, or in *croup.

laryngitis n. inflammation of the larynx and vocal folds, due to infection by bacteria or viruses or irritation by gases, chemicals, etc. The folds lose their vibrance (owing to swelling) and the voice becomes husky or is lost completely; breathing is harsh and difficult (see STRIDOR); and the cough is painful and honking. Obstruction of the airways may occasionally be serious, especially in children (see CROUP). The patient should rest his voice and remain in a warm moisture-laden atmosphere; steam inhalations for 15–20 minutes every 2–3 hours are traditionally beneficial. The patient should avoid cold air or fog and smoking.

laryngocele n. a condition in which an air sac communicates with the larynx. The sac forms a swelling in the neck that dilates on coughing or straining. The condition is probably congenital but is also noted in such people as glassblowers, who have chronically raised intralaryngeal pressure.

laryngofissure n. a surgical operation to open the larynx, enabling access for further procedures.

laryngology n. the study of diseases of the larynx and vocal folds.

laryngomalacia n. a condition characterized by paroxysmal attacks of breathing difficulty and *stridor. It occurs in small children and is caused by flaccidity

of the structure of the larynx. It usually resolves spontaneously by the age of two years.

laryngopharynx (hypopharynx) n. the part of the pharynx that lies below the hyoid bone.

laryngoscope n. an instrument (a type of *endoscope) for examining the larynx. See LARYNGOSCOPY.

laryngoscopy n. examination of the larynx. This may be done indirectly using a small mirror or directly using a laryngoscope.

laryngospasm n. involuntary closure of the larynx, obstructing the flow of air to the lungs.

laryngotomy n. surgical incision of the larynx. **Inferior laryngotomy**, in which an incision is made in the cricothyroid membrane beneath the larynx, is a life-saving operation for patients in whom there is obstruction to breathing at or above the larynx. See TRACHEOSTOMY.

laryngotracheobronchitis n. a severe and almost exclusively viral infection of the respiratory tract, especially of young children, in whom there may be a dangerous degree of obstruction either at the larynx (see CROUP) or main air passages (bronchi) due to the thickness and stickiness of the fluid (exudate) produced by the inflamed tissues. Symptoms normally start at night. Treatment is supportive until the condition resolves naturally. In mild and moderate cases the child may benefit from being kept in a humid atmosphere (e.g. a steamy room). Nebulized medications and oxygen can help in more severe cases. In extreme cases endotracheal *intubation may be necessary. The condition may recur.

larynx n. the organ responsible for the production of vocal sounds, also serving as an air passage conveying air from the pharynx to the lungs. It is situated in the front of the neck, above the trachea. It is made up of a framework of nine cartilages (see illustration) – the epiglottis, thyroid, cricoid, arytenoid (two), corniculate (two), and cuneiform (two) – bound together by ligaments and muscles and lined with mucous membrane. Within are a pair of *vocal cords, which function in the production of voice. —**laryngeal** *adj.*

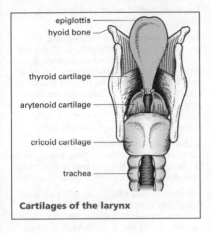

epiglottis
hyoid bone
thyroid cartilage
arytenoid cartilage
cricoid cartilage
trachea

Cartilages of the larynx

laser *n.* a device that produces a very thin beam of light in which high energies are concentrated (the word derives from light amplification by stimulated emission of radiation). In surgery, lasers can be used to operate on small areas of abnormality without damaging delicate surrounding tissue. For example, lasers are used to unblock coronary arteries narrowed by atheroma and to remove certain types of birthmark (see NAEVUS). Different types of laser are used in eye surgery for operations on the cornea, lens capsule, and retina (see ARGON LASER, DIODE LASER, EXCIMER LASER, YAG LASER). Lasers are also used in the treatment of *cervical intraepithelial neoplasia and in a specialized form (the **Nd:YAG laser**) for *endometrial ablation.

laser Doppler flowmeter an instrument for measuring blood flow through tissue (e.g. skin) utilizing a laser beam.

laser laparoscopy *see* LAPAROSCOPY.

laser palatoplasty *see* PALATOPLASTY.

LASIK laser in situ keratomileusis: a type of eye surgery that is especially useful for correcting severe degrees of *myopia (short-sightedness). A thin flap of cornea is raised, the bed (*stroma) is reshaped using an *excimer laser, and the flap is then re-

placed. *Compare* INTRASTROMAL KERATOMILEUSIS.

Lasix *n. see* FRUSEMIDE.

Lassa fever a serious virus disease confined to Central West Africa. After an incubation period of 3–21 days, headache, high fever, and severe muscular pains develop; difficulty in swallowing often arises. Death from kidney or heart failure occurs in over 50% of cases. Treatment with plasma from recovered patients is the best therapy, and the causative virus is susceptible to ribavirin.

latah *n.* a pattern of behaviour seen especially in certain cultures, such as that of Malaysia. After a psychological shock the affected individual becomes very anxious and very suggestible and shows excessive obedience and pathological imitation of the actions of another person (echopraxia).

latamoxef *n.* a type of *cephalosporin antibiotic active against many Gram negative bacilli (see GRAM'S STAIN). Trade name: **Moxalactam**.

latanoprost *n.* a *prostaglandin drug (an analogue of PGF$_2$) that both increases the drainage of aqueous humour from the eye and reduces the production of aqueous humour. It is used topically as a treatment for glaucoma. Trade name: **Xalatan**.

latent period (in neurology) the pause of a few milliseconds between the time that a nerve impulse reaches a muscle fibre and the time that the fibre starts to contract.

lateral *adj.* **1.** situated at or relating to the side of an organ or organism. **2.** (in anatomy) relating to the region or parts of the body that are furthest from the *median plane. **3.** (in radiology) in the *sagittal plane.

lathyrism *n.* a disease, characterized by muscular weakness and paralysis, found among people whose staple diet consists mostly of large quantites of *Lathyrus sativus*, a kind of chick pea, and/or vetches and pulses related to it. Except in mild cases complete recovery does not occur, despite administration of an adequate diet and physiotherapy.

laudanum *n.* a hydroalcoholic solution containing 1% morphine, prepared from macerated raw opium. It was formerly widely used as a narcotic analgesic, taken by mouth.

laughing gas *see* NITROUS OXIDE.

lavage *n.* washing out a body cavity, such as the colon or stomach, with water or a medicated solution. In cases of bowel obstruction the washing out can be done during the operation (**on-table lavage**).

laxative *n.* a drug used to stimulate or increase the frequency of bowel evacuation (also called a **cathartic** or **purgative**), or to encourage the passage of a softer or bulkier stool. The common laxatives are the stimulants castor oil, bisacodyl, and senna and its derivatives; magnesium sulphate and other mineral salts; and methylcellulose, ispaghula husk, and other bulking agents.

LD₅₀ the dose of a toxic compound that causes death in 50% of a group of experimental animals to which it is administered: used as a measure of the toxicity of drugs.

LDL low-density lipoprotein. *See* LIPOPROTEIN.

L-dopa *n.* *see* LEVODOPA.

lead¹ *n.* a soft bluish-grey metallic element that forms several poisonous compounds. Acute lead poisoning, which may follow inhalation of lead fumes or dust, causes abdominal pains, vomiting, and diarrhoea, with paralysis and convulsions and sometimes *encephalitis. In chronic poisoning a characteristic bluish marking of the gums ('lead line') is seen and the peripheral nerves are affected; there is also anaemia. Treatment is with *edetate. The use of lead in paints is now strictly controlled. Symbol: Pb.

lead² *n.* a portion of an electrocardiographic record that is obtained from a single electrode or a combination of electrodes placed on a particular part of the body (*see* ELECTROCARDIOGRAM, ELECTROCARDIOGRAPHY). In the conventional ECG, 12 leads are recorded. Each lead represents the electrical activity of the heart as 'viewed' from a different position on the body surface and may help to localize myocardial damage.

learning disability (learning difficulty) *see* MENTAL HANDICAP.

leather-bottle stomach *see* LINITIS PLASTICA.

Leber's congenital amaurosis a hereditary disease (inherited as an autosomal *recessive inherited condition) causing severe visual loss in infants. The back of the eye appears to be normal when examined with an *ophthalmoscope, but marked abnormalities are found on the ERG (*see* ELECTRORETINOGRAPHY). [T. Leber (1840–1917), German ophthalmologist]

Leber's optic atrophy a rare hereditary disorder, affecting young males, that is characterized by rapid loss of central vision due to neuroretinal degeneration.

lecithin *n.* one of a group of *phospholipids that are important constituents of cell membranes and are involved in the metabolism of fat by the liver. An example is **phosphatidylcholine**. Lecithins are present in the *surfactant that occurs in fetal lung tissue. The **lecithin-sphingomyelin ratio (LS ratio)** is used as a measure of fetal lung maturity; an LS ratio below 2 indicates a higher risk of *respiratory distress syndrome (RDS). In such cases cortisone may be given to stimulate fetal lung maturity and hence reduce the risk of RDS in the newborn.

lecithinase *n.* an enzyme from the small intestine that breaks *lecithin down into glycerol, fatty acids, phosphoric acid, and choline.

leech *n.* a type of worm that possesses suckers at both ends of its body. Leeches occur in tropical forests and grasslands and in water. Certain parasitic species suck blood from animals and humans, and their bites cause irritation and, in some cases, infection. Rarely, leeches are taken in with foul drinking water and pass from the mouth to the nose, where they provoke headache and nose bleeds. A leech can be detached from its host by applying salt; calamine lotion eases the irritation of the bites. Formerly widely used for letting blood, the medicinal leech (*Hirudo medicinalis*) may now be used following microsurgery (e.g. to replace a severed finger) to restore patency to blocked or collapsed blood vessels and thus encourage the growth of new capillaries. The anticoagulants in the saliva of this and other species are being investigated for the treatment and prevention of thrombosis. *See also* HIRUDIN.

Le Fort classification a classification of fractures involving the *maxilla (upper jaw) and *orbit. Type I involves the maxilla only, type II the anterior orbit, and type III the posterior orbit. [R. Le Fort (19th century), French surgeon]

Legg-Calvé-Perthes disease (Perthes disease, pseudocoxalgia) necrosis of the head of the femur (thigh bone) due to interruption of its blood supply (*see* OSTEOCHONDRITIS). Of unknown cause, it occurs most commonly in boys between the ages of 5 and 10 and causes aching and a limp. The head of the femur can collapse and become deformed, resulting in a short leg and restricted hip movement. Affected boys are kept under observation and their activities are restricted; surgery may be required in more severe cases. [A. T. Legg (1874–1939), US surgeon; J. Calvé (1875–1954), French orthopaedist; G. C. Perthes (1869–1927), German surgeon]

legionnaires' disease an infection of the lungs caused by the bacterium *Legionella pneumophila*, named after an outbreak at the American Legion convention in Pennsylvania in 1976. *Legionella* organisms are widely found in water; outbreaks of the disease have been associated with defective central heating, air conditioning, and other ventilating systems. Symptoms appear after an incubation period of 2–10 days: malaise and muscle pain are succeeded by a fever, dry cough, chest pain, and breathlessness. X-ray of the lungs shows patchy consolidation. Erythromycin provides the most effective therapy.

leio- *prefix denoting* smoothness. Example: **leiodermia** (abnormal smoothness of the skin).

leiomyoma *n.* a benign tumour of smooth muscle. Such tumours occur most commonly in the uterus (*see* FIBROID) but can also arise in the digestive tract, walls of blood vessels, etc. They may undergo malignant change (*see* LEIOMYOSARCOMA).

leiomyosarcoma *n.* a malignant tumour of smooth muscle, most commonly found in the uterus, stomach, small bowel, and at the base of the bladder. It is the second most common *sarcoma of soft tissues. This tumour is rare in children, occurring most commonly in the bladder, prostate, and stomach.

Leishman-Donovan body *see* LEISHMANIA. [Sir W. B. Leishman (1865–1926), British surgeon; C. Donovan (1863–1951), Irish physician]

Leishmania *n.* a genus of parasitic flagellate protozoans, several species of which cause disease in man (*see* LEISHMANIASIS). The parasite assumes a different form in each of its two hosts. In man, especially in *kala-azar patients, it is a small rounded structure, with no flagellum, called a **Leishman-Donovan body**, which is found within the cells of the lymphatic system, spleen, and bone marrow. In the insect carrier it is long and flagellated.

leishmaniasis *n.* a disease, common in the tropics and subtropics, caused by parasitic protozoans of the genus *Leishmania*, which are transmitted by the bite of sandflies. There are two principal forms of the disease: **visceral leishmaniasis**, in which the cells of various internal organs are affected (*see* KALA-AZAR); and **cutaneous leishmaniasis**, which affects the tissues of the skin. Cutaneous leishmaniasis itself has several different forms, depending on the region in which it occurs and the species of *Leishmania* involved. In Asia it is common in the form of *oriental sore. In America there are several forms of leishmaniasis (*see* CHICLERO'S ULCER, ESPUNDIA). Cutaneous leishmaniasis is treated with drugs containing antimony.

lemniscus *n.* a ribbon-like tract of nerve tissue conveying information from the spinal cord and brainstem upwards through the midbrain to the higher centres. On each side a **medial lemniscus** acts as a pathway from the spinal cord, while an outer **lateral lemniscus** commences higher up and is mainly concerned with hearing.

lens *n.* **1.** (in anatomy) the transparent crystalline structure situated behind the pupil of the eye and enclosed in a thin transparent **capsule**. It helps to refract incoming light and focus it onto the *retina. *See also* ACCOMMODATION. **2.** (in optics) a piece of glass shaped to refract rays of light in a particular direction. **Convex lenses** converge the light, and **concave lenses** diverge it; they are worn to correct faulty eyesight. *See also* BIFOCAL LENSES, CONTACT LENSES, TRIFOCAL LENSES.

lens implant *see* CATARACT.

lenticonus *n.* a condition in which the central part of the front surface of the lens of the eye (or sometimes, the back) has a much steeper curvature than normal and bulges forwards in a blunted cone. It is usually congenital.

lenticular nucleus (lentiform nucleus) *see* BASAL GANGLIA.

lentigo *n.* (*pl.* **lentigines**) a flat dark brown spot found mainly in the elderly on skin exposed to light. Lentigines have increased numbers of *melanocytes in the basal layer of the epidermis (freckles, by contrast, do not show an increase in these cells). In **lentigo maligna** (or **Hutchinson's lentigo**), which occurs on the cheeks of the elderly, the spot is larger than 2 cm in diameter and has variable pigmentation; it is an early malignant *melanoma that has not spread deeply.

leontiasis *n.* overgrowth of the skull bones, said to resemble the appearance of a lion's head: a rare feature of untreated *Paget's disease. Medical name: **leontiasis ossea**.

lepra reaction an aggravation of lumps on the skin caused by *leprosy, accompanied by fever and malaise.

leproma *n.* a lump on the skin characteristic of *leprosy.

lepromin *n.* a chemical prepared from lumps on the skin caused by lepromatous *leprosy.

leprosy (Hansen's disease) *n.* a chronic disease, caused by the bacterium *Mycobacterium leprae*, that affects the skin, mucous membranes, and nerves. It is confined mainly to the tropics and is transmitted by direct contact. After an incubation period of 1–30 years, symptoms develop gradually and mainly involve the skin and nerves. **Lepromatous (multibacillary) leprosy** is a contagious steadily progressive form of the disease characterized by the development of widely distributed lumps on the skin, thickening of the skin and nerves, and in serious cases by severe numbness of the skin, muscle weakness, and paralysis, which leads to disfigurement and deformity. Tuberculosis is a common complication. **Tuberculoid leprosy** is a benign, often self-limiting, form of leprosy causing discoloration and disfiguration of patches of skin (sparsely distributed) associated with localized numbness. **Indeterminate leprosy** is a form of the disease in which skin manifestations represent a combination of the two main types; tuberculoid and indeterminate leprosy are known as **paucibacillary leprosy**.

Like tuberculosis, leprosy should be treated with a combination of antibacterial drugs, to overcome the problem of resistance developing to a single drug; the WHO advocates a combination of rifampicin and dapsone for six months to treat paucibacillary leprosy and these drugs with the addition of clofazimine for multibacillary leprosy, this **multidrug therapy (MDT)** to be continued for two years. The WHO is conducting a trial in which ofloxacin is used in combination with other drugs to shorten the treatment time before cure. Reconstructive surgery can repair some of the damage caused by the disease. A vaccine is being developed and tested.

lept- (lepto-) *prefix denoting* **1.** slender; thin. **2.** small. **3.** mild; slight.

leptin *n.* a protein, produced by white *fat cells in adipose tissue, that is involved in controlling the amount of white adipose tissue laid down in the body. It acts on the brain, possibly as a signal to regulate appetite or energy expenditure. Mutations in the *ob* gene, which codes for leptin, are responsible for some cases of *obesity.

leptocyte *n.* a red blood cell (*erythrocyte) that is abnormally narrow. Leptocytes are seen in certain types of anaemia.

leptomeninges *pl. n.* the inner two *meninges: the arachnoid and pia mater.

leptomeningitis *n.* inflammation of the inner membranes (the *pia mater and *arachnoid) of the brain and spinal cord. *See also* MENINGITIS.

leptophonia *n.* weakness of the voice.

Leptospira *n.* a genus of spirochaete bacteria, commonly bearing hooked ends. They are not visible with ordinary light microscopy and are best seen using dark-ground microscopy. The parasitic species *L. icterohaemorrhagiae* is the main causative agent of Weil's disease (*see* LEPTOSPIROSIS), but many closely related species cause similar symptoms.

leptospirosis (Weil's disease) *n.* an infectious disease, caused by bacteria of the genus *Leptospira* (especially *L. icterohaemorrhagiae*), that occurs in rodents, dogs, and other mammals and may be transmitted to people whose work brings them into contact with these animals. The disease begins with a high fever and headache and may affect the liver (causing jaundice) or kidneys (resulting in renal failure); in some cases patients may go on to develop meningitis.

leptotene *n.* the first stage in the first prophase of *meiosis, in which the chromosomes become visible as single long threads.

leresis *n.* rambling speech, immature both in syntax and pronunciation. It is a feature of dementia.

Leriche's syndrome a condition in males characterized by absence of penile erection combined with absence of pulses in the femoral arteries and wasting of the buttock muscles. It is caused by occlusion of the abdominal aorta and iliac arteries. [R. Leriche (1879–1956), French surgeon]

lesbianism *n.* female *homosexuality: the condition in which a woman is sexually attracted to, or engages in sexual behaviour with, another woman. Lesbianism is not an illness. **—lesbian** *adj., n.*

Lesch-Nyhan disease a *sex-linked hereditary disease caused by an enzyme deficiency resulting in overproduction of uric acid. Affected boys are mentally retarded and suffer from *spasticity and gouty arthritis. They also have a compulsion for self-mutilation. [M. Lesch (1939–   ) and W. L. Nyhan Jr. (1926–   ), US physicians]

lesion *n.* a zone of tissue with impaired function as a result of damage by disease or wounding. Apart from direct physical injury, examples of primary lesions include abscesses, ulcers, and tumours; secondary lesions (such as crusts and scars) are derived from primary ones.

lethal gene a gene that, under certain conditions, causes the death of the individual carrying it. Lethal genes are usually *recessive: an individual will die only if both his parents carry the gene. If only one parent is affected, the lethal effects of the gene will be masked by the dominant *allele inherited from the normal parent.

lethargy *n.* mental and physical sluggishness: a degree of inactivity and unresponsiveness approaching or verging on the unconscious. The condition results from disease (such as sleeping sickness) or hypnosis.

Letterer-Siwe disease *see* RETICULOENDOTHELIOSIS. [E. Letterer (20th century) and S. A. Siwe (1897–1966), German physicians]

leuc- (leuco-, leuk-, leuko-) *prefix denoting* **1.** lack of colour; white. **2.** leucocytes.

leucine *n.* an *essential amino acid. *See also* AMINO ACID.

leucocidin *n.* a bacterial *exotoxin that selectively destroys white blood cells (leucocytes).

leucocyte (white blood cell) *n.* any blood cell that contains a nucleus. In health there are three major subdivisions: *granulocytes, *lymphocytes and *monocytes, which are involved in protecting the body against foreign substances and in antibody production. In disease, a variety of other types may appear in the blood, most notably immature forms of the normal red or white blood cells.

leucocytosis *n.* an increase in the number of white blood cells (leucocytes) in the blood. *See* BASOPHILIA, EOSINOPHILIA, LYMPHOCYTOSIS, MONOCYTOSIS.

leucocytospermia *n.* the presence of excess white blood cells (leucocytes) in the semen (more than 1 million/ml). It has an adverse effect on fertility.

leucoderma *n.* loss of pigment in areas of the skin, resulting in the appearance of white patches or bands.

leucolysin *n. see* LYSIN.

leucoma *n.* a white opacity occurring in the cornea. Most leucomas result from scarring after corneal inflammation or ulceration. Congenital types may be associated with other abnormalities of the eye.

leuconychia *n.* white discoloration of the nails, which may be total or partial. The cause is unknown.

leucopenia *n.* a reduction in the number of white blood cells (leucocytes) in the blood. *See* EOSINOPENIA, LYMPHOPENIA, NEUTROPENIA.

leucoplakia (leukoplakia) *n.* a thickened white patch on a mucous membrane, such as the mouth lining or vulva, that cannot be rubbed off. It is not a specific disease and is present in about 1% of the elderly. Occasionally leucoplakia can become malignant. **Hairy leucoplakia**, with a shaggy or hairy appearance, is a marker of AIDS. *See also* KHAT.

leucopoiesis *n.* the process of the production of white blood cells (leucocytes), which normally occurs in the blood-forming tissue of the *bone marrow. *See also* GRANULOPOIESIS, HAEMOPOIESIS, LYMPHOPOIESIS, MONOBLAST.

leucorrhoea *n.* a whitish or yellowish discharge of mucus from the vaginal opening. It may occur normally, the quantity usually increasing before and after menstruation. An abnormally large discharge may indicate infection of the lower reproductive tract, e.g. by the protozoan *Trichomonas vaginalis* (*see* VAGINITIS).

leucotomy *n.* the surgical operation of interrupting the pathways of white nerve fibres within the brain: it is the most common procedure in *psychosurgery. In the original form, **prefrontal leucotomy** (**lobotomy**), the operation involved cutting through the nerve fibres connecting the *frontal lobe with the *thalamus and the association fibres of the frontal lobe. This was often successful in reducing severe emotional tension. However, prefrontal leucotomy had serious side-effects and the procedure has now been abandoned.

Modern procedures use *stereotaxy and make selective lesions in smaller areas of the brain. Side-effects are uncommon and the operation is occasionally used for intractable pain, severe depression, obsessional neurosis, and chronic anxiety, where very severe emotional tension has not been relieved by other treatments.

leukaemia *n.* any of a group of malignant diseases in which the bone marrow and other blood-forming organs produce increased numbers of certain types of white blood cells (*leucocytes). Overproduction of these white cells, which are immature or abnormal forms, suppresses the production of normal white cells, red cells, and platelets. This leads to increased susceptibility to infection (due to *neutropenia), *anaemia, and bleeding (due to *thrombocytopenia). Other symptoms include enlargement of the spleen, liver, and lymph nodes.

Leukaemias are classified into **acute** or **chronic** varieties depending on the rate of progression of the disease. They are also classified according to the type of white cell that is proliferating abnormally; for example **acute lymphoblastic leukaemia** (*see* LYMPHOBLAST), **acute myeloblastic leukaemia** (*see* MYELOBLAST), and **hairy-cell leukaemia** (*see* HAIRY CELL). (*See also* MYELOID LEUKAEMIA.) Leukaemias are treated with radiotherapy or *cytotoxic drugs, which are aimed at suppressing the production of the abnormal cells.

leukoplakia *n. see* LEUCOPLAKIA.

leukotaxine *n.* a chemical, present in inflammatory exudates, that attracts white blood cells (leucocytes) and increases the permeability of blood capillaries. It is probably produced by injured cells.

leuprorelin *n. see* LHRH ANALOGUE.

levallorphan *n.* a drug that counteracts the depression in breathing caused by narcotic analgesics such as morphine without affecting their pain-relieving effects. It is administered by injection, usually before or at the same time as the analgesic. Trade name: **Lorfan**.

levamisole *n.* an *anthelmintic drug used to remove roundworms. It has also been found to have an unexpected effect in stimulating the immune system by increasing T-cell responsiveness and encouraging the activity of *phagocytes. It is effective in rheumatoid arthritis. The drug is administered by mouth; possible side-effects include joint pain and interference with blood-cell production, which limit its use.

levator n. **1.** a surgical instrument used for levering up displaced bone fragments in a depressed fracture of the skull. **2.** any muscle that lifts the structure into which it is inserted; for example, the **levator scapulis** helps to lift the shoulder blade.

levo- (laevo-) *prefix denoting* **1.** the left side. **2.** (in chemistry) levorotation.

levodopa (L-dopa) n. a naturally occurring amino acid (*see* DOPA) administered by mouth to treat *parkinsonism. Common side-effects are nausea, vomiting, loss of appetite, and involuntary facial movements; high doses may cause weakness, faintness, and dizziness. Trade names: **Brocadopa, Larodopa.** *See also* BENSERAZIDE.

levonorgestrel n. a synthetic female sex hormone – a *progestogen – used mainly in *oral contraceptives, either in combination with an oestrogen or as a progestogen-only preparation. It is also available in the form of capsules that are implanted beneath the skin in the upper arm. Side-effects of implants include prolonged bleeding and premenstrual tension. Trade names: **Microval, Norgeston, Norplant.**

levorphanol n. a narcotic analgesic, similar to *morphine, that is used to relieve severe pain. It is administered by mouth or injection and may cause nausea, vomiting, loss of appetite, constipation, and confusion. Dependence may develop. Trade name: **Dromoran.**

levulosuria n. *see* FRUCTOSURIA.

Leydig cells *see* INTERSTITIAL CELLS. [F. von Leydig (1821–1908), German anatomist]

Leydig tumour a tumour of the *interstitial (Leydig) cells of the testis. Such tumours often secrete testosterone, which in prepubertal boys causes *virilization.

LH *see* LUTEINIZING HORMONE.

Lhermitte's sign a tingling shocklike sensation passing down the arms or trunk when the neck is flexed. It is a nonspecific indication of disease in the cervical (neck) region of the spinal cord. [J. Lhermitte (1877–1959), French neurologist]

LHRH analogue any one of a group of analogues of **luteinizing hormone releasing hormone**, which stimulates the release of *luteinizing hormone (LH) from the pituitary gland (*see also* GONADO-TROPHIN-RELEASING HORMONE). LHRH analogues are more powerful than the naturally occurring hormone, initially increasing the secretion of LH by the pituitary: this acts to block the hormone receptors and to inhibit the release of further LH. LHRH analogues, which are also known as **GnRH analogues** (*see* GONADO-TROPHIN-RELEASING HORMONE), are effective in the treatment of endometriosis; administered by depot injection or nasal spray, they ensure ovarian suppression. They are also used to shrink fibroids and in the treatment of some types of infertility. Two LHRH analogues, **goserelin** (Zoladex) and **leuprorelin** (Prostap), are increasingly being used in the treatment of advanced prostate cancer. Both are given subcutaneously in depot form into the abdominal wall at monthly intervals. After causing an initial rise in plasma testosterone for approximately ten days the level then falls to the same low level as that achieved by castration. *See also* BUSERELIN, GONADO-RELIN.

libido n. the sexual drive: the term is often used to refer to the intensity of sexual desires. In psychoanalytic theory, the libido (like the death instinct) is said to be one of the fundamental sources of energy for all mental life. The normal course of development (*see* PSYCHOSEXUAL DEVELOPMENT) can be altered by fixation at one level and by regression.

Librium n. *see* CHLORDIAZEPOXIDE.

lice *pl. n. see* LOUSE, PEDICULOSIS.

lichenification n. thickening of the epidermis of the skin with exaggeration of the normal creases. The cause is abnormal scratching or rubbing of the skin.

lichenoid *adj.* describing any skin disease that resembles *lichen planus.

lichen planus an extremely itchy skin disease of unknown cause. Shiny flat-topped mauve spots may occur anywhere but are characteristically found on the inside of the wrists. It may take the form of a white lacy pattern in the mouth, which usually produces no symptoms. Trauma, such as a scratch, may induce a linear form of the disease (see KOEBNER PHENOMENON). Treatment with potent topical corticosteroids gives symptomatic relief.

lichen sclerosus et atrophicus a chronic skin disease affecting the anogenital area, especially in women, and characterized by sheets of thin ivory-white skin. In 20% of patients other skin areas are also affected.

lichen simplex chronicus (neurodermatitis) thickened eczematous skin that develops at the site of constant rubbing in susceptible individuals. Common sites are the nape of the neck in women and the lower legs in men. Stress is a relevant factor.

Lieberkühn's glands (crypts of Lieberkühn) simple tubular glands in the mucous membrane of the *intestine. In the small intestine they lie between the villi. They are lined with columnar *epithelium in which various types of secretory cells are found. In the large intestine Lieberkühn's glands are longer and contain more mucus-secreting cells. [J. N. Lieberkühn (1711–56), German anatomist]

lien n. see SPLEEN.

lien- (lieno-) prefix denoting the spleen. Example: **lienopathy** (disease of).

life table an actuarial presentation of the ages at which a group of males and/or females will die and from which mean **life expectancy** at any age can be estimated, based on the assumption that mortality patterns current at the time of preparation of the table will continue to apply.

ligament n. **1.** a tough band of white fibrous connective tissue that links two bones together at a joint. Ligaments are inelastic but flexible; they both strengthen the joint and limit its movements to certain directions. **2.** a sheet of peritoneum that supports or links together abdominal organs.

ligand n. a molecule that binds to another molecule, as in antigen–antibody and hormone–receptor bondings.

ligation n. the application of a *ligature.

ligature n. any material – for example, nylon, silk, catgut, or wire – that is tied firmly round a blood vessel to stop it bleeding or around the base of a structure (such as the *pedicle of a growth) to constrict it.

light adaptation reflex changes in the eye to enable vision either in normal light after being in darkness or in very bright light after being in normal light. The pupil contracts (see PUPILLARY REFLEX) and the pigment in the *rods is bleached. *Compare* DARK ADAPTATION.

lightening n. the sensation experienced, usually after the 36th week of gestation, by many pregnant women, particularly those carrying their first child, as the presenting part of the fetus enters the pelvis. This reduces the pressure on the diaphragm and the woman notices that it is easier to breathe. *Compare* ENGAGEMENT.

light reflex see PUPILLARY REFLEX.

lignocaine n. a widely used local *anaesthetic administered by injection for minor surgery and dental procedures. For the latter it is normally used in combination with adrenaline to achieve better and longer anaesthesia. It can also be applied directly to the eye, throat, and mouth as it is absorbed through mucous membranes. Lignocaine is also injected to treat conditions involving abnormal heart rhythm, particularly myocardial infarction. When used as a local anaesthetic, side-effects are uncommon. Trade names: **Xylocaine**, **Xylocard**.

limbic system a complex system of nerve pathways and networks in the brain, involving several different nuclei, that is involved in the expression of instinct and mood in activities of the endocrine and motor systems of the body. Among the brain regions involved are the *amygdala, *hippocampal formation, and *hypothalamus. The activities of the body that are governed are those concerned with self-preservation (e.g. searching for food, fighting) and preservation of the species (e.g. reproduction and the care of offspring), the expression of fear, rage, and pleasure, and the establishment of memory patterns. *See also* RETICULAR ACTIVATING SYSTEM.

limb lengthening an orthopaedic procedure for increasing the length of a limb (usually the leg). An *external fixator is attached to the bone. This can be a circular frame surrounding the bone, which was invented by the Russian surgeon Ilizarov, or a bar down one side of the limb. The bone is divided, and the gap produced is slowly widened by moving the two ends of the frame apart; if a bar fixator is used, its body has a screw thread that is turned to increase the distance between the two ends. New bone is produced in the widening gap as the bone is stretched (*see* CALLOTASIS). Limb lengthening is undertaken when there is inequality in the length of the legs; for example, following trauma or resulting from paralysis in childhood. Both legs can be lengthened to increase the height of a person of excessively short stature.

limbus *n.* (in anatomy) an edge or border; for example, the **limbus sclerae** is the junction of the cornea and sclera of the eye.

limen *n.* (in anatomy) a border or boundary. The **limen nasi** is the boundary between the bony and cartilaginous parts of the nasal cavity.

liminal *adj.* (in physiology) relating to the threshold of perception.

limosis *n.* abnormal hunger or an excessive desire for food.

linac *n. see* LINEAR ACCELERATOR.

lincomycin *n.* an *antibiotic used to treat infections caused by a narrow range of bacteria, including osteomyelitis. It is administered by mouth or injection and occasionally causes diarrhoea, nausea, and stomach pains. Trade name: **Lincocin**.

linctus *n.* a syrupy liquid medicine, particularly one used in the treatment of irritating coughs.

lindane *n.* an insecticide drug applied as a lotion or cream to kill such parasites as lice and the scabies mite, *Sarcoptes scabei*. Possible side-effects include skin irritation

and rashes, but these are rare. Trade names: **Esoderm, Lorexane**.

Lindau's tumour *see* HAEMANGIOBLASTOMA. [A. Lindau (1892–1958), Swedish pathologist]

linea *n.* (*pl.* **lineae**) (in anatomy) a line, narrow streak, or stripe. The **linea alba** is a tendinous line, extending from the xiphoid process to the pubic symphysis, where the flat abdominal muscles are attached.

linear accelerator (linac) a machine that accelerates particles to produce high-energy radiation, used in the treatment (radiotherapy) of malignant disease.

lingual *adj.* relating to, situated close to, or resembling the tongue (lingua). The lingual surface of a tooth is the surface adjacent to the tongue.

lingula *n.* **1.** the thin forward-projecting portion of the anterior lobe of the cerebellum, in the midline. **2.** a small section of the upper lobe of the left lung, extending downwards in front of the heart. **3.** a bony spur on the inside of the mandible, above the angle of the jaw. **4.** a small backward-pointing projection on each side of the sphenoid bone.

liniment *n.* a medicinal preparation that is rubbed onto the skin or applied on a surgical dressing. Liniments often contain camphor.

lining *n.* (in dentistry) a protective layer placed in a prepared tooth cavity before a restoration is inserted.

linitis plastica (leather-bottle stomach) diffuse infiltration of the stomach submucosa with malignant tissue, producing rigidity and narrowing. Diagnosis by endoscopy may be difficult but radiological changes are more marked.

linkage *n.* (in genetics) the situation in which two or more genes lie close to each other on a chromosome and are therefore very likely to be inherited together. The further two genes are apart the more likely they are to be separated by *crossing over during meiosis.

linoleic acid *see* ESSENTIAL FATTY ACID.

linolenic acid *see* ESSENTIAL FATTY ACID.

lint *n.* a material used in surgical dressings, made of scraped linen or a cotton substitute. It is usually fluffy one side and smooth the other.

liothyronine *n.* a hormone produced by the thyroid gland that is similar to *thyroxine and used to treat conditions of thyroid deficiency. It is administered by mouth or injection and has a rapid but short-lived effect. Trade name: **Tertroxin**.

lip- (lipo-) *prefix denoting* **1.** fat. **2.** lipid.

lipaemia *n.* the presence in the blood of an abnormally large amount of fat.

lipase (steapsin) *n.* an enzyme, produced by the pancreas and the glands of the small intestine, that breaks down fats into glycerol and fatty acids during digestion.

lipid *n.* one of a group of naturally occurring compounds that are soluble in solvents such as chloroform or alcohol, but insoluble in water. Lipids are important dietary constituents, not only because of their high energy value but also because certain vitamins and essential fatty acids are associated with them. The group includes *fats, the *steroids, *phospholipids, and *glycolipids.

lipidosis (lipoidosis) *n.* (*pl.* **-ses**) any disorder of lipid metabolism within the cells of the body. The **brain lipidoses** (*see* GAUCHER'S DISEASE, HUNTER'S SYNDROME, HURLER'S SYNDROME, TAY-SACHS DISEASE) are inborn defects causing the accumulation of lipids within the brain.

lipochondrodystrophy *n.* multiple congenital defects affecting lipid (fat) metabolism, cartilage and bone, skin, and the major internal organs, leading to mental retardation, dwarfism, and deformities of the bones.

lipochrome *n.* a pigment that is soluble in fat and therefore gives colour to fatty materials. An example is *carotene, the pigment responsible for the colour of egg yolks and butter.

lipodystrophy *n.* any disturbance of fat metabolism or of the distribution of fat in the body. In **inferior lipodystrophy** fat is absent from the legs; in **insulin lipodystrophy**, sometimes occurring in diabetics, it disappears from the areas at which insulin is injected.

lipofuscin *n.* a brownish pigment staining with certain fat stains. It is most common in the cells of heart muscle, nerves, and liver and is normally contained within the *lysosomes.

lipogenesis *n.* the process by which glucose and other substances, derived from carbohydrate in the diet, are converted to *fatty acids in the body.

lipogranulomatosis *n.* an abnormality of lipid metabolism causing deposition of yellowish nodules in the skin.

lipoic acid a sulphur-containing compound that can be readily interconverted to and from its reduced form, **dihydrolipoic acid**. Lipoic acid functions in carbohydrate metabolism as one of the *coenzymes in the oxidative decarboxylation of pyruvate and other α-keto acids.

lipoid factor one of the substances involved in the clotting of blood, which is important for the activation of plasma *thromboplastin.

lipoidosis *n.* *see* LIPIDOSIS.

lipolysis *n.* the process by which lipids, particularly triglycerides in fat, are broken down into their constituent fatty acids in the body by the enzyme *lipase. —**lipolytic** *adj.*

lipoma *n.* (*pl.* **lipomas** or **lipomata**) a common benign tumour composed of well-differentiated fat cells.

lipomatosis *n.* **1.** the presence of an abnormally large amount of fat occurring in the tissues. **2.** the presence of multiple *lipomas.

lipopolysaccharide *n.* a complex molecule containing both a lipid component and a polysaccharide component. Lipopolysaccharides are constituents of the cell walls of Gram-negative bacteria and are important in determining the antigenic properties of these bacteria.

lipoprotein *n.* one of a group of proteins, found in blood plasma and lymph, that are combined with fats or other lipids. Lipoproteins are important for the transport of lipids in the blood and lymph. *Cholesterol is transported in the bloodstream in the form of the **low-density lipoproteins (LDL**s). Cholesterol is removed from the bloodstream by means of special LDL receptors, which are inserted into the membranes of cells and bind the LDLs, which are then taken into the cells. Other forms of lipoprotein are **high-density lipoprotein (HDL)** and **very low-density lipoprotein (VLDL)**.

liposarcoma *n.* a rare malignant tumour of fat cells. It is most commonly found in the thigh and is rare under the age of 30 years. There are four main histological types: **well-differentiated, myxoid, pleomorphic,** and **round-cell liposarcomas,** the first two of which respond best to treatment, usually by surgery.

liposome *n.* a microscopic spherical membrane-enclosed vesicle or sac (20–30 nm in diameter) made artificially in the laboratory by the addition of an aqueous solution to a phospholipid gel. The membrane resembles a cell membrane and the whole vesicle is similar to a cell organelle. Liposomes can be incorporated into living cells and may be used to transport relatively toxic drugs into cancer cells, where they can exert their maximum effects. The cancerous organ is at a higher temperature than normal body temperature, so that when the liposome passes through its blood vessels the membrane melts and the drug is released. Liposomes are also undergoing clinical trials as vehicles in *gene therapy for cystic fibrosis.

liposuction *n.* a technique for removing unwanted collections of subcutaneous fat by using a powerful suction tube passed through the skin at different locations.

lipotrophin *n.* a hormone-like substance from the anterior pituitary gland that stimulates the transfer of fat from the body stores to the bloodstream.

lipotropic *adj.* describing a substance that promotes the transport of fatty acids from the liver to the tissues or accelerates the utilization of fat in the liver itself. An example of such a substance is the amino acid methionine.

lipping *n.* overgrowth of bone as seen in X-rays near a joint margin. This is a characteristic sign of degenerative or inflammatory joint disease and occurs most frequently and prominently in osteoarthritis. *See also* OSTEOPHYTE.

lipuria *n.* the presence of fat or oil droplets in the urine.

liquor *n.* (in pharmacy) any solution, usually an aqueous solution.

Lisch nodules pigmented *hamartomas of the iris of the eye seen in *tuberous sclerosis. [K. Lisch (1907–   ), Austrian ophthalmologist]

Listeria *n.* a genus of Gram-positive aerobic motile rodlike bacteria that are parasites of warm-blooded animals. The single species, *L. monocytogenes*, infects many domestic and wild animals. If it is transmitted to man, by eating infected animals or animal products, it may cause disease (**listeriosis**), especially in the frail, ranging from influenza-like symptoms to meningoencephalitis. In pregnant women it may terminate the pregnancy or damage the fetus.

lith- (litho-) *prefix denoting* a calculus (stone). Example: **lithogenesis** (formation of).

-lith *suffix denoting* a calculus (stone). Example: **faecalith** (a stony mass of faeces).

lithaemia *n. see* HYPERURICAEMIA.

lithiasis *n.* formation of stones (*see* CALCULUS) in an internal organ, such as the gall bladder (*see* GALLSTONE), urinary system, pancreas, or appendix.

lithium (lithium carbonate) *n.* a drug given by mouth to prevent episodes of manic-depressive psychosis or to treat mania. Side-effects include tremor, weakness, nausea, thirst, and excessive urination. Thyroid function can be interfered with, and changes in the kidney can appear after long-term lithium treatment. Excessive doses can cause an *encephalopathy and even death. The levels of lithium in the blood are therefore usually checked during long-term therapy. Trade names: **Camcolit, Litarex, Priadel**.

litholapaxy (lithotripsy) *n.* the operation of crushing a stone in the bladder, using an instrument called a **lithotrite**.

The small fragments of stone can then be removed by irrigation and suction.

lithonephrotomy *n.* surgical removal of a stone from the kidney. *See* NEPHRO-LITHOTOMY, PYELOLITHOTOMY.

lithopaedion *n.* a fetus that has died in the uterus or abdominal cavity and has become calcified.

lithotomy *n.* the surgical removal of a stone (calculus) from the urinary tract. *See* NEPHROLITHOTOMY, PYELOLITHOTOMY, URETEROLITHOTOMY.

lithotripsy *n.* **1.** the destruction of calculi (stones) by the application of shock waves. In **extracorporeal shock-wave lithotripsy (ESWL)**, used for destroying calculi in the upper urinary tract and gallstones, the shock waves are generated and transmitted by an external power source. The specialized machine (a **lithotripter**) consists of a sophisticated radiological system to localize the stone accurately by biplanar X-ray or ultrasound and a shock head or transducer to produce and focus the energy source. The prototype machines required the patient to be anaesthetized and immersed in a water bath for treatment, but the newer machines require neither water bath nor general anaesthesia. In **electrohydraulic lithotripsy (EHL)**, used for destroying urinary calculi, an electrically generated shock wave is transmitted to the stone by a contact probe delivered via a *nephroscope. **2.** *see* LITHOLAPAXY.

lithotrite *n.* a surgical instrument used for crushing a stone in the bladder. *See* LITHOLAPAXY.

lithotrophic *adj.* *see* AUTOTROPHIC.

lithuresis *n.* the passage of small stones or *gravel in the urine.

lithuria *n.* *see* HYPERURICURIA.

litre *n.* a unit of volume equal to the volume occupied by 1 kilogram of pure water at 4°C and 760 mmHg pressure. In *SI units the litre is treated as a special name for the cubic decimetre, but is not used when a high degree of accuracy is required (1 litre = 1.0000028 dm^3). For approximate purposes 1 litre is assumed to be equal to 1000 cubic centimetres (cm^3), therefore 1 millilitre (ml) is often taken to be equal to 1 cm^3. This practice is now deprecated.

Little's area the anterior region of the nasal septum (*see* NOSE), which is richly supplied with capillaries; it is a common site from which *nosebleeds arise. [J. L. Little (1836–85), US surgeon]

Little's disease a form of *cerebral palsy involving both sides of the body and affecting the legs more severely than the arms. [W. J. Little (1810–94), British surgeon]

Litzmann's obliquity *see* ASYNCLITISM. [K. C. T. Litzmann (1815–90), German obstetrician]

livedo *n.* a discoloured area or spot on the skin, often caused by local congestion of the circulation.

liver *n.* the largest gland of the body, weighing 1200–1600 g. Situated in the top right portion of the abdominal cavity, the liver is divided by fissures (**fossae**) into four lobes: the **right** (the largest lobe), **left**, **quadrate**, and **caudate lobes**. It is connected to the diaphragm and abdominal walls by five ligaments: the membranous **falciform** (which separates the right and left lobes), **coronary**, and **right** and **left triangular ligaments** and the fibrous **round ligament**, which is derived from the embryonic umbilical vein. Venous blood containing digested food is brought to the liver in the **hepatic portal vein** (*see* PORTAL SYSTEM). Branches of this vein pass in between the lobules and terminate in the **sinusoids** (see illustration).

Oxygenated blood is supplied in the **hepatic artery**. The blood leaves the liver via a central vein in each lobule, which drains into the *hepatic vein. The liver is supplied by parasympathetic nerve fibres from the vagus nerve, and by sympathetic fibres from the solar plexus. The liver has a number of important functions. It synthesizes *bile, which drains into the *gall bladder before being released into the duodenum. The liver is an important site of metabolism of carbohydrates, proteins, and fats. It regulates the amount of blood sugar, converting excess glucose to *glycogen; it removes excess amino acids by breaking them down into ammonia and finally *urea; and it stores and metabolizes fats. The liver also synthesizes *fibrinogen and *prothrombin (essential blood-clotting substances) and *heparin, an anticoagulant. It forms red blood cells in the fetus and is the site of production of plasma proteins. It has an important role in the detoxification of poisonous substances and it breaks down worn out red cells and other unwanted substances, such as excess oestrogen in the male (*see also* KUPFFER'S CELLS). The liver is also the site of *vitamin A synthesis; this vitamin is stored in the liver, together with vitamins B_{12}, D, and K.

The liver is the site of many important diseases, including *hepatitis, *cirrhosis, *amoebiasis, *hydatid disease, and *hepatomas.

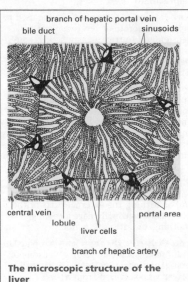

branch of hepatic portal vein
bile duct
sinusoids
central vein
lobule
liver cells
portal area
branch of hepatic artery

The microscopic structure of the liver

livid *adj.* denoting a bluish colour of the skin, such as that produced locally by a bruise or of the general complexion in ˄cyanosis.

living will a statement signed by a person that outlines the degree of life-saving treatment desired in case of incapacitation. It enables terminally ill patients to refuse resuscitation in the event of cardiac arrest.

Loa *n.* a genus of parasitic nematode worms (*see* FILARIA). The adult eye worm, *L. loa*, lives within the tissues beneath the skin, where it causes inflammation and swelling (*see* LOIASIS). The motile embryos, present in the blood during the day, may be taken up by bloodsucking *Chrysops* flies. Here they develop into infective larvae, ready for transmission to a new human host.

lobe *n.* a major division of an organ or part of an organ, especially one having a rounded form and often separated from other lobes by fissures or bands of connective tissue. For example, the brain, liver, and lung are divided into lobes. —**lobar** *adj.*

lobectomy *n.* the surgical removal of a lobe of an organ or gland, such as the lung, thyroid, or brain. Lobectomy of the lung may be performed for cancer or other disease of the lung; in some cases the operation can be done through an endoscope.

lobotomy (prefrontal leucotomy) *n. see* LEUCOTOMY.

lobule *n.* a subdivision of a part or organ that can be distinguished from the whole by boundaries, such as septa, that are visible with or without a microscope. For example, the **lobule of the liver** is a structural and functional unit seen in cross-section under a microscope as a column of cells drained by a central vein and bounded by a branch of the portal vein. The **lung lobule** is a practical subdivision of the lung tissue seen macroscopically in lung slices as outlined by incomplete septa of fibrous tissue. It is made up of three to five lung *acini.

lochia *n.* the material eliminated from the uterus through the vagina after the completion of labour. The first discharge, **lochia rubra (lochia cruenta)**, consists largely of blood. This is followed by **lochia serosa**, a brownish mixture of blood and mucus, and finally **lochia alba (lochia purulenta)**, a yellowish or whitish discharge containing microorganisms and cell fragments. Each stage may last for several days. —**lochial** *adj.*

locked-in syndrome *see* PERSISTENT VEGETATIVE STATE.

lockjaw n. see TETANUS.

locomotor ataxia see TABES DORSALIS.

loculus n. (in anatomy) a small space or cavity.

locum tenens a doctor who stands in temporarily for a colleague who is absent or ill and looks after the patients in his practice. Often shortened to **locum**.

locus n. **1.** (in anatomy) a region or site. The **locus caeruleus** is a small pigmented region in the floor of the fourth ventricle of the brain. **2.** (in genetics) the region of a chromosome occupied by a particular gene.

lofepramine n. a tricyclic *antidepressant that is administered by mouth or injection. Possible side-effects include flushing, sweating, dry mouth, blurred vision, difficulty in passing urine, and drowsiness. Trade name: **Gamanil**.

log- (logo-) prefix denoting words; speech.

logopaedics n. the scientific study of defects and disabilities of speech and of the methods used to treat them; speech therapy.

logorrhoea n. a rapid flow of voluble speech, often with incoherence, such as is encountered in *mania.

-logy (-ology) suffix denoting field of study. Example: **cytology** (study of cells).

loiasis n. a disease, occurring in West and Central Africa, caused by the eye worm *Loa loa. The adult worms live and migrate within the skin tissues, causing the appearance of transitory **calabar** swellings. These are probably an allergic reaction to the worms' waste products, and they sometimes lead to fever and itching. Worms often migrate across the eyeball just beneath the conjunctiva, where they cause irritation and congestion. Loiasis is treated with *diethylcarbamazine, which kills both the adults and larval forms.

loin n. the region of the back and side of the body between the lowest rib and the pelvis.

Lomotil n. see DIPHENOXYLATE.

longitudinal study see COHORT STUDY.

long-sightedness n. see HYPERMETROPIA.

loop n. **1.** a bend in a tubular organ, e.g. *Henle's loop in a kidney tubule. **2.** one of the patterns of dermal ridges in *fingerprints.

loperamide n. a drug used in the treatment of diarrhoea. It acts by reducing *peristalsis of the digestive tract and is administered by mouth; side-effects are rare, but include abdominal distension, drowsiness, and skin rash. Trade name: **Imodium**.

loprazolam n. a long-acting *benzodiazepine drug administered by mouth. Possible side-effects include addiction and rebound insomnia. Trade name: **Loprazolam**.

lorazepam n. a *benzodiazepine used to relieve moderate or severe anxiety and tension and to treat insomnia. It is administered by mouth and may cause drowsiness, dizziness, blurred vision, and nausea. Trade name: **Ativan**.

lordosis n. inward curvature of the spine. A certain degree of lordosis is normal in the lumbar and cervical regions of the spine: loss of this is a sign of ankylosing *spondylitis. Exaggerated lordosis may occur in adolescence, through faulty posture or as a result of disease affecting the vertebrae and spinal muscles. Compare KYPHOSIS.

lotion n. a medicinal solution for washing or bathing the external parts of the body. Lotions usually have a cooling, soothing, or antiseptic action.

Lou Gehrig's disease amyotrophic lateral *sclerosis. See also MOTOR NEURONE DISEASE. [Lou Gehrig (1903–41), US baseball player who suffered from it]

loupe n. a small magnifying hand lens used for examining the front part of the eye, usually with a pocket torch to provide illumination. In modern practice a slit-lamp microscope is used.

louse n. (pl. **lice**) a small wingless insect that is an external parasite of man. Lice attach themselves to hair and clothing using their well-developed legs and claws. Their flattened leathery bodies are resistant to crushing and their mouthparts are adapted for sucking blood. Lice thrive in overcrowded and unhygienic conditions; they can infest humans (*see* PEDICULOSIS) and they may transmit disease. *See also* PEDICULUS, PHTHIRUS.

lovastatin *n.* a drug that interferes with the synthesis of cholesterol in the liver and is used to reduce abnormally high blood cholesterol levels. Possible side-effects include muscle pain and weakness, liver damage, insomnia, headache, nausea, dyspepsia, diarrhoea, and abdominal cramps.

Løvset's manoeuvre rotation and traction of the trunk of the fetus during a breech birth to facilitate delivery of the arms and the shoulders. [J. Løvset (20th century), Norwegian obstetrician]

low-density lipoprotein (LDL) *see* LIPOPROTEIN.

low-molecular-weight heparin a type of *heparin that is more readily absorbed and requires less frequent administration than standard heparin preparations used as anticoagulant therapy to prevent deep-vein thrombosis following surgery or during kidney dialysis. It also produces less risk of bleeding. Preparations in use include **enoxaparin**.

lozenge *n.* a medicated tablet containing sugar. Lozenges should dissolve slowly in the mouth so that the medication is applied to the mouth and throat.

LSD *see* LYSERGIC ACID DIETHYLAMIDE.

lubb-dupp *n.* a representation of the normal heart sounds as heard through the stethoscope. Lubb (the first heart sound) coincides with closure of the mitral and tricuspid valves; dupp (the second heart sound) is due to closure of the aortic and pulmonary valves.

lucid interval temporary recovery of consciousness after a blow to the head, before relapse into coma. It is a sign of intracranial arterial bleeding.

Ludwig's angina severe inflammation caused by infection of both sides of the floor of the mouth, resulting in massive swelling of the neck. If untreated, it may obstruct the airways, necessitating tracheostomy. [W. F. von Ludwig (1770–1865), German surgeon]

lues *n.* a serious infectious disease such as syphilis.

lumbago *n.* low backache, of any cause or description. Severe lumbago, of sudden onset while bending or lifting, can be due either to a slipped disc or to a strained muscle or ligament. When associated with *sciatica it is often due to a prolapsed intervertebral disc.

lumbar *adj.* relating to the loin.

lumbar puncture a procedure in which cerebrospinal fluid is withdrawn by means of a hollow needle inserted into the *subarachnoid space in the region of the lower back (usually between the third and fourth lumbar vertebrae). The fluid thus obtained is examined for diagnostic purposes. The procedure is usually without risk to the patient, but in patients with raised intracranial pressure it may be hazardous. CT and MRI scanning prior to lumbar puncture have greatly reduced the risk of performing the test in patients with unsuspected raised intracranial pressure. *See also* QUECKENSTEDT TEST.

lumbar triangle a weak area in the abdomen bounded by the iliac crest (below), the external oblique muscle (in front), and the erector spinae muscle (behind). It can be the site of a **lumbar hernia**.

lumbar vertebrae the five bones of the *backbone that are situated between the thoracic vertebrae and the sacrum, in the lower part of the back. They are the largest of the unfused vertebrae and have stout processes for attachment of the strong muscles of the lower back. *See also* VERTEBRA.

lumbo- *prefix denoting* the loin; lumbar region.

lumbosacral *adj.* relating to part of the spine composed of the lumbar vertebrae and the sacrum.

lumen *n.* **1.** the space within a tubular or sac-like part, such as a blood vessel, the intestine, or the stomach. **2.** the *SI unit of luminous flux, equal to the amount of light emitted per second in unit solid angle of 1 steradian by a point source of 1 candela. Symbol: lm.

luminescence *n.* the emission of light from a substance after it has been irradi-

ated. *Fluorescence is a type of luminescence.

lumpectomy *n.* an operation for *breast
cancer in which the tumour and surrounding breast tissue are removed: muscles, skin, and lymph nodes are left intact
(*compare* MASTECTOMY). The procedure, usually followed by radiation, is indicated for
patients with a tumour less than 2 cm in
diameter and who have no metastases to
local lymph nodes or to distant organs.

lunate bone a bone of the wrist (*see*
CARPUS). It articulates with the capitate
and hamate bones in front, with the radius behind, and with the triquetral and
scaphoid at the sides.

lung *n.* one of the pair of organs of *respiration, situated in the chest cavity on either side of the heart and enclosed by a
serous membrane (*see* PLEURA). The lungs
are fibrous elastic sacs that are expanded
and compressed by movements of the rib
cage and diaphragm during *breathing.
They communicate with the atmosphere
through the *trachea, which opens into
the pharynx. The trachea divides into two
bronchi (*see* BRONCHUS), which enter the
lungs and branch into *bronchioles. These
divide further and terminate in minute

air sacs (*see* ALVEOLUS), the sites of gaseous
exchange. (See illustration.) Atmospheric
oxygen is absorbed and carbon dioxide
from the blood of the pulmonary capillaries is released into the lungs; in each case
down a concentration gradient (*see* PUL-
MONARY CIRCULATION). The total capacity of
the lungs in an adult male is about 5.5
litres, but during normal breathing only
about 500 ml of air is exchanged (*see also*
RESIDUAL VOLUME). Other functions of the
lung include water evaporation: an important factor in the fluid balance and heat
regulation of the body.

lung cancer cancer arising in the epithelium of the air passages (**bronchial
cancer**) or lung. It is a very common form
of cancer, particularly in Britain, and is
strongly associated with cigarette smoking and exposure to industrial air pollu-
tants (including asbestos). There are often
no symptoms in the early stages of the
disease, when diagnosis is made on X-ray
examination. Treatment includes surgical
removal of the affected lobe or lung (20%
of cases are suitable for surgery), radiotherapy, and chemotherapy.

lunula *n.* the whitish crescent-shaped
area at the base of a *nail.

The lungs and main air passages with details of the alveoli

lupus *n.* any of several chronic skin diseases. *See* LUPUS ERYTHEMATOSUS, LUPUS VERRUCOSUS, LUPUS VULGARIS.

lupus erythematosus (LE) a chronic inflammatory disease of connective tissue, affecting the skin and various internal organs (**systemic LE, SLE**). Typically, there is a red scaly rash on the face, affecting the nose and cheeks; arthritis; and progressive damage to the kidneys. Often the heart, lungs, and brain are also affected by progressive attacks of inflammation followed by the formation of scar tissue (fibrosis). In a milder form, known as **discoid LE (DLE)**, only the skin is affected. LE is an *autoimmune disease and can be diagnosed by the presence of abnormal antibodies in the bloodstream. The disease is treated with corticosteroids or immunosuppressive drugs.

lupus verrucosus a rare tuberculous infection of the skin – commonly the arm or hand – typified by warty lesions. It occurs in those who have been reinfected with tuberculosis.

lupus vulgaris tuberculous infection of the skin, usually due to direct inoculation of the tuberculosis bacillus into the skin. It is no longer common. This type of lupus often starts in childhood, with dark red patches on the nose or cheek. Unless treated lupus vulgaris spreads, ulcerates, and causes extensive scarring. Treatment is with antituberculous drugs.

lute *n.* (in dentistry) a thin layer of cement inserted into the minute space between a prepared tooth and a crown or inlay to hold it permanently in place.

lutein *n.* **1.** *see* XANTHOPHYLL. **2.** the yellow pigment of the corpus luteum.

luteinizing hormone (LH, interstitial cell stimulating hormone, ICSH) a hormone (*see* GONADOTROPHIN), synthesized and released by the anterior pituitary gland, that stimulates ovulation, *corpus luteum formation, progesterone synthesis by the ovary (*see also* MENSTRUAL CYCLE), and androgen synthesis by the interstitial cells of the testes.

luteo- *prefix denoting* **1.** yellow. **2.** the corpus luteum.

luteotrophic hormone (luteotrophin) *see* PROLACTIN.

lux *n.* the *SI unit of intensity of illumination, equal to 1 lumen per square metre. This unit was formerly called the metre candle. Symbol: lx.

luxation *n.* *see* DISLOCATION.

lyase *n.* one of a group of enzymes that catalyse the linking of groups by double bonds.

lycanthropy *n.* a very rare symptom of mental disorder in which an individual believes that he can change into a wolf.

Lyell's disease *see* STAPHYLOCOCCAL SCALDED SKIN SYNDROME. [A. Lyell (20th century), British dermatologist]

Lyme disease a disease caused by a spirochaete, *Borrelia burghdorferi*, and transmitted by certain ticks of the genus *Ixodes*. Following a 3–32-day incubation period, a slowly extending red rash develops in approximately 75% of cases; intermittent systemic symptoms include fever, malaise, headache and neck stiffness, and muscle and joint pains. Later, 60% of patients suffer intermittent attacks of arthritis, especially of the knees, each attack lasting months and recurring over several years. The spirochaete has been identified in synovium and synovial fluid. Neurological and cardiac involvement occurs in a smaller percentage of cases. Treatment is with tetracycline or penicillin.

lymph *n.* the fluid present within the vessels of the *lymphatic system. It consists of the fluid that bathes the tissues, which is derived from the blood and is drained by the lymphatic vessels. Lymph passes through a series of filters (*lymph nodes) and is ultimately returned to the bloodstream via the *thoracic duct. It is similar in composition to plasma, but contains less protein and some cells, mainly *lymphocytes.

lymphaden- (lymphadeno-) *prefix denoting* lymph node(s).

lymphadenectomy *n.* surgical removal of lymph nodes, an operation commonly performed when a cancer has invaded nodes in the drainage area of an organ infiltrated by a malignant growth.

lymphadenitis *n.* inflammation of lymph nodes, which become swollen, painful, and tender. Some cases may be chronic (e.g. tuberculous lymphadenitis) but most are acute and localized adjacent to an area of infection. The most commonly affected lymph nodes are those in the neck, in association with tonsillitis. The lymph nodes help to contain and combat the infection. Occasionally generalized lymphadenitis occurs as a result of virus infections. The treatment is that of the cause.

lymphadenoma *n.* an obsolete term for *lymphoma.

lymphangi- (lymphangio-) *prefix denoting* a lymphatic vessel.

lymphangiectasis *n.* dilatation of the lymphatic vessels, which is usually congenital and produces enlargement of various parts of the body (e.g. the leg in Milroy's disease). It may also be caused by obstruction of the lymphatic vessels. *See* LYMPHOEDEMA.

lymphangiography (lymphography) *n.* X-ray examination of the lymphatic vessels and lymph nodes after a contrast medium has been injected into them (*see* ANGIOGRAPHY). Its main uses are in the investigation of the extent and spread of cancer of the lymphatic system and in the investigation of lymphoedema. Alternatively, the lymphatic system can be imaged using a gamma camera following the injection of a radioactive tracer.

lymphangioma *n.* a localized collection of distended lymphatic vessels, which may result in a large cyst in the neck or armpit (**cystic hygroma**). This can be removed surgically.

lymphangiosarcoma *n.* a rare malignant tumour of the lymphatic vessels. It is most commonly seen in the chronically swollen (oedematous) arms of women who have had a mastectomy for breast cancer.

lymphangitis *n.* inflammation of the lymphatic vessels, which can be seen most commonly as red streaks in the skin adjacent to a focus of streptococcal infection. Occasionally a more chronic form results in *lymphoedema. The infected part is rested and the infection can be eliminated by an antibiotic (e.g. penicillin).

lymphatic 1. *n.* a lymphatic vessel. *See* LYMPHATIC SYSTEM. **2.** *adj.* relating to or transporting lymph.

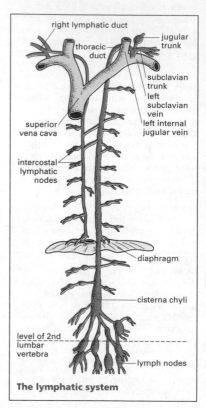

The lymphatic system

lymphatic system a network of vessels that conveys electrolytes, water, proteins, etc. – in the form of *lymph – from the tissue fluids to the bloodstream (see illustration). It consists of fine blind-ended lymphatic capillaries, which unite to form lymphatic vessels. At various points along the lymphatic vessels are *lymph nodes. Lymph drains into the capillaries and passes into the lymphatic vessels, which have valves to prevent backflow of lymph. The lymphatics lead to two large channels – the **thoracic duct** and the **right lymphatic duct** – which return the lymph to the bloodstream via the innominate veins.

lymph node one of a number of small swellings found at intervals along the lymphatic system. Groups of nodes are found in many parts of the body; for example, in the groin and armpit and behind the ear. They are composed of lymphoid tissue and act as filters for the lymph, preventing foreign particles from entering the bloodstream; they also produce lymphocytes.

lympho- *prefix denoting* lymph or the lymphatic system.

lymphoblast *n.* an abnormal cell present in the blood and the blood-forming organs in one type of leukaemia (**lymphoblastic leukaemia**). It has a large nucleus with very scanty cytoplasm and was once thought to be the precursor of the lymphocyte. —**lymphoblastic** *adj.*

lymphocele *n.* a collection of lymph in the tissues, which follows injury to, or operations upon, lymph nodes or ducts.

lymphocyte *n.* a variety of white blood cell (leucocyte), present also in the lymph nodes, spleen, thymus gland, gut wall, and bone marrow. With *Romanowsky stains, lymphocytes can be seen to have dense nuclei with clear pale-blue cytoplasm. Lymphocytes with scanty cytoplasm are **small lymphocytes**; those with abundant cytoplasm are **large lymphocytes**. There are normally $1.5–4.0 \times 10^9$ lymphocytes per litre of blood. They are involved in *immunity and can be subdivided into **B-lymphocytes** (or **B-cells**), which produce circulating antibodies, and **T-lymphocytes** (or **T-cells**), which are primarily responsible for cell-mediated immunity. T-lymphocytes can differentiate into *helper T-cells, cytotoxic T-cells (*see* KILLER CELL), or *suppressor T-cells. —**lymphocytic** *adj.*

lymphocytopenia *n. see* LYMPHOPENIA.

lymphocytosis *n.* an increase in the number of *lymphocytes in the blood. Lymphocytosis may occur in a wide variety of diseases, including chronic lymphocytic *leukaemia and infections due to viruses.

lymphoedema *n.* an accumulation of lymph in the tissues, producing swelling; the legs are most often affected. It may be due to a congenital abnormality of the lymphatic vessels (as in **Milroy's disease**,

congenital lymphoedema of the legs) or result from obstruction of the lymphatic vessels by a tumour, parasites, inflammation, or injury. Treatment consists of elastic support, by stockings or bandages, and diuretic drugs. A variety of surgical procedures have been devised but with little success.

lymphogranuloma venereum a sexually transmitted disease that is caused by *Chlamydia and is most common in tropical regions. An initial lesion on the genitals is followed by swelling and inflammation of the lymph nodes in the groin; the lymph vessels in the genital region may become blocked, causing thickening of the skin of that area. Early treatment with sulphonamides or tetracyclines is usually effective.

lymphography *n. see* LYMPHANGIOGRAPHY.

lymphoid tissue a tissue responsible for the production of lymphocytes and antibodies. It occurs as discrete organs, in the form of the lymph nodes, tonsils, thymus, and spleen, and also as diffuse groups of cells not separated from surrounding tissue. *See also* IMMUNE SYSTEM.

lymphokine *n.* a substance produced by lymphocytes that has effects on other cells involved in the immune system (*see* CYTOKINES). An example is *interleukin 2 (IL-2).

lymphoma *n.* a malignant tumour of the lymph nodes, including *Hodgkin's disease and **non-Hodgkin's lymphomas**. There is a broad spectrum of malignancy, with prognosis ranging from a few months to many years. The patient usually shows evidence of multiple enlarged lymph nodes and may have constitutional symptoms such as weight loss, fever, and sweating. Disease may be widespread, but in some cases is confined to a single area, such as the tonsil. Treatment is with drugs such as chlorambucil or combinations of cyclophosphamide, vincristine, and prednisone, sometimes with the addition of doxorubicin and/or bleomycin; response to these drugs is often dramatic. Localized disease may be treated with radiotherapy followed by drugs. Patients with non-Hodgkin's lymphoma who do not respond to chemotherapy may be considered for a bone-marrow transplant.

lymphopenia (lymphocytopenia) *n.* a decrease in the number of *lymphocytes in the blood, which may occur in a wide variety of diseases.

lymphopoiesis *n.* the process of the production of *lymphocytes, which occurs in the *bone marrow as well as in the lymph nodes, spleen, thymus gland, and gut wall. The precursor cell from which lymphocytes are derived has not yet been identified.

lymphorrhagia *n.* the escape of the lymph from lymphatic vessels that have been injured.

lymphosarcoma *n.* an old term for non-Hodgkin's *lymphoma.

lymphuria *n.* the presence in the urine of lymph.

lys- (lysi-, lyso-) *prefix denoting* lysis; dissolution.

lysergic acid diethylamide (LSD) a *psychedelic drug that is also a *hallucinogen. It has been used to aid treatment of psychological disorders. Side-effects include digestive upsets, dizziness, tingling, anxiety, sweating, dilated pupils, muscle incoordination and tremor. Alterations in sight, hearing and other senses occur, psychotic effects, depression, and confusion are common, and tolerance to the drug develops rapidly. Because of these toxic effects, LSD is no longer used clinically.

lysin *n.* a protein component in the blood that is capable of bringing about the destruction (lysis) of whole cells. Names are given to varieties of lysin with different targets; for example, **haemolysin** attacks red blood cells; **leucolysin** attacks white cells; and a **bacteriolysin** targets bacterial cells.

lysine *n.* an *essential amino acid. *See also* AMINO ACID.

lysis *n.* the destruction of cells through damage or rupture of the plasma membrane, allowing escape of the cell contents. *See also* AUTOLYSIS, LYSOZYME.

-lysis *suffix denoting* **1.** lysis; dissolution. **2.** remission of symptoms.

lysogenic *adj.* producing *lysis.

lysogeny *n.* an interaction between a *bacteriophage and its host in which a latent form of the phage (**prophage**) exists within the bacterial cell, which is not destroyed. Under certain conditions (e.g. irradiation of the bacterium) the phage can develop into an active form, which reproduces itself and eventually destroys the bacterial cell.

lysosome *n.* a particle in the cytoplasm of cells that contains enzymes responsible for breaking down substances in the cell and is bounded by a single membrane. Lysosomes are especially abundant in liver and kidney cells. Foreign particles (e.g. bacteria) taken into the cell are broken down by the enzymes of the lysosomes. When the cell dies, these enzymes are released to break down the cell's components.

lysozyme *n.* an enzyme found in tears and egg white. It catalyses the destruction of the cell walls of certain bacteria. Bacterial cells that are attacked by lysozyme are said to have been **lysed**.

maceration *n.* **1.** the softening of a solid by leaving it immersed in a liquid. **2.** (in obstetrics) the natural breakdown of a dead fetus within the uterus.

Macleod's syndrome (Swyer-James syndrome) pulmonary *emphysema affecting only one lung and beginning in childhood or in adolescence; it occurs secondarily to necrotising bronchitis, probably caused by a virus. [W. M. Macleod (1911–77), British physician]

macr- (macro-) *prefix denoting* large size. Example: **macrencephaly** (abnormally enlarged brain).

macrocephaly (megalocephaly) *n.* abnormal largeness of the head in relation to the rest of the body. *Compare* MICRO-CEPHALY.

macrocheilia *n.* hypertrophy of the lips: a congenital condition in which the lips are abnormally large. *Compare* MICRO-CHEILIA.

macrocyte (megalocyte) *n.* an abnormally large red blood cell (*erythrocyte), seen in certain anaemias. *See also* MACROCY-TOSIS. —**macrocytic** *adj.*

macrocytosis *n.* the presence of abnormally large red cells (**macrocytes**) in the blood. Macrocytosis is a feature of certain anaemias (**macrocytic anaemias**), including those due to deficiency of vitamin B$_{12}$ or folic acid, and also of anaemias in which there is an increase in the rate of red cell production.

macrodactyly *n.* abnormally large size of one or more of the fingers or toes.

macrodontia *n.* a condition in which the teeth are unusually large.

macrogamete *n.* the nonmotile female sex cell of the malarial parasite (*Plasmodium*) and other protozoans. The macrogamete is similar to the ovum of animals and larger than the male sex cell (*see* MICROGAMETE).

macrogametocyte *n.* a cell that under-

goes meiosis to form mature female sex cells (macrogametes) of the malarial parasite (*see* PLASMODIUM). Macrogametocytes are found in the blood of man but must be ingested by a mosquito before developing into macrogametes.

macrogenitosoma *n.* excessive bodily growth with marked enlargement of the genitalia. **Macrogenitosoma praecox** is a variant occurring in early childhood.

macroglia *n.* one of the two basic classes of *glia (the non-nervous cells of the central nervous system), divided into *astrocytes and *oligodendrocytes. *Compare* MICROGLIA.

macroglobulin *n.* **1. (immunoglobulin M, IgM)** a protein of the globulin series that is present in the blood and functions as an antibody, forming an effective first-line defence against bacteria in the bloodstream. *See also* IMMUNOGLOBULIN. **2.** an abnormal form of IgM (*see* PARAPROTEIN).

macroglobulinaemia *n.* the presence in the blood of excessive amounts of macroglobulin, produced by a malignant proliferation of the lymphocytes.

macroglossia *n.* an abnormally large tongue. It may be due to a congenital defect, such as thyroid deficiency (cretinism); to infiltration of the tongue with *amyloid or a tumour; or to obstruction of the lymph vessels.

macrognathia *n.* a condition in which one or both jaws are unusually large.

macromelia *n.* abnormally large size of the arms or legs. *Compare* MICROMELIA.

macronormoblast *n.* an abnormal form of any of the cells (*normoblasts) that form a series of precursors of red blood cells. Macronormoblasts are unusually large but have normal nuclei (*compare* MEGALOBLAST); they are seen in certain anaemias in which red cell production is impaired.

macrophage *n.* a large scavenger cell (a *phagocyte) present in connective tissue and many major organs and tissues, including the bone marrow, spleen, *lymph nodes, liver (*see* KUPFFER CELLS), and the central nervous system (*see* MICROGLIA). They are closely related to *monocytes. **Fixed macrophages (histiocytes)** are stationary within connective tissue; **free macrophages** wander between cells and aggregate at focal sites of infection, where they remove bacteria or other foreign bodies from blood or tissues. *See also* RETICULOENDOTHELIAL SYSTEM.

macropsia *n.* a condition in which objects appear larger than they really are. It is usually due to disease of the retina affecting the *macula but may also occur in spasm of *accommodation.

macroscopic *adj.* visible to the naked eye. *Compare* MICROSCOPIC.

macrosomia *n.* abnormally large size. In **fetal macrosomia** a large baby is associated with poorly controlled maternal diabetes. The increased size is due to excessive production of fetal insulin and thence to increased deposition of glycogen in the fetus.

macula *n.* (*pl.* **maculae**) a small anatomical area that is distinguishable from the surrounding tissue. The **macula lutea** is the yellow spot on the retina at the back of the eye, which surrounds the greatest concentration of cones (*see* FOVEA). Maculae occur in the saccule and utricle of the inner ear (see illustration). Tilting of the head causes the otoliths to bend the hair cells, which send impulses to the brain via the vestibular nerve. *See also* LABYRINTH.

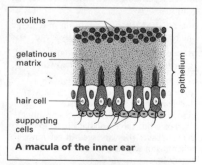

A macula of the inner ear

labels: otoliths; gelatinous matrix; hair cell; supporting cells; epithelium

macular degeneration a group of conditions affecting the *macula lutea of

the eye, resulting in a reduction or loss of central vision. **Age-related macular degeneration (AMD, ARMD)** is the most common cause of blindness in the elderly. Two types are commonly recognized. **Atrophic** (or **dry**) **AMD** results from chronic choroidal ischaemia: small blood vessels of the choroid, which lies beneath the retina, become constricted, reducing the blood supply to the macula. This gives rise to degenerative changes in the retinal pigment epithelium (RPE; *see* RETINA), clinically recognized by macular pigmentation and the deposition of *drusen. **Wet AMD** is associated with the growth of abnormal new blood vessels under the retina, derived from the choroid (*see* (CHOROIDAL) NEOVASCULARIZATION). These can leak fluid and blood into the RPE, which further reduces macular function. Laser surgery (*see* PHOTOCOAGULATION) can halt the degenerative process.

macule *n.* a flat circumscribed area of skin or an area of altered skin colour (e.g. a freckle). *Compare* PAPULE.

maculopapular *adj.* describing a rash that consists of both *macules and *papules.

maculopathy *n.* any abnormality of the *macula of the eye. For example, **bull's-eye maculopathy** describes the appearance of the macula in some toxic conditions (e.g. chloroquine toxicity) and in some hereditary disorders of the macula. *See also* EPIRETINAL MEMBRANE (CELLOPHANE MACULOPATHY).

madarosis *n.* **1.** a congenital deficiency of the eyelashes and eyebrows, which are sometimes absent altogether. **2.** a deficiency of the eyelashes alone, caused by chronic *blepharitis.

Madelung's disease the presence of multiple lipomas around the head and neck. [O. Madelung (1846–1926), German surgeon]

Madopar *n.* *see* BENSERAZIDE.

Madura foot an infection of the tissues and bones of the foot producing chronic inflammation (mycetoma), occurring in the tropics. It is caused by various filamentous fungi (including *Madurella*) and certain bacteria of the genera

Nocardia and *Streptomyces*. Medical name: **maduromycosis**.

Madurella *n.* a genus of widely distributed fungi. The species *M. grisea* and *M. mycetomi* cause the tropical infection *Madura foot.

maduromycosis *n.* *see* MADURA FOOT.

magenta *n.* *see* FUCHSIN.

maggot *n.* the wormlike larva of a fly, which occasionally infests human tissues (*see* MYIASIS). Formerly maggots were, in some cases, allowed to feed on dead and rotting tissues and so assist in the cleaning and healing of serious wounds. Interest in this ancient practice has revived in light of the growing resistance of bacteria to antibiotics: encouraging results were obtained in a recent clinical trial in which maggots were applied to refractory leg ulcers in patients unfit for surgery.

magic bullet *see* MONOCLONAL ANTIBODY.

magnesium *n.* a metallic element essential to life. The body of an average adult contains about 25 g of magnesium, concentrated mostly in the bones. Magnesium is necessary for the proper functioning of muscle and nervous tissue. It is required as a *cofactor for approximately 90 enzymes. A good source of magnesium is green leafy vegetables. Symbol: Mg.

magnesium carbonate a weak *antacid used to relieve indigestion and also pain due to stomach and duodenal ulcers; it is also used as a mild laxative. It is usually given with other compounds in mixtures, powders, and tablets.

magnesium hydroxide a magnesium salt with effects and uses similar to those of *magnesium carbonate. Trade name: **Milk of Magnesia**.

magnesium sulphate a magnesium salt given in mixtures or enemas to treat constipation (*see* LAXATIVE). It is also administered by injection to treat magnesium deficiency.

magnesium trisilicate a compound of magnesium with antacid and absorbent properties, used in the treatment of peptic ulcers and other digestive disorders.

magnetic resonance imaging (MRI) a diagnostic technique based on analysis of the absorption and transmission of high-frequency radio waves by the water molecules in tissues placed in a strong magnetic field (*see* NUCLEAR MAGNETIC RESONANCE). Using modern high-speed computers, this analysis can be used to 'map out' the variation in tissue signals in any plane and thus produce images of the tissues. It is particularly useful for examining the central nervous system and musculoskeletal system, and to a lesser extent the chest and abdomen. MRI can be used for the noninvasive diagnosis and treatment planning of a wide range of diseases, including cancer; it has the advantage that it does not use potentially harmful ionizing radiation, such as X-rays.

   The **magnetic resonance therapy scanner**, which utilizes split magnets and rapid *real time imaging, enables interventional procedures to be performed with great accuracy under MRI control. *See* INTERVENTIONAL RADIOLOGY, MINIMALLY INVASIVE SURGERY.

magnetic resonance spectroscopy (MRS) a diagnostic technique that utilizes the phenomenon of *nuclear magnetic resonance to obtain a biochemical profile of tissues. It is particularly useful for biochemical analysis of tissues, especially muscle, that are otherwise difficult to investigate and would require a biopsy.

magnetic resonance therapy scanner *see* MAGNETIC RESONANCE IMAGING.

MAGPI operation meatal advancement and glanuloplasty operation: a simple surgical procedure designed to correct minor to moderate degrees of coronal or subcoronal *hypospadias. This single-stage operation corrects any associated minor degrees of *chordee and transfers the urethral opening to the glans.

MAI complex a group of bacteria comprising *Mycobacterium avium* and *M. intracellulare*, which are responsible for *opportunistic infections of the lung. *See* MYCOBACTERIUM.

mal *n.* illness or disease.

mal- *prefix denoting* disease, disorder, or abnormality.

malabsorption *n.* a state in which absorption of one or more substances by the small intestine is reduced. It most commonly affects fat (causing *steatorrhoea), some vitamins (such as B_{12}, folic acid, vitamin D, and vitamin K), *electrolytes (such as calcium, potassium), iron, and amino acids. Symptoms (depending on the substances involved) include weight loss, diarrhoea, anaemia, swelling (oedema), and vitamin deficiencies. The commonest causes are *coeliac disease, *pancreatitis, *cystic fibrosis, *blind loop syndrome, or surgical removal of a length of small intestine.

malacia *n.* abnormal softening of a part, organ, or tissue, such as bone (*see* OSTEOMALACIA).

-malacia *suffix denoting* abnormal softening of a tissue. Example: **keratomalacia** (of the cornea).

maladie de Roger (Roger's disease) a form of congenital heart disease in which there is a small *ventricular septal defect. It usually causes no symptoms. [H. L. Roger (1809–91), French physician]

malaise *n.* a general feeling of being unwell. The feeling may be accompanied by identifiable physical discomfort and may indicate the presence of disease.

malar bone *see* ZYGOMATIC BONE.

malaria (ague, marsh fever, periodic fever, paludism) *n.* an infectious disease due to the presence of parasitic protozoa of the genus *Plasmodium (P. falciparum, P. malariae, P. ovale,* or *P. vivax*) within the red blood cells. The disease is transmitted by the *Anopheles* mosquito and is confined mainly to tropical and subtropical areas.

Parasites in the blood of an infected person are taken into the stomach of the mosquito as it feeds. Here they multiply and then invade the salivary glands. When the mosquito bites an individual, parasites are injected into the bloodstream and migrate to the liver and other organs, where they multiply. After an incubation period varying from 12 days (*P. falciparum*) to 10 months (some varieties of *P. vivax*), parasites return to the bloodstream and invade the red blood cells. Rapid multiplication of the parasites results in destruction of the red cells and the release of more parasites capable of infecting other red cells. This

causes a short bout of shivering, fever, and sweating, and the loss of healthy red cells results in anaemia. When the next batch of parasites is released symptoms reappear. The interval between fever attacks varies in different types of malaria: in **quartan malaria** (or **fever**), caused by *P. malariae,* it is three days; in **tertian malaria** (*P. ovale* or *P. vivax*) two days; and in **malignant tertian** (or **quotidian**) **malaria** (*P. falciparum*) – the most severe kind – from a few hours to two days (*see also* BLACKWATER FEVER). Preventive and curative treatment includes such drugs as *chloroquine, *proguanil, *mefloquine, and *pyrimethamine. A vaccine is being tested.

malathion *n.* an organophosphorous insecticide used to treat head and pubic lice and scabies. It is applied externally in the form of a lotion; possible side-effects are skin irritation and allergic reactions. Trade names: **Derbac-M, Prioderm, Soleo-M.**

malformation *n.* any variation from the normal physical structure, due either to congenital or developmental defects or to disease or injury.

malignant *adj.* **1.** describing a tumour that invades and destroys the tissue in which it originates and can spread to other sites in the body via the bloodstream and lymphatic system. If untreated such tumours cause progressive deterioration and death. *See* CANCER. **2.** describing any disorder that becomes life-threatening if untreated (e.g. **malignant hypertension**). *Compare* BENIGN.

malignant melanoma (MM) *see* MELANOMA.

malingering *n.* pretending to be ill, usually in order to avoid work or gain attention. It may be a sign of mental disorder (*see also* MUNCHAUSEN'S SYNDROME).

malleolus *n.* either of the two protuberances on each side of the ankle: the **lateral malleolus** at the lower end of the *fibula or the **medial malleolus** at the lower end of the *tibia.

mallet finger a condition in which a finger (usually the index finger) is bent downwards at the tip, due to *avulsion of the long extensor tendon from the bone.

Treatment is to hold the tip of the finger straight with a splint for at least six weeks.

malleus *n.* a hammer-shaped bone in the middle *ear that articulates with the incus and is attached to the eardrum. *See* OSSICLE.

Mallory bodies large irregular masses located in the hepatocytes of the liver. They are found in patients with alcoholic hepatitis, Wilson's disease, primary biliary cirrhosis, severe obesity, and hepatocellular carcinoma. [F. B. Mallory (1862–1941), US pathologist]

Mallory's triple stain a histological stain consisting of water-soluble aniline blue or methyl blue, orange G, and oxalic acid. Before the stain is applied the tissue is mordanted, then treated with acid fuchsin and phosphomolybdic acid. Nuclei stain red, muscle red to orange, nervous tissue lilac, collagen dark blue, and mucus and connective tissue become blue. [F. B. Mallory]

Mallory-Weiss syndrome tearing of the tissues around the junction of the oesophagus (gullet) and stomach as a result of violent vomiting or straining to vomit. It is associated with *haematemesis and perforation of the oesophagus. [G. K. Mallory (1926–), US pathologist; S. Weiss (1899–1942), US physician]

malnutrition *n.* the condition caused by an improper balance between what an individual eats and what he requires to maintain health. This can result from eating too little (**subnutrition** or **starvation**) but may also imply dietary excess or an incorrect balance of basic foodstuffs such as protein, fat, and carbohydrate. A deficiency (or excess) of one or more minerals, vitamins, or other essential ingredients may arise from *malabsorption of digested food or metabolic malfunction of one or more parts of the body as well as from an unbalanced diet.

malocclusion *n.* a condition in which there is an abnormal arrangement of the teeth, either within one jaw or in one jaw in relation to the other. If severe, it may require *orthognathic surgery.

Malpighian body the part of a *nephron comprising the blood capillaries of the glomerulus and its surrounding Bowman's capsule. [M. Malpighi (1628–94), Italian anatomist]

Malpighian layer the stratum germinativum: one of the layers of the *epidermis.

malposition *n.* (in obstetrics) an abnormal position of the fetal head when this is the presenting part in labour. The head is in such a position that the diameter of the skull in relation to the pelvic opening is greater than normal. This is likely to result in a prolonged and complicated labour.

malpractice *n.* professional misconduct: treatment falling short of the standards of skill and care that can reasonably be expected from a qualified medical practitioner.

malpresentation *n.* the condition in which the presenting part of the fetus (*see* PRESENTATION) is other than the head. Malpresentation is likely to complicate labour and may necessitate delivery by *Caesarean section.

malt *n.* a mixture of carbohydrates, predominantly maltose, produced by the breakdown of starch contained in barley or wheat grains. The cereal grain is allowed to germinate and the malt is extracted with hot water. Malt is used for brewing and distilling; it has been used as a source of nutrients in wasting diseases.

MALT mucosa-associated lymphoid tissue: an important part of the peripheral lymphoid system with special features of immune cell production. It is associated with the digestive tract and is concentrated in such areas as the *tonsils and *Peyer's patches.

Malta fever *see* BRUCELLOSIS.

maltase *n.* an enzyme, present in saliva and pancreatic juice, that converts maltose into glucose during digestion.

maltose *n.* a sugar that consists of two molecules of glucose. Maltose is formed from the digestion of starch and glycogen and is found in germinating cereal seeds.

malunion *n.* deformity of a bone resulting from *union of a fracture in which the bone ends are poorly aligned. Arthritis of adjoining joints may develop as a complication later. *Osteotomy may be needed to correct the deformity and prevent the complication.

mamilla *n. see* NIPPLE.

mamillary bodies two paired rounded swellings in the floor of the *hypothalamus, immediately behind the pituitary gland.

mamma *n. see* BREAST.

mammary gland the milk-producing gland of female mammals. *See* BREAST.

mammography *n.* X-ray examination of the female breast. Using low-energy X-rays, fine details of breast tissue can be visualized, particularly the presence of calcification or soft tissue masses enabling the early diagnosis of breast cancer. *See also* FORREST SCREENING.

mammoplasty *n.* plastic surgery of the breasts, in order to alter their shape or increase or decrease their size. In the case of sagging breasts skin and glandular tissue are removed and the remaining breast tissue is fixed in the normal position. After a mastectomy, or when the breasts are too small, a prosthesis (*see* BREAST IMPLANT) may be inserted to improve the contour.

mammothermography *n.* the technique of examining the breasts for the presence of abnormalities by *thermography.

M-AMSA (amsacrine) *n.* a *cytotoxic drug undergoing evaluation in the treatment of malignant disease. Side-effects include marrow suppression.

Manchester operation *see* DONALD-FOTHERGILL OPERATION.

mancinism *n.* the condition of being left-handed.

mandelic acid a drug that prevents bacterial growth and was formerly used (in the form of the ammonium or calcium salt) to treat infections of the urinary system (it has now largely been replaced by antibiotics). Mandelic acid is administered as a catheter solution.

mandible *n.* the lower jawbone. It consists of a horseshoe-shaped **body**, the upper surface of which bears the lower

teeth (*see* ALVEOLUS), and two vertical parts (**rami**). Each ramus divides into a **condyle** and a *coronoid process. The condyle articulates with the temporal bone of the cranium to form the **temporomandibular joint** (a hinge joint). *See also* MAXILLA, SKULL. —**mandibular** *adj.*

manganese *n.* a greyish metallic element, the oxide of which, when inhaled by miners in underventilated mines, causes brain damage and symptoms very similar to those of *parkinsonism. Minute quantities of the element are required by the body (*see* TRACE ELEMENT). Symbol: Mn.

mania *n.* a state of mind characterized by excessive cheerfulness and increased activity. The mood is euphoric and changes rapidly to irritability. Thought and speech are rapid to the point of incoherence and the connections between ideas may be impossible to follow. Behaviour is also overactive, extravagant, overbearing, and sometimes violent. Judgment is impaired, and therefore the sufferer may damage his own interests. There may be grandiose delusions. Treatment is usually with drugs, such as lithium or phenothiazines, and hospital admission is frequently necessary. *See also* AFFECTIVE DISORDER, MANIC-DEPRESSIVE PSYCHOSIS. —**manic** *adj.*

-mania *suffix denoting* obsession, compulsion, or exaggerated feeling for. Example: **pyromania** (for starting fires).

manic-depressive psychosis (bipolar disorder) a severe mental illness causing repeated episodes of *depression, *mania, or both. These episodes can be precipitated by upsetting events but are out of proportion to these causes. Sometimes chronic depression or chronic mania can result. There is a genetically inherited predisposition to the illness. Treatment is with *phenothiazine drugs for mania, and *antidepressant drugs or, in severe cases, *electroconvulsive therapy for depression. *Lithium and carbamazepine can prevent or reduce the frequency and severity of attacks, and the sufferer is usually well in the intervals between them.

manikin *n. see* HOMUNCULUS.

manipulation *n.* the use of the hands to produce a desired movement or therapeutic effect in part of the body. Both physiotherapists and osteopaths use manipulation to restore normal working to stiff joints.

mannitol *n.* a *diuretic administered by injection to supplement other diuretics in the treatment of fluid retention (oedema), to treat some kidney disorders, and to relieve pressure in brain injuries. Headache, chest pain, and dry mouth may occur following injection.

Mann-Whitney U test *see* SIGNIFICANCE.

manometer *n.* a device for measuring pressure in a liquid or gas. A manometer often consists of a U-tube containing mercury, water, or other liquid, open at one end and exposed to the fluid under pressure at the other end. The pressure can be read directly from a graduated scale. *See also* SPHYGMOMANOMETER.

manometry *n.* measurement of pressures within organs of the body. The technique is used to record changes within fluid-filled chambers (e.g. cerebral ventricles) or to indicate muscular activity in motile tubes, such as the oesophagus, rectum, or bile duct.

mantle *adj.* (in radiotherapy) *see* FIELD.

Mantoux test *see* TUBERCULIN. [C. Mantoux (1877–1947), French physician]

manubrium *n.* (*pl.* **manubria**) **1.** the upper section of the breastbone (*see* STERNUM). It articulates with the clavicles and the first costal cartilage; the second costal cartilage articulates at the junction between the manubrium and body of the sternum. **2.** the handle-like part of the *malleus (an ear ossicle), attached to the eardrum. —**manubrial** *adj.*

MAO *see* MONOAMINE OXIDASE.

MAO inhibitor a drug that prevents the activity of the enzyme *monoamine oxidase (MAO) in brain tissue and therefore affects mood. MAO inhibitors include isocarboxazid, *phenelzine, and *tranylcypromine. These drugs are *antidepressants, whose use is now restricted because of the severity of their side-effects. These include interactions with other drugs (e.g. ephedrine, amphetamine) and with foods containing *tyramine (e.g. cheese) to produce a sudden increase in blood pressure. *See also* MOCLOBEMIDE, SELEGILINE.

maple syrup urine disease an inborn defect of amino acid metabolism causing an excess of valine, leucine, isoleucine, and alloisoleucine in the urine, which has an odour like maple syrup. Treatment is dietary; if untreated, the condition leads to mental retardation and death in infancy.

maprotiline *n.* a drug used to treat all types of depression, including that associated with anxiety (*see* ANTIDEPRESSANT). It is administered by mouth and may cause drowsiness, dizziness, and tremor. Trade name: **Ludiomil**.

marasmus *n.* severe wasting in infants, when body weight is below 75% of that expected for age. The infant looks 'old', pallid, apathetic, lacks skin fat, and has subnormal temperature. The condition may be due to *malabsorption, wrong feeding, metabolic disorders, repeated vomiting, diarrhoea, severe disease of the heart, lungs, kidneys, or urinary tract, or chronic bacterial or parasitic disease (especially in tropical climates). Maternal rejection of an infant may cause marasmus through undereating. Acute infection may precipitate death. Treatment depends on the underlying cause, but initially very gentle nursing and the provision of nourishment and fluids by gradual steps is appropriate for all.

marble-bone disease *see* OSTEOPETROSIS.

Marburg disease (green monkey disease) a virus disease of vervet (green) monkeys transmitted to man by contact (usually in laboratories) with blood or tissues from an infected animal. It was first described in Marburg, Germany. Symptoms include fever, malaise, severe headache, vomiting, diarrhoea and bleeding from mucous membranes in the mouth and elsewhere. Treatment with antiserum and measures to reduce the bleeding are sometimes effective.

march fracture a fracture through the neck of the second or third metatarsal bone, associated with excessive walking.

Marcus Gunn jaw-winking syndrome a congenital condition characterized by drooping (*ptosis) of one eyelid. On opening or moving the mouth, the droopy lid elevates momentarily, resembling a wink. It is believed to be due to an abnormal innervation of the levator muscle by the trigeminal nerve. [R. Marcus Gunn (1850–1909), British ophthalmologist]

Marfan's syndrome an inherited disorder of connective tissue characterized by excessive tallness, abnormally long and slender fingers and toes (**arachnodactyly**), heart defects, and partial dislocation of the lenses of the eyes. [B. J. A. Marfan (1858–1942), French physician]

marijuana *n. see* CANNABIS.

Marion's disease obstruction of the outlet of the bladder caused by enlargement of the muscle cells in the neck of the bladder. [J. B. C. G. Marion (1869–1960), French surgeon]

Marjolin's ulcer a carcinoma that develops at the edge of a chronic *ulcer of the skin, usually a venous ulcer in the ankle region. [J. N. Marjolin (1780–1850), French surgeon]

marrow *n. see* BONE MARROW.

marsupialization *n.* an operative technique for curing a cyst. The cyst is opened, its contents removed, and the edges then stitched to the skin incision. The wound is kept open until it has healed by *granulation.

masculinization *n.* development of excess body and facial hair, deepening of the voice, and increase in muscle bulk (secondary male sexual characteristics) in a female due to a hormone disorder or to hormone therapy. *See also* VIRILISM, VIRILIZATION.

masochism *n.* sexual pleasure derived from the experience of pain. The word is sometimes used loosely for all forms of behaviour that lead to pain or humiliation. *See* SEXUAL DEVIATION. **—masochist** *n.* **—masochistic** *adj.*

massage *n.* manipulation of the soft tissues of the body with the hands. Massage is used to improve circulation, reduce oedema where present, prevent *adhesions in tissues after injury, reduce muscular spasm, and improve the tone of muscles. *See also* EFFLEURAGE, PETRISSAGE, TAPOTEMENT.

masseter *n.* a thick muscle in the cheek

extending from the zygomatic arch to the outer corner of the mandible. It is important for mastication and acts by closing the jaws.

mast- (masto-) *prefix denoting* the breast.

mastalgia *n.* pain in the breast.

mast cell a large cell in *connective tissue with many coarse cytoplasmic granules. These granules contain the chemicals *heparin, *histamine, and *serotonin, which are released during inflammation and allergic responses.

mastectomy *n.* surgical removal of a breast. **Simple mastectomy**, performed for extensive but not necessarily invasive tumours, involves simple removal of the breast; the skin and if possible the nipple may be retained and a prosthesis (*see* BREAST IMPLANT) may be inserted under the skin to give the appearance of normality. When breast cancer has spread to involve the lymph nodes, **radical mastectomy** may be performed. This classically involves removal of the breast with the skin and underlying pectoral muscles together with all the lymphatic tissue of the armpit. This treatment may be followed up with radiotherapy and/or chemotherapy. In modern surgical practice a modified radical mastectomy, preserving the pectoral muscles, is more usual than the classical technique. *See also* LUMPECTOMY.

mastication *n.* the process of chewing food.

mastitis *n.* inflammation of the breast, usually caused by bacterial infection via damaged nipples. It most often occurs as acute **puerperal mastitis**, which develops during the period of breast-feeding, about a month after childbirth, and sometimes involves the discharge of pus. Chronic **cystic mastitis** has a different cause and does not involve inflammation. The breast feels lumpy due to the presence of cysts, and the condition is thought to be caused by hormone imbalance.

mastoid *n.* the *mastoid process of the temporal bone. *See also* MASTOIDITIS.

mastoidectomy *n.* an operation to remove some or all of the air cells in the bone behind the ear (the *mastoid process of the temporal bone) when they have become infected (*see* MASTOIDITIS) or invaded by *cholesteatoma. *See also* ATTICOTOMY.

mastoiditis *n.* inflammation of the *mastoid process behind the ear and of the air space (**mastoid antrum**) connecting it to the cavity of the middle ear. It is usually caused by bacterial infection that spreads from the middle ear (*see* OTITIS (MEDIA)). Usually the infection responds to antibiotics, but surgery (*see* MASTOIDECTOMY) may be required in severe cases.

mastoid process a nipple-shaped process on the *temporal bone that extends downward and forward behind the ear canal and is the point of attachment of several neck muscles. It contains many air spaces (**mastoid cells**), which communicate with the cavity of the middle ear via an air-filled channel, the **mastoid antrum**. This provides a possible route for the spread of infection from the middle ear (*see* MASTOIDITIS).

masturbation *n.* physical self-stimulation of the male or female external genital organs in order to produce sexual pleasure, which may result in orgasm.

matched pair study *see* CASE CONTROL STUDY.

materia medica the study of drugs used in medicine and dentistry, including *pharmacognosy, *pharmacy, *pharmacology, and therapeutics.

maternal mortality rate the number of deaths due to complications of pregnancy, childbirth, and the puerperium expressed as a proportion of all births (i.e. including *stillbirths). Formerly the rate was expressed per 1000 births but with the low levels currently reported it is customary to use a base of a 100,000 births. Concern with maternal mortality resulted in Britain in a special confidential enquiry being held into every such death to try and pinpoint the possible shortfall in resources or care.

matrix *n.* **1.** (in histology) the substance of a tissue or organ in which more specialized structures are embedded; for example, the ground substance of connective tissue. **2.** (in radiology) the division of an image into rows and columns with equally sized elements (*pixels). The final image is completed by assigning a density to each of these elements. Increasing the number of pixels in the matrix improves the resolution of the final image. A typical value could be 256 rows × 256 columns.

matrix band a flexible strip that is placed round a tooth to restore a wall, thus simplifying insertion of a dental filling.

maturation *n.* the process of attaining full development. The term is applied particularly to the development of mature germ cells (ova and sperm).

maxilla *n.* (*pl.* **maxillae**) loosely, the upper jaw, which bears the upper teeth. Strictly, the maxilla is one of a pair of bones that partly form the upper jaw, the outer walls of the maxillary sinus, and the floor of the orbit. *See also* MANDIBLE, SKULL. —**maxillary** *adj.*

maxillary sinus (maxillary antrum) *see* PARANASAL SINUSES.

maxillofacial *adj.* describing or relating to the region of the face, jaws, and related structures.

maxwell *n.* a unit of magnetic flux equal to a flux of 1 gauss per square centimetre.

Mayo operation an overlapping repair of an umbilical hernia. [W. J. Mayo (1861–1939), US surgeon]

mazindol *n.* a drug that reduces the appetite and is used in the treatment of obesity. It is administered by mouth and may cause constipation, dry mouth, and insomnia. Trade name: **Teronac**.

McArdle's disease an *inborn error of metabolism in which a deficiency of the enzyme myophosphorylase prevents the breakdown of glycogen to lactate in exercising muscle. This results in fatigue, pain, and cramps in exercising muscles. The only treatment is avoidance of sustained or excessive exercise. [B. McArdle (20th century), British biochemist]

McBurney's point the point on the abdomen that overlies the anatomical position of the appendix and is the site of maximum tenderness in acute appendicitis. It lies one-third of the way along a line drawn from the anterior superior iliac spine (the projecting part of the hipbone) to the umbilicus. [C. McBurney (1845–1913), US surgeon]

McCormick toy test a hearing test used in preschool children in which the child must discriminate between similar speech sounds. The test consists of 14 toys that are paired because their names rhyme; for example, tree and key, plane and plate. Having first identified all the objects, the child is then asked in a quiet voice to indicate a particular toy (e.g. Can you find the key?).

MCU micturating cystourethrogram. *See* URETHROGRAPHY.

ME myalgic encephalomyelitis. *See* CHRONIC FATIGUE SYNDROME.

meals on wheels *see* SOCIAL SERVICES.

mean (arithmetic mean) *n.* the average of a group of observations calculated by adding their values and dividing by the number in the group. When one or more observations are substantially different from the rest, which can influence the arithmetic mean unduly, it is preferable to use the **geometric mean** (a similar calculation based on the logarithmic values of the observations) or – more commonly – the **median** (the middle observation of the series arranged in ascending order). A further method of obtaining an average value of a group is to identify the **mode** – the observation (or group of observations when these occur as a continuous quantitative *variable) that occurs most often in the series.

measles *n.* a highly infectious virus disease that tends to appear in epidemics every 2–3 years and mainly affects children. After an incubation period of 8–15 days, symptoms resembling those of a cold develop accompanied by a high fever. Small red spots with white centres (**Koplik's spots**) may appear on the inside of the cheeks. On the third to fifth day a blotchy slightly elevated pink rash develops, first behind the ears then on the face and elsewhere; it lasts 3–5 days. The patient is infectious throughout this period. In most cases the symptoms soon subside but patients are susceptible to pneumonia and middle ear infections. Complete recovery may take 2–4 weeks. Severe complica-

tions include encephalitis (one in 1000 cases) and *subacute sclerosing panencephalitis. Measles is a common cause of childhood mortality in malnourished children, particularly in the developing world. Vaccination against measles provides effective immunity (*see* MMR VACCINE). Medical names: **rubeola**, **morbilli**.

meat- (meato-) *prefix denoting* a meatus. Example: **meatotomy** (incision into the urethral meatus).

meatus *n.* (in anatomy) a passage or opening. The **auditory meatus** is the passage leading from the pinna of the outer *ear to the eardrum. A **nasal meatus** is one of three groovelike parts of the nasal cavity beneath each of the nasal conchae. The **urethral meatus** is the external opening of the urethra.

mebendazole *n.* an *anthelmintic drug used to get rid of roundworms, hookworms, threadworms, and whipworms. Side-effects may include stomach upsets. Trade name: **Vermox**. *See also* IMIDAZOLE.

mebhydrolin *n.* an *antihistamine drug used to treat allergic conditions, such as hay fever and urticaria. Trade name: **Fabahistin**.

mechanoreceptor *n.* a group of cells that respond to mechanical distortion, such as that caused by stretching or compressing a tissue, by generating a nerve impulse in a sensory nerve (*see* RECEPTOR). Touch receptors, *proprioceptors, and the receptors for hearing and balance all belong to this class.

mechanotherapy *n.* the use of mechanical equipment during physiotherapy to produce regularly repeated movements in part of the body. This is done to improve the functioning of muscles and joints.

Meckel's cartilage a cartilaginous bar in the fetus around which the *mandible develops. Part of Meckel's cartilage develops into the malleus (an ear ossicle) in the adult. [J. F. Meckel, the Younger (1781–1833), German anatomist]

Meckel's diverticulum *see* DIVERTICULUM.

meclozine *n.* an *antihistamine drug used mainly to prevent and treat nausea and vomiting, particularly in motion sickness, and also to relieve allergic reactions. It is administered by mouth.

meconism *n.* poisoning from the effects of eating or smoking *opium or the products derived from it, especially *morphine.

meconium *n.* the first stools of a newborn baby, which are sticky and dark green and composed of cellular debris, mucus, and bile pigments. The presence of meconium in the amniotic fluid during labour indicates fetal distress. *See also* (MECONIUM) ILEUS, (MECONIUM) PERITONITIS.

media (tunica media) *n.* **1.** the middle layer of the wall of a *vein or *artery. It is the thickest of the three layers, being composed of elastic fibres and smooth muscle fibres in alternating layers. **2.** the middle layer of various other organs or parts.

medial *adj.* relating to or situated in the central region of an organ, tissue, or the body.

median *adj.* **1.** (in anatomy) situated in or towards the plane that divides the body into right and left halves. **2.** (in statistics) *see* MEAN.

mediastinitis *n.* inflammation of the midline partition of the chest cavity (mediastinum), usually complicating a rupture of the oesophagus (gullet). **Sclerosing mediastinitis** often leads to *fibrosis, which may cause compression of other structures in the thorax, such as the superior vena cava, the bronchial tree, or the oesophagus.

mediastinoscopy *n.* examination of the *mediastinum, usually by means of an endoscope inserted through a small incision in the neck region. It can be used to assess the spread of intrathoracic tumours and for lymph node biopsy.

mediastinum *n.* the space in the thorax (chest cavity) between the two pleural sacs. The mediastinum contains the heart, aorta, trachea, oesophagus, and thymus gland and is divided into anterior, middle, posterior, and superior regions.

medical *adj.* **1.** of or relating to medicine, the diagnosis, treatment and prevention of disease. **2.** of or relating to conditions that require the attention of a

physician rather than a surgeon. For example, a **medical ward** of a hospital accommodates patients with such conditions.

medical assistant a health service worker who is not a registered medical practitioner (often a nurse or an ex-serviceman with experience as a senior medical orderly) working in association with a doctor to undertake minor treatments and preliminary assessments. In poorer countries, particularly in rural areas where qualified resources are short (e.g. China), agricultural workers receive limited training in health care and continue in a dual role as **barefoot doctors**; elsewhere, limited training concentrates more on environmental issues: the workers so trained are known as **sanitarians**.

medical audit a process by which doctors systematically review the procedures used for diagnosis, care, and treatment, examining how associated resources are used and investigating the effect care has on the outcome and quality of life for the patient. When this process is undertaken by doctors, nurses, and other health-care professionals, it is referred to as **clinical audit**.

medical certificate a certificate stating a doctor's diagnosis of a patient's medical condition, disability, or fitness to work.

medical committee **1.** (in a hospital) a group of doctors of consultant grade (some or all of the consultants on the hospital staff) who give medical viewpoints on affairs concerned with overall policies on patient care, resource allocation, and the running of the hospital. Representatives of other hospital professions (nursing, administration, planning, and junior doctors) are usually in attendance. It is generally divided into those specialist subgroups representing the broad divisions of hospital practice (medical, surgical, paediatric, etc.). Usually the chairmen of divisions form an executive committee for day-to-day decisions that are ratified at less frequent meetings of the medical committee. **2.** (**local medical committee**) (in Britain) a group of representatives of the general practitioners under contract with a single Health Authority. The members act as spokesmen for the local practitioners, by whom they are elected. Similar arrangements and responsibilities apply for the dentists, pharmacists, and opticians practising in the NHS outside hospitals.

medical jurisprudence the study or practice of the legal aspects of medicine. *See* FORENSIC MEDICINE.

Medical Officer of Health (formerly in Britain) the chief health executive of local government. The title is still used in many countries. *See* PUBLIC HEALTH PHYSICIAN.

Medical Research Council (MRC) a government-supported body that is an important source of funds for medical research.

medical social worker a social worker employed to assist patients with domestic problems that may arise through illness. *See also* SOCIAL SERVICES.

medicated *adj.* containing a medicinal drug: applied to lotions, soaps, sweets, etc.

medication *n.* **1.** a substance administered by mouth, applied to the body, or introduced into the body for the purpose of treatment. Medicated dressings are applied to wounds to prevent infection and allow normal healing. *See also* PREMEDICATION. **2.** treatment of a patient using drugs.

medicine *n.* **1.** the science or practice of the diagnosis, treatment, and prevention of disease. **2.** the science or practice of nonsurgical methods of treating disease. **3.** any drug or preparation used for the treatment or prevention of disease, particularly a drug that is taken by mouth.

medicochirurgical *adj.* of or describing matters that are related to both medicine and surgery. A medicochirurgical disorder is one that calls for treatment by both a physician and a surgeon.

medicolegal *adj.* relating to the legal aspects of the practice of medicine. There has been rapid expansion of the branch of the law relating to medicine due to the increasing number of court actions for accidents and injuries, many of them seeking compensation for negligence by doctors or hospitals.

Mediterranean fever **1.** *see* BRUCELLOSIS. **2.** *see* POLYSEROSITIS.

medium *n.* **1.** any substance, usually a broth, agar, or gelatin, used for the *culture of microorganisms or tissue cells. An **assay medium** is used to determine the concentration of a growth factor or chemical by measuring the amount of growth it produces in a particular microorganism; all other nutrients are present in amounts adequate for growth. **2.** *see* CONTRAST MEDIUM.

medroxyprogesterone *n.* a synthetic female sex hormone (*see* PROGESTOGEN) used to treat menstrual disorders, including amenorrhoea, to prevent miscarriage, and (in combination with an oestrogen) in *oral contraceptives. It is administered by mouth or injection. Trade names: **Farlutal**, **Provera**.

medulla *n.* **1.** the inner region of any organ or tissue when it is distinguishable from the outer region (the cortex), particularly the inner part of the kidney, adrenal glands, or lymph nodes. **2.** *see* MEDULLA OBLONGATA. **3.** the *myelin layer of certain nerve fibres. —**medullary** *adj.*

medulla oblongata (myelencephalon) the extension within the skull of the upper end of the spinal cord, forming the lowest part of the *brainstem. Besides forming the major pathway for nerve impulses entering and leaving the skull, the medulla contains centres that are responsible for the regulation of the heart and blood vessels, respiration, salivation, and swallowing. *Cranial nerves VI–XII leave the brain in this region.

medullary carcinoma a tumour whose consistency was thought to resemble that of bone marrow. **Medullary carcinoma of the thyroid** has associations with tumours of other organs (multiple endocrine neoplasia; *see* MENS) and is often familial: it arises from the *C cells of the thyroid and produces calcitonin.

medullated (myelinated) nerve fibre any nerve fibre that has a sheath of *myelin surrounding and insulating its axon.

medulloblastoma *n.* a malignant brain tumour (*see* CEREBRAL TUMOUR) that occurs during childhood. It is derived from cells

that have the apparent potential to mature into neurones and develops in the cerebellum, the part of the brain that is predominantly involved in the control of balance. The flow of cerebrospinal fluid (CSF) may become obstructed, causing *hydrocephalus. Symptoms include headaches, dizziness, and unsteadiness. Treatment involves surgery to remove most of the tumour and restore CSF flow, followed by radiotherapy directed using *stereotactic localization.
Medulloblastoma is the second most common form of cancer of childhood (after leukaemia); recent advances have improved the survival rate so that 40% of affected children live for more than five years.

mefenamic acid an anti-inflammatory drug (see NSAID) used to treat headache, toothache, rheumatic pain, and similar conditions. It is administered by mouth; side-effects include digestive upsets, drowsiness, and skin rashes. Trade name: **Ponstan**.

mefloquine n. a drug used in the prevention and treatment of malaria that is resistant to other drugs. It is administered by mouth; side-effects can include dizziness, rash, gastrointestinal problems, and psychological disturbances, and the drug should not be taken during pregnancy, by psychiatric patients, or with beta blockers. Trade name: **Lariam**.

mefruside n. a thiazide-like *diuretic used to treat high blood pressure and get rid of excess body fluid. It is administered by mouth. Possible side-effects include nausea and indigestion. Trade name: **Baycaron**.

mega- prefix denoting **1.** large size, or abnormal enlargement or distension. Example: **megacaecum** (of the caecum). **2.** a million. Example: **megavolt** (a million volts).

megacolon n. dilatation, and sometimes lengthening, of the colon. It is caused by obstruction of the colon, *Hirschsprung's disease, or longstanding constipation, or it may occur as a complication of ulcerative *colitis (**toxic megacolon**).

megakaryoblast n. a cell that gives rise to the platelet-forming cell *megakaryo-

cyte, found in the blood-forming tissue of the bone marrow. It is derived from a *haemopoietic stem cell and matures via an intermediate stage (**promegakaryocyte**) into a megakaryocyte.

megakaryocyte n. a cell in the bone marrow that produces *platelets. It is large (35–160 μm in diameter), with an irregular multilobed nucleus, and with *Romanowsky stains its abundant cytoplasm appears pale blue with fine reddish granules. See also THROMBOPOIESIS.

megal- (megalo-) prefix denoting abnormal enlargement. Example: **megalomelia** (of limbs).

megaloblast n. an abnormal form of any of the cells that are precursors of red blood cells (see ERYTHROBLAST). Megaloblasts are unusually large and their nuclei fail to mature in the normal way; they are seen in the bone marrow in certain anaemias (**megaloblastic anaemias**) due to deficiency of vitamin B_{12} or folic acid. —**megaloblastic** adj.

megalocephaly n. **1.** see MACROCEPHALY. **2.** overgrowth and distortion of skull bones (see LEONTIASIS).

megalocyte n. see MACROCYTE.

megalomania n. delusions of grandeur, such as being God, royalty, etc. It may be a feature of a schizophrenic or manic illness or of cerebral syphilis.

-megaly suffix denoting abnormal enlargement. Example: **splenomegaly** (of spleen).

megaureter n. gross dilatation of the *ureter. This occurs above the site of a long-standing obstruction in the ureter, which blocks the free flow of urine from the kidney. A common cause of megaureter is reflux of urine from the bladder into the ureters (see VESICOURETERIC REFLUX), but some of the most striking examples are found in so-called **idiopathic megaureter**. In this condition, which may affect one or both ureters, there is a segment of normal ureter of varying length at the extreme lower end of the bladder, above which the ureter is enormously dilated. Both reflux and idiopathic megaureter progress to urinary infection and/or renal impairment. Treatment is by corrective surgery.

megestrol *n.* a synthetic female sex hormone (*see* PROGESTOGEN) that is used in the treatment of metastatic breast cancer and metastatic endometrial cancer. Trade name: **Megace**.

meibomian cyst *n.* *see* CHALAZION.

meibomian glands (tarsal glands) small sebaceous glands that lie under the conjunctiva of the eyelids.

meibomianitis *n.* inflammation of the *meibomian glands of the eyelids.

meiosis (reduction division) *n.* a type of cell division that produces four daughter cells, each having half the number of chromosomes of the original cell. It occurs before the formation of sperm and ova and the normal (*diploid) number of chromosomes is restored after fertilization. Meiosis also produces genetic variation in the daughter cells, brought about by the process of *crossing over. Meiosis consists of two successive divisions, each divided into four stages (*see* PROPHASE, METAPHASE, ANAPHASE, TELOPHASE). (See illustration.) *Compare* MITOSIS. —**meiotic** *adj.*

Meissner's plexus (submucous plexus) a fine network of parasympathetic nerve fibres in the wall of the alimentary canal, supplying the muscles and mucous membrane. [G. Meissner (1829–1905), German physiologist]

melaena *n.* black tarry faeces due to the presence of partly digested blood from higher up the digestive tract. Melaena is not apparent unless at least 500 ml of blood has entered the gut. It often occurs after vomiting blood (*see* HAEMATEMESIS), having the same causes, but may be due to disease in the small intestine or upper colon, such as carcinoma or *angiodysplasia. *See also* HAEMORRHAGIC DISEASE OF THE NEWBORN (MELAENA NEONATORUM).

melan- (melano-) *prefix denoting* **1.** black coloration. **2.** melanin. Example: **melanaemia** (the presence in the blood of melanin).

melancholia *n.* *see* DEPRESSION, INVOLUTIONAL MELANCHOLIA.

melanin *n.* a dark-brown to black pigment occurring in the hair, the skin, and in the iris and choroid layer of the eyes. Melanin is contained within special cells

Prophase I leptotene

cytoplasm
chromosome — centriole
cell membrane — nuclear membrane

zygotene to pachytene

bivalent of homologous chromosomes

diplotene to diakinesis

chiasma

Metaphase I

one chromosome of each pair goes to each pole

Anaphase I

Telophase I

Metaphase II to Anaphase II

chromatids separate

Telophase II

four haploid nuclei

Stages in meiosis

(**chromatophores** or **melanophores**) and is produced by the metabolism of the amino acid tyrosine. Production of melanin by **melanocytes** in the epidermis of the skin is increased by the action of sunlight (producing tanning), which protects the underlying skin layers from the sun's radiation.

melanism (melanosis) *n.* an unusually pronounced darkening of body tissues caused by excessive production of the pigment *melanin. For example, melanism may affect the hair, the skin (after sunburn, during pregnancy, or in *Addison's disease), or the eye.

melanocyte *n.* any one of the cells, concentrated within the epidermis of skin, that produces the dark brown pigment *melanin.

melanocyte-stimulating hormone (MSH) a hormone synthesized and released by the pituitary gland. In amphibians MSH brings about colour changes in the skin but its physiological role in man is uncertain.

melanoma (malignant melanoma, MM) *n.* a highly malignant tumour of melanin-forming cells, the *melanocytes. Such tumours usually occur in the skin (excessive exposure to sunlight is a contributory factor) but are also found in the eye and the mucous membranes. They may contain melanin or be free of pigment (**amelanotic melanomas**). Spread of this cancer to other parts of the body, especially to the lymph nodes and liver, is common. In these cases melanin or its precursors (**melanogens**) may be excreted in the urine and the whole of the skin may be deeply pigmented. The prognosis is inversely related to the thickness of the tumour; almost all patients with tumours less than 0.76 mm survive following surgical excision.

melanonychia *n.* blackening of the nails with the pigment *melanin.

melanophore *n.* see MELANIN.

melanoplakia *n.* pigmented areas of *melanin in the mucous membrane lining the inside of the cheeks.

melanosis *n.* **1.** see MELANISM. **2.** a disorder in the body's production of the pig-

ment melanin. **3.** *cachexia associated with the spread of the skin cancer *melanoma. —**melanotic** *adj.*

melanuria *n.* the presence of dark pigment in the urine. This may be caused by the presence of melanin or its precursors, in some cases of *melanoma; it may alternatively be caused by metabolic disease, such as *porphyria.

melasma *n.* see CHLOASMA.

melatonin *n.* a hormone produced by the *pineal gland in darkness but not in bright light. Melatonin receptors in the brain, in a nucleus immediately above the *optic chiasma, react to this hormone and synchronize the nucleus to the 24-hour day/night rhythm, thus informing the brain when it is day and when it is night. Melatonin is a derivative of *serotonin, with which it works to regulate the sleep cycle, and is being used experimentally to treat jet lag, *SADS, and insomnia in shift workers and the elderly.

melioidosis *n.* a disease of wild rodents caused by the bacterium *Pseudomonas pseudomallei*. It can be transmitted to man, possibly by rat fleas, causing pneumonia, multiple abscesses, and septicaemia. It is often fatal.

Melkersson-Rosenthal syndrome a rare disorder characterized by the occurrence together of facial paralysis, enlargement of the glottis, and swollen lips, which is due to lymphatic *stasis and the consequent build-up of protein in the facial tissues. [E. Melkersson (1898–1932), Swedish physician; C. Rosenthal (20th century), German neurologist]

melomelus *n.* a fetus with one or more pairs of supernumery limbs.

melphalan *n.* a drug used to treat various types of cancer, including malignant melanoma, tumours of the breast and ovaries, and Hodgkin's disease. It is administered by mouth or injection. Side-effects include digestive upsets, mouth ulcers, and temporary hair loss. Trade name: **Alkeran.**

membrane *n.* **1.** a thin layer of tissue surrounding the whole or part of an organ or tissue lining a cavity, or separating adjacent structures or cavities. *See also*

BASEMENT MEMBRANE, MUCOUS MEMBRANE, SEROUS MEMBRANE. **2.** the lipoprotein envelope surrounding a cell (**plasma** or **cell membrane**). —**membranous** *adj.*

membrane bone a bone that develops in connective tissue by direct *ossification, without cartilage being formed first. The bones of the face and skull are membrane bones.

membranous labyrinth *see* LABYRINTH.

MEN multiple endocrine neoplasia. *See* MENS.

men- (meno-) *prefix denoting* menstruation.

menarche *n.* the start of the menstrual periods and other physical and mental changes associated with puberty. The menarche occurs when the reproductive organs become functionally active and may take place at any time between 10 and 18 years of age.

MENCAP a British voluntary association that promotes the welfare of the mentally handicapped and their families, through education, campaigning, and the provision of resources for projects.

mendelism *n.* the theory of inheritance based on *Mendel's laws.

Mendel's laws rules of inheritance based on the breeding experiments of the Austrian monk Gregor Mendel (1822–84), which showed that the inheritance of characteristics is controlled by particles now known as *genes. In modern terms they are as follows. (1) Each body (somatic) cell of an individual carries two factors (genes) for every characteristic and each gamete carries only one. It is now known that the genes are arranged on chromosomes, which are present in pairs in somatic cells and separate during gamete formation by the process of *meiosis. (2) Each pair of factors segregates independently of all other pairs at meiosis, so that the gametes show all possible combinations of factors. This law applies only to genes on different chromosomes; those on the same chromosome are affected by *linkage. *See also* DOMINANT, RECESSIVE.

Mendelson's syndrome inhalation of regurgitated stomach contents by an anaesthetized patient, which may result in death from anoxia or cause extensive lung damage or pulmonary *oedema with severe *bronchospasm. It is a well-recognized hazard of general anaesthesia in obstetrics and may be prevented by giving gastric-acid inhibitors (e.g. *cimetidine or *ranitidine) or sodium citrate before inducing anaesthesia. [C. L. Mendelson (1913–), US obstetrician]

Ménétrier's disease a disorder in which gross enlargement (*see* HYPERTROPHY) of the cells of the mucous membrane lining the stomach is associated with anaemia. [P. Ménétrier (1859–1935), French physician]

Ménière's disease a disease of the inner ear characterized by episodes of deafness, buzzing in the ears (*tinnitus), and *vertigo. Typically the attacks are preceded by a sensation of fullness in the ear. Symptoms last for several hours and between attacks the affected ear may return to normal, although hearing does tend to deteriorate gradually with repeated attacks. It is thought to be caused by the build-up of fluid in the inner ear. Drug treatments include *prochlorperazine to reduce vertigo in acute attacks and *betahistine as prophylactic treatment. Ototoxic drugs, such as *gentamicin, can be injected through the eardrum into the middle ear to reduce activity in the inner ear. Surgical procedures used include *grommet insertion, decompression or drainage of the *endolymphatic sac, *vestibular nerve section, and *labyrinthectomy. Medical name: **endolymphatic hydrops**. [P. Ménière (1799–1862), French physician]

mening- (meningo-) *prefix denoting* the meninges.

meninges *pl. n.* (*sing.* **meninx**) the three connective tissue membranes that line the skull and vertebral canal and enclose the brain and spinal cord (see illustration). The outermost layer – the *dura mater (pachymeninx) – is inelastic, tough, and thicker than the middle layer (the *arachnoid mater) and the innermost layer (the *pia mater). The inner two membranes are together called the **leptomeninges**; between them circulates the *cerebrospinal fluid.

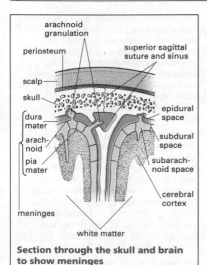

arachnoid
granulation

periosteum

superior sagittal
suture and sinus

scalp

skull

dura
mater

arach-
noid

pia
mater

epidural
space

subdural
space

subarach-
noid space

cerebral
cortex

meninges

white matter

**Section through the skull and brain
to show meninges**

meningioma n. a tumour arising from
the fibrous coverings of the brain and
spinal cord (*meninges). It is usually slow-
growing and produces symptoms by pressure on the underlying nervous tissue. In
the brain the tumour is a cause of focal
*epilepsy and gradually progressive neu-
rological disability. In the spinal cord it
may cause paraplegia and the *Brown-
Séquard syndrome. Some meningiomas
(**meningeal sarcomas**) are malignant and
can invade neighbouring tissues.
Treatment of the majority of cases is by
surgical removal if the tumour is accessible. The more malignant varieties may
also require additional radiotherapy. Some
patients have been known to have symptoms for as long as 30 years before the tumour has been discovered.

meningism n. stiffness of the neck
mimicking that found in meningitis. It is
most common in childhood and is usually
a symptom of chest infection or inflammation in the upper respiratory tract.
Examination of the *cerebrospinal fluid
reveals no abnormalities.

meningitis n. an inflammation of the
*meninges due to infection by viruses or
bacteria. Meningitis causes an intense
headache, fever, loss of appetite, intoler-

ance to light and sound, rigidity of muscles, especially those in the neck (*see also*
KERNIG'S SIGN), and in severe cases convulsions, vomiting, and delirium leading to
death. The most important causes of bacterial meningitis in young children are
Haemophilus influenzae and *Neisseria meningitidis* (the meningococcus); immunization
against *Haemophilus* meningitis is now
routine (*see* HIB VACCINE). In **meningococcal meningitis** (also known as **cerebrospinal fever** and **spotted fever**) the
symptoms appear suddenly and the bacteria can cause widespread meningococcal
infection culminating in **meningococcal
septicaemia**, with its characteristic haemorrhagic rash anywhere on the body.
Unless rapidly diagnosed and treated,
death can occur within a week.
  Bacterial meningitis is treated with
large doses of antibiotics administered as
soon as possible after diagnosis. With the
exception of herpes simplex *encephalitis
(which is treated with acyclovir), viral
meningitis does not respond to drugs but
normally has a relatively benign prognosis. *See also* LEPTOMENINGITIS, PACHYMENINGI-
TIS.

meningocele n. *see* NEURAL TUBE DEFECTS.

meningococcaemia n. the presence of
meningococci (bacteria of the species
Neisseria meningitidis) in the bloodstream.
See MENINGITIS.

meningococcus n. (pl **meningococci**)
the bacterium *Neisseria meningitidis*,
which can cause a serious form of septicaemia and is a common cause of *meningitis. —**meningococcal** adj.

meningoencephalitis n. inflammation
of the brain and its membranous coverings (the meninges) caused by bacterial or
viral infection. The disease may also involve the spinal cord, producing *myelitis
with paralysis of both legs, sometimes
called **meningomyelitis**.

meningoencephalocele n. *see* NEURAL
TUBE DEFECTS.

meningomyelitis n. *see* MENINGO-
ENCEPHALITIS.

meningomyelocele n. *see* NEURAL TUBE
DEFECTS.

meningovascular adj. relating to or affecting the meninges covering the brain and spinal cord and the blood vessels that penetrate them to supply the underlying neural tissues. The term is also used to describe secondary syphilitic infection of the nervous system.

meninx *n.* **1.** the thin layer of mesoderm that surrounds the brain of the embryo. It gives rise to most of the skull and the membranes that surround the brain. *See also* CHONDROCRANIUM. **2.** *see* MENINGES.

meniscectomy *n.* surgical removal of a cartilage (meniscus) in the knee. This is carried out when the meniscus has been torn or is diseased, to relieve pain and 'locking' of the knee joint. The operation can now be performed through an *arthroscope.

meniscus *n.* (in anatomy) a crescent-shaped structure, such as the fibrocartilaginous disc that divides the cavity of a synovial joint.

menopause (climacteric) *n.* the time in a woman's life when the ovaries cease to produce an egg cell every four weeks: menstruation ceases and the woman is no longer able to bear children. The menopause can occur at any age between the middle thirties and the middle fifties, most commonly between 45 and 55 (the median age is 51). Natural menopause can only be established in retrospect after 12 consecutive months of *amenorrhoea. Around the time of the menopause (the **perimenopause**) there are marked changes in the menstrual cycle. Menstruation may decrease gradually in successive periods or the intervals between the periods may lengthen; alternatively there may be a sudden and complete stoppage of the periods. There is a change in the balance of sex hormones in the body, which sometimes leads to hot flushes and other *vasomotor symptoms, palpitations, and dryness of the mucous membrane lining the vagina. Some women may also experience emotional disturbances. Some of these symptoms may be alleviated by *hormone replacement therapy. The term 'menopause' is also used for the postmenopausal period. —**menopausal** *adj.*

menorrhagia (epimenorrhagia) *n.* abnormally heavy bleeding at menstrua-tion, which may or may not be associated with abnormally long periods. Menorrhagia may be associated with hormonal imbalance (in which case it is described as **dysfunctional uterine bleeding**), pelvic inflammatory disease, tumours (especially fibroids) in the pelvic cavity, endometriosis, or the presence of an IUCD. In some cases no obvious pathology can be demonstrated.

MENS multiple endocrine neoplasia syndromes: a group of syndromes characterized by combinations of symptoms and signs caused by tumours and/or hyperplasia of more than one endocrine gland (**multiple endocrine neoplasia, MEN**). The tumours may involve the pituitary, thyroid, parathyroid, and adrenal glands and the pancreas, but some combinations predominate and are designated Types I, IIa, and IIb. *See also* APUD CELLS.

menses *n.* **1.** the blood and other materials discharged from the uterus at menstruation. **2.** *see* MENSTRUATION.

menstrual cycle the periodic sequence of events in sexually mature nonpregnant women by which an egg cell (ovum) is released from the ovary at four-weekly intervals until the change of life (*see* MENOPAUSE). The stages of the menstrual cycle are shown in the diagram. An ovum develops within a *Graafian follicle in the ovary. When mature, it bursts from the follicle and travels along the Fallopian tube to the uterus. A temporary endocrine gland – the corpus luteum – develops in the ruptured follicle and secretes the hormone *progesterone, which causes the lining of the uterus (endometrium) to become thicker and richly supplied with blood in preparation for pregnancy. If the ovum is not fertilized the cycle continues: the corpus luteum shrinks and the endometrium is shed at *menstruation. If fertilization does take place the fertilized ovum becomes attached to the endometrium and the corpus luteum continues to secrete progesterone, i.e. pregnancy begins.

menstruation (menses) *n.* the discharge of blood and of fragments of *endometrium from the vagina at intervals of about one month in women of child-bearing age (*see* MENARCHE,

| 1 | 2 | 3 | 4 | 5 | 6 | 7 | 8 | 9 | 10 | 11 | 12 | 13 | 14 | 15 | 16 | 17 | 18 | 19 | 20 | 21 | 22 | 23 | 24 | 25 | 26 | 27 | 28 |

days of cycle

follicle develops in ovary · growing follicle in ovary · ovum released from follicle during ovulation · mature follicle in ovary · degenerating follicle in ovary

menstruation — wall of uterus thickens to receive ovum

The menstrual cycle

MENOPAUSE). Menstruation is that stage of the *menstrual cycle during which the endometrium, thickened in readiness to receive a fertilized egg cell (ovum), is shed because fertilization has not occurred. The normal duration of discharge varies from three to seven days. In **anovular menstruation**, discharge takes place without previous release of an egg cell from the ovary. **Vicarious menstruation** is bleeding from a mucous membrane other than the endometrium when normal menstruation is due. **Retrograde menstruation** is the backflow of blood and endometrial cells through the Fallopian tubes (see ENDOMETRIOSIS). See also AMENORRHOEA, DYSMENORRHOEA, EPIMENORRHOEA, HYPOMENORRHOEA, MENORRHAGIA, OLIGOMENORRHOEA.

mental[1] *adj.* relating to or affecting the mind.

mental[2] *adj.* relating to the chin.

mental age a measure of the intellectual level at which an individual functions; for example, someone described as having a mental age of 6 years would be functioning at the level of an average 6-year-old child. This measure has largely been replaced by a comparison of the functioning of persons of the same age group (see INTELLIGENCE QUOTIENT, INTELLIGENCE TEST).

mental deficiency see MENTAL RETARDATION.

mental handicap delayed or incomplete intellectual development combined with some form of social malfunction, such as educational or occupational failure or inability to look after oneself. Good education alters the course of the handicap, for which the term **learning disability** (or **difficulty**) is now widely used. See also MENTAL RETARDATION.

Mental Health Act Commission a regulating body governed by the Mental Health Act 1983. Its members comprise some 90 psychiatrists, nurses, lawyers, members of other clinical professions, and lay people. They have the responsibilities of regularly visiting psychiatric hospitals (yearly for ordinary hospitals; more frequently for *special hospitals), reviewing psychiatric care, giving second opinions on the need for certain psychiatric treatments, and acting as a forum for the discussion of psychiatric issues.

Mental Health Acts the Acts of Parliament governing the care of the mentally disordered. The Mental Health Act 1959 provided the framework for England and Wales; similar Acts in 1960 and 1961 provided for Scotland and Northern Ireland. They abolished the old system of certification and established a legal framework for voluntary treatment of the mentally ill on the same basis as other patients. The Act also provides for *compulsory admission when the mentally disordered put themselves or other people into danger. It also enjoined local authorities to provide for the community treatment of mental disorder. The Mental Health (Amendment) Act of 1982 made further provisions for the protection of the civil rights of patients, the restriction of grounds for their detention and compulsory treatment, and for a commission to regulate aspects of the practice of psychiatry (*see* MENTAL HEALTH ACT COMMISSION). The provisions of the 1959 and 1982 Acts are now codified in a single statute, the Mental Health Act 1983, with amendments in 1996.

Mental Health Review Tribunal one of a number of tribunals, established under the Mental Health Act 1959 and now operating under the Mental Health Act 1983, to which applications may be made for the discharge from hospital of a person compulsorily detained there under provisions of the Act (*see* COMPULSORY ADMISSION). When a patient is subject to a restriction order an application may only be made after his first six months of detention. The powers of the tribunals, which comprise both legally and medically qualified members, include reclassifying unrestricted patients, recommending leave of absence for a patient, delaying discharge, and transferring patients to other hospitals.

mental illness a disorder of one or more of the functions of the mind (such as emotion, perception, memory, or thought), which causes suffering to the patient or others. If the sole problem is that the individual's behaviour as a whole is out of line with society's expectations, then the term 'illness' is not appropriate.

Mental illness should be distinguished from *mental retardation, in which an individual has a general failure of development of the normal intellectual capacities. It is broadly divided into *psychosis, in which the capacity for appreciating reality is lost, and *neurosis, in which insight is retained.

mental impairment (mostly in legal usage) the condition of significant or severe impairment of intellectual and social functioning associated with abnormally aggressive or seriously irresponsible behaviour.

mental retardation the state of those whose intellectual powers have failed to develop to such an extent that they are in need of care and protection and require special education. It is also known as **mental deficiency** and *mental handicap. The handicap may be classified according to the *intelligence quotient (IQ) as mild (IQ 50–70), moderate to severe (IQ 20–50), and profound (IQ less than 20). Mildly handicapped people often make a good adjustment to life after special help with education. The moderately and severely handicapped usually need much more help and most are permanently dependent on other people, while the profoundly handicapped usually need constant attention. There are very many causes of mental retardation, including *Down's syndrome, inherited metabolic disorders, brain injury, and gross psychological deprivation; some are preventable or treatable.

mental welfare officer (in Britain) formerly, an employee of a local authority with special training in and responsibility for people with mental illness. *See also* SOCIAL SERVICES.

mento- *prefix denoting* the chin.

mentum *n.* the chin.

mepacrine *n.* a drug used to treat various infestations, particularly giardiasis and taeniasis; it was formerly widely used to treat malaria but has now largely been replaced by safer drugs. It is administered by mouth. Digestive upsets and headache may occur and the skin often turns yellow.

meperidine *n. see* PETHIDINE.

meprobamate *n.* a mild *tranquillizer used to relieve anxiety and nervous tension. It is administered by mouth or injection; side-effects include digestive upsets, headache, and drowsiness. Trade name: **Equanil**.

meralgia paraesthetica painful tingling and numbness felt over the outer surface of the thigh when the lateral cutaneous nerve is trapped as it passes through the fibrous and muscular tissues of the groin.

mercaptopurine *n.* a drug that prevents the growth of cancer cells and is administered by mouth, chiefly in the treatment of some types of leukaemia (*see* ANTIMETABOLITE). It commonly reduces the numbers of white blood cells; mouth ulcers and digestive upsets may also occur. Trade name: **Puri-Nethol**.

mercurialism (hydrargyria) *n.* mercury poisoning. Metallic mercury is absorbed through the skin and alimentary canal, and its vapour is taken in through the lungs. Acute poisoning causes vomiting, severe abdominal pains, bloody diarrhoea, and kidney damage, with failure to produce urine. Treatment is with *dimercaprol. Chronic poisoning causes mouth ulceration, loose teeth, loss of appetite, and intestinal and renal disturbances, with anaemia and nervous irritability. Treatment is removing the patient from further exposure.

mercury *n.* a silvery metallic element that is liquid at room temperature. Its toxicity has caused a decline in the use of its compounds in medicine during this century; mercurial compounds were formerly used in the treatment of syphilis and as purgatives, teething pastes and powders, fungicides, and antiparasitic agents. Mercury is widely used in dentistry as a component of *amalgam fillings; when the mercury is combined with the filling alloy, it is nontoxic. Symbol: Hg. *See also* MERCURIALISM, PINK DISEASE.

merocrine (eccrine) *adj.* describing a type of *secretion in which the glandular cells remain intact during the process of secretion.

merozoite *n.* a stage in the life cycle of the malaria parasite (**Plasmodium*). Many merozoites are formed during the asexual division of the schizont (*see* SCHIZOGONY). The released merozoites may invade new red blood cells or new liver cells and continue the asexual phase with the production of yet more merozoites, effectively spreading the infection. Alternatively, merozoites invade red blood cells and begin the sexual cycle with the formation of male and female sex cells (*see* MICRO-GAMETOCYTE, MACROGAMETOCYTE).

mes- (meso-) *prefix denoting* middle or medial.

Mesa *see* MICROSURGICAL EPIDIDYMAL SPERM ASPIRATION.

mesaortitis *n.* inflammation of the middle layer (media) of the wall of the aorta, generally the result of late syphilis. Aneurysm formation may result. The infection can be eradicated with penicillin.

mesarteritis *n.* inflammation of the middle layer (media) of an artery, which is often combined with inflammation in all layers of the artery wall. It is seen in syphilis, polyarteritis, temporal arteritis, and Buerger's disease.

mescaline *n.* an alkaloid present in **mescal buttons** (the dried tops of the Mexican cactus *Lophophora williamsii*) that produces inebriation and vivid colourful hallucinations when ingested.

mesencephalon *n. see* MIDBRAIN.

mesenchyme *n.* the undifferentiated tissue of the early embryo that forms almost entirely from *mesoderm. It is loosely organized and the individual cells migrate to different parts of the body where they form most of the skeletal and connective tissue, the blood and blood system, and the visceral (smooth) muscles.

mesentery *n.* a double layer of *peritoneum attaching the stomach, small intestine, pancreas, spleen, and other abdominal organs to the posterior wall of the abdomen. It contains blood and lymph vessels and nerves supplying these organs. —**mesenteric** *adj.*

mesial *adj.* **1.** medial. **2.** relating to or situated in the *median line or plane. **3.** designating the surface of a tooth towards the midline of the jaw.

mesiodens *n.* an extra tooth that may occur in the midline of the palate, between the central incisors, and may interfere with their eruption.

mesmerism *n.* *hypnosis based on the ideas of the 18th-century physician Franz Mesmer, sometimes employing magnets and a variety of other equipment.

mesna *n.* a drug administered intravenously by injection or infusion to prevent the toxic effect of *ifosfamide and *cyclophosphamide on the bladder. It binds with the toxic metabolite acrolein in the urine.

mesoappendix n. the *mesentery of the appendix.

mesocolon n. the fold of peritoneum by which the colon is fixed to the posterior abdominal wall. Usually only the **transverse** and **sigmoid mesocolons** persist in the adult, attached to the transverse and sigmoid colon, respectively.

mesoderm n. the middle *germ layer of the early embryo. It gives rise to cartilage, muscle, bone, blood, kidneys, gonads and their ducts, and connective tissue. It separates into two layers – an outer **somatic** and an inner **splanchnic mesoderm**, separated by a cavity (**coelom**) that becomes the body cavity. The dorsal somatic mesoderm becomes segmented into a number of *somites. See also MESENCHYME. —**mesodermal** adj.

mesometrium n. the broad ligament of the uterus: a sheet of connective tissue that carries blood vessels to the uterus and attaches it to the abdominal wall.

mesomorphic adj. describing a *body type that has a well developed skeletal and muscular structure and a sturdy upright posture. —**mesomorph** n. —**mesomorphy** n.

mesonephros (Wolffian body) n. the second area of kidney tissue to develop in the embryo. Its excretory function only lasts for a very brief period before it degenerates. However, parts of it become incorporated into the male reproductive structures. Its duct – the **mesonephric** (or **Wolffian**) **duct** – persists in males as the epididymis and vas deferens, which conduct sperm from the testis. —**mesonephric** adj.

mesophilic adj. describing organisms, especially bacteria, that grow best at temperatures of about 25–45°C. Compare PSYCHROPHILIC, THERMOPHILIC.

mesosalpinx n. a fold of peritoneum that surrounds the Fallopian tubes. It is the upper part of the broad ligament that surrounds the uterus.

mesosome n. a structure occurring in some bacterial cells, formed by infolding of the cell membrane. Mesosomes are associated with the DNA and play a part in cell division.

mesotendon n. the delicate connective tissue membrane that surrounds a tendon.

mesothelioma n. a tumour of the pleura, peritoneum, or pericardium. The occurrence of pleural mesothelioma is often due to exposure to asbestos dust (see ASBESTOSIS), and workers in the asbestos industry who develop such tumours are entitled to industrial compensation. In other cases there is no history of direct exposure to asbestos at work, but the patients had been exposed to asbestos via the clothes of relatives who had had direct contact with asbestos, or they themselves had lived very close to an asbestos factory. There is no curative treatment for the disease, but moderately good results have occasionally been obtained from radical surgery for limited disease, from radiotherapy, and from chemotherapy.

mesothelium n. the single layer of cells that lines *serous membranes. It is derived from embryonic mesoderm. Compare EPITHELIUM.

mesovarium n. the *mesentery of the ovaries.

messenger RNA a type of RNA that carries the information of the *genetic code of the DNA from the cell nucleus to the ribosomes, where the code is translated into protein. See TRANSCRIPTION, TRANSLATION.

mestranol n. a synthetic female sex hormone (see OESTROGEN) used in combination with a progestogen to treat menopausal symptoms (see HORMONE REPLACEMENT THERAPY) and as a constituent of *oral contraceptive pills. Trade names: **Menophase, Norinyl-1**.

met- (meta-) prefix denoting **1.** distal to; beyond; behind. **2.** change; transformation.

metabolism n. **1.** the sum of all the chemical and physical changes that take place within the body and enable its continued growth and functioning. Metabolism involves the breakdown of complex organic constituents of the body with the liberation of energy, which is required for other processes (see CATABOLISM) and the building up of complex substances, which form the material of the tissues and organs, from simple ones (*see* ANABOLISM). *See also* BASAL METABOLISM. **2.** the sum of the biochemical changes undergone by a particular constituent of the body; for example, protein metabolism. —**metabolic** *adj.*

metabolite *n.* a substance that takes part in the process of *metabolism. Metabolites are either produced during metabolism or are constituents of food taken into the body.

metacarpal 1. *adj.* relating to the bones of the hand (*metacarpus). **2.** *n.* any of the bones forming the metacarpus.

metacarpus *n.* the five bones of the hand that connect the *carpus (wrist) to the *phalanges (digits).

metacentric *n.* a chromosome in which the centromere is at or near the centre of the chromosome. —**metacentric** *adj.*

metacercaria *n.* (*pl.* **metacercariae**) a mature form of the *cercaria larva of a fluke. Liver fluke metacercariae are enveloped by thin cysts and develop on various kinds of vegetation.

metachromasia (metachromatism) *n.* **1.** the property of a dye of staining certain tissues or cells a colour that is different from that of the stain itself. **2.** the variation in colour produced in certain tissue elements that are stained with the same dye. **3.** abnormal coloration of a tissue produced by a particular stain. —**metachromatic** *adj.*

Metagonimus *n.* a genus of small flukes, usually less than 3 mm in length, that are common as parasites of dogs and cats in the Far East, N Siberia, and the Balkan States. Adult flukes of *M. yokogawai* occasionally infect the duodenum of man if undercooked fish (the intermediate host) is eaten. They may cause inflammation and some ulceration of the intestinal lining, which produces a mild diarrhoea. Flukes can be easily removed with tetrachlorethylene.

metamorphopsia *n.* a condition in which objects appear distorted. It is usually due to a disorder of the retina affecting the *macula (the most sensitive part).

metamyelocyte *n.* an immature *granulocyte (a type of white blood cell), having a kidney-shaped nucleus (*compare* MYELOCYTE) and cytoplasm containing neutrophil, eosinophil, or basophil granules. It is normally found in the blood-forming tissue of the bone marrow but may appear in the blood in a wide variety of diseases, including acute infections. *See also* GRANULOPOIESIS.

metanephros *n.* the excretory organ of the fetus, which develops into the kidney and is formed from the rear portion of the *nephrogenic cord. It does not become functional until birth, since urea is transferred across the placenta to the mother.

metaphase *n.* the second stage of *mitosis and of each division of *meiosis, in which the chromosomes line up at the centre of the *spindle, with their centromeres attached to the spindle fibres.

metaphysis *n.* the growing portion of a long bone that lies between the *epiphyses (the ends) and the *diaphysis (the shaft).

metaplasia *n.* an abnormal change in the nature of a tissue. For instance, columnar epithelium lining the bronchi may be converted to squamous epithelium (**squamous metaplasia**): this may be an early sign of malignant change. **Myeloid metaplasia** is the development of bone marrow elements, normally found only within the marrow cavities of the bones, in organs such as the spleen and liver. This may occur after bone marrow failure.

metaraminol *n.* a *sympathomimetic drug that stimulates alpha receptors and is used to treat severe anaphylactic shock (*see* ANAPHYLAXIS). It is administered by injection. Trade name: **Aramine**.

metastasis *n.* the distant spread of malignant tumour from its site of origin. This occurs by three main routes: (1) through the bloodstream; (2) through the lymphatic system; (3) across body cavities, e.g. through the peritoneum. Highly malignant tumours have a greater potential for metastasis. Individual tumours may spread by one or all of the above routes, although *carcinoma is said classically to metastasize via the lymphatics and *sarcoma via the bloodstream. —**metastatic** adj.

metastasize vb. (of a malignant tumour) to spread by *metastasis.

metatarsal 1. adj. relating to the bones of the foot (*metatarsus). 2. n. any of the bones forming the metatarsus.

metatarsalgia n. aching pain in the metatarsal bones of the foot. Repeated injury, arthritis, and deformities of the foot are common causes, and corrective footwear and insoles may be prescribed.

metatarsus n. the five bones of the foot that connect the *tarsus (ankle) to the *phalanges (toes).

metathalamus n. a part of the *thalamus consisting of two nuclei through which impulses pass from the eyes and ears to be distributed to the cerebral cortex.

metencephalon n. part of the hindbrain, formed by the pons and the cerebellum and continuous below with the medulla oblongata. See BRAIN.

meteorism n. see TYMPANITES.

-meter suffix denoting an instrument for measuring. Example: **perimeter** (instrument for measuring the field of vision).

metformin n. a *biguanide drug that reduces blood sugar levels and is used to treat noninsulin-dependent *diabetes. It is administered by mouth and may cause loss of appetite and minor digestive upsets. Trade name: **Glucophage**. See also ORAL HYPOGLYCAEMIC DRUG.

methadone n. a potent narcotic *analgesic drug administered by mouth or injection to relieve severe pain and as a linctus to suppress coughs. It is also used to treat heroin addiction. Digestive upsets, drowsiness, and dizziness may occur, and prolonged use may lead to dependence. Trade name: **Physeptone**.

methaemalbumin n. a chemical complex of the pigment portion of haemoglobin (**haem**) with the plasma protein *albumin. It is formed in the blood in those anaemias in which red blood cells are destroyed and free haemoglobin is released into the plasma. In such conditions

methaemalbumin can be detected in both the blood and urine.

methaemoglobin n. a substance formed when the iron atoms of the blood pigment *haemoglobin have been oxidized from the ferrous to the ferric form (compare OXYHAEMOGLOBIN). The methaemoglobin cannot bind molecular oxygen and therefore it cannot transport oxygen round the body. The presence of methaemoglobin in the blood (**methaemoglobinaemia**) may result from the ingestion of oxidizing drugs or from an inherited abnormality of the haemoglobin molecule. Symptoms include fatigue, headache, dizziness and *cyanosis.

methanol n. see METHYL ALCOHOL.

methenamine n. see HEXAMINE.

methicillin n. a semisynthetic penicillin that was originally used to treat infections by penicillin-resistant staphylococci. It has been superseded for this purpose by *cloxacillin and *flucloxacillin but continues to be used to test the drug sensitivity of staphylococci. **Methicillin-resistant staphylococci (MRS)** can be responsible for increasing rates of infection in hospitals. Until now, such infections have responded to *vancomycin, but strains of bacilli have started to emerge that are resistant to both methicillin and vancomycin, giving rise to infections that are virtually untreatable by antibiotics. See also SUPERINFECTION.

methionine n. a sulphur-containing *essential amino acid. See also AMINO ACID.

methixene n. a drug with effects similar to those of *atropine, used to control the tremors and other symptoms in parkinsonism and to relieve spasm of smooth muscle in digestive disorders. It is administered by mouth; side-effects can include dry mouth, disturbed vision, flushing, and dizziness. Trade name: **Tremonil**.

methoserpidine n. a drug that lowers the blood pressure. It is administered by mouth; common side-effects include lethargy, drowsiness, and digestive upsets. Trade name: **Decaserpyl**.

methotrexate n. a drug that interferes with cell growth and is used to treat various types of cancer, including leukaemia (*see* ANTIMETABOLITE). It is administered by mouth or injection; common side-effects include mouth sores, digestive upsets, skin rashes, and hair loss. Trade name: **Maxtrex**.

methotrimeprazine *n.* a tranquillizing, sedative, and analgesic drug used to treat anxiety, tension, and agitation and to relieve moderate or severe pain. It is administered by mouth or by injection; common side-effects include drowsiness and weakness. Trade name: **Nozinan**.

methoxamine *n.* a *sympathomimetic drug that causes blood vessels to constrict and thus raises blood pressure. It is administered by injection to maintain the blood pressure during surgical operations. High doses may cause headache and vomiting. Trade name: **Vasoxine**.

methyclothiazide *n.* a thiazide *diuretic used in the treatment of high blood pressure (*hypertension) and oedema associated with congestive heart failure, cirrhosis, other drug therapy, and kidney dysfunction. It prevents reabsorption of sodium, chloride, and, to a lesser extent, potassium. It is administered by mouth; side-effects include loss of appetite, dizziness, and hypotension. Trade name: **Enduron**.

methyl alcohol (methanol) wood alcohol: an alcohol that is oxidized in the body much more slowly than ethyl alcohol and forms poisonous products. As little as 10 ml of pure methyl alcohol can produce permanent blindness, and 100 ml is likely to be fatal. The breakdown product formaldehyde is responsible for damage to the eyes; it is itself converted to formic acid, which causes acidosis and death from respiratory failure. *See also* METHYLATED SPIRITS.

methylamphetamine *n.* a drug with actions and side-effects similar to those of *amphetamine. It is administered by mouth to treat narcolepsy and parkinsonism and some depressive states, and to reduce appetite. It is also administered by injection in psychiatry, to restore the blood pressure in surgical procedures, and to treat drug overdosage. Its use is restricted to hospitals.

methylated spirits a mixture consisting mainly of ethyl alcohol with *methyl alcohol and petroleum hydrocarbons. The addition of pyridine gives it an objectionable smell, and the dye methyl violet is added to make it recognizable as unfit to drink. It is used as a solvent, cleaning fluid, and fuel.

methylcellulose *n.* a compound that absorbs water and is used as a bulk *laxative to treat constipation, to control diarrhoea, and in patients with a *colostomy. It is administered by mouth and usually has no side-effects. Trade name: **Celevac**.

methyldopa *n.* a drug that reduces blood pressure (*see* SYMPATHOLYTIC). It is administered by mouth or injection, and drowsiness commonly occurs during the first days of treatment. Trade names: **Aldomet, Dopamet, Hydromet, Medomet**.

methylene blue a blue dye used to stain bacterial cells for microscopic examination.

methyl green a basic dye used for colouring the stainable part of the cell nucleus (chromatin) and – with pyronin – for the differential staining of RNA and DNA, which give a red and a green colour respectively.

methylphenidate *n.* a *sympathomimetic drug that also stimulates the central nervous system. It is used to treat attention deficit disorder in children, to improve mental activity in convalescence and some depressive states, and to overcome lethargy associated with drug treatment. It is administered by mouth or injection; side-effects such as nervousness and insomnia may occur. Trade name: **Ritalin**.

methylprednisolone *n.* a glucocorticoid (*see* CORTICOSTEROID) used in the treatment of inflammatory conditions, such as rheumatoid arthritis, rheumatic fever, and allergic states, and for adrenocortical insufficiency. It is administered by mouth, intravenously, and intramuscularly; side-effects include *electrolyte imbalance, muscle weakness, and abdominal distension. Trade names: **Depo-Medrone, Medrone, Solu-Medrone**.

methyl salicylate oil of wintergreen: a liquid with *counterirritant and *analgesic properties, applied to the skin to relieve pain in lumbago, sciatica, and rheumatic conditions.

methyltestosterone *n.* a synthetic male sex hormone (*see* ANDROGEN) administered by mouth to treat sexual underdevelopment in men. It is also used to suppress lactation, to treat menstrual and menopausal disorders, and to treat breast cancer in women. Side-effects are those of *testosterone.

methylthiouracil *n.* a drug that inhibits thyroid activity, formerly administered by mouth to treat overactivity of the thyroid gland (*see* THYROTOXICOSIS). Side-effects may include rashes, digestive upsets, and headache, and *carbimazole is now preferred.

methyl violet (gentian violet) a dye used mainly for staining protozoans.

methysergide *n.* a drug used to prevent severe migraine attacks and to control diarrhoea associated with tumours in the digestive system. It is administered by mouth; common side-effects are digestive upsets, dizziness, and drowsiness. Trade name: **Deseril**.

metoclopramide *n.* a drug that antagonizes the actions of *dopamine; it is used to treat nausea, vomiting, indigestion, heartburn, and flatulence. It is administered by mouth or injection; high doses may cause drowsiness and muscle spasms. Trade names: **Gastromax**, **Maxolon**.

metolazone *n.* a *diuretic used to treat fluid retention (oedema) and high blood pressure. It is administered by mouth; side-effects include headache, loss of appetite, and digestive upsets, and blood potassium levels may be reduced. Trade name: **Metenix**, **Xuret**.

metoprolol *n.* a drug that controls the activity of the heart (*see* BETA BLOCKER) and is used to treat high blood pressure and angina. It is administered by mouth; the commonest side-effects are tiredness and digestive upsets. Trade names: **Betaloc**, **Lopresor**.

metr- (metro-) *prefix denoting* the uterus.

metre *n.* the *SI unit of length that is equal to 39.37 inches. It is formally defined as the length of the path travelled by light in vacuum during a time interval of 1/299 792 458 of a second. Symbol: m.

metritis *n.* inflammation of the uterus. *See also* ENDOMETRITIS, MYOMETRITIS.

metronidazole *n.* a drug used to treat infections of the urinary, genital, and digestive systems, such as trichomoniasis, amoebiasis, and giardiasis, and acute ulcerative gingivitis. It is administered by mouth or in suppositories; side-effects are rare but may include digestive upsets, drowsiness, and headache. Trade names: **Flagyl**, **Metrozol**.

metropathia haemorrhagica irregular episodes of bleeding from the uterus, without previous ovulation, due to excessive oestrogenic activity. It is associated with endometrial *hyperplasia and usually with follicular cysts of the ovary.

metrorrhagia *n.* bleeding from the uterus other than the normal menstrual periods. It may indicate serious disease and should always be investigated.

-metry *suffix denoting* measuring or measurement.

metyrapone *n.* a drug that interferes with the production of the hormones *cortisol and *aldosterone and is used in the treatment of *Cushing's syndrome. It is administered by mouth. Side-effects may include nausea, vomiting, low blood pressure, and allergic reactions. Trade name: **Metopirone**.

mexiletine *n.* an *anti-arrhythmic drug used in the treatment or prevention of severe heart irregularity arising in the lower chambers (ventricles). It is administered by mouth. Possible side-effects include nausea and vomiting, dizziness, and double vision. Trade name: **Mexitil**.

MHC major histocompatibility complex: a series of genes located on chromosome no. 6 that code for antigens, including the *HLA antigens, that are important in the determination of histocompatibility.

mianserin *n.* a drug used to relieve moderate or severe depression and anxiety. It is administered by mouth; side-effects are usually milder than with other potent antidepressants, the commonest being drowsiness. Trade names: **Bolvidon**, **Norval**.

MIBG meta-iodobenzylguanidine: a contrast medium. The labelled form can be used as a *tracer for the presence of a *phaeochromocytoma.

micelle *n.* one of the microscopic particles into which the products of fat digestion (i.e. fatty acids and monoglycerides), present in the gut, are dispersed by the action of *bile salts. Fatty material in this finely dispersed form is more easily absorbed by the small intestine.

miconazole *n.* a drug used to treat fungal infections, such as *ringworm of the scalp, body, and feet, and candidosis. It is administered by intravenous injection, intravaginally, and topically; side-effects include itching, skin rash, and nausea and vomiting. Trade names: **Daktarin, Gyno-daktarin**.

micr- (micro-) *prefix denoting* **1.** small size. **2.** one millionth part.

microaerophilic *adj.* describing microorganisms that grow best at very low oxygen concentrations (i.e. below the atmospheric level).

microaneurysm *n.* a minute localized swelling of a capillary wall, which is found in the retina of patients with diabetic *retinopathy. It is recognized as a small red dot when the interior of the eye is examined with an *ophthalmoscope.

microangiopathy *n.* damage to the walls of the smallest blood vessels. It may result from a variety of diseases, including diabetes mellitus, connective-tissue diseases, infections, and cancer. Some common manifestations of microangiopathy are kidney failure, haemolysis (damage to red blood cells), and purpura (bleeding into the skin). The treatment is that of the underlying cause.

microbe *n. see* MICROORGANISM.

microbiology *n.* the science of *microorganisms. Microbiology in relation to medicine is concerned mainly with the isolation and identification of the microorganisms that cause disease. —**microbiological** *adj.* —**microbiologist** *n.*

microblepharon (microblepharism) *n.* the condition of having abnormally small eyelids.

microbubbles *pl. n.* (in radiology) echo contrast agents: small gas bubbles that are introduced into the vascular system or the Fallopian tubes in order to enhance ultrasound images.

microcephaly *n.* abnormal smallness of the head in relation to the size of the rest of the body: a congenital condition in which the brain is not fully developed. *Compare* MACROCEPHALY.

microcheilia *n.* abnormally small size of the lips. *Compare* MACROCHEILIA.

Micrococcus *n.* a genus of spherical Gram-positive bacteria occurring in colonies. They are saprophytes or parasites. The species *M. tetragenus* (formerly *Gaffkya tetragena*) is normally a harmless parasite in man but it can become pathogenic, causing arthritis, endocarditis, meningitis, or abscesses in tissues. It occurs in groups of four.

microcyte *n.* an abnormally small red blood cell (*erythrocyte). *See also* MICROCYTOSIS. —**microcytic** *adj.*

microcytosis *n.* the presence of abnormally small red cells (**microcytes**) in the blood. Microcytosis is a feature of certain anaemias (**microcytic anaemias**), including iron-deficiency anaemias, certain *haemoglobinopathies, anaemias associated with chronic infections, etc.

microdactyly *n.* abnormal smallness or shortness of the fingers.

microdiscectomy *n.* surgical removal of all or part of a *prolapsed intervertebral disc using an *operating microscope, a very short incision, and very fine instruments that can be inserted between the individual vertebrae of the backbone. The procedure is used to relieve pressure on spinal nerve roots or on the spinal cord caused by protrusion of the pulpy matter of the disc (**nucleus pulposus**). This is a form of *minimally invasive surgery.

microdissection *n.* the process of dissecting minute structures under the microscope. Miniature surgical instruments, such as knives made of glass, are manipulated by means of geared connections that reduce the relatively coarse movements of the operator's fingers into microscopic movements. Using this technique it is possible to dissect the nuclei of cells and even to separate individual chromosomes. *See also* MICROSURGERY.

microdochectomy *n.* an exploratory operation on the mammary ducts, usually to detect (or exclude) the presence of a suspected tumour (adenoma).

microdontia *n.* a condition in which the teeth are unusually small.

microelectrode *n.* an extremely fine wire used as an electrode to measure the electrical activity in small areas of tissue. Microelectrodes can be used for recording the electrical changes that occur in the membranes of cells, such as those of nerve and muscle.

microfilaria *n.* (*pl.* **microfilariae**) the motile embryo of certain nematodes (*see* FILARIA). The slender microfilariae, 150–300 μm in length, are commonly found in the circulating blood or lymph of patients suffering an infection with any of the filarial worms, e.g. *Wuchereria*. They mature into larvae, which are infective, within the body of a bloodsucking insect, such as a mosquito.

microgamete *n.* the motile flagellate male sex cell of the malarial parasite (*Plasmodium*) and other protozoans. The microgamete is similar to the sperm cell of animals and smaller than the female sex cell (*see* MACROGAMETE).

microgametocyte *n.* a cell that undergoes meiosis to form 6–8 mature male sex cells (microgametes) of the malarial parasite (*see* PLASMODIUM). Microgametocytes are found in the blood of man but must be ingested by a mosquito before developing into microgametes.

microglia *n.* one of the two basic classes of *glia (the non-nervous cells of the central nervous system), having a mainly scavenging function (*see* MACROPHAGE). *Compare* MACROGLIA.

microglossia *n.* abnormally small size of the tongue.

micrognathia *n.* a condition in which one or both jaws are unusually small.

microgram *n.* one millionth of a gram. Symbol: μg.

micrograph (photomicrograph) *n.* a

photograph of an object as viewed through a microscope. An **electron micrograph** is photographed through an electron microscope; a **light micrograph** through a light microscope.

microgyria *n.* a developmental disorder of the brain in which the folds (convolutions) in its surface are small and its surface layer (cortex) is structurally abnormal. It is associated with mental and physical retardation.

microhaematocrit *n.* a measurement of the proportion of red blood cells in a volume of circulating blood. It is determined by taking a sample of the patient's blood in a fine tube and spinning it in a centrifuge until settling is complete. *See* PACKED CELL VOLUME.

micromanipulation *n.* the manipulation of extremely small structures under the microscope, as in *microdissection, or *microsurgery.

micromelia *n.* abnormally small size of the arms or legs. *Compare* MACROMELIA.

micrometastasis *n.* a secondary tumour that is undetectable by clinical examination or diagnostic tests but is visible under the microscope.

micrometer *n.* an instrument for making extremely fine measurements of thickness or length, often relying upon the movement of a screw thread and the principle of the *vernier.

micrometre *n.* one millionth of a metre (10^{-6} m). Symbol: μm.

microorganism (microbe) *n.* any organism too small to be visible to the naked eye. Microorganisms include *bacteria, some *fungi, *mycoplasmas, *protozoa, *rickettsiae, and *viruses.

microphotograph *n.* **1.** a photograph reduced to microscopic proportions. **2.** (loosely) a *photomicrograph.

microphthalmia *n.* a congenitally small eye, usually associated with a small eye socket.

micropipette *n.* an extremely fine tube from which minute volumes of liquid can be delivered. It can also be used to draw up minute quantities of liquid for examination. Using a micropipette it is possible to add or take away material from individual cells under the microscope.

micropsia *n.* a condition in which objects appear smaller than they really are. It is usually due to disease of the retina affecting the *macula but may occur in paralysis of *accommodation.

microscope *n.* an instrument for producing a greatly magnified image of an object, which may be so small as to be invisible to the naked eye. **Light** or **optical microscopes** use light as a radiation source for viewing the specimen and combinations of lenses to magnify the image; these are usually an *objective and an *eyepiece. *See also* ELECTRON MICROSCOPE, OPERATING MICROSCOPE, ULTRAMICROSCOPE. —**microscopical** *adj.* —**microscopy** *n.*

microscopic *adj.* **1.** too small to be seen clearly without the use of a microscope. **2.** of, relating to, or using a microscope.

microsome *n.* a small particle consisting of a piece of *endoplasmic reticulum to which ribosomes are attached. Microsomes are formed when homogenized cells are centrifuged. —**microsomal** *adj.*

microsonation *n.* the use of ultrasound waves generated inside the body from an extremely small source, such as the tip of a needle or a bubble within the tissues. This technique is used to obtain a picture of the fine structure of the neighbouring tissues. It is a specialized form of *ultrasonography.

Microsporum *n.* a genus of fungi causing *ringworm. *See also* DERMATOPHYTE.

microsurgery *n.* the branch of surgery in which extremely intricate operations are performed through highly refined *operating microscopes using miniaturized precision instruments (forceps, scissors, needles, etc.). The technique enables surgery of previously inaccessible parts of the eye, inner ear, spinal cord, and brain (e.g. for the removal of tumours and repair of cerebral aneurysms), as well as the reattachment of amputated fingers (necessitating the suturing of minute nerves and blood vessels) and the reversal of vasectomies.

microsurgical epididymal sperm

aspiration (Mesa) the removal of spermatozoa from the epididymis by needle *aspiration. This procedure, performed under anaesthetic, may be undertaken to assist conception in cases where the normal passage of sperm from the testis is obstructed, for example by blockage (through infection) of the ducts or by vasectomy. The extracted sperm are subjected to special treatment to select the strongest and most motile; these are then chemically treated to activate them and used for *in vitro fertilization.

microtome *n.* an instrument for cutting extremely thin slices of material that can be examined under a microscope. The material is usually embedded in a suitable medium, such as paraffin wax. A common type of microtome is a steel knife.

microvascular *adj.* involving small vessels. The term is often applied to techniques of *microsurgery for reuniting small blood vessels (the same techniques are applied frequently to nerve suture).

microvillus *n.* (*pl.* **microvilli**) one of a number of microscopic hairlike structures (about 5 μm long) projecting from the surface of epithelial cells (*see* EPITHELIUM). They serve to increase the surface area of the cell and are seen on absorptive and secretory cells. In some regions (particularly the intestinal tract) microvilli form a dense covering on the free surface of the cells: this is called a **brush border**.

microwave therapy a form of *diathermy using electromagnetic waves of extremely short wavelength. In modern apparatus the electric currents induced in the tissues have frequencies of up to 25,000 million cycles per second.

micturating cystourethrogram (MCU) *see* URETHROGRAPHY.

micturition *n.* *see* URINATION.

midazolam *n.* a *benzodiazepine drug used as a sedative for minor surgery, as a premedication, and to induce general anaesthesia. It is administered by injection. Possible side-effects include headache, dizziness, and difficulty in breathing. Trade name: **Hypnovel**.

midbrain (mesencephalon) *n.* the small portion of the *brainstem, excluding the pons and the medulla, that joins the hindbrain to the forebrain.

middle ear (tympanic cavity) the part of the *ear that consists of an air-filled space within the petrous part of the temporal bone. It is lined with mucous membrane and is connected to the pharynx by the *Eustachian tube and to the outer ear by the eardrum (*tympanic membrane). Within the middle ear are three bones – the auditory *ossicles – which transmit sound vibrations from the outer ear to the inner ear (*see* LABYRINTH).

midgut *n.* the middle portion of the embryonic gut, which gives rise to most of the small intestine and part of the large intestine. Early in development it is connected with the *yolk sac outside the embryo via the *umbilicus.

midstream specimen of urine (MSU) a specimen of urine that is subjected to examination for the presence of microorganisms. In order to obtain a specimen that is free of contamination, the periurethral area is cleansed and the patient is requested to discard the initial flow of urine before collecting the specimen in a sterile container.

midwifery *n.* the profession of providing assistance and medical care to women undergoing labour and childbirth. *See also* COMMUNITY MIDWIFE, OBSTETRICS. —**midwife** *n.*

mifepristone *n.* a drug used to produce an abortion within the first 63 days of pregnancy: it acts by blocking the action of *progesterone, which is essential for maintaining pregnancy. If a second drug, one of the prostaglandins (e.g. *gemeprost), is taken within 48 hours to complete the expulsion of the fertilized egg cell, the method is said to be 95% effective.

migraine *n.* a condition resulting from spasm and subsequent overdilatation of certain arteries in the brain, which causes a recurrent throbbing headache that characteristically affects one side of the head. There is sometimes forewarning of an attack (an **aura**) consisting of visual disturbance or numbness and/or weakness of the limbs, which clear up as the headache develops. It is often accompanied by pros-

tration, nausea and vomiting, and *photophobia. Effective preventive therapies now exist and drugs such as *sumatriptan may be used to treat acute attacks.

Mikulicz's disease damage to the lacrimal and salivary glands resulting in enlargement of these glands, narrowing of the corners of the eyes, conjunctivitis, and dryness of the mouth. The cause may be autoimmune disease or malignancy. [J. von Mikulicz Radecki (1850–1905), Polish surgeon]

miliaria *n. see* PRICKLY HEAT.

miliary *adj.* describing or characterized by very small nodules or lesions, resembling millet seed.

miliary tuberculosis acute generalized *tuberculosis characterized by lesions in affected organs, which resemble millet seeds.

milium *n.* (*pl.* **milia**) a white nodule in the skin, particularly on the face. Up to 2 mm in diameter, milia are tiny *keratin cysts occurring just beneath the outer layer (epidermis) of the skin. Milia are commonly seen in newborn babies around the nose; they disappear without active treatment.

milk *n.* the liquid food secreted by female mammals from the mammary gland. It is the sole source of food for the young of most mammals at the start of life. Milk is a complete food in that it has most of the nutrients necessary for life: protein, carbohydrate, fat, minerals, and vitamins. The composition of milk varies very much from mammal to mammal. Cows' milk contains nearly all the essential nutrients but is comparatively deficient in vitamins C and D. Human milk contains more sugar (lactose) and less protein than cows' milk.

milk rash a spotty red facial rash that is common during the first few months of life; it disappears without treatment.

milk teeth *Colloquial.* the primary teeth of young children. *See* DENTITION.

milli- *prefix denoting* one thousandth part.

milliampere *n.* one thousandth of an ampere (10^{-3} A). Symbol: mA.

milligram *n.* one thousandth of a gram. Symbol: mg.

millilitre *n.* one thousandth of a litre. Symbol: ml. *See* LITRE.

millimetre *n.* one thousandth of a metre (10^{-3} m). Symbol: mm.

Milroy's disease *see* LYMPHOEDEMA. [W. F. Milroy (1855–1942), US physician]

Minamata disease a form of mercury poisoning (from ingesting methyl mercury in contaminated fish) that caused 43 deaths in the Japanese coastal town of Minamata during 1953–56. The source of mercury was traced to an effluent containing mercuric sulphate from a local PVC factory. Symptoms include numbness, difficulty in controlling the limbs, and impaired speech and hearing.

MIND the National Association for Mental Health. It is a voluntary association, registered as a charity, that promotes the welfare of those with *mental illness through advice, education, campaigning, and the provision of resources.

mineralocorticoid *n.* *see* CORTICO-STEROID.

minim *n.* a unit of volume used in pharmacy, equivalent to one sixtieth part of a fluid *drachm.

minimally invasive surgery surgical intervention involving the least possible physical trauma to the patient, particularly surgery performed using an operating laparoscope or other endoscopy (*see* LAPAROSCOPY) passed through a tiny incision; it is known popularly as **keyhole surgery**. Several types of abdominal surgery, including gall bladder removal (*see* CHOLECYSTECTOMY) and extracorporeal shock-wave *lithotripsy for stones in the urinary or bile drainage system, are commonly performed in this way. Such methods usually allow the patient to resume normal activity much sooner than would be possible after more conventional procedures. *See also* INTERVENTIONAL RADIOLOGY.

minitracheostomy *n.* temporary *tracheostomy using a needle or fine-bore tube inserted through the skin.

minocycline *n.* a tetracycline antibiotic active against a wide range of bacteria and against rickettsial infections, mycoplasmal pneumonia, and relapsing fever. It is administered by mouth and by intravenous injection; side-effects include loss of appetite, skin rash, and dizziness. Trade name: **Minocin**.

minoxidil *n.* a peripheral vasodilator used in the treatment of high blood pressure (hypertension) when other drugs are not effective; it is administered by mouth in conjunction with a *diuretic. It is also applied to the scalp, in the form of a lotion, to restore hair growth. Side-effects include ECG changes and transient oedema. Trade names: **Loniten**, **Regaine**.

mio- *prefix denoting* **1.** reduction or diminution. **2.** rudimentary.

miosis (myosis) *n.* constriction of the pupil. This occurs normally in bright light, but persistent miosis is most commonly caused by certain types of eye drops used to treat glaucoma. *See also* MIOTIC. *Compare* MYDRIASIS.

miotic *n.* a drug that causes the pupil of the eye to contract. Miotics, such as *physostigmine and *pilocarpine, are used to counteract the dilation of the pupil caused by drugs such as ephedrine and phenylephrine and to reduce the pressure in the eye in the treatment of glaucoma.

miracidium *n.* (*pl.* **miracidia**) the first-stage larva of a parasitic *fluke. Miracidia hatch from eggs released into water with the host's excreta. They have *cilia and swim about until they reach a snail. The miracidia then bore into the snail's soft tissues and there continue their development as *sporocysts.

Mirena *n.* *see* IUS.

miscarriage *n.* *see* ABORTION.

miso- *prefix denoting* hatred. Example: **misopedia** (of children).

misoprostol *n.* a *prostaglandin drug used in the prevention and treatment of peptic ulcer caused by nonsteroidal anti-inflammatory drugs (*see* NSAID). It is administered by mouth. Possible side-effects include nausea, vomiting, diarrhoea, and abdominal pain. Trade names: **Cytotec**, **Napratec**.

missed case a person suffering from an infection in whom the symptoms and signs are so minimal that either there is no request for medical assistance or the doctor fails to make the diagnosis. The patient usually has partial immunity to the disease, but since the infecting organisms (pathogens) are of normal virulence, nonimmune contacts can be affected with the full manifestations of the illness. The period of infectivity is confined to the shortened duration of the illness (in contrast to a *carrier, in whom the pathogen is present without necessarily causing any ill effect). Alternatively the subject has had the disease but retains some of the pathogens (e.g. in the throat or bowel) and so acts as a continuing reservoir of infection.

Misuse of Drugs Act 1971 (in the UK) an Act of Parliament restricting the use of dangerous drugs. These **controlled drugs** include the natural *opiates and their synthetic substitutes, many stimulants (including amphetamine, cocaine, and pemoline), and hallucinogens such as LSD and cannabis. The Act specifies certain requirements for writing prescriptions for these drugs. The Misuse of Drugs (Notification of and Supply to Addicts) Regulations (1973) and the Misuse of Drugs Regulations, which are updated from time to time, also lay down who may supply controlled drugs. Five categories of persons are defined.

mite n. a free-living or parasitic arthropod belonging to a group (Acarina) that also includes the *ticks. Most mites are small, averaging 1 mm or less in length. A mite has no antennae or wings, and its body is not divided into a distinct head, thorax, and abdomen. Medically important mites include the many species causing dermatitis (e.g. *Dermatophagoides*) and the harvest mite (*see* TROMBICULA), which transmits scrub typhus.

mithramycin (plicamycin) n. an antibiotic that prevents the growth of cancer cells. It was formerly used for treating certain forms of cancer but is now used only to reduce high levels of calcium in the blood. Common side-effects are digestive upsets and mouth ulcers and, more seriously, nosebleeds and vomiting of blood.

mitochondrion (chondriosome) n. (pl. **mitochondria**) a structure, occurring in varying numbers in the cytoplasm of every cell, that is the site of the cell's

energy production. Mitochondria contain *ATP and the enzymes involved in the cell's metabolic activities; each is bounded by a double membrane, the inner being folded inwards to form projections (**cristae**). —**mitochondrial** adj.

mitogen n. any substance that can cause cells to begin division (*mitosis).

mitomycin C an antibiotic that inhibits the growth of cancer cells. It causes severe marrow suppression but is of use in the treatment of stomach and breast cancers. Trade name: **Mutamycin**.

mitosis n. a type of cell division in which a single cell produces two genetically identical daughter cells. It is the way in which new body cells are produced for both growth and repair. Division of the nucleus (**karyokinesis**) takes place in four stages (*see* PROPHASE, METAPHASE, ANAPHASE, TELOPHASE) and is followed by division of the cytoplasm (**cytokinesis**) to form the two daughter cells (see illustration). *Compare* MEIOSIS. —**mitotic** adj.

mitotic index the proportion of cells in a tissue that are dividing at a given time.

mitoxantrone n. a drug used in the treatment of certain cancers, including breast cancer, leukaemia, and lymphomas. Side-effects are usually mild. Trade name: **Novantrone**.

mitral incompetence failure of the *mitral valve to close, allowing a reflux of blood from the left ventricle of the heart to the left atrium. It most often results from scarring of the mitral valve by rheumatic fever, but it can also develop as a complication of myocardial infarction or cardiomyopathies. It may occur as a congenital defect. Its manifestations include breathlessness, atrial *fibrillation, embolism, enlargement of the left ventricle, and a systolic *murmur. Mild cases are symptomless and require no treatment, but in severe cases the affected valve should be replaced with an artificial one (**mitral prosthesis**).

mitral stenosis narrowing of the opening of the mitral valve: a result of chronic scarring that follows rheumatic fever. It may be seen alone or combined with *mitral incompetence. The symptoms are similar to those of mitral incompetence

cytoplasm
centrioles separate
nucleus
homologous chromosomes
centromere
cell membrane
Prophase

centriole
chromosomes attached to equatorial region
spindle
Metaphase

chromatids separate
Early anaphase

chromatids move towards the poles
Anaphase

cell constricts
Late anaphase

centriole replicates
cell divides into two
chromosomes disappear
nuclear membrane forms
Telophase

Stages in mitosis

except that the patient has a diastolic *murmur. Mild cases need no treatment, but severe cases are treated surgically by reopening the stenosis (**mitral valvotomy**) or by inserting an artificial valve (**mitral prosthesis**).

mitral valve (bicuspid valve) a valve in the heart consisting of two flaps (cusps) attached to the walls at the opening between the left atrium and left ventricle. It allows blood to pass from the atrium to the ventricle, but prevents any backward flow.

mittelschmerz n. pain in the lower abdomen experienced about midway between successive menstrual periods, i.e. when the egg cell is being released from the ovary. See also MENSTRUAL CYCLE.

mixed connective tissue disease a disease with features in common with systemic *lupus erythematosus, *polymyositis, and *scleroderma. Some authorities dispute its status as a separate entity.

ml abbrev. for millilitre. See LITRE.

MLC (MLR) mixed lymphocyte culture (or reaction): a test in which lymphocytes from prospective donor and recipient are cultured together in a test tube to assess the suitability of transplanting organs or bone marrow cells.

MLD minimal lethal dose: the smallest quantity of a toxic compound that is recorded as having caused death. See also LD$_{50}$.

MLR see MLC.

MM malignant melanoma (see MELANOMA).

mmHg a unit of pressure equal to 1 millimetre of mercury. 1 mmHg = 133.3224 pascals.

MMR vaccine a combined vaccine against measles, mumps, and German measles (rubella). It is currently recommended that this vaccine is given to all children between 13 and 15 months old with a booster dose at 3½–4 years. Specific contraindications include immunosuppression and allergy to eggs.

MND see MOTOR NEURONE DISEASE.

moclobemide n. an antidepressant drug that reversibly inhibits the enzyme monoamine oxidase. The adverse effects of existing *MAO inhibitors, which include severe reactions when cheese or other tyramine-containing foods are eaten by patients taking them, are less likely with reversible inhibitors.

modality *n.* **1.** a form of sensation, such as smell, hearing, tasting, or detecting temperature. Differences in modality are not due to differences in the structure of the nerves concerned, but to differences in the working of the sensory receptors and the areas of brain that receive the messages. **2.** one form of therapy as opposed to another, such as the modality of physiotherapy contrasted with that of radiotherapy.

mode *n.* see MEAN.

Modecate *n.* see FLUPHENAZINE.

modelling *n.* a technique used in *behaviour modification, whereby an individual learns a behaviour by observing someone else doing it. Together with *prompting, it is useful for introducing new behaviours to the individual.

modiolus *n.* the conical central pillar of the *cochlea in the inner ear.

MODS see MULTIPLE ORGAN DYSFUNCTION SYNDROME.

Moduretic *n.* see AMILORIDE.

MOF see MULTIPLE-ORGAN FAILURE.

Mogadon *n.* see NITRAZEPAM.

molar *n.* in the permanent *dentition, the sixth, seventh, or eighth tooth from the midline on each side in each jaw (see also WISDOM TOOTH). Permanent molars do not replace primary teeth. In the primary dentition, molars are the fourth and fifth teeth from the midline on each side in each jaw.

molarity *n.* the strength of a solution, expressed as the weight of dissolved substance in grams per litre divided by its molecular weight, i.e. the number of moles per litre. Molarity is indicated as 0.1 M, 1 M, 2 M, etc.

molar solution a solution in which the number of grams of dissolved substance per litre equals its molecular weight, i.e. a solution of molarity 1 M.

mole[1] *n.* the *SI unit of amount of substance, equal to the amount of substance that contains as many elementary units as there are atoms in 0.012 kilograms of carbon-12. The elementary units, which must be specified, may be atoms, molecules, ions, electrons, etc., or a specified group of such entities. One mole of a compound has a mass equal to its molecular weight expressed in grams. Symbol: mol.

mole[2] *n.* a nonmalignant collection of pigmented cells in the skin. Moles are rare in infancy, increase in numbers during childhood and especially in adolescence, but decline in numbers in old age. They vary widely in appearance, being flat or raised, smooth or hairy. Changes in the shape, colour, etc., of moles in adult life should be investigated as this may be an early sign of malignant *melanoma. Medical name: **pigmented naevus**. See also ATYPICAL MOLE SYNDROME.

molecular biology the study of the molecules that are associated with living organisms, especially proteins and nucleic acids.

molluscum contagiosum a common disease of the skin, mainly affecting children. Characterized by papules less than 5 mm in diameter, each with a central depression, the disease is caused by a *poxvirus and is spread by direct contact. Untreated, the papules disappear in 6–9 months.

mon- (mono-) *prefix denoting* one, single, or alone.

Mongolian blue spots blue-black pigmented areas seen at the base of the back and on the buttocks of babies. They are more common in Asian babies and usually fade during the first year of life. The spots are sometimes mistaken for bruising.

mongolism *n.* see DOWN'S SYNDROME.

Monilia *n.* the former name of the genus of yeasts now known as *Candida.

moniliasis *n.* an obsolete name for *candidosis.

monoamine oxidase (MAO) an enzyme that catalyses the oxidation of a large variety of monoamines, including adrenaline, noradrenaline, and serotonin.

Monoamine oxidase is found in most tissues, particularly the liver and nervous system. Drugs that act as inhibitors of this enzyme are widely used in the treatment of depression (see MAO INHIBITOR).

monoarthritis n. see ARTHRITIS.

monoblast n. the earliest identifiable cell that gives rise to a *monocyte. It is probably identical with the *myeloblast and matures via an intermediate stage (**promonocyte**). It is normally found in the blood-forming tissue of the *bone marrow but may appear in the blood in certain diseases, most notably in acute monoblastic *leukaemia.

monochromat n. a person who is completely colour-blind. There are two types. The **rod monochromat** appears to have totally defective *cones: he has very poor visual acuity as well as the inability to discriminate colours. The **cone monochromat** has normal visual acuity: his cones appear to respond normally to light but to be completely unable to discriminate colours. It is possible in this case that the defect does not lie in the cones themselves but in the integration of the nerve impulses as they pass from the cones to the brain. Both types of colour blindness are probably inherited.

monochromatic adj. denoting radiation, especially light, of the same frequency or wavelength.

monoclonal antibody an antibody produced artificially from a cell *clone and therefore consisting of a single type of immunoglobulin. Monoclonal antibodies are produced by fusing antibody-forming lymphocytes from mouse spleen with mouse myeloma cells. The resulting hybrid cells multiply rapidly (like cancer cells) and produce the same antibody as their parent lymphocytes. Monoclonal antibodies can be used for treating some malignant tumours (e.g. brain tumours), which can be targeted by these antibodies (known colloquially as 'magic bullets').

monocular adj. relating to or used by one eye only. Compare BINOCULAR.

monocyte n. a variety of white blood cell, 16–20 μm in diameter, that has a kidney-shaped nucleus and greyish-blue cytoplasm (when treated with *Romanowsky

stains). Its function is the ingestion of foreign particles, such as bacteria and tissue debris. There are normally $0.2–0.8 \times 10^9$ monocytes per litre of blood. —**monocytic** adj.

monocytosis n. an increase in the number of *monocytes in the blood. It occurs in a variety of diseases, including certain leukaemias (**monocytic leukaemias**) and infections due to some bacteria and protozoa.

monodactylism n. the congenital absence of all but one digit on each hand and foot.

monoiodotyrosine n. an iodine-containing substance produced in the thyroid gland from which the *thyroid hormones are derived.

monomania n. the state in which a particular delusion or set of delusions is present in an otherwise normally functioning person. See also PARANOIA.

mononeuritis n. disease affecting a single peripheral nerve. **Mononeuritis multiplex** is the separate involvement of two or more nerves. Compare POLYNEUROPATHY.

mononucleosis n. the condition in which the blood contains an abnormally high number of mononuclear leucocytes (*monocytes). See GLANDULAR FEVER (INFECTIOUS MONONUCLEOSIS).

monophobia n. an extreme fear of being alone.

monophyletic adj. describing a number of individuals, species, etc., that have evolved from a single ancestral group. Compare POLYPHYLETIC.

monoplegia n. paralysis of one limb. —**monoplegic** adj.

monoploid adj. see HAPLOID.

monorchism n. absence of one testis. This is usually due to failure of one testicle to descend into the scrotum before birth. The term is sometimes used for the condition in which one testicle has been removed surgically or destroyed by injury or disease. If the single testis is normal, no adverse effects result from the absence of the other.

monosaccharide n. a simple sugar having the general formula $(CH_2O)_n$. Monosaccharides may have between three and nine carbon atoms, but the most common number is five or six. Monosaccharides are classified according to the number of carbon atoms they possess. Thus **trioses** have three carbon atoms, **tetroses** four, **pentoses** five, and **hexoses** six. The most abundant monosaccharide is glucose (a hexose).

monosomy *n.* a condition in which there is one chromosome missing from the normal (*diploid) set. *Compare* TRISOMY. —**monosomic** *adj.*

monozygotic twins *see* TWINS.

mons *n.* (in anatomy) a rounded eminence. The **mons pubis** is the mound of fatty tissue lying over the pubic symphysis.

Mooren's ulcer a severe ulceration at the periphery of the cornea, characterized by an overhanging advancing edge and vascularization of the ulcer bed. It is usually very painful, progressive, and difficult to control. [A. Mooren (1829–99), German ophthalmologist]

Moraxella *n.* a genus of short rodlike Gram-negative aerobic bacteria, usually occurring in pairs. They exist as parasites in many warm-blooded animals. The species *M. lacunata* causes conjunctivitis.

morbid *adj.* diseased or abnormal; pathological.

morbidity *n.* the state of being diseased. The **morbidity rate** is the number of cases of a disease found to occur in a stated number of the population, usually given as cases per 100,000 or per million (the number may be smaller for common diseases). Annual figures for morbidity rate give the incidence of the disease, which is the number of new cases reported in the year. *See also* INCIDENCE RATE, PREVALENCE RATE.

morbilli *n. see* MEASLES.

morbilliform *adj.* describing a skin rash resembling that of measles.

morbus *n.* disease. The term is usually used as part of the medical name of a specific disease.

mordant *n.* (in microscopy) a substance,

such as alum or phenol, used to fix a *stain in a tissue.

moribund *adj.* dying.

moricizine *n.* a drug administered by mouth to treat life-threatening irregularity of the heartbeat (*arrhythmia). Possible side-effects include worsening of the arrhythmia and heart failure, and it is used only in cases in which these risks are thought to be justified.

morning sickness nausea and vomiting occurring during early pregnancy. In some women the symptoms disappear if a small amount of food is eaten before rising in the morning. *Compare* HYPEREMESIS GRAVIDARUM.

Moro reflex (startle reflex) a primitive reflex seen in newborn babies in response to the stimulus of a sudden noise or movement: the baby will fling its arms and legs wide and will appear to stiffen; the arms and legs are then drawn back into flexion. The Moro reflex should disappear spontaneously by four months. Its presence beyond this age is suggestive of an underlying neurological disorder, such as cerebral palsy. [E. Moro (1874–1951), German paediatrician]

morphine *n.* a potent analgesic and *narcotic drug used mainly to relieve severe and persistent pain. It is administered by mouth or injection; common side-effects are loss of appetite, nausea, constipation, and confusion. Morphine causes feelings of euphoria; *tolerance develops rapidly and *dependence may occur.

morpho- *prefix denoting* form or structure.

morphoea *n.* a localized form of *scleroderma characterized by firm ivory-coloured waxy plaques in the skin without any internal sclerosis. The plaques may often disappear spontaneously but resolution is slow.

morphogenesis *n.* the development of form and structure of the body and its parts.

morphology *n. see* ANATOMY.

-morphous *suffix denoting* form or structure (of a specified kind).

Morquio-Brailsford disease a defect of *mucopolysaccharide metabolism (*see* INBORN ERROR OF METABOLISM) that causes dwarfism with a *kyphosis, a short neck, *knock knees, and an angulated sternum in affected children. Intelligence is normal. [L. Morquio (1865–1935), Uruguayan physician; J. F. Brailsford (1888–1961), British radiologist]

mortality (mortality rate) *n.* the incidence of death in the population in a given period. The **annual mortality rate** is the number of registered deaths in a year, multiplied by 1000 and divided by the population at the middle of the year. *See also* INFANT MORTALITY RATE, MATERNAL MORTALITY RATE.

mortification *n. see* NECROSIS.

morula *n.* an early stage of embryonic development formed by *cleavage of the fertilized ovum. It consists of a solid ball of cells and is an intermediate stage between the zygote and *blastocyst.

mosaicism *n.* a condition in which the cells of an individual do not all contain identical chromosomes; there may be two or more genetically different populations of cells. Often one of the cell populations is normal and the other carries a chromosome defect such as *Down's syndrome or *Turner's syndrome. In affected individuals the chromosome defect is usually not fully expressed. —**mosaic** *adj.*

mosquito *n.* a small winged bloodsucking insect belonging to a large group – the *Diptera (two-winged flies). Its mouthparts are formed into a long proboscis for piercing the skin and sucking blood. Female mosquitoes transmit the parasites responsible for several major infectious diseases, such as *malaria. *See* ANOPHELES, AËDES, CULEX.

motile *adj.* being able to move spontaneously, without external aid: usually applied to a *microorganism or a cell (e.g. a sperm cell).

motion sickness (travel sickness) nausea, vomiting, and headache caused by motion during travel by sea, road, or air. The symptoms are due to overstimulation of the balance organs in the *inner ear by repeated small changes in the position of the body and are aggravated by move-

ments of the horizon. Sedative antihistamine drugs (*see* ANTIEMETIC) are effective in preventing motion sickness.

motor cortex the region of the *cerebral cortex that is responsible for initiating nerve impulses that bring about voluntary activity in the muscles of the body. It is possible to map out the cortex to show which of its areas is responsible for which particular part of the body. The motor cortex of the left cerebral hemisphere is responsible for muscular activity in the right side of the body.

motor nerve one of the nerves that carry impulses outwards from the central nervous system to bring about activity in a muscle or gland. *Compare* SENSORY NERVE.

motor neurone one of the units (*neurones) that goes to make up the nerve pathway between the brain and an effector organ, such as a skeletal muscle. An **upper motor neurone** has a cell body in the brain and an axon that extends into the spinal cord, where it ends in synapses. It is thus entirely within the central nervous system. A **lower motor neurone**, on the other hand, has a cell body in the spinal cord or brainstem and an axon that extends outwards in a cranial or spinal motor nerve to reach an effector.

motor neurone disease (MND) a progressive degenerative disease of the motor system occurring in middle age and causing muscle weakness and wasting. It primarily affects the cells of the anterior horn of the spinal cord, the motor nuclei in the brainstem, and the corticospinal fibres. There are three clinically distinct forms: **amyotrophic lateral sclerosis** (**ALS**, **Lou Gehrig's disease**), **progressive muscular atrophy**, and **progressive bulbar palsy**. Some forms of MND are familial (inherited). The drug riluzole has been licensed for the treatment of MND with upper motor neurone involvement, but its benefits are limited.

mould *n.* any multicellular filamentous fungus that commonly forms a rough furry coating on decaying matter.

moulding *n.* the changing of the shape of an infant's head during labour, brought about by the pressures to which it is subjected when passing through the birth canal.

mountain sickness *see* ALTITUDE SICKNESS.

mouth-to-mouth respiration a form of *artificial respiration, performed mouth-to-mouth, by blowing air into the victim's lungs to inflate them and then allowing exhalation to occur automatically. It is commonly known as the **kiss of life**. The operator should aim to produce roughly 20 cycles of respiration per minute, or more for a younger victim.

mouthwash *n.* an aqueous solution with antiseptic, astringent, or deodorizing properties used for rinsing of the mouth and teeth. Mouthwashes are used to prevent dental *caries (*see also* CHLORHEXIDINE, FLUORIDE) and to treat mild throat infections.

mouthwash test a simple noninvasive procedure that enables the detection of *carriers for single gene defects, e.g. *cystic fibrosis. Epithelial cells from the buccal cavity are obtained from a saline mouthwash: from these it is possible to isolate DNA, which is amplified by the *polymerase chain reaction to enable gene analysis.

moxibustion *n.* a form of treatment favoured in Japan, in which cones of sunflower pith or down from the leaves of the plant *Artemisia moxa* are stuck to the skin and ignited. The heat produced by the smouldering cones acts as a counter-irritant and is reputed to cure a variety of disorders.

MRC *see* MEDICAL RESEARCH COUNCIL.

MRI *see* MAGNETIC RESONANCE IMAGING.

MRS *see* MAGNETIC RESONANCE SPECTROSCOPY.

MRSA methicillin- (or multiple-)resistant *Staphylococcus aureus*: an increasingly common dangerous bacterium that is resistant to many antibiotics and is responsible for outbreaks of infection in hospitals. *See* METHICILLIN.

MS *see* MULTIPLE SCLEROSIS.

MSH *see* MELANOCYTE-STIMULATING HORMONE.

MSU *see* MIDSTREAM SPECIMEN OF URINE.

mucilage *n.* (in pharmacy) a thick aqueous solution of a gum used as a lubricant in skin preparations (*see also* GLYCERIN), for the production of pills, and for the suspension of insoluble substances. The most important mucilages are of acacia, tragacanth, and starch.

mucin *n.* the principal constituent of *mucus. Mucin is a *glycoprotein.

muco- *prefix denoting* **1.** mucus. **2.** mucous membrane.

mucociliary transport the process by which cilia (*see* CILIUM) move a thin film of *mucus from the upper and lower respiratory tracts towards the digestive tract. Particles of dust and microorganisms are trapped on the mucus and thereby removed from the respiratory tract.

mucocoele *n.* a space or organ distended with mucus. For example, it may occur in the gall bladder when the exit duct becomes obstructed so that the mucus secretions are retained and dilate the cavity of the organ. A mucocoele in the soft tissues arising from a salivary gland occurs when the duct is blocked or ruptured.

mucolytic *n.* an agent, such as carbocysteine or tyloxapol, that dissolves or breaks down mucus. Mucolytics are used to treat chest conditions involving excessive or thickened mucus secretions.

mucopolysaccharide *n.* one of a group of complex carbohydrates functioning mainly as structural components in connective tissue. Mucopolysaccharide molecules are usually built up of two repeating sugar units, one of which is an amino sugar. An example of a mucopolysaccharide is *chondroitin, occurring in cartilage.

mucopolysaccharidosis *n.* any one of a group of eight rare genetic diseases that are *inborn errors of metabolism in which the storage of complex carbohydrates is disordered. The two most common are *Hunter's syndrome and *Hurler's syndrome.

mucoprotein *n.* one of a group of proteins found in the *globulin fraction of blood plasma. Mucoproteins are globulins combined with a carbohydrate group (an amino sugar). They are similar to *glyco-proteins but contain a greater proportion of carbohydrate.

mucopurulent *adj.* containing mucus and pus. *See* MUCOPUS.

mucopus *n.* a mixture of *mucus and *pus.

Mucor *n.* a genus of mould fungi commonly seen on dead and decaying organic matter. They can be pathogenic in man.

mucosa *n. see* MUCOUS MEMBRANE. —**mucosal** *adj.*

mucous membrane (mucosa) the moist membrane lining many tubular structures and cavities, including the nasal sinuses, respiratory tract, gastrointestinal tract, biliary, and pancreatic systems. The surface of the mouth is lined by mucous membrane, the nature of which varies according to its site. The mucous membrane consists of a surface layer of *epithelium, which contains glands secreting *mucus, with underlying layers of connective tissue (lamina propria) and muscularis mucosae, which forms the inner boundary of the mucous membrane.

mucoviscidosis *n. see* CYSTIC FIBROSIS.

mucus *n.* a viscous fluid secreted by *mucous membranes. Mucus acts as a protective barrier over the membranes, a lubricant, and a carrier of enzymes. It consists chiefly of *glycoproteins, particularly **mucin**. —**mucous** *adj.*

MUGA scan (multiple-gated arteriography) a method of studying the left-ventricular function and wall motion of the heart by injecting the patient's red cells with radioactive technetium-99 to form an image of the blood pool within the heart at specific points in the cardiac cycle, using an ECG, *gamma camera, and computer.

Müllerian duct *see* PARAMESONEPHRIC DUCT. [J. P. Müller (1801–58), German physiologist]

multifactorial *adj.* describing a condition that is believed to have resulted from the interaction of genetic factors, usually polygenes, with an environmental factor or factors. Many disorders, e.g. spina bifida

and anencephaly, are thought to be multifactorial.

multifocal lenses lenses in which the power (*see* DIOPTRE) of the lower part gradually increases towards the lower edge. There is no dividing line on the lens as there is between the upper and lower segments of *bifocal lenses. The wearer can see clearly at any distance by lowering or raising his eyes.

multigravida *n.* a woman who has been pregnant at least twice.

multi-organ failure (MOF) the terminal stage of serious illness.

multipara *n.* a woman who has given birth to a live child after each of at least two pregnancies. *See also* GRAND MULTIPARITY.

multiple organ dysfunction syndrome (MODS) a common cause of death following severe injury, overwhelming infection, or immune deficiency states.

multiple personality disorder a psychiatric disorder in which the affected person has two or more distinct, and often contrasting, personalities. As each personality assumes dominance, it determines attitudes and behaviour and usually appears to be unaware of the other personality (or personalities). Transition is sudden and the mental states of the different personalities are normal. The condition is thought to be a late result of *child abuse. Treatment is by psychotherapy.

multiple sclerosis (MS, disseminated sclerosis) a chronic disease of the nervous system affecting young and middle-aged adults. The *myelin sheaths surrounding nerves in the brain and spinal cord are damaged, which affects the function of the nerves involved. The course of the illness is usually characterized by recurrent relapses followed by remissions, but a small proportion of patients run a chronic progressive course. The disease affects different parts of the brain and spinal cord, resulting in typically scattered symptoms. These include unsteady gait and shaky movements of the limbs (ataxia), rapid involuntary movements of the eyes (*nystagmus), defects in speech pronunciation (dysarthria), spastic weakness, and *retrobulbar neuritis. The underlying cause of the nerve damage remains unknown. Steroid treatment may be used in an acute relapse, and beta-*interferon therapy may reduce the relapse rate.

multisystem *adj.* describing a disease that affects many systems of the body.

multivariate analysis *see* CORRELATION.

mummification *n.* **1.** the conversion of dead tissue into a hard shrunken mass, chiefly by dehydration. **2.** (in dentistry) the application of a fixative to the dental pulp to prevent decomposition.

mumps *n.* a common virus infection mainly affecting school-age children. Symptoms appear 2–3 weeks after exposure: fever, headache, and vomiting may precede a typical swelling of the *parotid salivary glands. The gland on one side of the face often swells up days before the other but sometimes only one side is affected. The symptoms usually vanish within three days, the patient remaining infectious until the swelling has completely disappeared, but the infection may spread to other salivary glands and to the pancreas, brain (causing an aseptic meningitis), and testicles (after puberty mumps affecting the testicles can cause sterility). Vaccination against mumps provides effective immunity (*see* MMR VACCINE). Medical name: **infectious parotitis**.

Munchausen's syndrome a mental disorder in which the patient persistently tries to obtain hospital treatment, especially surgery, for an illness that is nonexistent: it is an extreme form of malingering. The disease may be described in vivid detail, and in some cases injury may be deliberately self-inflicted in an attempt to give the appearance of authenticity to the claims being made. In **Munchausen's syndrome by proxy**, the patient inflicts harm on others (often children) in order to attract medical attention. [Baron von Munchausen, a fictional character who told exaggerated stories]

murmur (bruit) *n.* a noise, heard with the aid of a stethoscope, that is generated by turbulent blood flow within the heart or blood vessels. Turbulent flow is produced by damaged valves, *septal defects,

narrowed arteries, or arteriovenous communications. Heart murmurs can also be heard in normal individuals, especially those who have hyperactive circulation, and frequently in normal children (**innocent murmurs**). Murmurs are classified as **systolic** or **diastolic** (heard in ventricular *systole or *diastole respectively); **continuous murmurs** are heard throughout systole and diastole.

Murphy's sign a sign of inflammation of the gall bladder: continuous pressure over the gall bladder while the patient is taking a deep breath will cause a catch in the breath at the point of maximum inhalation. [J. B. Murphy (1857–1916), US surgeon]

muscae volitantes *pl. n.* black spots seen floating before the eyes usually due to the presence of opacities in the vitreous humour as it becomes more fluid with age.

muscle *n.* a tissue whose cells have the ability to contract, producing movement or force (see illustration). Muscles possess mechanisms for converting energy derived from chemical reactions into mechanical energy. The major functions of muscles are to produce movements of the body, to maintain the position of the body against the force of gravity, to produce movements of structures inside the body, and to alter pressures or tensions of structures in the body. There are three types of muscle: *striated muscle, attached to the skeleton; *smooth muscle, which is found in such tissues as the stomach, gut, and blood vessels; and *cardiac muscle, which forms the walls of the heart.

muscle relaxant an agent that reduces tension in muscles. Drugs such as *dantrolene and *diazepam are used to relieve skeletal muscular spasms in various spastic conditions, parkinsonism, and tetanus. Other drugs, e.g. *alcuronium, *gallamine, *suxamethonium, and *tubocurarine, block the transmission of impulses at neuromuscular junctions and are used to relax voluntary muscles during the administration of anaesthetics in surgical operations.

muscle spindle a specialized receptor, sensitive to stretch, that is embedded between and parallel to the fibres of striated

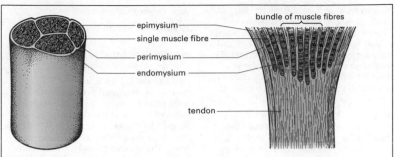

A voluntary muscle in transverse section (left) and in longitudinal section at its junction with a tendon (right)

muscles. These receptors are important for coordinated muscular movement. *See also* STRETCH RECEPTOR.

muscular dystrophy a group of muscle diseases, marked by weakness and wasting of selected muscles, in which there is a recognizable pattern of inheritance. The affected muscle fibres degenerate and are replaced by fatty tissue. The muscular dystrophies are classified according to the patient's age at onset, distribution of the weakness, the progression of the disease, and the mode of inheritance. Isolated cases may occur as a result of gene mutation. Confirmation of the diagnosis is based upon *electromyography and muscle biopsy.

One common form is **Duchenne's muscular dystrophy**, which is inherited as a *sex-linked recessive character and is nearly always restricted to boys. It usually begins before the age of four, with selective weakness and wasting of the muscles of the pelvic girdle and back. The child has a waddling gait and *lordosis of the lumbar spine. The calf muscles – and later the shoulders and upper limbs – often become firm and bulky. Although the disease cannot be cured, physiotherapy and orthopaedic measures can relieve the disability. The identification of the gene abnormality raises the possibility of *gene therapy in the future. *See also* BECKER MUSCULAR DYSTROPHY, DYSTROPHIA MYOTONICA (MYOTONIC DYSTROPHY).

muscularis *n.* a muscular layer of the wall of a hollow organ (such as the stom-

ach) or a tubular structure (such as the intestine or the ureter). The **muscularis mucosae** is the muscular layer of a mucous membrane complex, especially that of the stomach or intestine.

muscular rheumatism any aching pain in the muscles and joints. Commonly the symptoms are due to *fibrositis; wear and tear of the joints (*osteoarthritis); or to inflammation of the muscles associated with abnormal immune reactions (*polymyalgia rheumatica).

musculo- *prefix denoting* muscle.

musculocutaneous nerve a nerve of the *brachial plexus that supplies some muscles of the arm and the skin of the lateral part of the forearm.

mushroom *n.* the aerial fruiting (spore-producing) body of various fungi. Edible species include field mushrooms and cultivated mushrooms (*Agaricus campestris* and *A. bisporus*), the chanterelle (*Cantherellus cibarius*), and the parasol (*Lepiota procera*). However, great care must be taken in identifying edible fungi. Many species are poisonous, especially the death cap and panther cap (*see* AMANITA).

mustine (nitrogen mustard) *n.* a drug used to treat various types of cancer, including Hodgkin's disease and some types of leukaemia. It is administered by injection; common side-effects include nausea and vomiting, and the drug may damage the bone marrow, causing serious blood disorders.

mutagen *n.* an external agent that, when applied to cells or organisms, can increase the rate of *mutation. Mutagens usually only increase the number of mutants formed and do not cause mutations not found under natural conditions. Several kinds of radiation, many chemicals, and certain viruses can act as mutagens. *Compare* ANTIMUTAGEN.

mutant *n.* **1.** an individual in which a mutation has occurred, especially when the effect of the mutation is visible. **2.** a characteristic showing the effects of a mutation. —**mutant** *adj.*

mutation *n.* a change in the genetic material (*DNA) of a cell, or the change this causes in a characteristic of the individual, which is not caused by normal genetic processes. In a **point** (or **gene**) **mutation** there is a change in a single gene; in a **chromosome mutation** there is a change in the structure or number of the chromosomes. All mutations are rare events and may occur spontaneously or be caused by external agents (*mutagens). If a mutation occurs in developing sex cells (gametes) it may be inherited. Mutations in any other cells (**somatic mutations**) are not inherited.

mutism *n.* inability or refusal to speak; dumbness. Innate speechlessness most commonly occurs in those who have been totally deaf since birth (**deaf-mutism**). Inability to speak may result from brain damage (*see* APHASIA). It may also be caused by depression or psychological trauma, in which case the patient either does not speak at all or speaks only to particular persons or in particular situations. This latter condition is called **elective mutism**.

Treatment of mutism due to psychological causes is now increasingly by behavioural means, such as *prompting: people that the patient does not address are slowly introduced into the situation where the patient does speak. This may be done either alone or in combination with more traditional psychotherapy. —**mute** *adj.*, *n.*

mutualism *n.* the intimate but not necessarily obligatory association between two different species of organism in which there is mutual aid and benefit. *Compare* SYMBIOSIS.

my- (myo-) *prefix denoting* muscle.

myalgia *n.* pain in the muscles. —**myalgic** *adj.*

myalgic encephalomyelitis (ME) *see* CHRONIC FATIGUE SYNDROME.

myasthenia gravis a chronic disease marked by abnormal fatigability and weakness of selected muscles, which is relieved by rest or *anticholinesterase drugs. The degree of fatigue is so extreme that these muscles are temporarily paralysed. The muscles initially affected are those around the eyes, mouth, and throat, resulting in drooping of the upper eyelids (*ptosis), double vision, and *dysarthria. Myasthenia gravis is an *autoimmune disease in which autoantibodies bind to cholinergic receptors on muscle cells, which impairs the ability of the neurotransmitter acetylcholine to induce muscular contraction. It chiefly affects adolescents and young adults (usually women) and adults over 40. Drug treatment and surgical removal of the thymus lessen the severity of the symptoms. Steroid therapy or plasma exchange may be used to treat the more severely affected patients.

myc- (myco-, mycet(o)-) *prefix denoting* a fungus.

mycelium *n.* (*pl.* **mycelia**) the tangled mass of fine branching threads that make up the feeding and growing part of a *fungus.

mycetoma *n.* a chronic inflammation of tissues caused by a fungus. *See* MADURA FOOT.

Mycobacterium *n.* a genus of rodlike Gram-positive aerobic bacteria that can form filamentous branching structures. Some species are pathogenic to animals and man: *M. leprae* (**Hansen's bacillus**) causes *leprosy; *M. tuberculosis* (**Koch's bacillus**) causes *tuberculosis. *M. bovis* causes tuberculosis in cattle but can also infect the lungs, joints, and intestines of man. *M. paratuberculosis*, which causes Johne's disease in cattle, can also be transmitted in milk and is suspected of being a cause of Crohn's disease in man.

M. tuberculosis is by far the most common species responsible for infections of the lung. Other mycobacteria that infect the lung are variously described as atypical, anonymous, or *opportunistic – the favoured term since they usually require pre-existing lung damage or a defect in the patient's immunity before they can give rise to infection. The opportunistic mycobacteria that most commonly cause lung infections are *M. kansacii, M. xenopi, M. malmoense,* and a group known as the **MAI complex** (*M. avium, M. intracellulare*). Infections caused by all these organisms can mimic pulmonary tuberculosis but are much more difficult to treat since they are resistant to many of the antituberculosis drugs. The MAI organisms are particularly likely to cause superimposed infection in cases of AIDS.

mycology *n.* the science of fungi. *See also* MICROBIOLOGY. —**mycologist** *n.*

mycoplasma *n.* one of a group of minute nonmotile microorganisms that lack a rigid cell wall and hence display a variety of forms. They are regarded by most authorities as primitive bacteria. The group includes some species that cause severe respiratory disease in cattle, sheep, and goats; one of these, *Mycoplasma pneumoniae,* causes *atypical pneumonia in man. The group also includes the **pleuropneumonia-like organisms** (**PPLO**).

mycosis *n.* any disease caused by a fungus, including actinomycosis, aspergillosis, cryptococcosis, rhinosporidiosis, ringworm, and sporotrichosis.

mycosis fungoides a disease that is a variety of *reticulosis confined to the skin, with plaques and later nodules infiltrated with T-lymphocytes. It progresses very slowly and can be treated initially with topical corticosteroids, later with *PUVA and electron-beam therapy; chemotherapy is not helpful.

Mycota *n. see* UNDECENOIC ACID.

mydriasis *n.* widening of the pupil, which occurs normally in dim light. The commonest cause of prolonged mydriasis is drug therapy (*see* MYDRIATIC) or injury to the eye. *See also* CYCLOPLEGIA. *Compare* MIOSIS.

mydriatic *n.* a drug that causes the pupil of the eye to dilate. Examples are *atropine, *cyclopentolate, and *phenyl-

ephrine. Mydriatics are used to aid examination of the eye and to treat some eye inflammations such as iritis and cyclitis.

myectomy *n.* a surgical operation to remove part of a muscle.

myel- (myelo-) *prefix denoting* **1.** the spinal cord. **2.** bone marrow. **3.** myelin.

myelencephalon *n. see* MEDULLA OBLONGATA.

myelin *n.* a complex material formed of protein and *phospholipid that is laid down as a sheath around the *axons of certain neurones, known as **myelinated** (or **medullated**) **nerve fibres**. The material is produced and laid down in concentric layers by *Schwann cells at regular intervals along the nerve fibre (see illustrations). Myelinated nerves conduct impulses more rapidly than nonmyelinated nerves.

Schwann cell

axon of neurone

folds of Schwann cell wrap around axon

areas where myelin will form

Formation of a myelin sheath by a Schwann cell

node of Ranvier

Schwann cell

nucleus of Schwann cell

myelin sheath

axon

Longitudinal section through a myelinated nerve fibre

myelination *n.* the process in which *myelin is laid down as an insulating layer around the axons of certain nerves. Myelination of nerve tracts in the central nervous system is completed by the second year of life.

myelitis *n.* **1.** an inflammatory disease of the spinal cord. The most usual kind (**transverse myelitis**) most often occurs during the development of multiple sclerosis, but it is sometimes a manifestation of *encephalomyelitis, when it can occur as an isolated attack. The inflammation spreads more or less completely across the tissue of the spinal cord, resulting in a loss of its normal function to transmit nerve impulses up and down. It is as though the spinal cord had been severed: paralysis and numbness affects the legs and trunk below the level of the diseased tissue. **2.** inflammation of the bone marrow. *See* OSTEOMYELITIS.

myeloblast *n.* the earliest identifiable cell that gives rise to a *granulocyte, having a large nucleus and scanty cytoplasm. It is normally found in the blood-forming tissue of the bone marrow, but may appear in the blood in a variety of diseases, most notably in acute myeloblastic *leukaemia. *See also* GRANULOPOIESIS. —**myeloblastic** *adj.*

myelocele *n.* *see* NEURAL TUBE DEFECTS.

myelocyte *n.* an immature form of *granulocyte having a round nucleus (*compare* METAMYELOCYTE) and neutrophil, eosinophil, or basophil granules within its cytoplasm (*compare* PROMYELOCYTE). It is normally found in the blood-forming tissue of the bone marrow, but may appear in the blood in a variety of diseases, including infections, infiltrations of the bone marrow, and certain leukaemias. *See also* GRANULOPOIESIS.

myelofibrosis *n.* a chronic but progressive disease characterized by *fibrosis of the bone marrow, which leads to anaemia and the presence of immature red and white blood cells in the circulation. Other features include enlargement of the spleen and the presence of blood-forming (myeloid) tissue in abnormal sites, such as the spleen and liver. Its cause is unknown.

myelography *n.* a specialized method of X-ray examination to demonstrate the spinal canal that involves injection of a radiopaque contrast medium into the sub-

arachnoid space. The X-rays obtained are called **myelograms**. It is of importance in the recognition of tumours of the spinal cord and other conditions compressing the cord or the nerve roots. The former use of oil-based dyes in myelography was an occasional cause of *arachnoiditis. This complication is now avoided by the use of water-soluble contrast media. Myelography is now often combined with simultaneous CT scanning.

myeloid *adj.* **1.** like, derived from, or relating to bone marrow. **2.** resembling a *myelocyte. **3.** relating to the spinal cord.

myeloid leukaemia a variety of *leukaemia in which the type of blood cell that proliferates abnormally originates in the blood-forming (myeloid) tissue of the bone marrow. Myeloid leukaemias may be acute or chronic and may involve any one of the cells produced by the marrow.

myeloid tissue a tissue in the *bone marrow in which the various classes of blood cells are produced. *See also* HAEMOPOIESIS.

myeloma (multiple myeloma, myelomatosis) *n.* a malignant disease of the bone marrow, characterized by two or more of the following criteria: (1) the presence of an excess of abnormal malignant plasma cells in the bone marrow; (2) typical deposits in the bones on X-ray, giving the appearance of holes; (3) the presence in the serum of an abnormal gammaglobulin, usually IgG (an immunoglobulin; *see* PARAPROTEIN). *Bence-Jones protein may also be found in the serum or urine. The patient may complain of tiredness due to anaemia and of bone pain and may develop pathological fractures. Treatment is usually with such drugs as melphalan or cyclophosphamide, with local radiotherapy to particular areas of pain. Radiotherapy of the whole body is sometimes used in the primary treatment of myeloma. *See also* PLASMACYTOMA.

myelomalacia *n.* softening of the tissues of the spinal cord, most often caused by an impaired blood supply.

myelomatosis *n.* *see* MYELOMA.

myelomeningocele *n.* *see* NEURAL TUBE DEFECTS.

myelosuppression n. a reduction in blood-cell production by the bone marrow. It commonly occurs after chemotherapy and may result in anaemia, infection, and abnormal bleeding (see THROMBO-CYTOPENIA, NEUTROPENIA). —**myelosuppressive** adj.

myenteric reflex a reflex action of the intestine in which a physical stimulus causes the intestine to contract above and relax below the point of stimulation.

myenteron n. the muscular layer of the *intestine, consisting of a layer of circular muscle inside a layer of longitudinal muscle. These muscles are used in *peristalsis. —**myenteric** adj.

myiasis n. an infestation of a living organ or tissue by maggots. The flies normally breed in decaying animal and vegetable matter; myiasis therefore generally occurs only in regions of poor hygiene, and in most cases the infestations are accidental. Various genera may infect humans. *Gasterophilus, *Hypoderma, *Dermatobia, and Cordylobia affect the skin; Fannia invades the alimentary canal and the urinary system; *Phormia and *Wohlfahrtia can infest open wounds and ulcers; *Oestrus attacks the eyes; and Cochliomyia invades the nasal passages. Treatment of external myiases involves the destruction and removal of maggots followed by the application of antibiotics to wounds and lesions.

mylohyoid n. a muscle in the floor of the mouth, attached at one end to the mandible and at the other to the hyoid bone.

myo- prefix. see MY-.

myoblast n. a cell that develops into a muscle fibre. —**myoblastic** adj.

myocardial infarction death of a segment of heart muscle, which follows interruption of its blood supply (see CORONARY THROMBOSIS). Myocardial infarction is usually confined to the left ventricle. The patient experiences a 'heart attack': sudden severe chest pain, which may spread to the arms and throat. The main danger is that of ventricular *fibrillation, which accounts for most of the fatalities. Other *arrhythmias are also frequent; *ectopic beats in the ventricle are especially important as they predispose to ventricular fibrillation. Other complications include heart failure, rupture of the heart, phlebothrombosis, pulmonary embolism, pericarditis, shock, mitral incompetence, and perforation of the septum between the ventricles.

The best results from the management of patients with myocardial infarction follow mobile and hospital-based coronary care with facilities for the early detection, prevention, and treatment of arrhythmias and *cardiac arrest. Most survivors of myocardial infarction are able to return to a full and active life, including those who have been successfully resuscitated from cardiac arrest.

myocarditis n. acute or chronic inflammation of the heart muscle. It may be seen alone or as part of pancarditis (see ENDOMYOCARDITIS).

myocardium n. the middle of the three layers forming the wall of the heart (see also ENDOCARDIUM, EPICARDIUM). It is composed of *cardiac muscle and forms the greater part of the heart wall, being thicker in the ventricles than in the atria. —**myocardial** adj.

myoclonus n. a sudden spasm of the muscles. Occasional **myoclonic jerks** occur between seizures in patients with idiopathic *epilepsy, and myoclonus is a major feature of some progressive neurological illnesses with extensive degeneration of the brain cells (including the *spongiform encephalopathies). Myoclonic jerks on falling asleep (**nocturnal myoclonus**) occur in normal individuals. —**myoclonic** adj.

myocyte n. a muscle cell.

myodynia n. pain in the muscles.

myoepithelium n. a tissue consisting of cells of epithelial origin having a contractile cytoplasm. Myoepithelial cells play an important role in encouraging the secretion of substances into ducts.

myofibril n. one of numerous contractile filaments found within the cytoplasm of *striated muscle cells. When viewed under a microscope myofibrils show alternating bands of high and low refractive index, which give striated muscle its characteristic appearance.

myogenic *adj.* originating in muscle: applied to the inherent rhythmicity of contraction of some muscles (e.g. cardiac muscle), which does not depend on neural influences.

myoglobin *n.* *see* MYOHAEMOGLOBIN.

myoglobinuria *n.* *see* MYOHAEMOGLOBIN-URIA.

myogram *n.* a recording of the activity of a muscle. *See* ELECTROMYOGRAPHY.

myograph *n.* an instrument for recording the activity of muscular tissues. *See* ELECTROMYOGRAPHY.

myohaemoglobin (myoglobin) *n.* an iron-containing protein, resembling *haemoglobin, found in muscle cells. Like haemoglobin it contains a haem group, which binds reversibly with oxygen, and so acts as an oxygen reservoir within the muscle fibres.

myohaemoglobinuria (myoglobin-uria) *n.* the presence in the urine of the pigment myohaemoglobin.

myokymia *n.* prominent quivering of a few muscle fibres, not associated with any other abnormal features. It is a benign condition. *See also* FASCICULATION.

myology *n.* the study of the structure, function, and diseases of the muscles.

myoma *n.* a benign tumour of muscle. It may originate in smooth muscle (*see* LEIOMYOMA) or in striated muscle (*see* RHABDOMYOMA).

myomectomy *n.* an operation in which benign tumours (fibroids) are removed from the muscular wall of the uterus.

myometritis *n.* inflammation of the muscular wall (myometrium) of the uterus.

myometrium *n.* the muscular tissue of the uterus, which surrounds the *endometrium. It is composed of smooth muscle that undergoes small regular spontaneous contractions. The frequency and amplitude of these contractions alter in response to the hormones *oestrogen, *progesterone, and *oxytocin, which are present at particular stages of the menstrual cycle and pregnancy.

myoneural junction *see* NEUROMUSCULAR JUNCTION.

myopathy *n.* any disease of the muscles. The myopathies are usually subdivided into those that are inherited (*see* MUSCULAR DYSTROPHY) and those that are acquired. The acquired myopathies include *polymyositis and muscular diseases complicating endocrine disorders or carcinoma. All are typified by weakness and wasting of the muscles, which may be associated with pain and tenderness.

myopia (short-sightedness) *n.* the condition in which parallel light rays are brought to a focus in front of the retina (see illustration). Distant objects are blurred and cannot be made sharp by *accommodation. Myopia is corrected by wearing spectacles with concave lenses and can now be treated by surgery (*see* EXCIMER LASER, INTRASTROMAL KERATOMILEUSIS, RADIAL KERATOTOMY). *Compare* EMMETROPIA, LASIK, HYPERMETROPIA. —**myopic** *adj.*

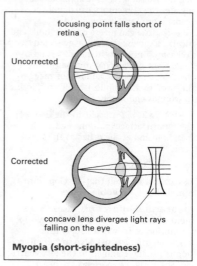

focusing point falls short of retina

Uncorrected

Corrected

concave lens diverges light rays falling on the eye

Myopia (short-sightedness)

myoplasm *n.* *see* SARCOPLASM.

myoplasty *n.* the plastic surgery of muscle, in which part of a muscle is partly detached and used to repair tissue defects or deformities in the vicinity of the muscle. It is frequently used in *flap surgery and anal operations (*anoplasty).

myosarcoma n. a malignant tumour of muscle. See also LEIOMYOSARCOMA, RHAB-DOMYOSARCOMA.

myosin n. the most abundant protein in muscle fibrils, having the important properties of elasticity and contractility. With actin, it comprises the principal contractile element of muscles. See STRIATED MUSCLE.

myosis n. see MIOSIS.

myositis n. any of a group of muscle diseases in which inflammation and degenerative changes occur. *Polymyositis is the most commonly occurring example, but myositis may be found in relation to systemic *connective-tissue diseases and a minority are caused by bacterial or parasitic infections.

myositis ossificans the formation of bone in a *muscle that occurs after dislocations or fractures, especially around the elbow. It is initially painful and swollen, and the joint then becomes very stiff, surrounded by a mass of new bone.

myotactic adj. relating to the sense of touch in muscles.

myotatic reflex see STRETCH REFLEX.

myotome n. that part of the segmented mesoderm in the early embryo that gives rise to all the skeletal muscle of the body. Visceral (smooth) muscles develop from unsegmented mesoderm (see MESENCHYME). See also SOMITE.

myotomy n. the dissection or surgical division of a muscle.

myotonia n. a disorder of the muscle fibres that results in abnormally prolonged contractions. The patient has difficulty in relaxing a movement (e.g. his grip) after any vigorous effort. It is a feature of a hereditary condition starting in infancy or early childhood (**myotonia congenita**) and of a form of muscular dystrophy (*dystrophia myotonica).

myotonic adj. relating to muscle tone.

myotonus n. **1.** a tonic muscular spasm. **2.** muscle tone.

myringa n. the eardrum (see TYMPANIC MEMBRANE).

myringitis n. inflammation of the eardrum. See OTITIS (MEDIA).

myringoplasty (tympanoplasty) n. surgical repair of a perforated eardrum by grafting.

myringotomy n. incision of the eardrum to create an artificial opening, either to allow infected fluid to drain from the middle ear in acute *otitis media or to remove fluid in *glue ear and permit the insertion of a *grommet.

myx- (myxo-) prefix denoting mucus.

myxoedema n. **1.** a dry firm waxy swelling of the skin and subcutaneous tissues found in patients with underactive thyroid glands (see HYPOTHYROIDISM). **2.** the clinical syndrome due to hypothyroidism in adult life, including coarsening of the skin, intolerance to cold, weight gain, and mental dullness. The symptoms are abolished with thyroxine treatment. —**myxoedematous** adj.

myxofibroma n. a benign tumour of fibrous tissue that contains myxomatous elements (see MYXOMA) or has undergone mucoid degeneration.

myxoid cyst a small cyst containing a thick sticky fluid. It develops over the end joint of a finger or toe and should not be cut out, because the cyst is usually in communication with the underlying joint.

myxoma n. a benign gelatinous tumour of connective tissue. **Atrial myxoma** is a tumour of the heart, usually of the left side, arising from the septum dividing the two upper chambers. Symptoms may include fever, lassitude, joint pains, and sudden loss of consciousness due to obstruction of the bloodflow. The tumour may be wrongly diagnosed as stenosis of the mitral valve as it can produce a similar murmur. Treatment requires surgical removal. —**myxomatous** adj.

myxosarcoma n. a *sarcoma containing mucoid material; it is the malignant counterpart of a *myxoma. It is doubtful whether myxosarcoma represents a true entity and it may be simply a variant of other sarcomas, such as a *liposarcoma or a *fibrosarcoma, with which it shares clinical features.

myxovirus *n.* one of a group of RNA-containing viruses that are associated with various diseases in animals and humans.

The **orthomyxoviruses** cause diseases of the respiratory tract, most notably influenza. The related **paramyxo-viruses** include the *respiratory syncytial virus (RSV) and the agents that cause measles, mumps, and parainfluenza.

nabilone *n.* a drug related to cannabis, used to control severe nausea and vomiting, especially when caused by anticancer drugs. Administered by mouth, it is thought to act on opiate receptors in the nervous system. Trade name: **Cesamet**.

nabothian follicle (nabothian cyst, nabothian gland) one of a number of cysts on the neck (cervix) of the uterus, near its opening to the vagina. The sacs, which contain mucus, form when the ducts of the glands in the cervix are blocked by a new growth of surface cells (epithelium) over an area damaged because of infection.

NAD (nicotinamide adenine dinucleotide) a *coenzyme that acts as a hydrogen acceptor in oxidation-reduction reactions, particularly in the *electron transport chain in cellular respiration. NAD and the closely related coenzyme **NADP (nicotinamide adenine dinucleotide phosphate)** are derived from nicotinic acid; they are reduced to **NADH** and **NADPH**, respectively.

nadolol *n.* a *beta blocker used in the treatment of angina pectoris and high blood pressure (hypertension). It is administered by mouth; side-effects include decreased heart rate, dizziness, and low blood pressure. Trade name: **Corgard**.

NADP (nicotinamide adenine dinucleotide phosphate) *see* NAD.

Naegele rule a method used to estimate the probable date of the onset of labour: nine months and seven days are added to the date of the first day of the last menstrual period. A correction is required if the woman does not have 28-day menstrual cycles. [F. K. Naegele (1777–1851), German obstetrician]

Naegele's obliquity *see* ASYNCLITISM.

Naegleria *n.* a genus of *amoebae that normally live in damp soil or mud. *Naegleria* species can, however, live as parasites in man and are believed to have caused some rare, but fatal, infections of the brain.

naevus *n.* (*pl.* **naevi**) a birthmark: a clearly defined malformation of the skin, present at birth. There are many different types of naevi. Some, including the strawberry naevus and port-wine stain, are composed of small blood vessels (*see* HAEMANGIOMA). The **strawberry naevus** (or **strawberry mark**) is a raised red lump usually appearing on the face and growing rapidly in the first month of life. These birthmarks slowly resolve and spontaneously disappear between the ages of five and ten. The **port-wine stain** (or **capillary naevus**) is a permanent purplish discoloration that may occur anywhere but usually appears on the upper half of the body. Laser treatment can reduce the discoloration. Occasionally a port-wine stain may be associated with a malformation of blood vessels over the brain, for example in the Sturge-Weber syndrome (*see* ANGIOMA).

It is not uncommon for a pale or white halo to develop around an ordinary pigmented naevus, especially on the trunk, forming a **halo naevus**. The pigmented naevus disappears over the course of a few months; this is followed by resolution of the pale area. A **blue naevus** is a small blue-grey papule appearing at birth or later in life, mainly on the extremities. Progression to malignant melanoma is very rare. A **naevus of Ota (oculodermal melanocytosis)** is a blue-grey pigmented area on the cheek, eyelid, or forehead with similar pigmentation of the sclera of an eye. It is associated with melanomas of the uvea, orbit, and brain as well as with glaucoma of the affected eye. *See also* MOLE².

Naga sore *see* TROPICAL ULCER.

NAI *see* NONACCIDENTAL INJURY.

nail *n.* a horny structure, composed of keratin, formed from the epidermis on the dorsal surface of each finger and toe (see illustration). The exposed part of the nail is the **body**, behind which is the **root**.

The whitish crescent-shaped area at the base of the body is called the **lunula**. Growth of the nail occurs at the end of the nail root by division of the germinative layer of the underlying *epidermis (which forms part of the **matrix**). The growing nail slides forward over the **nail bed**. The fold of skin that lies above the root is the **nail fold**; folds of skin on either side of the nail are the **nail walls**. The epidermis of the nail fold that lies next to the nail root is called the **eponychium** (forming the 'cuticle' at the base of the nail). Anatomical name: **unguis**.

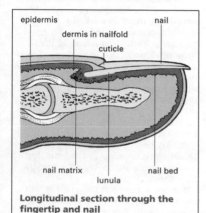

epidermis

nail

dermis in nailfold

cuticle

nail matrix

nail bed

lunula

Longitudinal section through the fingertip and nail

nalidixic acid a *quinolone antibiotic active against various bacteria and used to treat infections of the urinary and digestive systems. It is administered by mouth; common side-effects are nausea, vomiting, and skin reactions. Trade names: **Negram**, **Uriben**.

naloxone *n.* a drug that is a specific antidote to morphine and similar narcotic drugs. It is administered by intravenous or subcutaneous injection. As it is short-acting, repeated doses may be necessary. Trade name: **Narcan**.

naltrexone *n.* a narcotic antagonist drug that is used in the maintenance treatment of heroin- and other opiate-dependent patients. It is administered by mouth. Possible side-effects include abdominal cramps, nausea and vomiting,

sleep difficulties, and dizziness. Trade name: **Nalorex**.

nandrolone *n.* a synthetic male sex hormone with *anabolic effects. It is administered by injection and high doses may cause signs of *virilization in women. Trade name: **Deca-Durabolin**.

nano- *prefix denoting* **1.** extremely small size. **2.** one thousand-millionth part (10^{-9}).

nanometre *n.* one thousand-millionth of a metre $(10^{-9}$ m). One nanometre is equal to 10 angstrom. Symbol: nm.

nanophthalmos *n.* a congenitally small eye in which all the structures are proportionally reduced.

naphazoline *n.* a drug that constricts small blood vessels and is used to relieve congestion in rhinitis and sinusitis. It is administered as nasal drops and may cause slight irritation. Trade name: **Vasocon-A**.

napkin rash (nappy rash) a red skin rash within the napkin area, usually caused by chemical irritation (ammoniacal *dermatitis) or infection with *Candida*. Ammoniacal dermatitis is caused by skin contact with wet soiled nappies, the stool bacteria reacting with urine to form irritant ammonia. Treatment involves exposure to air, application of barrier creams, and frequent nappy changes. Candidal nappy rash is treated with antifungal creams. Other causes of napkin rash include eczema and psoriasis.

naprapathy *n.* a system of medicine based on the belief that a great many diseases are attributable to displacement of ligaments, tendons, and other connective tissues and that cure can be brought about only by manipulation to correct these displacements.

naproxen *n.* an analgesic drug that also reduces inflammation and fever (*see* NSAID). It is used to treat rheumatoid arthritis, ankylosing spondylitis, and gout. It is administered by mouth; side-effects may include digestive upsets and rashes. Trade names: **Naprosyn**, **Nycopren**.

narcissism *n.* an excessive involvement with oneself and one's self-importance. In Freudian terms it is a state in which the *ego has taken itself as a love object. Some degree of narcissism is present in most individuals, but when it is shown to an extreme degree it may be a symptom of schizophrenia, personality disorder, or other conditions. **—narcissistic** *adj.*

narco- *prefix denoting* narcosis; stupor.

narcolepsy *n.* an extreme tendency to fall asleep in quiet surroundings or when engaged in monotonous activities. The patient can be woken easily and is immediately alert. It is often associated with *cataplexy, and when falling asleep the patient may experience hallucinations or transient attacks of muscular paralysis. **—narcoleptic** *adj., n.*

narcosis *n.* a state of diminished consciousness or complete unconsciousness caused by the use of *narcotic drugs, which have a depressant action on the nervous system. The body's normal reactions to stimuli are diminished and the body may become sedated or completely anaesthetized.

narcotic *n.* a drug that induces stupor and insensibility and relieves pain. The term is used particularly for *morphine and other derivatives of opium (*see* OPIATE) but is also applied to other drugs that depress brain function (e.g. general anaesthetics and hypnotics). In legal terms a narcotic is any addictive drug subject to illegal use. Narcotics (i.e. morphine and morphine-like drugs) have been largely replaced as sleeping drugs because of their ability to cause *dependence and tolerance; they are still used for relief of severe pain (*see* ANALGESIC).

nares *pl. n.* (*sing.* **naris**) openings of the nose. The two **external** (or **anterior**) **nares** are the nostrils, leading from the nasal cavity to the outside. The two **internal** (or **posterior**) **nares** (**choanae**) are the openings leading from the nasal cavity into the pharynx.

nasal bone either of a pair of narrow oblong bones that together form the bridge and root of the nose. *See* SKULL.

nasal cavity the space inside the nose that lies between the floor of the cranium and the roof of the mouth. It is divided into two halves by a septum: each half communicates with the outside via the nostrils and with the nasopharynx through the posterior nares.

nasal concha (turbinate bone) any of three thin scroll-like bones that form the sides of the *nasal cavity. The **superior** and **middle nasal conchae** are part of the *ethmoid bone; the **inferior nasal conchae** are a separate pair of bones of the face. *See* SKULL.

nasion *n.* the point on the bridge of the nose at the centre of the suture between the nasal and frontal bones.

naso- *prefix denoting* the nose.

nasogastric tube a tube passed through the nose into the stomach, used to aspirate fluid from, or introduce material into, the stomach (*see* RYLE'S TUBE).

nasolacrimal *adj.* relating to the nose and the lacrimal (tear-producing) apparatus.

nasolacrimal duct the duct that passes through the hole (**nasolacrimal canal**) in the palatine bone of the skull. It drains the tears away from the *lacrimal apparatus into the inferior meatus of the nose.

nasopharynx (rhinopharynx) *n.* the part of the *pharynx that lies above the soft palate.

nates *pl. n.* the buttocks. **—natal** *adj.*

national census *see* OFFICE FOR NATIONAL STATISTICS.

National Health Service (in Britain) a comprehensive service offering therapeutic and preventive medical and surgical care including the prescription and dispensing of medicines, spectacles, and medical and dental appliances. Exchequer funds pay for the services of doctors, nurses, and other professionals, as well as residential costs in NHS hospitals, and meet a substantial part of the cost of the medicines and appliances. Legislation enacted in 1946 was implemented in 1948 and the services were subjected to substantial reorganization in 1974 and again in 1982, 1991, and 1996. In England overall responsibility is vested in the Secretary of State for Health assisted by a comprehensive department (*see* DEPARTMENT OF HEALTH). Administration was based on a system of delegation downwards and accountability upwards through a hierarchy of regions, each subdivided into a number of districts. In 1991 **District Health**

Authorities (**DHA**s) developed a new role as purchasers of health care, assessing the health needs of local populations and negotiating contracts with a range of health-care providers to meet those needs. **Family Health Service Authorities (FHSAs)** were responsible for the regulation, management, and funding of general practitioners, pharmacists, opticians, and dentists. In 1996 the **Regional Health Authorities** were replaced by eight NHS Executive regional offices (*see* DEPARTMENT OF HEALTH). In the same year, to ensure better coordination of purchasing across primary and secondary care, legislation was passed to require the merger of DHAs and FHSAs to form new **Health Authorities**.

Some of the special resources for patients with rarer complaints are shared on a regional or supraregional basis. Wherever possible, districts have common boundaries with local authorities in order to try and ensure liaison with the social service departments, which provide many important services to support the sick and aged (*see* SOCIAL SERVICES). However, many districts include part of more than one local authority since the division tends to be made on the basis of the *catchment area of a district general hospital.

Different arrangements apply in Northern Ireland, Wales, and Scotland (for which there is a separate Act), where the appropriate Secretary of State is responsible. In Wales and Scotland there is an intermediate tier by which districts are grouped into areas (*see* CHIEF ADMINISTRATIVE MEDICAL OFFICER).

National Insurance (in Britain) a compulsory scheme of insurance under the terms of which employers and employees make joint contributions so that those who have contributed for a qualifying period may claim benefits in times of sickness, injury, maternity leave, unemployment, and retirement; self-employed persons pay all their own contributions. Those who do not qualify under the terms of this insurance scheme may also receive financial payments in times of need, but only subject to a means test.

natriuresis *n.* the excretion of sodium in the urine, especially in greater than normal amounts.

natriuretic *n.* an agent that promotes the excretion of sodium salts in the urine. Most *diuretics are natriuretics.

natural killer cell (NK cell) a type of *lymphocyte that is able to kill virus infected cells and certain types of cancer cells. Patients with cancer typically have fewer of these cells in the blood. NK cells act independently of the antigen presentation and recognition mechanisms that are required for the activity of *killer cells (cytotoxic T-cells).

naturopathy *n.* a system of medicine that relies upon the use of only 'natural' substances for the treatment of disease, rather than drugs. Herbs, food grown without artificial fertilizers and prepared without the use of preservatives or colouring material, pure water, sunlight, and fresh air are all employed in an effort to rid the body of 'unnatural' substances, which are said to be at the root of most illnesses.

nausea *n.* the feeling that one is about to vomit, as experienced in seasickness and in morning sickness of early pregnancy. Actual vomiting often occurs subsequently.

navel *n. see* UMBILICUS.

navicular bone a boat-shaped bone of the ankle (*see* TARSUS) that articulates with the three cuneiform bones in front and with the talus behind.

nearthrosis *n. see* PSEUDARTHROSIS.

nebula *n.* a faint opacity of the cornea that remains after an ulcer has healed.

nebulizer *n.* an instrument used for applying a liquid in the form of a fine spray.

NEC *see* NECROTIZING ENTEROCOLITIS.

Necator *n.* a genus of *hookworms that live in the small intestine. The human hookworm, *N. americanus*, occurs in tropical Africa, Central and South America, India, and the Pacific Islands. The worm possesses two pairs of sharp cutting plates inside its mouth cavity, which enable it to feed on the blood and tissues of the gut wall. *Compare* ANCYLOSTOMA.

necatoriasis *n.* an infestation of the small intestine by the parasitic hookworm

437

negativism

Necator americanus. See also HOOKWORM DISEASE.

neck *n.* **1.** the part of the body that connects the head and the trunk. It is the region supported by the *cervical vertebrae. **2.** *see* CERVIX.

necro- *prefix denoting* death or dissolution.

necrobiosis *n.* a gradual process by which cells lose their function and die. **Necrobiosis lipoidica** is a disease in which degeneration of collagen produces sharply demarcated yellowish-brown plaques, especially on the shins of women. It is often, but not exclusively, associated with diabetes mellitus.

necrology *n.* the study of the phenomena of death, involving determination of the moment of death and the different changes that occur in the tissues of the body after death.

necromania *n.* morbid desire for a dead body or bodies. This may be necrophilism, but the attraction is sometimes not sexual. A bereaved person, for instance, who is not grieving normally, may occasionally treasure the body of a loved one.

necrophilism (necrophilia) *n.* sexual attraction to corpses. *See also* SEXUAL DEVIATION. **—necrophile** *n.*

necropsy *n. see* AUTOPSY.

necrosis (mortification) *n.* the death of some or all of the cells in an organ or tissue, caused by disease, physical or chemical injury, or interference with the blood supply (*see* GANGRENE). **Caseous necrosis** occurs in pulmonary tuberculosis, the lung tissue becoming soft, dry, and cheese-like.

necrospermia *n.* the presence of either dead or motionless spermatozoa in the semen. *See* INFERTILITY.

necrotizing enterocolitis (NEC) a serious disease affecting the bowel during the first three weeks of life; it is much more common in *preterm babies. The abdomen distends and blood and mucus appear in the stools; the bowel may perforate. Treatment is to rest the bowel and administer antibiotics. If the bowel becomes necrotic, surgery may be necessary. The cause is unknown but the dis-

ease may be the result of a reduced supply of oxygen to the bowel or infection.

necrotizing fasciitis bacterial infection of the layer of *fascia beneath the skin by *Streptococcus* Type A. There is tissue necrosis and toxin production causing shock and organ failure. Symptoms appear rapidly after initial infection; they include a rash with blistering and discoloration of the skin, pain and inflammation of lymph nodes, fever, drowsiness, diarrhoea, and vomiting. The elderly and those who have recently undergone surgery are particularly vulnerable to the infection, which requires prompt treatment with antibiotics (e.g. clindamycin) and excision of the involved tissue.

nedocromil *n.* an anti-inflammatory drug used to treat bronchitis and bronchial asthma. It is administered by metered-dose aerosol inhaler; possible side-effects include nausea and brief headaches. Trade name: **Tilade**.

needle *n.* a slender sharp-pointed instrument used for a variety of purposes. Needles used for sewing up tissue during surgery are of various designs, for specific operations; they are equipped with an eye for threading suture material or they have the suture material fused onto them (so-called **atraumatic needles**). Hollow needles are used to inject substances into the body (in hypodermic syringes), to obtain specimens of tissue (*see* PUNCTURE), or to withdraw fluid from a cavity (*see* ASPIRATION, BIOPSY). *See also* STOP NEEDLE.

needle-stick injury a common accidental injury to the fingers and hands of nurses and doctors by contaminated injection needles. It can result in transmitted infections (e.g. hepatitis, AIDS).

needling *n.* a form of *capsulotomy in which a sharp needle is used to make a hole in the capsule surrounding the lens of the eye. This technique has now largely been replaced by use of the *YAG laser.

negativism *n.* behaviour that is the opposite of that suggested by others. In **active negativism** the individual does the opposite of what he is asked (for example, he screws his eyes up when asked to open them). This is uncommon in adult life and is usually associated with other features of *catatonia. In **passive negativism** the person fails to cooperate (for example, he does not eat). This occurs in *schizophrenia and *depression.

Neisseria *n.* a genus of spherical Gram-negative aerobic nonmotile bacteria characteristically grouped in pairs. They are parasites of animals, and some species are normal inhabitants of the respiratory tract of man. The species *N. gonorrhoeae* (the **gonococcus**) causes *gonorrhoea. Gonococci are found within pus cells of urethral and vaginal discharge; they can be cultured only on serum or blood agar. *N. meningitidis* (the **meningococcus**) causes meningococcal *meningitis. Meningococci are found within pus cells of infected cerebrospinal fluid and blood or in the nasal passages of carriers. They too can only be cultured on serum or blood agar.

nematode (roundworm) *n.* any one of a large group of worms having an unsegmented cylindrical body, tapering at both ends. This distinguishes nematodes from other *helminths. Nematodes occur either as free-living forms in the sea, fresh water, and soil or as parasites of plants, animals, and man. *Hookworms and *threadworms infest the alimentary canal. *Filariae are found in the lymphatic tissues. The *guinea worm and *Onchocerca affect connective tissue. Some nematodes (e.g. threadworms) are transmitted from host to host by the ingestion of eggs; others (e.g. *Wuchereria) by the bite of a bloodsucking insect.

neo- *prefix denoting* new or newly formed.

neoadjuvant chemotherapy chemotherapy that is given before the treatment of a primary tumour with the aim of improving the results of surgery or radiotherapy and preventing the development of metastases. *Compare* ADJUVANT THERAPY.

neocerebellum *n.* the middle lobe of the *cerebellum, excluding the pyramid and uvula. In evolutionary terms it is the newest part, occurring only in mammals.

neologism *n.* (in psychiatry) the invention of words to which meanings are attached. It is common in childhood, but when it occurs in an adult it may be a symptom of a psychotic illness, such as *schizophrenia. It should be distinguished from *paraphasia, in which new meanings are attached to ordinary words.

neomycin *n.* an *aminoglycoside antibiotic used to treat infections caused by a wide range of bacteria, mainly those affecting the skin and eyes. It is usually applied in creams or drops with other antibiotics, but can also be given by mouth.

neonatal mortality rate *see* INFANT MORTALITY RATE.

neonatal screening *screening tests carried out on newborn babies to detect diseases that appear in the neonatal period, such as phenylketonuria (*see* GUTHRIE TEST). If these diseases are detected early enough, treatment may be instigated before any irreversible damage occurs to the baby.

neonate *n.* an infant at any time during the first four weeks of life. The word is particularly applied to infants just born or in the first week of life. —**neonatal** *adj.*

neopallium *n.* an enlargement of the wall of each cerebral hemisphere. In evolutionary terms it is the newest part of the cerebrum, formed by the development of new pathways for sight and hearing in mammals.

neoplasm *n.* any new and abnormal growth: any *benign or *malignant tumour.

neosphincter *n.* a substituted muscle or an implant for an absent or ineffective sphincter (*see* ARTIFICIAL SPHINCTER).

neostigmine *n.* a *parasympathomimetic drug that functions by inhibiting the enzyme cholinesterase (*see also* ANTICHOLINESTERASE). It is used mainly to diagnose and treat *myasthenia gravis and as an antidote to some *muscle-relaxant drugs, such as tubocurarine. It is also used to treat some intestinal disorders and glaucoma. Neostigmine is administered by mouth, injection, or in eye-drops; side-effects include digestive upsets and increased saliva flow. Trade name: **Prostigmin**.

neovascularization *n.* the abnormal formation of new and fragile blood vessels, usually in response to ischaemia. In

choroidal neovascularization, which occurs in such conditions as *macular degeneration and diabetic *retinopathy, abnormal vessels, derived from the *choroid, form a **choroidal neovascular membrane** in the space below the retinal pigment epithelium (*see* RETINA).

nephr- (nephro-) *prefix denoting* the kidney(s).

nephralgia *n.* pain in the kidney. The pain is felt in the loin and can be caused by a variety of kidney complaints.

nephrectomy *n.* surgical removal of a kidney. When performed for cancer of the kidney, the entire organ is removed together with its surrounding fat and the adjacent adrenal gland (**radical nephrectomy**). Removal of either the upper or lower pole of the kidney is termed **partial nephrectomy**.

nephritis (Bright's disease) *n.* inflammation of the kidney. Nephritis is a nonspecific term used to describe a condition resulting from a variety of causes. *See* GLOMERULONEPHRITIS.

nephroblastoma (Wilms' tumour) *n.* a malignant tumour arising from the embryonic kidney and occurring in young children, usually below the age of three and rarely over the age of eight. In some cases it involves both kidneys. Treatment consists of removing the kidney (*see* NEPHRECTOMY) and giving chemotherapy. Although almost half the cases have spread by the time diagnosis is made, this does not prevent a cure: the number of children that survive at least five years after diagnosis is improving, being currently around 75%. In some children the tumour is associated with an abnormality of chromosome number 13; in these cases other features, such as absence of the iris in the eye (*see* ANIRIDIA) and *hemihypertrophy, are present.

nephrocalcinosis *n.* the presence of calcium deposits in the kidneys. This can be caused by excess calcium in the blood, as caused by overactivity of the parathyroid glands, or it may result from an underlying abnormality of the kidney. The cause of nephrocalcinosis must be detected by full biochemical, radiological, and urological investigation so that appropriate treatment can be undertaken.

nephrogenic cord either of the paired ridges of tissue that run along the dorsal surface of the abdominal cavity of the embryo. Parts of it develop into the kidney, ovary, or testis and their associated ducts. Intermediate stages of these developments are the *pronephros, *mesonephros, and *metanephros.

nephrolithiasis *n.* the presence of stones in the kidney (*see* CALCULUS). Such stones can cause pain and blood in the urine, but they may produce no symptoms. Full investigation is undertaken to determine the underlying cause of stone formation. When stones are associated with urinary obstruction and infection they usually require surgical removal (*see* NEPHROLITHOTOMY, PYELOLITHOTOMY).

nephrolithotomy *n.* the surgical removal of a stone from the kidney by an incision into the kidney substance. It is normally performed in combination with an incision into the renal pelvis (*see* PYELOLITHOTOMY). *See also* PERCUTANEOUS NEPHROLITHOTOMY.

nephrology *n.* the branch of medicine concerned with the study, investigation, and management of diseases of the kidney. *See also* UROLOGY. —**nephrologist** *n.*

nephron *n.* the active unit of excretion in the kidney (see illustration). Blood, which is supplied by branches of the renal artery, is filtered through a knot of capillaries (**glomerulus**) into the cup-shaped **Bowman's capsule** so that water, nitrogenous waste, and many other substances (excluding colloids) pass into the **renal tubule**. Here most of the substances are reabsorbed back into the blood, the remaining fluid (*urine) passing into the collecting duct, which drains into the *ureter.

nephropathy *n.* disease of the kidney. *See also* BALKAN NEPHROPATHY.

nephropexy *n.* an operation to fix a mobile kidney. The kidney is fixed to the twelfth rib and adjacent posterior abdominal wall to prevent descent of the kidney on standing (*see* NEPHROPTOSIS).

nephroptosis *n.* abnormal descent of a

kidney into the pelvis on standing, which may occur if it is excessively mobile (for example, in thin women). If this is accompanied by pain and obstruction to free drainage of urine by the kidney, *nephropexy may be advised.

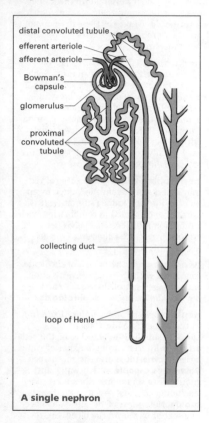

distal convoluted tubule
efferent arteriole
afferent arteriole
Bowman's capsule
glomerulus
proximal convoluted tubule
collecting duct
loop of Henle

A single nephron

nephrosclerosis n. hardening of the arteries and arterioles of the kidneys. **Arteriolar nephrosclerosis** is associated with *hypertension.

nephroscope n. an instrument (*endoscope) used for examining the interior of the kidney, usually passed into the renal pelvis through a track from the skin surface after needle *nephrostomy and dilatation of the tract over a guide wire. The nephroscope allows the passage of instruments under direct vision to remove calculi (see PERCUTANEOUS NEPHROLITHOTOMY) or disintegrate them by ultrasound probes or electrohydraulic shock waves (see LITHOTRIPSY).

nephroscopy n. inspection of the interior of the kidney with a *nephroscope.

nephrosis n. (in pathology) degenerative changes in the epithelium of the kidney tubules. The term is sometimes used loosely for the *nephrotic syndrome.

nephrostomy n. drainage of urine from the kidney by a tube (catheter) passing through the kidney via the skin surface. This is commonly used as a temporary procedure after operations on the kidney. Long-term urine drainage by nephrostomy may be complicated by the attendant problems of infection and obstruction of the catheter by debris. Nephrostomy is also performed to enable the passage of a *nephroscope.

nephrotic syndrome a condition in which there is great loss of protein in the urine, reduced levels of albumin in the blood, and generalized swelling of the tissues due to *oedema. It can be caused by a variety of disorders, most usually *glomerulonephritis. Treatment is with corticosteroids.

nephrotomy n. surgical incision into the substance of the kidney. This is usually undertaken to remove a kidney stone (see NEPHROLITHOTOMY).

nephroureterectomy (ureteronephrectomy) n. the surgical removal of a kidney together with its ureter. This operation is performed for cancer of the kidney pelvis or ureter. It is also undertaken when the kidney has been destroyed by *vesicoureteric reflux, to prevent subsequent continuing reflux into the stump of the ureter that would occur if the kidney alone were removed.

nerve n. a bundle of conducting *nerve fibres (see illustration) that transmit impulses from the brain or spinal cord to the muscles and glands (**motor nerves**) or inwards from the sense organs to the brain and spinal cord (**sensory nerves**). Most large nerves are **mixed nerves**, containing both motor and sensory nerve fibres running to and from a particular region of the body.

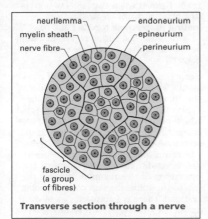

neurllemma
myelin sheath
nerve fibre
endoneurium
epineurium
perineurium

fascicle
(a group
of fibres)

Transverse section through a nerve

nerve block a method of producing *anaesthesia in part of the body by blocking the passage of pain impulses in the sensory nerves supplying it. A local anaesthetic, such as lignocaine, is injected into the tissues in the region of a nerve. In this way anaesthesia can be localized, so that minor operations can be performed without the necessity of giving a general anaesthetic. A *ring block is a common technique used for anaesthetizing a digit.

nerve cell *see* NEURONE.

nerve ending the final part (terminal) of one of the branches of a nerve fibre, where a *neurone makes contact either with another neurone at a synapse or with a muscle or gland cell at a neuromuscular or neuroglandular junction.

nerve entrapment syndrome any syndrome resulting from pressure on a nerve from surrounding structures. Examples include the *carpal tunnel syndrome and *meralgia paraesthetica.

nerve fibre the long fine process that extends from the cell body of a *neurone and carries nerve impulses. Bundles of nerve fibres running together form a *nerve. Each fibre has a sheath, which in medullated nerve fibres is a relatively thick layer containing the fatty insulating material *myelin.

nerve gas any gas that disrupts the normal functioning of nerves and thus of the muscles they supply. There are two groups, the **G agents** and the **V agents**. The latter are more than 300 times as deadly as mustard gas: one inhalation can kill by paralysing the respiratory muscles. V agents also act through the skin, therefore gas masks are ineffective protection against them.

nerve growth factor (NGF) a protein (*see* GROWTH FACTOR), consisting of two polypeptide chains, that is required for the development and longevity of some neurones, including those in the sympathetic nervous system and some central nervous system and sensory neurones. Nerve growth factor is necessary for axon growth and also for initiating new neuronal connections with other cells. The role of NGFs in preventing the degeneration of brain cells is being explored in research into Alzheimer's disease.

nerve impulse the electrical activity in the membrane of a *neurone that – by its rapid spread from one region to the next – is the means by which information is transmitted within the nervous system along the axons of the neurones. The membrane of a resting nerve is charged (**polarized**) because of the different concentrations of ions inside and outside the cell. When a nerve impulse is triggered, a wave of *depolarization spreads, and ions flow across the membrane (*see* ACTION POTENTIAL). Until the nerve has undergone *repolarization no further nerve impulses can pass.

nerve regeneration the growth of new nerve tissue, which occurs at a very slow rate (1–2 mm per day) after a nerve has been severed and is often partially or totally incomplete. *Microsurgery has improved the results by facilitating primary repair in the immediate aftermath of injury. *See also* AXONOTMESIS, NEUROTMESIS.

nervous breakdown a popular term applied to a range of emotional crises varying from a brief attack of 'hysterical' behaviour to a major psychoneurotic illness with severe long-term effects on the life of the sufferer. The term is also sometimes used as a euphemism for a frank psychiatric illness, such as *schizophrenia.

nervous system the vast network of cells specialized to carry information (in the form of *nerve impulses) to and from all parts of the body in order to bring about bodily activity. The brain and spinal cord together form the *central nervous system; the remaining nervous tissue is known as the *peripheral nervous system and includes the *autonomic nervous system, which is itself divided into the sympathetic and parasympathetic nervous systems. The basic functional unit of the nervous system is the *neurone (nerve cell).

Nesbit's operation an operation devised to surgically straighten a congenitally curved penis but now more frequently employed to correct the penile curvature caused by *Peyronie's disease. [R. M. Nesbit (20th century), US surgeon]

nettle rash see URTICARIA.

neur- (neuro-) *prefix denoting* nerves or the nervous system.

neural arch see VERTEBRA.

neural crest the two bands of ectodermal tissue that flank the *neural plate of the early embryo. Cells of the neural crest migrate throughout the embryo and develop into sensory nerve cells and peripheral nerve cells of the autonomic nervous system.

neuralgia *n.* a severe burning or stabbing pain often following the course of a nerve. **Postherpetic neuralgia** is an intense debilitating pain felt at the site of a previous attack of shingles. In **trigeminal neuralgia (tic douloureux)** there are brief paroxysms of searing pain felt in the distribution of one or more branches of the *trigeminal nerve in the face. Trigeminal neuralgia is managed principally by prescription of *carbamazepine. The facial pain of **migrainous neuralgia** lasts for 30–60 minutes and occurs at roughly the same time on successive days.

neural plate the strip of ectoderm lying along the central axis of the early embryo that forms the *neural tube and subsequently the central nervous system.

neural spine the spinous process situated on the neural arch of a *vertebra.

neural tube the embryological structure from which the brain and spinal cord develop. It is a hollow tube of ectodermal tissue formed when two edges of a groove in a plate of primitive neural tissue (**neural plate**) come together and fuse. Failure of normal fusion results in a number of congenital defects (*see* NEURAL TUBE DEFECTS).

neural tube defects a group of congenital abnormalities caused by failure of the *neural tube to form normally. In *spina bifida the bony arches of the spine, which protect the spinal cord and its coverings (the meninges), fail to close. More severe defects of fusion of these bones will result in increasingly serious neurological conditions. A **meningocele** is the protrusion of the meninges through the gap in the spine, the skin covering being vestigial. There is a constant risk of damage to the meninges, with resulting infection. Urgent surgical treatment to protect the meninges is therefore required. In a **meningomyelocele (myelomeningocele, myelocele)** the spinal cord and the nerve roots are exposed, often adhering to the fine membrane that overlies them. There is a constant risk of infection and this condition is accompanied by paralysis and numbness of the legs and urinary incontinence. *Hydrocephalus and the *Arnold-Chiari malformation are usually present. A failure of fusion at the cranial end of the neural tube (**cranium bifidum**) gives rise to comparable disorders. The bone defect is most often in the occipital region of the skull but it may occur in the frontal or basal regions. A protrusion of the meninges alone is known as a **cranial meningocele**. The terms **meningoencephalocele, encephalocele,** and **cephalocele** are used for the protrusion of brain tissue through the skull defect. This is accompanied by severe mental and physical disorders.

neurapraxia *n.* temporary loss of nerve function resulting in tingling, numbness, and weakness. It is usually caused by compression of the nerve and there is no structural damage involved. Complete recovery occurs. *Compare* AXONOTMESIS, NEUROTMESIS.

neurasthenia *n.* a set of psychological and physical symptoms, including fatigue, irritability, headache, dizziness, anxiety, and intolerance of noise. It can be caused by organic damage, such as a head injury, or it can be due to neurosis. —**neurasthenic** *adj.*, *n.*

neurectasis *n.* the surgical procedure for stretching a peripheral nerve.

neurectomy *n.* the surgical removal of the whole or part of a nerve.

neurilemma (neurolemma) *n.* the sheath of the *axon of a nerve fibre. The neurilemma of a medullated fibre contains *myelin laid down by Schwann cells. —**neurilemmal** *adj.*

neurilemmoma (neurinoma) *n.* a benign slow-growing tumour that arises from the neurilemma of a nerve fibre.

neurinoma *n.* *see* NEURILEMMOMA.

neuritis *n.* a disease of the peripheral nerves showing the pathological changes of inflammation. The term is also used in a less precise sense as an alternative to *neuropathy. *See also* RETROBULBAR NEURITIS.

neuroanatomy *n.* the study of the structure of the nervous system, from the gross anatomy of the brain down to the microscopic details of neurones.

neurobiotaxis *n.* the predisposition of a nerve cell to move towards the source of its stimuli during development.

neuroblast *n.* any of the nerve cells of the embryo that give rise to functional nerve cells (neurones).

neuroblastoma *n.* a malignant tumour composed of embryonic nerve cells. It may originate in any part of the sympathetic nervous system, most commonly in the medulla of the adrenal gland, and secondary growths are often widespread in other organs and in bones.

neurocranium *n.* the part of the skull that encloses the brain.

neurodermatitis *n.* *see* LICHEN SIMPLEX CHRONICUS.

neuroendocrine system the system of dual control of certain activities of the body by means of both nerves and circulating hormones. The functioning of the autonomic nervous system is particularly closely linked to that of the pituitary and adrenal glands. The system can give rise to

neuroendocrine tumours, which have special structural features and often produce active hormones. *See also* NEUROHORMONE, NEUROSECRETION.

neuroepithelioma *n.* a malignant tumour of the retina of the eye. It is a form of *glioma and may spread into the brain if not treated early.

neuroepithelium *n.* a type of epithelium associated with organs of special sense. It contains sensory nerve endings and is found in the retina, the membranous labyrinth of the inner ear, the mucous membrane lining the nasal cavity, and the taste buds. —**neuroepithelial** *adj.*

neurofibril *n.* one of the microscopic threads of cytoplasm found in the cell body of a *neurone and also in the *axoplasm of peripheral nerves.

neurofibroma (Schwannoma) *n.* a benign tumour growing from the fibrous coverings of a peripheral nerve: it is usually symptomless. When it develops from the sheath of a nerve root, it causes pain and may compress the spinal cord.

neurofibromatosis (von Recklinghausen's disease) *n.* a congenital disease, inherited as a *dominant characteristic, that is typified by numerous benign tumours growing from the fibrous coverings of nerves (*see* NEUROFIBROMA). Tumours may occur in the spinal canal, where they may press on the spinal cord. The tumours can be felt beneath the skin along the course of the nerves; they sometimes (but rarely) become malignant, giving rise to **neurofibrosarcomas**. Pigmented patches on the skin (*see* CAFÉ AU LAIT SPOTS) are commonly found. Neurofibromatosis is sometimes associated with *fibrous dysplasia and occasionally with the adrenal tumour *phaeochromocytoma, acoustic *neuroma, *glioma, or *meningioma.

neurogenesis *n.* the growth and development of nerve cells.

neurogenic *adj.* **1.** caused by disease or dysfunction of the nervous system. **2.** arising in nervous tissue. **3.** caused by nerve stimulation.

neuroglia *n.* *see* GLIA.

neurohormone *n.* a hormone that is

produced within specialized nerve cells and is secreted from the nerve endings into the circulation. Examples are the hormones oxytocin and vasopressin, produced within the nerve cells of the hypothalamus and released into the circulation in the posterior pituitary gland, and noradrenaline, released from *chromaffin tissue in the adrenal medulla.

neurohumour n. a *neurohormone or a *neurotransmitter.

neurohypophysis n. the posterior lobe of the *pituitary gland.

neurolemma n. see NEURILEMMA.

neurology n. the study of the structure, functioning, and diseases of the nervous system (including the brain, spinal cord, and all the peripheral nerves). —**neurological** adj. —**neurologist** n.

neuroma n. any tumour derived from cells of the nervous system. Such tumours are now usually categorized more specifically (e.g. *neurofibroma, *neurilemmoma). An **acoustic neuroma** is a slow-growing benign tumour of the sheath of the vestibular branch of the *vestibulocochlear nerve that arises in the auditory canal. It progresses to cause tinnitus and hearing loss.

neuromuscular junction (myoneural junction) the meeting point of a nerve fibre and the muscle fibre that it supplies. Between the enlarged end of the nerve fibre (**motor end-plate**) and the membrane of the muscle is a gap across which a *neurotransmitter must diffuse from the nerve to trigger contraction of the muscle.

neuromyelitis optica (Devic's disease) a condition that is closely related to multiple sclerosis. Typically there is a transverse *myelitis, producing paralysis and numbness of the legs and trunk below the inflamed spinal cord, and *retrobulbar (optic) neuritis affecting both optic nerves. The attacks of myelitis and optic neuritis may coincide or they may be separated by days or weeks. Recovery from the initial attack is often incomplete, but relapses appear to be less common than in conventional multiple sclerosis.

neurone (nerve cell) n. one of the basic functional units of the nervous system: a cell specialized to transmit electrical *nerve impulses and so carry information from one part of the body to another (see illustration). Each neurone has an enlarged portion, the **cell body** (**perikaryon**), containing the nucleus; from the body extend several processes (**dendrites**) through which impulses enter from their branches. A longer process, the nerve fibre (see AXON), extends outwards and carries impulses away from the cell body. This is normally unbranched except at the *nerve ending. The point of contact of one neurone with another is known as a *synapse.

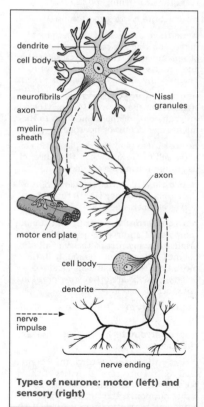

Types of neurone: motor (left) and sensory (right)

neuronophagia n. the process whereby

damaged or degenerating nerve cells finally disintegrate and are removed by scavenger cells (*phagocytes).

neuronoplasty *n.* reconstructive surgery for damaged or severed peripheral nerves.

neuropathic bladder a malfunctioning bladder due to partial or complete interruption of its nerve supply. Causes include injury to the spinal cord, spina bifida, multiple sclerosis, and diabetic neuropathy.

neuropathy *n.* any disease of the peripheral nerves, usually causing weakness and numbness. In a **mononeuropathy** a single nerve is affected and the extent of the symptoms depends upon the distribution of that nerve. In a **polyneuropathy** many or all of the nerves are involved and the symptoms are most profound at the extremities of the limbs.

neurophysiology *n.* the study of the complex chemical and physical changes that are associated with the activity of the nervous system.

neuropil *n.* nerve tissue that is visible microscopically as a mass of interwoven and interconnected nerve endings, dendrites, and other neurone components, rather than an ordered array of axons.

neuropsychiatry *n.* the branch of medicine concerned with the psychiatric effects of disorders of neurological function or structure. Increasingly, the correlation is being drawn between demonstrable brain changes and the resulting effects on the mind. It is the function of the growing speciality of neuropsychiatry to investigate this relationship.

neuroretinitis *n.* combined inflammation of the optic nerve and the retina.

neurosecretion *n.* any substance produced within, and secreted by, a nerve cell. Important examples are the hormone-releasing factors produced by the cells of the *hypothalamus and released into blood vessels of the pituitary gland, on which they act.

neurosis *n.* (*pl.* **neuroses**) any long-term mental or behavioural disorder in which contact with reality is retained and the condition is recognized by the sufferer as abnormal. A neurosis essentially features anxiety or behaviour exaggeratedly designed to avoid anxiety. Defence mechanisms against anxiety take various forms and may appear as phobias, obsessions, compulsions, or sexual dysfunctions. In recent attempts at classification, the disorders formerly included under the neuroses have been renamed. The general term is now **anxiety disorder**; hysteria has become *conversion disorder; amnesia, fugue, multiple personality, and depersonalization are *dissociative disorders; obsessional neurosis is now known as **obsessive–compulsive disorder** (*see* OBSESSION); and depressive neurosis has become **dysthymic disorder** (*see* DEPRESSION) in *DSM-IV. Psychoanalysis has proved of little value in curing these conditions and Freud's speculations as to their origins are not now widely accepted outside Freudian schools of thought. Neurotic disorders are probably best regarded as being the result of inappropriate early programming. *Behaviour therapy seems effective in some cases. —**neurotic** *adj.*

neurosurgery *n.* the surgical or operative treatment of diseases of the brain and spinal cord. This includes the management of head injuries, the relief of raised intracranial pressure and compression of the spinal cord, the eradication of infection, the control of intracranial haemorrhage, and the diagnosis and treatment of tumours. The development of neurosurgery has been supported by advances in anaesthetics, radiology, antiseptics, and scanning techniques.

neurosyphilis *n.* *syphilis affecting the nervous system.

neuroticism *n.* a dimension of personality derived from questionnaires and psychological tests. People with high scores in neuroticism are anxious and intense and more prone to develop *neurosis.

neurotmesis *n.* the complete severance of a peripheral nerve, which is associated with degeneration of the nerve fibres distal to the point of severance and slow *nerve regeneration. *Compare* AXONOTMESIS, NEURAPRAXIA.

neurotomy *n.* the surgical procedure of severing a nerve.

neurotoxic *adj.* poisonous or harmful to nerve cells.

neurotransmitter *n.* a chemical substance released from nerve endings to transmit impulses across *synapses to other nerves and across the minute gaps between the nerves and the muscles or glands that they supply. Outside the central nervous system the chief neurotransmitter is *acetylcholine; *noradrenaline is released by nerve endings of the sympathetic system. In the central nervous system, as well as acetylcholine and noradrenaline, *dopamine, *serotonin, *gamma-aminobutyric acid, the amino acid glutamate, and several other substances act as transmitters.

neurotrophic *adj.* relating to the growth and nutrition of neural tissue in the body.

neurotropic *adj.* growing towards or having an affinity for neural tissue. The term may be applied to viruses, chemicals, or toxins.

neutropenia *n.* a decrease in the number of *neutrophils in the blood. Neutropenia may occur in a wide variety of diseases, including certain hereditary defects, aplastic *anaemias, tumours of the bone marrow, *agranulocytosis, and acute leukaemias. It results in an increased susceptibility to infections.

neutrophil (polymorph) *n.* a variety of *granulocyte (a type of white blood cell) distinguished by a lobed nucleus and the presence in its cytoplasm of fine granules that stain purple with *Romanowsky stains. It is capable of ingesting and killing bacteria and provides an important defence against infection. There are normally $2.0–7.5 \times 10^9$ neutrophils per litre of blood.

newton *n.* the *SI unit of force, equal to the force required to impart to 1 kilogram an acceleration of 1 metre per second per second. Symbol: N.

nexus *n.* (in anatomy) a connection or link.

NGF *see* NERVE GROWTH FACTOR.

niacin *n. see* NICOTINIC ACID.

nicardipine *n.* a *calcium antagonist used to treat long-term angina. It is administered by mouth. Possible side-effects include nausea, chest pain, dizziness, headache, flushing, and palpitations. Trade name: **Cardene**.

niche *n.* (in anatomy) a recess or depression in a smooth surface.

niclosamide *n.* an *anthelmintic drug used to remove tapeworms. It is administered by mouth; unlike older treatments, it is free from side-effects. Trade name: **Yomesan**.

nicotinamide *n.* a B vitamin: the amide of *nicotinic acid.

nicotinamide adenine dinucleotide *see* NAD.

nicotine *n.* a poisonous alkaloid derived from *tobacco, responsible for the dependence of regular smokers on cigarettes. In small doses nicotine has a stimulating effect on the autonomic nervous system, causing in regular smokers such effects as raised blood pressure and pulse rate and impaired appetite. Large doses cause paralysis of the autonomic ganglia.

nicotinic acid (niacin) a B vitamin. Nicotinic acid is a derivative of pyridine and is interchangeable with its amide, **nicotinamide**. Both forms of the vitamin are equally active. Nicotinamide is a component of the coenzymes *NAD (nicotinamide adenine dinucleotide) and NADP, its phosphate. Nicotinic acid is required in the diet but can also be formed in small amounts in the body from the essential amino acid tryptophan. A deficiency of the vitamin leads to *pellagra. Good sources of nicotinic acid are meat, yeast extracts, and some cereals. Nicotinic acid is present in some cereals (e.g. maize) in a bound unavailable form. The adult recommended intake is 18 mg equivalent per day (1 mg equivalent is equal to 1 mg of available nicotinic acid or 60 mg tryptophan).

nicotinyl *n.* a drug that dilates blood vessels. It is similar to *nicotinic acid and is used to treat disorders due to poor circulation, such as chilblains and Raynaud's disease. It is administered by mouth; side-effects are rare, but temporary flushing of the face may occur. Trade name: **Ronicol**.

nictitation *n.* exaggerated and frequent blinking or winking of the eyes.

nidation *n. see* IMPLANTATION.

nidus *n.* a place in which bacteria have settled and multiplied because of particularly suitable conditions: a focus of infection.

nifedipine *n.* a *calcium antagonist used in the treatment of angina and high blood pressure (hypertension). It is administered by mouth; side-effects include dizziness, headache, and nausea. Trade names: **Adalat, Calcilat**.

night blindness the inability to see in dim light or at night. It is due to a disorder of the cells in the retina that are responsible for vision in dim light (*see* ROD), and can result from dietary deficiency of *vitamin A. If the vitamin deficiency is allowed to continue, its manifestations may progress to include *xerophthalmia and *keratomalacia. Night blindness may be caused by other retinal diseases, e.g. *retinitis pigmentosa. **Congenital stationary night blindness** is characterized by poor night vision from early childhood that does not get worse. Medical name: **nyctalopia**. *Compare* DAY BLINDNESS.

night sweat copious sweating during sleep. Night sweats may be an early indication of tuberculosis, AIDS, or other disease.

night terror the condition in which a child (usually aged 2–4 years) soon after falling asleep, starts screaming and appears terrified. The child cannot be comforted because he remains mentally inaccessible; the attack ceases when he wakes up fully and is never remembered. Attacks sometimes follow a stressful experience.

nikethamide *n.* an *analeptic drug used to raise the level of consciousness in comatose patients so that they can be encouraged to cough and bring up bronchial secretions. It is administered by mouth or injection. Possible side-effects include nausea, rapid and irregular heartbeat, dizziness, restlessness, and tremor.

Nile blue an oxazine chloride, used for staining lipids and lipid pigments. **Nile blue A (Nile blue sulphate)**, which stains

fatty acids, changes from blue to purplish at pH 10–11.

ninhydrin reaction a histochemical test for proteins, in which ninhydrin (triketohydrindene hydrate) is boiled with the test solution and gives a blue colour in the presence of amino acids and proteins.

nipple (mamilla, papilla) *n.* the protuberance at the centre of the *breast. In females the milk ducts open at the nipple.

niridazole *n.* an anthelmintic drug used particularly in the treatment of schistosomiasis. It is administered by mouth and side-effects may include agitation and confusion, abdominal discomfort, some digestive upset, and headache. Niridazole should not be used in patients with impaired liver function.

Nissl granules collections of dark-staining material, containing RNA, seen in the cell bodies of neurones on microscopic examination. [F. Nissl (1860–1919), German neuropathologist]

nit *n.* the egg of a *louse. The eggs of head lice are firmly cemented to the hair, usually at the back of the head; those of body lice are fixed to the clothing. Nits, 0.8 × 0.3 mm, are visible as light white specks.

nitrazepam *n.* a *hypnotic drug administered by mouth to treat insomnia and sleep disturbances. It is often preferred to other hypnotics since side-effects are less severe, though morning drowsiness can sometimes occur. Trade name: **Mogadon**.

nitric acid a strong corrosive mineral acid, HNO_3, the concentrated form of which is capable of producing severe burns of the skin. Swallowing the acid leads to intense burning pain and ulceration of the mouth and throat. Treatment is by immediate administration of alkaline solutions, followed by milk or olive oil.

nitric oxide an important member of the group of gaseous mediators, which – together with amine mediators (e.g. adrenaline, noradrenaline, histamine, acetylcholine) and lipid mediators (e.g. prostaglandins) – produce many physiological responses (e.g. smooth muscle relaxation). Nitric oxide is involved in the manifestations of sepsis and septic shock. Formula: NO.

nitrofurantoin *n.* a drug used to treat bacterial infections of the urinary system. It is administered by mouth and may cause nausea, vomiting, and skin rashes. Trade names: **Furadantin, Macrodantin.**

nitrogen *n.* a gaseous element and a major constituent of air (79 per cent). Nitrogen is an essential constituent of proteins and nucleic acids and is obtained by man in the form of protein-containing foods (atmospheric nitrogen cannot be utilized directly). Nitrogenous waste is excreted as *urea. Liquid nitrogen is used to freeze some specimens before pathological examination. Symbol: N.

nitrogen balance the relationship between the nitrogen taken into the body and that excreted, denoting the balance between the manufacture and breakdown of the body mass. A negative nitrogen balance, when excretion exceeds intake, is usual after injury or operations as the energy requirements of the body are met disproportionately from endogenous sources.

nitrogen mustard *See* MUSTINE.

nitroglycerin *n. see* GLYCERYL TRINITRATE.

nitroprusside *n.* a cyanide-containing drug used in the emergency treatment of high blood pressure. Given by controlled infusion into a vein, it is the most effective known means of reducing dangerously high pressure, but its effects and level in the blood must be closely monitored. Possible side-effects include nausea, vomiting, headache, palpitations, sweating, and chest pain.

nitrous oxide a colourless gas used as an *anaesthetic with good *analgesic properties. It is administered by inhalation, in conjunction with oxygen, and is used as a vehicle for potent anaesthetic vapours, such as halothane. A mixture of oxygen and nitrous oxide provides effective analgesia for some dental procedures and in childbirth; such a state is known as *relative analgesia. Nitrous oxide was formerly referred to as **laughing gas** because of its tendency to excite the patient when used alone.

NK cell *see* NATURAL KILLER CELL.

nm *abbrev. for* NANOMETRE.

NMR *see* NUCLEAR MAGNETIC RESONANCE.

Nocardia *n.* a genus of rodlike or filamentous Gram-positive nonmotile bacteria found in the soil. As cultures age, filaments form branches, but these soon break up into rodlike or spherical cells. Three or more spores may form in each cell; these germinate to form filaments. Some species are pathogenic: *N. asteroides* causes *nocardiosis and *N. madurae* is associated with the disease *Madura foot.

nocardiosis *n.* a disease caused by bacteria of the genus *Nocardia*, primarily affecting the lungs, skin, and brain, resulting in the formation of abscesses. Treatment involves antibiotics and sulphonamides.

noci- *prefix denoting* pain or injury.

nociceptive *adj.* describing nerve fibres, endings, or pathways that are concerned with the condition of pain.

nociceptor *n.* a *receptor that responds to the stimuli responsible for the sensation of pain. Nociceptors may be *interoceptors, responding to such stimuli as inflammation, or *exteroceptors, sensitive to heat, etc.

noct- (nocti-) *prefix denoting* night.

noctambulation *n. see* SOMNAMBULISM.

nocturia *n.* the passage of urine at night. In the absence of a high fluid intake, sleep is not normally interrupted by the need to pass urine. Nocturia usually occurs in elderly men with enlarged prostate glands, and is a common reason for patients to request *prostatectomy.

node *n.* a small swelling or knot of tissue. *See* ATRIOVENTRICULAR NODE, LYMPH NODE, SINOATRIAL NODE.

node of Ranvier one of the gaps that occur at regular intervals in the *myelin sheath of medullated nerve fibres, between adjacent *Schwann cells.

nodule *n.* a small swelling or aggregation of cells.

noma *n.* a gangrenous infection of the mouth that spreads to involve the face. It is rare in civilized communities and is usually found in debilitated or malnourished individuals. Noma is a severe form of *ulcerative gingivitis.

nonaccidental injury (NAI) injury inflicted on babies and young children; the perpetrator is usually an adult – often a parent or step-parent. Most commonly seen in babies aged six months or less, it usually takes the form of bruising, particularly on the face; bite marks; burns or scalds, particularly cigarette burns; and bone injuries, especially spiral fractures of the long bones in the limbs and skull fractures. Internal injuries may be fatal. Careful examination often reveals several injuries of different ages, indicating long-term abuse. NAI usually has serious consequences for the child, including *failure to thrive and behavioural problems.

Known colloquially as the **battered baby** (or **child) syndrome**, it may be precipitated by many factors, including relationship difficulties, social problems, and ill health, and is more common if the child is handicapped. It is often found that abusers suffered similar abuse themselves when young. Many abused children suffer further injury if discharged into the same environment with no support (*see also* RISK REGISTER). A child at considerable risk may need to be removed from the family home.

nondisjunction *n.* a condition in which pairs of homologous chromosomes fail to separate during meiosis or a chromosome fails to divide at *anaphase of mitosis or meiosis. It results in a cell with an abnormal number of chromosomes (*see* MONOSOMY, TRISOMY).

non-Hodgkin's lymphoma *see* LYMPHOMA.

noninvasive *adj.* **1.** denoting techniques of investigation or treatment that do not involve penetration of the skin by needles or knives. **2.** denoting tumours that do not spread into surrounding tissues (*see* BENIGN).

Nonne's syndrome (cerebellar syndrome) *see* (CEREBELLAR) ATAXIA. [M. Nonne (1861–1959), German neurologist]

nonsecretor *n.* a person in whose body fluids it is not possible to detect soluble

forms of the A, B, or O agglutinogens that determine blood group. *Compare* SECRETOR.

nonsteroidal anti-inflammatory drug *see* NSAID.

noradrenaline (norepinephrine) *n.* a hormone, closely related to *adrenaline and with similar actions, secreted by the medulla of the *adrenal gland and also released as a *neurotransmitter by sympathetic nerve endings. Among its many actions are constriction of small blood vessels leading to an increase in blood pressure, increased blood flow through the coronary arteries and a slowing of the heart rate, increase in the rate and depth of breathing, and relaxation of the smooth muscle in intestinal walls.

norepinephrine *n. see* NORADRENALINE.

norethisterone *n.* a synthetic female sex hormone (*see* PROGESTOGEN) administered by mouth to treat menstrual disorders, including amenorrhoea. Its main use, however, is in oral contraceptives, often in combination with an oestrogen. Trade name: **Primolut.**

norma *n.* a view of the skull from one of several positions, from which it can be described or measured. For example the **norma lateralis** is a side view of the skull; the **norma verticalis** is the view of the top of the skull.

normalization *n.* (in psychiatry) the process of making the living conditions of people with *mental handicap as similar as possible to those of people who are not handicapped. This includes moves to living outside institutions and encouragement to cope with work, pay, social life, sexuality, and civil rights.

normo- *prefix denoting* normality.

normoblast *n.* a nucleated cell that forms part of the series giving rise to the red blood cells and is normally found in the blood-forming tissue of the bone marrow. Normoblasts pass through three stages of maturation: **early** (or **basophilic**), **intermediate** (or **polychromatic**), and **late** (or **orthochromatic**) forms. *See also* ERYTHROBLAST, ERYTHROPOIESIS.

normocyte *n.* a red blood cell of normal size. A **normocytic anaemia** is one characterized by the presence of such cells. —**normocytic** adj.

normotensive adj. describing the state in which the arterial blood pressure is within the normal range. Compare HYPERTENSION, HYPOTENSION.

Norplant n. see LEVONORGESTREL.

Northern blot analysis a technique for identifying a specific form of messenger RNA in cells. It uses a gene *probe known to match the RNA being sought. Compare SOUTHERN BLOT ANALYSIS, WESTERN BLOT ANALYSIS.

nortriptyline n. a tricyclic *antidepressant drug that is used to relieve all types of depression. It is administered by mouth; side-effects may include dry mouth and drowsiness. Trade names: **Allegron, Aventyl.**

nose n. the organ of olfaction, which also acts as an air passage that warms, moistens, and filters the air on its way to the lungs. The **external nose** is a triangular projection in the front of the face that is composed of cartilage and covered with skin. It leads to the **nasal cavity (internal nose)**, which is lined with mucous membrane containing olfactory cells and is divided into two chambers (**fossae**) by the **nasal septum**. The lateral wall of each chamber is formed by the three scroll-shaped *nasal conchae, below each of which is a groovelike passage (**meatus**). The *paranasal sinuses open into these meatuses.

nosebleed n. bleeding from the nose, which may be caused by physical injury or may be associated with fever, high blood pressure, or blood disorders. The blood often comes from a vessel just inside the nostril, in which case the flow may be stopped by applying pressure on the side of the nose. Otherwise gauze packing may be effective in controlling the loss of blood. Medical name: **epistaxis.**

noso- prefix denoting disease.

nosocomial infection (hospital infection) an infection whose development is favoured by a hospital environment. It may develop in a hospitalized patient without having been present or incubating at the time of admission, or it may be acquired in hospital but only appears after discharge. Such infections include fungal and opportunist bacterial infections. They are aggravated by factors favouring the spread of organisms (cross-contamination) and by reduced resistance of individual patients, as well as by antibiotic-resistant strains of bacteria (see MRSA). The term also includes infections developing among hospital staff.

nosology n. the naming and classification of diseases.

Nosopsyllus n. a genus of fleas. The common rat flea of temperate regions, N. fasciatus, will, in the absence of rats, bite man and may therefore transmit plague or murine typhus from an infected rat population. The rat flea is also an intermediate host for the larval stage of two tapeworms, *Hymenolepis diminuta and H. nana.

nostrils n. see NARES.

notch n. (in anatomy) an indentation, especially one in a bone.

notifiable disease a disease that must be reported to the Health Authorities in order that speedy control and preventive action may be undertaken if necessary. In Great Britain such diseases must be notified to the proper officer for the control of communicable diseases (formerly to the Medical Officer of Health). They include diphtheria, dysentery, food poisoning, infective jaundice, malaria, measles, poliomyelitis, tuberculosis, typhoid, and whooping cough. The list varies for different countries, and some diseases are internationally notifiable through the *World Health Organization; these include cholera, plague, relapsing fever, typhus, and yellow fever.

notochord n. a strip of mesodermal tissue that develops along the dorsal surface of the early embryo, beneath the *neural tube. It becomes almost entirely obliterated by the development of the vertebrae, persisting only as part of the intervertebral discs.

NSAID (nonsteroidal anti-inflammatory drug) any one of a large group of drugs used for pain relief, particularly in rheumatic disease. NSAIDs act by inhibiting the **cyclo-oxygenase** enzymes (COX-1 and COX-2) responsible for controlling the formation of *prostaglandins, which are important mediators of inflammation. They include *aspirin, *azapropazone, *diflunisal, *ibuprofen, *ketoprofen, and *naproxen. Adverse effects include gastric bleeding and ulceration.

nucha *n.* the nape of the neck. —**nuchal** *adj.*

nuchal thickness scanning an ultrasound screening test performed during pregnancy at 10–14 weeks of gestation that looks specifically at the thickness of the skin at the back of the neck (the nuchal fold) of the fetus as an aid to the prenatal diagnosis of chromosomal defects. The thicker the nuchal fold, the higher the risk of the baby having a chromosomal defect. *See also* ULTRASOUND MARKER.

nuclear cardiology the study and diagnosis of heart disease by the intravenous injection of a *radionuclide. The radionuclide emits gamma rays, enabling a gamma camera and computer to form an image of the heart. *See* MUGA SCAN, THALLIUM SCAN.

nuclear magnetic resonance (NMR) the absorption and transmission of highfrequency radio waves by the nuclei of molecules when placed in a strong magnetic field. The effect is highly dependent on the concentration of hydrogen nuclei within each molecule, and is therefore particularly useful for analysing biological material. It has important applications in noninvasive diagnostic techniques (*see* MAGNETIC RESONANCE IMAGING, MAGNETIC RESONANCE SPECTROSCOPY).

nuclear medicine the use of *radionuclides (especially technetium-99) as *tracers to study the structure and function of organs of the body. The radionuclide is attached to a compound that is injected, inhaled, or ingested. When concentrated in the organ under investigation, the tracer can be imaged using a *gamma camera, revealing the structure or demonstrating the function of the organ. Alternatively, blood or urine samples may be analysed. *See also* NUCLEAR CARDIOLOGY.

nuclease *n.* an enzyme that catalyses the breakdown of nucleic acids by cleaving the bonds between adjacent nucleotides.

Examples are **ribonuclease**, which acts on RNA, and **deoxyribonuclease**, which acts on DNA.

nucleic acid either of two organic acids, *DNA or *RNA, present in the nucleus and in some cases the cytoplasm of all living cells. Their main functions are in heredity and protein synthesis.

nucleolus *n.* (*pl.* **nucleoli**) a dense spherical structure within the cell *nucleus that disappears during cell division. The nucleolus contains *RNA for the synthesis of *ribosomes and plays an important part in RNA and protein synthesis.

nucleoplasm (karyoplasm) *n.* the protoplasm making up the nucleus of a cell.

nucleoprotein *n.* a compound that occurs in cells and consists of nucleic acid and protein tightly bound together. *Ribosomes are nucleoproteins containing RNA; *chromosomes are nucleoproteins containing DNA.

nucleoside *n.* a compound consisting of a nitrogen-containing base (a *purine or *pyrimidine) linked to a sugar. Examples are *adenosine, *guanosine, *cytidine, *thymidine, and *uracil.

nucleotide *n.* a compound consisting of a nitrogen-containing base (a *purine or *pyrimidine) linked to a sugar and a phosphate group. Nucleic acids (DNA and RNA) are long chains of linked nucleotides (**polynucleotide** chains), which in DNA contain the purine bases adenine and guanine and the pyrimidines thymine and cytosine; in RNA, thymine is replaced by uracil.

nucleus *n.* **1.** the part of a *cell that contains the genetic material, *DNA. The DNA, which is combined with protein, is normally dispersed throughout the nucleus as *chromatin. During cell division the chromatin becomes visible as *chromosomes. The nucleus also contains *RNA, most of which is located in the *nucleolus. The nucleus is separated from the cytoplasm by a double membrane, the **nuclear envelope**. **2.** an anatomically and functionally distinct mass of nerve cells within the brain or spinal cord. **3.** the central part of the lens of the eye, which is harder than the outer cortex.

nude mouse a mouse born without a thymus and therefore no T-lymphocytes. Human tumours will often grow in these mice. For unknown reasons these mice are also hairless, hence the name.

nuisance *n.* any noxious substance, accumulating in refuse or as dust or effluent, that is deemed by British law to be injurious to health or offensive. It can also include dwellings, work premises, animals, and noise.

null hypothesis *see* SIGNIFICANCE.

nullipara *n.* a woman who has never given birth to an infant capable of survival.

nurse *n.* a person trained and experienced in nursing matters and entrusted with the care of the sick and the carrying out of medical and surgical routines. In Britain student nurses must receive a specified period of training in a hospital approved by the General Nursing Council and pass an examination before qualifying for registration with the UKCC (United Kingdom Central Council for Nursing, Midwifery, and Health Visiting) as a **general nurse**. In 1989 a new scheme for nurse education, known as **Project 2000**, was introduced by the UKCC. Student nurses gain a diploma in higher education as well as their registered nurse qualification. *See also* COMMUNITY MIDWIFE, DISTRICT NURSE, HEALTH VISITOR, PRACTICE NURSE, SCHOOL NURSE.

nutation *n.* the act of nodding the head.

nutrient *n.* a substance that must be consumed as part of the diet to provide a source of energy, material for growth, or substances that regulate growth or energy production. Nutrients include carbohydrates, fats, proteins, minerals, and vitamins.

nutrition *n.* **1.** the study of food in relation to the physiological processes that depend on its absorption by the body (growth, energy production, repair of body tissues, etc.). The science of nutrition includes the study of diets and of deficiency diseases. **2.** the intake of nutrients and their subsequent absorption and assimilation by the tissues. Patients who cannot be fed in a normal way can be given nutrients by tubes into the intestines (**enteral feeding**) or by infusion into a vein (**intravenous feeding**).

nux vomica the seed of the tree *Strychnos nux-vomica*, which contains the poisonous alkaloid *strychnine.

nyct- (nycto-) *prefix denoting* night or darkness.

nyctalopia *n.* *see* NIGHT BLINDNESS.

nyctophilia *n.* an intense preference for the darkness and an avoidance of activity in daylight hours. This is sometimes a form of social *phobia.

nyctophobia *n.* extreme fear of the dark. It is common in children and not unusual in normal adults.

nyctophonia *n.* speaking in the night but not in the daytime: a form of elective *mutism.

nymph *n.* **1.** an immature stage in the life history of certain insects, such as grasshoppers and *reduviid bugs. On emerging from the eggs, nymphs resemble the adult insects except that they are smaller, do not have fully developed wings, and are not sexually mature. **2.** the late larval stage of a tick.

nympho- *prefix denoting* **1.** the labia minora. **2.** female sexuality.

nymphomania *n.* an extreme degree of sexual promiscuity in a woman. *Compare* SATYRIASIS. —**nymphomaniac** *adj., n.*

nystagmus *n.* rapid involuntary movements of the eyes that may be from side to side, up and down, or rotatory. Nystagmus may be congenital and associated with poor sight; it also occurs in disorders of the part of the brain responsible for eye movements and their coordination and in disorders of the organ of balance in the ear or the associated parts of the brain. **Optokinetic nystagmus** occurs in normal people when they try to look at a succession of objects moving quickly across their line of sight. Jerking eye movements sometimes occur in normal people when tired, on concentrating their gaze in any direction. These are called **nystagmoid jerks** and they do not imply disease.

nystagmus block syndrome a type of

squint (convergent *strabismus) that results from the use of the convergence mechanism to block or dampen down *nystagmus in an attempt to improve visual acuity.

nystatin *n.* an antifungal drug used especially to treat yeast infections, such as candidosis. It is formulated, often in conjunction with other drugs (e.g. tetracycline in **Mysteclin** and **Trimovate**), as a cream for skin infections, as tablets for oral and intestinal infections, as pessaries or suppositories for vaginal or anal infections, or as eye drops for eye infections. Side-effects include mild digestive upsets. Trade name: **Nystan**.

O

oat cell a cell type of carcinoma of the bronchus. Oat cells are small round or oval cells with darkly staining nuclei and scanty indistinct cytoplasm. Oat-cell carcinoma is usually related to smoking and accounts for about one-quarter of bronchial carcinomas; it carries a poor prognosis. Also known as **small-cell lung cancer**, it is very sensitive to chemotherapy and radiotherapy.

obesity *n.* the condition in which excess fat has accumulated in the body, mostly in the subcutaneous tissues. Obesity is usually considered to be present when a person is 20% above the recommended weight for his/her height and build. The accumulation of fat is usually caused by the consumption of more food than is required for producing enough energy for daily activities. However, recent evidence indicates that a genetic element is involved. Hunger and satiety appear to be controlled by peptide messengers, encoded by specific genes and acting on the brain; an example is *leptin. Obesity is the most common nutritional disorder of recent years in Western societies: some patients may require surgical treatment to attain worthwhile weight reduction. —**obese** *adj.*

obex *n.* the curved lower margin of the fourth *ventricle of the brain, between the medulla oblongata and the cerebellum.

objective *n.* (in microscopy) the lens or system of lenses in a light microscope that is nearest to the object under examination and furthest from the *eyepiece. In many types of microscope interchangeable objectives with different powers of magnification are provided.

obligate *adj.* describing an organism that is restricted to one particular way of life; for example, an **obligate parasite** cannot exist without a host. *Compare* FACULTATIVE.

observer error *see* VALIDITY.

obsession *n.* a recurrent thought, feel-ing, or action that is unpleasant and provokes anxiety but cannot be got rid of. Although an obsession dominates the person, he (or she) realizes its senselessness and struggles to expel it. The obsession may be a vivid image, a thought, a fear (for example, of contamination), or an impulse (for example, to wash the hands repetitively). It is a feature of **obsessive–compulsive disorder** (*see also* NEUROSIS) and sometimes of depression and of organic states, such as encephalitis. It can be treated with behaviour therapy and also with psychotherapy and tranquillizers. *See also* ANANKASTIC. —**obsessional** *adj.*

obsessive–compulsive disorder *see* NEUROSIS, OBSESSION.

obstetrics *n.* the branch of medical science concerned with the care of women during pregnancy, childbirth, and the period of about six weeks following the birth, when the reproductive organs are recovering. *Compare* GYNAECOLOGY. —**obstetrical** *adj.* —**obstetrician** *n.*

obstipation *n. Chiefly US.* severe or complete constipation.

obstructive airways disease *see* BRONCHOSPASM.

obstructive sleep apnoea a serious condition in which airflow from the nose and mouth to the lungs is restricted during sleep. It is characteristically associated with loud snoring and a fall in the oxygen concentration in the blood, and it can lead to heart failure. In children the cause is usually enlargement of the tonsils and adenoids and treatment is by removing these structures. In adults the tonsils may be implicated but there are often other abnormalities of the *pharynx and the patients are often obese. Treatment may include weight reduction or nocturnal breathing support using a *ventilator; alternatively *tonsillectomy, *uvulopalatopharyngoplasty, or *tracheostomy may be required.

obtund *vb.* to blunt or deaden sensitivity; for example, by the application of a local anaesthetic, which reduces or causes complete loss of sensation in nearby nerves.

obturation *n.* obstruction of a body passage, usually by impaction of a foreign body, thickened secretions, or hard faeces.

obturator *n.* **1.** *see* OBTURATOR MUSCLE. **2.** a wire or rod within a cannula or hollow needle for piercing tissues or fitting aspirating needles. **3.** a removable form of denture that both closes a defect in the palate and also bears artificial teeth for cosmetic purposes. The defect may be congenital, as in a cleft palate, or result from the removal of a tumour.

obturator foramen a large opening in the *hip bone, below and slightly in front of the acetabulum. *See also* PELVIS.

obturator muscle either of two muscles that cover the outer surface of the anterior wall of the pelvis (the **obturator externus** and **obturator internus**) and are responsible for lateral rotation of the thigh and movements of the hip.

obtusion *n.* the weakening or blunting of normal sensations. This may be associated with disease.

occipital bone a saucer-shaped bone of the *skull that forms the back and part of the base of the cranium. At the base of the occipital are two **occipital condyles**: rounded surfaces that articulate with the first (atlas) vertebra of the backbone. Between the condyles is the **foramen magnum**, the cavity through which the spinal cord passes.

occiput *n.* the back of the head. —**occipital** *adj.*

occlusal *adj.* (in dental anatomy) denoting or relating to the biting surface of a premolar or molar tooth.

occlusal rim the occlusal extension of a denture base to allow analysis of jaw relations and to record jaw relations for the construction of *dentures, bridges, and extensive crowning.

occlusion *n.* **1.** the closing or obstruction of a hollow organ or part. **2.** (in dentistry) the relation of the upper and lower teeth when they are in contact. Maximum contact between the teeth is known as **intercuspal** (or **centric**) **occlusion**. *See also* MALOCCLUSION.

occult *adj.* not apparent to the naked eye; not easily determined or detected. For example **occult blood** is blood present in such small quantities, for example in the faeces, that it can only be detected microscopically or by chemical testing.

occupational disease any one of various specific diseases to which workers in certain occupations are particularly prone. **Industrial diseases**, associated with a particular industry or group of industries, fall within this category. Examples of such diseases include the various forms of *pneumoconiosis, which affect the lungs of workers continually exposed to dusty atmospheres; cataracts in glassblowers; decompression sickness in divers; poisoning from toxic metals in factory and other workers; and infectious diseases contracted from animals by farm workers, such as woolsorter's disease (*see* ANTHRAX). *See also* COSHH, PRESCRIBED DISEASE, INDUSTRIAL INJURIES DISABLEMENT BENEFIT.

occupational health service (OHS) a scheme by which employers provide a mainly preventive health service for employees during working hours. Specially trained doctors and nurses advise management on hazardous situations at work, including canteens, washrooms, etc. Advice is also given to management in relation to employees with prolonged or repeated sickness absence and on the potential for rehabilitation programmes for those with *disability. Instruction is given to the work force on simple first aid procedures and *health promotion programmes in relation to nutrition, exercise, and stress; there is also surveillance of equipment for coping with emergencies. Smaller employing units may band together and obtain such services from a common source or hire them on a sessional basis as required. With the approval of the *Health and Safety Executive, the OHS may conduct routine statutory tests on employees working with potentially hazardous substances, such as lead. *See also* COSHH.

occupational mortality rates and causes of death in relation to different jobs, occupational and socioeconomic groups, or *social class. Because some occupations have older incumbents than others (e.g. judges) allowance for age bias is made by comparing either **standardized mortality ratios** for those aged 15–64 years or related but less familiar indices, such as **comparative mortality figures** or **proportional mortality ratios**.

occupational therapy the treatment of physical and psychiatric conditions by encouraging patients to undertake specific selected activities that will help them to reach their maximum level of function and independence in all aspects of daily life. These activities are designed to make the best use of the patient's capabilities and are based on individual requirements. They range from woodwork, metalwork, and printing to pottery and other artistic activities, household management, social skills (for psychiatric patients), and leisure activities (for geriatic patients). Occupational therapy also includes assessment for mechanical aids and adaptations in the home.

ochronosis n. the presence of brown-black pigment in the skin, cartilage, and other tissues due to the abnormal accumulation of homogentisic acid that occurs in the metabolic disease *alcaptonuria.

oct- (octa-, octi-, octo-) prefix denoting eight.

ocular adj. of or concerned with the eye or vision.

oculist n. an old term for an *ophthalmologist.

oculo- prefix denoting the eye(s).

oculogyric adj. causing or concerned with movements of the eye.

oculomotor adj. concerned with eye movements.

oculomotor nerve the third *cranial nerve (III), which is composed of motor fibres distributed to muscles in and around the eye. Fibres of the parasympathetic system are responsible for altering the size of the pupil and the lens of the eye. Fibres outside the eye run to the upper eyelid and to muscles that turn the eyeball in different directions.

oculonasal adj. concerned with the eye and nose.

oculoplethysmography n. measurement of the pressure inside the eyeball. A rising or above-normal pressure is an important indication of the presence of *glaucoma.

odont- (odonto-) prefix denoting a tooth. Example: **odontalgia** (toothache).

odontoblast n. a cell that forms dentine. Odontoblasts line the pulp and have small processes that extend into the dentine.

odontogenic tumour any one of a group of rare tumours composed of dental tissue; the most important example is the *ameloblastoma.

odontoid process a toothlike process from the upper surface of the axis vertebra. See CERVICAL VERTEBRAE.

odontology n. the study of the teeth.

odontome n. an abnormal mass of calcified dental tissue, which usually represents a developmental abnormality. Compare HAMARTOMA.

-odynia suffix denoting pain in (a specified part).

odynophagia n. a sensation of pain behind the sternum as food or fluid is swallowed; particularly, the burning sensation experienced by patients with *oesophagitis when hot, spicy, or alcoholic liquid is swallowed.

oedema n. excessive accumulation of fluid in the body tissues: popularly known as **dropsy**. The resultant swelling may be local, as with an injury or inflammation, or more general, as in heart or kidney failure. In generalized oedema there may be collections of fluid within the chest cavity (**pleural effusions**), abdomen (see ASCITES), or within the air spaces of the lung (**pulmonary oedema**). It may result from heart or kidney failure, cirrhosis of the liver, acute nephritis, the nephrotic syndrome, starvation, allergy, or drugs (e.g. phenylbutazone or cortisone derivatives). In such cases the kidneys can usually be stimulated to get rid of the excess fluid by the administration of *diuretic drugs. **Subcutaneous oedema** commonly occurs in the legs and ankles due to the influence of gravity and (in women) before menstruation; the swelling subsides with rest and elevation of the legs. —**oedematous** *adj.*

Oedipus complex repressed sexual feelings of a child for its opposite-sexed parent, combined with rivalry towards the same-sexed parent: said, in Freudian psychoanalytic theory, to be a normal stage of development. The end of the Oedipus complex in children is marked by a loss of sexual feelings towards the opposite-sexed parent and an increase in identification with the same-sexed parent. Arrest of development at the Oedipal stage is said to be responsible for sexual deviations and other neurotic behaviour.

oesophag- (oesophago-) *prefix denoting* the oesophagus. Example: **oesophagectomy** (surgical removal of).

oesophageal ulcer *see* PEPTIC ULCER, OESOPHAGITIS.

oesophageal varices dilated veins in the lower oesophagus due to *portal hypertension. These may rupture and bleed, resulting in *haematemesis; serious bleeding may endanger life. Bleeding may be arrested by a compression balloon, by *sclerotherapy, by applying elastic bands via an endoscope, or by intravenous infusions of *vasopressin or *somatostatin.

oesophagitis *n.* inflammation of the oesophagus (gullet). Frequent regurgitation of acid and peptic juices from the stomach causes **reflux oesophagitis**, the commonest form, which may be associated with a hiatus *hernia. The main symptoms are heartburn, regurgitation of bitter fluid, and sometimes difficulty in swallowing; complications include bleeding, narrowing (*stricture) of the oesophageal canal, ulceration, and *Barrett's oesophagus. It is treated by antacid medicines, drugs to reduce acid secretion, weight reduction, and avoidance of bending; in severe cases surgery may be required. **Corrosive oesophagitis** is caused by the ingestion of caustic acid or alkali. It is often severe and may lead to perforation of the oesophagus or to extensive stricture formation. Treatment includes avoidance of food and administration of antibiotics; later dilatation of the stricture

may also be needed. **Infective oesophagitis** is most commonly due to a fungus (*Candida*) infection in debilitated patients, especially those being treated with antibiotics, corticosteroids, and immunosuppressive drugs, but is occasionally due to viruses (such as cytomegalovirus or herpesvirus). All these infections are common in patients with AIDS.

oesophagocele *n.* protrusion of the lining (mucosa) of the oesophagus (gullet) through a tear in its muscular wall.

oesophagogastroduodenoscopy (OGD) *n.* endoscopic examination of the upper alimentary tract using a fibreoptic or video instrument. *See also* GASTROSCOPE.

oesophagoscope *n.* an illuminated optical instrument used to inspect the interior of the oesophagus (gullet), dilate its canal (in cases of stricture), obtain material for biopsy, or remove a foreign body. It may be a rigid metal tube or a flexible fibreoptic or video-camera instrument (*see* GASTROSCOPE). —**oesophagoscopy** *n.*

Oesophagostomum *n.* a genus of parasitic nematodes occurring in Brazil, Africa, and Indonesia. It is a rare intestinal parasite of man, producing symptoms of dysentery in cases of heavy infection. The worms may also invade the tissues of the gut wall, giving rise to abscesses. The worms can be eliminated with anthelmintics.

oesophagostomy *n.* a surgical operation in which the oesophagus (gullet) is opened onto the neck. It is usually performed after operations on the throat as a temporary measure to allow feeding.

oesophagotomy *n.* surgical opening of the oesophagus (gullet) in order to inspect its interior or to remove or insert something.

oesophagus *n.* the gullet: a muscular tube, about 23 cm long, that extends from the pharynx to the stomach. It is lined with mucous membrane, whose secretions lubricate food as it passes from the mouth to the stomach. Waves of *peristalsis assist the passage of food.

Diseases of the oesophagus include *achalasis, carcinoma, hiatus hernia, *oesophageal varices, *oesophagitis, and *peptic ulcer. —**oesophageal** *adj.*

oestradiol *n.* the major female sex hormone produced by the ovary. *See* OESTROGEN.

oestriol *n.* one of the female sex hormones produced by the ovary. *See* OESTROGEN.

oestrogen *n.* one of a group of steroid hormones (including oestriol, oestrone, and oestradiol) that control female sexual development, promoting the growth and function of the female sex organs (*see* MENSTRUAL CYCLE) and female secondary sexual characteristics (such as breast development). Oestrogens are synthesized mainly by the ovary; small amounts are also produced by the adrenal cortex, testes, and placenta. In men excessive production of oestrogen gives rise to *feminization.

Naturally occurring and synthetic oestrogens, given by mouth or injection, are used to treat *amenorrhoea and menopausal symptoms (*see* HORMONE REPLACEMENT THERAPY), as well as androgen-dependent cancers (e.g. cancer of the prostate), and also to inhibit lactation. Synthetic oestrogens are a major constituent of *oral contraceptives. Side-effects of oestrogen therapy may include nausea and vomiting, headache and dizziness, irregular vaginal bleeding, fluid and salt retention, and feminization in men. Oestrogens should not be used in patients with a history of cancer of the breast, uterus, or genital tract. —**oestrogenic** *adj.*

oestrogen receptor a specific site on the surface of a cell that binds to *oestrogen; the binding triggers responses of the cell to the hormone. *Anti-oestrogens, used for treating breast cancer, act by preventing the binding of oestrogen to these *receptors.

oestrone *n.* one of the female sex hormones produced by the ovary. *See* OESTROGEN.

Oestrus *n.* a genus of widely distributed nonbloodsucking flies, occurring wherever sheep and goats are raised. The parasitic larvae of *O. ovis*, the sheep nostril fly, may occasionally and accidentally infect man. By means of large mouth hooks, it at-

taches itself to the conjunctiva of the eye, causing a painful *myiasis that may result in loss of sight. This is an occupational disease of shepherds. Larvae can be removed with forceps following anaesthesia.

Office for National Statistics (ONS) (in Britain) an executive agency of the Treasury that was formed in 1996 from a merger between the Central Statistical Office and the Office of Population Censuses and Surveys (OPCS). It is responsible for the compilation and publication of statistics relating to national and local populations, including their social and economic situation and contribution to the economy, and the demographic patterns of births, marriages, and deaths (including the medical cause of death). The ONS will continue the work of the former OPCS in organizing a **national census** at ten-yearly intervals based on the actual presence of individuals in a house or institution on a designated night (known as a **de facto census**). This contrasts with the approach in the US, where enumeration is based on official address (**de jure census**).

ofloxacin *n.* a *quinolone antibiotic used to treat urinary-tract and sexually transmitted infections and undergoing trials for multidrug therapy of leprosy. It is administered by mouth or injection; possible side effects include nausea, vomiting, and skin rashes. Trade name: **Tarivid**.

OGD *n. see* OESOPHAGOGASTRODUODENOSCOPY.

ohm *n.* the *SI unit of electrical resistance, equal to the resistance between two points on a conductor when a constant potential difference of 1 volt applied between these points produces a current of 1 ampere. Symbol: Ω.

-oid *suffix denoting* like; resembling. Example: **pemphigoid** (condition resembling pemphigus).

ointment *n.* a greasy material, usually containing a medicament, applied to the skin or mucous membranes.

olanzapine *n. see* ANTIPSYCHOTIC.

olecranon process the large process of the *ulna that projects behind the elbow joint.

oleic acid *see* FATTY ACID.

oleo- *prefix denoting* oil.

oleothorax *n.* the procedure of introducing paraffin wax extrapleurally so that the lung is allowed to collapse. This was sometimes formerly undertaken to allow closure of tuberculous cavities within the lung.

oleum *n.* (in pharmacy) an oil.

olfaction *n.* **1.** the sense of smell. **2.** the process of smelling. Sensory cells in the mucous membrane that lines the nasal cavity are stimulated by the presence of chemical particles dissolved in the mucus. *See* NOSE. —**olfactory** *adj.*

olfactory nerve the first *cranial nerve (I): the special sensory nerve of smell. Fibres of the nerve run upwards from smell receptors in the nasal mucosa high in the roof of the nose, through minute holes in the skull, join to form the olfactory tract, and pass back to reach the brain.

olig- (oligo-) *prefix denoting* **1.** few. **2.** a deficiency.

oligaemia *n. see* HYPOVOLAEMIA.

oligoarthritis *n. see* ARTHRITIS.

oligodactylism *n.* the congenital absence of some of the fingers and toes.

oligodendrocyte *n.* one of the cells of the *glia, responsible for producing the *myelin sheaths of the neurones of the central nervous system and therefore equivalent to the *Schwann cells of the peripheral nerves.

oligodendroglioma *n.* a tumour of the central nervous system derived from a type of *glia (the supporting tissue) rather than from the nerve cells themselves. *See also* GLIOMA.

oligodipsia *n.* a condition in which thirst is diminished or absent.

oligodontia *n.* the congenital absence of some of the teeth.

oligohydramnios *n.* a condition in which the amount of amniotic fluid bathing a fetus during pregnancy is abnormally small (0–200 ml in the third trimester). It is usually associated with retarded fetal growth and may indicate serious fetal kidney abnormalities. *See* POTTER SYNDROME.

oligomenorrhoea *n.* sparse or infrequent menstruation.

oligo-ovulation *n.* infrequent occurrence of ovulation.

oligospermia *n.* the presence of less than the normal amount of spermatozoa in the semen (*see* SEMINAL ANALYSIS). In oligospermia there are less than 20 million spermatozoa per ml with poor motility (**asthenospermia**) and often including many bizarre and immature forms (**teratospermia**). Treatment is directed to any underlying cause (such as *varicocele). *See also* ANDROLOGY, INFERTILITY.

oliguria *n.* the production of an abnormally small volume of urine. This may be a result of copious sweating associated with intense physical activity and/or hot weather. It can also be due to kidney disease, retention of water in the tissues (*see* OEDEMA), loss of blood, diarrhoea, or poisoning.

olive *n.* a smooth oval swelling in the upper part of the medulla oblongata on each side. It contains a mass of nerve cells, mainly grey matter (**olivary nucleus**). —**olivary** *adj.*

Ollier's disease *see* DYSCHONDROPLASIA. [L. L. X. E. Ollier (1830–1900), French surgeon]

-ology *suffix. see* -LOGY.

olsalazine *n.* a salicylate preparation used to treat mild ulcerative colitis. It is administered by mouth. Possible side-effects include nausea, vomiting, headache, joint pain, and skin rashes. Trade name: **Dipentum**.

om- (omo-) *prefix denoting* the shoulder.

-oma *suffix denoting* a tumour. Examples: **hepatoma** (of the liver); **lymphoma** (of the lymph nodes).

omentectomy *n.* the removal of all or part of the omentum (the fold of peritoneum between the stomach and other abdominal organs).

omentopexy *n.* an operation in which the *omentum is attached to some other tissue, usually the abdominal wall (in order to improve blood flow through the liver) or the heart (to increase the blood supply to the heart).

omentum (epiploon) *n.* a double layer of *peritoneum attached to the stomach and linking it with other abdominal organs, such as the liver, spleen, and intestine. The **great omentum** is a highly folded portion of the omentum, rich in fatty tissue, that covers the intestines in an apron-like fashion. It acts as a heat insulator and prevents friction between abdominal organs. The **lesser omentum** links the stomach with the liver. —**omental** *adj.*

omeprazole *n.* a *proton-pump inhibitor used to treat gastric and duodenal ulcers and the *Zollinger-Ellison syndrome. Omeprazole can be effective in cases that have failed to respond to H_2-receptor antagonists, such as *ranitidine. Administered by mouth, it is long-acting and need only be taken once a day. Possible side effects include nausea, diarrhoea, headache, constipation, and skin rashes. Trade name: **Losec**.

Ommaya reservoir a device inserted into the ventricles of the brain to enable the repeated injection of drugs into the cerebrospinal fluid. It is used, for example, in the treatment of malignant meningitis, particularly in children with leukaemia.

omphal- (omphalo-) *prefix denoting* the navel or umbilical cord.

omphalitis *n.* inflammation of the navel, especially in newborn infants.

omphalocele *n.* an umbilical *hernia.

omphalus *n. see* UMBILICUS.

Onchocerca *n.* a genus of parasitic worms (*see* FILARIA) occurring in central Africa and central America. The adult worms are found in fibrous nodules within the connective tissues beneath the skin and their presence causes disease (*see* ONCHOCERCIASIS). Various species of black fly, in which *Onchocerca* undergoes part of its development, transmit the infective larvae to man.

onchocerciasis *n.* a tropical disease of the skin and underlying connective tissue caused by the parasitic worm *Onchocerca*

volvulus. Fibrous nodular tumours grow around the adult worms in the skin; these may take several months to appear, and if secondary bacterial infection occurs they may degenerate into abscesses. The skin also becomes inflamed and itches. The migration of the *microfilariae into the eye can cause total or partial blindness – called **river blindness** in Africa. Onchocerciasis occurs in Africa and Central and South America. The drugs *suramin, *diethylcarbamazine, and – more recently – *ivermectin are used in treatment; if possible, the nodules are removed as and when they appear.

onco- *prefix denoting* **1.** a tumour. **2.** volume.

oncofetal antigen a protein normally produced only by fetal tissue but often produced by certain tumours. An example is *carcino-embryonic antigen (CEA), which has been used as a *tumour marker.

oncogene *n.* a gene in viruses (*v-onc*) and mammalian cells (*c-onc*) that can cause cancer. It results from the mutation of a normal gene. An oncogene is capable of both initiation and continuation of malignant transformation of normal cells. It probably produces proteins (*growth factors) regulating cell division that, under certain conditions, become uncontrolled and may transform a normal cell to a malignant state.

oncogenesis *n.* the development of a new abnormal growth (a benign or malignant tumour).

oncogenic *adj.* describing a substance, organism, or environment that is known to be a causal factor in the production of a tumour. Some viruses are considered to be oncogenic; these include the *papovaviruses, the *retroviruses, certain *adenoviruses and *herpesviruses, and the *Epstein-Barr virus. *See also* CARCINOGEN.

oncology *n.* the study and practice of treating tumours. It is often subdivided into medical, surgical, and radiation oncology. —**oncologist** *n.*

oncolysis *n.* the destruction of tumours and tumour cells. This may occur spontaneously or, more usually, in response to treatment with drugs or by radiotherapy.

oncometer *n.* an instrument for measuring the volume of blood circulating in one of the limbs. *See* PLETHYSMOGRAPHY.

oncosphere (hexacanth) *n.* the six-hooked larva of a *tapeworm. If ingested by a suitable intermediate host, such as a pig or an ox, the larva will use its hooks to penetrate the wall of the intestine. The larva subsequently migrates to the muscles, where it develops into a *cysticercus.

oncotic *adj.* **1.** characterized by a tumour or swelling. **2.** relating to an increase in volume or pressure.

oncotic pressure a pressure represented by the pressure difference that exists between the osmotic pressure of blood and that of the lymph or tissue fluid. Oncotic pressure is important for regulating the flow of water between blood and tissue fluid. *See also* OSMOSIS.

ondansetron *n.* a drug used to control severe nausea and vomiting, especially when it results from chemotherapy and radiotherapy. Ondansetron works by opposing the action of the neurotransmitter *serotonin (5-hydroxytryptamine) and is undergoing trials for its ability to improve memory in patients with Alzheimer's disease and to treat anxiety. Trade name: **Zofran**.

oneir- (oneiro-) *prefix denoting* dreams or dreaming.

oneirism *n.* day-dreaming. Obviously this is a normal phenomenon, but in excess it may impair the ability to cope with life. This is a feature of *schizoid and *asthenic personalities.

onomatomania *n.* the repeated intrusion of a specific word or a name into a person's thoughts: a form of *obsession.

onomatopoiesis *n.* inventing words that reflect the sound made by the object or event to be described. It is one of the principles guiding some schizophrenics in the production of *neologisms.

ONS *see* OFFICE FOR NATIONAL STATISTICS.

ontogeny *n.* the history of the development of an individual from the fertilized egg to maturity.

onych- (onycho-) *prefix denoting* the nail(s).

onychogryphosis *n.* thickening and lateral curvature of a nail, usually the big toenail.

onycholysis *n.* separation or loosening of part or all of a nail from its bed. The condition may occur in *psoriasis and in fungal infection of the skin and nail bed. It is commoner in women and may return to normal spontaneously.

onychomycosis *n.* fungus infection of the nails caused by *dermatophytes or *Candida. The nails become yellow, opaque, and thickened. *See also* RINGWORM.

O'nyong nyong fever (joint-breaker fever) a disease of East Africa and Malaysia, caused by an *arbovirus and transmitted to man by mosquitoes of the genus *Anopheles. The disease is similar to *dengue and symptoms include rigor, severe headache, an irritating rash, fever, and pains in the joints. The patient is given drugs to relieve the pain and fever.

oo- *prefix denoting* an egg; ovum.

oocyst *n.* a spherical structure, 50–60 μm in diameter, that develops from the zygote (*see* OOKINETE) of the malarial parasite (*Plasmodium*) on the outer wall of the mosquito's stomach. The oocyst steadily grows in size and its contents divide repeatedly to form *sporozoites, which are released into the body cavity of the mosquito when the oocyst bursts.

oocyte *n.* a cell in the ovary that undergoes *meiosis to form an ovum. **Primary oocytes** develop from *oogonia in the fetal ovary as they enter the early stages of meiosis. Only a fraction of the primary oocytes survive until puberty, and even fewer will be ovulated. At ovulation the first meiotic division is completed and a **secondary oocyte** and a **polar body** are formed. Fertilization stimulates the completion of the second meiotic division, which produces a second polar body and an ovum.

oocyte donation the transfer of oocytes from one woman to another. Possible recipients include women with primary or secondary ovarian failure or severe genetic disorders, and women in whom ovulation has been suppressed as an incidental result of drug treatment for another condition (e.g. cancer). Pregnancy

rates are higher than with *in vitro fertilization.

oogenesis *n.* the process by which mature ova (egg cells) are produced in the
ovary (see illustration). Primordial germ
cells multiply to form *oogonia, which
start their first meiotic division to become
*oocytes in the fetus. This division is not
completed until each oocyte is ovulated.
The second division is only completed on
fertilization. Each meiotic division is un-
equal, so that one large ovum is produced
with a much smaller polar body.

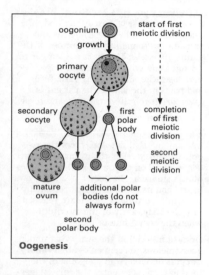

Oogenesis

oogonium *n.* (*pl.* **oogonia**) a cell produced at an early stage in the formation
of an ovum (egg cell). Primordial germ
cells that have migrated to the embryonic
ovary multiply to form numerous small
oogonia. After the fifth month of pregnancy they enter the early stages of the
first meiotic division to form the
*oocytes. *See also* OOGENESIS.

ookinete *n.* the motile elongated *zygote of the malarial parasite
(*Plasmodium*), formed after fertilization
of the *macrogamete. The ookinete bores
through the lining of the mosquito's
stomach and attaches itself to the outer
wall, where it later forms an *oocyst.

oophor- (oophoro-) *prefix denoting* the
ovary.

oophorectomy (ovariectomy) *n.* surgical removal of an ovary, performed, for
example, when the ovary contains tumours or cysts or is otherwise diseased. *See
also* OVARIOTOMY.

oophoritis (ovaritis) *n.* inflammation
of an ovary, either on the surface or
within the organ. Oophoritis may be associated with infection of the Fallopian
tubes (*see* SALPINGITIS) or the lower part of
the abdominal cavity. **Follicular oophoritis** is inflammation of the ovarian
(Graafian) follicles. A bacterial infection
usually responds to antibiotics.

oophoropexy *n.* the stitching of a displaced ovary to the wall of the pelvic cavity.

operant *adj.* describing a unit of behaviour that is defined by its effect on the environment. *See* CONDITIONING.

operating microscope a binocular
microscope commonly in use for microsurgery. The field of operation is illuminated through the objective lens by a
light source within the microscope (see
illustration). Many models incorporate a
beam splitter and a second set of eyepieces, to enable the surgeon's assistant to
view the operation.

operculum *n.* (*pl.* **opercula**) **1.** a plug of
mucus that blocks the cervical canal of
the uterus in a pregnant woman. When
the cervix begins to dilate at the start of
labour, the operculum, slightly stained
with blood, comes away as a discharge
('show'). **2.** (in embryology) a plug of fibrin
and blood cells that develops over the site
at which a developing fertilized ovum has
become embedded in the wall of the
uterus. **3.** (in neurology) one of the folded
and overlapping regions of cerebral cortex
that conceal the *insula on each side of
the brain. **4.** (in dentistry) a flap of gingival tissue that overlies the crown of a partially erupted tooth.

operon *n.* a group of closely linked
genes that regulate the production of enzymes in bacteria. An operon is composed
of one or more **structural genes**, which
determine the nature of the enzymes
made, and **operator** and **promoter gene**,

which control the working of the structural genes. The operator is itself controlled by a **regulator gene**, which is not part of the operon.

ophthalm- (ophthalmo-) *prefix denoting* the eye or eyeball. Examples: **ophthalmectomy** (surgical removal of); **ophthalmorrhexis** (rupture of); **ophthalmotomy** (incision into).

ophthalmia *n.* inflammation of the eye, particularly the conjunctiva (*see* CONJUNCTIVITIS). **Sympathetic ophthalmia** is a granulomatous *uveitis affecting all parts of the uveal tract of both eyes that may

develop after trauma or (more rarely) after eye surgery.

ophthalmia neonatorum a form of conjunctivitis occurring in newborn infants, who contract the disease as they pass through an infected birth canal. The two most common infections are gonorrhoea and *Chlamydia* (*see* INCLUSION CONJUNCTIVITIS); if untreated, the infection may cause permanent eye disease. Diagnosis should be confirmed on a culture swab, and treatment is with antibiotics.

ophthalmic *adj.* concerned with the eye.

eyepieces

prisms

magnification changer

objective

lamp

prism

filters

An operating microscope

ophthalmic nerve the smallest of the three branches of the *trigeminal nerve. It supplies sensory fibres to the eyeball, conjunctiva, and lacrimal gland, to a small region of the nasal mucous membrane, and to the skin of the nose, brows, and scalp.

ophthalmitis *n.* inflammation of the eye. *See* CONJUNCTIVITIS, UVEITIS.

ophthalmodynamometry *n.* measurement of the blood pressure in the vessels of the retina of the eye. A small instrument is pressed against the eye until the vessels are seen (through an *ophthalmoscope) to collapse. The pressure recorded by the instrument reflects the pressure within the vessels of the retina. In certain disorders of the blood circulation to the eye, the pressure in the vessels is reduced and the vessels can be made to collapse by a lower than normal pressure on the eyeball.

ophthalmologist *n.* a doctor who specializes in the diagnosis and treatment of eye diseases.

ophthalmology *n.* the branch of medicine that is devoted to the study and treatment of eye diseases. —**ophthalmological** *adj.*

ophthalmometer *n.* see KERATOMETER.

ophthalmoplegia *n.* paralysis of the muscles of the eye. **Internal ophthalmoplegia** affects the muscles inside the eye: the iris (which controls the size of the pupil) and also the ciliary muscle (which is responsible for *accommodation). **External ophthalmoplegia** affects the muscles moving the eye. **Chronic progressive external ophthalmoplegia** is a progressive disease of the extrinsic eye muscles leading to *ptosis and then paralysis of the muscles; eye movements become increasingly frozen in the primary position. Ophthalmoplegia may accompany *exophthalmos due to thyrotoxicosis. **Internuclear ophthalmoplegia**, due to a lesion in the brainstem, is commonly seen with multiple sclerosis.

ophthalmoscope *n.* an instrument for examining the interior of the eye (see illustration). There are two types. The **direct ophthalmoscope** enables a fine beam of light to be directed into the eye and at the same time allows the examiner to see the spot where the beam falls inside the eye. Examiner and subject are very close together. In the **indirect ophthalmoscope** an image of the inside of the eye is formed between the subject and the examiner; it is this image that the examiner sees. The examiner and subject are almost an arm's length apart. A **scanning laser ophthalmoscope** uses a scanning camera, rather than a human observer, to view the inside of the eye. —**ophthalmoscopy** *n.*

disc for changing lenses

An ophthalmoscope

ophthalmotomy *n.* the operation of making an incision in the eyeball.

ophthalmotonometer (tonometer) *n.* a small instrument for measuring the pressure inside the eye. There are several types. The **applanation tonometer** measures the force required to flatten a known area of the cornea after a drop of local anaesthetic has made the cornea numb. A greater force is required when the pressure inside the eye is increased, and vice versa.

-opia *suffix denoting* a defect of the eye or of vision. Example: **asthenopia** (eyestrain).

opiate *n.* one of a group of drugs derived from opium, which include *apomorphine, *codeine, *morphine, and *papaverine. Opiates depress the central nervous system: they relieve pain, suppress coughing, and stimulate vomiting. The most important opiate – morphine – and its synthetic derivative diamorphine (*see* HEROIN) are *narcotics, producing feelings of euphoria before inducing stupor. They are only used for severe pain since they cause *dependence.

opisth- (opistho-) *prefix denoting* **1.** dorsal; posterior. **2.** backwards.

opisthorchiasis *n.* a condition caused by the presence of the parasitic fluke *Opisthorchis* in the bile ducts. The infection is acquired through eating raw or undercooked fish that contains the larval stage of the parasite. Heavy infections can lead to considerable damage of the tissues of the bile duct and liver, progressing in advanced cases to *cirrhosis. Symptoms may include loss of weight, abdominal pain, indigestion, and sometimes diarrhoea. The disease, occurring in E Europe and the Far East, is treated with *chloroquine.

Opisthorchis *n.* a genus of parasitic flukes occurring in E Europe and parts of SE Asia. *O. felineus* is normally a parasite of fish-eating mammals but accidental infections of man have occurred. The adult flukes, which live in the bile ducts, can cause *opisthorchiasis.

opisthotonos *n.* the position of the body in which the head, neck, and spine are arched backwards. It is assumed involuntarily by patients with tetanus and strychnine poisoning.

opium *n.* an extract from the poppy *Papaver somniferum*, which has analgesic and narcotic action due to its content of *morphine. It has the same uses and side-effects as morphine and prolonged use may lead to *dependence. *See also* OPIATE.

opponens *n.* one of a group of muscles in the hand that bring the digits opposite to other digits. For example, the **opponens pollicis** is the principal muscle causing opposition of the thumb.

opportunistic *adj.* denoting a disease that occurs when the patient's immune system is impaired by, for example, an infection, another disease, or drugs. The infecting organism, which is also described as opportunistic, rarely causes the disease in healthy persons. Opportunistic infections, such as *Pneumocystis carinii* pneumonia and that caused by the MAI complex (*see* MYCOBACTERIUM), are common in patients with AIDS.

opposition *n.* (in anatomy) the position of the thumb in relation to the other fingers when it is moved towards the palm of the hand.

OPSI *opportunistic post-splenectomy infection: infection, particularly by encapsulated organisms, that occurs after surgical removal of the spleen (*see* SPLENECTOMY). It results from immune deficiency caused by loss of the spleen.

-opsia *suffix denoting* a condition of vision. Example: **erythropsia** (red vision).

opsoclonus *n.* a series of erratic eye movements in any direction, which is seen in people with disease of the cerebellum.

opsonic index a numerical measurement of the power of a person's serum to attack invading bacteria and prepare them for destruction by *phagocytes. It is measured by dividing the average number of bacteria in the blood per phagocyte in the presence of immune serum by the corresponding number in the presence of normal serum. A vaccine increases the opsonic index.

opsonin *n.* a serum component that attaches itself to invading bacteria and apparently makes them more attractive to *phagocytes and thus more likely to be engulfed and destroyed.

opsonization *n.* the process by which opsonins render bacteria more attractive to *phagocytes by attaching themselves to their outer surfaces and changing their physical and chemical composition.

opt- (opto-) *prefix denoting* vision or the eye.

optic *adj.* concerned with the eye or vision.

optical activity the property possessed by some substances of rotating the plane of polarization of polarized light. A compound that rotates the plane to the left is described as **laevorotatory** (or l-); one that rotates the plane to the right is described as **dextrorotatory** (or d-).

optic atrophy degeneration of the optic nerve. It may be secondary to disease within the eye or it may follow damage to the nerve itself resulting from injury or inflammation. It is visible as pallor of the optic nerve as viewed inside the eye with an ophthalmoscope.

optic chiasma (optic commissure) the X-shaped structure formed by the two optic nerves, which pass backwards from the eyeballs to meet in the midline beneath the brain, near the pituitary gland (see illustration). Nerve fibres from the nasal side of the retina of each eye cross over to join fibres from the lateral side of the retina of the opposite eye. The optic tracts resulting from the junction pass backwards to the occipital lobes.

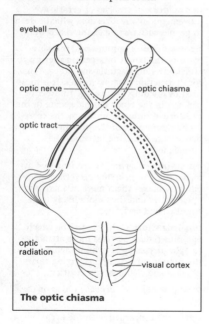

eyeball

optic nerve

optic chiasma

optic tract

optic radiation

visual cortex

The optic chiasma

optic cup either of the paired cup-shaped outgrowths of the embryonic brain that form the retina and iris of the eyes.

optic disc (optic papilla) the start of

the optic nerve, where nerve fibres from the rods and cones leave the eyeball. *See* BLIND SPOT.

optic foramen the groove in the top of the *orbit that contains the optic nerve and the ophthalmic artery.

optician *n.* a person who either makes and fits glasses (**dispensing optician**) or who can both test people for glasses and dispense glasses (**ophthalmic optician** or **optometrist**).

optic nerve the second *cranial nerve (II), which is responsible for vision. Each nerve contains about one million fibres that receive information from the rod and cone cells of the retina. It passes into the skull behind the eyeball to reach the *optic chiasma, after which the visual pathway continues to the cortex of the occipital lobe of the brain on each side.

optic neuritis *see* RETROBULBAR NEURITIS.

optometer (refractometer) *n.* an instrument for measuring the *refraction of the eye. An **autorefractor** calculates the required spectacle lens correction automatically. Because the design and use of optometers is very complex, errors of refraction are usually determined using a *retinoscope.

optometrist *n. see* OPTICIAN.

oral *adj.* **1.** relating to the mouth. **2.** taken by mouth: applied to medicines, etc.

oral cavity the mouth.

oral contraceptive the Pill: a preparation, consisting of one or more synthetic female sex hormones, taken by women to prevent conception. Most oral contraceptives are combined pills, consisting of an *oestrogen, which blocks the normal process of ovulation, and a *progestogen, which acts on the pituitary gland to block the normal control of the menstrual cycle. Progestogens also alter the lining of the uterus and the viscosity of mucus in its outlet, the cervix, so that conception is less likely should ovulation occur. These pills are taken every day for three weeks and then stopped for a week, during which time menstruation occurs. Side-effects may include headache, weight gain, nausea, skin changes, and depression. There is also a small risk that blood clots may form in the veins, especially those of the legs (which may lead to *pulmonary embolism), or that prolonged use of hormonal contraceptives may reduce fertility. The unwanted pregnancy rate is less than 1 per 100 woman-years. With progestogen-only pills (sometimes known as **minipills**) the unwanted pregnancy rate is slightly higher (1–2 per 100 woman-years) but there are fewer side-effects (due to the absence of oestrogen).

Other hormonal contraceptives include injections and implants (*see* CONTRACEPTION). *See also* POSTCOITAL CONTRACEPTION.

oral hypoglycaemic drug one of the group of drugs that reduce the level of glucose in the blood and are taken by mouth for the treatment of noninsulin-dependent (Type II) *diabetes mellitus. They include the *sulphonylurea group (e.g. *chlorpropamide, *glibenclamide, and *tolbutamide) and *metformin (a biguanide).

oral rehabilitation the procedure of rebuilding a dentition that has been mutilated as a result of disease, wear, or trauma.

oral rehydration therapy (ORT) the administration of an isotonic solution of various sodium salts, potassium chloride, glucose, and water to treat acute diarrhoea, particularly in children. In developing countries it is the mainstay of treatment for cholera. Once the diarrhoea has settled, normal feeding is gradually resumed. Preparations in clinical use include **Dioralyte** and **Rehidrat**.

Orbenin *n. see* CLOXACILLIN SODIUM.

orbicularis *n.* either of two circular muscles of the face. The **orbicularis oris**, around the mouth, closes and compresses the lips. The **orbicularis oculi**, around each orbit, is responsible for closing the eye.

orbit *n.* the cavity in the skull that contains the eye. It is formed from parts of the frontal, sphenoid, zygomatic, lacrimal, ethmoid, palatine, and maxillary bones. —**orbital** *adj.*

orbitotomy *n.* surgical removal of part of the orbital bones to gain access to the orbital space.

orchi- (orchido-, orchio-) *prefix denoting* the testis or testicle. Example: **orchioplasty** (plastic surgery of).

orchidalgia *n.* pain in the testicle. The pain may not be due to a primary condition of the testicle itself: it may be caused by a hernia in the groin, the presence of a stone in the lower ureter, or the presence of a *varicocele.

orchidectomy *n.* surgical removal of a testis, usually to treat such diseases as *seminoma (a malignant tumour of the testis). Removal of both testes (*castration) causes sterility.

orchidopexy *n.* the operation of mobilizing an undescended testis in the groin and fixing it in the scrotum. The operation should be performed well before puberty to allow the testis every chance of normal development (*see* CRYPTORCHIDISM).

orchidotomy *n.* an incision into the testis, usually done to obtain *biopsy material for histological examination, particularly in men with few or no sperm in their semen (*see* AZOOSPERMIA, OLIGOSPERMIA).

orchitis *n.* inflammation of the testis. This causes pain, redness, and swelling of the scrotum, and may be associated with inflammation of the epididymis (**epididymo-orchitis**). The condition may affect one or both testes; it is usually caused by infection spreading down the vas deferens but can develop in mumps. Mumps orchitis affecting both testes may result in sterility. Treatment of epididymo-orchitis is by local support and by administration of analgesics and antibiotics; mumps orchitis often responds to *corticosteroids.

orciprenaline *n.* a drug used to relieve bronchitis and asthma. It has the same actions and side-effects as *isoprenaline. Trade name: **Alupent**.

orf *n.* an infectious disease of sheep and goats caused by a parapoxvirus. Those bottle-feeding infected lambs may develop a painful nodule, 2–3 cm across, on the fingers or hands; it resolves spontaneously.

organ *n.* a part of the body, composed of more than one tissue, that forms a structural unit responsible for a particular function (or functions). Examples are the heart, lungs, and liver.

organelle *n.* a structure within a cell that is specialized for a particular function. Examples of organelles are the nucleus, endoplasmic reticulum, Golgi apparatus, lysosomes, and mitochondria.

organic *adj.* **1.** relating to any or all of the organs of the body. **2.** describing chemical compounds containing carbon, found in all living systems.

organic disorder a disorder associated with changes in the structure of an organ or tissue. *Compare* FUNCTIONAL DISORDER.

organism *n.* any living thing, which may consist of a single cell (*see* MICROORGANISM) or a group of differentiated but interdependent cells.

organo- *prefix denoting* organ or organic. Examples: **organogenesis** (formation of); **organopathy** (disease of).

organ of Corti (spiral organ) the sense organ of the *cochlea of the inner ear, which converts sound signals into nerve impulses that are transmitted to the brain via the cochlear nerve. [A. Corti (1822–88), Italian anatomist]

organ of Jacobson (vomeronasal organ) a small blind sac in the wall of the nasal cavity. In man it never develops properly and has no function, but in lower animals (e.g. snakes) it is one of the major organs of olfaction. [L. L. Jacobson (1783–1843), Danish anatomist]

organotrophic *adj. see* HETEROTROPHIC.

orgasm *n.* the climax of sexual excitement, which – in men – occurs simultaneously with *ejaculation. In women its occurrence is much more variable, being dependent upon a number of physiological and psychological factors.

oriental sore (Baghdad boil, Delhi boil, Aleppo boil) a skin disease, occurring in tropical and subtropical Africa and Asia, caused by the parasitic protozoan *Leishmania tropica* (*see* LEISHMANIASIS). The disease commonly affects children and takes the form of a slow-healing open sore or ulcer, which sometimes becomes secondarily infected with bacteria. Antibiotics are administered to combat the infection.

orientation *n.* (in psychology) awareness of oneself in time, space, and place. Orientation may be disturbed in such conditions as organic brain disease, toxic drug states, and concussion.

origin *n.* (in anatomy) **1.** the point of attachment of a muscle that remains relatively fixed during contraction of the muscle. *Compare* INSERTION. **2.** the point at which a nerve or blood vessel branches from a main nerve or blood vessel.

ornithine *n.* an *amino acid produced in the liver as a by-product during the conversion of ammonia to *urea.

Ornithodoros (Ornithodorus) *n.* a genus of soft *ticks, a number of species of which are important in various parts of the world in the transmission of *relapsing fever.

ornithosis *n. see* PSITTACOSIS.

oro- *prefix denoting* the mouth.

oroantral fistula a connection between the mouth and the maxillary sinus (antrum), usually as a sequel to tooth extraction. It may resolve or require surgical closure.

oropharynx *n.* the part of the *pharynx that lies between the soft palate and the hyoid bone (which is situated near the upper portion of the epiglottis).

Oroya fever *see* BARTONELLOSIS.

orphenadrine *n.* a drug that relieves spasm in muscle, used to treat all types of parkinsonism. It is administered by mouth or injection; side-effects may include dry mouth, sight disturbances, and difficulty in urination. Trade names: **Disipal**, **Norflex**.

ORT *see* ORAL REHYDRATION THERAPY.

ortho- *prefix denoting* **1.** straight. Example: **orthograde** (having straight posture). **2.** normal. Example: **orthocrasia** (normal reaction to drugs).

orthochromatic *adj.* describing or relating to a tissue specimen that stains normally.

orthodiagraph *n.* an X-ray photograph designed to give an undistorted picture of part of the body so that accurate measurements may be made from it.

orthodontic appliance an appliance used to move teeth as part of orthodontic treatment. A **fixed appliance** is fitted to the teeth by stainless steel bands or brackets that hold a special archwire, to perform complex tooth movements; it is used by dentists with specialist training (**orthodontists**). A **removable appliance** is a dental plate with appropriate retainers and springs to perform simple tooth movements; it is removed from the mouth for cleaning by the patient.

orthodontics n. the branch of dentistry concerned with the growth and development of the face and jaws and the treatment of irregularities of the teeth. See ORTHODONTIC APPLIANCE. —**orthodontic** adj.

orthognathic surgery surgical correction of severe *malocclusion, in which development of one or both jaws is abnormal, to improve facial appearance. It needs to be carried out in combination with orthodontic treatment and may involve surgery to one or both jaws.

orthopaedics n. the science or practice of correcting deformities caused by disease of or damage to the bones and joints of the skeleton. This specialized branch of surgery may involve operation, manipulation, traction, *orthoses, or *prostheses. —**orthopaedic** adj.

orthophoria n. the condition of complete balance between the alignment of the two eyes, such that perfect alignment is maintained even when one eye is covered. This theoretically normal state is in fact rarely seen, since in most people there is a minimal tendency for the eyes to deviate (see HETEROPHORIA).

orthopnoea n. breathlessness that prevents the patient from lying down, so that he has to sleep propped up in bed or sitting in a chair. —**orthopnoeic** adj.

orthoptics n. the practice of using non-surgical methods, particularly eye exercises, to treat abnormalities of vision and of coordination of eye movements (most commonly strabismus (squint) and amblyopia). Orthoptics also includes the detection and measurement of the degree of any such abnormalities. —**orthoptist** n.

orthoptoscope n. see AMBLYOSCOPE.

orthosis n. a surgical appliance that exerts external forces on part of the body to support joints or correct deformity.

orthostatic adj. relating to the upright position of the body: used when describing this posture or a condition caused by it. **Orthostatic hypotension**, for example, is low blood pressure found in some patients when they stand upright.

orthotics n. the science and practice of fitting surgical appliances to assist weakened joints.

Ortolani manoeuvre a test for *congenital dislocation of the hip in which, with the baby lying supine and the pelvis steadied with one hand, the examiner attempts to relocate a dislocated hip by gently abducting the hip while simultaneously pushing forward on the greater trochanter. If the hip is dislocated, it will relocate with a detectable and sometimes audible clunk. [M. Ortolani (20th century), Italian orthopaedic surgeon]

os¹ n. (pl. **ossa**) a bone.

os² n. (pl. **ora**) the mouth or a mouthlike part.

osche- (oscheo-) prefix denoting the scrotum. Example: **oscheocele** (a scrotal hernia).

oscilloscope n. a cathode-ray tube designed to display electronically a wave form corresponding to the electrical data fed into it. Oscilloscopes are used to provide a continuous record of many different measurements, such as the activity of the heart and brain. See ELECTROCARDIOGRAPHY, ELECTROENCEPHALOGRAPHY.

osculum n. (in anatomy) a small aperture.

Osgood-Schlatter disease inflammation and swelling at the site of insertion of the main quadriceps tendon at the top of the tibia, just below the knee (see APOPHYSITIS, OSTEOCHONDRITIS). It is common in adolescence and results from excessive physical activity. Most cases resolve with time and rest. [R. B. Osgood (1873–1956), US orthopaedist; C. Schlatter (1864–1934), Swiss surgeon]

-osis suffix denoting 1. a diseased condition. Examples: **nephrosis** (of the kidney); **lep-**

tospirosis (caused by *Leptospira* species). **2.** any condition. Example: **narcosis** (of stupor). **3.** an increase or excess. Example: **leucocytosis** (of leucocytes).

osm- (osmo-) *prefix denoting* **1.** smell or odour. **2.** osmosis or osmotic pressure.

osmic acid *see* OSMIUM TETROXIDE.

osmiophilic *adj.* describing a tissue that stains readily with osmium tetroxide.

osmium tetroxide (osmic acid) a colourless or faintly yellowish compound used to stain fats or as a *fixative in the preparation of tissues for microscopical study. Osmium tetroxide evaporates readily, the vapour having a toxic action on the eyes, skin, and respiratory tract.

osmole *n.* a unit of osmotic pressure equal to the molecular weight of a solute in grams divided by the number of ions or other particles into which it dissociates in solution.

osmoreceptor *n.* a group of cells in the *hypothalamus that monitor blood concentration. Should this increase abnormally, as in dehydration, the osmoreceptors send nerve impulses to the hypothalamus, which then increases the rate of release of *vasopressin from the posterior pituitary gland. Loss of water from the body in the urine is thus restricted until the blood concentration returns to normal.

osmosis *n.* the passage of a solvent from a less concentrated to a more concentrated solution through a *semipermeable membrane. This tends to equalize the concentrations of the two solutions. In living organisms the solvent is water and cell membranes function as semipermeable membranes, and the process of osmosis plays an important role in controlling the distribution of water. The **osmotic pressure** of a solution is the pressure by which water is drawn into it through the semipermeable membrane; the more concentrated the solution (i.e. the more solute molecules it contains), the greater its osmotic pressure. —**osmotic** *adj.*

osseointegration *n.* the process by which certain materials, such as titanium, may be introduced into living bone without producing a foreign-body reaction.

This allows a very tight and strong joint between the two structures. Osseointegration is used, for example, to fix recently developed types of dental *implants and *bone-anchored hearing aids.

osseous *adj.* bony: applied to the bony parts of the inner ear (cochlea, semicircular canals, labyrinth).

ossicle *n.* a small bone. The **auditory ossicles** are three small bones (the incus, malleus, and stapes) in the middle *ear. They transmit sound from the outer ear to the labyrinth (inner ear).

ossification (osteogenesis) *n.* the formation of *bone, which takes place in three stages by the action of special cells (osteoblasts). A meshwork of collagen fibres is deposited in connective tissue, followed by the production of a cementing polysaccharide. Finally the cement is impregnated with minute crystals of calcium salts. The osteoblasts become enclosed within the matrix as **osteocytes** (**bone cells**). In **intracartilaginous** (or **endochondral**) **ossification** the bone replaces cartilage. This process starts to occur soon after the end of the second month of embryonic life.
Intramembranous ossification is the formation of a *membrane bone (e.g. a bone of the skull). This starts in the early embryo and is not complete at birth (*see* FONTANELLE).

ost- (oste-, osteo-) *prefix denoting* bone. Examples: **ostalgia** (pain in); **osteocarcinoma** (carcinoma of); **osteonecrosis** (death of); **osteoplasty** (plastic surgery of).

ostectomy *n.* the surgical removal of a bone or a piece of bone. *See also* OSTEOTOMY.

osteitis *n.* inflammation of bone, due to infection, damage, or metabolic disorder. **Osteitis fibrosa cystica** refers to the characteristic cystic changes that occur in bones during long-standing *hyperparathyroidism. *See also* PAGET'S DISEASE (OF BONE) (OSTEITIS DEFORMANS).

osteo- *prefix. see* OST-.

osteoarthritis (osteoarthrosis) *n.* a degenerative disease of joints resulting from wear of the articular cartilage, which may lead to secondary changes in the underlying bone. It can be primary or it can occur secondarily to abnormal load to the joint or damage to the cartilage from inflammation or trauma. The joints are painful and stiff with restricted movement. Osteoarthritis is recognized on X-ray by narrowing of the joint space (due to loss of cartilage) and the presence of *osteophytes, *osteosclerosis, and cysts in the bone. The condition is treated with analgesics, by reducing the load to the joint by weight loss or the use of a walking stick, or surgically by *osteotomy, *arthrodesis, or *arthroplasty.

osteoarthropathy n. any disease of the bone and cartilage adjoining a joint. **Hypertrophic osteoarthropathy** is characterized by the formation of new bony tissue and occurs as a complication of chronic diseases of the chest, including pulmonary abscess, mesothelioma, and lung cancer.

osteoarthrosis n. see OSTEOARTHRITIS.

osteoarthrotomy n. surgical excision of the bone adjoining a joint.

osteoblast n. a cell, originating in the mesoderm of the embryo, that is responsible for the formation of *bone. See also OSSIFICATION.

osteochondritis n. **1.** necrosis of a bone due to interruption of its blood supply, which causes it to fragment and collapse before undergoing revascularization. See KIENBOCK'S DISEASE, KÖHLER'S DISEASE, LEGG-CALVÉ-PERTHES DISEASE. **2.** inflammation of an *apophysis from the pull of the attached tendon, usually occurring during the adolescent growth spurt. A fragment of bone may be avulsed (see AVULSION), producing a lump. See OSGOOD-SCHLATTER DISEASE, SEVER'S DISEASE.

osteochondritis dissecans separation of a small fragment (or fragments) of bone and cartilage from the surface of a joint, most frequently the knee, with resulting pain, swelling, and limitation of movement. If the condition persists, the fragment can be reattached or removed via an *arthrotomy or through an *arthroscope.

osteochondroma n. (pl. **osteochondromata**) a bone tumour composed of cartilage-forming cells. It appears as a painless mass, usually at the end of a long bone, and is most common between the ages of 10 and 25. As a small proportion of these tumours become malignant if untreated, they are excised.

osteochondrosis n. see OSTEOCHONDRITIS.

osteoclasia (osteoclasis) n. **1.** the deliberate breaking of a malformed or malunited bone, carried out by a surgeon to correct deformity. Also called: **osteoclasty**. **2.** dissolution of bone through disease (see OSTEOLYSIS).

osteoclasis n. **1.** remodelling of bone by *osteoclasts, during growth or the healing of a fracture. **2.** see OSTEOCLASIA.

osteoclast n. **1.** a large multinucleate cell that resorbs calcified bone. Osteoclasts are only found when bone is being resorbed and may be seen in small depressions on the bone surface. **2.** a device for fracturing bone for therapeutic purposes.

osteoclastoma n. a rare tumour of bone, caused by proliferation of *osteoclast cells.

osteocyte n. a bone cell: an *osteoblast that has ceased activity and has become embedded in the bone matrix.

osteodystrophy n. any generalized bone disease resulting from a metabolic disorder. **Renal osteodystrophy** is the characteristic change in bones occurring in chronic kidney failure.

osteogenesis n. see OSSIFICATION.

osteogenesis imperfecta (fragilitas ossium) a congenital disorder in which the bones are unusually brittle and fragile. No treatment is available, but the tendency to fracture sometimes diminishes at adolescence. There are four types, of varying severity, the worst being lethal at birth. The sclerae may be blue, and the teeth can be deformed.

osteogenic adj. arising in, derived from, or composed of any of the tissues that are concerned with the production of bone. An **osteogenic sarcoma** (see OSTEOSARCOMA) affects bone-producing cells.

osteology n. the study of the structure and function of bones and related structures.

osteolysis (osteoclasia) n. dissolution of bone through disease, commonly by infection or by loss of the blood supply (ischaemia) to the bone. In **acro-osteolysis** the terminal bones of the fingers or toes are affected: a common feature of some disorders involving blood vessels (including *Raynaud's disease), *scleroderma, and systemic *lupus erythematosus.

osteoma n. a benign bone tumour. A **cancellous osteoma** (**exostosis**) is an outgrowth from the end of a long bone, usually rising to a point. A **compact osteoma** (**ivory tumour**) is usually harmless but it may rarely compress surrounding structures, as within the skull. An **osteoid osteoma** is an overgrowth of bone-forming cells, usually causing pain in the middle of a long bone. Compact and osteoid osteomas are treated by surgical excision.

osteomalacia n. softening of the bones caused by a deficiency of *vitamin D, either from a poor diet or lack of sunshine or both. It is the adult counterpart of *rickets. Vitamin D is necessary for the uptake of calcium from food; the deficiency therefore leads to progressive decalcification of bony tissues, often causing bone pain. The condition may become irreversible if treatment with vitamin D is not given.

osteomyelitis n. inflammation of bone due to infection. **Acute osteomyelitis** occurs when bacteria enter the bone via the bloodstream and is more common in children. There is severe pain, tenderness, and redness over the involved bone, accompanied by general illness and high fever. Treatment is by antibiotics, and surgical drainage is often required. **Chronic osteomyelitis** may develop from partially treated acute osteomyelitis or after open fractures or surgery during which the bone is contaminated; tuberculosis is an occasional cause. Osteomyelitis can cause fracture and deformity of the bone.

osteopathy n. a system of diagnosis and treatment based on the theory that many diseases are associated with disorders of the musculoskeletal system. Diagnosis and treatment of these disorders involve palpation, manipulation, and massage. Osteopathy provides relief for many disorders of bones and joints, especially those

producing back pain. —**osteopath** n. —**osteopathic** adj.

osteopetrosis (Albers-Schönberg disease, marble-bone disease) n. a congenital abnormality in which bones become abnormally dense and brittle and tend to fracture. Affected bones appear unusually opaque to X-rays. In severe forms the bone marrow is obliterated, causing anaemia and infections. Treatment is by bone marrow transplantation. *See also* OSTEOSCLEROSIS.

osteophyte n. a projection of bone, usually shaped like a rose thorn, that occurs at sites of cartilage degeneration or destruction near joints and intervertebral discs. Osteophyte formation is an X-ray sign of *osteoarthritis but is not a cause of symptoms in itself.

osteoporosis n. loss of bony tissue, resulting in bones that are brittle and liable to fracture. Infection, injury, and *synovitis can cause localized osteoporosis of adjacent bone. Generalized osteoporosis is common in the elderly, and in women often follows the menopause. It is also a feature of *Cushing's disease and prolonged steroid therapy. Osteoporosis can be detected by *quantitative digital radiography and by *DEXA scans. A diet with adequate calcium, exercise, and hormone replacement therapy are preventative, and *biphosphonates can be used to reduce or halve further bone loss.

osteosarcoma (osteogenic sarcoma) n. a malignant bone tumour. It is usually seen in children and adolescents but can occur in adults of all ages, occasionally in association with *Paget's disease of bone. In children the usual site for the tumour is the leg, particularly the femur. Secondary growths (metastases) are common, most frequently in the lungs (though other sites, such as the liver, may also be involved). The symptoms are usually pain and swelling at the site of the tumour and there is often a history of preceding trauma, although it is doubtful whether this contributes to the cause. Treatment of disease localized to the primary site was traditionally by amputation of the limb; limb-sparing surgery is now possible with replacement of the diseased bone by a metal prosthesis. Many centres also give *adjuvant chemotherapy in an attempt to kill any microscopic tumour that might have already spread. The drugs used include doxorubicin, cisplatin, vincristine, cyclophosphamide, and methotrexate.

osteosclerosis *n.* an abnormal increase in the density of bone, as a result of poor blood supply, chronic infection, or tumour. The affected bone is more opaque to X-rays than normal bone. *See also* OSTEO-PETROSIS.

osteotome *n.* a surgical chisel designed to cut bone (see illustration).

An osteotome

osteotomy *n.* a surgical operation to cut a bone into two parts, followed by realignment of the ends to allow healing. The operation is performed to reduce pain and disability in an arthritic joint, for cases in which conservative treatment has failed. Osteotomy of the jaws is performed to improve severe discrepancies in jaw relation.

ostium *n.* (*pl.* **ostia**) (in anatomy) an opening. The **ostium abdominale** is the opening of the Fallopian tube into the abdominal cavity.

-ostomy *suffix. see* -STOMY.

ot- (oto-) *prefix denoting* the ear. Example: **ototomy** (surgical incision of).

otalgia *n.* pain in the ear. Apart from local causes it may be due to diseases of the jaw joints, neck, throat, or teeth.

OTC drug *see* OVER-THE-COUNTER DRUG.

otic *adj.* relating to the ear.

otic capsule the cup-shaped cartilage in the head of an embryo that later develops into the bony *labyrinth of the ear.

otitis *n.* inflammation of the ear. **Otitis externa** is inflammation of the canal between the eardrum and the external opening of the ear (the external auditory meatus). **Acute otitis media** is inflamma-

tion, usually due to viral or bacterial infection, of the middle ear (the chamber lying behind the eardrum and containing the three bony ossicles that conduct sound to the inner ear). Symptoms include pain and a high fever. Treatment is with antibiotics and sometimes also by surgical drainage (*myringotomy). **Secretory otitis media** is a chronic accumulation of fluid in the middle ear, causing hearing loss (*see* GLUE EAR). **Chronic suppurative otitis media** is chronic inflammation of the middle ear associated with perforations of the eardrum and in some instances with *cholesteatoma. The treatment involves surgical repair of perforations (*myringoplasty) or removal of the air cells in the mastoid bone (*mastoidectomy). **Labyrinthitis (otitis interna)** is inflammation of the inner ear causing vertigo, vomiting, loss of balance, and deafness.

otoacoustic emissions (Kemp echoes) tiny sounds that emerge from the inner ear shortly after the ear is exposed to an external sound. They are used as the basis for an objective test of hearing.

otoconium *n. see* OTOLITH.

otocyst *n.* a small cavity in the mesoderm of the head of an embryo that later develops into the membranous *labyrinth of the ear.

otolaryngology *n.* the study of diseases of the ears and larynx.

otolith (otoconium) *n.* one of the small particles of calcium carbonate associated with a macula in the *saccule or *utricle of the inner ear.

otology *n.* the study of diseases of the ear.

-otomy *suffix. see* -TOMY.

otomycosis *n.* a fungus infection of the ear, causing irritation and inflammation of the canal between the eardrum and the external opening of the ear (external auditory meatus). It is one of the causes of *otitis externa.

otoplasty (pinnaplasty) *n.* surgical repair or reconstruction of the ears after injury or in the correction of a congenital defect (such as 'bat ears').

otorhinolaryngology *n.* the study of ear, nose, and throat diseases (i.e. ENT disorders).

otorrhagia *n.* bleeding from the ear.

otorrhoea *n.* any discharge from the ear, commonly a purulent discharge in chronic middle ear infection (*otitis media).

otosclerosis (otospongiosis) *n.* a disorder causing deafness in adult life. An overgrowth of the bone of the inner ear leads to the third ear ossicle (the stapes) becoming fixed to the fenestra ovalis, which separates the middle and inner ears, so that sounds cannot be conducted to the inner ear. *Deafness is progressive and may become very severe, but treatment by surgery is highly effective (*see* FENESTRATION, STAPEDECTOMY). Nonsurgical treatments include fluoride tablets and the provision of suitable *hearing aids.

otoscope *n.* *see* AURISCOPE.

otospongiosis *n.* *see* OTOSCLEROSIS.

ototoxic *adj.* having a toxic effect on the organs of balance or hearing in the inner ear or on the vestibulocochlear nerve. Ototoxic drugs may be used in the treatment of *Ménière's disease.

ouabain *n.* a drug that stimulates the heart and is used to treat heart failure and other heart conditions. It is administered by mouth or injection and has the same actions and side-effects as *digitalis.

outbreeding *n.* the production of offspring by parents who are not closely related. *Compare* INBREEDING.

outer ear the pinna and the external auditory meatus of the *ear.

out-of-the-body experience a form of *derealization in which there is a sensation of leaving one's body and visions of travelling through tunnels into light or of journeys on another plane of existence. It typically occurs after anaesthesia or severe illness and is often attributed to *anoxia of the brain.

out-patient *n.* a patient who receives treatment at a hospital, either at a single attendance or at a series of attendances, but is not admitted to a bed in a hospital ward. Large hospitals have *clinics at which out-patients with various complaints can be given specialist treatment. *Compare* IN-PATIENT.

oval window *see* FENESTRA (OVALIS).

ovari- (ovario-) *prefix denoting* the ovary.

ovarian cancer a malignant tumour of the ovary, usually a carcinoma. Because of its wide-ranging pathology and an imperfect understanding of its causes, ovarian cancer is not readily detected in the early stages of development, when the tumour is small and produces few suspicious symptoms. The incidence of the disease reaches a peak in postmenopausal women; treatment involves surgery and most cases also require combined chemotherapy and/or radiotherapy (*see also* PACLITAXEL). In an attempt to facilitate a better understanding of the disease, and hence an earlier diagnosis and treatment, the World Health Organization (WHO) published in 1992 a revised Histological Classification of Ovarian Neoplasms and Tumour-like Lesions. An ultrasound screening test for ovarian cancer is being developed.

ovarian cyst a fluid-filled sac, one or more of which may develop in the ovary. Although most ovarian cysts are not malignant, they may reach a very large size, causing gross swelling of the abdomen and pressure on surrounding organs. The cyst may rotate on its stalk, thus cutting off its blood supply and causing severe abdominal pain and vomiting. In this case the cyst requires urgent surgical removal. Ovarian cysts that do become malignant may not be recognized until the tumour has advanced to a stage where treatment may be unsuccessful in eradicating the cancer. Screening programmes, based on ultrasound techniques, have been introduced in some areas to assist with the early detection of ovarian cysts and tumours.

ovariectomy *n.* *see* OOPHORECTOMY.

ovariotomy *n.* literally, incision of an ovary. However, the term commonly refers to surgical removal of an ovary (*oophorectomy).

ovaritis *n.* *see* OOPHORITIS.

ovary *n.* the main female reproductive organ, which produces ova (egg cells) and steroid hormones in a regular cycle (*see* MENSTRUAL CYCLE) in response to hormones (*gonadotrophins) from the anterior pituitary gland. There are two ovaries, situated in the lower abdomen, one on each side of the uterus (*see* REPRODUCTIVE SYSTEM). Each ovary contains numerous **follicles**, within which the ova develop (see illustration), but only a small proportion of them reach maturity (*see* GRAAFIAN FOLLICLE, OOGENESIS). The follicles secrete *oestrogen and small amounts of androgen. After ovulation a *corpus luteum forms at the site of the ruptured follicle and secretes progesterone. Oestrogen and progesterone regulate the changes in the uterus throughout the menstrual cycle and pregnancy. —**ovarian** *adj.*

developing primary follicle
maturing follicle
mature Graafian follicle
germinal epithelium
ovum
released ovum
ruptured follicle
corpus albicans
degenerating follicle
connective tissue
young corpus luteum
fully formed corpus luteum

Section of the ovary showing ova in various stages of maturation

overbite *n.* the vertical overlap of the upper incisor teeth over the lower ones.

overcompensation *n.* (in psychology) the situation in which a person tries to overcome a disability by making greater efforts than are required. This may result in the person becoming extremely efficient in what he (or she) is trying to achieve; alternatively, excessive overcompensation may be harmful to the person.

overjet *n.* the horizontal overlap of the upper incisor teeth in front of the lower ones.

overt *adj.* plainly to be seen or detected: applied to diseases with observable signs and symptoms, as opposed to those whose presence may not be suspected for years despite the fact that they cause insidious damage. An infectious disease becomes overt only at the end of an incubation period.

over-the-counter (OTC) drug a drug that may be purchased directly from a pharmacist without a doctor's prescription. Current government policy is to extend the range of OTC drugs: a number have already been derestricted (e.g. ibuprofen) and this trend is expected to increase, which will place an additional advisory responsibility on pharmacists.

ovi- (ovo-) *prefix denoting* an egg; ovum.

oviduct *n.* *see* FALLOPIAN TUBE.

ovulation *n.* the process by which an ovum is released from a mature *Graafian follicle. The fluid-filled follicle distends the surface of the ovary until a thin spot breaks down and the ovum floats out surrounded by a cluster of follicle cells (the cumulus oophoricus) and starts to travel down the Fallopian tube to the uterus. Ovulation is stimulated by the secretion of *luteinizing hormone by the anterior pituitary gland.

perivitelline space
zona pellucida
ooplasm
centrosome with two centrioles
nucleus
corona radiata

A mature ovum (magnification about X 600)

ovum (egg cell) *n.* the mature female sex cell (*see* GAMETE). The term is often applied to the secondary *oocyte although this is technically incorrect. The final stage of meiosis occurs only when the oocyte has been activated by fertilization.

oxalic acid an extremely poisonous acid, $C_2H_2O_4$. It is a component of some bleaching powders and is found in many plants, including sorrel and the leaves of rhubarb. Oxalic acid is a powerful local irritant; when swallowed it produces burning sensations in the mouth and throat, vomiting of blood, breathing difficulties, and circulatory collapse. Treatment is with calcium lactate or other calcium salts, lime water, or milk.

oxalosis *n.* an inborn defect of metabolism causing deposition of oxalate in the kidneys and elsewhere and eventually leading to renal failure.

oxaluria *n.* the presence in the urine of oxalic acid or oxalates, especially calcium oxalate. Excessive amounts of oxalates are excreted in *oxalosis.

oxatomide *n.* an *antihistamine drug used to treat hay fever. It is administered by mouth; possible side-effects include drowsiness and slowed reactions. Trade name: **Tinset**.

oxazepam *n.* a *benzodiazepine drug used to relieve anxiety and tension and for the treatment of alcoholism. It is administered by mouth and commonly causes drowsiness. *See also* TRANQUILLIZER.

oxethazaine *n.* a local anaesthetic of skin and mucous membranes, used in indigestion mixtures (e.g. **Mucaine**) to relieve heartburn and pain due to inflammation of the digestive system. Mild side-effects, including dry mouth and nausea, may occur.

oxidant *n.* (in biological systems) a molecule that serves as an electron acceptor. In human disease oxidants are derived from normal intracellular processes and released by inflammatory cells. They are counteracted by *antioxidants, such as beta-carotene.

oxidase *n. see* OXIDOREDUCTASE.

oxidoreductase *n.* one of a group of enzymes that catalyse oxidation-reduction reactions. This class includes the enzymes formerly known either as **dehydrogenases** or as **oxidases**.

oximeter *n.* an instrument for measuring the proportion of oxygenated haemoglobin (oxyhaemoglobin) in the blood.

oxprenolol *n.* a drug that controls the activity of the heart (*see* BETA BLOCKER), used to treat angina, high blood pressure, and abnormal heart rhythm. It is administered by mouth or injection; side-effects may include dizziness, drowsiness, headache, and digestive upsets. Trade name: **Trasicor**.

oxybutinin *n.* a drug administered orally to reduce frequency and urgency of passing urine associated with an unstable bladder or instability of the *detrusor muscle of the bladder wall. It acts by relaxing the bladder muscle.

oxycephaly (turricephaly) *n.* a deformity of the bones of the skull giving the head a pointed appearance. *See* CRANIOSYNOSTOSIS. —**oxycephalic** *adj.*

oxygen *n.* an odourless colourless gas that makes up one-fifth of the atmosphere. Oxygen is essential to most forms of life in that it combines chemically with glucose (or some other fuel) to provide energy for metabolic processes. In man oxygen is absorbed into the blood from air breathed into the lungs. Oxygen is administered therapeutically in various conditions in which the tissues are unable to obtain an adequate supply through the lungs (*see* OXYGENATOR, (OXYGEN) TENT). Symbol: O.

oxygenator *n.* a machine that oxygenates blood outside the body. It is used together with pumps to maintain the patient's circulation while he is undergoing open heart surgery (*see* HEART-LUNG MACHINE) or to improve the circulation of a patient with heart or lung disorders that lower the amount of blood oxygen.

oxygen deficit a physiological condition that exists in cells during periods of temporary oxygen shortage. During periods of violent exertion the body requires extra energy, which is obtained by the breakdown of glucose in the absence of oxygen, after the available oxygen has been used up. The breakdown products are acidic and cause muscle pain. The oxygen required to get rid of the breakdown products (called the oxygen deficit) must be made available after the exertion stops.

oxygen tent *see* TENT.

oxyhaemoglobin *n.* the bright-red substance formed when the pigment *haemoglobin in red blood cells combines reversibly with oxygen. Oxyhaemoglobin is the form in which oxygen is transported from the lungs to the tissues, where the oxygen is released. *Compare* METHAEMOGLOBIN.

oxymetazoline *n.* a *sympathomimetic drug administered as a nasal spray to treat nasal congestion. Possible side-effects include irritation of the nose, headache, fast pulse, and insomnia. Trade name: **Afrazine**.

oxymetholone *n.* a synthetic male sex hormone with *anabolic effects. Trade name: **Anapolon 50**.

oxyntic cells (parietal cells) cells of the *gastric glands that secrete hydrochloric acid in the fundic region of the stomach.

oxytetracycline *n.* an *antibiotic used to treat infections caused by a wide variety of bacteria. It is administered by mouth or injection or applied to the skin in a cream; side-effects are those of the other *tetracyclines. Trade names: **Imperacin, Terramycin**.

oxytocic *n.* any agent that induces or accelerates labour by stimulating the muscles of the uterus to contract. *See also* OXYTOCIN.

oxytocin *n.* a hormone, released by the pituitary gland, that causes contraction of the uterus during labour and stimulates milk flow from the breasts by causing contraction of muscle fibres in the milk ducts. Pituitary extract (**Syntocinon**) is used to induce uterine contractions and to control or prevent postpartum haemorrhage.

oxyuriasis *n.* *see* ENTEROBIASIS.

Oxyuris *n.* *see* THREADWORM.

ozaena *n.* a disorder of the nose in which the mucous membranes inside the nose become atrophied, with the production of an offensive discharge and crusts.

ozone *n.* a poisonous gas containing three oxygen atoms per molecule. Ozone is a very powerful oxidizing agent and is formed when oxygen or air is subjected to electric discharge. Ozone is found in the atmosphere at very high altitudes (the **ozone layer**) and is responsible for destroying a large proportion of the sun's ultraviolet radiation. Without this absorption by ozone the earth would be subjected to a lethal amount of ultraviolet radiation.

p53 *n.* a gene that mutates to form an important *oncogene for human *cancers. Recent trials of *gene therapy that involved replacing the oncogene with the normal version of the gene have had a limited success.

Pacchionian body *see* ARACHNOID VILLUS. [A. Pacchioni (1665–1726), Italian anatomist]

pacemaker *n.* **1.** a device used to produce and maintain a normal heart rate in patients who have *heart block. The unit consists of a battery that stimulates the heart through an insulated electrode wire attached to the surface of the ventricle (**epicardial pacemaker**) or lying in contact with the lining of the heart (**endocardial pacemaker**). A pacemaker may be used as a temporary measure with an external battery or it may be permanent, when the whole apparatus is surgically implanted under the skin. Some pacemakers stimulate the heart at a fixed rate; others sense when the natural heart rate falls below a predetermined value and then stimulate the heart (**demand pacemaker**). **2.** the part of the heart that regulates the rate at which it beats: the *sinoatrial node.

pachy- *prefix denoting* **1.** thickening of a part or parts. **2.** the dura mater.

pachydactyly *n.* abnormal enlargement of the fingers and toes, occurring either as a congenital abnormality or as part of an acquired disease (such as *acromegaly).

pachyglossia *n.* abnormal thickness of the tongue.

pachymeningitis *n.* inflammation of the dura mater, one of the membranes (meninges) covering the brain and spinal cord (*see* MENINGITIS).

pachymeninx *n.* the *dura mater, outermost of the three meninges.

pachymeter *n.* an instrument used to measure the thickness of the cornea. —**pachymetry** *n.*

pachyonychia congenita a rare genet-

ically determined skin disorder (*see* GENO-DERMATOSIS) characterized by thickening of the nails together with other ectodermal abnormalities.

pachysomia *n.* thickening of parts of the body, which occurs in certain diseases.

pachytene *n.* the third stage of the first prophase of *meiosis, in which *crossing over begins.

Pacinian corpuscles sensory receptors for touch in the skin, consisting of sensory nerve endings surrounded by capsules of membrane in 'onion-skin' layers. They are especially sensitive to changes in pressure and so detect vibration particularly well. [F. Pacini (1812–83), Italian anatomist]

pack *n.* a pad of folded moistened material, such as cotton-wool, applied to the body or inserted into a cavity.

packed cell volume (haematocrit) the volume of the red cells (erythrocytes) in blood, expressed as a fraction of the total volume of the blood. The packed cell volume is determined by centrifuging blood in a tube and measuring the height of the red-cell column as a fraction of the total.

paclitaxel *n.* a *cytotoxic anticancer drug formerly obtainable only from the bark of the Pacific yew tree but now synthesized; it has also been produced by biotechnological methods. Paclitaxel interacts with tubulin, a protein involved in cell division, and has been found to exercise control on the growth of certain cancers. Administered by intravenous infusion, it is used to treat ovarian and breast cancers that are resistant to standard therapies. Side-effects include numbness and tingling of the extremities, damage to bone marrow, and loss of hair. Trade name: **Taxol**.

PACS (picture archiving and communication system) an electronic system enabling the storage of X-ray and other images digitally on computer disk, for later retrieval and subsequent display on high-resolution monitors, via computer links (digital networks), at local or distant sites (*see* DIGITIZATION). PACS enables electronically stored images from one or more hospitals to be immediately available, through digital networks, as an aid to diagnosis and treatment. The system also allows the manipulation of images on screen.

pad *n.* cotton-wool, foam rubber, or other material used to protect a part of the body from friction, bruising, or other unwanted contact.

paed- (paedo-) *prefix denoting* children.

paederasty *n.* *sodomy with a boy or a young man.

paediatric dentistry the branch of dentistry concerned with the care and treatment of children's teeth.

paediatrics *n.* the general medicine of childhood. Handling the sick child requires a special approach at every age from birth (or premature birth) to adolescence and also a proper understanding of parents. It also requires detailed knowledge of genetics, obstetrics, psychological development, management of handicaps at home and in school, and effects of social conditions on child health. The preventive measures associated with all these aspects of paediatrics are the concern of *public health physicians and *community paediatricians. *See also* CHILD HEALTH CLINIC. —**paediatrician** *n.*

paedophilia *n.* sexual attraction to children (of either sex). Sexual activity with any children under the age of 16 is illegal in the UK. The condition is usually caused by psychological and social factors, which affect the development of sexuality. Paedophiles may seek treatment because of society's disapproval: *behaviour therapy can be used, or the sexual drive can be reduced by drug treatment. —**paedophile** *n.* —**paedophilic** *adj.*

Paget's disease 1. a chronic disease of bones, occurring in the elderly and most frequently affecting the skull, backbone, pelvis, and long bones. Affected bones become thickened and their structure disorganized: X-rays reveal patchy *sclerosis. There are often no symptoms, but pain,

deformity, and fracture can occur; when the skull is affected, blindness and deafness can occur. Treatment is with *biphosphonates or calcitonin. Medical name: **osteitis deformans**. 2. a malignant condition of the nipple, resembling eczema in appearance, associated with underlying infiltrating cancer of the breast. *See also* BREAST CANCER. 3. an uncommon condition of the vulva characterized by an epithelial lesion that histologically resembles the lesion of Paget's disease of the nipple. It may be associated with locally invasive *adenocarcinomas of the surrounding skin, as well as tumours at other sites. [Sir J. Paget (1814–99), British surgeon]

pain clinic a clinic that specializes in techniques of long-term pain relief, such as *transcutaneous electrical nerve stimulation (TENS). Pain clinics are usually directed by anaesthetists.

paint *n.* (in pharmacy) a liquid preparation that is applied to the skin or mucous membranes. Paints usually contain antiseptics, astringents, caustics, or analgesics.

palaeo- *prefix denoting* 1. ancient. 2. primitive.

palaeocerebellum *n.* the anterior lobe of the cerebellum. In evolutionary terms it is one of the earliest parts of the hindbrain to develop in mammals.

palaeopathology *n.* the study of the diseases of man and other animals in prehistoric times, from examination of their bones or other remains. By examining the bones of specimens of Neanderthal man it has been discovered that spinal arthritis was a disease that existed at least 50,000 years ago.

palaeostriatum *n. see* PALLIDUM.

palaeothalamus *n.* the anterior and central part of the *thalamus, older in evolutionary terms than the lateral part, the neothalamus, which is well developed in apes and man.

palate *n.* the roof of the mouth, which separates the mouth from the nasal cavity and consists of two portions. The **hard palate**, at the front of the mouth, is formed by processes of the maxillae and palatine bones and is covered by mucous membrane. The **soft palate**, further back, is a movable fold of mucous membrane that tapers at the back of the mouth to form a fleshy hanging flap of tissue – the **uvula**.

palatine bone either of a pair of approximately L-shaped bones of the face that contribute to the hard *palate, the nasal cavity, and the orbits. *See* SKULL.

palato- *prefix denoting* **1.** the palate. **2.** the palatine bone.

palatoplasty *n.* plastic surgery of the roof of the mouth, usually to correct cleft palate or other defects present at birth. **Laser palatoplasty** is carried out under local or general anaesthesia to shorten and/or stiffen the palate in the treatment of snoring.

palatorrhaphy *n. see* STAPHYLORRHAPHY.

pali- (palin-) *prefix denoting* repetition or recurrence.

palilalia *n.* a disorder of speech in which a word spoken by the individual is rapidly and involuntarily repeated. It is seen, with other tics, in the *Gilles de la Tourette syndrome. It is also encountered when encephalitis or other processes damage the *extrapyramidal system of the brain.

palindromic *adj.* relapsing: describing diseases or symptoms that recur or get worse.

palingraphia *n.* a disorder of writing in which words and letters are repeated. It is a feature of acquired brain disease, such as stroke.

paliphrasia *n.* repetition of phrases while speaking: a form of *stammering or a kind of *tic.

palliative *n.* a medicine that gives temporary relief from the symptoms of a disease but does not actually cure the disease. Palliatives are often used in the treatment of such diseases as cancer.

pallidectomy (pallidotomy) *n.* a neurosurgical operation to destroy or modify the effects of the globus pallidus (*see* BASAL GANGLIA). This operation was used for the relief of *parkinsonism and other conditions in which involuntary movements are prominent before the advent of modern drug therapies. The development of more accurate techniques to localize the globus

pallidus has led to a revival in the use of the operation.

pallidum (palaeostriatum) *n.* one of the dense collections of grey matter, deep in each cerebral hemisphere, that go to make up the *basal ganglia.

pallium *n.* the outer wall of the cerebral hemisphere as it appears in the early stages of evolution of the mammalian brain. In the modern brain it corresponds to the *cerebral cortex.

pallor *n.* abnormal paleness of the skin, due to reduced blood flow or lack of normal pigments. Pallor may be associated with an indoor mode of life; it may also indicate shock, anaemia, cancer, or other diseases.

palmitic acid *see* FATTY ACID.

palpation *n.* the process of examining part of the body by careful feeling with the hands and fingertips. Using palpation it is possible, in many cases, to distinguish between swellings that are solid and those that are cystic (*see* FLUCTUATION). Palpation is also used to discover the presence of a fetus in the uterus (*see* BALLOTTEMENT).

palpebral *adj.* relating to the eyelid (palpebra).

palpitation *n.* an awareness of the heartbeat. This is normal with fear, emotion, or exertion. It may also be a symptom of neurosis, arrhythmias, heart disease, and overactivity of the circulation (as in thyrotoxicosis).

palsy *n.* paralysis. This archaic word is retained in compound terms, such as *Bell's palsy, *cerebral palsy, and *Todd's palsy.

paludism *n. see* MALARIA.

pamidronate *n. see* BIPHOSPHONATES.

pan- (pant(o)-) *prefix denoting* all; every: hence (in medicine) affecting all parts of an organ or the body; generalized.

panacea *n.* a medicine said to be a cure for all diseases and disorders, no matter what their nature. Unfortunately panaceas do not exist, despite the claims of many patent medicine manufacturers.

Panadol *n. see* PARACETAMOL.

pancarditis *n. see* ENDOMYOCARDITIS.

Pancoast syndrome pain and paralysis involving the lower branches of the brachial plexus due to infiltration by a malignant tumour of the apical region of the lung. *Horner's syndrome may also be present. [H. K. Pancoast (1875–1939), US radiologist]

pancreas *n.* a compound gland, about 15 cm long, that lies behind the stomach. One end lies in the curve of the duodenum; the other end touches the spleen. It is composed of clusters (**acini**) of cells that secrete *pancreatic juice. This contains a number of enzymes concerned in digestion. The juice drains into small ducts that open into the **pancreatic duct**. This unites with the common *bile duct and the secretions pass into the duodenum. Interspersed among the acini are the *islets of Langerhans – isolated groups of cells that secrete the hormones *insulin and *glucagon into the bloodstream.

pancreas divisum a congenital abnormality in which the pancreas develops in two parts draining separately into the duodenum, the small ventral pancreas through the main ampulla and the larger dorsal pancreas through an accessory papilla. In rare instances this is associated with recurrent abdominal pain, probably due to inadequate drainage of the dorsal pancreas. Diagnosis is made by *ERCP.

pancreatectomy *n.* surgical removal of the pancreas. **Total pancreatectomy (Whipple's operation)** involves the entire gland and part of the duodenum. In **subtotal pancreatectomy** most of the gland is removed, usually leaving a small part close to the duodenum. In **partial pancreatectomy** only a portion of the gland is removed. The operations are performed for tumours in the gland or because of chronic or relapsing *pancreatitis. After total or subtotal pancreatectomy it is necessary to administer pancreatic enzymes with food to aid its digestion and insulin injections to replace that normally secreted by the gland.

pancreatic juice the digestive juice secreted by the *pancreas. Its production is stimulated by hormones secreted by the duodenum, which in turn is stimulated by contact with food from the stomach. If the duodenum produces the hormone *se-

cretin the pancreatic juice contains a large amount of sodium bicarbonate, which neutralizes the acidity of the stomach contents. Another hormone (*see* CHOLECYSTO-KININ) stimulates the production of a juice rich in digestive enzymes, including trypsinogen and chymotrypsinogen (which are converted to *trypsin and *chymotrypsin in the duodenum), *amylase, *lipase, and *maltase.

pancreatin *n.* an extract obtained from the *pancreas, containing the pancreatic enzymes. Pancreatin is administered to treat conditions in which pancreatic secretion is deficient; for example, in pancreatitis.

pancreatitis *n.* inflammation of the pancreas. **Acute pancreatitis** is a sudden illness in which the patient experiences severe pain in the upper abdomen and back, with shock; its cause is not always discovered, but it may be associated with gallstones or alcoholism. It may be mistaken for a perforated peptic ulcer but differs from this condition in that the level of the enzyme *amylase in the blood is raised. The main complication is the formation of a *pseudocyst. Treatment consists of intravenous feeding (no food or drink should be given by mouth), and *anticholinergic drugs. **Relapsing pancreatitis**, in which the above symptoms are recurrent and less severe, may be associated with gallstones or alcoholism; prevention is by removal of gallstones and avoidance of alcohol and fat. Operations may be done to improve drainage of the pancreatic duct. **Chronic pancreatitis** may produce symptoms similar to relapsing pancreatitis or may be painless; it leads to pancreatic failure causing *malabsorption and *diabetes mellitus. The pancreas often becomes calcified, producing visible shadowing on X-rays. The malabsorption is treated by a low-fat diet with pancreatic enzyme supplements, and the diabetes with insulin.

pancreatogram *n.* a radiographic image of the pancreatic ducts obtained by injecting a contrast medium into them by direct puncture under *ultrasound guidance, at the time of laparotomy or by *ERCP.

pancreatotomy *n.* surgical opening of

the duct of the pancreas in order to inspect the duct, to join the duct to the intestine, or to inject contrast material in order to obtain X-ray pictures of the duct system.

pancreozymin *n.* the name originally given to the fraction of the hormone *cholecystokinin that acts on the pancreas.

pancytopenia *n.* a simultaneous decrease in the numbers of red cells (*anaemia), white cells (*neutropenia), and platelets (*thrombocytopenia) in the blood. It occurs in a variety of disorders, including aplastic *anaemias, *hypersplenism, and tumours of the bone marrow.

panda sign a sign of bilateral periorbital *haematoma associated with injury to the anterior cranial fossa, the front of the skull cavity that supports the frontal lobes of the brain. The name derives from its similarity in appearance to the black eye patches of a panda.

pandemic *n.* an *epidemic so widely spread that vast numbers of people in different countries are affected. The Black Death, the epidemic plague that ravaged Europe in the fourteenth century and killed over one third of the population, was a classical pandemic. AIDS is currently considered to be pandemic. —**pandemic** *adj.*

panic disorder a condition featuring recurrent brief episodes of acute distress, mental confusion, and fear of impending death. The heart beats rapidly, breathing is deep and fast, and sweating occurs. Overbreathing (hyperventilation) often makes the attack worse. These panic attacks usually occur about twice a week but may be more frequent and they are especially common in people with *agoraphobia. The condition tends to run in families and appears to be an organic disorder with a strong psychological component. Treatment is with *antidepressant drugs. *Behaviour therapy can also be helpful.

panmixis *n.* random mating within a population, i.e. when there is no selection of partners on religious, racial, social, or other grounds.

panniculitis (Weber-Christian disease) *n.* inflammation of the layer of fat beneath the skin, leading to multiple tender nodules in the legs and trunk.

panniculus *n.* a membranous sheet of tissue. For example, the **panniculus adiposus** is the fatty layer of tissue underlying the skin.

pannus *n.* invasion of the outer layers of the cornea of the eye by tissue containing many blood vessels, which grows in from the conjunctiva. It is seen as a result of inflammation of the cornea or conjunctiva, particularly in *trachoma.

panophthalmitis *n.* inflammation involving the whole of the interior of the eye.

Panstrongylus *n.* a genus of large bloodsucking bugs (*see* REDUVIID). *P. megistus* is important in transmitting *Chagas' disease to man in Brazil.

pant- (panto-) *prefix. see* PAN-.

pantaloon hernia a double sac comprising the sac of an indirect (external) and a direct (internal) inguinal *hernia on the same side.

pantoprazole *n. see* PROTON-PUMP INHIBITOR.

pantothenic acid a B vitamin that is a constituent of *coenzyme A. It plays an important role in the transfer of acetyl groups in the body. Pantothenic acid is widely distributed in food and a deficiency is therefore unlikely to occur.

pantropic *adj.* describing a virus that can invade and affect many different tissues of the body, for example the nerves, skin, or liver, without showing a special affinity for any one of them.

papain *n.* a preparation that contains one or more protein-digesting enzymes. It is obtained from the pawpaw fruit and is used as a digestant.

Papanicolaou test (Pap test) *see* CERVICAL SMEAR. [G. N. Papanicolaou (1883–1962), Greek physician, anatomist, and cytologist]

papaverine *n.* an alkaloid, derived from opium, that relaxes smooth muscle. In combination with *morphine and *codeine (a mixture called **papaveretum**), it is administered by injection as a pre-anaesthetic medication. It may cause abnormal heart rate.

papilla n. (pl. **papillae**) any small nipple-shaped protuberance. Several different kinds of papillae occur on the *tongue, in association with the taste buds. The **optic papilla** is an alternative name for the *optic disc.

papillitis n. inflammation of the first part of the optic nerve (the optic disc or optic papilla), i.e. where the nerve leaves the eyeball.

papilloedema n. swelling of the first part of the optic nerve (the optic disc or optic papilla).

papilloma n. a benign nipple-like growth on the surface of skin or mucous membrane. Examples include **basal-cell papillomas** (see (SEBORRHOEIC) KERATOSIS) and **bladder papillomas**. —**papillomatous** adj.

papillomatosis n. a condition in which many *papillomas grow on an area of skin or mucous membrane.

papillotomy n. the operation of cutting the *ampulla of Vater to widen its outlet in order to improve bile drainage and allow the passage of stones from the common bile duct. It is usually performed using a diathermy wire through a *duodenoscope following *ERCP.

papovavirus n. one of a group of small DNA-containing viruses producing tumours in animals (subgroup **polyomaviruses**) and in animals and humans (subgroup **papillomaviruses**). See also HUMAN PAPILLOMAVIRUS.

Pappataci fever see SANDFLY FEVER.

papule n. a small raised spot on the skin, less than 5 mm in diameter.

papulo- prefix denoting a papule or pimple.

papulosquamous adj. describing a rash that is both papular and scaly.

para- prefix denoting **1.** beside or close to. Example: **paranasal** (near the nasal cavity). **2.** resembling. Example: **paradysentery** (a mild form of dysentery). **3.** abnormal. Example: **paralalia** (abnormal speech).

para-aminobenzoic acid a naturally occurring drug used in lotions and creams to prevent sunburn.

para-aminosalicylic acid (PAS) a drug, chemically related to aspirin, used – in conjunction with isoniazid or streptomycin – to treat various types of tuberculosis. It is administered by mouth and commonly causes nausea, vomiting, diarrhoea, and rashes.

paracentesis n. tapping: the process of drawing off excess fluid from a part of the body through a hollow needle or *cannula.

paracetamol (acetaminophen) n. an *analgesic drug that also reduces fever. It is used to treat mild or moderate pain, such as headache, toothache, and rheumatism. It is administered by mouth and may cause digestive upsets; overdosage causes liver damage. Trade names: **Calpol, Panadol, Panaleve**.

Paracoccidioides n. a genus of yeast-like fungi causing infection of the skin and mucous membranes. The species P. brasiliensis causes a chronic skin disease, South American *blastomycosis.

paracrine adj. describing a hormone that is secreted by an endocrine gland and affects the function of nearby cells, rather than being transported distally by the blood or lymph.

paracusis n. any abnormality of hearing.

paradidymis n. the vestigial remains of part of the embryonic *mesonephros that are found near the testis of the adult. Some of the mesonephric collecting tubules persist as the functional *vasa efferentia but the rest degenerate almost completely. A similar vestigial structure (the **paroophoron**) is found in females.

paradox n. (in *family therapy) a surprising interpretation or suggestion made in the course of therapy in order to demonstrate the relationship between a psychological symptom and a system of family relationships. For example, a child might be told to go on stealing from his parents because their concern about the symptom is all that is keeping their marriage intact.

paradoxical breathing breathing

movements in which the chest wall moves in on inspiration and out on expiration, in reverse of the normal movements. It may be seen in children with respiratory distress of any cause, which leads to indrawing of the intercostal spaces during inspiration. Patients with chronic airways obstruction also show indrawing of the lower ribs during inspiration, due to the distorted action of a depressed and flattened diaphragm. Crush injuries of the chest, with fractured ribs and sternum, can lead to a severe degree of paradoxical breathing.

paraesthesiae *pl. n.* spontaneously occurring abnormal tingling sensations, sometimes described as **pins and needles**. They may be symptoms of partial damage to a peripheral nerve, such as that caused by external pressure on the affected part, but can also result from damage to sensory fibres in the spinal cord. *Compare* DYSAESTHESIAE.

paraffin *n.* one of a series of hydrocarbons derived from petroleum. **Paraffin wax** (**hard paraffin**), a whitish mixture of solid hydrocarbons melting at 45–60°C, is used in medicine mainly as a base for ointments; it is also used for *embedding specimens for microscopical study. **Liquid paraffin** is a mineral oil, which has been used as a laxative.

paraganglion *n.* one of the small oval masses of cells found in the walls of the ganglia of the sympathetic nervous system, near the spinal cord. They are *chromaffin cells, like those of the adrenal gland, and may secrete adrenaline.

parageusia (parageusis) *n.* abnormality of the sense of taste.

paragonimiasis (endemic haemoptysis) *n.* a tropical disease that occurs principally in the Far East, caused by the presence of the fluke *Paragonimus westermani* in the lungs. The infection is acquired by eating inadequately cooked shellfish, such as crayfish and crabs. Symptoms resemble those of chronic *bronchitis, including the coughing up of blood and difficulty in breathing (dyspnoea). Paragonimiasis is treated with the drugs bithionol and chloroquine.

Paragonimus *n.* a genus of large tropi-cal parasitic *flukes that are particularly prevalent in the Far East. The adults of *P. westermani* live in the lungs of man, where they cause destruction and bleeding of the tissues (see PARAGONIMIASIS). However, they may also be found in other organs of the body. Eggs are passed out in the sputum and the larvae undergo their development in two other hosts, a snail and a crab.

paragranuloma *n.* an old term for one of the types of *Hodgkin's disease. It is now known as **lymphocyte-predominant Hodgkin's disease** and has the best prognosis of all the types.

paragraphia *n.* a disorder of writing, involving the omission or transposition of letters or of whole words. The appearance of this in adult life is usually due to damage to the brain. In childhood it usually reflects a developmental delay in learning to write correctly.

parainfluenza viruses a group of large RNA-containing viruses that cause infections of the respiratory tract producing mild influenza-like symptoms. They are included in the paramyxovirus group (see MYXOVIRUS).

paraldehyde *n.* a *hypnotic and *anti-convulsant drug used to induce sleep in mental patients and to control convulsions in tetanus. It is administered by mouth, injection, or in suppositories; side-effects may include digestive upsets and, in large doses, prolonged unconsciousness. Both *tolerance and *dependence may result from prolonged use of the drug.

paralysis *n.* muscle weakness that varies in its extent, its severity, and the degree of *spasticity or flaccidity according to the nature of the underlying disease and its distribution in the brain, spinal cord, peripheral nerves, or muscles. *See also* DIPLEGIA, HEMIPLEGIA, PARAPLEGIA, POLIO-MYELITIS. —**paralytic** *adj.*

paramedian *adj.* situated close to or beside the *median plane.

paramedical *adj.* describing or relating to the professions closely linked to the medical profession and working in conjunction with them. Such professions require expert knowledge and experience in certain fields, but no medical degree. Paramedical personnel in a hospital include the radiographers, physiotherapists, occupational therapists, and dietitians.

paramesonephric duct (Müllerian duct) either of the paired ducts that form adjacent to the mesonephric ducts (*see* MESONEPHROS) in the embryo. In the female these ducts develop into the Fallopian tubes, uterus, and part of the vagina. However, in the male they degenerate almost completely.

parameter *n.* (in medicine) a measurement of some factor, such as blood pressure, pulse rate, or haemoglobin level, that may have a bearing on the condition being investigated.

parametric test *see* SIGNIFICANCE.

parametritis (pelvic cellulitis) *n.* inflammation of the loose connective tissue and smooth muscle around the uterus (the parametrium). The condition may be associated with *puerperal infection.

parametrium *n.* the layer of connective tissue surrounding the uterus.

paramnesia *n.* a distorted memory, such as *confabulation or *déjà vu.

paramyoclonus multiplex a benign disorder of the nervous system that is characterized by brief and irregular twitchlike contractions of the muscles of the limbs and trunk.

paramyotonia congenita a rare constitutional disorder in which prolonged contraction of muscle fibres (*see* MYOTONIA) develops when the patient is exposed to cold. This may be due to a disorder of potassium metabolism.

paramyxovirus *n.* *see* MYXOVIRUS.

paranasal sinuses the air-filled spaces, lined with mucous membrane, within some of the bones of the skull. They open into the nasal cavity, via the meatuses, and are named according to the bone in which they are situated. They comprise the **frontal sinuses** and the **maxillary sinuses** (one pair of each), the **ethmoid sinuses** (consisting of many spaces inside the ethmoid bone), and the two **sphenoid sinuses**. (See illustration.)

paraneoplastic syndrome signs or symptoms that may occur in a patient with cancer but are not due directly to

local effects of the cancer cells. Removal of the cancer usually leads to resolution of the problem. An example is *myasthenia gravis secondary to a tumour of the thymus.

paranoia *n.* a mental disorder characterized by *delusions organized into a system, without hallucinations or other marked symptoms of mental illness. It is a rare chronic condition; most people with such delusions will in time develop signs of other mental illness.

The same term is sometimes used more loosely for a state of mind in which the individual has a strong belief that he is persecuted by others. His behaviour is therefore suspicious and isolated. This can be a result of *personality disorder as well as mental illnesses causing *paranoid states.

paranoid *adj.* **1.** describing a mental state characterized by fixed and logically elaborated *delusions. There are many causes, including paranoid *schizophrenia, *manic-depressive psychosis, organic psychoses such as *alcoholism, *paraphrenia, and severe emotional stress. **2.** describing a personality distinguished by such traits as excessive sensitivity to rejection by others, suspiciousness, hostility, and self-importance.

Paranasal sinuses projected to the surface

paraparesis *n.* weakness of both legs, resulting from disease of the nervous system.

paraphasia *n.* a disorder of language in which unintended syllables, words, or phrases are interpolated in the patient's speech. A severe degree of paraphasia results in speech that is a meaningless jumble of words and sounds, called **jargon aphasia**.

paraphimosis *n.* retraction and constriction of the foreskin behind the glans penis. This occurs in some patients with *phimosis on erection of the penis: the tight foreskin cannot be drawn back over the glans and becomes painful and swollen. Manual replacement of the foreskin can usually be achieved under local or general anaesthesia, but *circumcision is required to prevent a recurrence.

paraphrenia *n.* a mental disorder characterized by systematic *delusions and prominent *hallucinations but without any other marked symptoms of mental illness. The only loss of contact with reality is in areas affected by the delusions and hallucinations. It is typically seen in the elderly and deaf. Some sufferers, if followed up over a period of years, eventually show other symptoms of *schizophrenia. It is therefore debatable whether paraphrenia constitutes a separate entity.

paraplegia *n.* *paralysis of both legs, usually due to disease or injury of the spinal cord. It is often accompanied by loss of sensation below the level of the injury and disturbed bladder function. —**paraplegic** *adj., n.*

paraprotein *n.* an abnormal protein of the *immunoglobulin series. Paraproteins appear in malignant disease of the spleen, bone marrow, liver, etc. Examples of paraproteins are *myeloma globulins, *Bence-Jones protein, and *macroglobulin.

parapsoriasis *n.* a former name for the earliest phase of *mycosis fungoides.

parapsychology *n.* the study of *extrasensory perception, *psychokinesis, and other mental abilities that appear to defy natural law.

Paraquat *n. Trademark.* the chemical compound dimethyl dipyridilium, widely used as a weed-killer. When swallowed it exerts its most serious effects upon the lungs, the tissues of which it destroys after a few days. Paraquat poisoning is almost invariably fatal.

parasite *n.* any living thing that lives in (*see* ENDOPARASITE) or on (*see* ECTOPARASITE) another living organism (*see* HOST). The parasite, which may spend all or only part of its existence with the host, obtains food and/or shelter from the host and contributes nothing to its welfare. Some parasites cause irritation and interfere with bodily functions; others destroy host tissues and release toxins into the body, thus injuring health and causing disease. Human parasites include fungi, bacteria, viruses, protozoa, and worms. *See also* COMMENSAL, SYMBIOSIS. —**parasitic** *adj.*

parasiticide *n.* an agent that destroys parasites (excluding bacteria and fungi). *See also* ACARICIDE, ANTHELMINTIC, TRYPANOCIDE.

parasitology *n.* the study and science of parasites.

parasternal *adj.* situated close to the sternum. The **parasternal line** is an imaginary vertical line parallel to and midway between the lateral margin of the sternum and the vertical line through the nipple.

parasuicide *n.* a self-injuring act (such as an overdose of sleeping tablets) that is not motivated by a genuine wish to die. It differs from attempted *suicide in being common in young people who are distressed but not seriously mentally ill. However, many people who have acted in this way go on to attempt, or even to achieve, suicide. Help in sorting out their difficulties should therefore be given. *See also* SAMARITANS.

parasympathetic nervous system one of the two divisions of the *autonomic nervous system, having fibres that leave the central nervous system from the brain and the lower portion of the spinal cord and are distributed to blood vessels, glands, and the majority of internal organs. The system works in balance with the *sympathetic nervous system, the actions of which it frequently opposes.

parasympatholytic *n.* a drug opposing the effects of the *parasympathetic nervous system. The actions of parasympatholytic drugs are **anticholinergic** (i.e.

preventing acetylcholine from acting as a neurotransmitter); they include relaxation of smooth muscle, decreased secretion of saliva, sweat, and digestive juices, and dilation of the pupil of the eye. *Atropine and similar drugs have these effects; they are used in the treatment of peptic ulcers (e.g. *propantheline) and of parkinsonism (e.g. *benzhexol, *benztropine), to relieve spasm of smooth muscle (see SPASMOLYTIC), and as *mydriatics. Characteristic side-effects include dry mouth, thirst, blurred vision, dry skin, increased heart rate, and difficulty in urination.

parasympathomimetic n. a drug that has the effect of stimulating the *parasympathetic nervous system. The actions of parasympathomimetic drugs are **cholinergic** (resembling those of *acetylcholine) and include stimulation of skeletal muscle, *vasodilatation, depression of heart rate, increasing the tension of smooth muscle, increasing secretions (such as saliva), and constricting the pupil of the eye. They are used in the treatment of *myasthenia gravis (see ANTICHOLINESTERASE), glaucoma (see MIOTIC), and some heart and circulatory conditions (e.g. *carbachol) and to restore intestinal and bladder function after surgery (e.g. *bethanechol).

paratenon n. the tissue of a tendon sheath that fills up spaces round the tendon.

parathion n. an organic phosphorus compound, used as a pesticide, that causes poisoning when inhaled, ingested, or absorbed through the skin. Like several other organic phosphorus compounds, it attacks the enzyme *cholinesterase and causes excessive stimulation of the parasympathetic nervous system. The symptoms are headache, sweating, salivation, lacrimation, vomiting, diarrhoea, and muscular spasms. Treatment is by administration of *atropine.

parathormone n. see PARATHYROID HORMONE.

parathyroidectomy n. surgical removal of the parathyroid glands, usually as part of the treatment of *hyperparathyroidism.

parathyroid glands two pairs of yellowish-brown *endocrine glands that are situated behind, or sometimes embedded within, the *thyroid gland. They are stimulated to produce *parathyroid hormone by a decrease in the amount of calcium in the blood.

parathyroid hormone (parathormone) a hormone, synthesized and released by the parathyroid glands, that controls the distribution of calcium and phosphate in the body. A high level of the hormone causes transfer of calcium from the bones to the blood; a deficiency lowers blood calcium levels, causing *tetany. This condition may be treated by injections of the hormone. Compare CALCITONIN.

paratyphoid fever an infectious disease caused by the bacterium Salmonella paratyphi A, B, or C. Bacteria are spread in the faeces of patients or carriers, and outbreaks occur as a result of poor sanitation or unhygienic food-handling. After an incubation period of 1–10 days, symptoms, including diarrhoea, mild fever, and a pink rash on the chest, appear and last for about a week. Treatment with chloramphenicol is effective. Vaccination with *TAB provides temporary immunity against paratyphoid A and B.

pareidolia n. misperception of random stimuli as real things or people, as when faces are vividly seen in the flames of a fire.

parenchyma n. the functional part of an organ, as opposed to the supporting tissue (**stroma**).

parental order see SECTION 30 ORDER.

parenteral adj. administered by any way other than through the mouth: applied, for example, to the introduction of drugs or other agents into the body by injection.

paresis n. muscular weakness caused by disease of the nervous system. It implies a lesser degree of weakness than *paralysis, although the two words are often used interchangeably.

paries n. (pl. **parietes**) 1. the enveloping or surrounding part of an organ or other structure. 2. the wall of a cavity.

parietal adj. 1. of or relating to the inner walls of a body cavity, as opposed to the contents: applied particularly to the membranes lining a cavity (see PERITONEUM,

PLEURA). **2.** of or relating to the parietal bone.

parietal bone either of a pair of bones forming the top and sides of the cranium. *See* SKULL.

parietal cells *see* OXYNTIC CELLS.

parietal lobe one of the major divisions of each cerebral hemisphere (*see* CEREBRUM), lying behind the frontal lobe, above the temporal lobe, and in front of the occipital lobe. It is thus beneath the crown of the skull. It contains the *sensory cortex and *association areas.

parity *n.* a term used to indicate the number of pregnancies a woman has had that have each resulted in the birth of an infant capable of survival. *See also* GRAND MULTIPARITY.

parkinsonism *n.* a clinical picture characterized by tremor, rigidity and a poverty of spontaneous movements. The commonest symptom is tremor, which often affects one hand, spreading first to the leg on the same side and then to the other limbs. It is most pronounced in resting limbs, interfering with such actions as holding a cup. The patient has an expressionless face, an unmodulated voice, an increasing tendency to stoop, and a shuffling walk. Parkinsonism is a disease process affecting the basal ganglia of the brain and associated with a deficiency of the neurotransmitter *dopamine. Sometimes a distinction is made between **Parkinson's disease**, a degenerative disorder associated with ageing, and parkinsonism due to other causes. For example, it may be induced by the long-term use of *antipsychotic drugs and uncommonly it can be attributed to the late effects of *encephalitis or coal-gas poisoning or to *Wilson's disease. Relief of the symptoms may be obtained with anticholinergic drugs (*see* PARASYMPATHOLYTIC), dopamine-receptor agonists (*see* DOPAMINE), and *levodopa. [J. Parkinson (1755–1824), British physician]

paromomycin *n.* an antibiotic, active against intestinal bacteria and amoebae, used mainly to treat dysentery. It is administered by mouth; side-effects include stomach pains, itching, and heartburn.

paronychia (whitlow) *n.* an inflamed swelling of the *nail folds. **Acute paronychia** is usually caused by infection with *Staphylococcus aureus*. **Chronic paronychia** occurs mainly in those who habitually engage in wet work; it is associated with secondary infection with *Candida albicans*. It is vital to keep the hands dry in order to control chronic paronychia.

paroophoron *n.* the vestigial remains of part of the mesonephric duct (*see* MESONEPHROS) in the female, situated next to each ovary. It is associated with a similar structure, the **epoophoron**. Both are without known function.

parosmia *n.* any disorder of the sense of smell.

parotid gland one of a pair of *salivary glands situated in front of each ear. The openings of the parotid ducts (**Stensen's ducts**) are on the inner sides of the cheeks, opposite the second upper molar teeth.

parotitis *n.* inflammation of the parotid salivary glands. *See* MUMPS (INFECTIOUS PAROTITIS).

parous *adj.* having given birth to one or more children.

paroxetine *n.* an antidepressant drug that acts by prolonging the action of the neurotransmitter serotonin (5-hydroxytryptamine) in the brain (*see* SSRI). It is taken by mouth; side-effects may include dizziness, agitation, tremor, nausea, diarrhoea, and drowsiness. Trade name: **Seroxat**.

paroxysm *n.* **1.** a sudden violent attack, especially a spasm or convulsion. **2.** the abrupt worsening of symptoms or recurrence of disease. —**paroxysmal** *adj.*

parrot disease *see* PSITTACOSIS.

pars *n.* a specific part of an organ or other structure, such as any of parts of the pituitary gland.

Part III accommodation residential accommodation provided by local authorities, under the terms of Part III of the National Assistance Act 1948, for the vulnerable elderly who are in need of care and attention.

parthenogenesis *n.* reproduction in which an organism develops from an unfertilized ovum. It is common in plants and occurs in some lower animals (e.g. aphids).

partially sighted register (in Britain) a list of persons who have poor sight but are not technically blind. In general their sight is adequate to permit the performance of tasks for which some vision is essential. *Compare* BLIND REGISTER.

partogram *n.* a graphic record of the course of labour.

parturition *n.* childbirth. *See* LABOUR.

parvi- *prefix denoting* small size.

PAS *see* PARA-AMINOSALICYLIC ACID.

pascal *n.* the *SI unit of pressure, equal to 1 newton per square metre. Symbol: Pa.

Paschen bodies particles that occur in the cells of skin rashes in patients with *cowpox or *smallpox; they are thought to be the virus particles. [E. Paschen (1860–1936), German pathologist]

passive movement movement not brought about by a patient's own efforts. Passive movements are induced by manipulation of the joints by a physiotherapist. They are useful in maintaining function when a patient has nerve or muscle disorders that prevent voluntary movement.

paste *n.* (in pharmacy) a medicinal preparation of a soft sticky consistency, which is applied externally.

Pasteurella a genus of small rodlike Gram-negative bacteria that are parasites of animals and man. The species *P. multocida* usually infects animals but may be transmitted to man through bites or scratches.

pasteurization *n.* the treatment of milk by heating it to 65°C for 30 minutes, or to 72°C for 15 minutes, followed by rapid cooling, to kill such bacteria as those of tuberculosis and typhoid.

pastille *n.* a medicinal preparation containing gelatine and glycerine, usually coated with sugar, that is dissolved in the mouth so that the medication is applied to the mouth or throat.

Patau syndrome a chromosome disorder in which there are three no. 13 chromosomes (instead of the usual two),

causing mental retardation and defects in the heart, kidney, and scalp. Affected individuals rarely survive. [K. Patau (20th century), US geneticist]

patch test a test to discover which allergen is responsible for contact *dermatitis in a patient. Very low concentrations of common allergens (and any substances suspected of causing the dermatitis in the individual patient) are applied under a patch on the back. The patches are removed after 48 hours and the underlying skin is examined then and again after a further 48 hours. A positive test will show an eczematous reaction. The commonest allergens are nickel in women and chromium in men.

patella *n.* the lens-shaped bone that forms the kneecap. It is situated in front of the knee in the tendon of the quadriceps muscle of the thigh. *See also* SESAMOID BONE.

patellar reflex the knee jerk, in which stretching the muscle at the front of the thigh by tapping its tendon below the knee cap causes a *reflex contraction of the muscle, so that the leg kicks. This is a test of the connection between the sensory nerves attached to stretch receptors in the muscle, the spinal cord, and the motor neurones running from the cord to the thigh muscle, all of which are involved in the reflex. Disease or damage may result in absence of the reflex.

patent ductus arteriosus *see* DUCTUS ARTERIOSUS.

path- (patho-) *prefix denoting* disease. Example: **pathophobia** (morbid fear of).

pathogen *n.* a microorganism, such as a bacterium, that parasitizes an animal (or plant) or man and produces a disease.

pathogenic *adj.* capable of causing disease. The term is applied to a parasitic microorganism (especially a bacterium) in relation to its host. —**pathogenicity** *n.*

pathognomonic *adj.* describing a symptom or sign that is characteristic of or unique to a particular disease. The presence of such a sign or symptom allows positive diagnosis of the disease.

pathological *adj.* relating to or arising from disease.

pathological fracture a fracture through diseased or abnormal bone, usually resulting from a force insufficient to fracture a normal bone. Tumour, infection, congenital bone defects, and osteoporosis are among the causes.

pathology *n.* the study of disease processes with the aim of understanding their nature and causes. This is achieved by observing samples of blood, urine, faeces, and diseased tissue obtained from the living patient or at autopsy, by the use of X-rays, and by many other techniques. (See BIOPSY.) **Clinical pathology** is the application of the knowledge gained to the treatment of patients. —**pathologist** *n.*

-pathy *suffix denoting* **1.** disease. Example: **nephropathy** (of the kidney). **2.** therapy. Example: **osteopathy** (by manipulation).

pauciarthritis *n. see* ARTHRITIS.

pavementation (pavementing) *n.* the sticking of white blood cells to the linings of the finest blood vessels (capillaries) when inflammation occurs.

PCP *Pneumocystis carinii* pneumonia. See PNEUMOCYSTIS.

PCR *see* POLYMERASE CHAIN REACTION.

PDGF *see* GROWTH FACTOR.

peak expiratory flow rate (PEFR) the rate at which a person can expel air from the lungs: a reliable measure of lung reserves in tests of vital capacity.

peau d'orange a dimpled appearance of the skin over a breast tumour, resembling the surface of an orange. The skin is thickened and the openings of hair follicles and sweat glands are enlarged.

pecten *n.* **1.** the middle section of the anal canal, below the anal valves (*see* ANUS). **2.** a sharp ridge on the upper branch of the pubis (part of the hip bone). —**pectineal** *adj.*

pectoral *adj.* relating to the chest.

pectoral girdle *see* SHOULDER GIRDLE.

pectoral muscles the chest muscles (see illustration). The **pectoralis major** is a large fan-shaped muscle that works over the shoulder joint, drawing the arm forward across the chest and rotating it medially. Beneath it, the **pectoralis minor**

depresses the shoulder and draws the scapula down towards the chest.

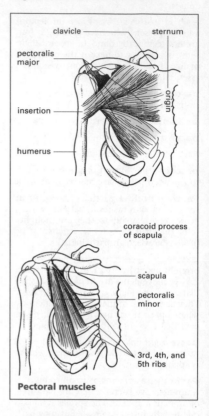

Pectoral muscles

pectoriloquy *n.* abnormal transmission of the patient's voice sounds through the chest wall so that they can be clearly heard through a stethoscope. Whispered sounds (**whispering pectoriloquy**) can be heard over the lung of a patient with pneumonia.

pectus *n.* the chest or breast.

pectus carinatum *see* PIGEON CHEST.

pectus excavatum *see* FUNNEL CHEST.

pedicle *n.* **1.** the narrow neck of tissue connecting some tumours to the normal tissue from which they have developed. **2.** (in plastic surgery) a narrow folded tube of skin by means of which a piece of skin used for grafting remains attached to its original site. A pedicle graft is used when the recipient site is unsuited to take an independent skin graft (for example, because of poor blood supply). *See also* FLAP, SKIN GRAFT. **3.** (in anatomy) any slender stemlike process.

pediculicide *n.* an agent that kills lice; examples include *benzyl benzoate, *carbaryl, *lindane, *malathion, and *permethrin.

Pediculoides (Pyemotes) *n.* a genus of widely distributed tiny predaceous mites. *P. ventricosus* occasionally attacks man and causes an allergic dermatitis called **grain itch**. This complaint most usually affects those people coming into contact with stored cereal products, such as hay and grain.

pediculosis *n.* an infestation with lice, which causes intense itching; continued scratching by the patient may result in secondary bacterial infection of the skin. **Head lice (pediculosis capitis)** are quite common in schoolchildren and do not indicate poor hygiene; they may be treated with *malathion, *carbaryl, or *permethrin lotions. By contrast, **body lice (pediculosis corporis)** affect vagabonds and refugees; help is required from social services. **Pubic lice** (*Phthirus pubis*, the crab louse) are commonly sexually transmitted and respond to the same treatment as head lice.

Pediculus *n.* a widely distributed genus of lice. There are two varieties of the species affecting humans: *P. humanus capitis*, the head louse; and *P. humanus corporis*, the body louse. The presence of these parasites can irritate the skin (*see* PEDICULOSIS), and in some parts of the world body lice are involved in transmitting *relapsing fever and *typhus.

pedometer *n.* a small portable device that records the number of paces walked, and thus the approximate distance covered. A pedometer is usually attached to the leg or hung at the belt.

peduncle *n.* a narrow process or stalk-like structure, serving as a support or a connection. For example, the **middle cer-**

ebellar peduncle connects the pons and cerebellum.

PEFR *see* PEAK EXPIRATORY FLOW RATE.

pellagra *n.* a nutritional disease due to a deficiency of *nicotinic acid (a B vitamin). Pellagra results from the consumption of a diet that is poor in either nicotinic acid or the amino acid tryptophan, from which nicotinic acid can be synthesized in the body. It is common in maize-eating communities. The symptoms of pellagra are scaly dermatitis on exposed surfaces, diarrhoea, and depression.

pellicle *n.* a thin layer of skin, membrane, or any other substance.

pelvic girdle (hip girdle) the bony structure to which the bones of the lower limbs are attached. It consists of the right and left *hip bones.

pelvic inflammatory disease (PID) an acute or chronic condition in which the uterus, Fallopian tubes, and ovaries are infected. The inflammation is the result of infection spreading from an adjacent infected organ (such as the appendix) or ascending from the vagina (as in the case of infection with *Chlamydia trachomatis*); it may also result from a blood-borne infection, such as tuberculosis. The main feature is lower abdominal pain that may, at times, be severe. An acute infection may respond to treatment with antibiotics, but in the chronic state, when pelvic *adhesions have developed, surgical removal of the diseased tissue may be necessary. Blocking of the Fallopian tubes is a common result of pelvic inflammatory disease; this can lead to *ectopic pregnancy or infertility.

pelvimetry *n.* the measurement of the four internal diameters of the pelvis (transverse, anteroposterior, left oblique, and right oblique). Pelvimetry helps in determining whether it will be possible for a fetus to be delivered in the normal way. Sufficient reduction of any one or more diameters may be an indication for Caesarean section.

pelvis *n.* (*pl.* **pelves**) **1.** the bony structure formed by the *hip bones, *sacrum, and *coccyx: the bony pelvis (see illustration). The hip bones are fused at the back to the sacrum to form a rigid structure that protects the organs of the lower abdomen and provides attachment for the bones and muscles of the lower limbs. **2.** the lower part of the abdomen. **3.** the cavity within the bony pelvis. **4.** any structure shaped like a basin, e.g. the expanded part of the ureter in the kidney (**renal pelvis**). —**pelvic** *adj.*

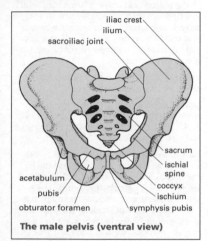

iliac crest
ilium
sacroiliac joint
sacrum
ischial spine
acetabulum
coccyx
pubis
ischium
obturator foramen
symphysis pubis

The male pelvis (ventral view)

pemoline *n.* a weak stimulant of the nervous system used to treat attention deficit disorder in children. It is administered by mouth. Possible side-effects include headache, irritability, dizziness, sweating, palpitations, loss of appetite, weight loss, and dry mouth. Trade name: **Volital**.

pemphigoid (bullous pemphigoid) *n.* a chronic itchy blistering disorder of the elderly. The blisters most commonly occur on the limbs and persist for several days, unlike those of *pemphigus. Pemphigoid is an *autoimmune disease and responds to treatment with corticosteroids or immunosuppressive drugs.

pemphigus (pemphigus vulgaris) *n.* a rare but serious *autoimmune skin disease marked by successive outbreaks of blisters. The blisters are superficial and do not remain intact for long; the mouth and other mucous membranes, as well as the skin, are usually affected. A number of milder variants of the disease exist.

Pena operation a recommended surgical treatment of congenital anal maldevelopment.

Pendred's syndrome goitre associated with congenital deafness due to deficiency of *peroxidase, an enzyme that is essential for the utilization of iodine. [V. Pendred (1869–1946), British physician]

penetrance *n.* the frequency with which the characteristic controlled by a gene is seen in the individuals possessing it. Complete penetrance occurs when the characteristic is seen in all individuals known to possess the gene. If a percentage of individuals with the gene do not show its effects, penetrance is incomplete. In this way a characteristic in a family may appear to 'skip' a generation.

-penia *suffix denoting* lack or deficiency. Example: **neutropenia** (of neutrophils).

penicillamine *n.* a drug that binds metals and therefore aids their excretion (*see* CHELATING AGENT). It is used to treat *Wilson's disease, poisoning by metals such as lead, copper, and mercury, and severe rheumatoid arthritis. It is administered by mouth and commonly causes digestive upsets and allergic reactions. Trade names: **Distamine**, **Pendramine**.

penicillin *n.* an *antibiotic that was derived from the mould *Penicillium rubrum* and first became available for treating bacterial infections in 1941. Since then, a number of naturally occurring penicillins have been developed to treat a wide variety of infections, notably **penicillin G** (**benzylpenicillin**), usually administered by injection but taken orally to treat dental abscesses, and **penicillin V** (**phenoxymethylpenicillin**), which is administered orally. There are few serious side-effects, but some patients are allergic to penicillin and develop such reactions as skin rashes, swelling of the throat, and fever. Similar drugs prepared from *Penicillium* moulds include *benethamine penicillin and *benzathine penicillin. All these penicillins are *beta-lactam antibiotics and are sensitive to penicillinase.

There are many antibiotics that are derived from the penicillins, including *amoxycillin, *ampicillin, *cloxacillin sodium, and *flucloxacillin; these are known as **semisynthetic penicillins**.

penicillinase *n.* an enzyme, produced by some bacteria, that is capable of antagonizing the antibacterial action of penicillin and other *beta-lactam antibiotics. Purified penicillinase may be used to treat reactions to penicillin. It is also used in diagnostic tests to isolate microorganisms from the blood of patients receiving penicillin.

Penicillium *n.* a genus of mouldlike fungi that commonly grow on decaying fruit, bread, or cheese. The species *P. rubrum* is the major natural source of the antibiotic *penicillin. Some species of *Penicillium* are pathogenic to man, causing diseases of the skin and respiratory tract.

penile prosthesis *see* PROSTHESIS.

penis *n.* the male organ that carries the *urethra, through which urine and semen are discharged (see illustration). Urination can occur in the normal hanging position. Most of the organ is composed of erectile tissue (*see* CORPUS CAVERNOSUM, CORPUS SPONGIOSUM), which becomes filled with blood under conditions of sexual excitement so that the penis is erected. In this position it can act as a sexual organ, capable of entering the vagina and ejaculating semen. *See also* GLANS, PREPUCE.

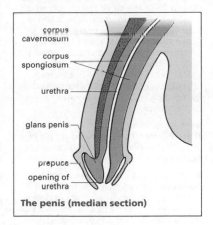

corpus cavernosum

corpus spongiosum

urethra

glans penis

prepuce

opening of urethra

The penis (median section)

pent- (penta-) *prefix denoting* five.

pentaerythritol *n.* a drug that dilates blood vessels and is used in the treatment of angina and other heart conditions. It is administered by mouth and may cause headache and indigestion. Trade name: **Mycardol**.

pentagastrin *n.* a synthetic hormone that has the same effects as *gastrin in stimulating the secretion of gastric juice from the stomach. It is injected to test for gastric secretion in the diagnosis of digestive disorders. Trade name: **Peptavlon**.

pentamidine *n.* a drug effective against protozoans and used in the treatment of *Pneumocystis carinii* pneumonia in AIDS patients, *trypanosomiasis, and *kala-azar. It is administered by injection or from an inhaler. Possible side-effects include low blood pressure, heart irregularity, low blood sugar (hypoglycaemia), low white blood cell count, and kidney damage. Trade names: **Pentam 300, Nebupent**.

pentazocine *n.* a potent *analgesic drug used to relieve moderate or severe pain. It is administered by mouth, injection, or in suppositories; side-effects include dizziness and digestive upsets. Trade name: **Fortral**.

pentose *n.* a simple sugar with five carbon atoms: for example, ribose and xylose.

pentosuria *n.* an inborn defect of sugar metabolism causing abnormal excretion of pentose in the urine. There are no serious ill-effects.

Pentothal *n. see* THIOPENTONE.

pepsin *n.* an enzyme in the stomach that begins the digestion of proteins by splitting them into peptones (*see* PEPTIDASE). It is produced by the action of hydrochloric acid on **pepsinogen**, which is secreted by the gastric glands. Once made, pepsin itself can act on pepsinogen to produce more pepsin.

pepsinogen *n. see* PEPSIN.

peptic *adj.* **1.** relating to pepsin. **2.** relating to digestion.

peptic ulcer a breach in the lining (mucosa) of the digestive tract produced by digestion of the mucosa by pepsin and acid. This may occur when pepsin and acid are present in abnormally high concentrations or when some other mechanism reduces the normal protective mechanisms of the mucosa; bile salts may play a part, especially in stomach ulcers. A peptic ulcer may be found in the oesophagus (**oesophageal ulcer**, which is associated with reflux *oesophagitis); the stomach (*see* GASTRIC ULCER); duodenum (*see* DUODENAL ULCER); jejunum (**jejunal ulcer**, usually in the *Zollinger-Ellison syndrome); in a Meckel's *diverticulum; and close to a *gastroenterostomy (**stomal ulcer, anastomotic ulcer, marginal ulcer**).

peptidase *n.* one of a group of digestive enzymes that split proteins in the stomach and intestine into their constituent amino acids. The group is divided into the *endopeptidases and *exopeptidases.

peptide *n.* a molecule consisting of two or more *amino acids linked by bonds between the amino group (–NH) and the carboxyl group (–CO). This bond is known as a **peptide bond**. *See also* POLYPEPTIDE.

peptone *n.* a large protein fragment produced by the action of enzymes on proteins in the first stages of protein digestion.

peptonuria *n.* the presence in the urine of *peptones, intermediate compounds formed during the digestion of proteins.

perception *n.* (in psychology) the process by which information about the world, as received by the senses, is analysed and made meaningful. Abnormalities of perception include *hallucinations, *illusions, and *agnosia.

percussion *n.* the technique of examining part of the body by tapping it with the fingers or an instrument (**plessor**) and sensing the resultant vibrations. With experience it is possible to detect the presence of abnormal solidification or enlargement in different organs and the presence of fluid, for example in the lungs.

percutaneous *adj.* through the skin: often applied to the route of administration of drugs in ointments, etc., which are absorbed through the skin.

percutaneous epididymal sperm aspiration *see* PESA.

percutaneous nephrolithotomy a technique of removing stones from the kidney via a *nephroscope passed into the kidney through a track from the skin sur-

face previously established by the presence of a catheter.

percutaneous transhepatic cholangiopancreatography (PTC) a method for outlining the bile ducts and pancreatic ducts with radiopaque dyes, which are introduced by a catheter inserted into the ducts from the surface of the skin. *See* CHOLANGIOGRAPHY.

perforation *n.* the creation of a hole in an organ, tissue, or tube. This may occur in the course of a disease (e.g. a *duodenal ulcer, colonic *diverticulitis, or stomach cancer), allowing the contents of the intestine to enter the peritoneal cavity, which causes acute inflammation (*peritonitis) with sudden severe abdominal pain and shock. Treatment is usually by surgical repair of the perforation, but conservative treatment with antibiotics may result in spontaneous healing. Perforation may also be caused accidentally by instruments – for example a gastroscope may perforate the stomach, a curette may perforate the uterus – or by injury, for example to the eardrum.

perfusion *n.* **1.** the passage of fluid through a tissue, especially the passage of blood through the lung tissue to pick up oxygen from the air in the alveoli, which is brought there by *ventilation, and release carbon dioxide. If ventilation is impaired deoxygenated venous blood is returned to the general circulation. If perfusion is impaired insufficient gas exchange takes place. **2.** the deliberate introduction of fluid into a tissue, usually by injection into the blood vessels supplying the tissue.

perfusion scan the demonstration of abnormal structures or blood supply of an organ by the perfusion of radioactive or radiopaque substances.

pergolide *n.* a drug that stimulates *dopamine receptors in the brain and is used in the treatment of *parkinsonism. It is administered by mouth. Possible side-effects include confusion, hallucinations, sleepiness, heart irregularity, nausea, breathing difficulties, and double vision. Trade name: **Celance**.

peri- *prefix denoting* near, around, or enclosing. Examples: **perianal** (around the anus); **pericardial** (around the heart); **peritonsillar** (around a tonsil).

periadenitis n. inflammation of tissues surrounding a gland.

perianal haematoma (external haemorrhoid) a small painful swelling beside the anus, occurring after a bout of straining to pass faeces or coughing. Perianal haematomas are caused by the rupture of a small vein in the anus. They often heal spontaneously but occasionally rupture. Rarely this is followed by abscess formation. If severe pain continues, surgical removal can be undertaken. *See also* HAEMORRHOIDS.

periapical adj. around an apex, particularly the apex of a tooth. The term is applied to bone surrounding the apex and to X-ray views of this area.

periarteritis nodosa *see* POLYARTERITIS NODOSA.

periarthritis n. inflammation of tissues around a joint capsule, including tendons and *bursae. **Chronic periarthritis**, which may be spontaneous or follow injury, is a common cause of pain and stiffness of the shoulder; it usually responds to local steroid injections or physiotherapy.

pericard- (pericardio-) *prefix denoting* the pericardium.

pericardiectomy (pericardectomy) n. surgical removal of the membranous sac surrounding the heart (pericardium). It is used in the treatment of chronic constrictive pericarditis and chronic pericardial effusion (*see* PERICARDITIS).

pericardiocentesis n. removal of excess fluid from within the sac (pericardium) surrounding the heart by means of needle *aspiration. *See* PERICARDITIS, HYDROPERICARDIUM.

pericardiolysis n. the surgical separation of *adhesions between the heart and surrounding structures within the ribcage (**adherent pericardium**). The operation has now fallen into disuse.

pericardiorrhaphy n. the repair of wounds in the membrane surrounding the heart (pericardium), such as those due to injury or surgery.

pericardiostomy n. an operation in which the membranous sac around the heart is opened and the fluid within drained via a tube. It is sometimes used in the treatment of septic pericarditis.

pericardiotomy (pericardotomy) n. surgical opening or puncture of the membranous sac (pericardium) around the heart. It is required to gain access to the heart in heart surgery and to remove excess fluid from within the pericardium.

pericarditis n. acute or chronic inflammation of the membranous sac (pericardium) surrounding the heart. Pericarditis may be seen alone or as part of pancarditis (*see* ENDOMYOCARDITIS). It has numerous causes, including virus infections, uraemia, and cancer. **Acute pericarditis** is characterized by fever, chest pain, and a pericardial friction rub. Fluid may accumulate within the pericardial sac (**pericardial effusion**). Rarely, chronic thickening of the pericardium (**chronic constrictive pericarditis**) develops. This interferes with activity of the heart and has many features in common with *heart failure, including oedema, pleural effusions, ascites, and engorgement of the veins. Constrictive pericarditis most often results from tubercular infection.

The treatment of pericarditis is directed to the cause. Pericardial effusions may be aspirated by a needle inserted through the chest wall. Chronic constrictive pericarditis is treated by surgical removal of the pericardium (**pericardiectomy**).

pericardium n. the membrane surrounding the heart, consisting of two portions. The outer **fibrous pericardium** completely encloses the heart and is attached to the large blood vessels emerging from the heart. The internal **serous pericardium** is a closed sac of *serous membrane: the inner visceral portion (**epicardium**) is closely attached to the muscular heart wall and the outer parietal portion lines the fibrous pericardium. Within the sac is a very small amount of fluid, which prevents friction as the two surfaces slide over one another as the heart beats. —**pericardial** adj.

pericardotomy n. *see* PERICARDIOTOMY.

perichondritis n. inflammation of cartilage and surrounding soft tissues, usually due to chronic infection. A common site is the external ear.

perichondrium *n.* the dense layer of fibrous connective tissue that covers the surface of *cartilage.

pericoronitis *n.* inflammation around the crown of a tooth, particularly a partially erupted third molar.

pericranium *n.* the *periosteum of the skull.

pericystitis *n.* inflammation in the tissues around the bladder, causing pain in the pelvis, fever, and symptoms of *cystitis. It usually results from infection in the Fallopian tubes or uterus, but can occasionally arise from severe infection in a *diverticulum of the bladder itself. Treatment of pericystitis is directed to the underlying cause and usually involves antibiotic therapy. Pericystitis associated with a pelvic abscess clears when the abscess is surgically drained.

periderm *n. see* EPITRICHIUM.

perihepatitis *n.* inflammation of the membrane covering the liver. It is usually associated with abnormalities of the liver (including liver abscess, cirrhosis, tuberculosis) or in chronic peritonitis.

perikaryon *n. see* CELL BODY.

perilymph *n.* the fluid between the bony and membranous *labyrinths of the ear.

perimenopause *n.* the period of time around the *menopause in which marked changes in the menstrual cycle occur, usually accompanied by hot flushes, and in which no 12 consecutive months of amenorrhoea have yet occurred.

perimeter *n.* an instrument for mapping the extent of the *visual field (see illustration). The patient fixes his gaze on a target in the centre of the inner surface of the hemisphere. Objects are presented on this surface and the patient says if he sees them. The area of the visual field can be defined and any gaps in the field can be detected. There are several types of perimeter. In the **static perimeter** the movable object is replaced by a system of tiny lights, set in a black background, that can be flashed briefly. If the patient has a field defect he will fail to see the lights

that flash in the area of the defect. Modern visual field testing uses computer-assisted **automated perimeters** to map out and analyse visual fields and thus detect very subtle field defects (**computerized perimetry**). Automated perimeters are commonly used in the diagnosis and follow-up of glaucoma. —**perimetry** *n.*

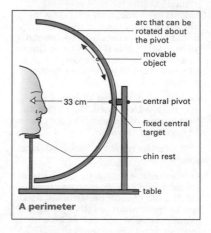

A perimeter

perimetritis *n.* inflammation of the membrane on the outer surface of the uterus. The condition may be associated with *parametritis.

perimetrium *n.* the *peritoneum of the uterus.

perimysium *n.* the fibrous sheath that surrounds each bundle of *muscle fibres.

perinatal *adj.* relating to the period starting a few weeks before birth and including the birth and a few weeks after birth.

perinatal mortality rate *see* INFANT MORTALITY RATE.

perineal descent abnormal bulging down of the *perineum as a result of weakness of the pelvic floor muscles. It often accompanies problems with defecation and micturition.

perineal pouch *see* ILEAL POUCH.

perineoplasty *n.* an operation designed to enlarge the vaginal opening by incising the hymen and part of the perineum (**Fenton's operation**).

perineorrhaphy n. the surgical repair of a damaged perineum. The damage is usually the result of a tear in the perineum sustained during childbirth.

perinephric abscess a collection of pus around the kidney, usually secondary to *pyonephrosis.

perinephritis n. inflammation of the tissues around the kidney. This is usually due to spread of infection from the kidney itself (*see* PYELONEPHRITIS, PYONEPHROSIS). The patient has pain in the loins, fever, and fits of shivering. Prompt treatment of the underlying renal infection is required to prevent progression to an abscess.

perineum n. the region of the body between the anus and the urethral opening, including both skin and underlying muscle. In females it is perforated by the vaginal opening. —**perineal** adj.

perineurium n. the sheath of connective tissue that surrounds individual bundles (fascicles) of nerve fibres within a large *nerve.

periocular adj. adjacent to the eyeball.

periodic acid–Schiff reaction (PAS reaction) a test for the presence of glycoproteins, polysaccharides, certain muco polysaccharides, glycolipids, and certain fatty acids in tissue sections. The tissue is treated with periodic acid, followed by *Schiff's reagent. A positive reaction is the development of a red or magenta coloration.

periodic fever *see* MALARIA.

periodontal adj. denoting or relating to the tissues surrounding the teeth.

periodontal abscess an abscess that arises in the periodontal tissues and is usually an acute manifestation of periodontal disease.

periodontal disease disease of the tissues that support and attach the teeth – the gums, periodontal membrane, and alveolar bone. It is caused by the metabolism of bacterial *plaque on the surfaces of the teeth adjacent to these tissues. Periodontal disease includes *gingivitis

and the more advanced stage of **periodontitis**, which results in the formation of spaces between the gums and the teeth (**periodontal pockets**), the loss of some fibres that attach the tooth to the jaw, and the loss of bone. The disease is widespread and is the most common cause of tooth loss in older people. Poor oral hygiene is a major contributory factor, but the resistance of the patient also has some influence; for example, the reduced resistance of AIDS patients may predispose to periodontal disease.

periodontal membrane (periodontal ligament) the ligament around a *tooth, by which it is attached to the bone.

periodontal pocket a space between the gingival tissues and tooth occurring in periodontitis. See PERIODONTAL DISEASE.

periodontium n. the tissues that support and attach the teeth: the gums (*see* GINGIVA), *periodontal membrane, alveolar bone, and *cementum.

periodontology n. the branch of dentistry concerned with the tissues that support and attach the teeth and the prevention and treatment of *periodontal disease.

periorbital adj. **1.** around the eye socket (*orbit). **2.** relating to the periosteum within the orbit.

periosteum n. a layer of dense connective tissue that covers the surface of a bone except at the articular surfaces. The outer layer of the periosteum is extremely dense and contains a large number of blood vessels. The inner layer is more cellular in appearance and contains osteoblasts and fewer blood vessels. The periosteum provides attachment for muscles, tendons, and ligaments.

periostitis n. inflammation of the membrane surrounding a bone (*see* PERIOSTEUM). **Acute periostitis** results from direct injury to the bone and is associated with a *haematoma, which may later become infected. The uncomplicated condition subsides quickly with rest and anti-inflammatory analgesics. **Chronic periostitis** sometimes follows but is more often due to an inflammatory disease, such as tuberculosis or syphilis, or to a chronic ulcer overlying the bone involved. Chronic peri-ostitis causes thickening of the underlying bone, which is evident on X-ray.

peripheral nervous system all parts of the nervous system lying outside the central nervous system (brain and spinal cord). It includes the *cranial nerves and *spinal nerves and their branches, which link the receptors and effector organs with the brain and spinal cord. *See also* AUTONOMIC NERVOUS SYSTEM.

periphlebitis n. inflammation of the tissues around a vein: seen as an extension of *phlebitis.

perisalpingitis n. inflammation of the peritoneal membrane on the outer surface of a Fallopian tube.

perisplenitis n. inflammation of the external coverings of the spleen.

peristalsis n. a wavelike movement that progresses along some of the hollow tubes of the body. It occurs involuntarily and is characteristic of tubes that possess circular and longitudinal muscles, such as the *intestines. It is induced by distension of the walls of the tube. Immediately behind the distension the circular muscle contracts. In front of the distension the circular muscle relaxes and the longitudinal muscle contracts, which pushes the contents of the tube forward. —**peristaltic** adj.

peritendineum n. the fibrous covering of a tendon.

peritendinitis n. see TENOSYNOVITIS.

peritomy n. an eye operation in which an incision of the conjunctiva is made in a complete circle around the cornea.

peritoneoscope n. see LAPAROSCOPE.

peritoneum n. the *serous membrane of the abdominal cavity (see illustration). The **parietal peritoneum** lines the walls of the abdomen, and the **visceral peritoneum** covers the abdominal organs. *See also* MESENTERY, OMENTUM. —**peritoneal** adj.

peritonitis n. inflammation of the *peritoneum. **Primary peritonitis** is caused by bacteria spread via the bloodstream: examples are **pneumococcal peritonitis** and **tuberculous peritonitis**. Symptoms are diffuse abdominal pain and swelling, with

fever and weight loss. Fluid may accumulate in the peritoneal cavity (*see* ASCITES) or the infection may complicate existing ascites. **Secondary peritonitis** is due to perforation or rupture of an abdominal organ (for example, a duodenal ulcer or the vermiform appendix), allowing access of bacteria and irritant digestive juices to the peritoneum. This produces sudden severe abdominal pain, first at the site of rupture but becoming generalized. Shock develops, and the abdominal wall becomes rigid; X-ray examination may reveal gas within the peritoneal cavity. Treatment is usually by surgical repair of the perforation, but in some cases conservative treatment using antibiotics and intravenous fluid may be used. *Subphrenic abscess is a possible complication. **Meconium peritonitis** occurs in newborn infants as a result of a perforated intestine; it is initially a sterile contamination of the peritoneum.

peritonsillar abscess see QUINSY.

peritrichous adj. describing bacteria in which the flagella cover the entire cell surface.

perityphlitis n. Archaic. inflammation of the tissues around the caecum.

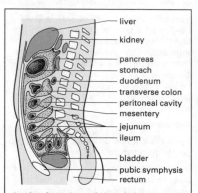

liver
kidney
pancreas
stomach
duodenum
transverse colon
peritoneal cavity
mesentery
jejunum
ileum
bladder
pubic symphysis
rectum

Sagittal section of the abdomen to show arrangement of the peritoneum

periureteritis n. inflammation of the tissues around a ureter. This is usually associated with inflammation of the ureter itself (*ureteritis) often behind an obstruction caused by a stone or stricture. Treatment is directed to relieving any obstruction of the ureter and controlling the infection with antibiotics.

PERLA pupils equal, react to light and accommodation: used in hospital notes.

perle *n.* a soft capsule containing medicine.

perleche *n.* dryness and cracking of the corners of the mouth, sometimes with infection. Perleche may be caused by persistent lip licking or by a vitamin-deficient diet.

permethrin *n.* a synthetic derivative of the naturally occurring insecticide pyrethrin that is applied externally to treat head lice and scabies. Trade name: **Lyclear**.

pernicious *adj.* describing diseases that are highly dangerous or likely to result in death if untreated. *See also* PERNICIOUS ANAEMIA.

pernicious anaemia a form of *anaemia resulting from deficiency of *vitamin B$_{12}$. This in turn results either from failure to produce the substance (*intrinsic factor) that facilitates absorption of B$_{12}$ from the bowel or from dietary deficiency of the vitamin. Pernicious anaemia is characterized by defective production of red blood cells and the presence of *megaloblasts in the bone marrow. In severe forms the nervous system is affected (*see* SUBACUTE COMBINED DEGENERATION OF THE CORD). The condition is treated by injections of vitamin B$_{12}$.

pernio *n.* the medical name for a chilblain (*see* CHILBLAINS).

perniosis *n.* *see* CHILBLAINS.

pero- *prefix denoting* deformity; defect. Example: **peromelia** (of the limbs).

peroneal *adj.* relating to or supplying the outer (fibular) side of the leg.

peroneus *n.* one of the muscles of the leg that arises from the fibula. The **peroneus longus** and **peroneus brevis** are situated at the side of the leg and inserted into the metatarsal bones of the foot. They help to turn the foot outwards.

peroxidase *n.* an enzyme, found mainly in plants but also present in leucocytes and milk, that catalyses the dehydrogenation (oxidation) of various substances in the presence of hydrogen peroxide (which acts as a hydrogen acceptor, being converted to water in the process).

peroxisome *n.* a small structure within a cell that is similar to a *lysosome but contains different enzymes, some of which may take part in reactions involving hydrogen peroxide.

perphenazine *n.* a phenothiazine *antipsychotic drug used to relieve anxiety, tension, and agitation and to prevent nausea and vomiting. It is administered by mouth or injection; side-effects are similar to those of *chlorpromazine. Trade name: **Fentazin**.

perseveration *n.* **1.** excessive persistence at a task that prevents the individual from turning his attention to new situations. It is a symptom of organic disease of the brain and sometimes of obsessional neurosis. **2.** the phenomenon in which an image continues to be perceived briefly in the absence of the object. This is a potentially serious neurological disorder.

persistent vegetative state (PVS) the condition of living like a vegetable, without consciousness or the ability to initiate voluntary action, as a result of brain damage. People in the vegetative state may sometimes give the appearance of being awake and conscious, with open eyes. They may make random movements of the limbs or head and may pick or rub with the fingers, but there is no response to any form of communication and no reason to suppose that there is any awareness of the environment.

The vegetative state must be distinguished from apparently similar conditions, such as the psychiatric state of *catatonia, in which consciousness is retained and from which full recovery is possible, and the **locked-in syndrome**, resulting from damage to the brainstem, in which the patient is conscious but unable to speak or make any movement of any part of the body, except for blinking and upward eye movements, which permit signalling.

personality *n.* (in psychology) an enduring disposition to act and feel in particular ways that differentiate one individual from another. These patterns of behaviour are sometimes conceptualized as different categories (see PERSONALITY DISORDER) and sometimes as different dimensions (see EXTROVERSION, NEUROTICISM).

personality disorder a deeply ingrained and maladaptive pattern of behaviour, persisting through many years. It is usually manifest by the time the individual is adolescent. The abnormality of behaviour must be sufficiently severe that it causes suffering, either to the patient or to other people (or to both). Some individuals with such personalities mature into happier people. Most forms of psychotherapy claim to be of therapeutic value, but the worth of any treatment remains debatable. See ANANKASTIC, AVOIDANT, BORDERLINE, DYSSOCIAL, HYSTERICAL, PARANOID, SCHIZOID.

perspiration *n.* *sweat or the process of sweating. **Insensible perspiration** is sweat that evaporates immediately from the skin and is therefore not visible; **sensible perspiration** is visible on the skin in the form of drops.

Perthes' disease *see* LEGG-CALVÉ-PERTHES DISEASE.

pertussis *n. see* WHOOPING COUGH.

pes *n.* (in anatomy) the foot or a part resembling a foot.

PESA (percutaneous epididymal sperm aspiration) a method of removing spermatozoa directly from the *epididymis, a new technique used in assisted conception. The sperm are then used to fertilize egg cells in vitro.

pes cavus *see* CLAW-FOOT.

pes planus *see* FLAT-FOOT.

pessary *n.* **1.** a plastic device, often ring-shaped, that fits into the vagina and keeps the uterus in position: used to treat *prolapse. The usual type is a **ring pessary** but occasionally a **Hodge pessary** is used. **2.** (or **vaginal suppository**) a plug or cylinder of cocoa butter or some other soft material containing a drug that is fitted into the vagina for the treatment of gynaecological disorders (e.g. vaginitis) or for the induction of labour (a **Prostin pessary** containing prostaglandin).

pesticide *n.* a chemical agent used to kill insects or other organisms harmful to crops and other cultivated plants. Some pesticides, such as *parathion and *dieldrin, have caused poisoning in human beings and livestock after accidental exposure.

petechiae *pl. n.* small round flat dark-red spots caused by bleeding into the skin or beneath the mucous membrane. Petechiae occur, for example, in the *purpuras.

pethidine (meperidine) *n.* a potent *analgesic drug with mild sedative action, used to relieve moderate or severe pain. It is administered by mouth or injection; side-effects may include nausea, dizziness, and dry mouth, and *dependence may occur with prolonged use.

petit mal *see* EPILEPSY.

Petri dish a flat shallow circular glass or plastic dish with a pillbox-like lid, used to hold solid agar or gelatin media for culturing bacteria. [J. R. Petri (1852–1921), German bacteriologist]

petrissage *n.* kneading: a form of *massage in which the skin is lifted up, pressed down and squeezed, and pinched and rolled. Alternate squeezing and relaxation of the tissues stimulates the local circulation and may have a pain-relieving effect in muscular disorders.

petrositis *n.* inflammation of the petrous part of the *temporal bone (which encloses the inner ear), usually due to an extension of *mastoiditis.

petrous bone *see* TEMPORAL BONE.

Peutz-Jeghers syndrome a hereditary disorder in which the presence of multiple *polyps in the lining of the small intestine (intestinal *polyposis) is associated with pigmented areas (similar to freckles) around the lips, on the inside of the mouth, and on the palms and soles. The polyps may bleed, resulting in anaemia, or may cause obstruction of the bowel. [J. L. A. Peutz (1886–1957), Dutch physician; H. J. Jeghers (1904–   ), US physician]

-pexy *suffix denoting* surgical fixation. Example: **omentopexy** (of the omentum).

Peyer's patches oval masses of *lymphoid tissue on the mucous membrane lining the small intestine. [J. C. Peyer (1653–1712), Swiss anatomist]

Peyronie's disease a dense fibrous plaque in the penis, which can be felt in the erectile tissue as an irregular hard lump. The penis curves or angulates at this point on erection and pain often results. The cause is unknown. The penis can be straightened surgically by means of *Nesbit's operation. [F. de la Peyronie (1678–1747), French surgeon]

pH a measure of the concentration of hydrogen ions in a solution, and therefore of its acidity or alkalinity. A pH of 7 indicates a neutral solution, a pH below 7 indicates acidity, and a pH in excess of 7 indicates alkalinity.

PHA *n. see* PHYTOHAEMAGGLUTININ.

phaco- (phako-) *prefix denoting* the lens of the eye.

phacoemulsification (phako-emulsification) *n.* the use of a high-frequency *ultrasound probe to break up a cataract so that it can be removed through a very small incision. This is now a popular method of performing cataract surgery.

phaeochromocytoma *n.* a small vascular tumour of the inner region (medulla) of the adrenal gland. By its uncontrolled and irregular secretion of the hormones *adrenaline and *noradrenaline, the tumour causes attacks of raised blood pressure, increased heart rate, palpitations, and headache. *See also* DEXAMETHASONE.

phag- (phago-) *prefix denoting* **1.** eating. **2.** phagocytes.

phage *n. see* BACTERIOPHAGE.

-phagia *suffix denoting* a condition involving eating.

phagocyte *n.* a cell that is able to engulf and digest bacteria, protozoa, cells and cell debris, and other small particles. Phagocytes include many white blood cells (*see* LEUCOCYTE) and *macrophages, which play a major role in the body's defence mechanism. —**phagocytic** *adj.*

phagocytosis *n.* the engulfment and digestion of bacteria and other foreign particles by a cell (*see* PHAGOCYTE). *Compare* PINOCYTOSIS.

phako- *prefix. see* PHACO-.

phalangeal cells rows of supporting cells between the sensory hair cells of the organ of Corti (*see* COCHLEA).

phalangectomy *n.* surgical removal of one or more of the small bones (phalanges) in the fingers or toes.

phalanges *n.* (*sing.* **phalanx**) the bones of the fingers and toes (digits). The first digit (thumb/big toe) has two phalanges. Each of the remaining digits has three phalanges. —**phalangeal** *adj.*

phalangitis *n.* inflammation of a finger or toe, causing swelling and pain. The condition may be caused by infection of the soft tissues, tendon sheaths, bone, or joints or by some rheumatic diseases, such as *psoriatic arthritis. *See also* DACTYLITIS.

phalanx *n. see* PHALANGES.

phalloplasty *n.* surgical reconstruction or repair of the penis. It is required for congenital deformity of the penis, as in *hypospadias or *epispadias, and sometimes also following injury to the penis with loss of skin.

phallus *n.* the embryonic penis, before the urethral duct has reached its final state of development.

phanero- *prefix denoting* visible; apparent.

phaneromania *n.* an excessively strong impulse to touch or rub parts of one's own body.

phantom limb the sensation that an arm or leg, or part of an arm or leg, is still attached to the body after it has been amputated. Pain may seem to come from the amputated part. This may arise because of stimulation of the amputation stump, which contains severed nerves that formerly carried messages from the removed portion.

phantom pregnancy *see* PSEUDOCYESIS.

phantom tumour a swelling, in the abdomen or elsewhere, caused by local muscular contraction or the accumulation of gases, that mimics a swelling caused by a tumour or other structural change. The condition is usually associated with emotional disorder, and the 'tumour' may disappear under anaesthesia.

pharmaceutical *adj.* relating to pharmacy.

pharmacist *n.* a person who is qualified by examination and registered and authorized to dispense medicines or to keep open a shop for the sale and dispensing of medicines.

pharmaco- *prefix denoting* drugs. Example: **pharmacophobia** (morbid fear of).

pharmacodynamics *n.* the interaction of drugs with cells. It includes such factors as the binding of drugs to cells, their uptake, and intracellular metabolism.

pharmacognosy *n.* the knowledge or study of pharmacologically active principles derived from plants.

pharmacokinetics *n.* the handling of a drug within the body, which includes its absorption, distribution in the body, metabolism, and excretion.

pharmacology *n.* the science of the properties of drugs and their effects on the body. —**pharmacological** *adj.*

pharmacomania *n.* an abnormal desire for taking medicines.

pharmacopoeia *n.* a book containing a list of the drugs used in medicine, with details of their formulae, methods of preparation, dosages, standards of purity, etc.

pharmacy *n.* **1.** the preparation and dispensing of drugs. **2.** premises registered to dispense medicines and sell poisons.

pharyng- (pharyngo-) *prefix denoting* the pharynx. Example: **pharyngopathy** (disease of).

pharyngeal arch (branchial or **visceral arch)** any of the paired segmented ridges of tissue in each side of the throat of the early embryo that correspond to the gill arches of fish. Each arch contains a cartilage, a cranial nerve, and a blood vessel. Between each arch there is a *pharyngeal pouch.

pharyngeal cleft (branchial or **visceral cleft)** any of the paired segmented clefts in each side of the throat of the

early embryo that correspond to the gills of fish. Soon after they have formed they close to form the *pharyngeal pouches, except for the first cleft, which persists as the external auditory meatus.

pharyngeal pouch (branchial or **visceral pouch)** any of the paired segmented pouches in the side of the throat of the early embryo. They give rise to the tympanic cavity, the parathyroid glands, the thymus, and probably the thyroid gland.

pharyngectomy *n.* surgical removal of part of the pharynx.

pharyngitis *n.* inflammation of the part of the throat behind the soft palate (pharynx). It produces *sore throat and may be associated with *tonsillitis.

pharyngocele *n.* a pouch or cyst opening off the pharynx (*see* BRANCHIAL CYST).

pharyngoplegia *n.* muscular paralysis of the pharynx.

pharyngoscope *n.* an *endoscope for the examination of the pharynx.

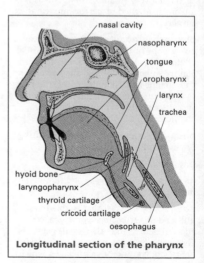

nasal cavity
nasopharynx
tongue
oropharynx
larynx
trachea
hyoid bone
laryngopharynx
thyroid cartilage
cricoid cartilage
oesophagus

Longitudinal section of the pharynx

pharynx *n.* a muscular tube, lined with mucous membrane, that extends from the beginning of the oesophagus (gullet) up to the base of the skull. It is divided into the *nasopharynx, *oropharynx, and *laryngopharynx (see illustration) and it communicates with the posterior *nares, *Eustachian tube, the mouth, larynx, and oesophagus. The pharynx acts as a passageway for food from the mouth to the oesophagus, and as an air passage from the nasal cavity and mouth to the larynx. It also acts as a resonating chamber for the sounds produced in the larynx. —**pharyngeal** *adj.*

phenazocine *n.* an *analgesic drug used for rapid relief of moderate or severe pain. It is administered by mouth or injection; side-effects may include digestive upsets and dizziness, and prolonged use may lead to *dependence. Trade name: **Narphen**.

phenazopyridine *n.* an *analgesic drug used to relieve pain in inflammatory conditions of the bladder and urinary tract, such as cystitis and urethritis. It is administered by mouth and occasionally causes digestive upsets; in patients with *glucose-6-phosphate dehydrogenase deficiency it may damage the red blood cells. Trade name: **Pyridium**.

phenelzine *n.* a drug used to relieve depression and anxiety (*see* MAO INHIBITOR). It is administered by mouth; side-effects include dizziness, drowsiness, tiredness, and digestive upsets. Trade name: **Nardil**.

phenindione *n.* an *anticoagulant drug used to treat thrombosis in the blood vessels of the heart and limbs. It is administered by mouth or injection; side-effects may include skin rashes, fever, and diarrhoea. Trade name: **Dindevan**.

pheniramine *n.* an *antihistamine used to treat allergic reactions such as hay fever and urticaria. It is administered by mouth or is applied to the skin in an ointment; side-effects may include drowsiness, digestive upsets, and skin reactions. Trade name: **Daneral**.

phenobarbitone *n.* a *barbiturate drug used to treat insomnia and anxiety and as an anticonvulsant in the treatment of epilepsy. It is administered by mouth or injection; side-effects may include drowsiness and skin sensitivity reactions, and dependence may result from continued use.

phenol (carbolic acid) *n.* a strong *disinfectant used for cleansing wounds, treating inflammations of the mouth, throat, and ear, and as a preservative in injections. It is administered as solution, ointments, and lotions and is highly toxic if taken by mouth.

phenolphthalein *n.* an irritant *laxative administered by mouth, usually given at night to act the following morning. Side-effects may include stomach cramps.

phenolsulphonphthalein *n.* a red dye administered by injection in a test for kidney function.

phenothiazines *pl. n.* a group of chemically related compounds with various pharmacological actions. Some (e.g. *chlorpromazine and *trifluoperazine) are *antipsychotic drugs; others (e.g. *piperazine) are anthelmintics.

phenotype *n.* **1.** the observable characteristics of an individual, which result from interaction between the genes he possesses (*genotype) and the environment. **2.** the expression in a person or on a cell of characteristics determined by genes that are not fully defined.

phenoxybenzamine *n.* a drug that dilates blood vessels (*see* ALPHA BLOCKER). It is used to reduce blood pressure and to treat conditions involving poor circulation, such as Raynaud's disease and chilblains. It is administered by mouth or injection and may cause dizziness and fast heartbeat. Trade name: **Dibenyline**.

phenoxymethylpenicillin (penicillin V) *n.* *see* PENICILLIN.

phensuximide *n.* an *anticonvulsant drug used to prevent or reduce absence seizures in epilepsy. It is administered by mouth; side-effects may include dizziness, drowsiness, nausea, and loss of appetite.

phentermine *n.* a *sympathomimetic drug that suppresses the appetite and is used in the treatment of obesity. It is administered by mouth; side-effects include dry mouth, nausea, and restlessness, and continued use produces *tolerance. Trade names: **Duromine, Ionamin**.

phentolamine *n.* a drug that dilates blood vessels (*see* ALPHA BLOCKER) and is used to reduce blood pressure in *phaeochromocytoma and to treat conditions of poor circulation such as Raynaud's disease and chilblains. It is administered by mouth or injection; side-effects include fast heartbeat and digestive upsets. Trade name: **Rogitine**.

phenylalanine *n.* an *essential amino acid that is readily converted to tyrosine. Blockade of this metabolic pathway gives rise to *phenylketonuria, which is associated with abnormally large amounts of phenylalanine and phenylpyruvic acid in the blood and retarded mental development.

phenylbutazone *n.* an *analgesic drug that reduces fever and inflammation and is used to relieve pain in rheumatic and related diseases. It is administered by mouth or injection; because of its adverse effect on the blood-forming tissues, its use has been restricted since 1984. Trade name: **Butazolidin**.

phenylephrine *n.* a drug that constricts blood vessels (*see* SYMPATHOMIMETIC). It is given by injection to increase blood pressure, in a nasal spray to relieve nasal congestion, and in eye drops to dilate the pupils. Irritation may occur when applied. Trade name: **Minims phenylephrine**.

phenylketonuria *n.* an inherited defect of protein metabolism (*see* INBORN ERROR OF METABOLISM) causing an excess of the amino acid phenylalanine in the blood, which damages the nervous system and leads to severe mental retardation. Screening of newborn infants by testing a blood sample for phenylalanine (*see* GUTHRIE TEST) enables the condition to be detected soon enough for dietary treatment to prevent any brain damage: the baby's diet contains proteins from which phenylalanine has been removed. The gene responsible for phenylketonuria is recessive, so that a child is affected only if both parents are carriers of the defective gene.

phenylpropanolamine *n.* a drug with actions similar to those of *ephedrine. It is used to relieve allergic conditions, such as asthma and hay fever, and nasal congestion, and is administered by mouth, injection, or by inhalation. Side-effects may include dizziness, headache, digestive disorders, sweating, and thirst.

phenylthiocarbamide (PTC) *n.* a sub-

stance that tastes bitter to some individuals but is tasteless to others. Response to PTC appears to be controlled by a single pair of genes (*alleles): ability to taste PTC is *dominant to the inability to taste it.

phenytoin *n.* an *anticonvulsant drug used to control major and focal epileptic seizures. It is administered by mouth or injection; the side-effects include gum hypertrophy, hirsutism, and skin rashes. Overdosage causes unsteadiness. Trade name: **Epanutin**.

phial *n.* a small glass bottle for storing medicines or poisons.

-philia *suffix denoting* morbid craving or attraction. Example: **nyctophilia** (for darkness).

phimosis *n.* narrowing of the opening of the foreskin, which cannot therefore be drawn back over the underlying glans penis. This predisposes to inflammation (*see* BALANITIS, BALANOPOSTHITIS), which results in further narrowing. Treatment is by surgical removal of the foreskin (*circumcision).

phleb- (phlebo-) *prefix denoting* a vein or veins. Example: **phlebectopia** (abnormal position of).

phlebectomy *n.* the surgical removal of a vein (or part of a vein), sometimes performed for the treatment of varicose veins in the legs (**varicectomy**).

phlebitis *n.* inflammation of the wall of a vein, which is most commonly seen in the legs as a complication of *varicose veins. A segment of vein becomes painful and tender and the surrounding skin feels hot and appears red. Thrombosis commonly develops (*see* THROMBOPHLEBITIS). Treatment consists of elastic support together with drugs, such as phenylbutazone, to relieve the inflammation and pain. Anticoagulants are not used (*compare* PHLEBOTHROMBOSIS). Phlebitis may also complicate sepsis (*see* PYLEPHLEBITIS) or cancer, especially of the stomach, bronchus, or pancreas. In pancreatic cancer the phlebitis may affect a variety of veins (**thrombophlebitis migrans**).

phlebography *n. see* VENOGRAPHY.

phlebolith *n.* a stone-like structure, usually found incidentally on abdominal X-ray, that results from deposition of calcium in a venous blood clot. It appears as a small round white opacity in the pelvic region. It does not produce symptoms and requires no treatment.

phlebosclerosis (venosclerosis) n. a rare degenerative condition, of unknown cause, that affects the leg veins of young men. The vein walls become thickened and feel like cords under the skin. It is not related to arteriosclerosis and needs no treatment.

phlebothrombosis n. obstruction of a vein by a blood clot, without preceding inflammation of its wall. It is most common within the deep veins of the calf of the leg – **deep vein thrombosis (DVT)** – in contrast to *thrombophlebitis, which affects superficial leg veins. Prolonged bed rest, heart failure, pregnancy, injury, and surgery predispose to thrombosis by encouraging sluggish blood flow. Many of these conditions are associated with changes in the clotting factors in the blood that increase the tendency to thrombosis; these changes also occur in some women taking oral contraceptives.

The affected leg may become swollen and tender. The main danger is that the clot may become detached and give rise to *pulmonary embolism. Regular leg exercises help to prevent deep vein thrombosis, and anticoagulant drugs (such as heparin and warfarin) are used in prevention and treatment. Large clots may be removed surgically in the operation of **thrombectomy** to relieve leg swelling.

Phlebotomus n. see SANDFLY.

phlebotomy (venesection) n. the surgical opening or puncture of a vein in order to remove blood (in the treatment of *polycythaemia) or to infuse fluids, blood, or drugs in the treatment of many conditions. It may also be required for cardiac *catheterization and *angiocardiography.

phlegm n. a nonmedical term for *sputum.

phlegmasia alba dolens see THROMBOPHLEBITIS.

phlegmon n. Archaic. inflammation of connective tissue, leading to ulceration.

phlycten n. a small pinkish-yellow nodule surrounded by a zone of dilated blood vessels that occurs in the conjunctiva or in the cornea. It develops into a small ulcer that heals without trace in the conjunctiva but produces some residual scarring in the cornea. Phlyctens, which are prone to recur, are thought to be due to a type of allergy to certain bacteria.

phobia n. a pathologically strong *fear of a particular event or thing. Avoiding the feared situation may severely restrict one's life and cause much suffering. The main kinds of phobia are **specific phobias** (isolated fears of particular things, such as sharp knives), *agoraphobia, *claustrophobia, **social phobias** of encountering people, and **animal phobias**, as of spiders, rats, or dogs (see also PREPAREDNESS). Treatment is with behaviour therapy, especially *desensitization, *graded self-exposure, and *flooding. *Psychotherapy and drug therapy are also useful.

-phobia suffix denoting morbid fear or dread.

phocomelia n. congenital absence of the upper arm and/or upper leg, the hands or feet or both being attached to the trunk by a short stump. The condition is extremely rare except as a side-effect of the drug *thalidomide taken during early pregnancy.

pholcodine n. a drug that suppresses coughs and reduces irritation in the respiratory system (see ANTITUSSIVE). It is administered by mouth in cough mixtures and sometimes causes nausea and drowsiness. Trade names: **Galenphol**, **Pholcomed**.

phon n. a unit of loudness of sound. The intensity of a sound to be measured is compared by the human ear to a reference tone of 2×10^{-5} pascal sound pressure and 1000 hertz frequency. The intensity of the reference tone is increased until it appears to be equal in loudness to the sound being measured; the loudness of this sound in phons is then equal to the number of decibels by which the reference tone has had to be increased.

phon- (phono-) prefix denoting sound or voice.

phonasthenia n. weakness of the voice, especially when due to fatigue.

phonation *n.* the production of vocal sounds, particularly speech.

phoniatrics *n.* the study of the voice and its disorders.

phonocardiogram *n.* *see* ELECTROCARDIOPHONOGRAPHY. —**phonocardiography** *n.*

phonosurgery *n.* surgery performed on the larynx externally or endoscopically to improve or modify the quality of the voice.

-phoria *suffix denoting* (in ophthalmology) an abnormal deviation of the eyes or turning of the visual axis. Example: **heterophoria** (tendency to squint).

Phormia *n.* a genus of non-bloodsucking flies, commonly known as blowflies. The maggot of *P. regina* normally breeds in decaying meat but it has occasionally been found in suppurating wounds, giving rise to a type of *myiasis.

phosgene *n.* a poisonous gas developed during World War I. It is a choking agent, acting on the lungs to produce *oedema, with consequent respiratory and cardiac failure.

phosphagen *n.* creatine phosphate (*see* CREATINE).

phosphataemia *n.* the presence of phosphates in the blood. Sodium, calcium, potassium, and magnesium phosphates are normal constituents.

phosphatase *n.* one of a group of enzymes capable of catalysing the hydrolysis of phosphoric acid esters. An example is glucose-6-phosphatase, which catalyses the hydrolysis of glucose-6-phosphate to glucose and phosphate. Phosphatases are important in the absorption and metabolism of carbohydrates, nucleotides, and phospholipids and are essential in the calcification of bone. **Acid phosphatase** is present in kidney, semen, serum, and the prostate gland. **Alkaline phosphatase** occurs in teeth, developing bone, plasma, kidney, and intestine.

phosphatidylcholine *n.* *see* LECITHIN.

phosphatidylserine *n.* a cephalin-like phospholipid containing the amino acid serine. It is found in brain tissue. *See also* CEPHALIN.

phosphaturia (phosphuria) *n.* the presence of an abnormally high concentration of phosphates in the urine, making it cloudy. The condition may be associated with the formation of stones (calculi) in the kidneys or bladder.

phosphocreatine *n.* creatine phosphate (*see* CREATINE).

phosphofructokinase *n.* an enzyme that catalyses the conversion of fructose-6-phosphate to fructose-1,6-diphosphate. This is an important reaction occurring during the process of *glycolysis.

phospholipid *n.* a *lipid containing a phosphate group as part of the molecule. Phospholipids are constituents of all tissues and organs, especially the brain. They are synthesized in the liver and small intestine and are involved in many of the body's metabolic processes. Examples of phospholipids are *cephalins, *lecithins, plasmalogens, and phosphatidylserine.

phosphonecrosis *n.* the destruction of tissues caused by excessive amounts of phosphorus in the system. The tissues likely to suffer in phosphorus poisoning are the liver, kidneys, muscles, bones, and the cardiovascular system.

phosphorus *n.* a nonmetallic element. Phosphorus compounds are major constituents in the tissues of both plants and animals. In man, phosphorus is mostly concentrated in *bone. However, certain phosphorus-containing compounds – for example adenosine triphosphate (*ATP) and *creatine phosphate – play an important part in energy conversions and storage in the body. In a pure state, phosphorus is toxic. Symbol: P.

phosphorylase *n.* any enzyme that catalyses the combination of an organic molecule (usually glucose) with a phosphate group (phosphorylation). Phosphorylase is found in the liver and kidney, where it is involved in the breakdown of glycogen to glucose-1-phosphate.

phot- (photo-) *prefix denoting* light.

photalgia *n.* pain in the eye caused by very bright light.

photoablation *n.* the use of light or lasers to destroy tissue.

photochemotherapy n. see PUVA.

photocoagulation n. the destruction of tissue by heat released from the absorption of light shone on it. In eye disorders the technique is used to destroy diseased retinal tissue, occurring, for example, as a complication of diabetes (diabetic *retinopathy) and *macular degeneration; and to produce scarring between the retina and choroid, thus binding them together, in cases of *retinal detachment. Photocoagulation of the retina is usually done with an *argon or *diode laser.

Photocoagulation is also a method of arresting bleeding by causing coagulation, usually using an infrared light source.

photodermatosis n. any of various skin diseases caused by exposure to light of varying wavelength (see PHOTOSENSITIVITY). The facial prominences and the 'V' of the neck are most commonly affected, the shadow areas behind the ears and below the chin being protected. A common photodermatosis is **polymorphic light eruption**, which affects 10% of the population. It appears with the first sunshine of spring and abates by late summer. The photodermatoses include certain *porphyrias, notably porphyria cutanea tarda. Photosensitivity reactions may also occur in those taking such drugs as tetracyclines, phenothiazines, frusemide, and NSAIDs.

photomicrograph n. an enlarged photographic record of an object taken through an optical or electron microscope. Compare MICROPHOTOGRAPH.

photomultiplier tube an electronic device that magnifies the light emitted from a *scintillator by accelerating electrons in a high-voltage field. The resulting signal can be used to display the scintillations on a TV screen. Such devices are commonly used in X ray *image intensifiers and *gamma cameras.

photophobia n. an abnormal intolerance of light, in which exposure to light produces intense discomfort of the eyes with tight contraction of the eyelids and other reactions aimed at avoiding the light. In most cases the light simply aggravates already existing discomfort from eye disease. Photophobia may be associated with dilation of the pupils as a result of

eye drops or with migraine, measles, German measles, or meningitis.

photophthalmia n. inflammation of the eye due to exposure to light. It is usually caused by the damaging effect of ultraviolet light on the cornea, for example in snow blindness.

photopic adj. relating to or describing conditions of bright illumination. For example, **photopic vision** is vision in bright light, in which the *cones of the retina are responsible for visual sensation. —**photopia** n.

photopsia n. the sensation of flashes of light caused by mechanical stimulation of the retina of the eye, usually due to traction by the attached vitreous humour when the eye is moved.

photoradiation n. a recently developed technique for the location and destruction of certain tumours that relies on the reaction to light of a substance that is derived from *haematoporphyrin (**haematoporphyrin derivative; HPD**). Injected into the body, HPD concentrates in tumour cells and glows when subjected to ultraviolet irradiation, thus allowing the tumour to be located. The tumour is then irradiated with red light, which breaks down HPD to release highly active oxygen that destroys the tumour cells without damaging surrounding normal tissue.

photoretinitis n. damage to the retina of the eye caused by looking at the sun without adequate protection for the eyes. The retina may be burnt by the intense light focused on it; this affects the central part of the visual field, which may be permanently lost (**sun blindness**).

photosensitivity n. abnormal reaction of the skin to sunlight. —**photosensitive** adj.

photosynthesis n. the process whereby green plants and some bacteria manufacture carbohydrates from carbon dioxide and water, using energy absorbed from sunlight by the green pigment chlorophyll. In green plants this complex process may be summarized thus:

$$6CO_2 + 6H_2O \rightarrow C_6H_{12}O_6 + 6O_2$$

phototaxis n. movement of a cell or organism in response to a stimulus of light.

photuria *n.* the excretion of phosphorescent urine, which glows in the dark, due to the presence of certain phosphorus-containing compounds derived from phosphates.

phren- (phreno-) *prefix denoting* **1.** the mind or brain. **2.** the diaphragm. **3.** the phrenic nerve.

-phrenia *suffix denoting* a condition of the mind. Example: **hebephrenia** (schizophrenia affecting young adults).

phrenic avulsion the surgical removal of a section of the *phrenic nerve, which paralyses the diaphragm. The procedure was used as a means of resting a lung infected with tuberculosis but is now obsolete.

phrenic crush surgical crushing of a portion of the *phrenic nerve. This paralyses the diaphragm on the side operated upon, which is then pushed upwards by the abdominal contents, thus pressing on the lung and partially collapsing it. This operation was formerly often combined with *pneumoperitoneum in the treatment of pulmonary tuberculosis but is now obsolete.

phrenic nerve the nerve that supplies the muscles of the diaphragm. On each side it arises in the neck from the third, fourth, and fifth cervical spinal roots and passes downwards between the lungs and the heart to reach the diaphragm. Impulses through the nerves from the brain bring about the regular contractions of the diaphragm during breathing.

phrenology *n.* the study of the bumps on the outside of the skull in order to determine a person's character. It is based on the mistaken theory that the skull becomes modified over the different functional areas of the cortex of the brain.

Phrygian cap the normal radiological appearance of the tip of the gall bladder, seen in a minority of cholecystograms (*see* CHOLECYSTOGRAPHY). Its name is derived from its resemblance to the characteristic Balkan headgear.

Phthirus *n.* a widely distributed genus of lice. The crab (or pubic) louse, *P. pubis*, is a common parasite of man that lives permanently attached to the body hair, particularly that of the pubic or perianal regions but also on the eyelashes and the hairs in the armpits. Crab lice are not known to transmit disease but their bites can irritate the skin (*see* PEDICULOSIS). An infestation may be acquired during sexual intercourse or from hairs left on clothing, towels, and lavatory seats.

phthisis *n.* **1.** any disease resulting in wasting of tissues. **Phthisis bulbi** is a shrunken eyeball that has lost its function due to disease or damage. **2.** a former name for pulmonary *tuberculosis.

phycomycosis *n.* a disease caused by parasitic fungi of the genera *Rhizopus*, *Absidia*, and *Mucor*. The disease affects the sinuses, the central nervous system, the lungs, and the skin tissues. The fungi are able to grow within the blood vessels of the lungs and nervous tissue, thus causing blood clots which cut off the blood supply (*see* INFARCTION). Treatment with the antibiotic *amphotericin B has proved effective.

phylogenesis *n.* the evolutionary history of a species or individual.

physi- (physio-) *prefix denoting* **1.** physiology. **2.** physical.

physical *adj.* (in medicine) relating to the body rather than to the mind. For example, a **physical sign** is one that a doctor can detect when examining a patient, such as abnormal dilation of the pupils or the absence of a knee-jerk reflex (*see also* FUNCTIONAL DISORDER, ORGANIC DISORDER).

physical medicine a medical specialty established by the Royal Society of Medicine in 1931. Initially the members pioneered clinics devoted to the diagnosis and management of rheumatic diseases, but later extended their interests to the *rehabilitation of patients with physical disabilities ranging from asthma and hand injuries to back trouble and poliomyelitis. The term has caused confusion in recent years, with many doctors preferring the description **rheumatology and rehabilitation** for this specialist activity. Since 1972, however, when the Royal College of Physicians approved it, physical medicine has become the generally accepted term. *See also* RHEUMATOLOGY.

physician *n.* a registered medical practitioner who specializes in the diagnosis and treatment of disease by other than surgical means. In the USA the term is applied to any authorized medical practitioner. *See also* DOCTOR.

physiological solution one of a group of solutions used to maintain tissues in a viable state. These solutions contain specific concentrations of substances that are vital for normal tissue function (e.g. sodium, potassium, calcium, chloride, magnesium, bicarbonate, and phosphate ions, glucose, and oxygen). An example of such a solution is *Ringer's solution.

physiology *n.* the science of the functioning of living organisms and of their component parts. —**physiological** *adj.* —**physiologist** *n.*

physiotherapy *n.* the branch of treatment that employs physical methods to promote healing, including the use of light, infrared and ultraviolet rays, heat, electric current, massage, manipulation, and remedial exercise.

physo- *prefix denoting* air or gas.

physostigmine (eserine) *n.* a *parasympathomimetic drug used mainly to constrict the pupil of the eye and to reduce pressure inside the eye in glaucoma. It is administered by injection, in eye drops, or in an ointment; side-effects include digestive upsets and salivation.

phyt- (phyto-) *prefix denoting* plants; of plant origin.

phytohaemagglutinin (PHA) *n.* a plant-derived alkaloid that stimulates T-lymphocytes to divide in the test tube.

phytomenadione *n.* a form of *vitamin K occurring naturally in green plants but usually synthesized for use as an antidote to overdosage with anticoagulant drugs. It promotes the production of prothrombin, essential for the normal coagulation of blood. Trade name: **Konakion**.

phytophotodermatitis *n.* an eruption of linear blisters occurring after exposure to light in people who have been in contact with certain plants, such as wild parsnip or cow parsley, to which they are sensitive.

phytotoxin *n.* any poisonous substance (toxin) produced by a plant, such as any of the toxins produced by fungi of the genus *Amanita.

pia (pia mater) *n.* the innermost of the three *meninges surrounding the brain and spinal cord. The membrane is closely attached to the surface of the brain and spinal cord, faithfully following each fissure and sulcus. It contains numerous finely branching blood vessels that supply the nerve tissue within. The subarachnoid space separates it from the arachnoid.

pian *n. see* YAWS.

pica *n.* the indiscriminate eating of non-nutritious or harmful substances, such as grass, stones, or clothing. It is common in early childhood but may also be found in mentally handicapped and psychotic patients. Although previously thought to be completely nonadaptive, some evidence suggests that some patients showing pica may have particular mineral deficiencies.

Pick's disease a rare cause of *dementia in middle-aged people. The damage is mainly in the frontal and temporal lobes of the brain, in contrast with the diffuse degeneration of *Alzheimer's disease. [A. Pick (1851–1924), Czech psychiatrist]

pico- *prefix denoting* one million-millionth (10^{-12}).

picornavirus *n.* one of a group of small RNA-containing viruses (pico = small, hence pico-RNA-virus). The group includes *Coxsackie viruses, *polioviruses, and *rhinoviruses.

picric acid (trinitrophenol) a yellow crystalline solid used as a dye and as a tissue *fixative.

picture archiving and communication system *see* PACS.

PID 1. *see* PELVIC INFLAMMATORY DISEASE. **2.** *see* PROLAPSED INTERVERTEBRAL DISC.

piedra *n.* a fungal disease of the hair in which the hair shafts carry hard masses of black or white fungus. The black fungus, *Piedraia hortai*, is found mainly in the tropics and the white variety, *Trichosporon cutaneum*, in temperate regions.

Pierre Robin syndrome a congenital disease in which affected infants have a very small lower jawbone (mandible) and a cleft palate. They are susceptible to feeding and respiratory problems. [Pierre Robin (1867–1950), French dentist]

piezoelectric *adj.* denoting or relating to an electrically generated pulse or polarity that is caused by pressure.

pigeon chest forward protrusion of the breastbone resulting in deformity of the chest. The condition is painless and harmless. Medical name: **pectus carinatum**.

pigeon toes an abnormal posture in which the toes are turned inwards. It is often associated with *knock-knee.

pigment *n.* a substance giving colour. Physiologically important pigments include the blood pigments (especially *haemoglobin), *bile pigments, and retinal pigment (*see* RHODOPSIN). The pigment *melanin occurs in the skin and in the iris of the eye. Important plant pigments include *chlorophyll and the *carotenoids.

pigmentation *n.* coloration produced in the body by the deposition of one pigment, especially in excessive amounts. Pigmentation may be produced by natural pigments, such as bile pigments (as in jaundice) or melanin, or by foreign material, such as lead or arsenic in chronic poisoning.

pigment epitheliopathy acute posterior multifocal placoid pigment epitheliopathy (APMPPE): an inflammatory disease of the retinal pigment epithelium (RPE; *see* RETINA), characterized by the presence of multiple cream-coloured irregular lesions scattered in the posterior segment of the eye. The disease occurs in young adults and usually affects both eyes. Visual acuity usually recovers with time.

pig-tail stents *see* STENT.

piles *n.* *see* HAEMORRHOIDS.

pili (fimbriae) *pl. n.* (*sing.* **pilus**, **fimbria**) hairlike processes present on the surface of certain bacteria. They are thought to be involved in adhesion of bacteria to other cells and in transfer of DNA during *conjugation.

pill *n.* **1.** a small ball of variable size, shape, and colour, sometimes coated with sugar, that contains one or more medicinal substances in solid form. It is taken by mouth. **2. the Pill** *see* ORAL CONTRACEPTIVE.

pillar *n.* (in anatomy) an elongated apparently supportive structure. For example, the **pillars of the fauces** are folds of mucous membrane on either side of the opening from the mouth to the pharynx.

pilo- *prefix denoting* hair. Example: **pilosis** (excessive development of).

pilocarpine *n.* a drug with actions and uses similar to those of *physostigmine. It is administered as eye drops and may cause digestive upsets and salivation if absorbed into the system. Trade name: **Minims pilocarpine**.

pilomotor nerves sympathetic nerves that supply muscle fibres in the skin, around the roots of hairs. Activity of the sympathetic nervous system causes the muscles to contract, raising the hairs and giving the 'gooseflesh' effect of fear or cold.

pilonidal sinus a short tract leading from an opening in the skin in or near the cleft at the top of the buttocks and containing hairs. The sinus may be recurrently infected, leading to pain and the discharge of pus. Treatment is by surgical opening and cleaning of the sinus.

pilosebaceous *adj.* relating to the hair follicles and their associated sebaceous glands.

pilus *n.* a hair. *See also* PILI.

pimel- (pimelo-) *prefix denoting* fat; fatty.

pimozide *n.* an *antipsychotic drug used to relieve hallucinations and delusions occurring in schizophrenia. It is administered by mouth; side-effects may include skin rashes, tremors, and abnormal movements. Trade name: **Orap**.

pimple *n.* a small inflamed swelling on the skin that contains pus. It may be the result of bacterial infection of a skin pore that has become obstructed with fatty secretions from the sebaceous glands. Pimples occurring in large numbers on the chest, back, and face are usually described as *acne, a common condition of adolescence.

pincement *n.* one of the techniques used in massage, in which pinches of the patient's flesh are taken between finger and thumb and twisted or rolled before release. This is said to improve the tone of the skin, improve circulation, and alleviate underlying pain.

pineal gland (pineal body) a pea-sized mass of nerve tissue attached by a stalk to the posterior wall of the third ventricle of the brain, deep between the cerebral hemispheres at the back of the skull. It functions as a gland, secreting the hormone *melatonin. The gland becomes calcified as age progresses, providing a useful landmark in X-rays of the skull. Anatomical name: **epiphysis**.

pinguecula *n.* a degenerative change in the conjunctiva of the eye, seen most commonly in the elderly and in those who live in hot dry climates. Thickened yellow triangles develop on the conjunctiva at the inner and outer margins of the cornea.

pink disease a severe illness of children of the teething age, marked by pink cold clammy hands and feet, heavy sweating, raised blood pressure, rapid pulse, photophobia, loss of appetite, and insomnia. Affected infants are very prone to secondary infection, which may be fatal. It has been suggested that the condition is an allergic reaction to mercury, since it used to occur when teething powders, lotions, and ointments containing mercury were used. Although there is no definite proof of this, the disease has virtually disappeared since all mercury-containing paediatric preparations have been banned. Medical names: **acrodynia, erythroedema, erythromelalgia**.

pink eye *see* CONJUNCTIVITIS.

pinna (auricle) *n.* the flap of skin and cartilage that projects from the head at the exterior opening of the external auditory meatus of the *ear (see illustration). In man the pinna is largely vestigial but it may be partly concerned with detecting the direction of sound sources.

pinnaplasty *n. see* OTOPLASTY.

pinocytosis *n.* the intake of small droplets of fluid by a cell by cytoplasmic engulfment. It occurs in many white blood cells and in certain kidney and liver cells. *Compare* PHAGOCYTOSIS.

pins and needles *see* PARAESTHESIAE.

pinta *n.* a skin disease, prevalent in tropical America, that seems to affect only the dark-skinned races. It is caused by the *spirochaete *Treponema carateum*, a microorganism similar to those causing *yaws and *syphilis. The disease is thought to be transmitted either by direct contact between individuals or by flies that carry the infective spirochaetes on their bodies. Symptoms include thickening and eventual loss of pigment of the skin, particularly on the hands, wrists, feet, and ankles. Pinta is rarely disabling or fatal and is treated successfully with *penicillin.

pinworm *n. see* THREADWORM.

piperazine *n.* a drug used to treat infestations by roundworms and threadworms. It is administered by mouth; side-effects do not usually occur, but continued treatment at high doses may cause nausea, vomiting, headache, tingling sensations, and rashes. Trade name: **Pripsen**.

piriform fossae two pear-shaped depressions that lie on either side of the opening to the larynx.

piroxicam *n.* a nonsteroidal anti-inflammatory drug (*see* NSAID) used to relieve pain and stiffness in osteoarthritis, rheumatoid arthritis, gout, and ankylosing spondylitis. It is administered by mouth; side-effects include dizziness, skin rash, and gastrointestinal symptoms. Trade name: **Feldene**.

pisiform bone the smallest bone of the wrist (*carpus); a pea-shaped bone that articulates with the triquetral bone and, indirectly by cartilage, with the ulna.

triangular fossa

helix

external auditory meatus

anthelix

concha

tragus

antitragus

lobule

The pinna

pit *n.* (in anatomy) a hollow or depression, such as any of the depressions on the surface of an embryo marking the site of future organs.

pithiatism *n.* the treatment of certain disorders by persuading the patient that all is well. Symptoms that disappear in these circumstances are regarded as manifestations of some psychological disturbance and are classified as hysterical symptoms.

pithing *n.* the laboratory procedure in which a part or the whole of the central nervous system of an experimental animal (such as a frog) is destroyed, usually by inserting a probe through the foramen magnum, in preparation for physiological or pharmacological experiments.

pitting *n.* the formation of depressed scars, as occurs on the skin following smallpox or acne. **Pitting oedema** is swelling of the tissues due to excess fluid in which fingertip pressure leaves temporary indentations in the skin.

pituicyte *n.* a type of cell found in the posterior lobe of the pituitary gland, similar in appearance to an *astrocyte, with numerous fine branches that end in contact with the lining membrane of the blood channels in the gland.

pituitary gland (hypophysis) the master endocrine gland: a pea-sized body attached beneath the *hypothalamus in a bony cavity at the base of the skull. It has an anterior lobe (**adenohypophysis**), which secretes *thyroid-stimulating hormone, *ACTH (adrenocorticotrophic hormone), the *gonadotrophins, *growth hormone, *prolactin, *lipotrophin, and *melanocyte-stimulating hormone. The secretion of all these hormones is regulated by specific **releasing hormones**, which are produced in the hypothalamus (*see also* GONADOTROPHIN-RELEASING HORMONE). The posterior lobe (**neurohypophysis**) secretes *vasopressin and *oxytocin, which are synthesized in the hypothalamus and transported to the pituitary, where they are stored before release.

pityriasis *n.* (originally) any of a group of skin diseases typified by the development of fine branlike scales. The term is now used only with a modifying adjective.

Pityriasis alba is a common condition in children in which pale scaly patches occur on the face; it may be related to atopic *eczema. **Pityriasis rosea** is a common skin rash, believed to be viral in origin, that starts with a single patch of spots (a **herald patch**) on the trunk and is followed by an eruption of oval pink scaly *macules. The spots are often aligned along the ribs. The rash clears completely in about eight weeks. **Pityriasis versicolor** is a common chronic infection of the skin caused by the fungus *Pityrosporum orbiculare*, which is a normal inhabitant of the scalp. In susceptible people it changes to a pathogenic form called *Malassezia furfur* and produces a persistent depigmented scaly rash on the trunk. Treatment with *selenium sulphide (Selsun) shampoo readily kills the organism but the skin may take months to regain its normal colour. *See also* DANDRUFF (PITYRIASIS CAPITIS).

Pityrosporum *n.* a genus of yeasts producing superficial infections of the skin. The species *P. orbiculare* is a normal inhabitant of the scalp but it can become pathogenic in susceptible individuals (*see* PITYRIASIS).

pivampicillin *n.* a broad-spectrum *penicillin-type antibiotic administered by mouth to treat bronchitis, pneumonia, skin infections, urinary infections, and gonorrhoea. Possible side-effects include allergic reactions, nausea, and vomiting. Trade name: **Pondocillin**.

pivmecillinam *n.* a *penicillin-type antibiotic used to treat urinary-tract and other infections. It is administered by mouth: possible side-effects include allergic reactions, nausea, and vomiting. Trade name: **Selexid**.

pivot joint *see* TROCHOID JOINT.

pixel *n.* the smallest element of an electronically produced image. A numerical value is ascribed to each pixel, which determines its relative density on the final image. A *matrix of pixels produces the final image.

pizotifen *n.* an antihistamine drug used to prevent severe migraine attacks. Administered by mouth, it acts by inhibiting the effects of *serotonin. Possible side-effects include dizziness, drowsiness, and weight gain. Trade name: **Sanomigran**.

placebo *n.* a medicine that is ineffective but may help to relieve a condition because the patient has faith in its powers. New drugs are tested against placebos in clinical trials: the drug's effect is compared with the **placebo response**, which occurs even in the absence of any pharmacologically active substance in the placebo.

placenta *n.* an organ within the uterus by means of which the embryo is attached to the wall of the uterus. Its primary function is to provide the embryo with nourishment, eliminate its wastes, and exchange respiratory gases. This is accomplished by the close proximity of the maternal and fetal blood systems within the placenta. It also functions as a gland, secreting *human chorionic gonadotrophin, *progesterone, and oestrogens, which regulate the maintenance of pregnancy. See also AFTERBIRTH. —**placental** *adj.*

placenta praevia a placenta situated wholly or partially in the lower and non-contractile part of the uterus. When this becomes elongated and stretched during the last few weeks of pregnancy, and the cervix becomes stretched either before or during labour, placental separation and haemorrhage will occur. The cause is not known. In the more severe degrees of placenta praevia, where the placenta is situated entirely before the presenting part of the fetus, delivery must be by Caesarean section. In lesser degrees of placenta praevia, vaginal delivery may be undertaken with safety.

placentography *n.* *radiography of the pregnant uterus in order to determine the position of the placenta. This method is now superseded by the use of ultrasound (see ULTRASONOGRAPHY).

placode *n.* any of the thickened areas of ectoderm in the embryo that will develop into nerve ganglia or the special sensory structures of the eye, ear, or nose.

plagiocephaly *n.* any distortion or lack of symmetry in the shape of the head, usually due to irregularity in the closure of the sutures between the bones of the skull.

plague *n.* **1.** any epidemic disease with a high death rate. **2.** an acute epidemic disease of rats and other wild rodents caused by the bacterium *Yersinia pestis*, which is transmitted to man by rat fleas. **Bubonic plague**, the most common form of the disease, has an incubation period of 2–6 days. Headache, fever, weakness, aching limbs, and delirium develop and are followed by acute painful swellings of the lymph nodes (see BUBO). In favourable cases the buboes burst after about a week, releasing pus, and then heal. In other cases bleeding under the skin, producing black patches, can lead to ulcers, which may prove fatal (hence the former name **Black Death**). In the most serious cases bacteria enter the bloodstream (**septicaemic plague**) or lungs (**pneumonic plague**); if untreated, these are nearly always fatal. Treatment with tetracycline, streptomycin, and chloramphenicol is effective; vaccination against the disease provides only partial protection.

plane *n.* a level or smooth surface, especially any of the hypothetical flat surfaces – orientated in various directions – used to divide the body; for example, the *coronal and *sagittal planes.

planoconcave *adj.* describing a structure, such as a lens, that is flat on one side and concave on the other.

planoconvex *adj.* describing a structure, such as a lens, that is flat on one side and convex on the other.

plantar *adj.* relating to the sole of the foot (**planta**). See also FLEXION.

plantar arch the arch in the sole of the foot formed by anastomosing branches of the plantar arteries.

plantar fasciitis (policeman's heel) inflammation of the point of attachment of the *fascia in the sole of the foot to the calcaneus (heel bone), causing pain and localized tenderness of the heel. Treatment is a pad under the heel, anti-inflammatory medication, or steroid injections.

plantar reflex a reflex obtained by drawing a bluntly pointed object along the outer border of the sole of the foot from the heel to the little toe. The normal **flexor response** is a bunching and downward movement of the toes. An upward movement of the great toe is called an **extensor response** (or **Babinski reflex**). In all persons over the age of 18 months this is a sensitive indication of disease in the brain or spinal cord.

plantar wart a *wart occurring on the sole of the foot.

plantigrade *adj.* walking on the entire sole of the foot: a habit of man and some animals.

plaque *n.* **1.** a layer that forms on the surface of a tooth, principally at its neck, composed of bacteria in an organic matrix. Under certain conditions the plaque may cause *gingivitis, *periodontal disease, or *dental caries. The purpose of oral hygiene is to remove plaque. **2.** a raised patch on the skin, formed by *papules enlarging or coalescing to form an area 2 cm or more across. **3.** a deposit, consisting of a fatty core covered with a fibrous cap, that develops on the inner wall of an artery in atherosclerosis (*see* ATHEROMA). **4.** any flat and often raised patch, for example on mucous membrane, resulting from local damage.

-plasia *suffix denoting* formation; development. Example: **hyperplasia** (excessive tissue formation).

plasm- (plasmo-) *prefix denoting* **1.** blood plasma. **2.** protoplasm or cytoplasm.

plasma (blood plasma) *n.* the straw-coloured fluid in which the blood cells are suspended. It consists of a solution of various inorganic salts of sodium, potassium, calcium, etc., with a high concentration of protein (approximately 70 g/l) and a variety of trace substances.

plasma cells antibody-producing cells found in bone-forming tissue and also in the epithelium of the lungs and gut. They develop in the bone marrow, lymph nodes, and spleen when antigens stimulate B-*lymphocytes to produce the precursor cells that give rise to them.

plasmacytoma *n.* a malignant tumour of plasma cells, often known as a 'solitary myeloma'. Although usually occurring as a single tumour in bone marrow, it may be multiple, in which case it is classified as a multiple myeloma. Less frequently it affects soft tissues, usually the upper air passages. All of these tumours may produce the abnormal gammaglobulins that are characteristic of myeloma, and they may progress to widespread myeloma. The soft-tissue tumours often respond to radiotherapy and to such drugs as melphalan and cyclophosphamide; the bone tumours are less responsive. Tumours originating in soft tissue may spread to bone, producing an appearance on X-ray identical to myeloma deposits; these secondary growths often resolve completely after radiological treatment.

plasmalogen *n.* a phospholipid, found in brain and muscle, similar in structure to *lecithin and *cephalin.

plasmapheresis *n.* a method of removing a quantity of plasma from the blood. Blood is withdrawn from the patient and allowed to settle in a container. The plasma is drawn off the top of the blood, and the blood cells are then transfused back into the patient.

plasmin (fibrinolysin) *n.* an enzyme that digests the protein fibrin. Its function is the dissolution of blood clots (*see* FIBRINOLYSIS). Plasmin is not normally present in the blood but exists as an inactive precursor, **plasminogen**.

plasminogen *n.* a substance normally present in the blood plasma that may be activated to form *plasmin. *See* FIBRINOLYSIS, TISSUE PLASMINOGEN ACTIVATOR.

plasmoditrophoblast (syncytiotrophoblast) *n.* that part of the *trophoblast that loses its cellular structure and becomes a *syncytium. This is the invasive part of the trophoblast, which erodes the maternal tissues and forms the villi of the placenta.

Plasmodium *n.* a genus of protozoans (*see* SPOROZOA) that live as parasites within the red blood cells and liver cells of man. The parasite undergoes its asexual development (*see* SCHIZOGONY) in man and completes the sexual phase of its development (*see* SPOROGONY) in the stomach and digestive glands of a bloodsucking *Anopheles* mosquito. Four species cause *malaria in man: *P. vivax, P. ovale, P. falciparum,* and *P. malariae.*

plasmolysis *n.* a process occurring in bacteria and plants in which the protoplasm shrinks away from the rigid cell wall when the cell is placed in a *hypertonic solution. Plasmolysis is due to withdrawal of water from the cell by *osmosis.

plaster n. adhesive tape used in shaped pieces or as a bandage to keep a dressing in place.

plaster model (in dentistry) an accurate cast of the teeth and jaws made from modified plaster of Paris. A pair of models are used to study the dentition, particularly before treatment. Models are also used to construct dentures, orthodontic appliances, or such restorations as crowns.

plaster of Paris a preparation of gypsum (calcium sulphate) that sets hard when water is added. It is used in various modified forms in dentistry to make *plaster models. It is also used in orthopaedics for preparing plaster *casts.

Plastibell device a plastic device that facilitates *circumcision while protecting the glans penis. It is widely used.

plastic lymph a transparent yellowish liquid produced in a wound or other site of inflammation, in which connective tissue cells and blood vessels develop during healing.

plastic surgery a branch of surgery dealing with the reconstruction of deformed or damaged parts of the body. It also includes the replacement of parts of the body that have been lost. If performed simply to improve appearances plastic surgery is called **cosmetic surgery**, but most plastic surgery involves the treatment and repair of disfigurement and disability caused by burns, major accidents, and cancer and the correction of congenital defects, such as cleft lip and cleft palate.

plastron n. the breastbone (*sternum) together with the costal cartilages attached to it.

-plasty suffix denoting plastic surgery. Example: **labioplasty** (of the lips).

platelet (thrombocyte) n. a disc-shaped cell structure, 1–2 μm in diameter, that is present in the blood. With *Romanowsky stains platelets appear as fragments of pale-blue cytoplasm with a few red granules. They have several functions, all relating to the arrest of bleeding (see BLOOD COAGULATION). There are normally $150–400 \times 10^9$ platelets per litre of blood. See also THROMBOPOIESIS.

platelet-derived growth factor (PDGF) see GROWTH FACTOR.

platy- prefix denoting broad or flat.

platyhelminth n. see FLATWORM.

platysma n. a broad thin sheet of muscle that extends from below the collar bone to the angle of the jaw. It depresses the jaw.

pledget n. a small wad of dressing material, such as lint, used either to cover a wound or sore or as a plug. It is also used during operations, mounted on an instrument, to wipe away blood or other fluids.

-plegia suffix denoting paralysis. Example: **hemiplegia** (of one side of the body).

pleio- (pleo-) prefix denoting 1. multiple. 2. excessive.

pleiotropy n. a situation in which a single gene is responsible for more than one effect in the *phenotype. The mutation of such a gene will therefore have multiple effects. —**pleiotropic** adj.

pleocytosis n. the presence of an abnormally large number of lymphocytes in the cerebrospinal fluid, which bathes the brain and spinal cord.

pleomastia (polymastia) n. multiple breasts or nipples. These are usually symmetrically arranged along a line between the mid point of the collar bone and the pelvis (the nipple line).

pleomorphism n. the condition in which an individual assumes a number of different forms during its life cycle. The malarial parasite (Plasmodium) displays pleomorphism.

pleoptics n. special techniques practised by orthoptists (see ORTHOPTICS) for developing normal function of the macula (the most sensitive part of the retina), in people whose macular function has previously been disturbed because of strabismus (squint).

plerocercoid n. a larval stage of certain tapeworms, such as *Diphyllobothrium *latum.* It differs from the *cysticercus (another larval form) in being solid and in lacking a cyst or bladder.

plessimeter (pleximeter) *n.* a small plate of bone, ivory, or other material pressed against the surface of the body and struck with a *plessor in the technique of *percussion.

plessor (plexor) *n.* a small hammer used to investigate nervous reflexes and in the technique of *percussion.

plethora *n.* any excess of any bodily fluid, especially blood (*see* HYPERAEMIA). —**plethoric** *adj.*

plethysmography *n.* the process of recording the changes in the volume of a limb caused by alterations in blood pressure. The limb is inserted into a fluid-filled watertight casing (**oncometer**) and the pressure variations in the fluid are recorded.

pleur- (pleuro-) *prefix denoting* **1.** the pleura. **2.** the side of the body.

pleura *n.* the covering of the lungs (**visceral pleura**) and of the inner surface of the chest wall (**parietal pleura**). (See illustration.) The covering consists of a closed sac of *serous membrane, which has a smooth shiny moist surface due to the secretion of small amounts of fluid. This fluid lubricates the opposing visceral and parietal surfaces so that they can slide painlessly over each other during breathing. —**pleural** *adj.*

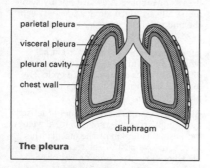

parietal pleura

visceral pleura

pleural cavity

chest wall

diaphragm

The pleura

pleural cavity the space between the visceral and parietal *pleura, which is normally very small as the pleural membranes are in close contact. The introduction of fluid (**pleural effusion**) or gas separates the pleural surfaces and increases the volume of the pleural space.

pleurectomy *n.* surgical removal of part of the *pleura, which is sometimes done to prevent further recurrences of spontaneous *pneumothorax or to remove diseased areas of pleura.

pleurisy *n.* inflammation of the *pleura, often due to pneumonia in the underlying lung. The normally shiny and slippery pleural surfaces lose their sheen and become slightly sticky, so that there is pain on deep breathing and a characteristic 'rub' can be heard through a stethoscope. Pleurisy is always associated with some other disease in the lung, chest wall, diaphragm, or abdomen.

pleurocele *n.* herniation of the pleura. *See* HERNIA.

pleurocentesis (thoracentesis, thoracocentesis) *n.* the insertion of a hollow needle into the *pleural cavity through the chest wall in order to withdraw fluid, blood, pus, or air.

pleurodesis *n.* the artificial production of pleurisy by chemical or mechanical means to obliterate the *pleural cavity, in order to prevent recurrent, usually malignant, pleural effusions.

pleurodynia *n.* severe paroxysmal pain arising from the muscles between the ribs. It is often thought to be of rheumatic origin.

pleurolysis (pneumolysis) *n.* surgical stripping of the parietal *pleura from the chest wall to allow the lung to collapse. The procedure was used in the days before effective antituberculous drugs to help tuberculosis to heal.

pleuropneumonia *n.* inflammation involving both the lung and pleura. *See* PLEURISY, PNEUMONIA.

pleuropneumonia-like organisms (PPLO) *n. see* MYCOPLASMA.

pleurotyphoid *n.* *typhoid fever involving the lungs.

pleximeter *n. see* PLESSIMETER.

plexor *n. see* PLESSOR.

plexus *n.* a network of nerves or blood vessels. *See* BRACHIAL PLEXUS.

PLF (serum) *p*lacental *f*ementin: a storage protein levels of which are used for monitoring placental function from conception until delivery.

plica *n.* a fold of tissue; for example, the **plica sublingualis**, the mucous fold in the floor of the mouth. —**plicate** *adj.*

plicamycin *n.* *see* MITHRAMYCIN.

plication *n.* a surgical technique in which the size of a hollow organ is reduced by taking tucks or folds in the walls.

ploidy *n.* the condition of having multiple the normal number of chromosomes for the species. An increase in ploidy in the cells of a malignant tumour usually indicates greater aggressiveness and ability to invade.

plombage *n.* **1.** a technique used in surgery for the correction of retinal detachment. A small piece of silicone plastic is sewn on the outside of the eyeball to produce an indentation over the retinal hole or tear to allow the retina to reattach. **2.** the insertion of plastic balls into the pleural cavity to cause collapse of the lung. This was done in the days before effective antituberculous drugs to help tuberculosis to heal.

plumbism *n.* lead poisoning. *See* LEAD[1].

pluri- *prefix denoting* more than one; several.

pneo- *prefix denoting* breathing; respiration.

pneum- *prefix.* *see* PNEUMO-.

pneumat- (pneumato-) *prefix denoting* **1.** the presence of air or gas. **2.** respiration.

pneumatization *n.* the presence of air-filled cavities in bone, such as the sinuses of the skull.

pneumatocele *n.* herniation of lung tissue. *See* HERNIA.

pneumatosis *n.* the occurrence of gas cysts in abnormal sites in the body. **Pneumatosis cystoides intestinalis** is the occurrence of multiple gas cysts in the

wall of the lower intestines. Its cause is unknown; it can be treated by *hyperbaric oxygenation.

pneumaturia *n.* the presence in the urine of bubbles of air or other gas, due to the formation of gas by bacteria infecting the urinary tract or to an abnormal connection (fistula) between the urinary tract and bowel.

pneumo- (pneum-) *prefix denoting* **1.** the presence of air or gas. Example: **pneumocolon** (within the colon). **2.** the lung(s). Example: **pneumogastric** (relating to the lungs and stomach). **3.** respiration.

pneumocephalus (pneumocele) *n.* the presence of air within the skull, usually resulting from a fracture passing through one of the air sinuses. There may be a leak of cerebrospinal fluid at the site of the fracture, manifested as a watery discharge from the nose. Pneumocephalus can be detected by plain X-rays of the skull, which show air and a fluid level inside a cavity, or by CT and MRI scanning.

pneumococcus *n.* (*pl.* **pneumococci**) the bacterium *Streptococcus pneumoniae*, which is associated with pneumonia. —**pneumococcal** *adj.*

pneumoconiosis *n.* a group of lung diseases caused by inhaling dust. The dust particles must be less than 0.5 μm in diameter to reach the depths of the lung and there is usually a long period after initial exposure before shadows appear on the chest X-ray and breathlessness develops. In practice industrial exposure to coal dust (*see* COAL-WORKER'S PNEUMOCONIOSIS), silica (*see* SILICOSIS), and asbestos (*see* ASBESTOSIS) produces most of the cases of pneumoconiosis. In Britain such cases are examined by the Medical Boarding Centres (Respiratory Diseases), on whose advice statutory compensation for industrial injury may be awarded.

Pneumocystis *n.* a genus of protozoans. The species *P. carinii* causes pneumonia in immunosuppressed patients, usually following intensive chemotherapy (*see also* AIDS). *Pneumocystis carinii* pneumonia (PCP) is fatal in 10–30% of cases if untreated, but it can be overcome with high doses of *co-trimoxazole or *pentamidine.

pneumocyte *n.* a type of cell that lines the walls separating the air sacs (*see* ALVEOLUS) in the lungs. Type I pneumocytes are flat and inconspicuous. Type II pneumocytes are cuboidal and secrete *surfactant.

pneumoencephalography *n.* a technique used in the X-ray diagnosis of disease within the skull. Air is introduced into the cavities (ventricles) of the brain to displace the cerebrospinal fluid, thus acting as a *contrast medium. X-ray photographs show the size and disposition of the ventricles and the subarachnoid spaces. The technique has largely been superseded by CT and MRI scanning.

pneumograph *n.* an instrument used to record the movements made during respiration.

pneumolysis *n.* *see* PLEUROLYSIS.

pneumon- (pneumono-) *prefix denoting* the lung(s). Example: **pneumonopexy** (surgical fixation to the chest wall).

pneumonectomy *n.* surgical removal of a lung, usually for cancer.

pneumonia *n.* inflammation of the lung caused by bacteria, in which the air sacs (*alveoli) become filled with inflammatory cells and the lung becomes solid (*see* CONSOLIDATION). The symptoms include those of any infection (fever, malaise, headaches, etc.), together with cough and chest pain. Pneumonias may be classified in different ways.
(1) According to the X-ray appearance. **Lobar pneumonia** affects whole lobes and is usually caused by *Streptococcus pneumoniae*, while **lobular pneumonia** refers to multiple patchy shadows in a localized or segmental area. When these multiple shadows are widespread, the term **bronchopneumonia** is used. In bronchopneumonia, the infection starts in a number of small bronchi and spreads in a patchy manner into the alveoli.
(2) According to the infecting organism. The most common organism is *Streptococcus pneumoniae*, but *Haemophilus influenzae*, *Staphylococcus aureus*, *Legionella pneumophila*, and *Mycoplasma pneumoniae* (among others) may all be responsible for the infection. *See also* ATYPICAL PNEUMONIA, VIRAL PNEUMONIA.
(3) According to the clinical and environmental circumstances under which the pneumonia is acquired. These infections are divided into **community-acquired pneumonia**, **hospital-acquired (nosocomial) pneumonia**, and pneumonias occurring in immunocompromised subjects (including those with AIDS). The organisms responsible for community-acquired pneumonia are totally different from those in the other groups.

Appropriate antibiotic therapy, based on the clinical situation and on microbiological studies, will result in complete recovery in the majority of patients.

pneumonitis *n.* inflammation of the lung that is confined to the walls of the air sacs (alveoli) and often caused by viruses or unknown agents. It may be acute and transient or chronic, leading to increasing respiratory disability. It does not respond to antibiotics but corticosteroids may be helpful. *Compare* PNEUMONIA.

pneumopericardium *n.* the presence of air within the membranous sac surrounding the heart. *See* HYDROPNEUMOPERICARDIUM.

pneumoperitoneum *n.* air or gas in the peritoneal or abdominal cavity, usually due to a perforation of the stomach or bowel. Pneumoperitoneum may be induced for diagnostic purposes (e.g. *laparoscopy). A former treatment of tuberculosis was the deliberate injection of air into the peritoneal cavity to allow the tuberculous lung to be rested (**artificial pneumoperitoneum**); this was frequently combined with *phrenic crush.

pneumoradiography *n.* X-ray examination of part of the body using a gas, such as air or carbon dioxide, as a contrast medium. The technique is now little used.

pneumoretinopexy *n.* a surgical technique in which an inert gas bubble is injected into the eye to press and seal breaks in the retina. When the retina is flat, a laser beam or *cryoretinopexy is applied to cause scarring and permanently seal the tear.

pneumothorax *n.* air in the *pleural cavity. Any breach of the lung surface or chest wall allows air to enter the pleural cavity, causing the lung to collapse. The leak can occur without apparent cause, in otherwise healthy people (**spontaneous pneumothorax**), or result from injuries to the chest (**traumatic pneumothorax**). In **tension pneumothorax** a breach in the lung surface acts as a valve, admitting air into the pleural cavity when the patient breathes in but preventing its escape when he breathes out. This air must be let out by surgical incision.

A former treatment for pulmonary tuberculosis – **artificial pneumothorax** – was the deliberate injection of air into the pleural cavity to collapse the lung and allow the tuberculous areas to heal.

pneumotonometer *n.* an instrument that blows a puff of air at the cornea to cause flattening and hence measure intraocular pressure. It is commonly used by optometrists in tests for glaucoma.

-pnoea *suffix denoting* a condition of breathing. Example: **dyspnoea** (breathlessness).

pock *n.* a small pus-filled eruption on the skin characteristic of *chickenpox and *smallpox rashes. *See also* PUSTULE.

pocket *n.* (in dentistry) *see* PERIODONTAL POCKET.

pod- *prefix denoting* the foot.

podagra *n.* gout of the foot, especially the big toe.

podalic version altering the position of a fetus in the uterus so that its feet will emerge first at birth. *See also* VERSION.

podopompholyx *n. see* POMPHOLYX.

-poiesis *suffix denoting* formation; production. Example: **haemopoiesis** (of blood cells).

poikilo- *prefix denoting* variation; irregularity.

poikilocyte *n.* an abnormally shaped red blood cell (*erythrocyte). Poikilocytes may be classified into a variety of types on the basis of their shape; for example elliptocytes (ellipsoid) and schistocytes (semilunar). *See also* POIKILOCYTOSIS.

poikilocytosis *n.* the presence of abnormally shaped red cells (*poikilocytes) in the blood. Poikilocytosis is particularly

marked in *myelofibrosis but can occur to some extent in almost any blood disease.

poikiloderma *n.* a condition in which the skin atrophies and becomes pigmented, giving it a mottled appearance.

poikilothermic *adj.* cold-blooded: being unable to regulate the body temperature, which fluctuates according to that of the surroundings. Reptiles and amphibians are cold-blooded. *Compare* HOMOIOTHERMIC. —**poikilothermy** *n.*

pointillage *n.* a procedure in massage in which the operator's fingers are pressed, fingertip first, deep into the patient's skin. This is done to manipulate underlying structures and break up adhesions that may have formed following injury.

poison *n.* any substance that irritates, damages, or impairs the activity of the body's tissues. In large enough doses almost any substance acts as a poison, but the term is usually reserved for substances, such as arsenic, cyanide, and strychnine, that are harmful in relatively small amounts.

Poisson distribution *see* FREQUENCY DISTRIBUTION. [S. D. Poisson (1781–1840), French mathematician]

polar body one of the small cells produced during the formation of an ovum from an *oocyte that does not develop into a functional egg cell.

poldine *n.* a drug, similar to *atropine, that inhibits gastric secretion and is used to treat such disorders as gastric and duodenal ulcers. It is administered by mouth; side-effects may include dry mouth, blurred vision, difficulty in urination, and fast heartbeat. Trade name: **Nacton**.

pole *n.* (in anatomy) the extremity of the axis of the body, an organ, or a cell.

poli- (polio-) *prefix denoting* the grey matter of the nervous system.

policeman's heel *see* PLANTAR FASCIITIS.

polioencephalitis *n.* a virus infection of the brain causing particular damage to the *grey matter of the cerebral hemispheres and the brainstem. The term is now usually restricted to infections of the brain by the poliomyelitis virus.

polioencephalomyelitis *n.* any virus infection of the central nervous system affecting the grey matter of the brain and spinal cord. *Rabies is the outstanding example.

poliomyelitis (infantile paralysis, polio) *n.* an infectious virus disease affecting the central nervous system. The virus is excreted in the faeces of an infected person and the disease is therefore most common where sanitation is poor. However, epidemics may occur in more hygienic conditions, where individuals have not acquired immunity to the disease during infancy. Symptoms commence 7–12 days after infection. In most cases paralysis does not occur: in **abortive poliomyelitis** only the throat and intestines are infected and the symptoms are those of a stomach upset or influenza; in **nonparalytic poliomyelitis** these symptoms are accompanied by muscle stiffness, particularly in the neck and back. **Paralytic poliomyelitis** is much less common. The symptoms of the milder forms of the disease are followed by weakness and eventual paralysis of the muscles: in **bulbar poliomyelitis** the muscles of the respiratory system are involved and breathing is affected.

There is no specific treatment, apart from measures to relieve the symptoms: cases of bulbar polio may require the use of a *respirator (ventilator). Immunization, using the *Sabin vaccine (taken orally) or the *Salk vaccine (injected), is highly effective.

poliovirus *n.* one of a small group of RNA-containing viruses causing *poliomyelitis. They are included within the *picornavirus group.

pollex *n.* (*pl.* **pollices**) the thumb.

pollinosis *n.* a more precise term than *hay fever for an allergy due to the pollen of grasses, trees, or shrubs.

poly- *prefix denoting* **1.** many; multiple. **2.** excessive. **3.** generalized; affecting many parts.

polyarteritis nodosa (periarteritis nodosa) a disease of unknown cause in which there is patchy inflammation of the walls of the arteries. It is one of the *connective-tissue diseases. Common manifestations are arthritis, neuritis, asthma, skin rashes, hypertension, kidney failure, and fever. The inflammation is suppressed by corticosteroid drugs (such as prednisolone).

polyarthritis *n.* rheumatic disease involving several to many joints, either together or in sequence, causing pain, stiffness, swelling, tenderness, and loss of function. *Rheumatoid arthritis is the most common cause.

polychromasia (polychromatophilia) *n.* the presence of certain blue red blood cells (*erythrocytes) seen in blood films stained with *Romanowsky stains, as well as the normal pink cells. The cells that appear blue are juvenile erythrocytes (*see* RETICULOCYTE).

polycoria *n.* a rare congenital abnormality of the eye in which there are one or more holes in the iris in addition to the pupil.

polycystic disease of the kidneys an inherited disorder, transmitted as an autosomal *dominant (the gene responsible is located on chromosome no. 16), in which the substance of both kidneys is largely replaced by numerous cysts. Symptoms – including *haematuria, urinary tract infection, and hypertension – appear between the ages of 20 and 40 and are associated with chronic kidney failure.

polycystic ovary syndrome (POS) a hormonal disorder characterized by incomplete development of *Graafian follicles in the ovary due to inadequate secretion of *luteinizing hormone; the follicles fail to ovulate and remain as multiple cysts distending the ovary. Further hormone imbalance results in obesity, hirsutism, and acne and the woman is infertile due to the lack of ovulation; this syndrome is known as the **Stein-Leventhal syndrome**. The treatment is administration of appropriate hormones.

polycythaemia *n.* an increase in the haemoglobin concentration of the blood. This may be due either to a decrease in the total volume of the plasma (**relative polycythaemia**) or to an increase in the total volume of the red cells (**absolute polycythaemia**). The latter may occur as a primary disease (*see* POLYCYTHAEMIA VERA) or as a secondary condition in association with various respiratory or circulatory disorders that cause deficiency of oxygen in the tissues and with certain tumours, such as carcinoma of the kidney.

polycythaemia vera (polycythaemia rubra vera, erythraemia, Vaquez-Osler disease) a disease in which the number of red cells in the blood is greatly increased (see also POLYCYTHAEMIA). There is often also an increase in the numbers of white blood cells and platelets. Symptoms include headache, thromboses, *cyanosis, *plethora, and itching. Polycythaemia vera may be treated by blood-letting, but more severe cases are best treated by radiotherapy or cytotoxic drugs. The cause of the disease is not known.

polydactylism n. see HYPERDACTYLISM.

polydipsia n. abnormally intense thirst, leading to the drinking of large quantities of fluid. This is a symptom typical of diabetes mellitus and diabetes insipidus.

polygene n. one of a number of genes that together control a single characteristic in an individual. Each polygene has only a slight effect and the expression of a set of polygenes is the result of their combined interaction. Characteristics controlled by polygenes are usually of a quantitative nature, e.g. height. See also MULTIFACTORIAL. —**polygenic** adj.

polymastia n. see PLEOMASTIA.

polymer n. a substance formed by the linkage of a large number of smaller molecules known as **monomers**. An example of a monomer is glucose, whose molecules link together to form glycogen, a polymer. Polymers may have molecular weights from a few thousands to many millions. Polymers made up of a single type of monomer are known as **homopolymers**; those of two or more monomers as **heteropolymers**.

polymerase chain reaction (PCR) a sensitive technique of molecular genetics in which the DNA of a single cell, treated with polymerase enzymes, is induced to replicate many times. This enables the DNA to be amplified in sufficient quantities to enable genetic analysis. The technique may be utilized in the course of preimplantation diagnosis of genetic disorders (see PRENATAL DIAGNOSIS) and also in the identification of viruses in tissue samples, e.g. *human papillomavirus in cervical smears.

polymorph (polymorphonuclear leucocyte) n. see NEUTROPHIL.

polymorphic light eruption see PHOTODERMATOSIS.

polymorphism n. (in genetics) a condition in which a chromosome or a genetic character occurs in more than one form, resulting in the coexistence of more than one morphological type in the same population.

polymyalgia rheumatica a rheumatic disease causing aching and progressive stiffness of the muscles of the shoulders and hips. These symptoms are typically associated with loss of appetite, fatigue, night sweats, and a raised *ESR. The condition is most common in the elderly, rarely occurring before the age of 50. The symptoms respond rapidly and effectively to corticosteroid treatment, which must usually be continued for several years. It is sometimes associated with temporal *arteritis.

polymyositis n. a generalized disease of the muscles that may be acute or chronic. It particularly affects the muscles of the shoulder and hip girdles, which are weak and tender to the touch. Microscopic examination of the affected muscles shows diffuse inflammatory changes, and relief of the symptoms is obtained with *corticosteroid drugs. The skin may be reddened and atrophic. See also DERMATOMYOSITIS.

polymyxin B an *antibiotic used to treat severe infections caused by Gram-negative bacteria. It is administered as a solution or ointment for ear and eye infections, often formulated with other drugs.

polyneuritis n. a disorder involving several of the peripheral nerves, usually in a symmetrical distribution. The term is often used interchangeably with *polyneuropathy although its specific use implies inflammation of the nerves.

polyneuropathy n. a disease involving multiple peripheral nerves. The symptoms first affect the tips of the fingers and toes (i.e. the extremities of the nerve fibres) and subsequently spread towards the trunk. The symptoms are usually roughly symmetrical. *See also* GUILLAIN-BARRÉ SYN-DROME (POSTINFECTIVE POLYNEUROPATHY), NEU-ROPATHY.

polynucleotide *n.* a long chain of linked *nucleotides, of which molecules of DNA and RNA are made.

polyopia *n.* the sensation of multiple images of one object. It is sometimes experienced by people with early cataract. *See also* DIPLOPIA.

polyorchidism *n.* a congenital abnormality resulting in more than two testes.

polyp (polypus) *n.* a growth, usually benign, protruding from a mucous membrane. Polyps are commonly found in the nose and sinuses, giving rise to obstruction, chronic infection, and discharge. They are often present in patients with allergic rhinitis, in whom they may develop in response to long-term antigenic stimulation. Other sites of occurrence include the ear, the stomach, and the colon, where they may eventually become malignant. **Juvenile polyps** occur in the intestine (usually colon or rectum) of infants or young people; sometimes they are multiple (**juvenile polyposis**). In the latter form there is a risk of malignant change (25% of cases) but most juvenile polyps are benign (*see also* POLYPOSIS, PEUTZ-JEGHERS SYNDROME). Polyps are usually removed surgically (*see* POLYPECTOMY).

polypectomy *n.* the surgical removal of a *polyp. The technique used depends upon the site and size of the polyp, but it is often done by cutting across the base using a wire loop (snare) through which is passed a coagulating *diathermy current.

polypeptide *n.* a molecule consisting of three or more amino acids linked together by *peptide bonds. *Protein molecules are polypeptides.

polyphagia *n.* gluttonous excessive eating.

polypharmacy *n.* treatment of a patient with more than one type of medicine.

polyphyletic *adj.* describing a number of individuals, species, etc., that have evolved from more than one ancestral group. *Compare* MONOPHYLETIC.

polyploid *adj.* describing cells, tissues, or individuals in which there are three or more complete sets of chromosomes. *Compare* DIPLOID, HAPLOID. —**polyploidy** *n.*

polypoid *adj.* having the appearance of a *polyp.

polyposis *n.* a condition in which numerous *polyps form in an organ or tissue. **Familial adenomatous polyposis** (**FAP**) is a hereditary disease (caused by a defective dominant gene) in which multiple *adenomas develop in the intestine, usually the large bowel or rectum, at an early age. As these polyps invariably become malignant, patients are usually advised to undergo total removal of the affected bowel. *See also* PEUTZ-JEGHERS SYNDROME. *Compare* PSEUDOPOLYPOSIS.

polypus *n.* *see* POLYP.

polyradiculitis (polyradiculopathy) *n.* any disorder of the peripheral nerves (*see* NEUROPATHY) in which the brunt of the disease falls on the nerve roots where they emerge from the spinal cord. An abnormal allergic response in the nerve fibres is thought to be the cause of this condition. The *Guillain-Barré syndrome is an example.

polyribosome *n.* *see* POLYSOME.

polysaccharide *n.* a *carbohydrate formed from many monosaccharides joined together in long linear or branched chains. Polysaccharides have two important functions: (1) as storage forms of energy; for example *glycogen in animals and man and *starch in plants, and (2) as structural elements; for example *muco-polysaccharides in animals and man and *cellulose in plants.

polyserositis *n.* inflammation of the membranes that line the chest, abdomen, and joints, with accumulation of fluid in the cavities. Commonly the condition is inherited and intermittent and is termed **familial Mediterranean fever**. If complicated by infiltration of major organs by a glycoprotein (*see* AMYLOIDOSIS) the disease usually proves fatal. Regular administration of colchicine will prevent the attacks in 95% of patients.

polysome (polyribosome) *n.* a structure that occurs in the cytoplasm of cells and consists of a group of *ribosomes linked together by *messenger RNA molecules: formed during protein synthesis.

polysomnograph *n.* a record of measurements of various bodily parameters during sleep. It is used in the diagnosis of sleep disorders, such as *obstructive sleep apnoea.

polyspermia *n.* **1.** excessive formation of semen. **2.** *see* POLYSPERMY.

polyspermy (polyspermia) *n.* fertilization of a single ovum by more than one spermatozoon: the development is abnormal and the embryo dies.

polythelia *n.* a congenital excess of nipples (*see* PLEOMASTIA).

polyuria *n.* the production of large volumes of urine, which is dilute and of a pale colour. The phenomenon may be due simply to excessive liquid intake or to disease, particularly diabetes mellitus, diabetes insipidus, and kidney disorders.

pompholyx *n.* *eczema of the hands (*see also* CHEIROPOMPHOLYX) and feet (**podopompholyx**). Because the horny layer of the skin in these parts is so thick the vesicles typical of eczema cannot rupture; they therefore persist in the skin, looking like sago grains. There is intense itching until the skin eventually peels. There may be secondary infection due to scratching. Pompholyx is commonest in early adulthood and attacks occur suddenly, lasting some weeks. The disease may be recurrent or persist as a chronic condition.

pons *n.* **1.** *see* PONS VAROLII. **2.** any portion of tissue that joins two parts of an organ.

pons Varolii (pons) the part of the *brainstem that links the medulla oblongata and the thalamus, bulging forwards in front of the cerebellum, from which it is separated by the fourth ventricle. It contains numerous nerve tracts between the cerebral cortex and the spinal cord and several nuclei of grey matter. From its front surface the *trigeminal nerves emerge.

pontic *n.* (in dentistry) *see* BRIDGE.

popliteus *n.* a flat triangular muscle at the back of the knee joint, between the femur and tibia, that helps to flex the knee. —**popliteal** *adj.*

porcelain *n.* (in dentistry) a ceramic material that is used to construct tooth-coloured crowns, inlays, or veneers.

pore *n.* a small opening; for example, **sweat pores** are the openings of the sweat glands on the surface of the skin.

porencephaly *n.* an abnormal communication between the lateral *ventricle and the surface of the brain. This is usually a consequence of brain injury or cerebrovascular disease; uncommonly it may be a developmental defect, when it would most likely affect both lateral ventricles.

porocephaliasis *n.* a rare infestation of the nasal cavities, windpipe, lungs, liver, or spleen by the nymphs of the parasitic arthropod *Porocephalus*. Man becomes infected on consumption of water or uncooked vegetables contaminated with the parasite's eggs. There may be some abdominal pain while the parasite is in the gut but in many cases there are no symptoms. Porocephaliasis has been occasionally reported in negroes of central Africa.

Porocephalus *n.* a genus of wormlike arthropods occurring mainly in tropical Africa and India. The legless adults are parasites in the lungs of snakes. The eggs, which are ejected with the snake's bronchial secretions, may be accidentally swallowed by man. The larva bores through the gut wall and usually migrates to the liver, where it develops into a nymph (*see* POROCEPHALIASIS).

porphin *n.* a complex nitrogen-containing ring structure and parent compound of the *porphyrins.

porphobilinogen *n.* a pigment that appears in the urine of individuals with acute *porphyria, causing it to darken if left standing.

porphyria *n.* one of a group of rare disorders due to *inborn errors of metabolism in which there are deficiencies in the enzymes involved in the biosynthesis of haem. The accumulation of the enzyme's substrate gives rise to symptoms of the disorder. The defect may be primarily in the liver (**hepatic porphyria**) or in the bone marrow (**erythropoietic porphyria**) or both. The prominent features include the excretion of *porphyrins and their derivatives in the urine, which may change colour on standing (*see* PORPHOBILINOGEN); sensitivity of the skin to sunlight causing chronic inflammation or blistering; inflammation of the nerves (neuritis); mental disturbances; and attacks of abdominal pain. The commonest porphyria is **porphyria cutanea tarda**, which affects up to 1 in 5000 people in some countries. It is a hereditary or acquired hepatic porphyria in which light-exposed areas of the skin become blistered and fragile. **Acute intermittent porphyria** is a hereditary hepatic porphyria characterized by recurrent attacks of acute abdominal pain, severe constipation, and psychotic behaviour. Factors triggering attacks include alcohol and many drugs.

porphyrin *n.* one of a number of pigments derived from *porphin, which are widely distributed in living things. All porphyrins form chelates with iron, magnesium, zinc, nickel, copper, and cobalt. These chelates are constituents of *haemoglobin, *myohaemoglobin, the *cytochromes, and chlorophyll, and are thus important in many oxidation/reduction reactions in all living organisms. *See also* PROTOPORPHYRIN IX.

porphyrinuria *n.* the presence in the urine of breakdown products of the red blood pigment haemoglobin (porphyrins), sometimes causing discoloration. *See* PORPHYRIA, PORPHOBILINOGEN.

porta *n.* the aperture in an organ through which its associated vessels pass. Such an opening occurs in the liver (**porta hepatis**).

portacaval anastomosis (portacaval shunt) **1.** a surgical technique in which the hepatic portal vein is joined to the inferior vena cava. Blood draining from the abdominal viscera is thus diverted past the liver. It is used in the treatment of *portal hypertension, since – by lowering the pressure within the veins of the stomach and oesophagus – it prevents serious bleeding into the gastrointestinal tract. **2.** any of the natural communications between the branches of the hepatic portal

vein in the liver and the inferior vena cava.

portal *adj.* **1.** relating to the portal vein or system. **2.** relating to a porta.

portal hypertension a state in which the pressure within the hepatic *portal vein is increased, causing enlargement of the spleen, enlargement of veins in the oesophagus (gullet) (which may rupture to cause severe bleeding), and accumulation of fluid in the peritoneal cavity (ascites). The commonest cause is *cirrhosis, but other diseases of the liver or thrombosis of the portal vein will also produce it. Treatment is by *diuretic drugs, by surgery to join the portal vein to the inferior vena cava (bypassing the liver; *see* PORTACAVAL ANASTOMOSIS), or by implanting a *stent within the liver to join portal tract veins to a hepatic vein tributary (**TIPSS – transcutaneous intrahepatic portosystemic shunt**).

portal system a vein or group of veins that terminates at both ends in a capillary bed. The best known is the **hepatic portal system**, which consists of the *portal vein and its tributaries (see illustration). Blood is drained from the spleen, stomach, pancreas, and small and large intestines into veins that merge to form the portal vein leading to the liver. Here the portal vein branches, ending in many small capillaries called *sinusoids. These permit the passage into the liver cells of nutrients absorbed by blood from the intestines.

portal vein a short vein, about 8 cm long, forming part of the hepatic *portal system. It receives many tributaries, including the splenic vein from the spleen and pancreas, the gastric vein from the stomach, the mesenteric vein from the small and large intestines, and the rectal vein from the rectum and anus.

port-wine stain *see* NAEVUS.

POS *see* POLYCYSTIC OVARY SYNDROME.

positron *n.* an electrically charged particle, released in some radioactive decays, that has the same mass as an electron but opposite charge. It has a very short lifetime as it quickly reacts with an electron to produce *gamma rays.

positron emission tomography

(PET) a technique of *nuclear medicine used to evaluate the activity of tissues by measuring their uptake of injected 2-deoxyglucose labelled with radioactive fluorine. As this substance is metabolized after uptake it emits positrons, which collide with electrons and are annihilated with the production of gamma rays. Metabolic activity is reduced in damaged tissues and emission of gamma radiation from these areas is absent or reduced considerably. Using a tomographic *gamma camera, the accurate position and source of positron annihilation within the body can be determined. In this way functional activity of the tissues can be compared with anatomical images obtained by CT or MRI scanning. Originally used to study activity in the brain, it is now also used for investigating the chest and abdomen. *See also* TOMOGRAPHY. *Compare* COMPUTERIZED TOMOGRAPHY (CT).

posology *n.* the science of the dosage of medicines.

posset *n.* a small amount of milk that is regurgitated, usually with some wind, by many babies after feeding.

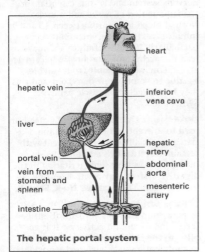

The hepatic portal system

Possum *n.* a device that enables severely paralysed patients to use typewriters, adding machines, telephones, and a wide variety of other machines. Modern Possums are operated by micro-switches that require only the slightest movement in any limb. The original device worked by blowing and sucking a mouthpiece. The name derives from **Patient-Operated Selector Mechanism (POSM)**.

post- *prefix denoting* **1.** following; after. Example: **postepileptic** (after an epileptic attack). **2.** (in anatomy) behind. Example: **postoral** (behind the mouth).

postcentral *adj.* **1.** situated behind any centre. **2.** situated behind the central fissure of the brain.

postcibal *adj.* occurring after eating.

postcoital contraception prevention of pregnancy after intercourse has taken place. This can be achieved by three methods, which aim to prevent implantation of the fertilized ovum in the uterus: (1) the **Yuzpe method**, which consists of spaced oral doses of oestrogen and progestogen taken within 72 hours of unprotected intercourse; (2) a single oral dose of the antiprogesterone drug, *mifepristone, taken within 72 hours of unprotected intercourse; and (3) insertion of an *IUCD within five days of unprotected intercourse.

postcoital test a test used in the investigation of infertility. A specimen of cervical mucus, taken 6–24 hours after coitus, is examined under a microscope The appearance of 10 or more progressively motile spermatozoa per high-power field in the specimen indicates that there is no abnormal reaction between spermatozoa and mucus. The test should be undertaken in the postovulatory phase of the menstrual cycle.

posterior *adj.* situated at or near the back of the body or an organ. The **posterior chamber** of the eye is the rear section, behind the lens, which is filled with vitreous humour.

postero- *prefix denoting* posterior. Example: **posterolateral** (behind and at the side of).

posteroanterior *adj.* from the back to the front. In radiology it denotes a view in the *coronal plane.

postganglionic *adj.* describing a neurone in a nerve pathway that starts at a ganglion and ends at the muscle or gland that it supplies. In the sympathetic nervous system, postganglionic fibres are *adrenergic, unlike those in the parasympathetic system, which are *cholinergic. *Compare* PREGANGLIONIC.

postgastrectomy syndrome *see* DUMPING SYNDROME.

posthetomy *n.* an obsolete term for *circumcision.

posthitis *n.* inflammation of the foreskin. This usually occurs in association with inflammation of the glans penis (**balanitis**; *see* BALANOPOSTHITIS). Pain, redness, and swelling of the foreskin occurs due to bacterial infection. Treatment is by antibiotic administration, and subsequent *circumcision prevents further attacks.

posthumous birth **1.** delivery of a child by *Caesarean section after the mother's death. **2.** birth of a child after the father's death.

postmature *adj.* describing a baby born after 42 weeks of gestation (calculated from the first day of the last menstrual period). Such a birth can be associated with maternal diabetes or with *anencephaly in the fetus. —**postmaturity** *n.*

postmenopause *n.* the period of a woman's life after the *menopause. The term 'menopause' is often used in reference to the postmenopausal period.

post mortem Latin: after death. *See* AUTOPSY.

postnatal depression *see* BABY BLUES, PUERPERAL DEPRESSION.

postoperative *adj.* following operation: referring to the condition of a patient or to the treatment given at this time.

postpartum *adj.* relating to the period of a few days immediately after birth.

postprandial *adj.* occurring after eating.

post-processing *n.* (in radiology) the electronic manipulation of digitally acquired images (*see* DIGITIZATION) following an examination in order to improve diagnostic accuracy.

post-traumatic stress disorder (PTSD) an anxiety disorder caused by the major personal stress of a serious or frightening event, such as an injury, assault, rape, or exposure to warfare or a disaster involving many casualties. The reaction may be immediate or delayed for months. The sufferer experiences the persistent recurrence of images or memories of the event, together with nightmares, insomnia, a sense of isolation, guilt, irritability, and loss of concentration. Emotions may be deadened or depression may develop. The condition usually settles with time, but support and skilled counselling may be needed. More severe cases may be treated by *cognitive therapy and/or *behaviour therapy.

postural muscles (antigravity muscles) muscles (principally extensors) that serve to maintain the upright posture of the body against the force of gravity.

postviral fatigue syndrome *see* CHRONIC FATIGUE SYNDROME.

potassium *n.* a mineral element and an important constituent of the human body. It is the main base ion of intracellular fluid. Together with *sodium, it helps to maintain the electrical potential of the nervous system and is thus essential for the functioning of nerve and muscle. Normal blood levels are between 3.5 and 5 mmols/litre. High concentrations occur particularly in kidney failure and may lead to *arrhythmia and finally to cardiac arrest. Low values result from fluid loss, e.g. due to vomiting or diarrhoea, and this may lead to general muscle paralysis. Symbol: K.

potassium chloride a salt of potassium used to prevent and treat potassium deficiency, especially during treatment with certain diuretics. It is administered by mouth or injection; some irritation in the digestive system may occur after oral administration. Trade names: **Nu-K**, **Slow-K**.

potassium hydroxyquinoline a salt of potassium that has antifungal, antibacterial, and deodorant activities. It is applied to the skin in creams or lotions (e.g. in combination with *benzoyl peroxide as **Quinoderm** or **Quinoped**) to treat skin infections and occasionally causes skin irritation.

potassium permanganate a salt of potassium used for disinfecting and cleansing wounds and as a general skin *antiseptic. It irritates mucous membranes and is poisonous if taken into the body.

Potter syndrome a congenital condition characterized by absence of kidneys, resulting in decreased amniotic fluid (see OLIGOHYDRAMNIOS) and compression of the fetus. Babies have poorly developed lungs, a characteristic wrinkled and flattened facial appearance, and leg deformities and do not usually survive. [E. L. Potter (1901–   ), US pathologist]

Pott's disease *tuberculosis of the backbone. Untreated, it can lead to a hunchback deformity. Treatment is antituberculous chemotherapy and occasionally surgery. [P. Pott (1714–88), British surgeon]

pouch n. **1.** (in anatomy) a small sac-like structure, especially occurring as an outgrowth of a larger structure. The **pouch of Douglas** is a pouch of peritoneum occupying the space between the rectum and uterus. **2.** (in surgery) a sac created from a loop of intestine and used to replace a section of rectum that has been surgically removed, for example for ulcerative colitis (see ILEAL POUCH), or to replace the bladder after *cystectomy.

poultice (fomentation) n. a preparation of hot moist material applied to any part of the body to increase local circulation, alleviate pain, or soften the skin to allow matter to be expressed from a boil. Poultices containing kaolin retain heat for a considerable period during use.

Poupart's ligament see INGUINAL LIGAMENT. [F. Poupart (1661–1708), French anatomist]

powder n. (in pharmacy) a medicinal preparation consisting of a mixture of two or more drugs in the form of fine particles.

pox n. **1.** an infectious disease causing a skin rash. **2.** a rash of pimples that become pus-filled, as in *chickenpox and *smallpox.

poxvirus n. one of a group of large DNA-containing viruses including those that cause *smallpox (variola) and *cow-

pox (vaccinia) in man, and pox and tumours in animals.

PPLO see MYCOPLASMA.

practice nurse a trained nurse caring for the patients of one or more general practitioners in the consulting room and on domiciliary consultations. In Britain, practice nurses are usually employed directly by GPs, who can claim the standard contribution from the Health Authority. However, they may also be employed by community trusts as *district nurses.

Prader-Willi syndrome a congenital condition in which obesity is associated with mental retardation and small genitalia; diabetes mellitus frequently develops in affected individuals. [A. Prader and H. Willi (20th century), Swiss paediatricians]

pravastatin n. a drug used to reduce abnormally high levels of cholesterol in the blood. Its actions and side-effects are similar to those of *lovastatin. Trade name: **Lipostat**.

praziquantel n. an *anthelmintic drug used to eliminate tapeworms, schistosomes, liver flukes, and lung flukes. It is administered by mouth. Possible side-effects include nausea, abdominal discomfort, fever, sweating, and drowsiness. Trade name: **Biltricide**.

prazosin n. a drug used in the treatment of high blood pressure (hypertension) by reducing peripheral vascular resistance (see ALPHA BLOCKER). It is administered by mouth; common side-effects include dizziness, headache, palpitations, and nausea. Trade name: **Hypovase**.

pre- prefix denoting **1.** before; preceding. Example: **premenstrual** (before menstruation); **prenatal** (before birth). **2.** (in anatomy) in front of; anterior to. Example: **precardiac** (in front of the heart); **prepatellar** (in front of the patella).

pre-agonal adj. relating to the phenomena that precede the moment of death. See also AGONAL.

precancerous adj. describing a nonmalignant condition that is known to become malignant if left untreated. *Leukoplakia of the vulva is known to be a precancerous condition. *See also* METAPLASIA.

precipitin *n.* any antibody that combines with its antigen to form a complex that comes out of solution and is seen as a precipitate. The antibody-antigen reaction is specific; the precipitin reaction is therefore a useful means of confirming the identity of an unknown antigen or establishing that a serum contains antibodies to a known disease. This test may be performed in watery solution or in a semisolid medium such as agar gel. *See also* AGGLUTINATION.

precipitinogen *n.* any antigen that is precipitated from solution by a *precipitin.

precision attachment (in dentistry) a special machined joint that holds certain types of partial *dentures in place. The attachment is in two parts, one fixed to the denture and the other fixed to a crown on one of the teeth abutting the denture.

precocious puberty the development at an early age of the physical and physiological changes associated with *puberty. In girls this is usually taken as development of breasts or pubic hair before the age of six or menstruation before the age of eight. In boys development of pubic hair or other adult sexual features below the age of nine is considered to be precocious. In girls 90% of cases have no underlying abnormalities, but in boys approximately half have a serious underlying cause, of which malignant testicular tumours and malignant adrenal tumours are the most common.

precocity *n.* an acceleration of normal development. The intellectually precocious child has a high IQ and may become isolated from his contemporaries or frustrated at school. Mental illness is less common than in those who develop normally. —**precocious** *adj.*

precordium *n.* the region of the thorax immediately over the heart. —**precordial** *adj.*

precuneus *n.* an area of the inner surface of the cerebral hemisphere on each side, above and in front of the *corpus callosum. *See* CEREBRUM.

predisposition *n.* a tendency to be affected by a particular disease or kind of disease. Such a tendency may be hereditary or may arise because of such factors as lack of vitamins, food, or sleep. *See also* DIATHESIS.

prednisolone *n.* a synthetic *corticosteroid used to treat rheumatic diseases and inflammatory and allergic conditions. It is administered by mouth, injected into joints, or applied in creams, lotions, and ointments (to treat skin conditions). Sideeffects are those of *cortisone. Trade names: **Deltacortril, Deltastab, Precortisyl, Prednesol**.

prednisone *n.* a synthetic *corticosteroid used to treat rheumatic diseases, severe allergic conditions, inflammatory conditions, and leukaemia. It is administered by mouth and the side-effects are those of *cortisone. Trade name: **Decortisyl**.

pre-eclampsia (pregnancy-induced hypertension) *n.* high blood pressure (greater than 140/90 mmHg) developing during pregnancy in a woman whose blood pressure was previously normal. It is often accompanied by excessive fluid retention and less often by the presence of protein in the urine. *See also* ECLAMPSIA.

prefrontal lobe the region of the brain at the very front of each cerebral hemisphere (*see* FRONTAL LOBE). The functions of the lobe are concerned with emotions, memory, learning, and social behaviour. Nerve tracts in the lobe are cut during the operation of prefrontal *leucotomy.

preganglionic *adj.* describing fibres in a nerve pathway that end in a ganglion, where they form synapses with *postganglionic fibres that continue the pathway to the effector organ, muscle or gland.

pre-gangrene *n.* the penultimate stage of vascular insufficiency before *gangrene sets in; the term is usually applied to *ischaemia of the lower limb.

pregnancy *n.* the period during which a woman carries a developing fetus, normally in the uterus (*compare* ECTOPIC PREGNANCY). Pregnancy lasts for approximately 266 days, from *conception until the baby is born, or 280 days from the first day of the last menstrual period (*see* NAEGELE

RULE). During pregnancy menstruation is absent, there may be a great increase in appetite, and the breasts increase in size; the woman may also experience *morning sickness. These and other changes are brought about by a hormone (*progesterone) produced at first by the ovary and later by the *placenta. Definite evidence of pregnancy is provided by various *pregnancy tests, by the detection of the heartbeat of the fetus, and by ultrasound. Medical name: **cyesis**. See also PSEUDOCYESIS (PHANTOM PREGNANCY). —**pregnant** adj.

pregnancy-induced hypertension (PIH) see PRE-ECLAMPSIA.

pregnancy test any of several methods used to demonstrate whether or not a woman is pregnant. Most pregnancy tests are based on the detection of a hormone, *human chorionic gonadotrophin (HCG), in the urine. The sample of urine is mixed with serum containing antibodies to HCG and marker particles (sheep red cells or latex particles) coated with HCG. In the absence of pregnancy, the antibodies will cause *agglutination of the marker particles. If the urine is from a pregnant woman, the antibodies will be absorbed and no agglutination will occur. These tests may be positive for pregnancy as early as 30 days after the date of the last normal period and are 98% accurate. Newer tests using *monoclonal antibodies (**beta HCG**) are more easily interpreted. When carried out on serum rather than urine, these tests give even earlier positive results.

pregnanediol n. a steroid that is formed during the metabolism of the female sex hormone *progesterone. It occurs in the urine during pregnancy and certain phases of the menstrual cycle.

pregnenolone n. a steroid synthesized in the adrenal glands, ovaries, and testes. Pregnenolone is an important intermediate product in steroid hormone synthesis and can – depending on the pathways followed – be converted to corticosteroids (glucocorticoids or mineralocorticoids), androgens, or oestrogens.

preimplantation diagnosis see PRENATAL DIAGNOSIS.

premature beat see ECTOPIC BEAT.

premature birth birth of a baby weighing less than 2.5 kg (5½ lb). Usually this is indicative of *preterm birth but it can also be caused by *intrauterine growth retardation (IUGR). Birth weights of less than 500 g are almost invariably incompatible with life.

premature ejaculation emission of semen (and consequent loss of erection) during the initial stages of preparation for sexual intercourse, before insertion into the vagina or immediately afterwards.

premedication n. drugs administered to a patient before an operation (usually one in which an anaesthetic is used). Premedication usually comprises injection of a sedative, to calm the patient down, together with a drug, such as *atropine, to dry up the secretions of the lungs (which might otherwise be inhaled during anaesthesia).

premenstrual tension a condition of nervousness, irritability, emotional disturbance, headache, and/or depression affecting some women for up to about ten days before menstruation. The condition is associated with the accumulation of salt and water in the tissues. It usually disappears soon after menstruation begins. The hormone progesterone is believed to be a causative element and a deficiency of essential fatty acids has also been observed.

premenstruum n. the stage of the *menstrual cycle immediately preceding menstruation.

premolar n. either of the two teeth on each side of each jaw behind the canines and in front of the molars in the adult *dentition.

premyelocyte n. see PROMYELOCYTE.

prenatal diagnosis (antenatal diagnosis) diagnostic procedures carried out on pregnant women in order to discover genetic or other abnormalities in the developing fetus. Ultrasound scanning (see ULTRASONOGRAPHY) remains the cornerstone of prenatal diagnosis. Other procedures include estimation of the level of *alphafetoprotein in the mother's serum and the amniotic fluid; chromosome and enzyme analysis of fetal cells obtained by *amniocentesis or, at an earlier stage of pregnancy, by *chorionic villus sampling (CVS); and examination of fetal blood obtained by *fetoscopy or *cordocentesis. If the results indicate that the child is likely or certain to be born with severe malformation or abnormality, the possibility of abortion is discussed by the doctors involved with the parents.

Until recently, prenatal genetic diagnosis was dependent on CVS and amniocentesis, but it may now be extended to the earliest stages of embryonic development, before implantation occurs (**preimplantation diagnosis**). Access to these early embryos requires the removal and *in vitro fertilization of egg cells: three days after fertilization one or two cells are aspirated from the six- to eight-cell embryo; alternatively, tissue is removed from an embryo at five or six days, when it has reached the *blastocyst stage. Isolated cells can then be genetically analysed, using the *polymerase chain reaction amplification technique to produce enough DNA for genetic diagnosis. Even before pregnancy, this technique can be used to enable a prospective mother to be identified as the carrier of a gene defect, by means of the *mouthwash test. When a defect is detected, *genetic counselling is offered.

preoperative *adj.* before operation: referring to the condition of a patient or to treatment, such as sedation, given at this time.

preparedness *n.* (in psychology) a quality of some stimuli that makes them much more likely to give rise to a pathological fear. For example, animals or high places are much more likely to become the subject of a *phobia than are plants or clothes. One theory is that individuals are genetically predisposed to *conditioning of fear to objects that have been a biological threat during the evolution of mankind.

prepatellar bursitis *see* HOUSEMAID'S KNEE.

prepubertal *adj.* relating to or occurring in the period before puberty.

prepuce (foreskin) *n.* the fold of skin that grows over the end (glans) of the penis. On its inner surface modified sebaceous glands (**preputial glands**) secrete a lubricating fluid over the glans. The accumulation of this secretion is known as *smegma. The foreskin is often surgically removed in infancy (*see* CIRCUMCISION). The fold of skin that surrounds the clitoris is also called the prepuce. —**preputial** *adj.*

preputial glands modified sebaceous glands on the inner surface of the *prepuce.

prepyramidal *adj.* **1.** situated in the middle lobe of the cerebellum, in front of the *pyramid. **2.** describing nerve fibres in tracts that descend from the cerebral cortex to the spinal cord, before the crossing over that occurs at the pyramid of the medulla oblongata.

presby- (presbyo-) *prefix denoting* old age.

presbyacusis *n.* the progressive sensorineural *deafness that occurs with age.

presbyopia *n.* difficulty in reading at the usual distance (about one foot from the eyes) and in performing other close work, due to the decline with age in the ability of the eye to alter its focus to see close objects clearly. This is caused by gradual loss of elasticity of the lens of the eye which thus becomes progressively less able to increase its curvature in order to focus on near objects.

prescribed disease one of a number of illnesses (currently 48) arising as a result of employment requiring close contact with a hazardous substance or circumstance. Examples include poisoning by such chemicals as mercury or benzene, decompression sickness in divers, and infections such as *anthrax in those handling wool. Some diseases that occur widely in the population may be prescribed in relation to a specific occupation (e.g. deafness in those working with pneumatic drills or tuberculosis in mortuary attendants). *See also* COSHH.

prescription *n.* a written direction from a registered medical practitioner to a pharmacist for preparing and dispensing a drug.

presenility *n.* premature ageing of the mind and body, so that a person shows the reduction in mental and physical abilities normally found only in old age. *See also* DE-MENTIA, PROGERIA. —**presenile** *adj.*

present *vb.* **1.** (of a patient) to come forward for examination and treatment because of experiencing specific symptoms (**presenting symptoms**). **2.** (in obstetrics) *see* PRESENTATION.

presentation *n.* the part of the fetus that is closest to the birth canal and can be felt on inserting a finger into the vagina. Normally the head presents (**cephalic presentation**). However, the buttocks may present (*see* BREECH PRESENTATION) or, if the fetus lies transversely across the uterus, the shoulder or arm may present. In *placenta praevia the placenta may lie in front of the presenting fetal part. These abnormal presentations may cause complications during childbirth, and attempts may be made to correct them.

pressor *n.* an agent that raises blood pressure. *See* VASOCONSTRICTOR.

pressure index (PI) the ratio of the pressure in the posterior tibial artery to that in the brachial artery, which reflects the degree of arterial obstruction in the artery of the lower limb.

pressure point a point at which an artery lies over a bone on which it may be compressed by finger pressure, to arrest haemorrhage beyond. For example, the femoral artery may be compressed against the pelvic bone in the groin.

pressure sore *see* BEDSORE.

presymptomatic *adj.* describing or relating to a symptom that occurs before the typical symptoms of a disease. *See also* PRODROMAL.

presystole *n.* the period in the cardiac cycle just preceding systole.

preterm birth birth of a baby before 37 weeks (259 days) of gestation (calculated from the first day of the mother's last menstrual period); a birth at less than 23 weeks is at present incompatible with life. Such factors as *pre-eclampsia, multiple pregnancies (e.g. twins), maternal infection, and *cervical incompetence may all result in preterm births, but in the majority of cases the cause is unknown. Conditions affecting preterm babies may

include *respiratory distress syndrome, feeding difficulties, inability to maintain normal body temperature, *apnoea, infection, *necrotizing enterocolitis, and brain haemorrhages. Supportive treatment is provided in an incubator in a neonatal unit; many infants survive with no residual handicap but the shorter the gestation period, the more serious are the problems to be overcome.

prevalence rate a measure of morbidity based on current sickness in a population, estimated either at a particular time (**point prevalence**) or over a stated period (**period prevalence**). It can be expressed either in terms of sick people (persons) or episodes of sickness per 1000 individuals at risk. *Compare* INCIDENCE RATE.

preventive dentistry the branch of dentistry concerned with the prevention of dental disease. It includes dietary counselling, advice on oral hygiene, and the application of *fluoride and *fissure sealants to the teeth.

preventive medicine the branch of medicine whose main aim is the prevention of disease. This is a wide field, in which workers tackle problems ranging from the immunization of persons against infectious diseases, such as diphtheria or whooping cough, to finding methods of eliminating *vectors, such as malaria carrying mosquitoes. *See also* WORLD HEALTH ORGANIZATION.

preventive resin restoration a hybrid between a *fissure sealant and a conventional *filling that is used to treat early dental caries involving dentine on the occlusal surfaces of posterior teeth.

Priadel *n.* *see* LITHIUM.

priapism *n.* persistent painful erection of the penis that requires decompression. A prolonged erection (i.e. of greater than six hours duration), resulting from administration of *papaverine or a similar drug, can be successfully treated by draining the blood from the corpora cavernosa of the penis with a 19 SWG butterfly needle and instilling a *vasoconstrictor (e.g. aramine). Priapism may also occur in patients with sickle-cell trait and those undergoing *haemodialysis. An unrelieved priapism results in eventual fibrosis of the spongy tissue of the corpora and no further erections are possible.

prickle cells cells with cytoplasmic processes that form intercellular bridges. The germinative layer of the *epidermis is sometimes called the prickle cell layer.

prickly heat an itchy rash of small raised red spots. It occurs usually on the face, neck, back, chest, and thighs. Infants and obese people are susceptible to prickly heat, which is most common in hot moist weather. It is caused by blockage of the sweat ducts and the only treatment is removal of the patient to a cool (air-conditioned) place. Medical name: **miliaria**.

prilocaine n. a local *anaesthetic used particularly in ear, nose, and throat surgery and in dentistry. It is applied in a solution to mucous membranes or injected; high doses of the drug may cause methaemoglobinaemia and cyanosis. Prilocaine is also a constituent of *EMLA cream. Trade name: **Citanest**.

primaquine n. a drug used in the treatment of malaria. It is administered by mouth, usually in combination with other antimalarial drugs, such as *chloroquine. High doses may cause blood disorders (such as methaemoglobinaemia or haemolytic anaemia) and digestive upsets.

primary health care health care provided by a *general practitioner or other health professional who has first contact with a patient seeking medical treatment. Primary health care services provided by the NHS include the general dental, ophthalmic, and pharmaceutical services, as well as the family doctor service, together with those community services outside the hospital service. *See also* COMMUNITY HEALTH, DOMICILIARY SERVICES, GENERAL DENTAL SERVICES, HEALTH CENTRE. *Compare* SECONDARY HEALTH CARE, TERTIARY HEALTH CARE.

primary teeth the first set of teeth, which develop in infancy. These teeth are normally shed just before the eruption of their permanent successors. In the absence of permanent successors they can remain functional for many years. *See* DENTITION.

prime vb. (in chemotherapy) to administer small doses of a *cytotoxic drug prior to high-dose chemotherapy and/or radiotherapy. This causes proliferation of the primitive bone marrow cells and aids subsequent regeneration of the bone marrow.

prime mover *see* AGONIST.

primidone n. an *anticonvulsant drug used to treat major epilepsy. It is administered by mouth; common side-effects, which are usually transient, include drowsiness, muscle incoordination, digestive upsets, vertigo, and sight disturbances. Trade name: **Mysoline**.

primigravida n. a woman experiencing her first pregnancy.

primipara n. a woman who has given birth to one infant capable of survival.

primitive streak the region of the embryo that proliferates rapidly, producing mesoderm cells that spread outwards between the layers of ectoderm and endoderm.

primordial adj. (in embryology) describing cells or tissues that are formed in the early stages of embryonic development.

P–R interval the interval on an *electrocardiogram between the onset of atrial activity and ventricular activity. It represents the time required for the impulse from the *sinoatrial node to reach the ventricles.

prion n. an abnormal form of a constituent protein (PrP) of brain cells. Prions are produced by mutations in the gene that codes for PrP and are very stable: they are not removed by the normal cellular processes of degradation and are resistant to radiation. They are believed to interact with normal PrP in such a way as to convert it to the abnormal form, which accumulates in the brain. Prions are now widely accepted as being the causal agents of a range of serious diseases including *Creutzfeldt-Jakob disease, Gerstmann-Straussler syndrome, and *kuru, all of which are *spongiform encephalopathies. Different mutations in the PrP gene are believed to be responsible for the different forms of these so-called **prion diseases**.

pro- prefix denoting **1.** before; preceding. **2.** a precursor. **3.** in front of.

probability n. see SIGNIFICANCE.

proband n. see PROPOSITUS.

probang *n.* a long flexible rod with a small sponge, ball, or tuft at the end, used to remove obstructions from the larynx or oesophagus (gullet). A probang is also used to apply medication to these structures.

probe *n.* **1.** a thin rod of pliable metal, such as silver, with a blunt swollen end. The instrument is used for exploring cavities, wounds, *fistulae, and sinus channels. **2.** (**gene probe**) a radioactively labelled cloned section of DNA that is used to detect identical sections of nucleic acid by means of pairing between complementary bases. *See* NORTHERN BLOT ANALYSIS, SOUTHERN BLOT ANALYSIS.

probenecid *n.* a drug that reduces the level of uric acid in the blood (*see* URICOSURIC DRUG) and is used chiefly in the treatment of gout. It is administered by mouth; mild side-effects, such as digestive upsets, dizziness, and skin rashes, may occur. Trade name: **Benemid**.

probucol *n.* a drug used to lower *cholesterol levels in the blood in patients with primary hypercholesterolaemia who have not responded to diet, weight reduction, and exercise. It acts by increasing the breakdown of low-density *lipoproteins and inhibits cholesterol synthesis. It is administered by mouth; side-effects include headache, skin rash, diarrhoea, and abdominal pain. Trade name: **Lurselle**.

procainamide *n.* a drug that slows down the activity of the heart and is used to control abnormal heart rhythm. It is administered by mouth or injection; side-effects may include digestive upsets, dizziness, and allergic reactions. Trade name: **Pronestyl**.

procaine (procaine hydrochloride) *n.* a local *anaesthetic administered by injection for *spinal anaesthesia. It was formerly used in dentistry. Side-effects are uncommon, but allergic reactions may occur.

procaine penicillin G an *antibiotic, consisting of penicillin and procaine, used to treat infections caused by organisms sensitive to penicillin. It is injected into muscle so that the penicillin is released slowly and remains effective for some time. Trade names: **Bicillin, Triplopen**.

procarbazine *n.* a drug that inhibits growth of cancer cells by preventing cell division and is used to treat such cancers as Hodgkin's disease. It is administered by mouth; common side-effects include loss of appetite, nausea, vomiting, diarrhoea, and mouth sores. Trade name: **Natulan**.

process *n.* (in anatomy) a thin prominence or protuberance; for example, any of the processes of a vertebra.

prochlorperazine *n.* a phenothiazine *antipsychotic drug used to treat schizophrenia and other mental disorders, migraine, vertigo, nausea, and vomiting. It is administered by mouth, injection, or in suppositories; possible side-effects include drowsiness and dry mouth, and high doses may cause tremors and abnormal muscle movements. Trade name: **Stemetil**.

procidentia *n.* the complete downward displacement (*prolapse) of an organ, especially the uterus (**uterine procidentia**), which protrudes from the vaginal opening. Uterine procidentia may result from injury to the floor of the pelvic cavity, invariably the result of childbirth.

proct- (procto-) *prefix denoting* the anus and/or rectum.

proctalgia (proctodynia) *n.* pain in the rectum or anus. In **proctalgia fugax** severe pain suddenly affects the rectum and may last for minutes or hours; attacks may be days or months apart. There is no structural disease and the pain is probably due to muscle spasm (*see* IRRITABLE BOWEL SYNDROME). Relief is sometimes obtained from a bowel action, inserting a finger into the rectum, or from a hot bath, but it may be prevented by measures used in treating the irritable bowel syndrome.

proctatresia *n. see* IMPERFORATE ANUS.

proctectasia *n.* enlargement or widening of the rectum, usually due to long-standing constipation (*see* DYSCHEZIA).

proctectomy *n.* surgical removal of the rectum. It is usually performed for cancer of the rectum and may require the construction of a permanent opening in the colon (*see* COLOSTOMY). If the anus is left, an *ileal pouch can be constructed to replace the rectum.

proctitis *n.* inflammation of the rectum.

Symptoms are ineffectual straining to empty the bowels (*tenesmus), diarrhoea, and often bleeding. Proctitis is invariably present in ulcerative *colitis and sometimes in *Crohn's disease, but may occur independently (**idiopathic proctitis**). Rarer causes include damage by irradiation (for example in radiation therapy for cervical cancer), by *lymphogranuloma venereum, or after a colostomy has rendered the rectum nonfunctional (**disuse proctitis**).

proctocele (rectocele) n. bulging or pouching of the rectum, usually a forward protrusion of the rectum into the posterior wall of the vagina in association with prolapse of the uterus. It is repaired by posterior *colporrhaphy.

proctoclysis n. an infusion of fluid into the rectum: formerly used to replace fluid but rarely employed now.

proctocolectomy n. a surgical operation in which the rectum and colon are removed. In **panproctocolectomy** the whole rectum and colon are removed, necessitating either a permanent opening of the ileum (see ILEOSTOMY) or the construction of an *ileal pouch. This is usually performed for ulcerative *colitis.

proctocolitis n. inflammation of the rectum and colon, usually due to ulcerative *colitis. See also PROCTITIS.

proctodeum n. the site of the embryonic anus, marked by a depression lined with ectoderm. The membrane separating it from the hindgut breaks down in the third month of gestation. Compare STOMODEUM.

proctodynia n. see PROCTALGIA.

proctogram an X-ray photograph of the rectum taken after the introduction into it of a contrast medium. A **defecating proctogram** demonstrates problems of abnormal defecation.

proctology n. the study of disorders of the rectum and anus.

proctorrhaphy n. a surgical operation to stitch tears of the rectum or anus.

proctoscope n. an illuminated instrument through which the lower part of the rectum and the anus may be inspected and minor procedures (such as injection

therapy for haemorrhoids) carried out. —**proctoscopy** n.

proctosigmoiditis n. inflammation of the rectum and the sigmoid (lower) colon. See also PROCTOCOLITIS.

proctotomy n. incision into the rectum or anus to relieve *stricture (narrowing) of these canals or to open an imperforate (closed) anus.

procyclidine n. a drug, similar in its effects to *atropine, used to reduce muscle tremor and rigidity in parkinsonism. It is administered by mouth or injection; common side-effects include dry mouth, blurred vision, and giddiness. Trade names: **Arpicolin, Kemadrin**.

prodromal adj. relating to the period of time between the appearance of the first symptoms of an infectious disease and the development of a rash or fever. A **prodromal rash** is one preceding the full rash of an infectious disease.

prodrome n. a symptom indicating the onset of a disease.

proenzyme (zymogen) n. the inactive form in which certain enzymes (e.g. digestive enzymes) are originally produced and secreted. The existence of this inactive form prevents the enzyme from breaking down the cells in which it was made. Once the proenzyme has been secreted it is converted to the active form.

proerythroblast n. the earliest recognizable precursor of the red blood cell (erythrocyte). It is found in the bone marrow and has a large nucleus and a cytoplasm that stains deep blue with *Romanowsky stains. See also ERYTHROBLAST, ERYTHROPOIESIS.

profunda adj. describing blood vessels that are deeply embedded in the tissues they supply.

profundaplasty n. surgical enlargement of the junction of the femoral artery and its deep branch, a common operation to relieve narrowing by atherosclerosis at this point.

progeria n. a very rare condition in which all the signs of old age appear and progress in a child, so that 'senility' is reached before puberty.

progesterone n. a steroid hormone secreted by the *corpus luteum of the ovary, the placenta, and also (in small amounts) by the adrenal cortex and testes. It is responsible for preparing the inner lining (endometrium) of the uterus for pregnancy. If fertilization occurs it maintains the uterus throughout pregnancy and prevents the further release of eggs from the ovary. See also MENSTRUAL CYCLE, PROGESTOGEN.

progestogen n. one of a group of naturally occurring or synthetic steroid hormones, including *progesterone, that maintain the normal course of pregnancy. Progestogens are used to treat premenstrual tension, *amenorrhoea, and abnormal bleeding from the uterus. Because they prevent ovulation, progestogens are a major constituent of *oral contraceptives and other forms of hormonal *contraception. Synthetic progestogens may be taken by mouth but the naturally occurring hormone must be given by intramuscular injection or subcutaneous implant, as it is rapidly broken down in the liver.

proglottis n. (pl. **proglottids** or **proglottides**) one of the segments of a *tapeworm. Mature segments, situated at the posterior end of the worm, each consist mainly of a branched uterus packed with eggs.

prognathism n. the state of one jaw being markedly larger than the other and therefore in front of it. —**prognathic** adj.

prognosis n. an assessment of the future course and outcome of a patient's disease, based on knowledge of the course of the disease in other patients together with the general health, age, and sex of the patient.

progressive supranuclear palsy a progressive neurological disorder resulting from degeneration of the motor neurones, basal ganglia, and brainstem. Starting in late middle age, it is characterized by a staring facial expression due to impaired ability to move the eyes up and down, progressing to difficulties in swallowing, speech, balance, and movement and general spasticity.

proguanil n. a drug that kills malaria parasites and is used in the prevention

and treatment of malaria. It is administered by mouth and rarely causes side-effects. Trade name: **Paludrine**.

proinsulin n. a substance produced in the pancreas from which the hormone *insulin is derived.

projection n. (in psychology) the attribution of one's own qualities to other people. This is one of the *defence mechanisms; people who cannot tolerate their own feelings (e.g. anger) may cope by imagining that other people have those feelings (e.g. are persecuting).

projective test a way of measuring aspects of personality, in which the subject is asked to talk freely about ambiguous objects. His responses are then analysed. Examples are the *Rorschach test and the Thematic Apperception Test (in which the subject invents stories about a set of pictures).

prokinetic agent an agent that induces movement, especially intestinal activity.

prolactin (lactogenic hormone, luteotrophic hormone, luteotrophin) n. a hormone, synthesized and stored in the anterior pituitary gland, that stimulates milk production after childbirth and also stimulates production of *progesterone by the *corpus luteum in the ovary. In both sexes excessive secretion of prolactin gives rise to abnormal production of milk (galactorrhoea).

prolapse n. downward displacement of an organ or tissue from its normal position, usually the result of weakening of the supporting tissues. Prolapse of the uterus and/or vagina is, in most cases, caused by stretching and/or tearing of the supporting tissues during childbirth. The cervix may be visible at the vaginal opening or the uterus and vagina may be completely outside the opening (procidentia). Treatment is by surgical shortening of the supporting ligaments and narrowing of the vagina and vaginal orifice (see COLPORRHAPHY, COLPOPERINEORRHAPHY). In prolapse of the rectum, the rectum descends to lie outside the anus.

prolapsed intervertebral disc (PID) a 'slipped disc': protrusion of the pulpy inner material of an *intervertebral disc through the fibrous outer coat, causing pressure on adjoining nerve roots, ligaments, etc. The condition often results from sudden twisting or bending of the backbone. Pressure on a nerve root causes *sciatica, and if severe may damage the nerve's function, leading to abnormalities or loss of sensation, muscle weakness, or loss of tendon reflexes. 70–80% of patients improve with conservative treatment of rest and analgesics, and traction may help. If these fail, the protruding portion of the disc is surgically removed (see LAMINECTOMY, MICRODISCECTOMY).

proline *n.* an *amino acid found in many proteins.

promazine *n.* a phenothiazine *antipsychotic drug used to relieve agitation, confusion, severe pain, anxiety, nausea, and vomiting and in the treatment of alcoholism and drug withdrawal symptoms. It is administered by mouth or injection; common side-effects are drowsiness and dizziness. Trade name: **Sparine**.

promegakaryocyte *n.* an immature cell, found in the bone marrow, that develops into a *megakaryocyte.

promethazine *n.* a powerful *antihistamine drug used to treat allergic conditions and – because of its sedative action – insomnia. It is also used as an *antitussive in cough mixtures. Promethazine is administered by mouth or injection; side-effects include drowsiness, dizziness, and confusion. Trade names: **Avomine**, **Phenergan**.

prominence *n.* (in anatomy) a projection, such as a projection on a bone.

promontory *n.* (in anatomy) a projecting part of an organ or other structure.

promoter (in oncogenesis) *n.* a substance that, in conjunction with an *initiator, leads to the production of a cancer.

prompting *n.* a technique used in *behaviour modification to elicit a response not previously present. The subject is made to engage passively in the required behaviour by instructions or by being physically put through the movements. The behaviour can then be rewarded (see REINFORCEMENT). This is followed by **fading**, in which the prompting is gradu-

ally withdrawn and the reinforcement maintained.

promyelocyte (premyelocyte) *n.* one of the series of cells that gives rise to the *granulocytes (a type of white blood cell). It has abundant cytoplasm that, with *Romanowsky stains, appears blue with reddish granules (compare MYELOBLAST, MYELOCYTE). Promyelocytes are normally found in the blood-forming tissue of the bone marrow but may appear in the blood in a variety of diseases. See also GRANULOPOIESIS.

pronation *n.* the act of turning the hand so that the palm faces downwards. In this position the bones of the forearm (radius and ulna) are crossed. Compare SUPINATION.

pronator *n.* any muscle that causes pronation of the forearm and hand; for example, the **pronator teres**, a two-headed muscle arising from the humerus and ulna, close to the elbow, and inserted into the radius.

prone *adj.* **1.** lying with the face downwards. **2.** (of the forearm) in the position in which the palm of the hand faces downwards (see PRONATION). Compare SUPINE.

pronephros *n.* the first kidney tissue that develops in the embryo. It is not functional and soon disappears. Compare MESONEPHROS, METANEPHROS.

pronucleus *n.* (pl. **pronuclei**) the nucleus of either the ovum or spermatozoon after fertilization but before the fusion of nuclear material. The pronuclei are larger than the normal nucleus and have a diffuse appearance.

propantheline *n.* a drug that decreases activity of smooth muscle (see PARASYMPATHOLYTIC) and is used to treat certain disorders of the digestive system, including stomach and duodenal ulcers, and enuresis (bed wetting). It is administered by mouth or injection; side-effects include dry mouth and blurred vision. Trade name: **Pro-Banthine**.

properdin *n.* a group of substances in blood plasma that, in combination with *complement and magnesium ions, is capable of destroying certain bacteria and viruses. The properdin complex occurs naturally, rather than as the result of previous exposure to microorganisms, and its activity is not directed against any particular species. *Compare* ANTIBODY.

proper officer *see* PUBLIC HEALTH PHYSICIAN.

prophase *n.* the first stage of *mitosis and of each division of *meiosis, in which the chromosomes become visible under the microscope. The first prophase of meiosis ocurs in five stages (*see* LEPTOTENE, ZYGOTENE, PACHYTENE, DIPLOTENE, DIAKINESIS).

prophylactic *n.* an agent that prevents the development of a condition or disease. An example is *glyceryl trinitrate, which is used to prevent attacks of angina.

prophylaxis *n.* any means taken to prevent disease, such as immunization against diphtheria or whooping cough, or *fluoridation to prevent dental decay in children. —**prophylactic** *adj.*

propositus (proband) *n.* the first individual studied in an investigation of several related patients with an inherited or familial disorder.

propranolol *n.* a drug (*see* BETA BLOCKER) used to treat abnormal heart rhythm, angina, and high blood pressure and also taken to relieve anxiety. It is administered by mouth or injection; common side-effects include digestive upsets, insomnia, and lassitude. Trade name: **Inderal**.

proprietary name (in pharmacy) the trade name of a drug: the name assigned to it by the firm that manufactured it. For example, Zantac is the proprietary name for ranitidine.

proprioceptor *n.* a specialized sensory nerve ending (*see* RECEPTOR) that monitors internal changes in the body brought about by movement and muscular activity. Proprioceptors located in muscles and tendons transmit information that is used to coordinate muscular activity (*see* STRETCH RECEPTOR, TENDON ORGAN). *See also* MECHANORECEPTOR.

proptometer *n. see* EXOPHTHALMOMETER.

proptosis *n.* forward displacement of an organ, especially the eye (*see* EXOPHTHALMOS).

propylthiouracil *n.* a drug that reduces thyroid activity and is used to treat *thyrotoxicosis and to prepare patients for surgical removal of the thyroid gland. It is administered by mouth; side-effects may include rashes and digestive upsets.

prorennin *n. see* RENNIN.

Proscar *n. see* FINASTERIDE.

prosencephalon *n.* the forebrain.

prosop- (prosopo-) *prefix denoting* the face. Example: **prosopodynia** (pain in).

prospective study **1.** a forward-looking review of a group of individuals in relation to morbidity. **2.** *see* COHORT STUDY.

prostaglandin *n.* one of a group of hormone-like substances present in a wide variety of tissues and body fluids (including the uterus, brain, lungs, kidney, and semen). Prostaglandins have many actions; for example, they cause contraction of smooth muscle (including that of the uterus), dilation of blood vessels, and are mediators in the process of inflammation (aspirin and other *NSAIDs act by blocking their production). They are also involved in the production of mucus in the stomach, which provides protection against acid gastric juice; use of NSAIDs reduces this effect and predisposes to peptic ulceration, the principal side-effect of these drugs. There are nine classes of prostaglandins (PGA–I), within which individual prostaglandins are denoted by numerals (e.g. PGE_1). Synthetic prostaglandins are used to induce labour or produce abortion (*see* DINOPROST, GEMEPROST), to treat peptic ulcers (*see* MISOPROSTOL), and in the treatment of newborn babies with congenital heart disease (*see* ALPROSTADIL) and of glaucoma (*see* LATANOPROST).

prostate cancer a malignant tumour (*carcinoma) of the prostate gland, a common form of cancer in elderly men. It may progress slowly over many years and give symptoms similar to those of benign enlargement of the prostate (*see* PROSTATE GLAND). Usually it has invaded locally, spread to regional lymph nodes, and metastasized to bone before clinical presentation. The tumour is associated with increased production of an enzyme, *prostatic specific antigen. Drug treatment aimed at suppressing the production or effects of androgen, on which the tumour is dependent, includes oestrogen therapy and the administration of *anti-androgens and *LHRH analogues. Surgical treatment includes radical *prostatectomy and *orchidectomy.

prostatectomy *n.* surgical removal of the prostate gland. The operation is necessary to relieve retention of urine due to enlargement of the prostate or to cure the symptoms of frequency and poor urinary flow due to the same cause. The operation can be performed through the bladder (**transvesical prostatectomy**) or through the surrounding capsule of the prostate (**retropubic prostatectomy**). In the operation of **transurethral prostatectomy** (or **transurethral resection**) some or all the obstructing prostate can be removed through the urethra using a resectoscope (*see* RESECTION). **Radical** (or **total**) **prostatectomy** is undertaken for the treatment of prostate cancer that is confined to the gland. It entails removal of the prostate together with its capsule and the seminal vesicles. Continuity of the urinary tract is achieved by anastomosing the bladder to the divided urethra.

The prostate gland and associated structures (median view)

prostate gland a male accessory sex gland that opens into the urethra just below the bladder and vas deferens (see illustration). During ejaculation it secretes an alkaline fluid that forms part of the *semen. The prostate may become enlarged in elderly men (**benign prostatic hypertrophy; BPH**). This obstructs the neck of the bladder, impairing urination.

The bladder dilates and the increased pressure is transmitted through the ureters to the kidney nephrons, leading to damage and impaired function of the kidneys. Treatment is by transurethral *resection of the prostate (*see also* PROSTATECTOMY) or by means of drugs (*finasteride or alpha blockers).

prostatic specific antigen (PSA) an enzyme produced by the glandular epithelium of the prostate. Increased quantities are secreted when the gland enlarges and levels of PSA in the blood are significantly elevated in cancer of the prostate, although there is no clear 'cut-off' level for normality. PSA levels tend to be much higher in advanced prostate cancer and the rate of fall on treatment is a good prognostic indicator of response.

prostatitis *n.* inflammation of the prostate gland. This may be due to bacterial infection and can be either acute or chronic. In acute prostatitis the patient has all the symptoms of a urinary infection, including pain in the perineal area, temperature, and shivering. Treatment is by antibiotic administration. In chronic prostatitis the urinary symptoms are variable; if urinary obstruction develops, transurethral *prostatectomy is indicated.

prostatorrhoea *n.* an abnormal discharge of fluid from the prostate gland. This occurs in some patients with acute *prostatitis, who complain of a profuse discharge from the urethra. The discharge is usually thin and watery and is often sterile on culture. The discharge usually subsides when the underlying prostatitis is controlled.

prosthesis (*pl.* **prostheses**) *n.* any artificial device that is attached to the body as an aid. Prostheses include bridges, dentures, artificial parts of the face, artificial limbs, hearing aids and cochlear implants, implanted pacemakers, and many other substitutes for parts of the body that are missing or nonfunctional. **Penile prostheses** are malleable, semirigid, or inflatable rods inserted into the corpora cavernosa of the penis to produce rigidity sufficient for vaginal penetration in men with impotence. —**prosthetic** *adj.*

prosthetic dentistry (prosthodontics) the branch of dentistry that is concerned with the provision of *dentures, *bridges, and implant-retained prostheses.

prosthodontics *n. see* PROSTHETIC DENTISTRY.

protamine *n.* one of a group of simple proteins that can be conjugated with nucleic acids to form nucleoproteins. Protamine can also be combined with *insulin and zinc to form **protamine zinc insulin**, which − when injected − is absorbed much more slowly than ordinary insulin and thus reduces the frequency of injections.

protanopia *n.* a defect in colour vision in which affected individuals are insensitive to red light and confuse reds, yellows, and greens. *Compare* DEUTERANOPIA, TRITANOPIA.

protease *n.* any enzyme that catalyses the splitting of a protein. *See also* PROTEOLYTIC ENZYME.

protease inhibitor any one of a new class of drugs undergoing clinical evaluation for the treatment of *AIDS. Used in combination with other antiviral agents, they act by inhibiting the action of protease, an enzyme produced by HIV that cleaves two precursor proteins into smaller fragments. These fragments are required for viral growth, infectivity, and replication.

protein *n.* one of a group of organic compounds of carbon, hydrogen, oxygen, and nitrogen (sulphur and phosphorus may also be present). The protein molecule is a complex structure made up of one or more chains of *amino acids, which are linked by peptide bonds. Proteins are essential constituents of the body; they form the structural material of muscles, tissues, organs, etc., and are equally important as regulators of function, as enzymes and hormones. Proteins are synthesized in the body from their constituent amino acids, which are obtained from the digestion of protein in the diet. Excess protein, not required by the body, can be converted into glucose and used as an energy source.

proteinuria *n.* the presence of protein in the urine. This may indicate the presence of damage to, or disease of, the kidneys. *See also* ALBUMINURIA.

proteolysis *n.* the process whereby complex protein molecules, obtained from the diet, are broken down by digestive enzymes in the stomach and small intestine into their constituent amino acids, which are then absorbed into the bloodstream. *See* ENDOPEPTIDASE, EXOPEPTIDASE. —**proteolytic** *adj.*

proteolytic enzyme a digestive enzyme that causes the breakdown of protein. *See* ENDOPEPTIDASE, EXOPEPTIDASE.

proteose *n.* a product of the hydrolytic decomposition of protein.

Proteus *n.* a genus of rodlike Gram-negative flagellate highly motile bacteria common in the intestines and in decaying organic material. All species can decompose urea. Some species may cause disease in man: *P. vulgaris* can cause urinary tract infections.

prothrombin *n.* a substance, present in blood plasma, that is the inactive precursor from which the enzyme *thrombin is derived during the process of *blood coagulation. *See also* COAGULATION FACTORS.

prothrombin time (PT) the time taken for blood clotting to occur in a sample of blood to which calcium and thromboplastin have been added. A prolonged PT (compared with a control sample) indicates a deficiency of *coagulation factors, which − with calcium and thromboplastin − are required for the conversion of prothrombin to thrombin to occur in the final stages of blood coagulation. Measurement of PT is used to control anticoagulant therapy (e.g. with warfarin).

proto- *prefix denoting* **1.** first. **2.** primitive; early. **3.** a precursor.

protodiastole *n.* the short period in the cardiac cycle between the end of systole and the closure of the *aortic valve marking the start of diastole.

proton pump the enzyme in the *oxyntic (parietal) cells of the stomach that causes acid secretion by producing hydrogen ions in exchange for potassium ions.

proton-pump inhibitor a drug that reduces gastric acid secretion by blocking the *proton-pump within the *oxyntic (parietal) cells. Proton-pump inhibitors include **lansoprazole**, *omeprazole, and

pantoprazole; they are used for treating gastric and duodenal ulcers, reflux oesophagitis and the hypersecretion caused by *gastrinoma.

proto-oncogene *n.* a gene in a normal cell that is of identical structure to certain viral genes. Some are important regulators of cell division and damage may change them into *oncogenes.

protopathic *adj.* describing the ability to perceive only strong stimuli of pain, heat, etc. Compare EPICRITIC.

protoplasm *n.* the material of which living cells are made, which includes the cytoplasm and nucleus. —**protoplasmic** *adj.*

protoplast *n.* a bacterial or plant cell without its cell wall.

protoporphyrin IX the most common type of *porphyrin found in nature. It is a constituent of haemoglobin, myohaemoglobin, most of the cytochromes, and the commoner chlorophylls.

protozoa *pl. n.* a group of microscopic single-celled organisms. Most protozoa are free-living but some are important disease-causing parasites of man; for example, *Plasmodium, *Leishmania, and *Trypanosoma cause *malaria, *kala-azar, and *sleeping sickness respectively. See also AMOEBA.

protozoan *n.* a microorganism of the group *protozoa.

protozoology *n.* the study of *protozoa.

protriptyline *n.* a tricyclic *antidepressant drug used to treat moderate or severe depression, especially in apathetic and withdrawn patients. It is administered by mouth; side-effects include dry mouth, blurred vision, fast heartbeat, digestive disturbances, and skin rashes. Trade name: **Concordin**.

protrusion *n.* (in dentistry) **1.** forward movement of the lower jaw. **2.** a *malocclusion in which some of the teeth are further forward than usual. Compare RETRUSION.

protuberance *n.* (in anatomy) a rounded projecting part, e.g. the projecting part of the chin (**mental protuberance**).

provitamin *n.* a substance that is not itself a vitamin but can be converted to a vitamin in the body. An example is β-carotene, which can be converted into vitamin A.

proximal *adj.* (in anatomy) situated close to the origin or point of attachment or close to the median line of the body. Compare DISTAL.

Prozac *n.* see FLUOXETINE.

prune belly syndrome a hereditary condition, occurring exclusively in males, characterized by a deficiency of abdominal muscles, complex malformation of the urinary tract, and bilateral undescended testes. The lungs may be underdeveloped. The name derives from the typically wrinkled appearance of the skin over the abdomen.

prurigo *n.* an intensely itchy eruption of small papules. **Besnier's prurigo** is a type of chronic atopic *eczema that is lichenified (see LICHENIFICATION). **Nodular prurigo** is a condition of unknown cause, although it is usually found in atopic individuals (see ATOPY). Very severe itching characterizes these nodules, which mostly occur on the distal limbs. **Prurigo of pregnancy** occurs in 1 in 300 women in the middle trimester of pregnancy, affecting mainly the abdomen and the extensor surfaces of the limbs. It may recur in later pregnancies.

pruritus *n.* itching. Mediated by histamine and other vasoactive chemicals, it is the predominant symptom of atopic *eczema, *lichen planus, and many other skin diseases. It also occurs in the elderly and may be a manifestation of psychological illness. Perineal itching is common: itching of the vulva in women (**pruritus vulvae**) may be accompanied by itching of the anal region (**pruritus ani**), although the latter is more common in men. Causes of perineal itching include poor hygiene, *candidosis, *threadworms, and itchy skin diseases (such as eczema). Pruritus also occurs as a symptom of certain systemic disorders, such as chronic renal failure, *cholestasis, and iron deficiency. Treatment of pruritus is determined by the cause.

prussic acid see HYDROCYANIC ACID.

PSA *see* PROSTATIC SPECIFIC ANTIGEN.

psammoma *n.* a tumour containing gritty sandlike particles (**psammoma bodies**). It is typical of cancer of the ovary but may also be found in the meninges (the membranes surrounding the brain).

psellism *n.* a deficiency of articulation of speech, such as *stammering.

pseud- (pseudo-) *prefix denoting* superficial resemblance to; false.

pseudarthrosis (nearthrosis) *n.* a 'false' joint, formed around a displaced bone end after dislocation. Congenital hip dislocation may result in a pseudarthrosis. A pseudoarthrosis also forms when a fracture fails to unite and the bone ends are separated by fibrous tissue.

pseudoagglutination *n.* the misleading appearance of clumping that occurs during an antiserum-antigen test as a result of incorrect temperature or acidity of the solutions used.

pseudocholinesterase *n.* an enzyme found in the blood and other tissues that – like *cholinesterase – breaks down acetylcholine, but much more slowly. Not being localized at nerve endings, it plays little part in the normal breakdown of acetylcholine in synapses and at neuromuscular junctions.

pseudocoxalgia *n. see* LEGG-CALVÉ-PERTHES DISEASE.

pseudocrisis *n* a false crisis: a sudden but temporary fall of temperature in a patient with fever. The pseudocrisis is followed by a return to the fever.

pseudocryptorchidism *n.* apparent absence of the testes. This is quite common in young boys, who retract their testes into the groin due to involuntary or reflex contraction of the cremasteric muscle of the suspensory cord. The condition is only important in that it needs to be distinguished from true failure of descent of the testes into the scrotum, which requires early surgical treatment (*see* CRYPTORCHIDISM).

pseudocyesis (phantom pregnancy, false pregnancy) *n.* a condition in which a nonpregnant woman exhibits symptoms of pregnancy, e.g. enlarged abdomen, increased weight, morning sickness, and absence of menstruation. The condition usually has an emotional basis.

pseudocyst *n.* a fluid-filled space without a proper wall or lining, within an organ. A **pancreatic pseudocyst** may develop in cases of chronic pancreatitis or as a complication of acute pancreatitis. As the pseudocyst, which is filled with enzyme-rich pancreatic juice, slowly expands it may cause episodes of abdominal pain accompanied by a rise in the level of enzymes in the blood. It may be felt by abdominal examination or seen by radiology or ultrasound examination. Treatment is by surgical drainage, usually by the technique of joining the pseudocyst to the stomach (*marsupialization).

pseudodementia *n.* **1.** a condition in which symptoms of *dementia, including memory disorders, are caused by depression rather than organic brain disease. It is most commonly seen in elderly depressed individuals. **2.** *see* GANSER STATE.

pseudogout *n.* joint pain and swelling, resembling gout, caused by crystals of calcium pyrophosphate in the synovial membrane and fluid. *See also* CHONDROCALCINOSIS.

pseudohermaphroditism *n.* a congenital abnormality in which the external genitalia of a male or a female resemble those of the opposite sex; for example, a woman would have enlarged labia and clitoris, resembling a scrotum and penis respectively.

pseudohypertrophy *n.* increase in the size of an organ or structure caused by excessive growth of cells that have a packing or supporting role but do not contribute directly to its functioning. The result is usually a decline in the efficiency of the organ although it becomes larger. —**pseudohypertrophic** *adj.*

pseudohypoparathyroidism *n.* a syndrome of mental retardation, restricted growth, and bony abnormalities due to a genetic defect that causes lack of response to the hormone secreted by the *parathyroid glands. Treatment with calcium and vitamin D can reverse most of the features.

pseudologia fantastica the telling of elaborate and fictitious stories as if they were true. Often some facts are woven into the tissue of lies. While not necessarily a symptom of illness, it is sometimes a feature of chronic mental illness and of personality disorders, particularly psychopathy.

pseudomembrane *n.* a false membrane, consisting of a layer of exudate on the surface of the skin or a mucous membrane. In diphtheria a pseudomembrane forms in the throat.

Pseudomonas *n.* a genus of rodlike motile pigmented Gram-negative bacteria. Most live in soil and decomposing organic matter; they are involved in recycling nitrogen, converting nitrates to ammonia or free nitrogen. The species *P. aeruginosa* is pathogenic to man, occurring in pus from wounds; it is associated with urinary tract infections. *P. pseudomallei* is the causative agent of *melioidosis.

pseudomutuality *n.* a disorder of communication within a family in which a superficial pretence of closeness and reciprocal understanding belies a lack of real feeling. It has been alleged, but not proved, to be a factor in the backgrounds of schizophrenics.

pseudomyxoma *n.* a mucoid tumour of the peritoneum, often seen in association with *myxomas of the ovary. In **pseudomyxoma peritonei** material from a myxoma, usually in the ovary, is spilled into the peritoneal cavity and continues to be produced within the abdomen, often to massive proportions.

pseudoneuritis *n.* a condition that resembles *retrobulbar neuritis but is not due to inflammation. The most usual cause is blockage of blood vessels in the optic nerve (**ischaemic optic neuropathy**).

pseudo-obstruction *n.* obstruction of the alimentary canal without mechanical narrowing of the bowel. It is usually associated with abnormality of the nerve supply to the muscles of the bowel. *See also* ILEUS, HIRSCHSPRUNG'S DISEASE.

pseudophakia *n.* the state of the eye after the natural lens has been replaced by a plastic lens implanted inside the eye, approximately in the position previously occupied by the natural lens. This is the current form of surgery for *cataract.

pseudoplegia *n.* paralysis of the limbs not associated with organic abnormalities. *See also* CONVERSION DISORDER.

pseudopodium *n.* (*pl.* **pseudopodia**) a temporary and constantly changing extension of the body of an amoeba or an amoeboid cell (*see* PHAGOCYTE). Pseudopodia engulf bacteria and other particles as food and are responsible for the movements of the cell.

pseudopolyposis *n.* a condition in which the bowel lining (mucosa) is covered by elevated or protuberant plaques (**pseudopolyps**) that are not true *polyps but abnormal growths of inflamed mucosa. It is usually found in patients with chronic ulcerative *colitis. The pseudopolyps may be seen with the *sigmoidoscope or the *colonoscope (through which they may be sampled for microscopic examination) or by barium enema examination.

pseudopseudohypoparathyroidism *n.* a condition in which all the symptoms of *pseudohypoparathyroidism are present but the patient's response to parathyroid hormone is normal. It is often found in families affected with pseudohypoparathyroidism.

pseudotumour cerebri *see* BENIGN INTRACRANIAL HYPERTENSION.

pseudoxanthoma elasticum a hereditary disease in which elastic fibres (*see* ELASTIC TISSUE) become calcified. The skin becomes lax and yellowish nodules develop in affected areas; this is accompanied by degenerative changes in the blood vessels and *angioid streaks in the retina.

psilosis *n.* *see* SPRUE.

psittacosis (parrot disease, ornithosis) *n.* an endemic infection of birds, especially parrots, budgerigars, canaries, finches, pigeons, and poultry, caused by a small intracellular bacterium, *Chlamydia psittaci*. The birds are often asymptomatic carriers. The infection is transmitted to humans by inhalation from handling the birds or by contact with feathers, faeces, or cage dust, but person-to-person transmission also occurs. The symptoms include fever, dry cough, severe muscle pain, and headache; occasionally a severe generalized systemic illness results. The condition responds to tetracycline or erythromycin.

psoas (psoas major) *n.* a muscle in the groin that acts jointly with the iliacus muscle to flex the hip joint (see illustration). A smaller muscle, **psoas minor**, has the same action but is often absent.

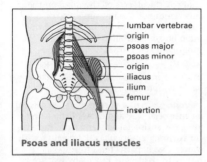

	lumbar vertebrae
	origin
	psoas major
	psoas minor
	origin
	iliacus
	ilium
	femur
	insertion

Psoas and iliacus muscles

psoralen *n. see* PUVA.

psoriasis *n.* a chronic skin disease in which scaly pink patches form on the elbows, knees, scalp, and other parts of the body. Psoriasis is one of the commonest skin diseases in Britain, affecting about 2% of the population, but its cause is not known. The disorder often runs in families, the commonest time of onset being in adolescence. It sometimes occurs in association with arthritis (*see* PSORIATIC ARTHRITIS). Occasionally the disease may be very severe, affecting much of the skin and causing considerable disability in the patient. While psychological stress may cause an exacerbation of psoriasis, the only significant event that precipitates the disease is a preceding streptococcal infection. Drugs, such as lithium or beta blockers, may occasionally be responsible.

Although there is as yet no cure, treatment of psoriasis has improved greatly in recent years. Tar and *dithranol may still be used and topical corticosteroids remain popular. The vitamin D analogues, e.g. *calcipotriol, are highly effective, while *PUVA is an effective treatment for moderately severe disease. Systemic therapy, such as *methotrexate, *retinoids, or *cyclosporin, is reserved for the worst cases.

psoriatic arthritis arthritis associated with *psoriasis. It occurs in only a small minority of patients with psoriasis but may be painful and disabling. It often affects small joints, such as the terminal joints of the fingers and toes, or the spine (*spondylitis) and the sacroiliac joints (*sacroiliitis).

psych- (psycho-) *prefix denoting* **1.** the mind; psyche. **2.** psychology.

psyche *n.* the mind or the soul; the mental (as opposed to the physical) functioning of the individual.

psychedelic *adj.* describing drugs that induce changes in the level of consciousness of the mind. Psychedelic drugs, which include *lysergic acid diethylamide (LSD) and *cannabis, are *hallucinogens and are used legally only for experimental purposes.

psychiatrist *n.* a medically qualified physician who specializes in the study and treatment of mental disorders.

psychiatry *n.* the study of mental disorders and their diagnosis, management, and prevention. —**psychiatric** *adj.*

psychic *adj.* **1.** of or relating to the *psyche. **2.** relating to parapsychological phenomena. **3.** describing a person who is endowed with extrasensory or psychokinetic powers.

psychoanalysis *n.* a school of psychology and a method of treating mental disorders based upon the teachings of Sigmund Freud (1856–1939). Psychoanalysis employs the technique of *free association in the course of intensive *psychotherapy in order to bring repressed fears and conflicts to the conscious mind, where they can be dealt with (*see* REPRESSION). It stresses the dynamic interplay of unconscious forces and the importance of sexual development in childhood for the development of personality. —**psychoanalyst** *n.* —**psychoanalytic** *adj.*

psychodrama *n.* a form of group psychotherapy in which individuals acquire insight into themselves by acting out situations from their past with other group members. *See* GROUP THERAPY.

psychogenic *adj.* having an origin in the mind rather than in the body. The term is applied particularly to symptoms and ill-nesses.

psychogeriatrics *n.* the branch of psy-chiatry that deals with the mental disor-ders of old people. —**psychogeriatric** *adj.*

psychokinesis *n.* a supposed ability of some individuals to alter the state or posi-tion of an object by the power of the mind alone, without any physical inter-vention. *See also* PARAPSYCHOLOGY.

psycholinguistics *n.* *see* COGNITIVE PSY-CHOLOGY.

psychologist *n.* a person who is engaged in the scientific study of the mind. A psy-chologist may work in a university, in in-dustry, in schools, or in a hospital. A **clinical psychologist** has been trained in aspects of the assessment and treatment of the ill and handicapped. He or she usu-ally works in a hospital, often as one of a multidisciplinary team. An **educational psychologist** has been trained in aspects of the cognitive and emotional develop-ment of children. He or she usually works in close association with schools and ad-vises on the management of children.

psychology *n.* the scientific study of be-haviour and its related mental processes. Psychology is concerned with such mat-ters as memory, rational and irrational thought, intelligence, learning, personal-ity, perceptions, and emotions and their relationship to behaviour. Schools of psy-chology differ in their philosophy and methods. They include the introspectionist Freudian, Jungian, and Adlerian schools and the gestaltist, behaviourist, and cogni-tive schools; contemporary psychology tends strongly towards the latter (*see* COG-NITIVE PSYCHOLOGY). Many practical psychol-ogists profess not to belong to any school; some take an eclectic position. The branches of psychology, on the other hand, are functional or professional sub-specialities based on practical considera-tions. They include abnormal, analytic, applied, clinical, comparative, developmen-tal, educational, experimental, geriatric, industrial, infant, physiological, and social psychology. —**psychological** *adj.*

psychometrics *n.* the measurement of individual differences in psychological functions (such as intelligence and person-ality) by means of standardized tests. —**psychometric** *adj.*

psychomotor *adj.* relating to muscular and mental activity. The term is applied to disorders in which muscular activities are affected by cerebral disturbance.

psychomotor epilepsy *see* EPILEPSY.

psychoneuroimmunology *n.* the study of the effects of the mind on the functioning of the immune system, espe-cially in relation to the influence of the mind on susceptibility to disease and the progression of a disease.

psychoneurosis *n.* a *neurosis that is manifest in psychological rather than or-ganic symptoms.

psychopath *n.* a person who behaves in an antisocial way and shows little or no guilt for antisocial acts and little capacity for forming emotional relationships with others. Psychopaths tend to respond poorly to treatment but many mature as they age. *See also* DYSSOCIAL. —**psycho-pathic** *adj.* —**psychopathy** *n.*

psychopathology *n.* **1.** the study of mental disorders, with the aim of explain-ing and describing aberrant behaviour. *Compare* PSYCHIATRY. **2.** the symptoms, col-lectively, of a mental disorder. —**psycho-pathological** *adj.*

psychopharmacology *n.* the study of the effects of drugs on mental processes and behaviour, particularly *psychotropic drugs.

psychophysiology *n.* the branch of psychology that records physiological measurements, such as the electrical resis-tance of the skin, the heart rate, the size of the pupil, and the electroencephalo-gram, and relates them to psychological events. —**psychophysiological** *adj.*

psychosexual development the process by which an individual becomes more mature in his sexual feelings and behaviour. Gender identity, sex-role behav-iour, and choice of sexual partner are the three major areas of development. The phrase is sometimes used specifically for a sequence of stages, supposed by psycho-analytic psychologists to be universal, in which oral, anal, phallic, latency, and geni-tal stages successively occur. These stages reflect the parts of the body on which sexual interest is concentrated during childhood development.

psychosis *n.* one of a group of mental disorders that feature loss of contact with reality. The psychoses include *schizophrenia, major disorders of *affect (*see* MANIC-DEPRESSIVE PSYCHOSIS), major *paranoid states, and organic mental disorders. Psychotic disorders manifest some of the following: *delusions, *hallucinations, severe thought disturbances, abnormal alteration of mood, poverty of thought, and grossly abnormal behaviour. Many cases of psychotic illness respond well to *antipsychotic drugs in that these drugs, while they are being taken, often induce a state of docility, acquiescence, apparent mental normality, and conformity with social norms. —**psychotic** *adj.*

psychosomatic *adj.* relating to or involving both the mind and body: usually applied to illnesses that are caused by the interaction of mental and physical factors. Certain physical illnesses, including asthma, eczema, and peptic ulcer, are thought to be in part a response to psychological and social stresses. Psychological treatments sometimes have a marked effect, but are usually much less effective than physical treatments for such illnesses.

psychosurgery *n.* surgery on the brain to relieve psychological symptoms. The procedure is irreversible and is therefore reserved for the most severe and intractable of symptoms, particularly severe chronic anxiety, depression, and untreatable pain. Side-effects can be severe but are less common with modern selective operations. —**psychosurgical** *adj.*

psychotherapy *n.* psychological (as opposed to physical) methods for the treatment of mental disorders and psychological problems. There are many different approaches to psychotherapy, including *psychoanalysis, *client-centred therapy, *group therapy, and *family therapy. These approaches share the views that the relationship between therapist and client is of prime importance, that the goal is to help personal development and self-understanding generally rather than only to remove symptoms, and that

the therapist does not direct the client's decisions. They have all been very widely applied to differing clinical conditions but are of little or no value as treatments of mental illness. *See also* BEHAVIOUR THERAPY, COGNITIVE THERAPY, COUNSELLING. —**psychotherapeutic** *adj.* —**psychotherapist** *n.*

psychoticism *n.* a dimension of personality derived from psychometric tests, which appears to indicate a degree of emotional coldness and some cognitive impairment.

psychotropic *adj.* describing drugs that affect mood. *Antidepressants, *sedatives, *stimulants, and *tranquillizers are psychotropic.

psychro- *prefix denoting* cold.

psychrophilic *adj.* describing organisms, especially bacteria, that grow best at temperatures of 0–25°C. *Compare* MESOPHILIC, THERMOPHILIC.

PTC **1.** *see* PERCUTANEOUS TRANSHEPATIC CHOLANGIOPANCREATOGRAPHY. **2.** *see* PHENYLTHIOCARBAMIDE.

pterion *n.* the point on the side of the skull at which the sutures between the *parietal, *temporal, and *sphenoid bones meet.

pteroylglutamic acid *see* FOLIC ACID.

pterygium *n.* a triangular overgrowth of the cornea, usually the inner side, by thickened and degenerative conjunctiva. It is most commonly seen in people from dry hot dusty climates, and only rarely interferes with vision.

pterygo- *prefix denoting* the pterygoid process of the sphenoid bone. Example: **pterygomaxillary** (of the pterygoid process and the maxilla).

pterygoid process either of two large processes of the *sphenoid bone.

ptomaine *n.* any of various substances produced in decaying foodstuffs and responsible for the unpleasant taste and smell of such foods. These compounds – which include putrescine, cadaverine, and neurine – were formerly thought to be responsible for food poisoning, but although they are often associated with toxic bacteria they themselves are harmless.

ptosis (blepharoptosis) *n.* drooping of the upper eyelid, for which there are several causes. It may be due to a disorder of the third cranial nerve (*oculomotor nerve), in which case it is likely to be accompanied by paralysis of eye movements causing double vision and an enlarged pupil. When part of *Horner's syndrome, ptosis is accompanied by a small pupil and an absence of sweating on that side of the face. It may be due to *myasthenia gravis, in which the ptosis increases with fatigue and is part of a more widespread fatiguable weakness. Ptosis may also occur as an isolated congenital feature or as part of a disease of the eye muscles, when it is associated with weak or absent eye movements.

-ptosis *suffix denoting* a lowered position of an organ or part; prolapse. Example: **colpoptosis** (of the vagina).

PTSD *see* POST-TRAUMATIC STRESS DISORDER.

ptyal- (ptyalo-) *prefix denoting* saliva. Example: **ptyalorrhoea** (excessive flow of).

ptyalin *n.* an enzyme (an *amylase) found in saliva.

ptyalism (sialorrhoea) *n.* the excessive production of saliva: a symptom of certain nervous disorders, poisoning (by mercury, mushrooms, or organophosphates), or infection (rabies). *Compare* DRY MOUTH.

ptyalith *n.* a stone (*calculus) in a salivary gland or duct.

ptyalography *n. see* SIALOGRAPHY.

puberty *n.* the time at which the onset of sexual maturity occurs and the reproductive organs become functional. This is manifested in both sexes by the appearance of *secondary sexual characteristics (e.g. deepening of the voice in boys; growth of breasts in girls) and in girls by the start of *menstruation. These changes are brought about by an increase in sex hormone activity due to stimulation of the ovaries and testes by pituitary hormones. *See also* ANDROGEN, OESTROGEN, PRECOCIOUS PUBERTY. —**pubertal** *adj.*

pubes *n.* **1.** the body surface that overlies the pubis, at the front of the pelvis. It is covered with **pubic hair**. **2.** *see* PUBIS. —**pubic** *adj.*

pubiotomy *n.* an operation to divide the pubic bone near the symphysis, the front midline where the left and right pubic bones meet. Pubiotomy is performed during childbirth if it is found necessary to increase the size of an abnormally small pelvis to allow passage of the child and a Caesarean section is contraindicated. It is also done to facilitate access to the base of the bladder and the urethra during complex urological procedures (e.g. *urethroplasty).

pubis *n.* (*pl.* **pubes**) a bone forming the lower and anterior part of each side of the *hip bone (*see also* PELVIS). The two pubes meet at the front of the pelvis at the **pubic symphysis**. *See also* PUBES.

Public Health Inspector (in Britain) the former title of the Environmental Health Officer.

Public Health Laboratory (in Britain) a regional service, with headquarters at Colindale Avenue, London, to assist with the investigation and control of infections. Such laboratories are a separate organization from hospital laboratories, but they can be located within a hospital and can contribute to the day-to-day diagnosis of hospital in-patients and out-patients.

public health medicine the branch of medicine concerned with assessing needs and trends in health and disease of populations as distinct from individuals. Formerly known as **community medicine** or **social medicine**, it includes *epidemiology, *health promotion, *health service planning and evaluation, communicable disease control, and environmental hazards. *See also* PUBLIC HEALTH PHYSICIAN.

public health nurse *see* HEALTH VISITOR.

public health physician (in Britain) a doctor of consultant status with special postgraduate training in public health medicine. Formerly known as **community physicians**, they undertake public health functions in the *National Health Service, either as **Directors of Public Health** or as consultants in public health. In some districts the Director of Public Health may act as **proper officer** to the appropriate local authority, giving epidemiological and other medical advice to the *Environmental Health Officer. More usually, however, there are specific posts as *consultants for communicable disease control (CCDC), who undertake the role of proper officer.

pudendal nerve the nerve that supplies the lowest muscles of the pelvic floor and the anal sphincter. It is often damaged in childbirth, causing incontinence.

pudendum *n.* (*pl.* **pudenda**) the external genital organs, especially those of the female (*see* VULVA). —**pudendal** *adj.*

puerperal *adj.* relating to childbirth or the period that immediately follows it.

puerperal depression a state of pathological sadness that sometimes affects a woman soon after the birth of her baby. The condition usually starts suddenly and without warning on the second or third day after delivery and usually resolves in about two months. In most cases the depression is not severe, but in about one case in 1000 it becomes serious enough to require admission to hospital. In these cases careful supervision and treatment are essential as there is a risk that the woman may kill herself or her baby.

puerperal infection infection of the female genital tract arising as a complication of childbirth.

puerperal pyrexia a temperature of 38°C occurring on any two days within 14 days of childbirth or miscarriage.

puerperium *n.* the period of up to about six weeks after childbirth, during which the uterus returns to its normal size (i.e. involution takes place).

Pulex *n.* a genus of widely distributed *fleas. P. irritans*, the human flea, is a common parasite of man and its bite may give rise to intense irritation and bacterial infection. It is an intermediate host for larvae of the tapeworms *Hymenolepis* and *Dipylidium*, which it can transmit to man, and it may also be involved in the transmission of plague.

pulmo- (pulmon(o)-) *prefix denoting* the lung(s).

pulmonary *adj.* relating to, associated with, or affecting the lungs.

pulmonary artery the artery that conveys blood from the heart to the lungs for oxygenation: the only artery in the body containing deoxygenated blood. It leaves the right ventricle and passes upwards for 5 cm before dividing into two, one branch going to each lung. Within the lungs each pulmonary artery divides into many branches, which end in capillaries in the alveolar walls. *See also* PULMONARY CIRCULATION.

pulmonary capillary wedge pressure (PCWP) pressure of blood in the left atrium of the heart, which indicates the adequacy of the pulmonary circulation. It is measured using a catheter wedged in the most distal segment of the pulmonary artery. *See also* SWAN-GANZ CATHETER.

pulmonary circulation a system of blood vessels effecting transport of blood between the heart and lungs. Deoxygenated blood leaves the right ventricle by the pulmonary artery and is carried to the alveolar capillaries of the lungs. Gaseous exchange occurs, with carbon dioxide leaving the circulation and oxygen entering. The oxygenated blood then passes into small veins leading to the pulmonary veins, which leave the lungs and return blood to the left atrium of the heart. The oxygenated blood can then be pumped around the body via the *systemic circulation.

pulmonary embolism obstruction of the *pulmonary artery or one of its branches by an *embolus, usually a blood clot derived from *phlebothrombosis of the leg veins. Large pulmonary emboli result in acute heart failure or sudden death. Smaller emboli cause death of sections of lung tissue, pleurisy, and haemoptysis (coughing of blood). Minor pulmonary emboli respond to the *anticoagulant drugs heparin and warfarin. Major pulmonary embolism is treated by *embolectomy or by dissolution of the blood clot with an infusion of *streptokinase. Recurrent pulmonary embolism may result in *pulmonary hypertension.

pulmonary hypertension a condition in which there is raised blood pressure within the blood vessels supplying the lungs (the pulmonary artery blood pressure is normally much lower than the pressure within the aorta and its branches). Pulmonary hypertension may complicate pulmonary embolism, *septal defects, heart failure, diseases of the mitral valve, and chronic lung diseases. It may also develop without any known cause (**primary pulmonary hypertension**). The right ventricle enlarges and heart failure, fainting, and chest pain occur. The treatment is that of the cause; drugs used to control *hypertension are ineffective.

pulmonary stenosis congenital narrowing of the outlet of the right ventricle of the heart to the pulmonary artery. The defect may be in the pulmonary valve (**valvular stenosis**) or in the outflow tract of the right ventricle below the valve (**infundibular stenosis**). It may be isolated or combined with other heart defects (e.g. *tetralogy of Fallot). Severe pulmonary stenosis may produce angina pectoris, faintness, and heart failure. The defect is corrected by surgery.

pulmonary tuberculosis see TUBERCULOSIS.

pulmonary vein a vein carrying oxygenated blood from the lung to the left atrium. See PULMONARY CIRCULATION.

pulp n. **1.** a soft mass of tissue (for example, of the *spleen, in which there is both **red pulp** and **white pulp**). **2.** the mass of connective tissue in the **pulp cavity**, at the centre of a *tooth. It is surrounded by dentine except where it communicates with the rest of the body at the apex. The pulp within the crown portion of the pulp cavity is described as **coronal pulp**; that within the root canal is the **radicular pulp**. **3.** the fleshy cushion on the flexor surface of the fingertip.

pulp capping the procedure of covering an exposed tooth pulp following trauma with a medicament (usually based on calcium hydroxide), which is then covered with a temporary or permanent *restoration.

pulpitis n. inflammation of the pulp of a tooth: a frequent cause of toothache.

pulpotomy n. a procedure in which part of the pulp of a tooth damaged by trauma or caries is cut back and then covered with a medicament and *restoration.

pulse n. a series of pressure waves within an artery caused by contractions of the left ventricle and corresponding with the heart rate (the number of times the heart beats per minute). It is easily detected on such superficial arteries as the radial artery near the wrist and the carotid artery in the neck. The average adult pulse rate at rest is 60–80 per minute, but exercise, injury, illness, and emotion may produce much faster rates.

pulseless disease see TAKAYASU'S DISEASE.

pulsus paradoxus a large fall in systolic blood pressure and pulse volume when the patient breathes in. It is seen in constrictive *pericarditis, pericardial effusion, and asthma.

pulvinar n. the expanded posterior end of the *thalamus.

punch-drunk syndrome a group of symptoms consisting of progressive *dementia, tremor of the hands, and epilepsy. It is a consequence of repeated blows to the head that have been severe enough to cause *concussion.

punctum n. (pl. **puncta**) (in anatomy) a point or small area, especially the **puncta lacrimalia** – the two openings of the tear ducts in the inner corners of the upper and lower eyelids (see LACRIMAL APPARATUS).

puncture **1.** n. a wound made accidentally or deliberately by a sharp object or instrument. Puncture wounds need careful treatment as a small entry hole in the skin can disguise serious injury in an underlying organ or tissue. Punctures are also performed for diagnostic purposes using a hollow needle, in order to withdraw a sample of tissue or fluid for examination; needle punctures are used especially for obtaining tissue samples for the liver, bone marrow, or breast. See also LUMBAR PUNCTURE. **2.** vb. to pierce a tissue with a sharp instrument or needle.

pupil n. the circular opening in the centre of the *iris, through which light passes into the lens of the eye. —**pupillary** adj.

pupillary reflex (light reflex) the reflex change in the size of the pupil according to the amount of light entering the eye. Bright light reaching the retina stimulates nerves of the *parasympathetic nervous system, which cause the pupil to contract. In dim light the pupil opens, due to stimulation of the *sympathetic nervous system. *See also* IRIS.

purgation *n.* the use of drugs to stimulate intestinal activity and clear the bowels. *See* LAXATIVE.

purgative *n. see* LAXATIVE.

purine *n.* a nitrogen-containing compound with a two-ring molecular structure. Examples of purines are adenine and guanine, which form the *nucleotides of nucleic acids, and uric acid, which is the end-product of purine metabolism.

Purkinje cells nerve cells found in great numbers in the cortex of the cerebellum. The cell body is flask-shaped, with numerous dendrites branching from the neck and extending fanwise among other cells towards the surface and a long axon that runs from the base deep into the cerebellum (see illustration). [J. E. Purkinje (1787–1869), Bohemian physiologist]

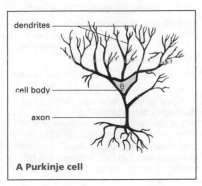

dendrites

cell body

axon

A Purkinje cell

Purkinje fibres *see* ATRIOVENTRICULAR BUNDLE.

purpura *n.* a skin rash resulting from bleeding into the skin from small blood vessels (capillaries); the individual purple spots of the rash are called **petechiae**. Purpura may be due either to defects in the capillaries (**nonthrombocytopenic purpura**) or to a deficiency of blood platelets (**thrombocytopenic purpura**).

See HENOCH-SCHÖNLEIN PURPURA, IDIOPATHIC THROMBOCYTOPENIC PURPURA, THROMBOCYTOPENIA.

purulent *adj.* forming, consisting of, or containing pus.

pus *n.* a thick yellowish or greenish liquid formed at the site of an established infection. Pus contains dead white blood cells, both living and dead bacteria, and fragments of dead tissue. *See also* MUCOPUS, SEROPUS.

push-bang technique a technique for removing a stone from the ureter. It consists of 'pushing' the stone back into the renal pelvis, where it can be destroyed by *lithotripsy ('bang').

pustule *n.* a small pus-containing blister on the skin.

putamen *n.* a part of the lenticular nucleus (*see* BASAL GANGLIA).

putrefaction *n.* the process whereby proteins are decomposed by bacteria. This is accompanied by the formation of amines (such as **putrescine** and **cadaverine**) having a strong and very unpleasant smell.

putrescine *n.* an amine formed during *putrefaction.

PUVA (photochemotherapy) psoralen + ultraviolet A: the combination of **psoralen**, a light-sensitive drug, and exposure to long-wave (315–400 nm) ultraviolet light (UVA). It was used in the East in ancient times, using natural sunlight as the light source, for the treatment of *vitiligo. PUVA was introduced into Western medicine in 1973, principally for treating *psoriasis; a number of other conditions also respond. The psoralen is usually taken as tablets but may be administered in a bath. The UVA is administered by means of specially designed light cabinets containing large numbers of fluorescent tubes.

PVS *see* PERSISTENT VEGETATIVE STATE.

py- (pyo-) *prefix denoting* pus; a purulent condition. Example: **pyoureter** (pus in a ureter).

pyaemia *n.* blood poisoning by pus-forming bacteria released from an abscess. The widespread formation of abscesses may develop, with fatal results. *Compare* SAPRAEMIA, SEPTICAEMIA, TOXAEMIA.

pyarthrosis *n.* an infected joint filled with pus. Drainage, combined with antibiotic treatment, is necessary, though the joint may already be severely damaged if diagnosis is late.

pyel- (pyelo-) *prefix denoting* the pelvis of the kidney. Example: **pyelectasis** (dilation of).

pyelitis *n.* inflammation of the pelvis of the kidney (the part of the kidney from which urine drains into the ureter). This is usually caused by a bacterial infection, which may develop in any condition causing obstruction to the flow of urine. The patient experiences pain in the loins, shivering, and a high temperature. Treatment is by the administration of a suitable antibiotic, together with analgesics and a high fluid intake. Any underlying abnormality of the urinary system must be relieved to prevent further attacks.

pyelocystitis *n.* inflammation of the renal pelvis and urinary bladder (*see* PYELITIS, CYSTITIS).

pyelogram *n. see* INTRAVENOUS PYELOGRAM, PYELOGRAPHY.

pyelography (urography) *n.* X-ray examination of the kidneys using *radiopaque contrast material. In **intravenous pyelography (excretion urography)** the contrast medium is injected into a vein and is concentrated and excreted by the kidneys (*see* INTRAVENOUS PYELOGRAM). In **retrograde pyelography**, fine catheters are passed up the ureter to the kidneys at *cystoscopy and contrast material is injected directly into the renal pelvis to allow X-ray examination. The X-ray pictures obtained from these procedures are called **pyelograms**.

pyelolithotomy *n.* surgical removal of a stone from the kidney through an incision made in the pelvis of the kidney. The incision is usually made into the posterior surface of the pelvis (**posterior pyelotomy**) to gain access to the stone, which can then be lifted clear.

pyelonephritis *n.* bacterial infection of the kidney substance. In **acute pyelonephritis**, the patient has pain in

the loins, a high temperature, and shivering fits. Treatment is by the administration of an appropriate antibiotic, and a full urological investigation is conducted to determine any underlying abnormality and prevent recurrence. In **chronic pyelonephritis**, the kidneys become small and scarred and kidney failure ensues. *Vesicoureteric reflux in childhood is one of the causes.

pyeloplasty *n.* an operation to relieve obstruction at the junction of the pelvis of the kidney and the ureter. *See* HYDRONEPHROSIS, DIETL'S CRISIS.

pyelotomy *n.* surgical incision into the pelvis of the kidney. This operation is usually undertaken to remove a stone (*see* PYELOLITHOTOMY) but is also necessary when surgical drainage of the kidney is required by a catheter or tube.

Pyemotes *n. see* PEDICULOIDES.

pyg- (pygo-) *prefix denoting* the buttocks.

pykno- *prefix denoting* thickness or density.

pyknolepsy *n. Obsolete.* a very high frequency of absence seizures (*see* EPILEPSY).

pyknosis *n.* the process in which the cell nucleus is thickened into a dense mass, which occurs when cells die. —**pyknotic** *adj.*

pyl- (pyle-) *prefix denoting* the portal vein.

pylephlebitis (portal pyaemia) *n.* septic inflammation and thrombosis of the hepatic portal vein. This is a rare result of the spread of infection within the abdomen (as from appendicitis). The condition causes severe illness, with fever, liver abscesses, and *ascites. Treatment is by antibiotic drugs and surgical drainage of abscesses.

pylethrombosis *n.* obstruction of the portal vein by a blood clot (*see* THROMBOSIS). It can result from infection of the umbilicus in infants, pylephlebitis, cirrhosis of the liver, and liver tumours. *Portal hypertension is a frequent result.

pylor- (pyloro-) *prefix denoting* the pylorus. Example: **pyloroduodenal** (of the pylorus and duodenum).

pylorectomy *n.* a surgical operation in

which the muscular outlet of the stomach (*pylorus) is removed. *See* ANTRECTOMY, PYLOROPLASTY.

pyloric stenosis narrowing of the muscular outlet of the stomach (*pylorus). This causes delay in passage of the stomach contents to the duodenum, which leads to repeated vomiting (sometimes of food eaten more than 24 hours earlier), and sometimes visible distension and movement of the stomach. If the condition persists the patient loses weight, becomes dehydrated, and develops *alkalosis. **Congenital hypertrophic pyloric stenosis** occurs in babies about 3–5 weeks old (particularly boys) in which the thickened pyloric muscle can be felt as a nodule. Treatment is by the surgical operation of *pyloromyotomy (Ramstedt's operation). Recovery is usually complete and the condition does not recur. Pyloric stenosis in adults is caused either by a *peptic ulcer close to the pylorus or by a cancerous growth invading the pylorus. Stenosis from peptic ulceration may be treated by healing the ulcer with an *antisecretory drug and dilating the pylorus with a *balloon, or by surgical removal or bypass (*see* GASTROENTEROSTOMY). Surgery is required for cancerous obstruction.

pyloromyotomy (Ramstedt's operation) *n.* a surgical operation in which the muscle around the outlet of the stomach (pylorus) is divided down to the lining (mucosa) in order to relieve congenital *pyloric stenosis.

pyloroplasty *n.* a surgical operation in which the outlet of the stomach (pylorus) is widened by a form of reconstruction. It is done to allow the contents of the stomach to pass more easily into the duodenum, particularly after *vagotomy to treat peptic ulcers (which would otherwise cause delay in gastric emptying).

pylorospasm *n.* closure of the outlet of the stomach (pylorus) due to muscle spasm, leading to delay in the passage of stomach contents to the duodenum and vomiting. It is usually associated with duodenal or pyloric ulcers.

pylorus *n.* the lower end of the *stomach, which leads to the duodenum. It terminates at a ring of muscle – the **pyloric sphincter** – which contracts to close the

opening by which the stomach communicates with the duodenum. —**pyloric** *adj.*

pyo- *prefix. see* PY-.

pyocele *n.* a swelling caused by an accumulation of pus in a part of the body.

pyocolpos *n.* the presence of pus in the vagina.

pyocyanin *n.* an antibiotic substance produced by the bacterium *Pseudomonas aeruginosa* and active principally against Gram-positive bacteria.

pyoderma gangrenosum an acute destructive ulcerating process of the skin, especially the legs. It may be associated with ulcerative *colitis or *Crohn's disease or with *rheumatoid arthritis or other forms of arthritis affecting many joints. Treatment is with high doses of corticosteroids or other *immunosuppressives.

pyogenic *adj.* causing the formation of pus. Pyogenic bacteria include *Staphylococcus aureus, Streptococcus hemolyticus,* and *Neisseria gonorrhoeae.*

pyogenic granuloma a common rapidly growing nodule on the surface of the skin; it resembles a redcurrant or, if large, a raspberry. It is composed of small blood vessels and therefore bleeds readily after the slightest injury. It never becomes malignant and is treated by *curettage and cautery.

pyometra *n.* the presence of pus in the uterus.

pyometritis *n.* inflammation of the uterus, with the formation of pus.

pyomyositis *n.* bacterial or fungal infection of a muscle resulting in painful inflammation.

pyonephrosis *n.* obstruction and infection of the kidney resulting in pus formation. A kidney stone is the usual cause of the obstruction, and the kidney becomes distended by pus and destroyed by the inflammation, which extends into the kidney substance itself and sometimes into the surrounding tissues (*see* PERINEPHRITIS). Treatment is urgent *nephrectomy under antibiotic cover.

pyopneumothorax *n.* pus and gas or air in the *pleural cavity. The condition can arise if gas is produced by gas-forming bacteria as part of an *empyema or if air is introduced during attempts to drain the pus from an empyema. Alternatively a *hydropneumothorax may become infected.

pyorrhoea *n.* a former name for *periodontal disease.

pyosalpingitis *n.* inflammation of a Fallopian tube, with the formation of pus.

pyosalpingo-oophoritis *n.* inflammation of an ovary and Fallopian tube, with the formation of pus.

pyosalpinx *n.* the accumulation of pus in a Fallopian tube.

pyosis *n.* the formation and discharge of pus.

pyothorax *n. see* EMPYEMA.

pyr- (pyro-) *prefix denoting* **1.** fire. **2.** a burning sensation. **3.** fever.

pyramid *n.* **1.** one of the conical masses that make up the medulla of the *kidney, extending inwards from a base inside the cortex towards the pelvis of the kidney. **2.** one of the elongated bulging areas on the anterior surface of the *medulla oblongata in the brain, extending downwards to the spinal cord. **3.** one of the divisions of the vermis of the *cerebellum in the middle lobe. **4.** a protrusion of the medial wall of the vestibule of the middle ear.

pyramidal cell a type of neurone found in the *cerebral cortex, with a pyramid-shaped cell body, a branched dendrite extending from the apex towards the brain surface, several dendrites extending horizontally from the base, and an axon running in the white matter of the hemisphere (see illustration).

pyramidal system a collection of nerve tracts within the *pyramid of the medulla oblongata, en route from the cerebral cortex to the spinal cord. Within the pyramid fibres cross from one side of the brain to the opposite of the spinal cord; this is called the **decussation of the pyramids**.

pyrantel *n.* an *anthelmintic drug used to treat infestations with intestinal worms, especially roundworms and threadworms. It is administered by

mouth. Side-effects occur only with large doses and include headache, dizziness, skin rash, and fever. Trade names: **Antiminth**, **Combantrin**.

pyrazinamide *n.* a drug administered by mouth, usually in combination with other drugs, to treat tuberculosis. Side-effects may include digestive upsets, joint pains, gout, fever, and rashes, and high doses may cause liver damage. Trade name: **Zinamide**.

pyret- (pyreto-) *prefix denoting* fever.

pyrexia *n. see* FEVER.

pyridostigmine *n.* an *anticholinesterase drug used in the treatment of *myasthenia gravis. It is administered by mouth or injection; side-effects may include nausea, vomiting, abdominal pain, diarrhoea, sweating, and increased salivation. Trade name: **Mestinon**.

pyridoxal phosphate a derivative of vitamin B_6 that is an important *coenzyme in certain reactions of amino-acid metabolism. *See* TRANSAMINATION.

pyridoxine *n. see* VITAMIN B_6.

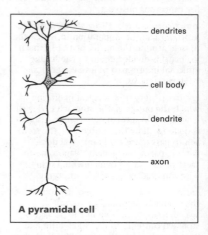

A pyramidal cell

pyrimethamine *n.* a drug administered by mouth for the prevention and treatment of *malaria, either alone or in combination with dapsone (in **Maloprim**); it is also used in the treatment of *toxoplasmosis. Possible side-effects include loss of appetite and vomiting, and prolonged use may interfere with red blood cell production. Trade name: **Daraprim**.

pyrimidine *n.* a nitrogen-containing compound with a ring molecular structure. The commonest pyrimidines are cytosine, thymine, and uracil, which form the *nucleotides of nucleic acids.

pyrogen *n.* any substance or agent producing fever. —**pyrogenic** *adj.*

pyromania *n.* an excessively strong impulse to set things on fire. —**pyromaniac** *adj., n.*

pyrosis *n.* another term (chiefly US) for *heartburn.

pyruvic acid (pyruvate) a compound, derived from carbohydrates, that may be oxidized via a complex series of reactions in the *Krebs cycle to yield carbon dioxide and energy in the form of ATP.

pyuria *n.* the presence of pus in the urine, making it cloudy. This is a sign of bacterial infection in the urinary tract.

qat *n. see* KHAT.

Q fever an acute infectious disease of many animals, including cattle, sheep, goats, deer, and dogs, that is caused by a *rickettsia, *Coxiella burnetii*; it can be transmitted to man primarily through inhalation of infected particles or consumption of contaminated unpasteurized milk but also via ticks, which can act as vectors. After an incubation period of up to three weeks a severe influenza-like illness develops, sometimes with pneumonia. The disease lasts about two weeks; treatment with tetracyclines or chloramphenicol is effective. *See also* TYPHUS.

qinghaosu *n.* a Chinese herbal drug used for 2000 years to treat *malaria. The active ingredient is a sesquiterpene lactone that greatly reduces the number of malarial parasites in the blood. Trials of the drug have recently started in the West.

QRS complex the element of an *electrocardiogram that precedes the *S–T segment and indicates ventricular contraction.

Q–T interval the interval on an *electrocardiogram that contains the deflections that are produced by ventricular contraction.

quadrantanopia *n.* absence or loss of one quarter of the *visual field (i.e. upper nasal (inner), upper temporal (outer), lower nasal (inner), or lower temporal (outer)).

quadrate lobe one of the lobes of the *liver.

quadratus *n.* any of various four-sided muscles. The **quadratus femoris** is a flat muscle at the head of the femur, responsible for lateral rotation of the thigh.

quadri- *prefix denoting* four. Example: **quadrilateral** (having four sides).

quadriceps *n.* one of the great extensor muscles of the legs. It is situated in the thigh and is subdivided into four distinct portions: the **rectus femoris** (which also flexes the thigh), **vastus lateralis**, **vastus medialis**, and **vastus intermedius** (see illustration).

- pelvic bone
- rectus femoris
- vastus lateralis
- vastus medialis
- common tibial tendon

- head of femur
- vastus intermedius
- cut end of rectus femoris

Components of the quadriceps femoris

quadriplegia (tetraplegia) *n.* paralysis affecting all four limbs. —**quadriplegic** *adj., n.*

quantitative digital radiography a method of detecting *osteoporosis. A narrow X-ray beam is directed at the area of interest (usually the spine and hip), which enables a measurement to be made of its calcium content (density). In this way the likelihood of fracture can be assessed and preventive measures considered, e.g. *hormone replacement therapy.

quarantine n. the period for which a person (or animal) is kept in isolation in order to prevent the spread of a contagious disease. The original quarantine was a period of 40 days, but different diseases now have different quarantine periods.

quartan fever see MALARIA.

Queckenstedt test a part of the routine *lumbar puncture procedure. It is used to determine whether or not the flow of cerebrospinal fluid is blocked in the spinal canal. [H. H. G. Queckenstedt (1876–1918), German physician]

quellung reaction a reaction in which antibodies against the bacterium *Streptococcus pneumoniae* combine with the bacterial capsule, which becomes swollen and visible to light microscopy.

quickening n. the first movement of a fetus in the uterus felt by the mother. Quickening is usually experienced after about 16 weeks of pregnancy although it may occur earlier.

quiescent adj. describing a disease that is in an inactive or undetectable phase.

quinestradol n. a synthetic female sex hormone (see OESTROGEN) administered by mouth to treat inflammation of the vagina, particularly after the menopause. Side-effects do not usually occur. Trade name: **Pentovis**.

quinestrol n. a synthetic female sex hormone (see OESTROGEN) used to inhibit lactation in mothers not breast feeding. It is administered by mouth and side-effects are uncommon, though nausea and vomiting sometimes occur. Trade name: **Estrovis**.

quinidine n. a drug that slows down the activity of the heart and is administered by mouth to control abnormal and increased heart rhythm. Digestive upsets and symptoms of *cinchonism may occur as side-effects. Trade names: **Kinitard, Kinidin Durules**.

quinine n. a drug used to prevent and treat *malaria, now largely replaced by more effective less toxic drugs except in cases of malaria due to *Plasmodium falciparum*. It is administered by mouth or injection; large doses can cause severe poisoning, symptoms of which include headache, fever, vomiting, confusion and damage to the eyes and ears (see CINCHONISM). Small doses of quinine are used to treat muscular cramps.

quinism n. the symptoms of overdosage or too prolonged treatment with quinine. See CINCHONISM.

quinolone n. one of a group of chemically related synthetic antibiotics that includes *ciprofloxacin, *nalidixic acid, and *ofloxacin. These drugs act by inactivating an enzyme, DNA gyrase, that is necessary for replication of the microorganisms and are often useful for treating infections with organisms that have become resistant to other antibiotics. They are administered by mouth. Possible side-effects include nausea, vomiting, diarrhoea, abdominal pain, headache, dizziness, and itching. Confusion, joint pains, skin troubles, and tendinitis occasionally occur.

quinsy n. pus in the space between the tonsil and the wall of the pharynx. The patient has severe pain with difficulty opening the mouth (*trismus) and swallowing. Treatment is with antibiotics. Surgical incision of the abscess may be necessary to release the collection of pus. Medical name: **peritonsillar abscess**.

quotidian fever see MALARIA.

Q wave the downward deflection on an *electrocardiogram that indicates the beginning of ventricular contraction.

rabbit fever *see* TULARAEMIA.

rabies (hydrophobia) *n.* an acute virus disease of the central nervous system that affects all warm-blooded animals and is usually transmitted to man by a bite from an infected dog. Symptoms appear after an incubation period ranging from 10 days to over a year and include malaise, fever, difficulty in breathing, salivation, periods of intense excitement, and painful muscle spasms of the throat induced by swallowing. In the later stages of the disease the mere sight of water induces convulsions and paralysis; death occurs within 4–5 days.

Daily injections of rabies vaccine, together with an injection of rabies antiserum, may prevent the disease from developing in a person bitten by an infected animal. —**rabid** *adj.*

racemose *adj.* resembling a bunch of grapes. The term is applied particularly to a compound gland the secretory part of which consists of a number of small sacs.

rachi- (rachio-) *prefix denoting* the spine.

rachis *n. see* BACKBONE.

rachischisis *n. see* SPINA BIFIDA.

rachitic *adj.* afflicted with rickets.

rad *n.* a former unit of absorbed dose of ionizing radiation. It has been replaced by the *gray.

radial *adj.* relating to or associated with the radius (a bone in the forearm).

radial artery a branch of the brachial artery, beginning at the elbow and passing superficially down the forearm to the styloid process of the radius at the wrist. It then winds around the wrist and enters the palm of the hand, sending out branches to the fingers.

radial keratotomy an operation for short-sightedness (myopia). Deep cuts into the tissue of the cornea are placed radially around the outer two-thirds of the cornea; this flattens the curvature of the central

part of the cornea and reduces the myopia. This procedure, used only for slight degrees of myopia, is being superseded by *excimer laser treatment.

radial nerve an important mixed sensory and motor nerve of the arm, forming the largest branch of the *brachial plexus. It extends downwards behind the humerus, supplying muscles of the upper arm, to the elbow, which it supplies with branches, and then runs parallel with the radius. It supplies sensory branches to the base of the thumb and a small area of the back of the hand.

radial reflex flexion of the forearm (and sometimes also of the fingers) that occurs when the lower end of the radius is tapped. It is due to contraction of the brachioradialis muscle, which is stimulated by tapping its point of insertion in the radius.

radiation *n.* energy in the form of waves or particles, especially **electromagnetic radiation**, which includes (in order of increasing wavelength), *gamma rays, *X-rays, *ultraviolet rays, visible light, and infrared rays (radiant heat), and the particles.

radiation sickness an acute illness caused by extreme exposure to rays emitted by radioactive substances, e.g. X-rays or gamma rays. Very high doses cause death within hours from destructive lesions of the central nervous system. Lower doses, which may still prove fatal, cause immediate symptoms of nausea, vomiting, and diarrhoea followed after a week or more by bleeding and other symptoms of damage to the bone marrow, loss of hair, and bloody diarrhoea.

radical treatment vigorous treatment that aims at the complete cure of a disease rather than the mere relief of symptoms. *Compare* CONSERVATIVE TREATMENT.

radicle *n.* (in anatomy) **1.** a small *root. **2.** the initial fibre of a nerve or the origin of a vein. —**radicular** *adj.*

radiculitis n. inflammation of the root of a nerve. See POLYRADICULITIS.

radio- prefix denoting **1.** radiation. **2.** radioactive substances.

radioactivity n. disintegration of the nuclei of certain elements, with the emission of energy in the form of alpha, beta, or gamma rays. As particles are emitted the elements 'decay' into other elements. Naturally occurring radioactive elements include radium and uranium. There are many artificially produced isotopes, including iodine-131 and cobalt-60, which are used in radiotherapy. See RADIOISOTOPE. —**radioactive** adj.

radioautography n. see AUTORADIOGRAPHY.

radiobiology n. the study of the effects of radiation on living cells and organisms. Studies of the behaviour of cancer cells exposed to radiation have important applications in *radiotherapy, revealing why some tumours fail to respond to the treatment; this had led to the development of new radiotherapeutic techniques that make tumours more susceptible to attack by radiation.

radiodermatitis n. inflammation of the skin after exposure to ionizing radiation. This may occur after a short dose of heavy radiation (radiotherapy or atomic explosions) or to prolonged exposure to small doses, as may happen accidentally to X-ray workers. The skin becomes dry, hairless, and atrophied, losing its colouring.

radiograph n. an image produced on a film by X-rays: an X-ray picture. See RADIOGRAPHY.

radiographer n. **1.** (**diagnostic radiographer**) a person who is trained in the technique of taking X-ray pictures of parts of the body. **2.** (**therapeutic radiographer**) a person who is trained in the technique of treatment by *radiotherapy.

radiography n. diagnostic radiology: the technique of examining the body by directing *X-rays through it to produce images (**radiographs**) on photographic plates or fluorescent screens. Radiography is used in the diagnosis of such disorders as broken bones, gastric ulcers, and stones in the gall bladder or kidney, when inspection from outside the body is insufficient for diagnosis. It is also widely used in dentistry for detecting dental caries, periodontal disease, periapical disease, the presence and position of unerupted teeth, and disease of the jaws.

radioimmunoassay n. a technique using radioactive *tracers to estimate the levels of natural substances in the blood through their ability to act as antigens or antibodies and bind to the radioactively labelled material. It is widely used in the estimation of hormone levels.

radioimmunolocalization n. a method of identifying the site of a tumour (e.g. colorectal cancer) that relies on its uptake of radioactive isotopes attached to an appropriate anticancer immune cell.

radioisotope n. an *isotope of an element that emits alpha, beta, or gamma radiation during its decay into another element. Artificial radioisotopes, produced by bombarding elements with beams of neutrons, are widely used in medicine as *tracers and as sources of radiation for the different techniques of *radiotherapy.

radiologist n. a doctor specialized in the interpretation of X-rays and other scanning techniques for the diagnosis of disease.

radiology n. the branch of medicine that is concerned with the use of radiation, including X-rays, and radioactive substances in the diagnosis and treatment of disease. See also INTERVENTIONAL RADIOLOGY, RADIOGRAPHY (DIAGNOSTIC RADIOLOGY), RADIOTHERAPY (THERAPEUTIC RADIOLOGY).

radionecrosis n. necrosis (death) of tissue, commonly bone or skin, whose ability to heal has been markedly reduced by previous radiation, such as radiotherapy. It can be induced by subsequent injury or surgery.

radionuclide n. a substance containing a radioactive atomic nucleus that is used as a *tracer for diagnosis in nuclear medicine.

radiopaque adj. having the property of absorbing, and therefore being opaque to, X-rays. Radiopaque materials, such as those containing iodine or barium, are used as *contrast media in radiography. Metallic foreign bodies in tissues are also radio-opaque and can be detected by radiography.

radio pill a capsule containing a miniature radio transmitter that can be swallowed by a patient. During its passage through the digestive tract it transmits information about internal conditions (acidity, etc.) that can be monitored by means of a radio receiver near the patient.

radiosensitive *adj.* describing certain forms of cancer cell that are particularly susceptible to radiation and are likely to be dealt with successfully by radiotherapy.

radiosensitizer *n.* a substance that increases the sensitivity of cells to radiation. The presence of oxygen and other compounds with a high affinity for electrons will increase radiosensitivity.

radiotherapist *n.* a doctor who specializes in treatment with radiotherapy.

radiotherapy *n.* therapeutic radiology: the treatment of disease with penetrating radiation, such as X-rays, beta rays, or gamma rays, which may be produced by machines or given off by radioactive isotopes. Beams of radiation may be directed at a diseased part from a distance (*see* TELE-CURIETHERAPY), or radioactive material, in the form of needles, wires, or pellets, may be implanted in the body. Many forms of cancer are destroyed by radiotherapy.

radium *n.* a radioactive metallic element that emits alpha and gamma rays during its decay into other elements. The gamma radiation is employed in *radiotherapy for the treatment of cancer. Because *radon, a radioactive gas, is released from radium, the metal must be enclosed in gas-tight containers during use. Radium is stored in lead-lined containers, which give protection from the radiation. Symbol: Ra. *See also* THORIUM-X.

radius *n.* the outer and shorter bone of the forearm (*compare* ULNA). It partially revolves about the ulna, permitting *pronation and *supination of the hand. The head of the radius articulates with the *humerus. The lower end articulates both with the scaphoid and lunate bones of the *carpus (wrist) and with the ulna (via the **ulnar notch** on the side of the bone).
—**radial** *adj.*

radix *n.* *see* ROOT.

radon *n.* a radioactive gaseous element that is produced during the decay of *radium. Sealed in small capsules called **radon seeds**, it is used in *radiotherapy for the treatment of cancer. It emits alpha and gamma radiation. Symbol: Rn.

rale *n.* *see* CREPITATION.

Ramsay Hunt syndrome a form of *herpes zoster affecting the facial nerve, associated with facial paralysis and loss of taste. It also produces pain in the ear and other parts supplied by the nerve. [J. R. Hunt (1872–1937), US neurologist]

Ramstedt's operation *see* PYLOROMY-OTOMY. [W. C. Ramstedt (1867–1963), German surgeon]

ramus *n.* (*pl.* **rami**) **1.** a branch, especially of a nerve fibre or blood vessel. **2.** a thin process projecting from a bone, e.g. the rami of the *mandible.

Randall's plaque the initial deposit of calcium-loaded material on a renal *pyramid that develops into a kidney stone. [A. Randall (20th century), US urologist]

randomized controlled trial *see* INTERVENTION STUDY.

random sample a subgroup of a total population (the so-called **universe**) selected by a random process ensuring that each member of the universe has an equal chance of being included in the sample. It is sometimes **stratified** so that separate samples are drawn from each of several layers of the universe, usually on the basis of age, sex, and *social class. Selection is sometimes facilitated by identifying, in advance, groups of individuals (e.g. townships or neighbourhoods) whom it is deemed will together represent the whole (a so-called **sampling frame**).

ranitidine *n.* an *antihistamine drug that inhibits gastric secretion and is used in the treatment of gastric and duodenal ulcers and reflux oesophagitis. It is administered by mouth, intravenously, and intramuscularly; side-effects include headache, rash, and drowsiness. Trade name: **Zantac**.

ranula *n.* a cyst found under the tongue, formed when the duct leading from a salivary or mucous gland is obstructed and distended.

raphe n. a line, ridge, seam, or crease in a tissue or organ, especially the line that marks the junction of two embryologically distinct parts that have fused to form a single structure in the adult. For example, the **raphe of the tongue** is the furrow that passes down the centre of the dorsal surface of the tongue.

rarefaction n. thinning of bony tissue sufficient to cause decreased density of bone to X-rays, as in osteoporosis.

rash n. a temporary eruption on the skin, usually typified by reddening – either discrete red spots or generalized reddening – which may be accompanied by itching. A rash may be a local skin reaction or the outward sign of a disorder affecting the body. Rashes commonly occur with infectious diseases, such as chickenpox and measles.

raspatory n. a filelike surgical instrument used for scraping the surface of bone (see illustration).

A rib raspatory

raspberry tumour an *adenoma of the umbilicus.

rat-bite fever (sodokosis) a disease, contracted from the bite of a rat, due to infection by either the bacterium *Spirillum minus*, which causes ulceration of the skin and recurrent fever, or by the fungus *Streptobacillus moniliformis*, which causes inflammation of the skin, muscular pains, and vomiting. Both infections respond well to penicillin.

rationalization n. (in psychiatry) the explanation of events or behaviour in terms that avoid giving the true reasons. For example, a patient may explain not going to a party in terms of being too tired whereas he did not go because he was afraid of meeting new people.

rauwolfia n. the dried root of the shrub

Rauwolfia serpentina, which contains several alkaloids, including *reserpine. Rauwolfia and its alkaloids lower blood pressure and depress activity of the central nervous system. They were formerly used as tranquillizers in the treatment of mental illness but have been replaced by more effective and reliable drugs.

Raynaud's disease a condition of unknown cause in which the arteries of the fingers are unduly reactive and enter spasm (**angiospasm** or **vasospasm**) when the hands are cold. This produces attacks of pallor, numbness, and discomfort in the fingers. A similar condition (**Raynaud's phenomenon**) may result from atherosclerosis, connective-tissue diseases, ingestion of ergot derivatives, or the frequent use of vibrating tools. Gangrene or ulceration of the fingertips may result from lack of blood to the affected part. Warm gloves and antispasmodic drugs (such as phenoxybenzamine) may relieve the condition. In unresponsive cases *sympathectomy is of value. [M. Raynaud (1834–81), French physician]

reaction formation (in psychoanalysis) a *defence mechanism by which unacceptable unconscious ideas are replaced by the opposite conscious attitude. For instance, a man might make an ostentatious show of affection to a person for whom he has an unconscious hatred.

reactive adj. describing mental illnesses that are precipitated by events in the psychological environment.

reagin n. a type of *antibody, formed against an allergen, that has special affinity for cell membranes and remains fixed in various tissues. Subsequent contact with the allergen causes damage to the tissues when the antigen-antibody reaction occurs. The damaged cells, particularly *mast cells, release histamine and serotonin, which are responsible for the local inflammation of an allergy or the very severe effects of anaphylactic shock (see ANAPHYLAXIS). Reagins belong to the IgE class of *immunoglobulins.

real-time imaging the rapid acquisition and manipulation of ultrasound information from a scanning probe by electronic circuits to enable images to be produced on TV screens almost instantaneously. The operator can accurately place the scanning probe on the region of interest in order to observe its structure and appreciate moving structures within it (*see* DOPPLER ULTRASOUND). Using similar techniques, the instantaneous display of other imaging modalities, such as CT scanning and magnetic resonance imaging, can now be achieved.

reamer *n.* an instrument used in *endodontics to prepare the walls of a root canal for *root canal treatment.

receptaculum *n.* the dilated portion of a tubular anatomical part. The **receptaculum** (or **cisterna**) **chyli** is the dilated end of the *thoracic duct, into which lymph vessels from the lower limbs and intestines drain.

receptor *n.* **1.** a cell or group of cells specialized to detect changes in the environment and trigger impulses in the sensory nervous system. All sensory nerve endings act as receptors, whether they simply detect touch, as in the skin, or chemical substances, as in the nose and tongue, or sound or light, as in the ear and eye. *See* EXTEROCEPTOR, INTEROCEPTOR, MECHANORECEPTOR, PROPRIOCEPTOR. **2.** a specialized area of a cell membrane, consisting of a specially adapted protein, that can bind with a specific hormone (e.g. *oestrogen receptors), neurotransmitter (e.g. *adrenergic receptors), drug, or other chemical, thereby initiating a change within the cell.

recess *n.* (in anatomy) a hollow chamber or a depression in an organ or other part.

recessive *adj.* describing a gene (or its corresponding characteristic) whose effect is shown in the individual only when its *allele is the same, i.e. when two such alleles are present (the **double recessive** condition). Many hereditary diseases (including cystic fibrosis) are due to the presence of a defective gene as a double recessive. They are said to show **autosomal recessive** inheritance, since the gene is carried on an autosome (any chromosome other than a sex chromosome). *Compare* DOMINANT. —**recessive** *n.*

recipient *n.* a person who receives something from a *donor, such as a blood transfusion or a kidney transplant.

recombinant DNA DNA that contains genes from different sources that have been combined by the techniques of *genetic engineering rather than by breeding experiments. Genetic engineering is therefore also known as **recombinant DNA technology**.

record linkage the means by which information about health events from several different sources (e.g. hospital attendance, vaccination, and consultation with general practitioners) are all related to a specific individual in a common file or more usually a computerized record. This contrasts with data in which events only are recorded (*see* HOSPITAL IN-PATIENT ENQUIRY) and two separate individuals treated for the same disease cannot be distinguished from one individual treated on two separate occasions.

recrudescence *n.* a fresh outbreak of a disorder in a patient after a period during which its signs and symptoms had died down and recovery seemed to be taking place.

recruitment *n.* **1.** (in physiology) the phenomenon whereby an increase in the strength of a stimulus or repetition of the stimulus will stimulate increasing numbers of nerve cells to respond. **2.** the **loudness recruitment test**: a test of hearing used to distinguish deafness due to disease of the *cochlea (in the inner ear) from other causes of deafness. In cochlear deafness, while quiet sounds are heard with difficulty in the deaf ear compared with the normal one, louder sounds are heard equally well in both ears.

rect- (recto-) *prefix denoting* the rectum. Examples: **rectouterine** (relating to the rectum and uterus); **rectovesical** (relating to the rectum and bladder).

rectocele *n. see* PROCTOCELE.

rectosigmoid *n.* the region of the large intestine around the junction of the sigmoid colon and the rectum.

rectum *n.* the terminal part of the large *intestine, about 12 cm long, which runs from the sigmoid colon to the anal canal. Faeces are stored in the rectum before defecation. —**rectal** *adj.*

rectus *n.* any of several straight muscles.

The **rectus muscles of the orbit** are some of the extrinsic *eye muscles. **Rectus abdominis** is a long flat muscle that extends bilaterally along the entire length of the front of the abdomen. The rectus muscles acting together serve to bend the trunk forwards; acting separately they bend the body sideways. The **rectus femoris** forms part of the *quadriceps.

recurrent adj. (in anatomy) describing a structure, such as a nerve or blood vessel, that turns back on its course, forming a loop.

red blood cell see ERYTHROCYTE.

redia n. (pl. **rediae**) the third-stage larva of a parasitic *fluke. Rediae develop within the body of a freshwater snail and undergo a process of asexual reproduction, giving rise to many fourth-stage larvae called *cercariae. See also MIRACIDIUM, SPOROCYST.

reduction n. (in surgery) the restoration of a displaced part of the body to its normal position by manipulation or operation. The fragments of a broken bone are reduced before a splint is applied; a dislocated joint is reduced to its normal seating; or a hernia is reduced when the displaced organ or tissue is returned to its usual anatomical site.

reduction division the first division of *meiosis, in which the chromosome number is halved. The term is sometimes used as a synonym for the whole of meiosis.

reduplication n. doubling of the heart sounds, which may be heard in healthly individuals and shows variation with respiration due to the slightly asynchronous closure of the heart valves.

reduviid n. any one of a group of winged insects (Reduviidae) whose mouthparts – adapted for piercing and sucking – take the form of a long proboscis that is tucked beneath the head when not in use. Some South American genera, notably *Panstrongylus*, *Rhodnius*, and *Triatoma* – the kissing bugs, are nocturnal bloodsucking insects that transmit the parasite causing *Chagas' disease in man.

Reduvius n. a genus of predatory bloodsucking reduviid bugs. *R. personatus*, widely distributed in Europe, normally preys upon insects but occasionally attacks man. Its bite causes various allergic symptoms, including rash, nausea, and palpitations.

Reed-Sternberg cell see STERNBERG-REED CELL.

referred pain (synalgia) pain felt in a part of the body other than where it might be expected. An abscess beneath the diaphragm, for example, may cause a referred pain in the shoulder area, while heart disorders may cause pain in the left arm and fingers. The confusion arises because sensory nerves from different parts of the body share common pathways when they reach the spinal cord.

reflex n. an automatic or involuntary activity brought about by relatively simple nervous circuits, without consciousness being necessarily involved. Thus a painful stimulus such as a pinprick will bring about the reflex of withdrawing the finger before the brain has had time to send a message to the muscles involved. See CONDITIONED REFLEX, PATELLAR REFLEX, PLANTAR REFLEX, PUPILLARY REFLEX, ROOTING REFLEX.

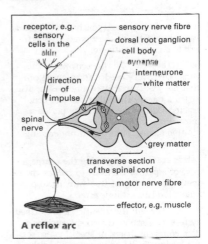

receptor, e.g. sensory cells in the skin
sensory nerve fibre
dorsal root ganglion
cell body
synapse
interneurone
white matter
direction of impulse
spinal nerve
grey matter
transverse section of the spinal cord
motor nerve fibre
effector, e.g. muscle

A reflex arc

reflex arc the nervous circuit involved in a *reflex, being at its simplest a sensory nerve with a receptor, linked at a synapse in the brain or spinal cord with a motor nerve, which supplies a muscle or gland (see illustration). In a simple reflex (such

as the *patellar reflex) only two neurones
may be involved, but in other reflexes
there may be several *interneurones in
the arc.

reflux *n.* a backflow of liquid, against its
normal direction of movement. *See also*
(REFLUX) OESOPHAGITIS, VESICOURETERIC RE-
FLUX.

refraction *n.* **1.** the change in direction
of light rays when they pass obliquely
from one transparent medium to another,
of a different density. Refraction occurs as
light enters the eye, when it passes from
air to the media of the eye, i.e. cornea,
aqueous humour, lens, and vitreous humour, to come to a focus on the retina.
Errors of refraction, in which light rays
do not come to a focus on the retina due
to defects in the refracting media or
shape of the eyeball, include astigmatism
and long- and short-sightedness. **2.** determination of the power of refraction of
the eye. This gives the degree to which the
eye differs from normal, which will determine whether or not the patient needs
glasses and, if so, how strong they should
be.

refractometer *n.* *see* OPTOMETER.

refractory *adj.* unresponsive: applied to a
condition that fails to respond satisfactorily to a given treatment.

refractory period (in neurology) the
time of recovery needed for a nerve cell
that has just transmitted a nerve impulse
or for a muscle fibre that has just contracted. During the refractory period a
normal stimulus will not bring about excitation of the cell, which is undergoing
*repolarization.

refrigeration *n.* lowering the temperature of a part of the body to reduce the
metabolic activity of its tissues or to provide a local anaesthetic effect.

regimen *n.* (in therapeutics) a prescribed
systematic form of treatment, such as a
diet, course of drugs, or special exercises,
for curing disease or improving health.

Regional Health Authority *see*
NATIONAL HEALTH SERVICE.

regional ileitis *see* CROHN'S DISEASE.

regional specialty *see* CATCHMENT AREA.

registrar *n.* (in a hospital) *see* CONSULTANT.

regression *n.* **1.** (in psychiatry) reversion
to a more immature level of functioning.
The term may be applied to the state of a
patient in hospital who becomes inconti-
nent and demanding. It may also be applied to a single psychological function;
for example, psychoanalysts speak of the
*libido regressing to an early stage of de-
velopment. **2.** the stage of a disease during which the signs and symptoms
disappear and the patient recovers.

regurgitation *n.* **1.** the bringing up of
undigested material from the stomach to
the mouth (*see* VOMITING). **2.** the flowing
back of a liquid in a direction opposite to
the normal one, as when blood surges
back through a defective valve in the
heart after the heart has contracted.

rehabilitation 1. (in *physical medicine) the treatment of an ill, injured, or
disabled patient with the aim of restoring
normal health and function or to prevent
the disability from getting worse. **2.** any
means for restoring the independence of a
patient after diseases or injury, including
employment retraining.

reimplantation *n.* *see* REPLANTATION.

reinforcement *n.* (in psychology) the
strengthening of a conditioned reflex (*see*
CONDITIONING). In classical conditioning
this takes place when a conditioned stimulus is presented at the same time as – or
just before – the unconditioned stimulus.
In operant conditioning it takes place
when a pleasurable event (or **reinforcer**),
such as a reward, follows immediately
after some behaviour. The **reinforcement
schedule** governs how often and when
such behaviour is rewarded. Different
schedules produce different effects on behaviour.

Reissner's membrane the membrane
that separates the scala vestibuli and the
scala media of the *cochlea of the ear. [E.
Reissner (1824–78), German anatomist]

Reiter's syndrome a condition characterized by inflammation of the urethra
(*see* URETHRITIS), conjunctivitis, and arthritis. Horny areas may develop on the skin.
No causative agent has been positively
identified, although a virus may be impli-

cated. [H. Reiter (1881–1969), German physician]

rejection *n.* (in transplantation) the destruction by immune mechanisms of a tissue grafted from another individual. Antibodies, complement, clotting factors, and platelets are involved in the failure of the graft to survive. *Homograft rejection is a vigorous response that can be modified by drugs, such as cyclosporin A; *heterograft rejection is a violent acute response that is at present beyond therapeutic control.

relapse *n.* a return of disease symptoms after recovery had apparently been achieved or the worsening of an apparently recovering patient's condition during the course of an illness.

relapsing fever an infectious disease caused by bacteria of the genus *Borrelia*, which is transmitted by ticks or lice and results in recurrent fever. The first episode of fever occurs about a week after infection: it is accompanied by severe headache and aching muscles and joints and lasts 2–8 days. Subsequent attacks are milder and occur at intervals of 3–10 days; untreated, the attacks may continue for up to 12 weeks. Treatment with antibiotics, such as tetracycline or erythromycin, is effective.

relative analgesia a sedation technique, used particularly in dentistry, in which a mixture of *nitrous oxide and oxygen is given. The patient remains conscious throughout; the technique is used to supplement local anaesthesia in nervous patients.

relative density *see* SPECIFIC GRAVITY.

relaxant *n.* an agent that reduces tension and strain, particularly in muscles (*see* MUSCLE RELAXANT).

relaxation *n.* (in physiology) the diminution of tension in a muscle, which occurs when it ceases to contract: the state of a resting muscle.

relaxation therapy treatment by teaching a patient to decrease his anxiety by reducing the tone in his muscles. This can be used by itself to help people cope with stressful situations or as a part of *desensitization to specific fears.

relaxin *n.* a hormone, secreted by the placenta in the terminal stages of pregnancy, that causes the cervix (neck) of the uterus to dilate and prepares the uterus for the action of *oxytocin during labour.

reline *n.* the procedure by which the fitting surface of a denture is rebased to make it fit a jaw that has undergone resorption since the denture was originally made. The procedure is often necessary for dentures that were fitted immediately after extraction of the teeth.

rem *n.* roentgen equivalent man: a former unit dose of ionizing radiation equal to the dose that gives the same biological effect as that due to one roentgen of X-rays. The rem has been replaced by the *sievert.

REM rapid eye movement: describing a stage of *sleep during which the muscles of the eyeballs are in constant motion behind the eyelids. People woken up during this stage of sleep generally report that they were dreaming at the time.

remedial profession any profession (including occupational therapy, physiotherapy, and speech therapy) in which the therapists use their skills to assist those with *disability to achieve living and working standards as near normal as possible.

remission *n.* **1.** a lessening in the severity of symptoms or their temporary disappearance during the course of an illness. **2.** a reduction in the size of a cancer and the symptoms it is causing.

remittent fever *see* FEVER.

Remploy *n.* (in Britain) a nationally financed system of sheltered employment for those with severe *disability in specially designed workshops managed and financed by the Department of Employment. Limited numbers of able-bodied craftsmen are included on the payroll to assist with administration and supervision and also to carry out tasks that would be potentially dangerous for those with disability. Goods produced (especially furniture and luggage) are sold on the open market.

renal *adj.* relating to or affecting the kidneys.

renal artery either of two large arteries arising from the abdominal aorta and supplying the kidneys. Each renal artery divides into an anterior and a posterior branch before entering the kidney.

renal cell carcinoma *see* HYPERNEPHROMA.

renal function tests tests for assessing the function of the kidneys. These include measurements of the specific gravity of urine, creatinine *clearance time, and blood urea levels; intravenous *pyelography; and renal angiography.

renal transplantation *see* TRANSPLANTATION.

renal tubule (uriniferous tubule) the fine tubular part of a *nephron, through which water and certain dissolved substances are reabsorbed back into the blood.

reni- (reno-) *prefix denoting* the kidney.

renin *n.* an enzyme released into the blood by the kidney in response to stress. It reacts with a substrate from the liver to produce *angiotensin, which causes constriction of blood vessels and thus an increase in blood pressure. Excessive production of renin results in the syndrome of renal *hypertension.

rennin *n.* an enzyme produced in the stomach that coagulates milk. It is secreted by the gastric glands in an inactive form, **prorennin**, which is activated by hydrochloric acid. Rennin converts caseinogen (milk protein) into insoluble casein in the presence of calcium ions. This ensures that the milk remains in the stomach, exposed to protein-digesting enzymes, for as long as possible. The largest amounts of rennin are present in the stomachs of young mammals.

renography *n.* the radiological study of the kidneys by a *gamma camera following the intravenous injection of a radioactive substance, which is concentrated and excreted by the kidneys. The radioactive isotope (usually *technetium-99) emits gamma rays, which are recorded by the camera positioned over the kidneys. The resultant graph of each kidney gives information regarding function and rate of drainage.

reovirus *n.* one of a group of small RNA-containing viruses that infect both respiratory and intestinal tracts without producing specific or serious diseases (and were therefore termed respiratory enteric orphan viruses). *Compare* ECHOVIRUS.

repetitive strain injury (RSI) pain with associated loss of function in a limb resulting from its repeated movement or sustained static loading. *Tenosynovitis and *tendovaginitis of the wrist associated with typing or operating a word processor is the injury most frequently encountered. When an industrial cause is identified and negligence of the employer proven, financial compensation is indicated.

replacement bone a bone that is formed by replacing cartilage with bony material.

replantation *n.* **1.** a developing specialty for the reattachment of severed limbs (or parts of limbs) and other body parts (e.g. the nose). It employs techniques of *microsurgery to rejoin nerves and vessels. **2.** (or **reimplantation**) (in dentistry) the reinsertion of a tooth into its socket after its accidental or deliberate removal. —**replant** *vb.*

A adenine
C cytosine
G guanine
T thymine

parent molecule

parent strand

complementary base pairs

new strand

replicated molecules

Replication of a DNA molecule

replication *n.* the process by which *DNA makes copies of itself when the cell divides. The two strands of the DNA molecule unwind and each strand directs the synthesis of a new strand complementary to itself (see illustration).

repolarization *n.* the process in which the membrane of a nerve cell returns to its normal electrically charged state after a nerve impulse has passed. During the passage of a nerve impulse a temporary change in the molecular structure of the membrane allows a surge of ions across the membrane (*see* ACTION POTENTIAL). During repolarization ions diffuse back to restore the charge and the nerve becomes ready to transmit further impulses. *See* REFRACTORY PERIOD.

repositor *n.* an instrument used to return a displaced part of the body – for instance, a prolapsed uterus – to its normal position.

repression *n.* (in *psychoanalysis) the process of excluding an unacceptable wish or an idea from conscious mental life. The repressed material may give rise to symptoms. One goal of psychoanalysis is to return repressed material to conscious awareness so that it may be dealt with rationally.

reproduction rate *see* FERTILITY RATE.

reproductive system the combination of organs and tissues associated with the process of reproduction. In males it includes the testes, vasa deferentia, prostate gland, seminal vesicles, urethra, and penis; in females it includes the ovaries, Fallopian tubes, uterus, vagina, and vulva. (See illustration.)

resection *n.* surgical removal of a portion of any part of the body. For example, a section of diseased intestine may be removed and the healthy ends sewn together. A **submucous resection** is removal of part of the cartilage septum (central division) of the nose that has become deviated, usually by injury. **Transurethral resection of the prostate** (**TUR** or **TURP**) – an operation performed when the prostate gland becomes enlarged – involves removal of portions of the gland through the urethra using an instrument called a **resectoscope.**

resectoscope *n.* a type of surgical instrument (an *endoscope) used in resection of the prostate or in the removal of bladder tumours.

reserpine *n.* a drug extracted from *rauwolfia. Administered by mouth or injection, it has been used to lower high blood pressure. Side-effects often include mental depression, nasal congestion, and digestive upsets.

reserve volume the extra volume of air that an individual could inhale or exhale if he is not breathing to the limit of his capacity

residual volume the volume of air

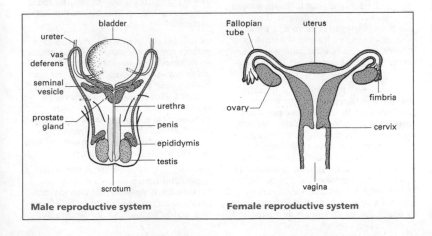

Male reproductive system   **Female reproductive system**

that remains in the lungs after the individual has breathed out as much as he can. This volume is increased in *emphysema.

resistance n. **1.** the degree of *immunity that the body possesses: a measure of its ability to withstand disease. **2.** the degree to which a disease or disease-causing organism remains unaffected by antibiotics or other drugs.

resolution n. **1.** the stage during which inflammation gradually disappears. **2.** the degree to which individual details can be distinguished by the eye, as through a *microscope.

resorcinol n. a drug that causes the skin to peel. It has been used in skin ointments to treat such conditions as acne, but with prolonged use the drug is absorbed into the body, causing underactivity of the thyroid gland (myxoedema) and convulsions.

resorption n. loss of substance through physiological or pathological means.

respiration n. the process of gaseous exchange between an organism and its environment. This includes both **external respiration**, which involves *breathing, in which oxygen is taken up by the capillaries of the lung *alveoli and carbon dioxide is released from the blood, and **internal respiration**, during which oxygen is released to the tissues and carbon dioxide absorbed by the blood. Blood provides the transport medium for the gases between the lungs and tissue cells. In addition, it contains a pigment, *haemoglobin, with special affinity for oxygen. Once inside the cell oxygen is utilized in metabolic processes resulting in the production of energy (see ATP), water, and waste materials (including carbon dioxide). See also LUNG. —**respiratory** adj.

respirator n. **1.** a device used to maintain the breathing movements of paralysed patients. In the **positive-pressure respirator** air is blown into the patient's lungs via a tube passed either through the mouth into the trachea or through a *tracheostomy. Air is released from the lungs when the pressure from the respirator is relaxed. The **iron lung** is a type of respirator in which the patient is enclosed, except for the head, in an airtight container in which the air pressure is decreased and

increased mechanically. This draws air into and out of the lungs, through the normal air passages. The **cuirass respirator** works on a similar principle, but leaves the limbs free. **2.** a face mask for administering oxygen or other gas or for filtering harmful fumes, dust, etc. See also ARTIFICIAL RESPIRATION.

respiratory distress syndrome (hyaline membrane disease) the condition of a newborn infant in which the lungs are imperfectly expanded. Initial inflation and normal expansion of the lungs requires the presence of a substance (*surfactant) that reduces the surface tension of the air sacs (alveoli) and prevents collapse of the small airways. Without surfactant the airways collapse, leading to inefficient and 'stiff' lungs. The condition is most common and serious among preterm infants, in whom surfactant is liable to be deficient. Breathing is rapid, laboured, and shallow, and microscopic examinations of lung tissue in fatal cases has revealed the presence of *hyaline material in the collapsed air sacs. The condition is treated by careful nursing, intravenous fluids, and oxygen, with or without positive pressure by a *respirator. Recently, surfactant administered at birth has produced encouraging results.

respiratory quotient (RQ) the ratio of the volume of carbon dioxide transferred from the blood into the alveoli to the volume of oxygen absorbed into the alveoli. The RQ is usually about 0.8 because more oxygen is taken up than carbon dioxide excreted.

respiratory syncytial virus (RSV) a paramyxovirus (see MYXOVIRUS) that causes infections of the nose and throat. It is a major cause of bronchiolitis and pneumonia in young children. In tissue cultures infected with the virus, cells merge together to form a conglomerate (**syncytium**). RSV is thought to have a role in *cot deaths. Vulnerable children can be treated with *ribavirin, but most children just require supportive measures.

respiratory system the combination of organs and tissues associated with *breathing. It includes the nasal cavity, pharynx, larynx, trachea, bronchi, bronchioles, and lungs and also the diaphragm and other muscles associated with breathing movements.

response n. the way in which the body or part of the body reacts to a *stimulus. For example, a nerve impulse may produce the response of a contraction in a muscle that the nerve supplies.

response prevention a form of *behaviour therapy given for severe *obsessions. Patients are encouraged to abstain from rituals and repetitive acts while they are in situations that arouse anxiety. For example, a hand-washing ritual might be treated by stopping washing while being progressively exposed to dirt. The anxiety then declines, and with it the obsessions.

restenosis n. recurrent *stenosis, especially in a heart valve or an artery after corrective surgery.

restiform body a thick bundle of nerve fibres that conveys impulses from tracts in the spinal cord to the cortex of the anterior and posterior lobes of the cerebellum.

resting cell a cell that is not undergoing division. See INTERPHASE.

restoration n. (in dentistry) any type of dental *filling or *crown, which is aimed at restoring a tooth to its normal form, function, and appearance. A **sealant restoration** (or **preventive resin restoration**) is a combination of a *fissure sealant and a small filling.

rest pain pain, usually experienced in the feet, that indicates an extreme degree of *ischaemia.

restriction enzyme (restriction endonuclease) an enzyme, obtained from bacteria, that cuts DNA into specific short segments. Restriction enzymes are widely used in *genetic engineering.

resuscitation n. the restoration of a person who appears to be dead. It depends upon the revival of cardiac and respiratory function. See also ARTIFICIAL RESPIRATION, MOUTH-TO-MOUTH RESPIRATION.

retainer n. (in dentistry) **1.** a component of a partial *denture that keeps it in place. **2.** an *orthodontic appliance that holds the teeth in position at the end of

active treatment. **3.** a component of a *bridge that is fixed to a natural tooth.

retardation n. the slowing up of a process. **Psychomotor retardation** is a marked slowing down of activity and speech, which can reach a degree where a patient can no longer care for himself. It is a symptom of severe *depression. The term *mental retardation implies a delay in intellectual development rather than a qualitative defect.

retching n. repeated unavailing attempts to vomit.

rete n. a network of blood vessels, nerve fibres, or other strands of interlacing tissue in the structure of an organ. The **rete testis** is a network of tubules conducting sperm from the seminiferous tubules of the *testis to the vasa efferentia.

retention n. inability to pass urine, which is retained in the bladder. The condition may be acute and painful or chronic and painless. The commonest cause is enlargement of the prostate gland in men, although many other conditions may result in obstruction of bladder outflow. Retention is relieved by catheter drainage of the bladder, after which the underlying problem is dealt with. See also INTERMITTENT SELF-CATHETERIZATION.

retention defect (in psychology) a memory defect in which items that have been registered in the memory are lost from storage. It is a feature of *dementia.

reticular activating system the system of nerve pathways in the brain concerned with the level of consciousness – from the states of sleep, drowsiness, and relaxation to full alertness and attention. The system integrates information from all of the senses and from the cerebrum and cerebellum and determines the overall activity of the brain and the autonomic nervous system and patterns of behaviour during waking and sleeping.

reticular fibres microscopic, almost nonelastic, branching fibres of *connective tissue that join together to form a delicate supportive meshwork around blood vessels, muscle fibres, glands, nerves, etc. They are composed of a collagen-like protein (**reticulin**) and are particularly common in lymph nodes, the spleen, liver, kidneys, and muscles.

reticular formation a network of nerve pathways and nuclei throughout the *brainstem, connecting motor and sensory nerves to and from the spinal cord, the cerebellum and the cerebrum, and the cranial nerves. It is estimated that a single neurone in this network may have synapses with as many as 25,000 other neurones.

reticulin *n.* a protein that is the major constituent of *reticular fibres.

reticulocyte *n.* an immature red blood cell (erythrocyte). Reticulocytes may be detected and counted by staining living red cells with certain basic dyes that result in the formation of a blue precipitate (**reticulum**) within the reticulocytes. They normally comprise about 1% of the total red cells and are increased (**reticulocytosis**) whenever the rate of red cell production increases.

reticulocytosis *n.* an increase in the proportion of immature red blood cells (reticulocytes) in the bloodstream. It is a sign of increased output of new red cells from the bone marrow.

reticuloendothelial system (RES) a community of cells – *phagocytes – spread throughout the body. It includes *macrophages and *monocytes. The RES is concerned with defence against microbial infection and with the removal of worn-out blood cells from the bloodstream. *See also* SPLEEN.

reticuloendotheliosis (histiocytosis X) *n.* overgrowth of cells of the *reticuloendothelial system, causing either isolated swelling of the bone marrow (**eosinophilic granuloma**) or destruction of the bones of the skull (**Hand-Schüller-Christian disease**). The most acute form, starting in infancy and usually rapidly fatal, is associated with tumours containing histiocytes in the internal organs (**Letterer-Siwe disease**).

reticulosis *n.* abnormal overgrowth, usually malignant, of any of the cells of the lymphatic glands or the immune system. *See* LYMPHOMA, HODGKIN'S DISEASE, BURKITT'S LYMPHOMA, MYCOSIS FUNGOIDES.

reticulum *n.* a network of tubules or blood vessels. *See* ENDOPLASMIC RETICULUM, SARCOPLASMIC RETICULUM.

retin- (retino-) *prefix denoting* the retina. Example: **retinopexy** (fixation of a detached retina).

retina *n.* the light-sensitive layer that lines the interior of the eye. The outer part of the retina (**retinal pigment epithelium; RPE**), next to the *choroid, is pigmented to prevent the passage of light. The inner part, next to the cavity of the eyeball, contains *rods and *cones (light-sensitive cells) and their associated nerve fibres (see illustration). A large number of cones is concentrated in a depression in the retina at the back of the eyeball called the *fovea. —**retinal** *adj.*

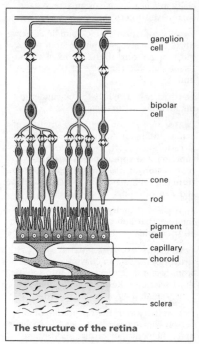

The structure of the retina

retinaculum *n.* (*pl.* **retinacula**) a thickened band of tissue that serves to hold various tissues in place. For example, **flexor retinacula** are found over the flexor tendons in the wrist and ankle.

retinal (retinene) *n.* the aldehyde of retinol (*vitamin A). *See also* RHODOPSIN.

retinal artery occlusion blockage of an artery supplying blood to the retina, usually as a result of *thrombosis or *embolism. The central retinal artery enters the eye at the optic disc and then divides into branches to supply different parts of the retina. Blockage of the central retinal artery (**central retinal artery occlusion**) usually results in sudden painless loss of vision. Blockage of one of the branches of the central retinal artery (**branch retinal artery occlusion**), usually by emboli, results in *ischaemia of the retina supplied by the occluded vessel and related visual field loss.

retinal detachment (detached retina) separation of the inner nervous layer of the *retina from the outer pigmented layer (retinal pigment epithelium) to which it is attached. It commonly occurs when one or more holes in the retina allow fluid from the vitreous cavity of the eyeball to accumulate under the retina. Vision is lost in the affected part of the retina. The condition can be treated surgically by creating patches of scar tissue between the retina and the choroid by application of extreme cold (*see* CRYO-SURGERY) or heat (*see* PHOTOCOAGULATION); this, combined with *plombage, allows reattachment of the retina.

retinal vein occlusion blockage of a vein carrying blood from the retina. Small branch veins carry blood from different parts of the retina and drain into the central retinal vein, which leaves the eye at the optic disc. Blockage of the central retinal vein (**central retinal vein occlusion**) usually results in sudden painless reduction of vision. Distended veins, haemorrhages, and *cotton-wool spots are seen in the retina and the optic disc may become swollen. Blockage of a branch of the central retinal vein (**branch retinal vein occlusion**) results in painless reduction of vision in the affected area, where engorged veins, haemorrhages, and cotton-wool spots may be seen.

retinene *n. see* RETINAL.

retinitis *n.* inflammation of the retina. In practice, the term is often used for conditions now known not to be inflammatory; for example, *retinitis pigmentosa. For such conditions the term *retinopathy is becoming more widely used.

retinitis pigmentosa a hereditary condition characterized by progressive degeneration of the *retina due to malfunctioning of the retinal pigment epithelium. It starts in childhood with *night blindness and limited peripheral vision and may progress to complete loss of vision.

retinoblastoma *n.* a rare malignant tumour of the retina, occurring in infants.

retinoid *n.* any one of a group of drugs derived from vitamin A. They bind to one or more of six specific receptors that are found on many cells. On the skin they act to cause drying and peeling and a reduction in oil (sebum) production. These effects can be useful in the treatment of severe *acne, *psoriasis, *ichthyosis, and other skin disorders. Retinoids include *isotretinoin, *tretinoin, **acitretin**, and **tazarotene**; they are administered by mouth or applied as a cream. Possible side-effects, which may be serious, include severe fetal abnormalities (if taken by pregnant women), toxic effects on babies (if taken by breastfeeding mothers), liver and kidney damage, excessive drying, redness and itching of the skin, and muscle pain and stiffness.

retinol *n. see* VITAMIN A.

retinopathy *n.* any of various disorders of the retina resulting in impairment or loss of vision. It is usually due to damage to the blood vessels of the retina, occurring (for example) as a complication of diabetes (**diabetic retinopathy**), high blood pressure, or AIDS (**AIDS retinopathy**). In diabetic retinopathy, haemorrhaging or exudation may occur, either from damaged vessels into the retina or from new abnormal vessels (*see* NEOVASCULARIZATION) into the vitreous humour. Unless treated, this may lead to permanent loss of vision. Treatment may require laser surgery (*see* PHOTOCOAGULATION).

retinoscope *n.* an instrument used to determine the power of spectacle lens required to correct errors of *refraction of the eye. It is held in the hand and casts a beam of light into the subject's eye. The examiner looks along the beam and sees the reflection in the subject's pupil. By interpreting the way the reflection moves when he moves the instrument, and by altering this by lenses held in his other hand near the subject's eye, he is able to detect long- or short-sightedness or astigmatism and to determine its degree. —**retinoscopy** n.

retraction n. **1.** (in obstetrics) the quality of uterine muscle fibres of remaining shortened after contracting during labour. This results in a gradual progression of the fetus downwards through the pelvis. The basal portion of the uterus becomes thicker and pulls up the dilating cervix over the presenting part. **2.** (in dentistry) the drawing back of one or more teeth into a better position by an *orthodontic appliance.

retraction ring a depression in the uterine wall marking the junction between the actively contracting muscle fibres of the upper segment of the uterus and the muscle fibres of the lower segment. This depression is not always visible and is normal. In obstructed labour (e.g. contracted pelvis or malposition of the fetus resulting in shoulder presentation), the muscle fibres of the upper segment become shorter and thicker; the muscle fibres of the lower segment, on the other hand, become elongated and thinner. The junction between the two becomes more distinct as it rises into the abdomen from the pelvis. This abnormal ring is known as **Bandl's ring** and is a sign of impending rupture of the lower segment of the uterus, which becomes progressively thinner as Bandl's ring rises upwards. Immediate action to relieve the obstruction is then necessary, usually in the form of Caesarean section.

retractor n. a surgical instrument used to expose the operation site by drawing aside the cut edges of skin, muscle, or other tissues. There are several types of retractors for different operations (see illustration).

retro- *prefix denoting* at the back or behind. Examples: **retrobulbar** (at the back of the eyeball); **retroperitoneal** (behind the peritoneum).

retrobulbar neuritis (optic neuritis)

inflammation of the optic nerve behind the eye, causing increasingly blurred vision. When the inflammation involves the first part of the nerve and can be seen at the optic disc, it is called **optic papillitis**. Retrobulbar neuritis is one of the symptoms of multiple sclerosis but it can also occur as an isolated lesion, in the absence of any other involvement of the nervous system, with the patient recovering vision completely.

retroflexion n. the bending backward of an organ or part of an organ, especially the abnormal bending backward of the upper part of the uterus (i.e. the part furthest from the cervix).

retrograde *adj.* going backwards, or moving in the opposite direction to the normal. (*See* (RETROGRADE) PYELOGRAPHY.) **Retrograde amnesia** is a failure to remember events immediately preceding an illness or injury.

retrography n. writing in which letters are reversed so that they appear as mirror images. Adoption of this as a consistent style is usually a matter of voluntary choice or is *hysterical; very occasionally it follows brain damage. Mirror-image reversals of single letters are common in children learning to write and in older children whose language abilities are impaired.

retrolental fibroplasia *see* FIBROPLASIA.

wound retractor

abdominal retractor

Retractors

retroperitoneal fibrosis (RPF) a condition in which a dense plaque of fibrous tissue develops behind the peritoneum adjacent to the abdominal aorta. The ureters become encased and hence obstructed, causing acute *anuria and renal failure.

The obstruction can be relieved by *nephrostomy or the insertion of double J *stents. In the acute phase steroid administration may help, but in established RPF *ureterolysis is required.

retroperitoneal space the region between the posterior parietal *peritoneum and the front of the *lumbar vertebrae. It contains important structures, including the kidneys, adrenal glands, pancreas, lumbar spinal nerve roots, sympathetic ganglia and nerves, and the abdominal *aorta and its major branches.

retropulsion n. a compulsive tendency to walk backwards. It is a symptom of *parkinsonism.

retrospective study 1. a backward-looking review of the characteristics of a group of individuals in relation to morbidity, embracing some aspects of *cross-sectional and/or *case control studies. The term is sometimes loosely used as a synonym for such studies. **2.** see COHORT STUDY.

retroversion n. an abnormal position of the uterus in which it is tilted backwards, with the base lying in the *pouch of Douglas, against the rectum, instead of on the bladder. It occurs in about 20% of women.

retrovirus n. an RNA-containing virus that can convert its genetic material into DNA by means of the enzyme *reverse transcriptase, which enables it to become integrated into the DNA of its host's cells. Retroviruses have been implicated in the development of some cancers and are associated with conditions characterized by an impaired immune system (*HIV is a retrovirus). They are also used as *vectors in gene therapy.

retrusion n. (in dentistry) **1.** backward movement of the lower jaw. **2.** a malocclusion in which some of the teeth are further back than usual. Compare PROTRUSION.

Rett's syndrome a disorder affecting young girls, in which *stereotyped movements and social withdrawal appear during early childhood. Intellectual development is often impaired and special educational help is needed. [A. Rett (20th century), Austrian paediatrician]

revascularization n. **1.** the regrowth of blood vessels following disease or injury so that normal blood supply to an organ, tissue, or part is restored. **2.** the surgical restoration of blood flow to a part by replacing a diseased blood vessel with a graft. See CORONARY REVASCULARIZATION.

reverse transcriptase an enzyme, found mainly in *retroviruses, that catalyses the synthesis of DNA from RNA. It enables the viral RNA to be integrated into the host DNA.

Reye's syndrome a rare disorder occurring in childhood. It is characterized by the symptoms of *encephalitis combined with evidence of liver failure. Often, the symptoms develop in the apparent recovery phase of a viral infection. Treatment is aimed at controlling cerebral *oedema and correcting metabolic abnormalities in order to allow spontaneous recovery, but there is still a significant mortality and there may be residual brain damage. The cause is not known, but *aspirin has been implicated and this drug should not be used in children below the age of 12 unless specifically indicated. [R. D. K. Reye (1912–77), Australian histopathologist]

rhabdomyoma n. a rare benign tumour of skeletal muscle or heart muscle.

rhabdomyosarcoma n. a rare malignant tumour originating in, or showing the characteristics of, striated muscle. **Pleomorphic rhabdomyosarcoma** occurs in late middle age, in the muscles of the limbs. **Embryonal rhabdomyosarcomas**, affecting infants, children, and young adults, are classified as **botryoid** (in the vagina, bladder, ear, etc.), **embryonal** (most common in the head and neck, particularly the orbit); and **alveolar** (at the base of the thumb). The pleomorphic and alveolar types respond poorly to treatment; botryoid tumours are treated with a combination of radiotherapy, surgery, and drugs. The embryonal type, if treated at an early stage, can often be cured with a combination of radiotherapy and drugs (including vincristine, actinomycin D, and cyclophosphamide).

rhagades pl. n. cracks or long thin scars in the skin, particularly around the mouth or other areas of the body subjected to constant movement. The fissures around the mouth and nose of babies with congenital syphilis eventually heal to form rhagades.

rheo- *prefix denoting* **1.** a flow of liquid. **2.** an electric current.

rhesus factor (Rh factor) a group of *antigens that may or may not be present on the surface of the red blood cells; it forms the basis of the rhesus blood group system. Most people have the rhesus factor, i.e. they are **Rh-positive**. People who lack the factor are termed **Rh-negative**. Incompatibility between Rh-positive and Rh-negative blood is an important cause of blood transfusion reactions and *haemolytic disease of the newborn. *See also* BLOOD GROUP.

rheumatic fever (acute rheumatism) a disease affecting mainly children and young adults that arises as a delayed complication of infection of the upper respiratory tract with haemolytic streptococci (*see* STREPTOCOCCUS). The main features are fever, arthritis progressing from joint to joint, reddish circular patches on the skin, small painless nodules formed on bony prominences such as the elbow, abnormal involuntary movements of the limbs and head (Sydenham's *chorea), and inflammation of the heart muscle, its valves, and the membrane surrounding the heart. The condition may progress to **chronic rheumatic heart disease**, with scarring and chronic inflammation of the heart and its valves leading to heart failure, murmurs, and damage to the valves. The initial infection is treated with antibiotics (e.g. penicillin) and bed rest, with aspirin to relieve the joint pain. Following an acute attack, long-term prophylaxis with penicillin is often recommended to prevent a relapse. Rheumatic fever is becoming much less common in developed countries, probably as a result of antibiotic use.

rheumatism *n.* any disorder in which aches and pains affect the muscles and joints. *See* RHEUMATOID ARTHRITIS, RHEUMATIC FEVER, OSTEOARTHRITIS, GOUT.

rheumatoid arthritis the second most common form of *arthritis (after *osteoarthritis). It typically involves the joints of the fingers, wrists, feet, and ankles, with later involvement of the hips, knees,

shoulders, and neck. It is a disease of the synovial lining of joints; the joints are initially painful, swollen, and stiff and are usually affected symmetrically. As the disease progresses the ligaments supporting the joints are damaged and there is erosion of the bone, leading to deformity of the joints. Tendon sheaths can be affected, leading to tendon rupture. Onset can be at any age, and there is a considerable range of severity. Women are at greater risk. Rheumatoid arthritis is an *autoimmune disease, and most patients show the presence of **rheumatoid factor** in their serum. There are characteristic changes on X-ray.

Treatment is with a variety of drugs, including anti-inflammatory analgesics, steroids, *methotrexate, and *gold injections. Surgical treatment is by excision of the synovium in early cases or by *fusion or joint replacement once bony changes have occurred. (*See also* HIP REPLACEMENT.) The condition may resolve spontaneously, but is usually relapsing and remitting with steady progression. It may finally burn itself out, leaving severely deformed joints.

rheumatology *n.* the medical specialty concerned with the diagnosis and management of disease involving joints, tendons, muscles, ligaments, and associated structures. *See also* PHYSICAL MEDICINE. **—rheumatologist** *n.*

rhexis *n.* the breaking apart of a blood vessel, organ, or tissue.

Rh factor *see* RHESUS FACTOR.

rhin- (rhino-) *prefix denoting* the nose.

rhinencephalon *n.* the parts of the brain, collectively, that in early stages of evolution were concerned mainly with the sense of smell. The rhinencephalon includes the olfactory nerve, olfactory tract, and the regions now usually classified as belonging to the *limbic system.

rhinitis *n.* inflammation of the mucous membrane of the nose. It may be caused by virus infection (**acute rhinitis**; *see* COMMON COLD) or an allergic reaction (**allergic rhinitis**; *see* HAY FEVER). In **atrophic rhinitis** the mucous membrane becomes thinned and fragile. In **perennial** (or **vasomotor**) **rhinitis** there is overgrowth of, and increased secretion by, the membrane.

rhinolith *n.* a stone (calculus) in the nose.

rhinology *n.* the branch of medicine concerned with disorders of the nose and nasal passages.

rhinomycosis *n.* fungal infection of the lining of the nose.

rhinophyma *n.* a bulbous craggy swelling of the nose, usually in men. It is a complication of *rosacea and in no way related to alcohol intake. Paring by plastic surgery may be necessary for cosmetic purposes.

rhinoplasty *n.* surgery to alter the shape of the nose, sometimes using tissue (skin, cartilage, or bone) from elsewhere in the body or artificial implants.

rhinorrhoea *n.* a persistent watery mucous discharge from the nose, as in the common cold.

rhinoscleroma *n.* the formation of nodules in the interior of the nose and *nasopharynx, which become thickened. It is caused by bacterial infection (with *Klebsiella rhinoscleromatis*).

rhinoscopy *n.* examination of the interior of the nose.

rhinosinusitis *n.* inflammation of the lining of the nose and paranasal sinuses. Rhinosinusitis is a common condition caused by allergies, infection, immune deficiencies, *mucociliary transport abnormalities, trauma, drugs, or tumours. *See* RHINITIS, SINUSITIS.

rhinosporidiosis *n.* an infection of the mucous membranes of the nose, larynx, eyes, and genitals that is caused by the fungus *Rhinosporidium seeberi* and is characterized by the formation of tiny *polyps. It occurs most commonly in Asia.

rhinovirus *n.* any one of a group of RNA-containing viruses that cause respiratory infections in man resembling the common cold. They are included in the *picornavirus group.

Rhipicephalus *n.* a genus of hard *ticks widely distributed in the tropics. The dog tick (*R. sanguineus*) can suck the blood of man and is commonly involved in the

transmission of diseases caused by rickettsiae (*see* TYPHUS).

rhiz- (rhizo-) *prefix denoting* a root. Example: **rhizonychia** (the root of a nail).

rhizotomy *n.* a surgical procedure in which selected nerve roots are cut at the point where they emerge from the spinal cord. In **posterior rhizotomy** the posterior (sensory) nerve roots are cut for the relief of intractable pain in the organs served by these nerves. An **anterior rhizotomy** – the cutting of the anterior (motor) nerve roots – is sometimes done for the relief of severe muscle spasm.

Rhodnius *n.* a genus of large bloodsucking bugs (*see* REDUVIID). *R. prolixus* is important in the transmission of *Chagas' disease in Central America and the northern part of South America.

rhodopsin (visual purple) *n.* a pigment in the retina of the eye, within the *rods, consisting of **retinal** – an aldehyde of retinol (*vitamin A) – and a protein. The presence of rhodopsin is essential for vision in dim light. It is bleached in the presence of light and this stimulates nervous activity in the rods.

rhombencephalon *n. see* HINDBRAIN.

rhomboid *n.* either of two muscles (**rhomboid major** and **rhomboid minor**) situated in the upper part of the back, between the backbone and shoulder blade. They help to move the shoulder blade backwards and upwards.

rhonchus *n.* (*pl.* **rhonchi**) an abnormal musical noise produced by air passing through narrowed bronchi. It is heard through a stethoscope, usually when the patient breathes out.

rhythm method a contraceptive method in which sexual intercourse is restricted to the **safe period** at the beginning and end of the *menstrual cycle. The safe period is calculated either on the basis of the length of the menstrual cycle or by reliance on the change of body temperature that occurs at ovulation. A third possible indicator (*see* BILLINGS METHOD) is the change that occurs with ovulation in the stickiness of the mucus at the neck (cervix) of the uterus. The method depends for its reliability on the woman having uniform regular periods and its failure rate is higher than with mechanical methods, approaching 25 pregnancies per 100 woman-years.

rib *n.* a curved, slightly twisted, strip of bone forming part of the skeleton of the thorax, which protects the heart and lungs. There are 12 pairs of ribs. The head of each rib articulates with one of the 12 thoracic vertebrae of the backbone; the other end is attached to a section of cartilage (*see* COSTAL CARTILAGE). The first seven pairs – the **true ribs** – are connected directly to the sternum by their costal cartilages. The next three pairs – the **false ribs** – are attached indirectly: each is connected by its cartilage to the rib above it. The last two pairs of ribs – the **floating ribs** – end freely in the muscles of the body wall. Anatomical name: **costa**.

ribavirin *n.* an antiviral drug effective against a range of DNA and RNA viruses, including the herpes group, *respiratory syncytial virus, and those causing *hepatitis, several strains of influenza, and *Lassa fever. It is administered by a small-particle aerosol inhaler and sometimes by intravenous injection. Possible side-effects include breathing difficulty, bacterial pneumonia, and *pneumothorax. Unfortunately, it antagonizes the action of *zidovudine against HIV. Trade name: **Virazole**.

riboflavin *n. see* VITAMIN B₂.

ribonuclease *n.* an enzyme, located in the *lysosomes of cells, that splits RNA at specific places in the molecule.

ribonucleic acid *see* RNA.

ribose *n.* a pentose sugar (i.e. one with free carbon atoms) that is a component of *RNA and several coenzymes. Ribose is also involved in intracellular metabolism.

ribosome *n.* a particle, consisting of RNA and protein, that occurs in cells and is the site of protein synthesis in the cell (*see* TRANSLATION). Ribosomes are either attached to the *endoplasmic reticulum or free in the cytoplasm as *polysomes. —**ribosomal** *adj.*

ribozyme *n.* an RNA molecule that can act as an enzyme, catalysing changes to its own molecular structure (before the dis-

covery of ribozymes it was assumed that all enzymes were proteins). Since replication of DNA and RNA cannot occur without enzymes, and since protein enzymes can only be produced by DNA coding, the question arose as to how nucleic acid molecules were able to replicate in the early stages of evolution. The discovery of ribozymes appears to resolve the enigma. Research is currently being undertaken to exploit the ability of genetically engineered ribozymes to destroy the RNA of HIV (the AIDS virus).

ricin *n.* a highly toxic albumin obtained from castor-oil seeds (*Ricinus communis*) that inhibits protein synthesis and becomes attached to the surface of cells, resulting in gastroenteritis, hepatic congestion and jaundice, and cardiovascular collapse. It is lethal to most species, even in minute amounts (1 μg/kg body weight); it is most toxic if injected intravenously or inhaled as fine particles. Ricin is being investigated as a treatment for certain lymphomas, which depends on its delivery to the exact site of the tumour in order to avoid destruction of healthy cells (*see* IMMUNOTOXIN).

rickets *n.* a disease of childhood in which the bones do not harden due to a deficiency of *vitamin D. Without vitamin D, not enough calcium salts are deposited in the bones to make them rigid: consequently they become soft and malformed. This is particularly noticeable in the long bones, which become bowed, and in the front of the ribcage, where a characteristic rickety 'rosary' may become apparent. The deficiency of vitamin D may be dietary or due to lack of exposure to sunlight, which is important in the conversion of vitamin D to its active form. In the UK rickets is more common in Asian immigrant families.

Renal rickets is due to impaired kidney function causing bone-forming minerals to be excreted in the urine, which results in softening of the bones.

rickettsiae *pl. n.* (*sing.* **rickettsia**) a group of very small nonmotile spherical or rodlike parasitic organisms. They resemble bacteria in their cellular structure and method of asexual reproduction, but – like viruses – they cannot reproduce outside the bodies of their hosts. Rickettsiae infect arthropods (ticks, mites, etc.), through whom they can be transmitted to mammals (including man), in which they can cause severe illness. The species *Rickettsia akari* causes *rickettsial pox, *R. conorii*, *R. prowazekii*, *R. tsutsugamushi*, and *R. typhi* cause different forms of *typhus, *R. rickettsii* causes *Rocky Mountain spotted fever, and *Coxiella burnetii* causes *Q fever. —**rickettsial** *adj*.

rickettsial pox a disease of mice caused by the microorganism *Rickettsia akari* and transmitted to man by mites: it produces chills, fever, muscular pain, and a rash similar to that of *chickenpox. The disease is mild and runs its course in 2–3 weeks. *See also* TYPHUS.

ridge *n*. **1.** (in anatomy) a crest or a long narrow protuberance, e.g. on a bone. **2.** (in dental anatomy) *see* ALVEOLUS.

rifampicin *n*. an *antibiotic used to treat various infections, particularly tuberculosis. It is administered by mouth; digestive upsets and sensitivity reactions sometimes occur. Trade names: **Rifadin**, **Rimactane**.

Rift Valley fever a virus disease of East Africa transmitted from animals to man by mosquitoes and causing symptoms resembling those of *influenza.

rigidity *n*. (in neurology) resistance to the passive movement of a limb that persists throughout its range. It is a symptom of *parkinsonism. A smooth resistance is called **plastic** or **lead-pipe rigidity** while intermittent resistance is called **cogwheel rigidity**. *Compare* SPASTICITY.

rigor *n*. **1.** an abrupt attack of shivering and a sensation of coldness, accompanied by a rapid rise in body temperature. This often marks the onset of a fever and may be followed by a feeling of heat, with copious sweating. **2.** *see* RIGOR MORTIS.

rigor mortis the stiffening of a body that occurs within some eight hours of death, due to chemical changes in muscle tissue. It starts to disappear after about 24 hours.

rima *n*. (in anatomy) a cleft. The **rima glottidis** (or glottis) is the space between the vocal folds.

rimiterol *n*. a drug, similar to *isoprena-line, that is used as a *bronchodilator to relieve asthma and chronic bronchitis. It is administered by inhalation; side-effects, following large doses, may include dizziness, fainting, tremor, anxiety, and fast heart rate. Trade name: **Pulmadil**.

ring *n*. (in anatomy) *see* ANNULUS.

ring block a circumferential ring of local anaesthetic solution used to block the nerves of a digit for purposes of minor surgery (*see* NERVE BLOCK). Precautions are necessary to avoid vascular damage leading to gangrene.

Ringer's solution (Ringer's mixture) a clear colourless *physiological solution of sodium chloride (common salt), potassium chloride, and calcium chloride prepared with recently boiled pure water. The osmotic pressure of the solution is the same as that of blood serum. Ringer's solution is used for maintaining organs or tissues alive outside the animal or human body for limited periods. Sterile Ringer's solution may be injected intravenously to treat dehydration. [S. Ringer (1835–1910), British physiologist]

ringworm (tinea) *n*. a fungus infection of the skin, the scalp, or the nails. Ringworm is caused by the dermatophyte fungi – species of *Microsporum*, *Trichophyton*, and *Epidermophyton* – and also affects animals, a source of infection for man. It can be spread by direct contact or via infected materials. The lesions of ringworm may be ringlike (as its name suggests) and may cause intense itching. The commonest form of ringworm is **athlete's foot (tinea pedis)**, which affects the skin between the toes. Another common type is ringworm of the scalp (**tinea capitis**), of which there is a severe form – *favus. Ringworm also affects the groin and thighs (**tinea cruris**: *see* DHOBIE ITCH) and the skin under a beard (**tinea barbae**). The disease is treated with antifungal agents taken by mouth (such as itraconazole or terbinafine) or applied locally (there is now a wide choice of topical agents).

Rinne's test a test to determine whether *deafness is conductive or sensorineural. A vibrating tuning fork is held first in the air, close to the ear, and then with its base placed on the bone (mastoid process) behind the ear. If the sound conducted by air is heard louder than the sound conducted by bone the test is positive and the deafness sensorineural; a negative result, when the sound conducted by bone is heard louder, indicates conductive deafness. [H. A. Rinne (1819–68), German otologist]

risk factor an attribute, such as a habit (e.g. cigarette smoking) or exposure to some environmental hazard, that leads the individual concerned to have a greater likelihood of developing an illness. The relationship is one of probability and as such can be distinguished from a *causal agent.

risk register a list of infants who have experienced some event in their obstetric and/or perinatal history known to be correlated with a higher than average likelihood of serious abnormality; a similar listing is kept of children (and other vulnerable groups) whose social circumstances render them liable to abuse. Such children are subjected to extra surveillance from health and/or social services. Problems associated with risk registers include limiting the designation of predisposing conditions so as to contain the number on the register within reasonable proportions and ensuring that children not on the register receive adequate surveillance.

risperidone *n.* an atypical *antipsychotic drug used in the treatment of schizophrenia and other psychoses in patients unresponsive to conventional antipsychotics. Side-effects, which are fewer and less severe than those of the older antipsychotics, include nausea, anxiety, headache, and fatigue. Trade name: **Risperdal**.

risus sardonicus an abnormal grinning expression resulting from involuntary prolonged contraction of facial muscles, as seen in *tetanus.

Ritter's disease *see* STAPHYLOCOCCAL SCALDED SKIN SYNDROME. [G. Ritter von Rittershain (1820–83), German physician]

river blindness *see* ONCHOCERCIASIS.

RNA (ribonucleic acid) a *nucleic acid, occurring in the nucleus and cytoplasm of cells, that is concerned with synthesis of proteins (*see* MESSENGER RNA, RIBOSOME, TRANSFER RNA, TRANSLATION). In some viruses RNA is the genetic material. The RNA molecule is a single strand made up of units called *nucleotides.

Rocky Mountain spotted fever (spotted fever, tick fever) a disease of rodents and other small mammals in the USA caused by the microorganism *Rickettsia rickettsii* and transmitted to man by ticks. Symptoms include fever, muscle pains, and a profuse reddish rash like that of measles. If untreated the disease may be fatal, but treatment with tetracycline or chloramphenicol is effective. *See also* TYPHUS.

rod *n.* one of the two types of light-sensitive cells in the *retina of the eye (*compare* CONE). The human eye contains about 125 million rods, which are necessary for seeing in dim light. They contain a pigment, *rhodopsin (or visual purple), which is broken down (bleached) in the light and regenerated in the dark. Breakdown of visual purple gives rise to nerve impulses; when all the pigment is bleached (i.e. in bright light) the rods no longer function. *See also* DARK ADAPTATION, LIGHT ADAPTATION.

rodent ulcer *see* BASAL CELL CARCINOMA.

roentgen *n.* a unit of exposure dose of X- or gamma-radiation equal to the dose that will produce 2.58×10^{-4} coulomb on all the ions of one sign, when all the electrons released in a volume of air of mass 1 kilogram are completely stopped.

role playing acting out another person's expected behaviour, usually in a contrived situation, in order to understand that person better. It is used in family psychotherapy, in teaching social skills to patients, and also in the training of psychiatric (and other) staff.

Romaña's sign an early clinical sign of *Chagas' disease, appearing some three weeks after infection. There is considerable swelling of the eyelids of one or both eyes. This may be due to the presence of the parasites causing the disease but it may also be an allergic reaction to the repeated bites of their insect carriers. [C. Romaña (20th century), Brazilian physician]

Romanowsky stains a group of stains

used for microscopical examination of blood cells, consisting of variable mixtures of thiazine dyes, such as azure B, with eosin. Romanowsky stains give characteristic staining patterns, on the basis of which blood cells are classified. The group includes the stains of Leishmann, Wright, May-Grünwald, Giemsa, etc. [D. L. Romanowsky (1861–1921), Russian physician]

Romberg's sign a finding on examination suggesting either a sensory disorder affecting those nerves that transmit information to the brain about the position of the limbs and joints and the tension in the muscles or a failure of the brain (cerebellum) to process this information. The patient is asked to stand upright. Romberg's sign is positive if he maintains his posture when his eyes are open but sways and falls when his eyes are closed. [M. Romberg (1795–1873), German neurologist]

rongeur *n.* powerful biting forceps for cutting tissue, particularly bone.

root *n.* **1.** (in neurology) a bundle of nerve fibres at its emergence from the spinal cord. The 31 pairs of *spinal nerves have two roots on each side, an anterior root containing motor nerve fibres and a posterior root containing sensory fibres. The roots merge outside the cord to form mixed nerves. **2.** (in dentistry) the part of a *tooth that is not covered by enamel and is normally attached to the alveolar bone by periodontal fibres. **3.** the origin of any structure, i.e. the point at which it diverges from another structure. Anatomical name: **radix.**

root canal treatment (in *endodontics) the procedure of removing the remnants of the pulp of a tooth, cleaning and shaping the canal inside the tooth, and filling the root canal (*see* ROOT FILLING). The entire treatment usually extends over several visits. It is used to treat toothache and apical abscesses.

root filling 1. the final stage of *root canal treatment, in which the prepared canal inside a tooth root is filled with a suitable material. **2.** the material used to fill the canal in the root, usually a core of *gutta-percha with a thin coating of sealing cement.

root induction (in *endodontics) a procedure to allow continued root formation in an immature tooth with a damaged pulp. *See* APEXOGENESIS.

rooting reflex a primitive reflex present in newborn babies: if the cheek is stroked near the mouth, the infant will turn its head to the same side to suckle.

Rorschach test a test to measure aspects of personality, consisting of ten inkblots, half of which are in various colours and the other half in black and white. The responses to the different inkblots are used to derive hypotheses about the subject. The use of the test for the diagnosis of brain damage or schizophrenia is no longer generally supported. *See also* PROJECTIVE TEST. [H. Rorschach (1884–1922), Swiss psychiatrist]

rosacea *n.* a chronic inflammatory disease of the face in which the skin becomes abnormally flushed. At times it becomes pustular and there may be an associated *keratitis. The disease occurs in both sexes and at all ages but is most common in women in their thirties; the cause is unknown. Treatment with oral tetracycline or topical metronidazole is very effective.

roseola (roseola infantum) *n.* a condition of young children in which a fever lasting for three or four days is followed by a rose-coloured maculopapular rash that fades after two days. The commonest exanthematous fever in young children, it is caused by human herpesvirus 6.

rostellum *n.* (*pl.* **rostella**) a mobile and retractable knob bearing hooks, present on the head (scolex) of certain *tapeworms, e.g. *Taenia* and *Echinococcus*.

rostrum *n.* (*pl.* **rostra**) (in anatomy) a beaklike projection, such as that on the sphenoid bone. —**rostral** *adj.*

rotator *n.* a muscle that brings about rotation of a part. The **rotatores** are small muscles situated deep in the back between adjacent vertebrae. They help to extend and rotate the vertebrae.

Rothera's test a method of testing urine for the presence of acetone or acetoacetic acid: a sign of *diabetes mellitus. Strong ammonia is added to a sample of urine saturated with ammonium sulphate crystals and containing a small quantity of sodium nitroprusside. A purple colour confirms the presence of acetone or aceto-acetic acid. [A. C. H. Rothera (1880–1915), Australian biochemist]

Roth spot a pale area surrounded by haemorrhage sometimes seen in the retina, with the aid of an *ophthalmo-scope, in those who have bacterial endo-carditis, septicaemia, or leukaemia. [M. Roth (1839–1915), Swiss physician]

roughage *n.* *see* DIETARY FIBRE.

rouleau *n.* (*pl.* **rouleaux**) a cylindrical structure in the blood formed from sev-eral red blood cells piled one upon the other and adhering by their rims.

round window *see* FENESTRA (ROTUNDA).

roundworm *n.* *see* NEMATODE.

RPE retinal pigment epithelium. *See* RETINA.

-rrhagia (-rrhage) *suffix denoting* exces-sive or abnormal flow or discharge from an organ or part. Examples: **haemorrhage** (excessive bleeding); **menorrhagia** (exces-sive menstrual flow).

-rrhaphy *suffix denoting* surgical sewing; suturing. Example: **herniorrhaphy** (of a hernia).

-rrhexis *suffix denoting* splitting or rup-ture of a part.

-rrhoea *suffix denoting* a flow or discharge from an organ or part. Example: **rhinor-rhoea** (from the nose).

RSI *see* REPETITIVE STRAIN INJURY.

RSV *see* RESPIRATORY SYNCYTIAL VIRUS.

rubber dam (in dentistry) a sheet of rubber used to isolate one or more teeth during treatment.

rubefacient *n.* an agent that causes red-dening and warming of the skin. Rubefacients are often used as *counter-irritants for the relief of muscular pain.

rubella *n.* *see* GERMAN MEASLES.

rubeola *n.* *see* MEASLES.

rubidium-81 *n.* an artificial radioactive isotope that has a half-life of about four hours and decays into the radioactive gas

*krypton-81m, emitting radiations as it does so. Symbol: ^{81}Rb.

rubor *n.* redness: one of the classical signs of inflammation in a tissue, the other three being *calor (heat), *dolor (pain) and *tumor (swelling). The redness of inflamed tissue is due to the increase in size of the small blood vessels in the area, which therefore contain more blood.

rubrospinal tract a tract of *motor neurones that extends from the midbrain down to different levels in the spinal cord, carrying impulses that have trav-elled from the cerebral and cerebellar cor-tex via the nucleus ruber (red nucleus). The tract plays an important part in the control of skilled and dextrous move-ments.

ruga *n.* (*pl.* **rugae**) a fold or crease, espe-cially one of the folds of mucous mem-brane that line the stomach.

rumination *n.* (in psychiatry) an obses-sional type of thinking in which the same thoughts or themes are experienced repet-itively, to the exclusion of other forms of mental activity. The patient commonly feels depressed and guilty after rumina-tion. Rumination may be distinguished from morbid preoccupation in that the thoughts are irrational and resisted by the patient; they often involve abhorrent or aggressive feelings about events in the re-mote past and are accompanied by a lack of confidence in memory.

rupture **1.** *n.* *see* HERNIA. **2.** *n.* the burst-ing apart or open of an organ or tissue; for example, the splitting of the mem-branes enclosing an infant during child-birth. **3.** *vb.* (of tissues, etc.) to burst apart or open.

Russell-Silver syndrome a congenital condition characterized by short stature, a triangular face with a small mandible (lower jaw), and asymmetry of the body. [W. Russell (1852–1940), British pathologist; H. K. Silver (1918–), US paediatrician]

Russian spring-summer encephalitis an influenza-like viral disease that affects the brain and nervous system and occurs in Russia and central Europe. It is trans-mitted to man either through the bite of forest-dwelling ticks of the species

Ixodes persulcatus or by drinking the milk of infected goats. Infection of the meninges results in paralysis of the limbs and of the muscles of the neck and back. The disease, which is often fatal, can be prevented by vaccination.

Ryle's tube a thin flexible tube of rubber or plastic, inserted through the mouth or nose of a patient and used for withdrawing fluid from the stomach or giving a test meal. [J. A. Ryle (1889–1950), British physician]

S

Sabin vaccine an oral vaccine against poliomyelitis, prepared by culture of the virus under special conditions so that it loses its virulence (i.e. it becomes attenuated) but retains its ability to stimulate antibody production. [A. B. Sabin (1906–93), US bacteriologist]

sac *n.* a pouch or baglike structure. Sacs can enclose natural cavities in the body, e.g. in the lungs (*see* ALVEOLUS) or in the *lacrimal apparatus of the eye, or they can be pathological, as in a hernia.

saccades *pl. n.* voluntary rapid movements of the eyes, usually when changing the point of fixation on an object (e.g. when reading).

sacchar- (saccharo-) *prefix denoting* sugar.

saccharide *n.* a carbohydrate. *See also* DISACCHARIDE, MONOSACCHARIDE, POLYSACCHARIDE.

saccharine *n.* a sweetening agent. Saccharine is 400 times as sweet as sugar and has no energy content. It is very useful as a sweetener in diabetic and lowcalorie foods. Saccharine is destroyed by heat and is not therefore used in cooking.

Saccharomyces *n. see* YEAST.

saccule (sacculus) *n.* the smaller of the two membranous sacs within the vestibule of the ear: it forms part of the membranous *labyrinth. It is filled with fluid (endolymph) and contains a *macula. This responds to gravity and relays information to the brain about the position of the head.

saccus *n.* a sac or pouch. The **saccus endolymphaticus** is the small sac connected to the saccule and utricle of the inner ear by the *endolymphatic duct.

sacralization *n.* abnormal fusion of the fifth lumbar vertebra with the sacrum.

sacral nerves the five pairs of *spinal nerves that emerge from the spinal column in the sacrum. The nerves carry sensory and motor fibres from the upper and lower leg and from the anal and genital regions.

sacral vertebrae the five vertebrae that are fused together to form the *sacrum.

sacro- *prefix denoting* the sacrum. Examples: **sacrococcygeal** (relating to the sacrum and coccyx); **sacrodynia** (pain in); **sacroiliac** (relating to the sacrum and ilium).

sacroiliitis *n.* inflammation of the sacroiliac joint. Involvement of both joints is a common feature of ankylosing *spondylitis and associated rheumatic diseases, including *Reiter's syndrome and *psoriatic arthritis. The resultant low back pain and stiffness may be alleviated by rest and anti-inflammatory analgesics.

sacrum *n.* (*pl.* **sacra**) a curved triangular element of the *backbone consisting of five fused vertebrae (**sacral vertebrae**). It articulates with the last lumbar vertebra above, the coccyx below, and the hip bones laterally. *See also* VERTEBRA. —**sacral** *adj.*

saddle joint a form of *diarthrosis (freely movable joint) in which the articulating surfaces of the bones are reciprocally saddle-shaped. It occurs at the carpometacarpal joint of the thumb.

sadism *n.* sexual excitement in response to inflicting or thinking about inflicting pain upon other people. *See also* MASOCHISM, SEXUAL DEVIATION. —**sadist** *n.* —**sadistic** *adj.*

SADS (seasonal affective disorder syndrome) a disorder in which the mood of the affected person is said to change according to the season of the year. Typically, with the onset of winter, there is depression, general slowing of mind and body, excessive sleeping, and overeating. These symptoms resolve with the coming of spring. The phenomenon may partly account for the known seasonal variation in suicide rates. SADS is not yet generally accepted as a clinical entity and the prevalence is unknown. There is evidence that mood is related to light, which suppresses the release of the hormone *melatonin from the pineal gland. Exposure to additional light during the day is said sometimes to relieve symptoms.

safe period the days in each *menstrual cycle when conception is least likely. Ovulation generally occurs at the midpoint of each cycle, and in women with regular periods it is possible to calculate the days at the beginning and end of the cycle when coitus is unlikely to result in pregnancy. *See* RHYTHM METHOD.

safranin (safranine) *n.* a group of water- and alcohol-soluble basic dyes used to stain cell nuclei and as counterstains for Gram-negative bacteria.

sagittal *adj.* describing the dorsoventral plane that extends down the long axis of the body, dividing it into right and left halves (see illustration).

sagittal suture *see* SUTURE.

Saint's triad the association between *gallstones, colonic diverticula (*see* DIVERTICULUM), and hiatus *hernia. In a patient with dyspepsia it is important to identify which of these conditions, if any, is causing the symptoms. [C. F. M. Saint (1886–1973), South African surgeon]

salaam attacks *see* INFANTILE SPASMS.

salbutamol *n.* a drug that stimulates beta-adrenergic receptors (*see* SYMPATHOMIMETIC); it is used as a *bronchodilator to relieve asthma, chronic bronchitis, and emphysema. It is administered by mouth, injection, or inhalation; side-effects may include dizziness, tremor, and fast heart rate, particularly after large doses. Trade name: **Ventolin**.

salicylic acid a drug that causes the skin to peel and destroys bacteria and fungi. It is applied to the skin to treat ulcers, dandruff, eczema, psoriasis, warts, and corns. Skin sensitivity reactions may occur after continued use.

salicylism *n.* poisoning due to an overdose of aspirin or other salicylate containing compounds. The main symptoms are headache, dizziness, ringing in the ears (tinnitus), disturbances of vision, vomiting,

and – in severe cases – delirium and collapse. There is often severe *acidosis.

saline (normal saline) *n.* a solution containing 0.9% sodium chloride. Saline may be used clinically as a diluent for drugs administered by injection and as a plasma substitute.

Sagittal plane of section through the body

saliva *n.* the alkaline liquid secreted by the *salivary glands and the mucous membrane of the mouth. Its principal constituents are water, mucus, buffers, and enzymes (e.g. amylase). The functions of saliva are to keep the mouth moist, to aid swallowing of food, to minimize changes of acidity in the mouth, and to digest starch. *See also* DRY MOUTH. —**salivary** *adj.*

salivary gland a gland that produces *saliva. There are three pairs of salivary glands: the *parotid glands, *sublingual glands, and *submandibular glands (see illustration). They are stimulated by reflex action, which can be initiated by the taste, smell, sight, or thought of food.

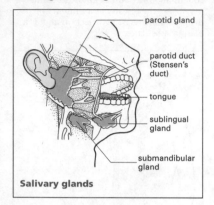

- parotid gland
- parotid duct (Stensen's duct)
- tongue
- sublingual gland
- submandibular gland

Salivary glands

salivary stone *see* SIALOLITH.

salivation *n.* the secretion of saliva by the salivary glands of the mouth, increased in response to the chewing action of the jaws or to the thought, taste, smell, or sight of food. A small but regular flow of saliva is maintained to promote cleanliness in the mouth even when food is not being eaten. *See also* PTYALISM.

Salk vaccine a vaccine against poliomyelitis, formed by treating the virus with formalin, which prevents it from causing disease but does not impair its ability to stimulate antibody production. It is administered by injection. [J. E. Salk (1914–95), US bacteriologist]

salmeterol *n.* a *sympathomimetic bronchodilator drug used to treat severe asthma. It is administered by metered-dose aerosol inhaler. Possible side-effects include a paradoxical worsening of the condition and a lowering of the blood potassium level. Trade name: **Serevent**.

Salmonella *n.* a genus of motile rodlike Gram-negative bacteria that inhabit the intestines of animals and man and cause disease. They ferment glucose, usually with the formation of gas. The species *S. paratyphi* causes *paratyphoid fever, and *S. typhi* causes *typhoid fever. Other

species of *Salmonella* cause *food poisoning, gastroenteritis, and septicaemia.

salmonellosis *n.* an infestation of the digestive system by bacteria of the genus *Salmonella. See also* FOOD POISONING.

salping- (salpingo-) *prefix denoting* **1.** the Fallopian tube. **2.** the auditory tube (meatus).

salpingectomy *n.* the surgical removal of a Fallopian tube. The operation involving both tubes is a permanent and completely effective method of contraception (*see* STERILIZATION) since it prevents the egg cells passing from the ovaries to the uterus.

salpingitis *n.* inflammation of a tube, most commonly applied to inflammation of one or both of the Fallopian tubes caused by bacterial infection spreading from the vagina or uterus or carried in the blood. In **acute salpingitis** there is a sharp pain in the lower abdomen, which may be mistaken for appendicitis, and the infection may spread to the membrane lining the abdominal cavity (*see* PERITONITIS). In severe cases the tubes may become blocked with scar tissue and the patient will be unable to conceive. The condition is treated with antibiotics and later, if necessary, by the surgical removal of the diseased tube(s).

salpingography *n.* *radiography of one or both Fallopian tubes after a *radio-opaque substance has been introduced into them via an injection into the uterus. **Standardized selective salpingography** enables occluded tubes, visualized by salpingography, to be restored to patency by means of tubal *catheterization.

salpingolysis *n.* a surgical operation carried out to restore patency to blocked Fallopian tubes; it involves the *division and removal of adhesions around the ovarian ends of the tubes.

salpingo-oophoritis *n.* inflammation of a Fallopian tube and an ovary.

salpingostomy *n.* the operation performed to restore free passage through a blocked Fallopian tube. The blocked portion of the tube is removed surgically and the continuity is then restored. It is performed in women who have been sterilized previously by tubal occlusion (*see* STERILIZATION) and in others whose Fallopian tubes have become blocked as a result of pelvic infection.

salt depletion excessive loss of sodium chloride (common salt) from the body. This may result from sweating, persistent vomiting or diarrhoea, or loss of fluid in wounds. The main symptoms are muscular weakness and cramps. Miners and workers in hot climates are particularly at risk, and salt tablets are often taken as a preventive measure.

Salter and Harris classification *see* EPIPHYSIS. [R. Salter and R. I. Harris (20th century), Canadian orthopaedic surgeons]

salvage procedure measures to palliate the worst effects of a tumour but with no aim to effect a cure.

Salvarsan *n. see* ARSENIC.

Salzmann's degeneration a noninflammatory condition of the cornea resulting in yellow-white nodules under the epithelium in the central area. These may cause symptoms if the epithelium over them breaks down or if they occur in the visual axis. [M. Salzmann (1862–1954), German ophthalmologist]

Samaritans *n.* a British voluntary organization providing a telephone service for the suicidal and despairing. Started in 1953 by the Rev. Chad Varah in the cellars of a London church (St Stephen, Walbrook) with one telephone, it now has 187 branches throughout the country manned by some 22,000 volunteers. It offers a non-professional, confidential, and (if required) anonymous service at all hours. Samaritans will listen for as long as they are needed (sometimes called the listening therapy) and the service is free. They offer little advice, believing that their clients will be helped to make their own decisions by talking to someone who cares. They also offer a befriending service to support exceptionally distressed clients through a serious crisis.

sampling frame *see* RANDOM SAMPLE.

sanatorium *n.* **1.** a hospital or institution for the rehabilitation and convalescence of patients of any kind. **2.** an institution for patients who have suffered from pulmonary tuberculosis.

sandfly *n.* a small hairy fly of the widely distributed genus *Phlebotomus*. Adult sandflies rarely exceed 3 mm in length and have long slender legs. The blood-sucking females of certain species transmit various diseases, including *leishmaniasis, *sandfly fever, and *bartonellosis.

sandfly fever (Pappataci fever) a viral disease transmitted to man by the bite of the sandfly *Phlebotomus papatasii*. Sandfly fever occurs principally in countries surrounding the Persian Gulf and the tropical Mediterranean; it occurs during the warmer months, does not last long, and is never fatal. Symptoms resemble those of influenza. There is no specific treatment apart from aspirin and codeine to relieve the symptoms.

sandwich therapy a combination of treatments in which one type of therapy is 'sandwiched' between exposures to another therapy. For example, surgical removal of a tumour may be 'sandwiched' between pre- and postoperative courses of radiotherapy. *See also* COMBINED THERAPY.

SANE a British charity whose role is to raise the awareness of mental health issues. It also initiates research into serious mental illness and offers telephone support for those with mental health problems and for those caring for them.

sangui- (sanguino-) *prefix denoting* blood.

sanguineous *adj.* **1.** stained, containing, or covered with blood. **2.** (of tissues) containing more than the normal quantity of blood.

sanies *n.* a foul-smelling watery discharge from a wound or ulcer, containing serum, blood, and pus.

sanitarian *n. see* MEDICAL ASSISTANT.

saphena *n. see* SAPHENOUS VEIN.

saphena varix an abnormal dilatation of the terminal section of the long *saphenous vein in the groin.

saphenous nerve a large branch of the *femoral nerve that arises in the upper thigh, travels down on the inside of the leg, and supplies the skin from the knee to below the ankle with sensory nerves.

saphenous vein (saphena) either of two superficial veins of the leg, draining blood from the foot. The **long saphenous vein** – the longest vein in the body – runs from the foot, up the medial side of the leg, to the groin, where it joins the femoral vein. The **short saphenous vein** runs up the back of the calf to join the popliteal vein at the back of the knee.

sapr- (sapro-) *prefix denoting* **1.** putrefaction. **2.** decaying matter.

sapraemia *n.* blood poisoning by toxins of saprophytic bacteria (bacteria living on dead or decaying matter). *Compare* PYAEMIA, SEPTICAEMIA, TOXAEMIA.

saprophyte *n.* any free-living organism that lives and feeds on the dead and putrefying tissues of animals or plants. *Compare* PARASITE. —**saprophytic** *adj.*

sarc- (sarco-) *prefix denoting* **1.** flesh or fleshy tissue. **2.** muscle.

sarcocele *n.* an obsolete term for a fleshy tumour (sarcoma) of the testis.

Sarcocystis *n.* a genus of parasitic protozoans (*see* SPOROZOA) that infect birds, reptiles, and herbivorous mammals. *S. lindemanni*, which occasionally infects man, forms cylindrical cysts (**sarcocysts**) in the muscle fibres. In heavy infections these cysts can cause tissue degeneration and therefore provoke muscular pain and weakness. Sarcocysts have, in the few positively diagnosed cases, been located in the heart muscles, arm muscles, and larynx.

sarcoid **1.** *adj.* fleshy. **2.** *n.* a fleshy tumour.

sarcoidosis (Boeck's disease) *n.* a chronic disorder of unknown cause in which the lymph nodes in many parts of the body are enlarged and small fleshy nodules (*see* GRANULOMA) develop in the lungs, liver, and spleen. The skin, nervous system, eyes, and salivary glands are also commonly affected (*see* UVEOPAROTITIS), and the condition has features similar to *tuberculosis. Recovery is complete with minimal after-effects in two-thirds of all cases.

sarcolemma *n.* the cell membrane that encloses a muscle cell (muscle fibre).

sarcoma *n.* any *cancer of connective tissue. These tumours may occur in any part of the body, as they arise in the tissues that make up an organ rather than being restricted to a particular organ. They can arise in fibrous tissue, muscle, fat, bone, cartilage, synovium, blood and lymphatic vessels, and various other tissues. *See also* CHONDROSARCOMA, FIBROSARCOMA, LEIOMYOSARCOMA, LIPOSARCOMA, LYMPHANGIOSARCOMA, OSTEOSARCOMA, RHABDOMYOSARCOMA. —**sarcomatous** *adj.*

sarcoma botryoides *see* CARCINOSARCOMA.

sarcomatosis *n.* *sarcoma that has spread widely throughout the body, most commonly through the bloodstream. It is treated with drugs, typically one or a combination of the following: cyclophosphamide, ifosfamide, vincristine, actinomycin D, methotrexate, or doxorubicin. The prognosis is very poor.

sarcomere *n.* one of the basic contractile units of which *striated muscle fibres are composed.

Sarcophaga *n.* a genus of widely distributed non-bloodsucking flies, the flesh flies. Maggots are normally found in carrion or excrement but occasionally females will deposit their eggs in wounds or ulcers giving off a foul-smelling discharge; the presence of the maggots causes a serious *myiasis. Rarely, maggots may be ingested with food and give rise to an intestinal myiasis.

sarcoplasm (myoplasm) *n.* the cytoplasm of muscle cells.

sarcoplasmic reticulum an arrangement of membranous vesicles and tubules found in the cytoplasm of striated muscle fibres. The sarcoplasmic reticulum plays an important role in the transmission of nervous excitation to the contractile parts of the fibres.

Sarcoptes *n.* a genus of small oval mites. The female of *S. scabiei*, the scabies mite, tunnels into the skin, where it lays its eggs. The presence of the mites causes severe irritation, which eventually leads to *scabies.

sarcostyle *n.* a bundle of muscle fibrils.

sartorius *n.* a narrow ribbon-like muscle at the front of the thigh, arising from the anterior superior spine of the ilium and extending to the tibia, just below the knee. The longest muscle in the body, the sartorius flexes the leg on the thigh and the thigh on the abdomen.

satyriasis *n.* an extreme degree of promiscuous heterosexual activity in men. *Compare* NYMPHOMANIA.

saucerization *n.* **1.** an operation in which tissue is cut away from a wound to form a saucer-like depression. It is carried out to facilitate healing and is commonly used to treat injuries or disorders in which bone is infected. **2.** the concave appearance of the upper surface of a vertebra that has been fractured by compression.

Sayre's jacket a plaster of Paris cast shaped to fit around and support the backbone. It is used in cases where the vertebrae have been severely damaged by disease, such as tuberculosis. [L. A. Sayre (1820–1900), US surgeon]

scab *n.* a hard crust of dried blood, serum, or pus that develops during the body's wound-healing process over a sore, cut, or scratch.

scabicide *n.* a drug that kills the mites causing *scabies.

scabies *n.* a skin infection caused by the mite *Sarcoptes scabiei*. Scabies is typified by severe itching (particularly at night), red papules, and often secondary infection. The female mite tunnels in the skin to lay her eggs and the newly hatched mites pass from person to person by close contact. The intense itching represents a true allergic reaction to the mite, its eggs, and its faeces. Commonly infected areas are the penis, nipples, and the finger webs. Treatment is by application of a scabicide, usually *permethrin, *lindane, or *malathion, to all areas of the body from the neck down; benzyl benzoate may be used but is more irritant. All members of a family need treatment, but clothing and bedding need not be disinfected.

scala *n.* one of the spiral canals of the *cochlea. The **scala media** (**cochlear duct**) is the central membranous canal, containing the sensory apparatus of the cochlea; the **scala vestibuli** and **scala tympani** are the two bony canals of the cochlea.

scald *n.* a *burn produced by a hot liquid or vapour, such as boiling water or steam.

scale 1. *n.* any of the flakes of dead epidermal cells shed from the skin. **2.** *vb.* to scrape deposits of calculus (tartar) from the teeth (*see* SCALER).

scalenus *n.* one of four paired muscles of the neck (**scalenus anterior, medius, minimus,** and **posterior**), extending from the cervical (neck) vertebrae to the first and second ribs. They are responsible for raising the first and second ribs in inspiration and for bending the neck forward and to either side.

scalenus syndrome (thoracic outlet syndrome) the group of symptoms caused by compression of the subclavian artery and the lower roots of the brachial plexus against the fibrous and bony structures of the outlet of the upper thoracic vertebrae. Loss of sensation, wasting, and vascular symptoms may be found in the affected arm, which may also be painful.

scaler *n.* an instrument for removing calculus from the teeth. It may be a hand instrument or one energized by rapid ultrasonic vibrations.

scalpel *n.* a small pointed surgical knife used by surgeons for cutting tissues. It has a straight handle and usually detachable disposable blades of different shapes.

scan 1. *n.* examination of the body or a part of the body using *ultrasonography, *computerized tomography (CT), *magnetic resonance imaging (MRI), or scintigraphy (*see* SCINTIGRAM). **2.** *n.* the image obtained from such an examination. **3.** *vb.* to examine the body using any of these techniques.

scanning laser ophthalmoscope *see* OPHTHALMOSCOPE.

scanning speech a disorder of articulation in which the syllables are inappropriately separated and equally stressed. It is caused by disease of the cerebellum or its connecting fibres in the brainstem.

scaphocephaly *n.* an abnormally long

and narrow skull due to premature closure of the suture between the two parietal bones, along the top of the skull. —**scaphocephalic** *adj.*

scaphoid bone a boat-shaped bone of the wrist (*see* CARPUS). It articulates with the trapezium and trapezoid bones in front, with the radius behind, and with the capitate and lunate medially. It is commonly injured by falls on the wrist.

scaphoid fracture a fracture of the scaphoid bone in the wrist, usually caused by a fall onto the outstretched hand. There is pain and swelling, and movements of the wrist and thumb are painful. Diagnosis is by X-ray, but the fracture may not initially be visible. Treatment is with a cast. Due to the anatomy of its blood supply, healing can take a long time, and bone grafting (*see* GRAFT) and internal fixation may be required for non-*union.

scapul- (scapulo-) *prefix denoting* the scapula.

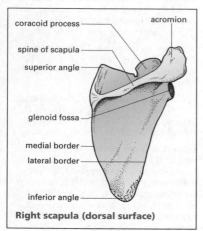

coracoid process
acromion
spine of scapula
superior angle
glenoid fossa
medial border
lateral border
inferior angle

Right scapula (dorsal surface)

scapula *n.* (*pl.* **scapulas** or **scapulae**) the shoulder blade: a triangular bone, a pair of which form the back part of the shoulder girdle (see illustration). The **spine** on its dorsal (back) surface ends at the **acromion process** at the top of the shoulder. This process turns forward and articulates with the collar bone (*clavicle) at the **acromioclavicular joint**; it overhangs

the **glenoid fossa**, into which the humerus fits to form the socket of the shoulder joint. The **coracoid process** curves upwards and forwards from the neck of the scapula and provides attachment for ligaments and muscles. —**scapular** *adj.*

scar *n. see* CICATRIX.

scarification *n.* the process of making a series of shallow cuts or scratches in the skin to allow a substance to penetrate the body. This was commonly performed during vaccination against smallpox; the vaccine was administered as a droplet left in contact with the scarified area.

scarlatina *n. see* SCARLET FEVER.

scarlet fever a highly infectious disease caused by a strain of *Streptococcus bacteria that produces toxins. Symptoms begin 2–4 days after exposure and include fever, tonsillitis, and a characteristic widespread scarlet rash. The tongue is also affected; initially covered by a thick white material, it then becomes bright red (the "strawberry tongue"). Treatment with antibiotics shortens the course of the disease and reduces the risk of secondary complications, which include kidney and ear inflammation. Medical name: **scarlatina**. *Compare* GERMAN MEASLES.

Scarpa's triangle *see* FEMORAL TRIANGLE. [A. Scarpa (1747–1832), Italian anatomist and surgeon]

scat- (scato-) *prefix denoting* faeces.

scatter diagram (in statistics) *see* CORRELATION.

SCC *see* SQUAMOUS CELL CARCINOMA.

Scheuermann's disease *osteochondritis involving one or more of the vertebrae. The condition often arises in adolescence and causes spinal pain and *kyphosis. It usually resolves spontaneously without deformity, causing sclerotic change in the affected bone. [H. W. Scheuermann (1877–1960), Danish surgeon]

Schick test a test to determine whether a person is susceptible to diphtheria. A small quantity of diphtheria toxin is injected under the skin; a patch of reddening and swelling shows that the person has no immunity and – if at particular risk – should be immunized. [B. Schick (1877–1967), US paediatrician]

Schiff's reagent aqueous *fuchsin solution decolourized with sulphur dioxide. A blue coloration develops in the presence of aldehydes. [H. Schiff (1834–1915), German chemist]

Schilling test a test used to assess a patient's capacity to absorb vitamin B_{12} from the bowel. Radioactive vitamin B_{12} is given by mouth and urine collected for 24 hours. A normal individual will excrete at least 10% of the original dose over this period; a patient with *pernicious anaemia will excrete less than 5%. [R. F. Schilling (1919–   ), US physician]

schindylesis *n.* a form of *synarthrosis (immovable joint) in which a crest of one bone fits into a groove of another.

-schisis *suffix denoting* a cleft or split.

schism *n.* a disorder of relationships within a family, in which parents quarrel and children are made to take sides. It was proposed as a cause of later schizophrenia in the children, but is more likely to be a nonspecific cause of psychological vulnerability.

schisto- *prefix denoting* a fissure; split.

schistoglossia *n.* fissuring of the tongue. Congenital fissures are transverse, whereas those due to disease (such as syphilis) are usually longitudinal.

Schistosoma (Bilharzia) *n.* a genus of blood *flukes, three species of which are important parasites of man causing one of the most serious of tropical diseases (*see* SCHISTOSOMIASIS). *S. japonicum* is common in the Far East; *S. mansoni* is widespread in Africa, the West Indies, and South and Central America; and *S. haematobium* occurs in Africa and the Middle East.

schistosomiasis (bilharziasis) *n.* a tropical disease caused by blood flukes of the genus *Schistosoma. Eggs present in the stools or urine of infected people undergo part of their larval development within freshwater snails living in water contaminated with human sewage. The disease is contracted when *cercaria larvae, released from the snails, penetrate the skin of anyone bathing in infected water. Adult flukes eventually settle in the blood vessels of the intestine (*S. mansoni* and *S. japonicum*) or the bladder (*S. haematobium*); the release of their spiked eggs causes anaemia, inflammation, and the formation of scar tissue. Additional intestinal symptoms are diarrhoea, dysentery, enlargement of the spleen and liver, and cirrhosis of the liver. If the bladder is affected, blood is passed in the urine and cystitis and cancer of the bladder may develop. The disease is treated with various drugs, including stibophen and other antimony-containing preparations, praziquantel, and niridazole.

schiz- (schizo-) *prefix denoting* a split or division.

schizogony *n.* a phase of asexual reproduction in the life cycle of a sporozoan (protozoan parasite) that occurs in the liver or red blood cells. The parasite grows and divides many times to form a **schizont**, which contains many *merozoites. The eventual release of merozoites of *Plasmodium*, the malaria parasite, from the blood cells produces fever in the patient.

schizoid personality a personality characterized by solitariness, emotional coldness to others, inability to experience pleasure, lack of response to praise and criticism, withdrawal into a fantasy world, excessive introspection, and eccentricity of behaviour. Some schizophrenics have this personality before their illness, but most schizoid personalities do not become schizophrenic. *See* PERSONALITY DISORDER.

schizont *n.* one of the stages that occurs during the asexual phase of the life cycle of a sporozoan. *See* SCHIZOGONY.

schizonticide *n.* any agent used for killing *schizonts.

schizophrenia *n.* a severe mental disorder (or group of disorders) characterized by a disintegration of the process of thinking, of contact with reality, and of emotional responsiveness. *Delusions and *hallucinations (especially of voices) are usual features, and the patient usually feels that his thoughts, sensations, and actions are controlled by, or shared with, others. He becomes socially withdrawn and loses energy and initiative. The main types of schizophrenia are **simple**, in which increasing social withdrawal and personal ineffectiveness are the major changes; **hebephrenic**, which starts in adolescence or young adulthood (see HEBEPHRENIA); **paranoid**, characterized by prominent delusions; and **catatonic**, with marked motor disturbances. The latter form is now rare.

Schizophrenia commonly – but not inevitably – runs a progressive course. The prognosis has improved with *antipsychotic drugs and with vigorous psychological and social management and rehabilitation. There are strong genetic factors in the causation, and environmental stress can precipitate illness. —**schizophrenic** adj.

schizotypal adj. describing a condition characterized by cold aloof feelings, eccentricities of behaviour, odd ways of thinking and talking, and occasional short periods of intense illusions, hallucinations, or delusion-like ideas. The condition, known as **borderline schizophrenia**, is similar to some aspects of *schizophrenia and is more common in people who are genetically related to schizophrenics.

Schlemm's canal a channel in the eye, at the junction of the cornea and the sclera, through which the aqueous humour drains. [F. Schlemm (1795–1858), German anatomist]

Schmorl's node (or nodule) a lucent area seen on X-ray of the backbone that denotes extrusion of some nucleus pulposus from an *intervertebral disc into the body of a vertebra. [C. G. Schmorl (1861–1932), German pathologist]

Schönlein-Henoch purpura see HENOCH-SCHÖNLEIN PURPURA.

school health service (in Britain) a service concerned with the early detection of physical, intellectual, and emotional abnormalities in schoolchildren and their subsequent treatment and surveillance. The service was formerly based on an ideal of three examinations at 5, 11, and 15 years by doctors and nurses specially employed by the Local Education Authority (LEA). It has now been changed to a system of selective examinations based on recommendations by teachers, *school nurses, or parental requests. The service is now the responsibility of the local community trust, but ascertainment and responsibility for allocation to *special schools remain the responsibility of the LEA.

school nurse a member of the *school health service who conducts routine examinations and/or treats minor ailments. *Health visitors may sometimes work in this capacity but State Registered and State Enrolled Nurses may also perform these tasks.

Schwann cells the cells that lay down the *myelin sheath around the axon of a medullated nerve fibre. Each cell is responsible for one length of axon, around which it twists as it grows, so that concentric layers of membrane envelop the axon. The gap between adjacent Schwann cells forms a *node of Ranvier. [T. Schwann (1810–82), German anatomist and physiologist]

Schwannoma n. see NEUROFIBROMA.

sciatica n. pain felt down the back and outer side of the thigh, leg, and foot. It is usually caused by degeneration of an intervertebral disc, which protrudes laterally to compress a lower lumbar or an upper sacral spinal nerve root. The onset may be sudden, brought on by an awkward lifting or twisting movement. The back is stiff and painful. There may be numbness and weakness in the leg. Bed rest will often relieve the pain but surgical treatment is occasionally necessary.

sciatic nerve the major nerve of the leg and the nerve with the largest diameter. It runs down behind the thigh from the lower end of the spine; above the knee joint it divides into two main branches, the **tibial** and **common peroneal nerves**, which are distributed to the muscles and skin of the lower leg.

SCID see SEVERE COMBINED IMMUNE DEFICIENCY.

scintigram n. a diagram showing the distribution of radioactive *tracer in a part of the body, produced by recording the flashes of light given off by a *scintillator as it is struck by radiation of different intensities. This technique is called **scintigraphy**. By scanning the body, section by section, a 'map' of the radioactivity in various regions is built up, aiding the diagnosis of cancer or other disorders. Such a record is known as a **scintiscan**.

scintillation counter a device to measure and record the fluorescent flashes in a *scintillator exposed to high-energy radiation.

scintillator n. a substance that produces a fluorescent flash when struck by high-energy radiation, such as beta or gamma rays. In medicine the most commonly used scintillator is a crystal of thallium-activated sodium iodide, which forms the basis of a *gamma camera. See also SCINTI-GRAM.

scintiscan n. see SCINTIGRAM.

scirrhous adj. describing carcinomas that are stony hard to the touch. Such a carcinoma (for example of the breast) is known as a **scirrhus**.

scissor leg a disability in which one leg becomes permanently crossed over the other as a result of spasticity of its *adductor muscles or deformity of the hips. The condition occurs in children with brain damage and in adults after strokes. A *tenotomy sometimes reduces the degree of disability.

scissura (scissure) n. a cleft or splitting, such as the splitting of the tip of a hair or the splitting open of tissues when a hernia forms.

scler- (sclero-) prefix denoting 1. hardening or thickening. 2. the sclera. 3. sclerosis.

sclera (sclerotic coat) n. the white fibrous outer layer of the eyeball. At the front of the eye it becomes the cornea. See EYE. —**scleral** adj.

sclerectomy n. an operation in which a portion of the sclera (the thick white layer of the eyeball) is removed.

scleritis n. inflammation of the sclera (the white of the eye).

scleroderma n. thickening of the skin, either localized (see MORPHOEA) or generalized, resulting in waxy ivory-coloured areas. Treatment is unsatisfactory, but spontaneous resolution may occur. The cause is unknown, but scleroderma may well be an *autoimmune disease.

*Systemic sclerosis is a related multisystem disorder.

scleromalacia n. thinning of the sclera (white of the eye) as a result of inflammation. Sometimes the sclera fades away completely in an area, and the underlying dark-bluish tissue (usually the ciliary body) bulges beneath the conjunctiva. This state is known as **scleromalacia perforans**.

sclerosis n. hardening of tissue, usually due to scarring (fibrosis) after inflammation or to ageing. It can affect the lateral columns of the spinal cord and the medulla of the brain (**amyotrophic lateral sclerosis** or **Lou Gehrig's disease**), causing progressive muscular paralysis (see MOTOR NEURONE DISEASE). It can also occur in scattered patches throughout the brain and spinal cord (see MULTIPLE SCLEROSIS) or in the walls of the arteries (see ARTERIOSCLEROSIS, ATHEROSCLEROSIS). See also TUBEROUS SCLEROSIS.

sclerotherapy n. treatment of varicose veins by the injection of an irritant solution. This causes thrombophlebitis, which encourages obliteration of the varicose vein by thrombosis and subsequent scarring. Sclerotherapy is also used for treating haemorrhoids and oesophageal varices.

sclerotic 1. (sclerotic coat) n. see SCLERA. **2.** adj. affected with *sclerosis.

sclerotome n. **1.** a surgical knife used in the operation of *sclerotomy. **2.** (in embryology) the part of the segmented mesoderm (see SOMITE) in the early embryo that gives rise to all the skeletal tissue of the body. The vertebrae and ribs retain the segmented structure, which is lost in the skull and limbs.

sclerotomy n. an operation in which an incision is made in the sclera (white of the eye).

scolex n. (pl. **scolices**) the head of a *tapeworm. The presence of suckers and/or hooks on the scolex enables the worm to attach itself to the wall of its host's gut.

scoliosis n. lateral (sideways) deviation of the backbone, caused by congenital or acquired abnormalities of the vertebrae, muscles, and nerves. Treatment may require spinal braces and, in cases of severe deformity, surgical correction by fusion or *osteotomy. *See also* KYPHOSIS, KYPHO-SCOLIOSIS.

-scope *suffix denoting* an instrument for observing or examining. Example: **gastroscope** (instrument for examining the stomach).

scopolamine *n.* *see* HYOSCINE.

scorbutic *adj.* affected with scurvy.

scoring system any of various methods in which the application of an agreed numerical scale is used as a means of estimating the degree of a clinical situation, e.g. the severity of an injury, the degree of patient recovery, or the extent of malignancy. Examples include the *Glasgow scoring system and the *injury scoring system.

scoto- *prefix denoting* darkness.

scotoma *n.* (*pl.* **scotomata**) a small area of abnormally less sensitive or absent vision in the visual field, surrounded by normal sight. All people have a *blind spot in the visual field of each eye due to the small area inside the eye occupied by the optic disc, which is not sensitive to light. Similar islands of total visual loss in other parts of the field are referred to as **absolute scotomata**. A **relative scotoma** is a spot where the vision is decreased but still present.

scotometer *n.* an instrument used for mapping defects in the visual field. *See also* CAMPIMETRY, PERIMETER.

scotopic *adj.* relating to or describing conditions of poor illumination. For example, **scotopic vision** is vision in dim light in which the *rods of the retina are involved (*see* DARK ADAPTATION).

screening test a test carried out on a large number of apparently healthy people to separate those who probably have a specified disease from those who do not. Examples are the *Guthrie test, *cervical smears, and *Forrest screening. Limitations depend on the severity and *frequency distribution of the disease and the efficiency and availability of treatment. Other factors to be taken into account are the safety, convenience, cost,

and *sensitivity of the test. *See also* GENETIC SCREENING.

scrofula *n.* *tuberculosis of lymph nodes, usually those in the neck, causing the formation of abscesses. Untreated, these burst through the skin and form running sores, which leave scars when they heal. Treatment with antituberculous drugs is effective. The disease, which is now rare, most commonly affects young children. —**scrofulous** *adj.*

scrofuloderma *n.* tuberculosis of the skin in which the skin breaks down over suppurating tuberculous glands, with the formation of irregular-shaped ulcers with blue-tinged edges. Treatment is with antituberculous drugs, to which scrofuloderma responds better than *lupus vulgaris, another type of skin tuberculosis.

scrototomy *n.* an operation in which the scrotum is surgically explored, usually undertaken to investigate patients with probable obstructive *azoospermia.

scrotum *n.* the paired sac that holds the testes and epididymides outside the abdominal cavity. Its function is to allow the production and storage of spermatozoa to occur at a lower temperature than that of the abdomen. Further temperature control is achieved by contraction or relaxation of muscles in the scrotum. —**scrotal** *adj.*

scrub typhus (tsutsugamushi disease) a disease, widely distributed in SE Asia, caused by the parasitic microorganism *Rickettsia tsutsugamushi* and transmitted to man through the bite of mites. Only larval mites of the genus *Trombicula* are involved as vectors. Symptoms include headache, chills, high temperature (104°F), a red rash over most of the body, a cough, and delirium. A small ulcer forms at the site of the bite. Scrub typhus is treated with tetracycline and other broad-spectrum antibiotics. *See also* RICKETTSIAE, TYPHUS.

scrum-pox *n.* a form of *herpes simplex found in rugby players and wrestlers. It is caused by abrasive contact.

scruple *n.* a unit of weight used in pharmacy. 1 scruple = 1.295 g (20 grains). 3 scruples = 1 drachm.

sculpting *n.* a technique of family psychotherapy, in which all the family members are seen together and one member is asked to arrange the others' physical positions to express their relationships and feelings. *See also* GROUP THERAPY.

scurvy *n.* a disease that is caused by a deficiency of *vitamin C (ascorbic acid). Unlike most animals, humans cannot synthesize ascorbic acid and must obtain it from fresh fruit and vegetables. The first sign of scurvy is swollen bleeding gums, and a rash of tiny bleeding spots around the hair follicles is characteristic. This may be followed by subcutaneous bleeding and the opening of previously healed wounds. Scurvy may result from food faddism or alcoholism; elderly men who live alone are at special risk. Treatment with vitamin C soon reverses the effects.

scybalum *n.* a lump or mass of hard faeces.

seasickness *n. see* MOTION SICKNESS.

seasonal affective disorder syndrome *see* SADS.

seat-belt syndrome thoracic injuries that arise from violent contact with a restraining seat belt in motor vehicle accidents occurring at high speeds.

sebaceous cyst 1. (wen) a pale or flesh-coloured dome shaped cyst that commonly occurs in adults, especially on the face, neck, or trunk. It is firm, with a central dot, and contains keratin, not sebum; such cysts are therefore more correctly referred to as **epidermoid cysts**. They are usually removed surgically. **2.** a cyst of the sebaceous glands occurring in multiple form in a rare inherited condition, **steatocystoma multiplex.**

sebaceous gland any of the simple or branched glands in the *skin that secrete an oily substance, *sebum. They open into hair follicles and their secretion is produced by the disintegration of their cells. Some parts of the skin have many sebaceous glands, others few. Activity varies with age: the glands are most active at puberty.

seborrhoea *n.* excessive secretion of sebum by the *sebaceous glands. The glands are enlarged, especially on the nose

and central face. The condition predisposes to acne and is common at puberty, usually lasting for a few years. Seborrhoea may be associated with a kind of *eczema (seborrhoeic eczema). —**seborrhoeic** *adj.*

sebum *n.* the oily substance secreted by the *sebaceous glands and reaching the skin surface through small ducts that lead into the hair follicles. Sebum provides a thin film of fat over the skin, which slows the evaporation of water; it also has an antibacterial effect.

second *n.* the *SI unit of time, equal to the duration of 9,192,631,770 periods of the radiation corresponding to the transition between two hyperfine levels of the ground state of the caesium-133 atom. This unit is now the basis of all time measurements. Symbol: s.

secondary health care health care provided by medical specialists or hospital staff members for a patient whose primary care was provided by the *general practitioner who first diagnosed or treated the patient. For example, a general practitioner who accepts a patient with an unusual skin condition provides primary care but if he refers the patient to a dermatologist, the skin specialist becomes the source of secondary care. *Compare* TERTIARY HEALTH CARE.

secondary prevention the avoidance or alleviation of the serious consequences of disease by early detection. Best known methods include routine examinations, as in *child health clinics and the *school health service, or *screening tests applied to populations that are regarded as having a high risk of contracting specific diseases.

secondary sexual characteristics the physical characteristics that develop after puberty as a result of sexual maturation. In boys they include the growth of facial and pubic hair and the breaking of the voice. In girls they include the growth of pubic hair and the development of the breasts.

second messenger an organic molecule that acts within a cell to initiate the response to a signal carried by a chemical messenger (e.g. a hormone) that does not itself enter the cell. Examples of second messengers are *inositol triphosphate and cyclic *AMP.

secretin *n.* a hormone secreted from the small intestine (duodenum) when acidified food leaves the stomach. It stimulates the secretion of relatively enzyme-free alkaline juice by the pancreas (*see* PANCREATIC JUICE) and of bile by the liver.

secretion *n.* **1.** the process by which a gland isolates constituents of the blood or tissue fluid and chemically alters them to produce a substance that it discharges for use by the body or excretes. The principal methods of secretion – *apocrine, *holocrine, and *merocrine – are illustrated in the diagram. **2.** the substance that is produced by a gland.

merocrine   apocrine

holocrine

Methods of secretion

secretor *n.* a person in whose saliva and other body fluids are found traces of the water-soluble A, B, or O agglutinogens that determine *blood group.

section **1.** *n.* (in surgery) the act of cutting (the cut or division made is also called a section). For example, an **abdominal section** is performed for surgical exploration of the abdomen (*see* LAPAROTOMY). A **transverse section** is a cut made at right angles to a structure's long axis. *See also* CAESAREAN SECTION. **2.** *n.* (in microscopy) a thin slice of the specimen to be examined under a microscope. **3.** *vb.* to issue an order for *compulsory admission to a psychiatric hospital under the appropriate section of the *Mental Health Act.

section 30 order (parental order) a court order made under the Human Fertilization and Embryology Act 1990 that enables a married couple to be regarded as the legal parents of a child born to a *surrogate mother commissioned by that couple. Application must be made within six months of the child's birth and the child's home must be with the husband and wife at the time of the application.

Section 47 a section of the National Assistance Act 1948 that enables a local authority to arrange for the compulsory removal to a place of care of a person who is unwilling to go voluntarily from his or her own home. Individuals who are suffering from a grave chronic disease, or are physically incapacitated, or are living in insanitary conditions because of old age or infirmity can be removed if they are unable to care for themselves and do not receive care and attention from others. A proper officer (*see* PUBLIC HEALTH PHYSICIAN) and another registered medical practitioner (usually the patient's general practitioner) must certify that removal is in the interests of the patient or that it would prevent injury to the health of, or serious nuisance to, other people.

security object a particular item that brings comfort and a sense of security to a young child, often for a number of years. Security objects are usually associated in some way with bed and are often made of soft material. A scrap of an old blanket or of a former night garment, a teddy bear, even an old nappy may be chosen as a comforter and these are often pressed to the face as the child settles down to sleep. There is no reason to suppose that security objects are in any way undesirable, at any age.

sedation *n.* the production of a restful state of mind, particularly by the use of drugs (*see* SEDATIVE).

sedative *n.* a drug that has a calming effect, relieving anxiety and tension. Sedatives are *hypnotic drugs administered at lower doses than those needed for sleep (drowsiness is a common side-effect). *See also* TRANQUILLIZER.

sedimentation rate the rate at which solid particles sink in a liquid under the influence of gravity. *See also* ESR (ERYTHRO-CYTE SEDIMENTATION RATE).

segment *n.* (in anatomy) a portion of a tissue or organ, usually distinguishable from other portions by lines of demarcation. For example, the uterus consists of **upper** and **lower segments**. The **anterior segment** of the eye is the front portion, including the cornea, anterior chamber, iris, and lens. *See also* SOMITE.

Seidel sign a bright green flow of liquid seen when fluorescein dye is applied to the cornea and viewed with cobalt blue light. It indicates leakage of aqueous humour. [E. Seidel (1882–1948), German ophthalmologist]

Seldinger technique the retrograde passage of a catheter into the aorta via a puncture in the femoral artery. It is used to outline the aorta and its major branches, including the blood vessels of the lower extremities. [S. I. Seldinger (1921–), Swedish radiologist]

selegiline *n.* a selective *MAO inhibitor used in the treatment of parkinsonism. Administered by mouth, selegiline is thought to retard the breakdown of *dopamine. Possible side-effects include faintness on standing up, nausea, involuntary movements, and confusion. Trade name: **Eldepryl**.

selenium *n.* a *trace element that is an essential component of the enzyme glutathione peroxidase, which catalyses the oxidation of *glutathione by hydrogen peroxide. It thus has important *antioxidant properties. Dietary deficiency of selenium results in *cardiomyopathy. Symbol: Se.

selenium sulphide a selenium compound with antifungal properties, used to treat *dandruff and scalp infections. It is administered in a shampoo. Trade names: **Lenium, Selsun**.

sella turcica a depression in the body of the sphenoid bone that encloses the pituitary gland.

semeiology *n. see* SYMPTOMATOLOGY.

semen (seminal fluid) *n.* the fluid ejaculated from the penis at sexual climax. Each ejaculate may contain 300–500 million spermatozoa suspended in a fluid secreted by the *prostate gland and *seminal vesicles with a small contribution from *Cowper's glands. It contains fructose, which provides the spermatozoa with energy, and *prostaglandins, which affect the muscles of the uterus and may therefore assist transport of the spermatozoa. —**seminal** *adj.*

semi- *prefix denoting* half.

semicircular canals three tubes that form part of the membranous *labyrinth of the ear. They are concerned with balance and each canal registers movement in a different plane. At the base of each canal is a small swelling (an **ampulla**), which contains a *crista. When the head moves the fluid (endolymph) in the canals presses on the cristae, which register the movement and send nerve impulses to the brain.

semilunar cartilage one of a pair of crescent-shaped cartilages in the knee joint situated between the femur and tibia.

semilunar valve either of the two valves in the heart situated at the origin of the aorta (**aortic valve**) and the pulmonary artery (**pulmonary valve**). Each consists of three flaps (cusps), which maintain the flow of blood in one direction.

seminal analysis analysis of a specimen of semen, which should be obtained after five days of abstinence from coitus, in order to assess male fertility. Normal values are as follows: volume of ejaculate: 2–6.5 ml; liquefaction complete in 30 minutes; sperm concentration: 20–200 million spermatozoa per ml (**sperm count** refers to the total number of spermatozoa in the ejaculate); motility: 60% moving progressively at 30 minutes to 3 hours; abnormal forms: less than 20%. Analysis of three separate specimens is necessary before confirming the presence of an abnormal result.

seminal vesicle either of a pair of male accessory sex glands that open into the vas deferens before it joins the urethra. The seminal vesicles secrete most of the liquid component of *semen.

seminiferous tubule any of the long convoluted tubules that make up the bulk of the *testis.

seminoma *n.* a malignant tumour of the testis, appearing as a swelling, often painless, in the scrotum. It tends to occur in an older age group than the *teratomas. The treatment for localized disease is surgery involving removal of the testis (*see* ORCHIDECTOMY). Secondary tumours in the lungs can be treated with chemotherapy and radiotherapy to the draining lymph nodes. A similar tumour occurs in the ovary (*see* DYSGERMINOMA).

semipermeable membrane a membrane that allows the passage of some molecules but not others. *Cell membranes are semipermeable. Semipermeable membranes are used clinically in *haemodialysis for patients with kidney failure.

semiprone *adj.* describing the position of a patient lying face downwards, but with one or both knees flexed to one side so that the body is not lying completely flat. *Compare* PRONE, SUPINE.

senescence *n.* the condition of ageing, which is often marked by a decrease in physical and mental abilities. —**senescent** *adj.*

senile dementia loss of the intellectual faculties often associated with behavioural deterioration, beginning for the first time in old age. *See also* DEMENTIA.

senior house officer *see* CONSULTANT.

senna *n.* the dried fruits of certain shrubs of the genus *Cassia*, used as an irritant *laxative to relieve constipation and to empty the bowels before X-ray examination. It is administered by mouth; side-effects do not usually occur, but severe diarrhoea may follow large doses. Trade name: **Senokot**.

sensation *n.* a feeling: the result of messages from the body's sensory receptors registering in the brain as information about the environment. Messages from *exteroceptors are interpreted as specific sensations – smell, taste, temperature, pain, etc. – in the conscious mind. Messages from *interoceptors, however, rarely reach the consciousness to produce sensation.

sense *n.* one of the faculties by which the qualities of the external environment are appreciated – sight, hearing, smell, taste, or touch.

sense organ a collection of specialized cells (*receptors), connected to the nervous system, that is capable of responding to a particular stimulus from either outside or inside the body. Sense organs can detect light (the eyes), heat, pain, and touch (the skin), smell (the nose), and taste (the taste buds).

sensibility *n.* the ability to be affected by, and respond to, changes in the surroundings (*see* STIMULUS). Sensibility is a characteristic of cells of the nervous system.

sensitive *adj.* possessing the ability to respond to a *stimulus. The cells of the retina, for example, are sensitive to the stimulus of light and respond by sending nerve impulses to the brain. Other *receptors are sensitive to different specific stimuli, such as pressure or the presence of chemical substances.

sensitivity *n.* **1.** (in microbiology) the degree to which a disease-causing organism responds to treatment by *antibiotics or other drugs. **2.** (in preventive medicine) a measure of the reliability of a *screening test based on the proportion of people with a specific disease who react positively to the test (the higher the sensitivity the fewer false negatives). This contrasts with **specificity**, which is the proportion of people free from disease who react negatively to the test (i.e. the higher the specificity the fewer the false positives). Though these are theoretically independent variables, most screening tests are so designed that if the sensitivity is increased the specificity is reduced and the number of false positives may rise to wasteful proportions.

sensitization *n.* **1.** alteration of the responsiveness of the body to the presence of foreign substances. In the development of an *allergy, an individual becomes sensitized to a particular allergen and reaches a state of *hypersensitivity. The phenomena of sensitization are due to the production of antibodies. **2.** (in behaviour therapy) a form of *aversion therapy in which anxiety-producing stimuli are associated with the unwanted behaviour. In **covert sensitization** the behaviour and an unpleasant feeling (such as disgust) are evoked simultaneously by verbal cues.

sensory *adj.* relating to the input division of the nervous system, which carries information from *receptors throughout the body towards the brain and spinal cord.

sensory cortex the region of the *cerebral cortex responsible for receiving incoming information relayed by sensory nerve pathways from all parts of the body. Different areas of cortex correspond to different parts of the body and to the various senses. *Compare* MOTOR CORTEX.

sensory deprivation the state in which there is a major reduction in incoming sensory information. Prolonged sensory deprivation is damaging as the body depends for health and normal function on constant stimulation. The main input sensory channels are the eyes, ears, skin, and nose. If input from all of these is blocked, there is loss of the sense of reality, distortion of time and imagined space, hallucinations, bizarre thought patterns, and other indications of neurological dysfunction. Even minimal sensory deprivation in early childhood can have a serious effect on the future personality. An eye covered for a few months in infancy remains effectively blind for life. Early deprivation of normal hearing can produce severe intellectual and educational damage. Deprivation of the normal contact and stimulation provided for the baby by the mother can cause personality disturbance in later life.

sensory nerve a nerve that carries information inwards, from an outlying part of the body towards the central nervous system. Different sensory nerves convey information about temperature, pain, touch, taste, etc., to the brain. *Compare* MOTOR NERVE.

separation anxiety a state of distress and fear at the prospect of leaving secure surroundings, such as is experienced by some children when they must leave parents to go to school. It is often caused by insecure *attachment.

sepsis *n.* the putrefactive destruction of tissues by disease-causing bacteria or their toxins.

sept- (septi-) *prefix denoting* **1.** seven. **2.** (or **septo-**) a septum, especially the nasal septum. **3.** sepsis.

septal defect a hole in the partition (septum) between the left and right halves of the heart. This abnormal communication is congenital due to an abnormality of heart development in the fetus. It may be found between the two atria (*see* ATRIAL SEPTAL DEFECT) or between the ventricles (*see* VENTRICULAR SEPTAL DEFECT). A septal defect permits abnormal circulation of blood from the left side of the heart, where pressures are higher, to the right. This abnormal circulation is called a **shunt** and results in excessive blood flow through the lungs. *Pulmonary hypertension develops and *heart failure may occur with large shunts. A heart *murmur is normally present. Large defects are closed surgically but small defects do not require treatment.

septic *adj.* relating to or affected with *sepsis.

septicaemia *n.* widespread destruction of tissues due to absorption of disease-causing bacteria or their toxins from the bloodstream. The term is also used loosely for any form of *blood poisoning. *Compare* PYAEMIA, SAPRAEMIA, TOXAEMIA.

septic arthritis infection in a joint. The joint is swollen, hot, and tender, and movement is very restricted and painful. The infecting organism can enter the joint via the bloodstream or from a penetrating injury. Treatment is by *arthrotomy or arthroscopy, irrigation of the joint, and antibiotics. If untreated, the articular cartilage is destroyed, leaving a stiff and deformed joint.

Septrin *n.* *see* CO-TRIMOXAZOLE.

septum *n.* (*pl.* **septa**) a partition or dividing wall within an anatomical structure. For example, the **atrioventricular septum** divides the atria of the heart from the ventricles. —**septal** *adj.* —**septate** *adj.*

sequela *n.* (*pl.* **sequelae**) any disorder or pathological condition that results from a preceding disease or accident.

sequestration *n.* **1.** the formation of a fragment of dead bone (*see* SEQUESTRUM) and its separation from the surrounding tissue. **2.** (in development) a separated part of an organ; a developmental anomaly.

sequestrectomy *n.* surgical removal of a *sequestrum.

sequestrum *n.* (*pl.* **sequestra**) a portion of dead bone formed in an infected bone in chronic *osteomyelitis. It is surrounded by an envelope (**involucrum**) of sclerotic bone and fibrous tissue and can be seen as a dense area within the bone on X-ray. It can cause irritation and the formation of pus, which may discharge through a *sinus, and is usually surgically removed (**sequestrectomy**).

ser- (sero-) *prefix denoting* **1.** serum. **2.** serous membrane.

serine *n.* *see* AMINO ACID.

seroconvert *vb.* to produce specific antibodies in response to the presence of an antigen (e.g. a vaccine or a virus). In *AIDS patients **seroconversion** occurs within 4–6 weeks of the initial HIV infection. It is marked by a sore throat, swollen lymph nodes, fever, aches and pains, and fatigue. *n.*

serofibrinous *adj.* describing an exudate of serum that contains a high proportion of the protein fibrin.

serology *n.* the study of blood serum and its constituents, particularly their contribution to the protection of the body against disease. *See* AGGLUTINATION, COMPLEMENT FIXATION, PRECIPITIN. —**serological** *adj.*

sero-negative arthritis *see* (ANKYLOSING) SPONDYLITIS.

seropus *n.* a mixture of serum and pus, which forms, for example, in infected blisters.

serosa *n.* *see* SEROUS MEMBRANE.

serositis *n.* inflammation of a *serous membrane, such as the lining of the thoracic cavity (pleura). *See* POLYSEROSITIS.

serotherapy *n.* the use of serum containing known antibodies (*see* ANTISERUM) to treat a patient with an infection or to confer temporary passive *immunity upon a person at special risk. The use of antisera prepared in animals carries its own risks (for example, a patient may be-

come hypersensitive to horse protein); the risk is reduced if the serum is taken from an immune human being.

serotonin (5-hydroxytryptamine) *n.* a compound widely distributed in the tissues, particularly in the blood platelets, intestinal wall, and central nervous system. Serotonin is thought to play a role in inflammation similar to that of *histamine and it is involved in the genesis of a migrainous headache. It also acts as a *neurotransmitter, and its levels in the brain are believed to have an important influence on mood. *See also* SSRI.

serotype *n.* a category into which material is placed based on its serological activity, particularly in terms of the antigens it contains or the antibodies that may be produced against it. Thus bacteria of the same species may be subdivided into serotypes that produce slightly different antigens. The serotype of an infective organism is important when treatment or prophylaxis with a vaccine is being considered.

serous *adj.* **1.** relating to or containing serum. **2.** resembling serum or producing a fluid resembling serum.

serous membrane (serosa) a smooth transparent membrane, consisting of *mesothelium and underlying elastic fibrous connective tissue, lining certain large cavities of the body. The *peritoneum of the abdomen, *pleura of the chest, and *pericardium of the heart are all serous membranes. Each consists of two portions: the **parietal** portion lines the walls of the cavity, and the **visceral** portion covers the organs concerned. The two are continuous, forming a closed sac with the organs essentially outside the sac. The inner surface of the sac is moistened by a thin fluid derived from blood serum, which allows frictionless movement of organs within their cavities. *Compare* MUCOUS MEMBRANE.

serpiginous *adj.* describing a creeping or extending skin lesion, especially one with a wavy edge.

serratus *n.* any of several muscles arising from or inserted by a series of processes that resemble the teeth of a saw. An example is the **serratus anterior**, a muscle situated between the ribs and shoulder blade in the upper and lateral parts of the thorax. It is the chief muscle responsible for pushing and punching movements.

sertindole *n.* *see* ANTIPSYCHOTIC.

Sertoli cells cells found in the walls of the seminiferous tubules of the *testis. Compared with the germ cells they appear large and pale. They anchor and probably nourish the developing germ cells, especially the *spermatids, which become partly embedded within them. A **Sertoli-cell tumour** is a rare testicular tumour causing *feminization. [E. Sertoli (1842–1910), Italian histologist]

sertraline *n.* an antidepressant drug that acts by prolonging the action of the neurotransmitter serotonin (5-hydroxytryptamine) in the brain (*see* SSRI). It is taken by mouth; side-effects may include dizziness, agitation, tremor, nausea, diarrhoea, and drowsiness. Trade name: **Lustral**.

serum (blood serum) *n.* the fluid that separates from clotted blood or blood plasma that is allowed to stand. Serum is essentially similar in composition to *plasma but lacks fibrinogen and other substances that are used in the coagulation process.

serum hepatitis *see* HEPATITIS.

serum sickness a reaction that sometimes occurs 7–12 days after injection of a quantity of foreign serum, such as horse serum used in the preparation of antitetanus injections. The usual symptoms are rashes, fever, joint pains, and enlargement of the lymph nodes. The reaction is due to the presence of antigenic material still in the circulation by the time that the body has started producing antibodies against it; it is therefore a form of delayed *hypersensitivity reaction. The condition is rarely serious.

sesamoid bone an oval nodule of bone that lies within a tendon and slides over another bony surface. The patella (kneecap) and certain bones in the hand and foot are sesamoid bones.

sessile *adj.* (of a tumour) attached directly by its base without a peduncle (stalk).

seton *n.* a form of treatment in which a thread is passed through a *fistula and tied in a loop. The seton acts as a wick to drain off pus and can be tightened to open the track. This method can be used to treat high anal fistulas because it has a reduced risk of causing incontinence.

severe combined immune deficiency (SCID) a rare disorder that usually manifests itself within the first three months of life by severe bacterial, fungal, and viral infection. It is due to reduced numbers of T- and B-*lymphocytes – white blood cells necessary for fighting infection. Some cases are caused by *adenosine deaminase (ADA) deficiency. The only treatment currently available is a bone-marrow transplant.

severe disablement allowance a state benefit payable to those under state retirement age who have not been able to work for at least 28 weeks because of illness or disablement and who do not qualify for *incapacity benefit because they have not paid enough National Insurance contributions. Claimants must normally undergo the 'all-work' test used to claim incapacity benefit.

Sever's disease *apophysitis caused by pulling at the point of insertion of the Achilles tendon into the calcaneus (heel bone), causing heel pain. [J. W. Sever (20th century), US orthopaedic surgeon]

sexarche *n.* the age when a person first engages in sexual intercourse.

sex chromatin *chromatin found only in female cells and believed to represent a single X chromosome in a nondividing cell. It can be used to discover the sex of a baby before birth by examination of cells obtained by *amniocentesis or *chorionic villus sampling. There are two main kinds: (1) the **Barr body**, a small object that stains with basic dyes, found on the edge of the nucleus just inside the nuclear membrane; (2) a drumstick-like appendage to the nucleus in neutrophils (a type of white blood cell).

sex chromosome a chromosome that is involved in the determination of the sex of the individual. Women have two *X chromosomes; men have one X chromosome and one *Y chromosome. *Compare* AUTOSOME.

sex hormone any steroid hormone, produced mainly by the ovaries or testes, that is responsible for controlling sexual development and reproductive function. *Oestrogens and *progesterone are the female sex hormones; *androgens are the male sex hormones.

sex-limited *adj.* describing characteristics that are expressed differently in the two sexes but are controlled by genes not on the sex chromosomes, e.g. baldness in men.

sex-linked *adj.* describing genes (or the characteristics controlled by them) that are carried on the sex chromosomes, usually the *X chromosome. The genes for certain disorders, such as *haemophilia, are carried on the X chromosome; these genes and disorders are described as **X-linked**. Since these sex-linked genes are *recessive, men are more likely to have the diseases since they have only one X chromosome; women can carry the genes but their harmful effects are usually masked by the dominant (normal) alleles on their second X chromosome.

sexology *n.* the study of sexual matters, including anatomy, physiology, behaviour, and techniques.

sex ratio the proportion of males to females in a population, usually expressed as the number of males per 100 females. The **primary sex ratio**, at the time of fertilization, is in theory 50% male. The **secondary sex ratio**, found at birth, usually indicates slightly fewer girls than boys.

sexual abuse *see* CHILD ABUSE, PAEDOPHILIA.

sexual deviation any sexual behaviour regarded as abnormal by society. The deviation may relate to the sexual object (as in *fetishism) or the activity engaged in (for example, *sadism and *exhibitionism). The activity is sexually pleasurable.

The definition of what is normal varies with different cultures, and treatment is appropriate only when the deviation causes suffering. Some people may find that *counselling helps them to adjust to their deviation. Others may wish for treatment to change the deviation: *aversion

therapy may be used, also *conditioning normal sexual fantasies to pleasurable behaviour. The only helpful effect of drugs is to reduce sexual drive generally.

sexually transmitted disease (STD) any disease transmitted by sexual intercourse, formerly known as **venereal disease**. STDs include *AIDS, *syphilis, *gonorrhoea, some *Chlamydia infections, genital *herpes, and *soft sore. The medical specialty concerned with STDs is **genitourinary medicine**.

SFD small for dates: *see* INTRAUTERINE GROWTH RETARDATION.

SGOT serum glutamic oxaloacetic transaminase. *See* GLUTAMIC OXALOACETIC TRANSAMINASE.

SGPT serum glutamic pyruvic transaminase. *See* GLUTAMIC PYRUVIC TRANSAMINASE.

shaking palsy an archaic name for *parkinsonism.

shaping *n.* a technique of *behaviour modification used in the teaching of complex skills or in encouraging rare forms of behaviour. At first the therapist rewards actions that are similar to the desired behaviour; thereafter the therapist rewards successively closer approximations, until eventually only the desired behaviour is rewarded and thereby learned.

sheath *n.* **1.** (in anatomy) the layer of connective tissue that envelops structures such as nerves, arteries, tendons, and muscles. **2.** a *condom.

Sheehan's syndrome a condition in which *amenorrhoea and infertility follow a major haemorrhage in pregnancy. It is caused by necrosis (death) of the anterior lobe of the pituitary gland as a direct result of the haemorrhage reducing the blood supply to the gland. *Compare* ASHERMAN SYNDROME. [H. L. Sheehan (20th century), British pathologist]

sheltered housing specially converted (or adapted) accommodation, often in the form of a flatlet, designed to meet the special needs of the elderly who are capable of a degree of self-care. A warden is generally in attendance. The extent to which meals and other services are provided on a continuous basis varies; so too in Britain does the *per capita* payment from the appropriate social service department.

Sheridan-Gardiner test a test for detecting visual handicap in children who are too young to be able to read the *Snellen chart. A series of cards, each marked with a single letter of a specific size, are held up at a distance of 6 metres from the child being tested. The child is provided with an identification card containing a selection of letters and is asked to point to the letter that is the same as the one on the card in the distance. The test is suitable for children between the ages of two and seven.

Shigella *n.* a genus of nonmotile rodlike Gram-negative bacteria normally present in the intestinal tract of warm-blooded animals and man. They ferment carbohydrates without the formation of gas. Some *Shigella* species are pathogenic. *S. dysenteriae* is associated with bacillary *dysentery.

shigellosis *n.* an infestation of the digestive system by bacteria of the genus *Shigella*, causing bacillary *dysentery.

shingles *n.* herpes zoster (*see* HERPES).

shock *n.* the condition associated with circulatory collapse, when the arterial blood pressure is too low to maintain an adequate supply of blood to the tissues. The patient has a cold sweaty pallid skin, a weak rapid pulse, irregular breathing, dry mouth, dilated pupils, and a reduced flow of urine.

   Shock may be due to a decrease in the volume of blood, as occurs after internal or external *haemorrhage, burns, dehydration, or severe vomiting or diarrhoea. It may be caused by reduced activity of the heart, as in coronary thrombosis, myocardial infarction, or pulmonary embolism. It may also be due to widespread dilation of the veins so that there is insufficient blood to fill them. This may be caused by the presence of bacteria in the bloodstream (**bacteraemic** or **toxic shock**), a severe allergic reaction (**anaphylactic shock**: *see* ANAPHYLAXIS), overdosage with such drugs as narcotics or barbiturates, or the emotional shock due to a personal tragedy or disaster (**neurogenic shock**). Sometimes shock may result from a combination of any of these causes, as in

*peritonitis. The treatment of shock is determined by the cause.

short-sightedness *n.* *see* MYOPIA.

shoulder *n.* the ball-and-socket joint (*see* ENARTHROSIS) between the glenoid cavity of the *scapula and the upper end (head) of the humerus. It is a common site of dislocation. The joint is surrounded by a capsule closely associated with many tendons: it is the site of many strains and inflammations ('cuff injuries').

shoulder girdle (pectoral girdle) the bony structure to which the bones of the upper limbs are attached. It consists of the right and left *scapulas (**shoulder blades**) and clavicles (collar bones).

shunt *n.* a passage connecting two anatomical channels and diverting blood or other fluid (e.g. cerebrospinal fluid) from one to the other. It may occur as a congenital abnormality (as in *septal defects of the heart) or be surgically created. *See also* ANASTOMOSIS.

sial- (sialo-) *prefix denoting* **1.** saliva. **2.** a salivary gland.

sialadenitis *n.* inflammation of a salivary gland.

sialagogue *n.* a drug that promotes the secretion of saliva. *Parasympathomimetic drugs have this action.

sialic acid an amino sugar. Sialic acid is a component of some *glycoproteins, *gangliosides, and bacterial cell walls.

sialography (ptyalography) *n.* X-ray examination of the salivary glands, after introducing a quantity of radiopaque material into the ducts of the salivary glands in the mouth. It enables the presence of degenerative disease or obstructive calculi to be detected.

sialolith *n.* a stone (calculus) in a salivary gland or duct, most often the duct of the submandibular gland. The flow of saliva is obstructed, causing swelling and intense pain. Treatment is by surgery or – more recently – by means of a lithotripter (*see* LITHOTRIPSY).

sialorrhoea *n.* *see* PTYALISM.

Siamese twins (conjoined twins) identical twins that are physically joined together at birth. The condition ranges from twins joined only by the umbilical blood vessels (**allantoido-angiopagous twins**) to those in whom conjoined heads or trunk are inseparable.

sib *n. see* SIBLING.

sibilant *adj.* whistling or hissing. The term is applied to certain high-pitched abnormal sounds heard through a stethoscope.

sibling (sib) *n.* one of a number of children of the same parents, i.e. a brother or sister.

sickle-cell disease (drepanocytosis) a hereditary blood disease that mainly affects people of African ancestry but also occurs in the Mediterranean region and reaches high frequencies in parts of Saudi Arabia and India. It occurs when the sickle-cell gene has been inherited from both parents and is characterized by the production of an abnormal type of *haemoglobin – **sickle-cell haemoglobin (Hbs)** – which precipitates in the red cells when the blood is deprived of oxygen, forming crystals that distort the cells into the characteristic sickle shape: this process is known as **sickling**. Sickle cells are rapidly removed from the circulation, leading to anaemia and jaundice. There is no satisfactory treatment; the highest mortality is in childhood but some patients may live to an age of 60–70 years.

The carrier condition (**sickle-cell trait**) occurs when the defective gene is inherited from only one parent. It generally causes no symptoms but confers some protection from malaria, which accounts for the high frequency of the gene in malarious areas. If a general anaesthetic is to be given to a patient with this condition, the anaesthetist should be alerted.

sickness benefit (in the UK) a former benefit paid, under the Social Security Act 1975, to those who did not qualify for statutory sick pay. It was replaced by *incapacity benefit in 1995.

side-effect *n.* an unwanted effect produced by a drug in addition to its desired therapeutic effects. Side-effects are often undesirable and may be harmful.

sidero- *prefix denoting* iron.

sideroblast *n.* a red blood cell precursor (*see* ERYTHROBLAST) in which iron-containing granules can be demonstrated by suitable staining techniques. Sideroblasts may be seen in normal individuals and are absent in iron deficiency. A certain type of anaemia (**sideroblastic anaemia**) is characterized by the presence of abnormal **ringed sideroblasts**. —**sideroblastic** *adj.*

siderocyte *n.* a red blood cell in which granules of iron-containing protein (**Pappenheimer bodies**) can be demonstrated by suitable staining techniques. These granules are normally removed by the spleen and siderocytes are characteristically seen when the spleen is absent.

sideropenia *n.* iron deficiency. This may result from dietary inadequacy; increased requirement of iron by the body, as in pregnancy or childhood; or increased loss of iron from the body, usually due to chronic bleeding. The most important manifestation of iron deficiency is *anaemia, which is readily corrected by iron therapy.

siderosis *n.* the deposition of iron oxide dust in the lungs, occurring in silver finishers, arc welders, and haematite miners. Iron oxide itself is inert, but pulmonary *fibrosis may develop if fibrogenic dusts such as silica are also inhaled.

SIDS sudden infant death syndrome: *see* COT DEATH.

siemens *n.* the *SI unit of electrical conductance, equal to the conductance between two points on a conductor when a potential difference of 1 volt between these points causes a current of 1 ampere to flow between them. Symbol: S.

sievert *n.* the *SI unit of dose equivalent, being the dose equivalent when the absorbed dose of ionizing radiation multiplied by the stipulated dimensionless factors is $1 \, J \, kg^{-1}$. As different types of radiation cause different effects in biological tissue a weighted absorbed dose, called the dose equivalent, is used in which the absorbed dose is modified by multiplying it by dimensionless factors stipulated by the International Commission on Radiological Protection. The sievert has replaced the *rem. Symbol: Sv.

sigmoid- *prefix denoting* the sigmoid colon. Example: **sigmoidotomy** (incision into).

sigmoid colon (sigmoid flexure) the S-shaped terminal part of the descending *colon, which leads to the rectum.

sigmoidectomy *n.* removal of the sigmoid colon by surgery. It is performed for tumours, severe *diverticular disease, or for an abnormally long sigmoid colon that has become twisted (*see* VOLVULUS).

sigmoidoscope *n.* an instrument inserted through the anus in order to inspect the interior of the rectum and sigmoid colon. In its commonest form it consists of a steel, chrome, or plastic tube, 25 cm long and 3 cm in diameter, with some form of illumination and a bellows to inflate the bowel, but flexible fibre-optic instruments ("flexiscopes"), 60 cm long, are increasingly being used.

sigmoidoscopy *n.* examination of the rectum and sigmoid colon with a *sigmoidoscope. It is used to investigate diarrhoea or rectal bleeding, particularly to detect colitis or cancer of the rectum.

sign *n.* an indication of a particular disorder that is observed by a physician but is not apparent to the patient. *Compare* SYMPTOM.

significance *n.* (in statistics) a relationship between two groups of observations indicating that the difference between them is unlikely to have occurred by chance alone. An assumption is made that there is no difference between the two populations from which the two groups come (**null hypothesis**). This is tested, and a calculation indicating that there is a **probability** of less than 5% (P<0.05) that the observed difference or a larger one could have arisen by chance is regarded as being **statistically significant** and the null hypothesis is rejected. Some tests are **parametric**, based on the assumption that the range of observations are distributed by chance in a **normal** or **Gaussian distribution**, where 95% lie within two *standard deviations of the *mean (**Student's t test** to compare means). Nonparametric tests (**Mann-Whitney U tests**) make no assumptions about distribution patterns. *See also* FREQUENCY DISTRIBUTION, STANDARD ERROR.

sign of Dance (signe de Dance) a depression elicited by palpation of the right lower quadrant of the abdomen, which is characteristic of *intussusception. [J. B. H. Dance (1797–1832), French physician]

sildenafil *n.* a drug administered orally for the treatment of erectile impotence. During sexual stimulation, it causes smooth muscle relaxation and increased blood flow to the corpus cavernosum of the penis, which results in erection. Side-effects include headache, facial flushing, dyspepsia, nasal congestion, and dizziness. Because of severe adverse reactions, the drug is contraindicated in patients taking nitrate-based drugs, such as glyceryl trinitrate. Trade name: **Viagra**.

silicosis *n.* a lung disease – a form of *pneumoconiosis – produced by inhaling silica dust particles. It affects workers in hard-rock mining and tunnelling, quarrying, stone dressing, sand blasting, and boiler scaling. Silica stimulates *fibrosis of lung tissue, which produces progressive breathlessness and considerably increased susceptibility to tuberculosis.

silver nitrate a salt of silver with *astringent, *caustic, and *disinfectant properties. Available as a stick, it is used mainly to destroy warts. Application discolours the skin bluish-black.

simethicone (activated dimethicone) *n.* a silicone-based material with antifoaming properties, used in the treatment of flatulence and often incorporated into antacid remedies.

Simmond's disease loss of sexual function, loss of weight, and other features of failure of the pituitary gland (*hypopituitarism) caused by trauma or tumours or occurring in women after childbirth complicated by bleeding (postpartum haemorrhage). [M. Simmonds (1885–1925), German physician]

Sims's position the left-sided knees-up position commonly assumed by patients undergoing examinations of the anus and rectum or vagina. [J. M. Sims (1813–83), US gynaecologist]

simulator *n.* an X-ray device used in radiotherapy to plan accurately the exact position of the final exposure of radiation before treatment begins.

Simulium *n.* *see* BLACK FLY.

simvastatin *n.* a drug used to reduce abnormally high levels of cholesterol in the blood. Its actions and side-effects are similar to those of *lovastatin. Trade name: **Zocor**.

sinew *n.* a tendon.

singer's nodule a pearly white nodule that may develop on the vocal folds of people who use their voice excessively or in those with poor vocal technique.

single photon emission computed tomography *see* SPECT SCANNING.

singultus *n.* *see* HICCUP.

sinistr- (sinistro-) *prefix denoting* left or the left side.

sino- (sinu-) *prefix denoting* **1.** a sinus. **2.** the sinus venosus.

sinoatrial node (SA node) the pacemaker of the heart: a microscopic area of specialized cardiac muscle located in the upper wall of the right atrium near the entry of the vena cava. Fibres of the SA node are self-excitatory, contracting rhythmically at around 70 times per minute. Following each contraction, the impulse spreads throughout the atrial muscle and into fibres connecting the SA node with the *atrioventricular node. The SA node is supplied by fibres of the autonomic nervous system; impulses arriving at the node accelerate or decrease the heart rate.

sinus *n.* **1.** an air cavity within a bone, especially any of the cavities within the bones of the face or skull (*see* PARANASAL SINUS). **2.** any wide channel containing blood, usually venous blood. **Venous sinuses** occur, for example, in the dura mater and drain blood from the brain. **3.** a pocket or bulge in a tubular organ, especially a blood vessel; for example, the *carotid sinus. **4.** (**sinus tract**) an infected tract leading from a focus of infection to the surface of the skin or a hollow organ. *See* PILONIDAL SINUS.

sinus arrhythmia a normal variation in the heart rate, which accelerates slightly on inspiration and slows on expiration. It is common in healthy individuals.

sinusitis *n.* inflammation of one or more of the mucous-membrane-lined air spaces in the facial bones that communicate with the nose (the paranasal sinuses). It is often associated with inflammation of the nasal lining (*rhinitis) and may be acute or chronic (*see* RHINOSINUSITIS). Symptoms may include pain, purulent discharge from the nose, nasal obstruction, and disturbances of the sense of smell. Many cases are self-limiting. Others require treatment with antibiotics, decongestants, or steroid nose drops. A few cases need surgery, such as sinus washouts, *antrostomy, or *functional endoscopic sinus surgery (FESS).

sinusoid *n.* a small blood vessel found in certain organs, such as the adrenal gland and liver. Large numbers of sinusoids occur in the liver. They receive oxygen-rich blood from the hepatic artery and nutrients from the intestines via the portal vein. Oxygen and nutrients diffuse through the capillary walls into the liver cells. The sinusoids are drained by the hepatic veins. *See also* PORTAL SYSTEM.

sinus venosus a chamber of the embryonic heart that receives blood from several veins. In the adult heart it becomes part of the right atrium.

siphonage *n.* the transfer of liquid from one container to another by means of a bent tube. The procedure is used in gastric *lavage, when the stomach is filled with water through a funnel and rubber tube, and the tube is then bent downwards to act as a siphon and empty the stomach of its contents.

Siphunculina *n.* a genus of flies. *S. funicola*, the eye fly of India, feeds on the secretions of the tear glands and in landing on or near the eyes contributes to the spread of *conjunctivitis.

sirenomelia *n.* *see* SYMPODIA.

SIRS *see* SYSTEMIC INFLAMMATORY RESPONSE SYNDROME.

sito- *prefix denoting* food.

sitz bath a fairly shallow hip bath in which the person is seated. Sitz baths of cold and hot water, rapidly alternated, were formerly used for the treatment of a variety of sexual disorders.

SI units (Système International d'Unités) the internationally agreed system of units now in use for all scientific purposes. Based on the metre-kilogram-second system, SI units have seven base units and two supplementary units. Measurements of all other physical quantities are expressed in derived units, consisting of two or more base units. Tables 1 and 2 (Appendix) list the base

skull

mandible

cervical vertebrae

clavicle

scapula

ribs

sternum

humerus

thoracic vertebrae

lumbar vertebrae

ulna

ilium

sacrum

radius

metacarpals

phalanges

carpals

coccyx

femur

patella

tibia

fibula

tarsals

phalanges

metatarsals

The skeleton

units and the derived units having special names; all these units are defined in the dictionary.

Decimal multiples of SI units are expressed using specified prefixes; where possible a prefix representing 10 raised to a power that is a multiple of three should be used. Prefixes are listed in Table 3 (Appendix).

Sjögren's syndrome an autoimmune condition affecting the salivary and lacrimal glands, resulting in a *dry mouth and dryness of the eyes. In the systemic form of the disease other glands may be affected, causing dryness of the airways, vagina, or skin, as well as the joints (producing a relatively mild form of arthritis) and muscles (which ache), and there may be tiredness and lethargy. Sjögren's syndrome may also occur secondarily to other conditions (e.g. rheumatoid arthritis).

Symptomatic treatment, including saliva and tear substitutes, is available. [H. S. C. Sjögren (20th century), Swedish ophthalmologist]

skatole (methyl indole) *n.* a derivative of the amino acid tryptophan, excreted in the urine and faeces.

skeletal muscle *see* STRIATED MUSCLE.

skeleton *n.* the rigid framework of connected *bones that gives form to the body, protects and supports its soft organs and tissues, and provides attachments for muscles and a system of levers essential for locomotion. The 206 named bones of the body are organized into the **axial skeleton** (of the head and trunk) and the **appendicular skeleton** (of the limbs). (See illustration.) —**skeletal** *adj.*

skew *n.* a disorder of relationships within a family, in which one parent is

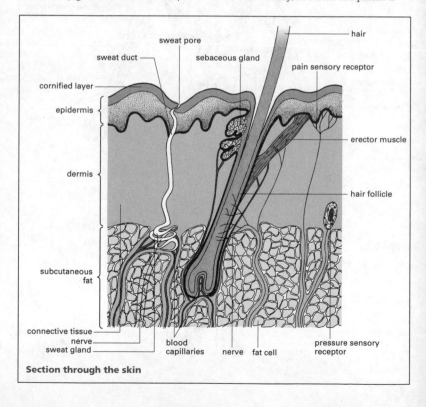

Section through the skin

overpowering and the other is submissive and there is a general avoidance of anxiety-provoking situations. It was proposed as a specific cause of schizophrenia in the children, but this has not been confirmed.

skew deviation a neurological condition of the eyes in which one eye turns down while the other turns up. It is seen in disorders of the *cerebellum or *brainstem.

skia- *prefix denoting* shadow.

skiagram *n.* an obsolete term for an X-ray photograph. —**skiagraphy** *n.*

skier's thumb (gamekeeper's thumb) rupture and consequent instability of the ligament on the inside of the thumb between the metacarpal and proximal (first) phalanx, caused by forced abduction of the thumb. Treatment is by surgical repair of the ligament.

skin *n.* the outer covering of the body, consisting of an outer layer, the *epidermis, and an inner layer, the *dermis (see illustration). Beneath the dermis is a layer of fatty tissue. The skin has several functions. The epidermis protects the body from injury and also from invasion by parasites. It also helps to prevent the body from becoming dehydrated. The combination of erectile hairs, *sweat glands, and blood capillaries in the skin form part of

the temperature-regulating mechanism of the body. When the body is too hot, loss of heat is increased by sweating and by the dilation of the capillaries. When the body is too cold the sweat glands are inactive, the capillaries contract, and a layer of air is trapped over the epidermis by the erected hairs. The skin also acts as an organ of excretion (by the secretion of *sweat) and as a sense organ (it contains receptors that are sensitive to heat, cold, touch, and pain). The layer of fat that lies underneath the dermis can act as a reservoir of food and water. Anatomical name: **cutis**.

skin graft a portion of healthy skin cut from one area of the body and used to cover a part that has lost its skin, usually as a result of injury, burns, or operation. A skin graft is normally taken from another part of the body of the same patient (an *autograft), but occasionally skin may be grafted from one person to another as a temporary healing measure (a *homograft). The full thickness of skin may be taken for a graft (*see* FLAP) or the surgeon may use three-quarters thickness, thin sheets of skin (*see* THIERSCH'S GRAFT), or a pinch skin graft. The type used depends on the condition and size of the damaged area to be treated. The skin graft may be free or attached by a *pedicle.

Side view of the skull

ski-stick injury a penetrating injury by a ski stick.

skull *n.* the skeleton of the head and face, which is made up of 22 bones. It can be divided into the cranium, which encloses the brain, and the face (including the lower jaw (mandible)). (See illustration.) The **cranium** consists of eight bones. The frontal, parietals (two), occipital, and temporals (two) form the vault of the skull (**calvaria**) and are made up of two thin layers of compact bone separated by a layer of spongy bone (**diploë**). The remaining bones of the cranium – the sphenoid and ethmoid – form part of its base. The 14 bones that make up the face are the nasals, lacrimals, inferior nasal conchae, maxillae, zygomatics, and palatines (two of each), the vomer, and the mandible. All the bones of the skull except the mandible are connected to each other by immovable joints (*see* SUTURE). The skull contains cavities for the eyes (*see* ORBIT) and nose (*see* NASAL CAVITY) and a large opening at its base (**foramen magnum**) through which the spinal cord passes.

SLE systemic lupus erythematosus. *See* LUPUS ERYTHEMATOSUS.

sleep *n.* a state of natural unconsciousness, during which the brain's activity is not apparent (apart from the continued maintenance of basic bodily functions, such as breathing) but can be detected by means of an electroencephalogram (EEG). Different stages of sleep are recognized by different EEG wave patterns. Drowsiness is marked by short irregular waves; as sleep deepens the waves become slower, larger, and more irregular. This slow-wave sleep is periodically interrupted by episodes of paradoxical, or *REM (rapid-eye-movement), sleep, when the EEG pattern is similar to that of an awake and alert person. Dreaming occurs during REM sleep. The two states of sleep alternate in cycles of from 30 to 90 minutes, REM sleep constituting about a quarter of the total sleeping time.

sleep apnoea cessation of breathing during sleep, which may be **obstructive**, due to frustrated efforts to breathe against blocked upper airways (*see* OBSTRUCTIVE SLEEP APNOEA), or **central**, in which there is no evidence of any voluntary effort.

sleeping sickness (African trypanosomiasis) a disease of tropical Africa caused by the presence in the blood of the parasitic protozoans *Trypanosoma gambiense* or *T. rhodesiense*. The parasites are transmitted to man through the bite of *tsetse flies. Initial symptoms include fever, headache, and chills, followed later by enlargement of the lymph nodes, anaemia, and pains in the limbs and joints. After a period of several months or even years, the parasites invade the minute blood vessels supplying the central nervous system. This causes drowsiness and lethargy, and ultimately – if untreated – the patient dies. Rhodesian sleeping sickness is the more virulent form of the disease. The drugs *suramin, *pentamidine, and *eflornithine are used to treat the early curable stages of sleeping sickness; drugs containing arsenic (*see* TRYPARSAMIDE) are administered after the brain is affected. Eradication of tsetse flies helps prevent spread of the infection.

sleep-walking *n. see* SOMNAMBULISM.

sling *n.* a bandage arranged to support and rest an injured limb so that healing is not hindered by activity. The most common sling is a *triangular bandage tied behind the neck to support the weight of a broken arm. The arm is bent at the elbow and held across the body.

slipped disc a colloquial term for a *prolapsed intervertebral disc.

slit lamp a device for providing a narrow beam of light, used in conjunction with a special microscope. It can be used to examine minutely the structures within the eye, one layer at a time.

slough *n.* dead tissue, such as skin, that separates from healthy tissue after inflammation or infection.

slow virus one of a group of infective disease agents that resemble *viruses in some of their biological properties but whose physical properties (e.g. sensitivity to radiation) suggest that they may not contain nucleic acid. They are now more commonly known as *prions.

SMA *see* SPINAL MUSCULAR ATROPHY.

small for dates (SFD) *see* INTRAUTERINE GROWTH RETARDATION.

smallpox *n* an acute infectious virus disease causing high fever and a rash that scars the skin. It is transmitted chiefly by direct contact with a patient. Symptoms commence 8–18 days after exposure and include headache, backache, high fever, and vomiting. On the third day, as the fever subsides, red spots appear on the face and spread to the trunk and extremities. Over the next 8–9 days all the spots (macules) change to pimples (papules), then to pea-sized blisters that are at first watery (vesicles) but soon become pus-filled (pustules). The fever returns, often causing delirium. On the eleventh or twelfth day the rash and fever abate. Scabs formed by drying out of pustules fall off 7–20 days later, leaving permanent scars. The patient remains infectious until all scabs have been shed. Most patients recover but serious complications, such as nephritis or pneumonia, may develop. Treatment with thiosemicarbazone is effective. An attack usually confers immunity; immunization against smallpox has now totally eradicated the disease. Medical name: **variola**. *See also* ALASTRIM, COWPOX.

smear *n.* a specimen of tissue or other material taken from part of the body and smeared on a microscope slide for examination. *See* CERVICAL SMEAR.

smegma *n.* the secretion of the glands of the foreskin (*prepuce), which accumulates under the foreskin and has a white cheesy appearance. It becomes readily infested by a harmless bacterium that resembles the tubercle bacillus.

Smith's fracture a fracture just above the wrist, across the lower end of the radius, resulting in forward displacement of the hand and wrist below the fracture. It is the reverse of *Colles' fracture. [R. W. Smith (1807–73), Irish surgeon]

smooth muscle (involuntary muscle) muscle that produces slow long-term contractions of which the individual is unaware. Smooth muscle occurs in hollow organs, such as the stomach, intestine, blood vessels, and bladder. It consists of spindle-shaped cells within a network of connective tissue (see illustration) and is

under the control of the autonomic nervous system. *Compare* STRIATED MUSCLE.

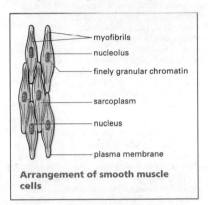

Arrangement of smooth muscle cells

snare *n.* an instrument consisting of a wire loop designed to remove polyps, tumours, and other projections of tissue, particularly those occurring in body cavities (see illustration). The loop is used to encircle the base of the tumour and is then pulled tight. *See also* DIATHERMY.

A nasal snare

sneeze **1.** *n.* an involuntary violent reflex expulsion of air through the nose and mouth provoked by irritation of the mucous membrane lining the nasal cavity. **2.** *vb.* to produce a sneeze.

Snellen chart the commonest chart used for testing sharpness of distant vision (*see* VISUAL ACUITY). It consists of rows of capital letters, called **test types**, the letters of each row becoming smaller down the chart. The large letter at the top is of such a size that it can be read by a person with normal sight from a distance of 60 metres. A normally sighted person can read successive lines of letters from 36, 24, 18, 12, 9, 6, and 5 metres respectively. There is sometimes a line for 4 metres. The subject sits 6 metres from the chart and one eye is tested at a time. If he can only read down as far as the 12-metre line the visual acuity is expressed as 6/12. Normally sighted people can read the 6-metre line, i.e. normal acuity is 6/6, and many people read the 5-metre line with ease. A smaller chart on the same principle is available for testing near vision. In North America the test is done at a distance of 20 feet: 20/20 vision is the same as 6/6. [H. Snellen (1834–1908), Dutch ophthalmologist]

snoring *n.* noisy breathing while asleep due to vibration of the soft palate, uvula, pharyngeal walls, or epiglottis. In children it is often associated with enlargement of the tonsils and adenoids. Treatments of snoring include weight loss, tobacco and alcohol avoidance, adenoidectomy, tonsillectomy, nasal airway surgery, *uvulopalatopharyngoplasty, and laser *palatoplasty.

snow blindness a painful disorder of the cornea of the eye due to excessive exposure to ultraviolet light reflected from the snow. Recovery usually follows within 24 hours of covering the eyes.

snuffles *n.* **1.** partial obstruction of breathing in infants, caused by the common cold. **2.** (formerly) discharge through the nostrils associated with necrosis of the nasal bones: seen in infants with congenital syphilis.

social class any one of the subdivisions of the population made by the Office for National Statistics based on occupation, as indicated in the ten-yearly census. Such groupings are intended to stratify the population according to standard of living and income (all married women and children up to school-leaving age are classified in accordance with the occupation of husband/father). Five classes are recognized: I professional/self-employed; II administrative; III (non-manual) clerical and (manual) skilled manual workers; IV semi-skilled; V unskilled. An alternative subdivision into **socio-economic groups** is believed by many sociologists to reflect employment grades more accurately, but it is more complicated and tends to be less generally applied.

social medicine *see* PUBLIC HEALTH MEDICINE.

social services advice and practical help with problems due to social circumstances. Every local authority is responsible for establishing and staffing a social service department, although block exchequer grants monitored by the *Department of Social Security meet some of the costs. An increasing proportion of the **social workers** in these departments are professionally trained. The present policy is to train generic social workers, but there are special social workers with medical and psychiatric training who are seconded for work in hospitals (*see* MEDICAL SOCIAL WORKER). Social workers assess the eligibility of clients for such social services as care assistants and meals on wheels or refer them to the appropriate statutory or voluntary services; difficulties may sometimes arise when the hospital *catchment area is not coterminous with the local authority. In relation to mental health, social workers may obtain court orders for *compulsory admission where necessary and provide surveillance and support for those being treated at home or in designated hostel accommodation, including those discharged from hospital. (*See also* AFTERCARE.) **Case work** involves identifying the cause of the client's problem and, where appropriate, advising how best to correct it and/or adapt to the circumstances.

social worker *see* SOCIAL SERVICES.

socio-economic group *see* SOCIAL CLASS.

socket *n.* (in anatomy) a hollow or depression into which another part fits, such as the cavity in the alveolar bone of the jaws into which the root of a tooth fits. *See also* DRY SOCKET.

sodium *n.* a mineral element and an important constituent of the human body (average sodium content of the adult body is 4000 mmol). Sodium controls the volume of extracellular fluid in the body and maintains the acid-base balance. It also helps maintain electrical potentials in the nervous system and is thus necessary for the functioning of nerves and muscles. Sodium is contained in most foods and is well absorbed, the average daily intake in the UK being 200 mmol. The amount of sodium in the body is controlled by the kidneys. An excess of sodium leads to the soma

condition of **hypernatraemia**, which often results in *oedema. This may develop in infants fed on bottled milk, which has a much higher sodium content than human milk. Since babies are less able to remove sodium from the body than adults the feeding of a high-sodium diet to babies is dangerous and may lead to dehydration. Sodium is also implicated in hypertension: a high-sodium diet is thought to increase the risk of hypertension in later life. Symbol: Na.

sodium bicarbonate a salt of sodium that neutralizes acid and is used to treat stomach and digestive disorders, *acidosis, and sodium deficiency. It is administered by mouth or injection; high doses may cause digestive upsets. See also ANTACID.

sodium chloride common salt: a salt of sodium that is present in all tissues and is important in maintaining the *electrolyte balance of the body. Sodium chloride infusions are the basis of fluid replacement therapy after operations and for conditions associated with salt depletion, including shock and dehydration. Sodium chloride is also a basic constituent of *oral rehydration therapy.

sodium fluoride a salt of sodium used to prevent tooth decay. It is administered by mouth or applied to the teeth as paste or solution. Taken by mouth, it may cause digestive upsets and large doses may cause fluorine poisoning. See also FLUORIDATION. Trade name: **Fluor-a-day**.

sodium fusidate an *antibiotic used mainly to treat infections caused by *Staphylococcus. It is administered by mouth or injection or applied in an ointment for skin infections; common side-effects are mild digestive upsets. Trade name: **Fucidin**.

sodium hydroxide (caustic soda) a powerful alkali in widespread use as a cleaning agent. It attacks the skin, causing severe chemical burns that are best treated by washing the area with large quantities of water. When swallowed it causes burning of the mouth and throat, which should be treated by giving water, milk, or other fluid to dilute the stomach contents and by gastric lavage.

sodium hypochlorite a salt of sodium used in solution as an antiseptic and disinfectant. In dentistry a 0.5–5.0% solution is used for washing out infected root canals.

sodium nitrite a sodium salt used, with sodium thiosulphate, to treat cyanide poisoning. It is administered by injection and may cause digestive upsets, dizziness, headache, fainting, and cyanosis. It also has effects similar to *glyceryl trinitrate and has been used to treat angina.

sodium salicylate a drug with actions and side-effects similar to those of *aspirin. It is used mainly to treat rheumatic fever.

sodium thiosulphate a salt of sodium used, with *sodium nitrite, to treat cyanide poisoning. It is administered by intravenous injection.

sodium valproate an *anticonvulsant drug used to treat all types of epilepsy. It is administered by mouth; side-effects may include digestive upsets, drowsiness, muscle incoordination, and impaired liver function. It should be used with caution in pregnant women because of a risk of abnormalities developing in the fetus. Trade name: **Epilim**.

sodokosis n. see RAT-BITE FEVER.

sodomy n. sexual intercourse using the anus. This may be homosexual, heterosexual, or between man and beast. See also SEXUAL DEVIATION.

soft sore (chancroid) a sexually transmitted disease caused by the bacterium Haemophilus ducreyi, resulting in enlargement and ulceration of lymph nodes in the groin. Treatment with sulphonamides is effective.

solarium n. a room in which patients are exposed to either sunlight or artificial sunlight (a blend of visible light and infrared and ultraviolet radiation directed from special lamps).

solar plexus (coeliac plexus) a network of sympathetic nerves and ganglia high in the back of the abdomen.

soleus n. a broad flat muscle in the calf of the leg, beneath the *gastrocnemius muscle. The soleus flexes the foot, so that the toes point downwards.

soma n. **1.** the entire body excluding the

germ cells. **2.** the body as distinct from the mind.

somat- *prefix denoting* **1.** the body. **2.** somatic.

somatic *adj.* **1.** relating to the nonreproductive parts of the body. A somatic mutation cannot be inherited. **2.** relating to the body wall (i.e. excluding the viscera), e.g. somatic *mesoderm. *Compare* SPLANCHNIC. **3.** relating to the body rather than the mind.

somatization disorder (Briquet's syndrome) a psychiatric disorder characterized by multiple recurrent changing physical symptoms in the absence of physical disorders that could explain them. The disorder is chronic and is often accompanied by depression and anxiety. It can disrupt personal and family relationships and lead to unnecessary medical and surgical treatment. It is sometimes treated with *cognitive therapy, *psychotherapy, and/or *antidepressants.

somatoform disorders a group of disorders in which there is a history of repeated physical complaints with no physical basis. They include *somatization disorder and hypochondriasis (*see* HYPOCHONDRIA). Also included (in DSM-IV but not in ICD-10) is *conversion disorder.

somatomedin *n.* a protein hormone, produced by the liver in response to stimulation by growth hormone, that stimulates protein synthesis and promotes growth. It is biochemically similar to *insulin and has some actions similar to insulin; it is therefore sometimes said to have **insulin-like activity** (**ILA**) or is referred to as **insulin-like growth factor** (**IGF**).

somatopleure *n.* the body wall of the early embryo, which consists of a simple layer of ectoderm lined with mesoderm. The amnion is a continuation of this structure outside the embryo. *Compare* SPLANCHNOPLEURE.

somatostatin (growth-hormone-release inhibiting factor) a hormone, produced by the hypothalamus and some extraneural tissues, including the gastrointestinal tract and pancreas (*see* ISLETS OF LANGERHANS), that inhibits *growth hormone (somatotrophin) release by the pitui-

tary gland. Both growth-hormone releasing hormone and somatostatin are controlled by complex neural mechanisms related to sleep rhythms, stress, neurotransmitters, blood glucose, and exercise. Its inhibitory effect on gastrointestinal secretions is used to reduce flow from *fistulae from the pancreas or bowel to the body surface. Its effect on reducing abdominal blood flow is used to reduce bleeding from *oesophageal varices.

somatostatinoma *n.* a rare tumour of the *islets of Langerhans that produces somatostatin, causing severe effects on gastrointestinal motility. It is an example of an *apudoma.

somatotrophin *n.* *see* GROWTH HORMONE.

somatotype *n.* *see* BODY TYPE.

somite *n.* any of the paired segmented divisions of *mesoderm that develop along the length of the early embryo. The somites differentiate into voluntary muscle, bones, connective tissue, and the deeper layers of the skin (*see* DERMATOME, MYOTOME, SCLEROTOME).

somnambulism (noctambulation) *n.* sleep-walking: walking about and performing other actions in a semiautomatic way during sleep without later memory of doing so. It is common during childhood and may persist into adult life. It can also arise spontaneously or as the result of stress or hypnosis. —**somnambulistic** *adj.*

somniloquence *n.* talking in one's sleep. *See also* SOMNAMBULISM.

somnolism *n.* a hypnotic trance. *See* HYPNOSIS.

sonography *n.* *see* ULTRASONOGRAPHY.

sonoplacentography *n.* the technique of using *ultrasound waves to determine the position of the placenta during pregnancy. This has an advantage over using X-rays in that the fetus is not subjected to possibly harmful radiation.

soporific *n.* *see* HYPNOTIC.

sorbitol *n.* a carbohydrate with a sweet taste, used by diabetics as a substitute for cane sugar. It is also used in disorders of carbohydrate metabolism and in drip feeding. It is administered by mouth or injection; large doses taken by mouth may cause digestive upsets.

sordes *pl. n.* the brownish encrustations that form around the mouth and teeth of patients suffering from fevers.

sore *n.* a lay term for any ulcer or other open wound of the skin or mucous membranes, which may be caused by injury or infection. *See also* BEDSORE, SOFT SORE.

sore throat pain at the back of the mouth, commonly due to bacterial or viral infection of the tonsils (*tonsillitis) or the pharynx (*pharyngitis). If infection persists the lymph nodes in the neck may become tender and enlarged (cervical adenitis).

sotalol *n.* a drug (*see* BETA BLOCKER) used to treat abnormal heart rhythm, angina, and high blood pressure and to relieve symptoms in *thyrotoxicosis. It is administered by mouth or injection; side-effects may include digestive upsets, tiredness, and dizziness. Trade names: **Beta-Cardone**, **Sotacor**.

souffle *n.* a soft blowing sound heard through the stethoscope, usually produced by blood flowing in vessels.

sound (in surgery) **1.** *n.* a long rodlike instrument, often with a curved end, used to explore body cavities (such as the bladder) or to dilate *strictures in the urethra or other canals. **2.** *vb.* to explore a cavity using a sound.

Southern blot analysis a technique for identifying a specific form of DNA in cells. The DNA is extracted from the cells and restriction enzymes used to cut it into small fragments. The fragments are separated and a gene *probe known to match the DNA fragment being sought is used. *Compare* NORTHERN BLOT ANALYSIS, WESTERN BLOT ANALYSIS. [E. M. Southern (1938–), US biologist]

Southey's tubes fine-calibre tubes for insertion into subcutaneous tissue to drain excess fluid. They are rarely used in practice today. [R. Southey (1835–99), British physician]

space maintainer an orthodontic appliance that maintains an existing space in the dentition.

Spanish fly the blister beetle, *Lytta vesicatoria*: source of the irritant and toxic chemical compound *cantharidin.

sparganosis *n.* a disease caused by the migration of certain tapeworm larvae (*see* SPARGANUM) in the tissues beneath the skin, between the muscles, and occasionally in the viscera and brain. The larvae, which normally develop in frogs and reptiles, are accidentally transferred to man by eating the uncooked flesh of these animals or by drinking water contaminated with minute crustaceans infected with the tapeworm larvae. The larvae cause inflammation, swelling, and fibrosis of the tissues. Treatment of the condition, common in the Far East, involves intravenous injections of neosalvarsan and surgical removal of the larvae.

sparganum *n.* the larvae of certain tapeworms, including species of *Diphyllobothrium* and *Spirometra*, which may accidentally infect man (*see* SPARGANOSIS). They are actually *plerocercoids, but the generic name *Sparganum* is sometimes given to them since they fail to develop into adults and definite classification of the species is not possible from the larvae alone.

spasm *n.* a sustained involuntary muscular contraction, which may occur either as part of a generalized disorder, such as a *spastic paralysis, or as a local response to an otherwise unconnected painful condition. **Carpopedal spasm** affects the muscles of the hands and feet and is caused by a reduction in the blood calcium level (often transitory, as in hyperventilation).

spasmo- *prefix denoting* spasm.

spasmodic *adj.* occurring in spasms or resembling a spasm.

spasmolytic *n.* a drug that relieves spasm of smooth muscle; examples are *aminophylline and *papaverine. Spasmolytics may be used as *bronchodilators to relieve spasm in bronchial muscle, to stimulate the heart in the treatment of angina, or to relieve colic due to spasm of the digestive system.

spasmus nutans a combination of symptoms including a slow nodding movement of the head, *nystagmus (involuntary movements of the eyes), and spasm of the neck muscles. It affects infants and it normally disappears within a year or two.

spastic colon *see* IRRITABLE BOWEL SYNDROME.

spasticity *n.* resistance to the passive movement of a limb that is maximal at the beginning of the movement and gives way as more pressure is applied. It is a symptom of damage to the corticospinal tracts in the brain or spinal cord. It is usually accompanied by weakness in the affected limb (*see* SPASTIC PARALYSIS). *Compare* RIGIDITY.

spastic paralysis weakness of a limb or limbs associated with increased reflex activity. This results in resistance to passive movement of the limb (*see* SPASTICITY). It is caused by disease affecting the nerve fibres of the corticospinal tract, which in health not only initiate movement but also inhibit the stretch reflexes to allow the movements to take place. *See* CEREBRAL PALSY.

spatula *n.* an instrument with a blunt blade used to spread ointments or plasters and, particularly in dentistry, to mix materials. A flat spatula is used to depress the tongue during examination of the oropharynx.

spatulation *n.* the technique of widening the orifice of an anatomical tube prior to joining it up, which makes the join more secure and less prone to narrowing.

special hospitals hospitals for the care of mentally ill patients who are also dangerous and must therefore be kept securely. There are four in the UK: Broadmoor, Rampton, Ashworth, and Carstairs. Most (but not all) patients are there compulsorily under a hospital order made by a court according to the *Mental Health Act.

special school (in Britain) an education establishment for disabled children. The discovery and assessment (**ascertainment**) of those needing to attend a special school may occur long before school age (2 years or younger); the responsibility for deciding who attends a special school lies with the local education authority. Special schools exist for each of the following 11 groups of disabled children: blind, partially sighted, deaf, partially deaf, delicate (those with such medical disabilities as congenital heart disease or cystic fibrosis), educationally subnormal, mentally handicapped (in which learning potential is limited and independent living may prove impossible), maladjusted (those with behavioural difficulties), physically disabled (by such conditions as poliomyelitis, muscular dystrophy, or limb absence from thalidomide), epileptic, and those with speech defects. Some special schools cater for combinations of two or more of these disabilities. Special education for the blind and for those with other severe disabilities may start as early as 2 years, deaf children requiring special education from the date of discovery.

species *n.* the smallest unit used in the classification of living organisms. Members of the same species are able to interbreed and produce fertile offspring. Similar species are grouped together within one *genus.

specific **1.** *n.* a medicine that has properties especially useful for the treatment of a particular disease. **2.** *adj.* (of a disease) caused by a particular microorganism that causes no other disease. **3.** *adj.* of or relating to a species.

specific gravity the ratio, more correctly known as **relative density**, of the density of a substance at 20°C to the density of water at its temperature of maximum density (4°C). Measurement of the specific gravity of urine is one of the tests of renal function.

specificity *n.* (in screening tests) *see* SENSITIVITY.

Spect scanning single photon emission computed tomography scanning: the production of a cross-sectional image of an organ or part of the body from a *gamma camera that is constructed to allow a complete rotation around the patient being scanned. Using computer tomographic reconstruction, cross-sectional *radionuclide scans can be produced in a similar way to CT scanning (*see* COMPUTERIZED TOMOGRAPHY). This has found particular use in bone scanning.

spectinomycin *n.* an *antibiotic used to treat various infections, particularly gonorrhoea. It is administered by injection;

side-effects may include nausea, dizziness, fever, and rash. Trade name: **Trobicin**.

spectrograph *n.* an instrument (a *spectrometer or *spectroscope) that produces a photographic record (**spectrogram**) of the intensity and wavelength of electromagnetic radiations.

spectrometer *n.* any instrument for measuring the intensity and wavelengths of visible or invisible electromagnetic radiations. *See also* SPECTROSCOPE.

spectrophotometer *n.* an instrument (a spectrometer) for measuring the intensity of the wavelengths of the components of light (visible or ultraviolet).

spectroscope *n.* an instrument used to split up light or other radiation into components of different wavelengths. The simplest spectroscope uses a prism, which splits white light into the rainbow colours of the visible spectrum.

specular reflection (in *ultrasonics) the reflection of sound waves from the surface of an internal structure, which can be used to produce a picture of the surface as a sonogram (*see* ULTRASONOGRAPHY). A specular reflection contrasts with vaguer diffuse echoes produced by minor differences in tissue density.

speculum *n.* (*pl.* **specula**) a metal instrument for inserting into and holding open a cavity of the body, such as the vagina, rectum, or nasal orifice, in order that the interior may be examined (see illustration).

speech therapy the rehabilitation of patients who are unable to speak coherently because of congenital causes, accidents, or illness (e.g. stroke). Speech therapists have special training in this field but are not medically registered.

sperm *n.* *see* SPERMATOZOON.

sperm- (spermi(o)- spermo-) *prefix denoting* sperm or semen.

spermat- (spermato-) *prefix denoting* **1.** sperm. **2.** organs or ducts associated with sperm.

spermatic artery either of two arteries that originate from the abdominal aorta and travel downwards to supply the testes.

spermatic cord the cord, consisting of the *vas deferens, nerves, and blood vessels, that runs from the abdominal cavity to the testicle in the scrotum. The *inguinal canal, through which the spermatic cord passes, becomes closed after the testes have descended.

spermatid *n.* a small cell produced as an intermediate stage in the formation of spermatozoa. Spermatids become embedded in *Sertoli cells in the testis. They are transformed into spermatozoa by the process of spermiogenesis (*see* SPERMATOGENESIS).

Cusco's

Fergusson's

Sims's

Vaginal specula

spermatocele *n.* a cystic swelling in the scrotum containing sperm. The cyst arises from the epididymis (the duct conveying sperm from the testis) and can be felt as a lump above the testis. Needle *aspiration of the cyst reveals a milky opalescent fluid that contains sperm. Treatment is by surgical removal.

spermatocyte n. a cell produced as an intermediate stage in the formation of spermatozoa (see SPERMATOGENESIS). Spermatocytes develop from spermatogonia in the walls of the seminiferous tubules of the testis; they are known as either **primary** or **secondary spermatocytes** according to whether they are undergoing the first or second division of meiosis.

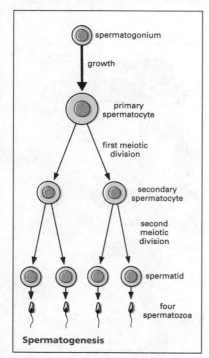

Spermatogenesis

spermatogenesis n. the process by which mature spermatozoa are produced in the testis (see illustration). *Spermatogonia, in the outermost layer of the seminiferous tubules, multiply throughout reproductive life. Some of them divide by meiosis into *spermatocytes, which produce haploid *spermatids. These are transformed into mature spermatozoa by the process of **spermiogenesis**. The whole process takes 70–80 days.

spermatogonium n. (pl. **spermatogonia**) a cell produced at an early stage in the formation of spermatozoa (see SPERMATOGENESIS). Spermatogonia first appear in the testis of the fetus but do not multiply significantly until after puberty. They act as stem cells in the walls of the seminiferous tubules, dividing continuously by mitosis and giving rise to *spermatocytes.

spermatorrhoea n. the involuntary discharge of semen without orgasm. Semen is usually produced by ejaculation at orgasm and does not normally discharge at other times. If, however, the mechanism of ejaculation is lost, spermatorrhoea may occur.

A spermatozoon

spermatozoon (sperm) n. (pl. **spermatozoa**) a mature male sex cell (see GAMETE). The tail of a sperm enables it to swim, which is important as a means for reaching and fertilizing the ovum (although muscular movements of the uterus may assist its journey from the vagina). See also ACROSOME, FERTILIZATION.

spermaturia n. the presence of spermatozoa in the urine. Spermatozoa are occasionally seen on microscopic examination of the urine and their presence is not abnormal. If present in large numbers, the urine becomes cloudy, usually towards the end of micturition. Abnormal ejaculation into the bladder on orgasm (retrograde ejaculation) may occur after *prostatectomy or other surgical procedures or in neurological conditions that destroy the ability of the bladder neck to close on ejaculation.

sperm count see SEMINAL ANALYSIS.

spermicide n. an agent that kills spermatozoa. Creams and jellies containing chemical spermicides are used – in conjunction with a *diaphragm – as contraceptives. —**spermicidal** adj.

spermiogenesis n. the process by which spermatids become mature spermatozoa within the seminiferous tubules of the testis. See SPERMATOGENESIS.

spheno- prefix denoting the sphenoid bone. Examples: **sphenomaxillary** (relating to the sphenoid and maxillary bones); **sphenopalatine** (relating to the sphenoid bone and palate).

sphenoid bone a bone forming the base of the cranium behind the eyes. It consists of a **body**, containing air spaces continuous with the nasal cavity (see PARANASAL SINUS); two **wings** that form part of the orbits; and two **pterygoid processes** projecting down from the point where the two wings join the body. See SKULL.

spherocyte n. an abnormal form of red blood cell (*erythrocyte) that is spherical rather than disc-shaped. In blood films spherocytes appear smaller and stain more densely than normal red cells. They are characteristically seen in some forms of haemolytic anaemia. Spherocytes tend to

be removed from the blood as they pass through the spleen. See also SPHEROCYTOSIS.

spherocytosis n. the presence in the blood of abnormally shaped red cells (*spherocytes). Spherocytosis may occur as a hereditary disorder (**hereditary spherocytosis**) or in certain haemolytic *anaemias.

sphincter n. a specialized ring of muscle that surrounds an orifice. Contractions of the sphincter partly or completely close the orifice. Sphincters are found, for example, around the anus (**anal sphincter**) and at the opening between the stomach and duodenum (**pyloric sphincter**).

sphincter- prefix denoting a sphincter.

sphincterectomy n. **1.** the surgical removal of any sphincter muscle. **2.** the complete division of a sphincter.

sphincterotomy n. **1.** surgical division, usually partial, of any sphincter muscle. See also ANAL FISSURE. **2.** surgical removal of part of the iris in the eye at the border of the pupil.

sphingomyelin n. a *phospholipid that contains sphingosine, a fatty acid, phosphoric acid, and choline. Sphingomyelins are found in large amounts in brain and nerve tissue.

sphingosine n. a lipid alcohol that is a constituent of sphingomyelin and cerebrosides.

sphygmo- prefix denoting the pulse.

sphygmocardiograph n. an apparatus for producing a continuous record of both the heartbeat and the subsequent pulse in one of the blood vessels. The recording can be shown on a moving tape or on an electronic screen.

sphygmograph n. an apparatus for producing a continuous record of the pulse in one of the blood vessels, showing the strength and rate of the beats.

sphygmomanometer n. an instrument for measuring *blood pressure in the arteries. It consists of an inflatable cuff connected via a rubber tube to a column of mercury with a graduated scale. The cuff is applied to a limb (usually the arm) and inflated to exert pressure on a large artery until the blood flow stops. The pressure is

arachnoid
septum
central canal
grey commissure
grey matter
white commissure
anterior (ventral) median fissure
blood vessel
subdural space

posterior (dorsal) root
posterior (dorsal) horn
white matter
lateral horn
meninges
anterior (ventral) horn
cell bodies of motor neurones
dura mater
pia mater
anterior (ventral) root

Transverse section through the spinal cord

then slowly released and, with the aid of a stethoscope to listen to the pulse, it is possible to determine both the systolic and diastolic pressures (which can be read on the scale).

sphygmophone *n.* a device to record the heartbeat or pulse in the form of amplified sound waves played through a loudspeaker or earphones.

sphygmoscope *n.* a device for showing the heartbeat or pulse as a visible signal, especially a continuous wave signal on a cathode-ray tube.

spica *n.* a bandage wound spirally around an injured limb. At each turn it is given a twist so that the slack material is taken up at the overlap.

spicule *n.* a small splinter of bone.

spina bifida (rachischisis) a developmental defect in which the newborn baby has part of the spinal cord and its coverings exposed through a gap in the backbone. The symptoms may include paralysis of the legs, incontinence, and mental retardation from the commonly associated brain defect, *hydrocephalus. Spina bifida is associated with an abnormally high level of *alpha-fetoprotein in the amniotic fluid surrounding the embryo. The condition can be diagnosed at about the

16th week of pregnancy by a maternal blood test and confirmed by amniocentesis and ultrasound, so making termination of the pregnancy possible. Recent evidence suggests that the risk of spina bifida is reduced if extra *folic acid is included in the diet of pregnant women in the first three months of pregnancy. *See also* NEURAL TUBE DEFECTS.

spina bifida occulta a defect in the bony arch of the spine that (unlike spina bifida) has a normal skin covering; there may be an overlying hairy patch. The condition is usually an incidental finding on X-ray and it is not associated with neurological involvement.

spinal accessory nerve *see* ACCESSORY NERVE.

spinal anaesthesia 1. suppression of sensation, usually in the lower part of the body, by the injection of a local anaesthetic into the spaces surrounding the spinal cord. There are two types used for surgery: **subarachnoid** and **epidural.** In the latter the anaesthetic is injected between the dura and the surrounding bony vertebral foramen, using a special blunt needle with a side-hole to reduce the chance of penetrating the dura. In the former a very fine needle is used to reduce the amount of cerebrospinal fluid that escapes as the needle penetrates the dura. Both techniques have complications, especially the subarachnoid route (headache, sepsis, paraplegia). The injection site for subarachnoid spinal anaesthetics is most often in the lumbar region of the vertebral column, the needle being inserted between the vertebrae (anywhere between the second and fifth). For epidural anaesthetics, the sacral and caudal regions are often used. The extent of the area anaesthetized depends upon the amount and strength of local anaesthetic injected. Dilute local anaesthetic solutions are used when the sensory nerves are targeted rather than the motor nerves. In many instances a fine catheter is passed through the needle to enable repeated or continuous injections of anaesthetic solution. Spinal anaesthesia is useful in patients whose condition makes them unsuitable for a general anaesthetic, perhaps because of chest infection; for certain obstetric procedures; to reduce the requirements for general anaesthetic drugs; or in circumstances where a skilled anaesthetist is not readily available to administer a general anaesthetic. The technique is more commonly used in Scandinavia and the USA than in Britain. **2.** loss of sensation in part of the body as a result of injury or disease to the spinal cord. The area of the body affected depends upon the site of the lesion: the lower it is in the cord the less the sensory disability.

spinal column see BACKBONE.

spinal cord the portion of the central nervous system enclosed in the vertebral column, consisting of nerve cells and bundles of nerves connecting all parts of the body with the brain. It contains a core of grey matter surrounded by white matter (see illustration). It is enveloped in three layers of membrane, the *meninges, and extends from the medulla oblongata in the skull to the level of the second lumbar vertebra. From it arise 31 pairs of *spinal nerves.

spinal muscular atrophy (SMA) a hereditary condition in which cells of the spinal cord die and the muscles in the arms and legs become progressively weaker. The gene responsible has been located: in affected children it is inherited as a double *recessive. SMA usually devel-

ops between the ages of 2 and 12. Eventually the respiratory muscles are affected and death usually results from respiratory infection. Most affected individuals are wheelchair-bound by the age of 20 and few survive beyond the age of 30. **Infantile spinal muscular atrophy** is an acute aggressive form of the condition (see WERDNIG-HOFFMANN DISEASE).

vertebrae

spinal cord

cervical nerves 1–8

thoracic nerves 1–12

sacral 1–5

coccygeal 1

lumbar nerves 1–5

sacral nerves 1–5

coccygeal nerve

Origins of the spinal nerves (one side only)

spinal nerves the 31 pairs of nerves that leave the spinal cord and are distributed to the body, passing out from the vertebral canal through the spaces between the arches of the vertebrae (see illustration). Each nerve has two *roots, an anterior, carrying motor nerve fibres, and a posterior, carrying sensory fibres. Immediately after the roots leave the spinal cord they merge to form a mixed spinal nerve on each side.

spinal shock a state of *shock accompanied by temporary paralysis of the lower extremities that results from injury to the spine and is often associated with *ileus. If the spinal cord is transected, permanent motor paralysis persists below the level of spinal-cord division.

spindle *n.* a collection of fibres seen in a cell when it is dividing. The fibres radiate from the two ends (**poles**) and meet at the centre (the **equator**) giving a structure shaped like two cones placed base to base. It plays an important part in chromosome movement in *mitosis and *meiosis and is also involved in division of the cytoplasm.

spine *n.* **1.** a sharp process of a bone. **2.** the vertebral column (*see* BACKBONE). —**spinal** *adj.*

spino- *prefix denoting* **1.** the spine. **2.** the spinal cord.

spinocerebellar degeneration any of a group of inherited disorders of the cerebellum and corticospinal tracts in the brain. They are characterized by *spasticity of the limbs and cerebellar *ataxia.

spiral bandage a bandage wound round a part of the body, overlapping the previous section at each turn.

spiral CT scanning (helical CT scanning) a development of conventional CT scanning (*see* COMPUTERIZED TOMOGRAPHY) in which the X-ray tube rotates continuously around the patient as he or she passes through the scanner. This allows the acquisition of images throughout a specified volume of tissue. Since these images are digitally acquired (*see* DIGITIZATION), they can be *post-processed to produce images in numerous planes, without further exposure of the patient.

spiral organ *see* ORGAN OF CORTI.

Spirillum *n.* a genus of highly motile rigid spiral-shaped bacteria usually found in fresh and salt water containing organic matter. They bear tufts of flagella at one or both ends of the cell. Most species are saprophytes, but *S. minus* causes *rat-bite fever.

spiro- *prefix denoting* **1.** spiral. **2.** respiration.

spirochaete *n.* any one of a group of spiral-shaped bacteria that lack a rigid cell wall and move by means of muscular flexions of the cell. The group includes the genera *Borrelia, *Leptospira, and *Treponema.

spirograph *n.* an instrument for recording breathing movements. The record (a tracing) obtained is called a **spirogram**. —**spirography** *n.*

spirometer *n.* an instrument for measuring the volume of air inhaled and exhaled. It is used in tests of *ventilation. —**spirometry** *n.*

spironolactone *n.* a synthetic corticosteroid that inhibits the activity of the hormone *aldosterone and is used as a potassium-sparing *diuretic to treat heart failure, high blood pressure, and fluid retention (oedema). It is administered by mouth; side-effects may include headache, stomach upsets, and drowsiness and since 1988 its use has been restricted as it was found to cause carcinomas in animals. Trade name: **Aldactone**.

Spitz-Holter valve a one-way valve used to drain cerebrospinal fluid in order to control *hydrocephalus. The device is inserted into the ventricles of the brain and passes via a subcutaneous tunnel to drain into either the right atrium or the peritoneum.

splanch- (splanchno-) *prefix denoting* the viscera.

splanchnic *adj.* relating to the viscera, e.g. splanchnic *mesoderm. *Compare* SOMATIC.

splanchnic nerves the series of nerves in the sympathetic system that are distributed to the blood vessels and viscera, passing forwards and downwards from the chain of sympathetic ganglia near the spinal cord to enter the abdomen and branch profusely.

splanchnocranium *n.* the part of the skull that is derived from the *pharyngeal arches, i.e. the mandible (lower jaw).

splanchnopleure *n.* the wall of the embryonic gut, which consists of a layer of endoderm with a layer of mesoderm outside it. The yolk sac is a continuation of this structure. *Compare* SOMATOPLEURE.

spleen *n.* a large dark-red ovoid organ situated on the left side of the body below and behind the stomach. It is enclosed within a fibrous capsule that extends into the spongy interior – the **splenic pulp** – to form a supportive framework. The pulp consists of aggregates of *lymphoid tissue (**white pulp**) within a meshwork of *reticular fibres packed with red blood cells (**red pulp**). The spleen is a major component of the *reticuloendothelial system, producing lymphocytes in the newborn and containing *phagocytes, which remove worn-out red blood cells and other foreign bodies from the bloodstream. It also acts as a reservoir for blood and, in the fetus, as a source of red blood cells. Anatomical name: **lien. —splenic** *adj.*

splen- (spleno-) *prefix denoting* the spleen. Example: **splenorenal** (relating to the spleen and kidney).

splenectomy *n.* surgical removal of the spleen. This is sometimes necessary in the emergency treatment of bleeding from a ruptured spleen and in the treatment of some blood diseases. Splenectomy in children may diminish the immune response to infections.

splenitis *n.* inflammation of the spleen. *See also* PERISPLENITIS.

splenium *n.* the thickest part of the *corpus callosum, rounded and protruding backwards over the thalami, the pineal gland, and the midbrain.

splenomegaly *n.* enlargement of the spleen. It most commonly occurs in *malaria, *schistosomiasis, and other disorders caused by parasites; in infections; in blood disorders, including some forms of anaemia and lack of platelets (*thrombocytopenia); in *leukaemia; and in *Hodgkin's disease. *See also* HYPERSPLENISM.

splenorenal anastomosis a method of treating *portal hypertension by joining the splenic vein to the left renal vein. *Compare* PORTACAVAL ANASTOMOSIS.

splenunculus *n.* a small sphere of splenic tissue occurring at a site other

than the spleen. Splenunculi are present in many people.

splint *n.* a rigid support to hold broken bones in position until healing has occurred.

splinter haemorrhage a linear haemorrhage below the nails, usually the result of trauma but also occurring in such conditions as subacute bacterial *endocarditis or severe rheumatoid arthritis.

splitting *n.* a *defence mechanism by which people deal with an emotional conflict by viewing some people as all good and others as all bad: they fail to integrate themselves or other people into complex but coherent images.

spondyl- (spondylo-) *prefix denoting* a vertebra or the spine.

spondylitis *n.* inflammation of the synovial joints of the backbone. **Ankylosing spondylitis** is a **sero-negative arthritis**, one of a group of arthritides that do not exhibit rheumatoid factors in the serum. 90% of cases carry the tissue-type antigen HLA B27 (*see* HLA SYSTEM). Ankylosing spondylitis predominantly affects young males and the inflammation affects the joint capsules and their attached ligaments and tendons, principally the intervertebral joints and sacroiliac joints (*see* SACROILIITIS). The resultant pain and stiffness are treated by analgesics and regular daily exercises. The disorder can lead to severe deformities of the spine (*see* KYPHOSIS, ANKYLOSIS).

spondylolisthesis *n.* a forward shift of one vertebra upon another, due to a defect in the bone or in the joints that normally bind them together. This may be congenital or develop after injury. The vertebral displacement is most likely to occur in the lumbar (lower back) or cervical (neck) regions of the backbone. The majority of cases in which pain is present are treated with rest and a surgical belt or corset; in a small minority, showing severe disability or pressure on nerve roots, surgical fusion may be required.

spondylosis *n.* a spinal condition resulting from degeneration of the intervertebral discs in the cervical, thoracic, or lumbar regions. Symptoms include pain and restriction of movement. Spondylosis produces a characteristic appearance on X-ray, including narrowing of the space occupied by the disc and the presence of *osteophytes; these features of the disease (**radiological spondylosis**) may not be accompanied by any signs and symptoms. Pain is relieved by wearing a collar (when the neck region is affected) or a surgical belt (for the lower spine), which prevents movement. Very severe cases sometimes require surgical fusion.

spondylosyndesis *n.* surgical fusion of the intervertebral joints of the backbone.

spongiform encephalopathy any one of a group of rapidly progressive degenerative neurological diseases that include scrapie in sheep, bovine spongiform encephalopathy (BSE) in cattle, and *kuru and *Creutzfeldt-Jakob disease in humans. In humans the spongiform encephalopathies are characterized by rapidly progressive dementia associated with myoclonic jerks (see MYOCLONUS); on pathological examination the brains of affected individuals show a characteristic cystic degeneration. The diseases are thought to be caused by unconventional transmissible agents (see PRION).

spongioblast *n.* a type of cell that forms in the early stages of development of the nervous system, giving rise to *astrocytes and *oligodendrocytes.

spongioblastoma *n. see* GLIOBLASTOMA.

spontaneous *adj.* arising without apparent cause or outside aid. The term is applied in medicine to certain conditions, such as pathological fractures, that arise in the absence of outside injury; also to recovery from a disease without the aid of specific treatment.

sporadic *adj.* describing a disease that occurs only occasionally or in a few isolated places. *Compare* ENDEMIC, EPIDEMIC.

spore *n.* a small reproductive body produced by plants and microorganisms. Some kinds of spores function as dormant stages of the life cycle, enabling the organism to survive adverse conditions. Other spores are the means by which the organism can spread vegetatively. *See also* ENDOSPORE.

sporicide *n.* an agent that kills spores

(e.g. bacterial spores). Some disinfectants that liberate chlorine are sporicides, but most other germicides are ineffective since spores are very resistant to chemical action. —**sporicidal** *adj.*

sporocyst *n.* the second-stage larva of a parasitic *fluke, found within the tissues of a freshwater snail. A sporocyst develops from a first stage larva (see MIRACIDIUM) and gives rise either to the next larval stage (see REDIA) or daughter sporocysts. The latter develop directly into the final larval stage (see CERCARIA) without the intermediate redia stage.

sporogony *n.* the formation of *sporozoites during the life cycle of a sporozoan. The contents of the zygote, formed by the fusion of sex cells, divide repeatedly and eventually release a number of sporozoites. *Compare* SCHIZOGONY.

sporotrichosis *n.* a chronic infection of the skin and superficial lymph nodes that is caused by the fungus *Sporothrix schenckii* and results in the formation of abscesses and ulcers. It occurs mainly in the tropics.

Sporozoa *n.* a group of parasitic protozoans that includes *Plasmodium*, the malaria parasite. Most sporozoans do not have cilia or flagella. Sporozoan life cycles are complex and usually involve both sexual and asexual stages. Some sporozoans are parasites of invertebrates, and the parasites are passed to new hosts by means of spores. Sporozoans that parasitize vertebrates are transmitted from host to host by invertebrates, which act as intermediate hosts. For example, the mosquito *Anopheles* is the intermediate host of *Plasmodium*.

sporozoite *n.* one of the many cells formed as a result of *sporogony during the life cyle of a sporozoan. In *Plasmodium* sporozoites are formed by repeated divisions of the contents of the *oocyst inside the body of the mosquito. The released sporozoites ultimately pass into the insect's salivary glands and await transmission to a human host at the next blood meal.

sports injury any injury related to the practice of a sport, often resulting from the overuse and stretching of muscles, tendons, and ligaments.

sports medicine a developing specialty concerned with the treatment of *sports injuries and measures designed to prevent or minimize them (e.g. in the design of sports equipment).

spotted fever *see* MENINGITIS, ROCKY MOUNTAIN SPOTTED FEVER, TYPHUS.

sprain *n.* injury to a ligament, caused by sudden overstretching. As the ligament is not severed it gradually heals, but this may take several months. Sprains should be treated by cold compresses (ice-packs) at the time of injury, and later by restriction of activity.

Sprengel's deformity a congenital abnormality of the scapula (shoulder blade), which is small and positioned high in the shoulder. It is caused by failure of the normal development and descent of this bone. [O. G. K. Sprengel (1852–1915), German surgeon]

sprue (psilosis) *n.* deficient absorption of food due to disease of the small intestine. **Tropical sprue** is seen in people from temperate regions who stay in tropical climates for weeks or months. It is characterized by diarrhoea (usually *steatorrhoea), an inflamed tongue (glossitis), anaemia, and weight loss; the lining of the small intestine is inflamed and atrophied, probably because of infection. Treatment with antibiotics and *folic acid is usually effective, but the condition often improves spontaneously on return to a temperate climate. *See also* COELIAC DISEASE (NONTROPICAL SPRUE), MALABSORPTION.

spud *n.* a blunt needle used for removing foreign bodies embedded in the cornea of the eye.

spur *n.* a sharp projection, especially one of bone.

sputum *n.* material coughed up from the respiratory tract. Its characteristics, including colour, consistency, volume, smell, and the appearance of any solid material within it, often provide important information affecting the diagnosis and management of respiratory disease. Pathological examination of sputum for microorganisms and for abnormal cells may add further information.

squalene *n.* an unsaturated hydrocarbon

(a terpene), synthesized in the body, from which *cholesterol is derived.

squama *n.* (*pl.* **squamae**) **1.** a thin plate of bone. **2.** a scale, such as any of the scales from the cornified layer of the *epidermis.

squamo- *prefix denoting* **1.** the squamous portion of the temporal bone. **2.** squamous epithelium.

squamous bone *see* TEMPORAL BONE.

squamous cell carcinoma (SCC) the second commonest form of skin cancer (after *basal cell carcinoma), occurring usually in late-middle and old age. Sunlight is the commonest cause but other environmental carcinogens may be responsible. SCC is mainly found on areas exposed to light and is three times more common in men than in women. SCC grows faster than basal cell carcinoma; it spreads locally at first but later may spread to sites distant from its origin (*see* METASTASIS). Treatment is usually by surgical excision or radiotherapy.

squamous epithelium *see* EPITHELIUM.

squint *n.* *see* STRABISMUS.

SSPE *see* SUBACUTE SCLEROSING PANENCEPHALITIS.

SSRI (selective serotonin reuptake inhibitor) any one of a group of *antidepressant drugs that exert their action by blocking the reabsorption of the neurotransmitter *serotonin by the nerve endings in the brain. Their effect is to increase levels of serotonin in the brain. The group includes *citolapram, *fluoxetine, *fluvoxamine, *paroxetine, and *sertraline. Side-effects include agitation and nausea.

stadium *n.* (*pl.* **stadia**) a stage in the course of a disease; for example, the **stadium invasionis** is the period between exposure to infection and the onset of symptoms.

stage *vb.* (in oncology) to classify a primary tumour, by its size and the presence or absence of metastases, in order to plan treatment. In addition to clinical examination, a variety of imaging and surgical techniques may be employed to provide a more accurate assessment. *See also* TNM CLASSIFICATION.

staghorn calculus a branched stone forming a cast of the collecting system of the kidney and therefore filling the calyces and pelvis. The stone is usually associated with infected urine, the commonest organism being *Proteus vulgaris*. The combination of obstruction and infection can cause *pyonephrosis and, if neglected, a *perinephric abscess.

stagnant loop syndrome *see* BLIND LOOP SYNDROME.

stain 1. *n.* a dye used to colour tissues and other specimens for microscopical examination. In an **acid stain** the colour is carried by an acid radical and the stain is taken up by parts of the specimen having a basic (alkaline) reaction. In a **basic stain** the colour, carried by a basic radical, is attracted to parts of the specimen having an acidic reaction. **Neutral stains** have neither acidic nor basic affinities. A **contrast stain** is used to give colour to parts of a tissue not affected by a previously applied stain. A **differential stain** allows different elements in a specimen to be distinguished by staining them in different colours. **2.** *vb.* to treat a specimen for microscopical study with a stain.

Stamey procedure an operation devised to cure stress incontinence of urine in women in which specially designed needles are employed to sling or hitch up the neck of the bladder to the anterior abdominal wall with unabsorbable suture material. *See also* COLPOSUSPENSION. [T. A. Stamey, US surgeon]

stammering (stuttering) *n.* halting articulation with interruptions to the normal flow of speech and repetition of the initial consonants of words or syllables (*compare* CLUTTERING). It usually first appears in childhood and the symptoms are most severe when the stammerer is under any psychological stress. It is not a symptom of organic disease and it will usually respond to the re-education of speech by a trained therapist. Medical name: **dysphemia. —stammerer** *n.*

standard deviation (in statistics) a measure of the scatter of observations about their arithmetic *mean, which is calculated from the square root of the **variance** of the readings in the series. The arithmetic sum of the amounts by which each observation varies from the mean must be zero, but if these variations are squared before being summated, a positive value is obtained: the mean of this value is the variance. In practice a more reliable estimate of variance is obtained by dividing the sum of the squared deviations by one *less* than the total number of observations. *See also* SIGNIFICANCE.

standard error (of a *mean) the extent to which the means of several different samples would vary if they were taken repeatedly from the same population. Differences between means are said to have statistical *significance when they are greater than twice the standard error of those means, since the probability of this difference or a larger one occurring by chance is less than 5%.

stanozolol *n.* an *anabolic steroid used to treat the effects of deep vein thrombosis and systemic sclerosis. Trade name: **Stromba**.

St Anthony's fire an old colloquial name for the inflammation of the skin associated with ergot poisoning. *See* ERGOTISM.

stapedectomy *n.* surgical removal of the third ear ossicle (stapes), enabling it to be replaced with a prosthetic bone in the treatment of *otosclerosis.

stapes *n.* a stirrup-shaped bone in the middle *ear that articulates with the incus and is attached to the membrane of the fenestra ovalis. *See* OSSICLE.

staphylectomy *n.* surgical removal of the uvula (the back of the soft palate).

staphylococcal scalded skin syndrome (Lyell's disease, Ritter's disease) a potentially serious condition of young infants in which the skin becomes reddened and tender and then peels off, giving the appearance of a scald. The area of skin loss may be quite extensive. The underlying cause is an infection by certain bacteria of the genus *Staphylococcus*. It is contagious and may occur in clusters. Treatment is by antibiotics, but careful nursing is essential to prevent skin damage. Medical name: **toxic epidermal necrolysis.**

Staphylococcus n. a genus of Gram-positive nonmotile spherical bacteria occurring in grapelike clusters. Some species are saprophytes; others parasites. Many species produce *exotoxins. The species *S. aureus* is commonly present on skin and mucous membranes; it causes boils and internal abscesses. More serious infections caused by staphylococci include pneumonia, bacteraemia, osteomyelitis, and enterocolitis. —**staphylococcal** adj.

staphyloma n. abnormal bulging of the cornea or sclera (white) of the eye. **Anterior staphyloma** is a bulging scar in the cornea to which a part of the iris is attached. It is usually the site of a healed corneal ulcer that has penetrated right through the cornea; the iris blocks the hole and prevents the further leakage of fluid from the front chamber of the eye. In **ciliary staphyloma** the sclera bulges over the ciliary body as a result of high pressure inside the eyeball. A bulging of the sclera at the back of the eye (**posterior staphyloma**) occurs in some severe cases of short-sightedness.

staphylorrhaphy (palatorrhaphy, uraniscorrhaphy) n. surgical suture of a cleft palate.

staple n. (in surgery) a piece of metal used to join up pieces of tissue. Staples can be used as an alternative to *sutures for an *anastomosis; stapling machines have been produced for this purpose. *See also* ENDOSTAPLER.

starch n. the form in which *carbohydrates are stored in many plants and a major constituent of the diet. Starch consists of linked glucose units and occurs in two forms, α-**amylose** and **amylopectin.** In α-amylose the units are in the form of a long unbranched chain; in amylopectin they form a branched chain. The presence of starch can be detected using iodine: α-amylose gives a blue colour with iodine; amylopectin a red colour. Starch is digested by means of the enzyme *amylase. *See also* DEXTRIN.

Starling's law a law stating that a muscle, including the heart muscle, responds to increased stretching at rest by an increased force of contraction when stimulated. [E. H. Starling (1866–1927), British physiologist]

startle reflex *see* MORO REFLEX.

starvation n. *see* MALNUTRITION.

stasis n. stagnation or cessation of flow; for example, of blood or lymph whose flow is obstructed or of the intestinal contents when onward movement (peristalsis) is hindered.

-stasis *suffix denoting* stoppage of a flow of liquid; stagnation. Example: **haemostasis** (of blood).

static reflex the reflex maintenance of muscular tone for posture.

status asthmaticus a severe attack of asthma, which often follows a period of poorly controlled asthma. Patients are distressed and very breathless and may die from respiratory failure if not vigorously treated with inhaled oxygen, nebulized or intravenous bronchodilators, and corticosteroid therapy; sedatives are absolutely contraindicated. These patients need hospital care in an intensive care unit.

status epilepticus the occurrence of repeated epileptic seizures without any recovery of consciousness between them. Its control is a medical emergency, since prolonged status epilepticus may lead to the patient's death or long-term disability.

status lymphaticus enlargement of the thymus gland and other parts of the lymphatic system, formerly believed to be a predisposing cause to sudden death in infancy and childhood associated with hypersensitivity to drugs or vaccines.

STD *see* SEXUALLY TRANSMITTED DISEASE.

steapsin n. *see* LIPASE.

stearic acid *see* FATTY ACID.

steat- (steato-) *prefix denoting* fat; fatty tissue.

steatoma n. any cyst or tumour of a sebaceous gland.

steatopygia n. the accumulation of large quantities of fat in the buttocks. In the Hottentots of Africa this is a normal condition, thought to be an adaptation that allows fat storage without impeding heat loss from the rest of the body.

steatorrhoea *n.* the passage of abnormally increased amounts of fat in the faeces (more than 5 g/day) due to reduced absorption of fat by the intestine (*see* MALABSORPTION). The faeces are pale, smell offensive, may look greasy, and are difficult to flush away.

steatosis *n.* infiltration of *hepatocytes with fat. This may occur in pregnancy, alcoholism, malnutrition, obesity, hepatitis C infection, or with some drugs.

stellate fracture a star-shaped fracture of the kneecap caused by a direct blow. The bone may be either split or severely shattered; if the fragments are displaced, the bone may need to be surgically repaired or rarely removed (**patellectomy**).

stellate ganglion a star-shaped collection of sympathetic nerve cell bodies in the root of the neck, from which sympathetic nerve fibres are distributed to the face and neck and to the blood vessels and organs of the thorax.

Stellwag's sign apparent widening of the distance between the upper and lower eyelids (the palpebral fissure) due to retraction of the upper lid and protrusion of the eyeball. It is a sign of exophthalmic *goitre. [C. Stellwag von Carion (1823–1904), Austrian ophthalmologist]

stem cell an immortal cell that is able to produce all the cells within an organ. The term is most usually applied to the *haemopoietic stem cells of the bone marrow.

steno- *prefix denoting* **1.** narrow. Example: **stenocephaly** (narrowness of the head). **2.** constricted.

stenopaeic *adj.* (in ophthalmology) describing an optical device consisting of an opaque disc punctured with a fine slit or hole (or holes), which is placed in front of the eye in the same position as glasses and enables sharper vision in cases of gross long- or short-sightedness or astigmatism. It sharpens the image formed on the retina because it confines the light reaching the eye to one or more fine beams. The same principle is used in the pin-hole camera.

stenosis *n.* the abnormal narrowing of a passage or opening, such as a blood vessel or heart valve. *See* AORTIC; CAROTID-ARTERY, MITRAL, PULMONARY, and PYLORIC STENOSIS.

stenostomia (stenostomy) *n.* the abnormal narrowing of an opening, such as the opening of the bile duct.

Stensen's duct the long secretory duct of the *parotid salivary gland. [N. Stensen (1838–86), Danish physician]

stent *n.* a splint placed inside a duct or canal, such as the ureter, urethra, oesophagus, or bile duct, or an artery. It may be used at operation to aid healing of an anastomosis, or placed across an obstruction to maintain an open lumen, e.g. in a bile duct obstructed by a tumour or stricture or in an artery after *angioplasty to prevent restenosis. **Double J** (or **pig-tail**) **stents** are slender catheters with side holes that are passed over a guide wire either through an endoscope or at open operation to drain urine from the kidney pelvis to the bladder via the ureter. On removal of the guide wire both the upper and lower extremities of the stent assume a J-shape, hence preventing both upward and downward migration. They are commonly used to splint a damaged ureter and to relieve obstruction.

sterco- *prefix denoting* faeces.

stercobilin *n.* a brownish-red pigment formed during the metabolism of the *bile pigments biliverdin and bilirubin, which are derived from haemoglobin. Stercobilin is subsequently excreted in the urine or faeces.

stercolith *n.* a stone formed of dried compressed faeces.

stercoraceous *adj.* composed of or containing faeces.

stereognosis *n.* the ability to recognize the three-dimensional shape of an object by touch alone. This is a function of the *association areas of the parietal lobe of the brain. *See also* AGNOSIA.

stereoisomers *pl. n.* compounds having the same molecular formula but different three-dimensional arrangements of their atoms. The atomic structures of stereoisomers are mirror images of each other.

stereopsis n. see STEREOSCOPIC VISION.

stereoscopic vision (stereopsis) perception of the shape, depth, and distance of an object as a result of having *binocular vision. The brain receives two distinct images from the eyes, which it interprets as a single three-dimensional image.

stereotactic localization the accurate localization of structures within the body by using three-dimensional measurements. It enables the accurate positioning within the body of radiotherapy beams or sources for the treatment of tumours and of localizing wires for the biopsy of small tumours. See also STEREOTAXY (STEREOTACTIC SURGERY).

stereotaxy (stereotactic surgery) n. a surgical procedure in which a deep-seated area in the brain is operated upon after its position has been established very accurately by three-dimensional measurements. The operation may be performed using an electrical current or by heat, cold, or mechanical techniques. See also LEUCOTOMY.

stereotypy n. the constant repetition of a complex action, which is carried out in the same way each time. It is seen in *catatonia and infantile *autism; sometimes it is an isolated symptom in mental retardation. It is more common in patients who live in institutions where they are bored and unstimulated. It can prevent a patient from carrying on normal life, and sometimes causes physical injury to the patient. Drugs, such as *phenothiazines, and behaviour therapy are sometimes used in treating the condition.

sterile adj. **1.** (of a living organism) barren; unable to reproduce its kind (see STERILITY). **2.** (of inanimate objects) completely free from bacteria, fungi, viruses, or other microorganisms that could cause infection.

sterility n. inability to have children, either due to *infertility or (in someone who has been fertile) deliberately induced by surgical procedures as a means of contraception (see STERILIZATION). Sterility may also be an incidental result of an operation or drug treatment undertaken for other reasons, such as removal of the uterus (*hysterectomy) because of cancer.

sterilization n. **1.** a surgical operation or any other process that induces *sterility in men or women. In women, hysterectomy and bilateral oophorectomy (surgical removal of both ovaries) are 100% effective and permanent. Alternatively, the Fallopian tubes may be removed (see SALPINGECTOMY) or divided and/or ligated. These operations can be performed through the abdomen or the vagina. The modern technique (**tubal occlusion**) is to occlude (close) permanently the inner (lower) half of the Fallopian tube through a *laparoscope. The occluding device is usually a clip (the **Hulka-Clemens** or **Filshie clips**) or a small plastic ring (**Falope ring**); *diathermy coagulation carries greater dangers (e.g. bowel burns) and is now little used. A more recent method is the use of a rapid-setting plastic introduced into the tubes through a *hysteroscope. Men are usually sterilized by *vasectomy. See also CASTRATION. **2.** the process by which all types of microorganisms (including spores) are destroyed. This is achieved by the use of heat, radiation, chemicals, or filtration. See also AUTOCLAVE.

stern- (sterno-) prefix denoting the sternum. Example: **sternocostal** (relating to the sternum and ribs).

Sternberg-Reed cell (Reed-Sternberg cell) a large binucleate cell that is characteristic of *Hodgkin's disease. [C. Sternberg (1872–1935), Austrian pathologist; D. Reed Mendenhall (1874–1964), US pathologist]

sternebra n. (pl. **sternebrae**) one of the four parts that fuse during development to form the body of the sternum.

sternocleidomastoid muscle see STERNOMASTOID MUSCLE.

sternohyoid n. a muscle in the neck, arising from the sternum and inserted into the hyoid bone. It depresses the hyoid bone.

sternomastoid muscle (sternocleidomastoid muscle) a long muscle in the neck, extending from the mastoid process to the sternum and clavicle. It serves to rotate the neck and flex the head.

sternomastoid tumour a small painless nonmalignant swelling in the lower half of the *sternomastoid muscle, appearing a few days after birth. It occurs when the neck of the fetus is in an abnormal position in the uterus, which interferes with the blood supply to the affected muscle, and it is most common after breech births. The tumour may cause a slight tilt of the head towards the tumour and turning of the face to the other side. This can be corrected by physiotherapy aimed at increasing all movements of the body, but without stretching the neck.

sternotomy *n.* surgical division of the breastbone (sternum), performed to allow access to the heart and its major vessels.

sternum *n.* (*pl.* **sterna**) the breastbone: a flat bone, 15–20 cm long, extending from the base of the neck to just below the diaphragm and forming the front part of the skeleton of the thorax. The sternum articulates with the collar bones (*see* CLAVICLE) and the costal cartilages of the first seven pairs of ribs. It consists of three sections: the middle and longest section – the **body** or **gladiolus** – is attached to the *manubrium at the top and the *xiphoid (or ensiform) process at the bottom. The manubrium slopes back from the body so that the junction between the two parts forms an angle (**angle of Louis** or **sternal angle**). —**sternal** *adj.*

steroid *n.* one of a group of compounds having a common structure based on the **steroid nucleus**, which consists of three six-membered carbon rings and one five-membered carbon ring. The naturally occurring steroids include the male and female sex hormones (*androgens and *oestrogens), the hormones of the adrenal cortex (*see* CORTICOSTEROID), *progesterone, *bile salts, and *sterols. Synthetic steroids have been produced for therapeutic purposes.

sterol *n.* one of a group of *steroid alcohols. The most important sterols are *cholesterol and *ergosterol.

stertor *n.* a snoring type of noisy breathing heard in deeply unconscious patients.

steth- (stetho-) *prefix denoting* the chest.

stethoscope *n.* an instrument used for listening to sounds within the body, such as those in the heart and lungs (*see* AUSCUL-

TATION). A simple stethoscope usually consists of a diaphragm or an open bell-shaped structure (applied to the body) connected by rubber or plastic tubes to earpieces for the examiner. More complicated devices may contain electronic amplification systems to aid diagnosis.

sthenia *n.* a state of normal or greater than normal strength. *Compare* ASTHENIA. —**sthenic** *adj.*

stibophen *n.* a sodium-containing salt of antimony used to treat *schistosomiasis. It is administered by injection; side-effects may include digestive upsets, slow heart rate, and anaemia.

stigma *n.* (*pl.* **stigmata**) **1.** a mark that characterizes a particular disease, such as the *café au lait spots characteristic of neurofibromatosis. **2.** any spot or lesion on the skin.

stilboestrol *n.* a synthetic female sex hormone (*see* OESTROGEN) used as *hormone replacement therapy to relieve vaginal atrophy; it is given as pessaries. It is sometimes taken by mouth to treat breast and prostate cancer; side-effects include nausea and vomiting, fluid retention, and in men breast enlargement and impotence. Trade names: **Apstil, Tampovagan**.

stilet (stylet, stylus) *n.* **1.** a slender probe. **2.** a wire placed in the lumen of a catheter to give it rigidity while the instrument is passed along a body canal (such as the urethra).

stillbirth *n.* birth of a fetus that shows no evidence of life (heartbeat, respiration, or independent movement) at any time later than 24 weeks after conception. Under the Stillbirth (Definition) Act 1992, there is a legal obligation to notify all stillbirths to the appropriate authority. The number of such births expressed per 1000 births (live and still) is known as the **stillbirth rate**. In legal terms, viability is deemed to start at the 24th week of pregnancy and a fetus born dead before this time is known as an *abortion or miscarriage. However, some fetuses born alive before the 24th week may now survive as a result of improved perinatal care.

Still's disease chronic arthritis developing in children before the age of 16. There are several different forms of arthritis affecting children, and some authorities confine the diagnosis of Still's disease to the following: a disease of childhood marked by arthritis (often involving several joints) with a swinging fever and a transitory red rash. There is sometimes severe illness affecting the entire body and the condition may be complicated by enlargement of the spleen and lymph nodes and inflammation of the pericardium and iris. [Sir G. F. Still (1868–1941), British physician]

stimulant *n.* an agent that promotes the activity of a body system or function. *Amphetamine and *caffeine are stimulants of the central nervous system.

stimulator *n.* any apparatus designed to stimulate nerves and muscles for a variety of purposes. It can be used to stimulate particular areas of the brain or to block pain (as in *transcutaneous electrical nerve stimulation).

stimulus *n.* (*pl.* **stimuli**) any agent that provokes a response, or particular form of activity, in a cell, tissue, or other structure, which is said to be sensitive to that stimulus.

stippling *n.* a spotted or speckled appearance, such as is seen in the retina in certain eye diseases or in abnormal red blood cells stained with basic dyes.

stirrup *n.* (in anatomy) *see* STAPES.

stitch *n.* **1.** a sharp localized pain, commonly in the abdomen, associated with strenuous physical activity (such as running), especially shortly after eating. It is a form of cramp. **2.** *see* SUTURE.

stock culture *see* CULTURE.

Stokes-Adams syndrome (Adams-Stokes syndrome) attacks of temporary loss of consciousness that occur when blood flow ceases due to ventricular *fibrillation or to *asystole. This syndrome may complicate *heart block. It is treated by means of a battery-operated *pacemaker. [W. Stokes (1804–78) and R. Adams (1791–1875), Irish physicians]

stoma *n.* (*pl.* **stomata**) **1.** (in anatomy) the mouth or any mouthlike part. **2.** (in surgery) the artificial opening of a tube (e.g. the colon or ileum) that has been brought to the abdominal surface (*see*

COLOSTOMY, ILEOSTOMY). **Stoma therapists** are nurses specially trained in the care of these artificial openings and the appliances used with them. **—stomal** *adj.*

stomach *n.* a distensible saclike organ that forms part of the alimentary canal between the oesophagus (gullet) and the duodenum (see illustration). It communicates with the former by means of the **cardiac orifice** and with the latter by the **pyloric sphincter**. The stomach lies just below the diaphragm, to the right of the spleen and partly under the liver. Its function is to continue the process of digestion that begins in the mouth. *Gastric juice, secreted by gastric glands in the mucosa, contains hydrochloric acid and the enzyme *pepsin, which contribute to chemical digestion. This – together with the churning action of the muscular layers of the stomach – reduces the food to a semiliquid partly digested mass that passes on to the duodenum.

stomat- (stomato-) *prefix denoting* the mouth.

stomatitis *n.* inflammation of the mucous lining of the mouth.

stomatology *n.* the branch of medicine concerned with diseases of the mouth.

stomodeum *n.* the site of the embryonic mouth, marked by a depression lined with ectoderm from which the teeth develop. The membrane separating it from the foregut breaks down by the end of the first month of pregnancy. *Compare* PROCTODEUM.

-stomy (-ostomy) *suffix denoting* a surgical opening into an organ or part. Example: **colostomy** (into the colon).

stone *n.* *see* CALCULUS.

stool *n.* *faeces discharged from the anus.

stop needle a surgical needle with a shank that has a protruding collar to stop it when the needle has been pushed a prescribed distance into the tissue. A stop needle has the eye at the tip.

strabismus (heterotropia) *n.* squint: any abnormal alignment of the two eyes. The strabismus is most commonly horizontal – **convergent strabismus (or es-**

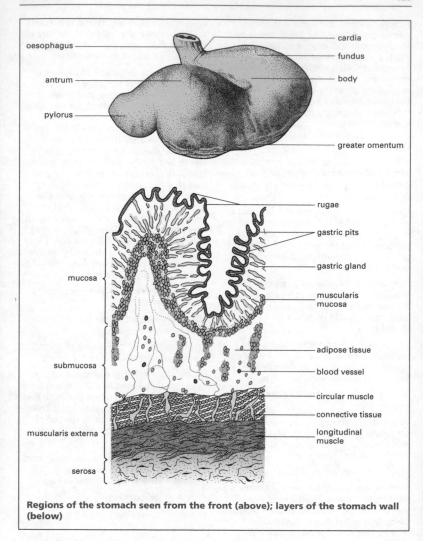

oesophagus

cardia

fundus

antrum

body

pylorus

greater omentum

rugae

gastric pits

gastric gland

mucosa

muscularis
mucosa

submucosa

adipose tissue

blood vessel

circular muscle

connective tissue

muscularis externa

longitudinal
muscle

serosa

**Regions of the stomach seen from the front (above); layers of the stomach wall
(below)**

otropia) or **divergent strabismus** (**exotropia**) – but it may be vertical (**hypertropia**, in which the eye looks upwards, or
hypotropia, in which it looks downwards). In rare cases both eyes look towards the same point but one is twisted
clockwise or anticlockwise in relation to
the other (**cyclotropia**). Double vision is

possible, but the image from the deviating
eye usually becomes ignored. In cyclotropia the image is not separated from
the normal one but rotated across it. Most
strabismus is **concomitant**, i.e. the abnormal alignment of the two eyes remains
fairly constant, in whatever direction the
person is looking. This is usual with child-

hood squints. Strabismus acquired by injury or disease is usually **incomitant**, i.e. the degree of misalignment varies in different directions of gaze. See also COVER TEST, DEVIATION, DIVERGENCE, HETEROPHORIA.

strain 1. n. excessive stretching or working of a muscle, resulting in pain and swelling of the muscle. Compare SPRAIN. **2.** n. a group of organisms, such as bacteria, obtained from a particular source or having special properties distinguishing them from other members of the same species. **3.** vb. to damage a muscle by overstretching.

strain gauge a sensitive instrument for measuring tension and alterations in pressure. It is extensively used in medical instruments.

strangulated adj. describing a part of the body whose blood supply has been interrupted by compression of a blood vessel, as may occur in a loop of intestine trapped in a *hernia.

strangulation n. the closure of a passage, such as the main airway to the lungs (resulting in the cessation of breathing), a blood vessel, or the gastrointestinal tract.

strangury n. severe pain in the urethra referred from the base of the bladder and associated with an intense desire to pass urine. It occurs when the base of the bladder is irritated by a stone or an indwelling catheter. It is also noted in patients with an invasive cancer of the base of the bladder or severe *cystitis or *prostatitis, when the strong desire to urinate is accompanied by the painful passage of a few drops of urine.

Strassman procedure an operation to correct a double uterus (see UTERUS DIDELPHYS). It has now largely been replaced by techniques involving the use of a *hysteroscope. [P. F. Strassman (1866–1938), German obstetrician and gynaecologist]

stratum n. a layer of tissue or cells, such as any of the layers of the *epidermis of the skin (the **stratum corneum** is the outermost layer).

strawberry mark (strawberry naevus) see NAEVUS.

streak n. (in anatomy) a line, furrow, or narrow band. See also PRIMITIVE STREAK.

Streptobacillus n. a genus of Gram-negative aerobic nonmotile rodlike bacteria that tend to form filaments. The single species, S. moniliformis, is a normal inhabitant of the respiratory tract of rats but causes *rat-bite fever in man.

streptococcal toxic shock syndrome a bacterial disease characterized by fever, shock, and multiple organ failure. It is similar to the *toxic shock syndrome caused by staphylococci, but in these cases the infecting organisms are *Streptococcus Type A bacteria. See also NECROTIZING FASCIITIS.

Streptococcus n. a genus of Gram-positive nonmotile spherical bacteria occurring in chains. Most species are saprophytes; some are pathogenic. Many pathogenic species are **haemolytic**, i.e. they have the ability to destroy red blood cells in blood agar. This provides a useful basis for classifying the many different strains. Strains of S. pyogenes (the β-haemolytic streptococci) are associated with many infections, including *scarlet fever, and produce many *exotoxins. Strains of the α-haemolytic streptococci are associated with bacterial *endocarditis. The species S. pneumoniae (formerly Diplococcus pneumoniae) – the **pneumococcus** – is associated with pneumonia. It occurs in pairs, surrounded by a capsule (see QUELLUNG REACTION). S. mutans has been shown to cause dental caries. See also LANCEFIELD CLASSIFICATION, STREPTOKINASE. —**streptococcal** adj.

streptodornase n. an enzyme produced by some haemolytic bacteria of the genus Streptococcus that is capable of liquefying pus. See also STREPTOKINASE.

streptokinase n. an enzyme produced by some haemolytic bacteria of the genus *Streptococcus that is capable of liquefying blood clots (see also FIBRINOLYTIC). It is injected to treat blockage of blood vessels, including infarction and pulmonary embolism. It is also used in combination with streptodornase, applied topically or taken by mouth or injection, to liquefy pus and relieve inflammation. Side-effects may include digestive upsets, haemorrhage, and fever. Trade names: **Kabikinase**, **Streptase**.

streptolysin n. an *exotoxin that is produced by strains of *Streptococcus* bacteria and destroys red blood cells.

Streptomyces *n.* a genus of aerobic mouldlike bacteria. Most species live in the soil, but some are parasites of animals, humans, and plants; in humans they cause *Madura foot. They are important medically as a source of such antibiotics as *streptomycin, *neomycin, *actinomycin, and *chloramphenicol.

streptomycin *n.* an *antibiotic, derived from the bacterium *Streptomyces griseus*, that is effective against a wide range of bacterial infections; it is administered by intramuscular injection. In tuberculosis therapy streptomycin is given in conjunction with other drugs (e.g. *isoniazid) because bacteria soon become resistant to it. Side-effects causing ear and kidney damage may develop in some patients.

stress *n.* any factor that threatens the health of the body or has an adverse effect on its functioning, such as injury, disease, or worry. The existence of one form of stress tends to diminish resistance to other forms. Constant stress brings about changes in the balance of hormones in the body.

stretch receptor a cell or group of cells found between muscle fibres that responds to stretching of the muscle by transmitting impulses to the central nervous system through the sensory nerves. Stretch receptors are part of the *proprioceptor system necessary for the performance of coordinated muscular activity.

stretch reflex (myotatic reflex) the reflex contraction of a muscle in response to its being stretched.

stria *n.* (*pl.* **striae**) (in anatomy) a streak, line, or thin band. The **striae gravidarum** (stretch marks) are the lines that appear on the skin of the abdomen of pregnant women, due to excessive stretching of the elastic fibres. Red or purple during pregnancy, they become white after delivery. The **stria terminalis** is a white band that separates the thalamus from the ventricular surface of the caudate nucleus in the brain.

striated muscle a tissue comprising the bulk of the body's musculature. It is also known as **skeletal muscle**, because it is attached to the skeleton and is responsible for the movement of bones, and **voluntary muscle**, because it is under voluntary control. Striated muscle is composed of parallel bundles of multinucleate fibres (each containing many **myofibrils**), which reveal cross-banding when viewed under the microscope. This effect is caused by the alternation of **actin** and **myosin** protein filaments within each myofibril (see illustration). According to the 'sliding filament' theory, When muscle contraction takes place, the two sets of filaments slide past each other, so reducing the length of each unit (**sarcomere**) of the myofibril. The sliding is caused by a series of cyclic reactions, requiring ATP, resulting in a change in orientation of projections on the myosin filaments; each projection is first attached to an actin filament but contracts and releases it to become reattached at a different site.

Structure of striated muscle

stricture *n.* a narrowing of any tubular structure in the body, such as the oesophagus (gullet), bowel, ureter, or urethra. A stricture may result from inflammation, muscular spasm, growth of a tumour within the affected part, or from pressure on it by neighbouring organs. For example, a **urethral stricture** is a fibrous narrowing of the urethra, usually resulting from injury or inflammation. The patient has increasing difficulty in passing urine and may develop *retention. The site and length of the stricture is assessed by *urethrography and urethroscopy, and treatment is by periodic dilatation of the urethra using *sounds, *urethrotomy, or *urethroplasty. Strictures in the alimentary canal are dilated by *balloon or *stricturoplasty.

stricturoplasty n. an operation in which a stricture (usually in the small intestine) is widened by cutting it.

stridor n. the noise heard on breathing in when the trachea or larynx is obstructed. It tends to be louder and harsher than *wheeze.

strobila n. (pl. **strobilae**) the entire chain of segments that make up the body of an adult *tapeworm.

stroke (apoplexy) n. a sudden attack of weakness affecting one side of the body. It is the consequence of an interruption to the flow of blood to the brain. The primary disease is in the heart or blood vessels and the effect on the brain is secondary. An **ischaemic stroke** occurs when the flow of blood is prevented by clotting (see THROMBOSIS) or by a detached clot that lodges in an artery (see EMBOLISM). A **haemorrhagic stroke** results from rupture of an artery wall (see CEREBRAL HAEMORRHAGE). Prolonged reduction of blood pressure may result in similar brain damage. A stroke can vary in severity from a passing weakness or tingling in a limb (see TRANSIENT ISCHAEMIC ATTACK) to a profound paralysis, coma, and death.

stroma n. the connective tissue basis of an organ, as opposed to the functional tissue (**parenchyma**). For example, the stroma of the erythrocytes is the spongy framework of protein strands within a red blood cell in which the blood pigment haemoglobin is packed; the stroma of the cornea is the transparent fibrous tissue making up the main body of the cornea.

Strongyloides n. a genus of small slender nematode worms that live as parasites inside the small intestines of mammals. S. stercoralis infects the human small intes-

tine (see STRONGYLOIDIASIS); its larvae, which are passed out in the stools, develop quickly into infective forms.

strongyloidiasis (strongyloidosis) n. an infestation of the small intestine with the parasitic nematode worm Strongyloides stercoralis, common in humid tropical regions. Larvae, present in soil contaminated with human faeces, penetrate the skin of a human host and may produce an itching rash. They migrate to the lungs, where they cause tissue destruction and bleeding, and then via the windpipe and gullet to the intestine. Adult worms burrow into the intestinal wall and may cause ulceration, diarrhoea, abdominal pain, nausea, anaemia, and weakness. Treatment involves use of the drug *thiabendazole.

strontium n. a yellow metallic element, absorption of which causes bone damage when its atoms displace calcium in bone. The radioactive isotope **strontium-90**, which emits beta rays, is used in radiotherapy for the *contact therapy of skin and eye tumours. Symbol: Sr.

struma n. (pl. **strumae**) a swelling of the thyroid gland (see GOITRE). **Riedel's struma** is a rare chronic inflammation of the thyroid (see THYROIDITIS), which becomes firm and enlarged and is eventually destroyed.

strychnine n. a poisonous alkaloid produced in the seeds of the East Indian tree Strychnos nux-vomica. In small doses it was formerly widely used in 'tonics'. Poisoning causes painful muscular spasms similar to those of tetanus; the back becomes arched (the posture known as **opisthotonos**) and death is likely to occur from spasm in the respiratory muscles.

S–T segment the segment on an *electrocardiogram that represents the interval preceding the last phase of the *cardiac cycle, when the heart recovers from contraction. The S–T segment is usually raised by acute *ischaemia of the heart muscle; it usually returns to normal with recovery.

Student's t test see SIGNIFICANCE. [Pseudonym of W. S. Gosset (1876–1937), British statistician]

stupe n. any piece of material, such as a wad of cottonwool, soaked in hot water (with or without medication) and used to apply a poultice.

stupor *n.* a condition of near unconsciousness, with apparent mental inactivity and reduced ability to respond to stimulation.

Sturge-Weber syndrome *see* ANGIOMA. [W. A. Sturge (1850–1919) and F. P. Weber (1863–1962), British physicians]

stuttering *n.* *see* STAMMERING.

St Vitus' dance an archaic name for Sydenham's *chorea.

Stycar tests Standard Tests for Young Children and Retardates: tests to detect visual problems in children between the ages of six months and five years. They consist of a series of standardized balls, toys, or letters. The tests were developed by the paediatrician Mary Sheridan.

stye *n.* acute inflammation of a gland at the base of an eyelash, caused by bacterial infection. The gland becomes hard and tender and a pus-filled cyst develops at its centre. Styes are treated by bathing in warm water or removal of the eyelash involved. Medical name: **hordeolum**.

stylet *n.* *see* STILET.

stylo- *prefix denoting* the styloid process of the temporal bone. Example: **stylomastoid** (relating to the styloid and mastoid processes).

styloglossus *n.* a muscle that extends from the tongue to the styloid process of the temporal bone. It serves to draw the tongue upwards and backwards.

stylohyoid *n.* a muscle that extends from the styloid process of the temporal bone to the hyoid bone. It serves to draw the hyoid bone backwards and upwards.

styloid process 1. a long slender downward-pointing spine projecting from the lower surface of the *temporal bone of the skull. It provides attachment for muscles and ligaments of the tongue and hyoid bone. 2. any of various other spiny projections; occurring, for example, at the lower ends of the ulna and radius.

stylus *n.* 1. a pencil-shaped instrument, commonly used for applying external

medication; for example, to apply silver nitrate to warts. 2. *see* STILET.

styptic *n.* *see* HAEMOSTATIC.

sub- *prefix denoting* 1. below; underlying. Examples: **subcostal** (below the ribs); **sublingual** (below the tongue); **submandibular** (below the mandible). 2. partial or slight.

subacute *adj.* describing a disease that progresses more rapidly than a *chronic condition but does not become *acute.

subacute combined degeneration of the cord the neurological disorder complicating a deficiency of *vitamin B_{12} and pernicious anaemia. There is selective damage to the motor and sensory nerve fibres in the spinal cord, resulting in *spasticity of the limbs and a sensory *ataxia. It may also be accompanied by damage to the peripheral nerves and the optic nerve and by dementia. It is treated by giving vitamin B_{12} injections.

subacute sclerosing panencephalitis (SSPE) a rare and late complication of *measles characterized by a slow progressive neurological deterioration that is usually fatal. It can occur four to ten years after the initial infection.

subarachnoid haemorrhage bleeding into the subarachnoid space surrounding the brain, which causes severe headache with stiffness of the neck. The usual source of such a haemorrhage is a cerebral *aneurysm that has burst. The diagnosis is confirmed by CT scan or by finding blood-stained cerebrospinal fluid at *lumbar puncture. Identification of the site of the aneurysm, upon which decisions about treatment will be based, is achieved by cerebral *angiography.

subarachnoid space the space between the arachnoid and pia *meninges of the brain and spinal cord, containing circulating cerebrospinal fluid and large blood vessels. Several large spaces within it are known as **cisternae**.

subclavian artery either of two arteries supplying blood to the neck and arms. The right subclavian artery branches from the innominate artery; the left subclavian arises directly from the aortic arch.

subclavian steal syndrome diversion of blood from the vertebral artery to the subclavian artery when the latter is blocked proximally. It causes attacks of diminished consciousness (*syncope).

subclinical *adj.* describing a disease that is suspected but is not sufficiently developed to produce definite signs and symptoms in the patient.

subconscious *adj.* **1.** describing mental processes of which a person is not aware. **2.** (in psychoanalysis) denoting the part of the mind that includes memories, motives, and intentions that are momentarily not present in consciousness but can more or less readily be recalled to awareness. *Compare* UNCONSCIOUS.

subcutaneous *adj.* beneath the skin. A **subcutaneous injection** is given beneath the skin. **Subcutaneous tissue** is loose connective tissue, often fatty, situated under the dermis.

subdural *adj.* below the dura mater (the outermost of the meninges); relating to the space between the dura mater and arachnoid. *See also* HAEMATOMA.

subglottis *n.* that part of the *larynx that lies below the vocal folds.

subinvolution *n.* failure of the uterus to revert to its normal size during the six weeks following childbirth.

sublimation *n.* the replacement of socially undesirable means of gratifying motives or desires by means that are socially acceptable. *See also* DEFENCE MECHANISM, REPRESSION.

subliminal *adj.* subconscious: beneath the threshold of conscious perception.

sublingual gland one of a pair of *salivary glands situated in the lower part of the mouth, one on either side of the tongue. The sublingual glands are the smallest salivary glands; each gland has about 20 ducts, most of which open into the mouth directly above the gland.

subluxation *n.* partial *dislocation of a joint, so that the bone ends are misaligned but still in contact.

submandibular gland (submaxillary gland) one of a pair of *salivary glands situated below the parotid glands. Their ducts (**Wharton's ducts**) open in two papillae under the tongue, on either side of the frenulum.

submaxillary gland *see* SUBMANDIBULAR GLAND.

submentovertical (SMV) *adj.* denoting an X-ray view of the base of the skull.

submucosa *n.* the layer of loose connective (*areolar) tissue underlying a mucous membrane; for example, in the wall of the intestine. —**submucosal** *adj.*

subphrenic abscess a collection of pus in the space below the diaphragm, usually on the right side, between the liver and diaphragm. Causes include postoperative infection (particularly after the stomach or bowel have been opened) and perforation of an organ (e.g. perforated peptic ulcer). Prompt treatment by antibiotics may be effective, but more frequently the abscess requires surgical drainage.

substitution *n.* **1.** (in psychoanalysis) the replacement of one idea by another: a form of *defence mechanism. **2.** (**symptom substitution**) the supposed process whereby removing one psychological symptom leads to another symptom appearing if the basic psychological cause has not been removed. It is controversial whether this happens.

substitution therapy treatment by providing a less harmful alternative to a drug or remedy that a patient has been receiving. It is used when the patient has become addicted to a drug or is placing too much reliance upon a particular remedy. The patient is weaned off the 'hard' drug to which he has become addicted by the gradual substitution of a nonaddictive drug with a similar or a sedative effect.

substrate *n.* the specific substance or substances on which a given *enzyme acts. For example, starch is the substrate for salivary amylase; RNA is the substrate for ribonuclease.

subsultus *n.* abnormal twitching or tremor of muscles, such as may occur in feverish conditions.

subtertian fever a form of *malaria resulting from repeated infection by *Plasmodium falciparum* and characterized by continuous fever.

subthalamic nucleus a collection of grey matter, shaped like a biconvex lens, lying beneath the *thalamus and close to the *corpus striatum, to which it is connected by nerve tracts. It has connections with the cerebral cortex and several other nuclei nearby.

subzonal insemination (Suzi) a method of assisting conception in cases of infertility caused by the inability of the spermatozoa to penetrate the barriers surrounding the ovum. Using *in vitro fertilization techniques, a small number of spermatozoa (no more than six) are injected through the *zona pellucida into the perivitelline space (which surrounds the egg membrane). If fertilization subsequently occurs, the blastocyst is implanted in the mother's uterus.

succus *n.* any juice or secretion of animal or plant origin.

succus entericus (intestinal juice) the clear alkaline fluid secreted by the glands of the small intestine. It contains mucus and digestive enzymes, including *enteropeptidase, *erepsin, *lactase, and *sucrase.

succussion *n.* a splashing noise heard when a patient who has a large quantity of fluid in a body cavity, such as the pleural cavity, moves suddenly or is deliberately shaken.

sucralfate *n.* an aluminium-containing drug that forms a protective coating over the stomach or duodenal lining. Administered by mouth, sucralfate is used in the treatment of peptic ulcer. A fairly common side-effect is constipation. Trade name: **Antepsin**.

sucrase *n.* an enzyme, secreted by glands in the small intestine, that catalyses the hydrolysis of sucrose into its components (glucose and fructose).

sucrose *n.* a carbohydrate consisting of glucose and fructose. Sucrose is the principal constituent of cane sugar and sugar beet; it is the sweetest of the natural dietary carbohydrates. The increasing consumption of sucrose in the last 50 years has coincided with an increase in the incidence of dental caries, diabetes, coronary heart disease, and obesity.

suction *n.* the use of reduced pressure to remove unwanted fluids or other material through a tube for disposal. Suction is often used to clear secretions from the airways of newly born infants to aid breathing. During surgery, suction tubes are used to remove blood from the area of operation and to decompress the stomach (**nasogastric suction**) and the pleural space of air and blood (**chest suction**).

Sudan stains a group of azo compounds used for staining fats. The group includes **Sudan I, Sudan II, Sudan III, Sudan IV**, and **Sudan black**.

sudden infant death syndrome (SIDS) *see* COT DEATH.

Sudek's atrophy (reflex sympathetic dystrophy) pain, swelling, stiffness, and skin changes in a part of the body, most often the hand or foot, caused by overactivity of the sympathetic nervous system following trauma or surgery or occasionally arising spontaneously; a Colles' fracture is frequently the precipitating cause. In more severe cases the condition progresses over a few months with increasing stiffness, cool shiny skin, and osteoporosis; severe pain may persist. Treatment is physiotherapy and sympathetic nerve blocks, often using *guanethidine. The condition can last many months, and in the most severe cases the patient is left with a useless painful limb. [P. H. M. Sudek (1866–1938), German surgeon]

sudor *n.* *see* SWEAT.

sudorific *n.* *see* DIAPHORETIC.

suffocation *n.* cessation of breathing as a result of drowning, smothering, etc., leading to unconsciousness or death (*see* ASPHYXIA).

suffusion *n.* the spreading of a flush across the skin surface, caused by changes in the local blood supply.

sugar *n.* any *carbohydrate that dissolves in water, is usually crystalline, and has a sweet taste. Sugars are classified chemically as *monosaccharides or *disaccharides. Table sugar is virtually 100% pure *sucrose and contains no other nutrient; brown sugar is less highly refined sucrose. Sugar is used as both a sweetening and preserving agent. *See also* FRUCTOSE, GLU-COSE, LACTOSE.

suggestion *n.* (in psychology) the process of changing people's beliefs, attitudes, or emotions by telling them that they will change. It is sometimes used as a synonym for *hypnosis. *See also* AUTOSUGGESTION.

suicide *n.* self-destruction as a deliberate act. Distinction is usually made between **attempted suicide**, when death is averted although the person concerned intended to kill himself (or herself), and *parasuicide, when the attempt is made for reasons other than actually killing oneself. In the UK 4547 people killed themselves in 1991 (3494 of whom were men). Some 22% of these suicides were caused by overdoses and 29% by toxic gases.

sulcus *n.* (*pl.* **sulci**) **1.** one of the many clefts or infoldings of the surface of the brain. The raised outfolding on each side of a sulcus is termed a **gyrus**. **2.** any of the infoldings of soft tissue in the mouth, for example between the cheek and the alveolus.

sulfametopyrazine *n.* *see* SULPHONAMIDE.

sulphacetamide *n.* a drug of the *sulphonamide group that is used in eye drops to treat such infections as conjunctivitis. Transient irritation may occur with higher doses. Trade names: **Albucid**, **Ocusol**.

sulphadiazine *n.* *see* SULPHONAMIDE.

sulphadimidine *n.* *see* SULPHONAMIDE.

sulpha drug *see* SULPHONAMIDE.

sulphamethoxazole *n.* a drug of the *sulphonamide group. It is taken by mouth and is effective in the treatment of infections of the respiratory tract (including bronchitis), the urinary and gastrointestinal tracts, and the skin. The drug is combined with trimethoprim in *co-trimoxazole (Bactrim, Septrin).

sulphasalazine *n.* a drug of the *sulphonamide group, used in the treatment of ulcerative colitis. It is given by mouth or in the form of suppositories. The most common side-effects are nausea, loss of appetite, and raised temperature. Trade name: **Salazopyrin**.

sulphinpyrazone *n.* a *uricosuric drug given by mouth for the treatment of chronic gout. The main side-effects are nausea and abdominal pain; the drug may also activate a latent duodenal ulcer and it should not be taken by patients with impaired kidney function. Trade name: **Anturan**.

sulphonamide (sulpha drug) *n.* one of a group of drugs, derived from sulphanilamide (a red dye), that prevent the growth of bacteria (i.e. they are bacteriostatic). Sulphonamides are usually given by mouth and are effective against a variety of infections. Because many sulphonamides are rapidly excreted and very soluble in the urine, they are used to treat infections of the urinary tract, especially in combination with other drugs (such as *trimethoprim).

A variety of side-effects may occur with sulphonamide treatment, including nausea, vomiting, headache, and loss of appetite; more severe effects include *cyanosis, blood disorders, skin rashes, and fever. Because of increasing bacterial resistance to sulphonamides, and with the development of more effective less toxic antibiotics, the clinical use of these drugs has declined. Those still used include *sulphacetamide, *sulphamethoxazole, *sulphasalazine, **sulphadimidine**, **sulphadiazine**, and **sulfametopyrazine**.

sulphone *n.* one of a group of drugs closely related to the *sulphonamides in structure and therapeutic actions. Sulphones possess powerful activity against the bacteria that cause leprosy and tuberculosis. The best known sulphone is *dapsone.

sulphonylurea *n.* one of a group of *oral hypoglycaemic drugs, derived from a *sulphonamide, that are used in the treatment of noninsulin-dependent diabetes mellitus; they act by stimulating the islet cells in the pancreas to produce more insulin. The group includes *chlorpropamide, *tolazamide, *glibenclamide, and *tolbutamide.

sulphur *n.* a nonmetallic element that is active against fungi and parasites. It is a constituent of ointments and other preparations used in the treatment of skin disorders and infections (such as psoriasis and dermatitis).

sulphuric acid a powerful corrosive acid, H_2SO_4, widely used in industry. Swallowing the acid causes severe burning of the mouth and throat and difficulty in breathing, speaking, and swallowing. The patient should drink large quantities of milk or water or white of egg; gastric lavage should not be delayed. Skin or eye contact should be treated by flooding the area with water.

sumatriptan n. a drug that stimulates *serotonin receptors and is effective in the treatment of acute *migraine by rapidly reversing the dilatation of blood vessels in the head that causes the migraine headache. It is administered by mouth or by subcutaneous injection. Possible side-effects include dizziness, drowsiness, fatigue, chest pain, and a rise in blood pressure. Trade name: **Imigran**.

sunburn n. damage to the skin by excessive exposure to the sun's rays. Sunburn may vary from reddening of the skin to the development of large painful fluid-filled blisters, which may cause shock if they cover a large area (see BURN). Fair-skinned red-haired people are more susceptible to sunburn than others. Severe sunburn in childhood is a risk factor for the development of malignant *melanoma in later life.

sunstroke n. see HEATSTROKE.

super- prefix denoting **1.** above; overlying. **2.** extreme or excessive.

superciliary adj. of or relating to the eyebrows (supercilia).

superego n. (in psychoanalysis) the part of the mind that functions as a moral conscience or judge. It is also responsible for the formation of ideals for the *ego. The superego is the result of the incorporation of parental injunctions into the child's mind.

superfecundation n. the fertilization of two or more ova of the same age by spermatozoa from different males. See SUPERFETATION.

superfetation n. the fertilization of a second ovum some time after the start of

pregnancy, resulting in two fetuses of different maturity in the same uterus.

superficial adj. (in anatomy) situated at or close to a surface. Superficial blood vessels are those close to the surface of the skin.

superinfection n. an infection arising during the course of another infection and caused by a different microorganism, which is usually resistant to the drugs used to treat the primary infection. The infective agent may be a normally harmless inhabitant of the body that becomes pathogenic when other harmless types are removed by the drugs or it may be a resistant variety of the primary infective agent, such as *MRSA (see also METHICILLIN).

superior adj. (in anatomy) situated uppermost in the body in relation to another structure or surface.

supernumerary n. (in dentistry) an additional tooth.

superovulation n. **1.** controlled hyperstimulation of the ovary to produce more follicles with oocytes. Usually induced by drugs (e.g. *clomiphene), it is performed in *in vitro fertilization and other procedures of assisted conception in order to improve the pregnancy rates. **2.** uncontrolled hyperstimulation of the ovary (**ovarian hyperstimulation syndrome**), an abnormal response of the ovaries leading to multiple follicle production. It may be associated with abdominal pain, ascites, oliguria, or even renal failure. Thromboembolism is the most dangerous complication.

supination n. the act of turning the hand so that the palm is uppermost. Compare PRONATION.

supinator n. a muscle of the forearm that extends from the elbow to the shaft of the radius. It supinates the forearm and hand.

supine adj. **1.** lying on the back or with the face upwards. **2.** (of the forearm) in the position in which the palm of the hand faces upwards. Compare PRONE.

supportive adj. (of treatment) aimed at reinforcing the patient's own defence mechanisms in overcoming a disease or disorder.

suppository n. a medicinal preparation in solid form suitable for insertion into the rectum or vagina. **Rectal suppositories** may contain simple lubricants (e.g. glycerin); drugs that act locally in the rectum or anus (e.g. corticosteroids, local anaesthetics); or drugs that are absorbed and act at other sites (e.g. *bronchodilators). **Vaginal suppositories** are used in the treatment of some gynaecological disorders (see PESSARY).

suppression n. **1.** the cessation or complete inhibition of any physiological activity. **2.** treatment that removes the outward signs of an illness or prevents its progress. **3.** (in psychology) a *defence mechanism by which a person consciously and deliberately ignores an idea that is unpleasant to him.

suppressor gene a gene that prevents the expression of another (non-allelic) gene.

suppressor T-cell a type of T-*lymphocyte that prevents an immune response by B-cells or other T-cells to an antigen.

suppuration n. the formation of pus.

supra- prefix denoting above; over. Examples: **supraclavicular** (above the clavicle); **suprahyoid** (above the hyoid bone); **suprarenal** (above the kidney).

supraglottis n. that part of the *larynx that lies above the vocal folds and includes the *epiglottis.

supraorbital adj. of or relating to the area above the eye orbit.

supraorbital reflex the closing of the eyelids when the supraorbital nerve is struck, due to contraction of the muscle surrounding the orbit (orbicularis oculi muscle).

supraregional specialty see CATCHMENT AREA.

suprarenal glands see ADRENAL GLANDS.

supratonsillar fossa a pharyngeal recess that is situated above the upper pole of the palatine *tonsil. It is a 'hidden' site of tumour origin.

supravital staining the application of a *stain to living tissue, particularly blood cells, removed from the body.

suramin n. a nonmetallic drug used in the treatment of *trypanosomiasis. It is usually given by slow intravenous injection. Side-effects, which vary in intensity and frequency and are related to the nutritional state of the patient, include nausea, vomiting, shock, and loss of consciousness.

surfactant n. a wetting agent. **Pulmonary surfactant**, secreted by type II *pneumocytes, is a complex mixture of compounds (including lipids, protein, and carbohydrates) that prevents the air sacs (alveoli) of the lungs from collapsing by reducing surface tension. In its absence, as in the immature lungs of premature babies, *atelectasis and *respiratory distress syndrome will develop.

surgeon n. a qualified medical practitioner who specializes in surgery. See DOCTOR.

surgery n. the branch of medicine that treats injuries, deformities, or disease by operation or manipulation. See also CRYOSURGERY, MICROSURGERY. —**surgical** adj.

surgical neck the constriction of the shaft of the *humerus, below the head. It is frequently the point at which fracture of the humerus occurs.

surgical spirit methylated spirit, usually with small amounts of castor oil and oil of wintergreen, used to sterilize the skin before surgery, injections, etc.

surrogate n. **1.** (in psychology) a person or object in someone's life that functions as a substitute for another person. In the treatment of sexual problems, when the patient does not have a partner to cooperate in treatment, a surrogate provided by the therapist acts as a sexual partner who gives service to the patient up to and including intercourse. According to psychoanalysts, people and objects in dreams can be surrogates for important individuals in a person's life. **2.** (in reproduction) see SURROGATE MOTHER.

surrogate mother a woman who becomes pregnant (by artificial insemination or embryo insertion) following an arrangement made with another party (usually a couple unable themselves to have children) in which she agrees to hand over the child she carries to that party when it is born. Such an arrangement is made on the understanding that no payment is involved between either parties. Certain activities in connection with surrogacy are regulated by the Surrogacy Arrangements Act 1985: it is unlawful for any form of advertisement to be employed, and for commercial agencies to commission surrogate mothers.

susceptibility *n.* lack of resistance to disease. It is partly a reflection of general health but is also influenced by vaccination or other methods of increasing resistance to specific diseases.

suspensory bandage a bandage arranged to support a hanging part of the body. Examples include a sling used to hold an injured lower jaw in position and a bandage used to support the scrotum in various conditions of the male genital organs.

suspensory ligament a ligament that serves to support or suspend an organ in position. For example, the suspensory ligament of the lens is a fibrous structure attached to the ciliary processes (*see* CILIARY BODY) by means of which the lens of the eye is held in position.

sustentaculum *n.* any anatomical structure that supports another structure. —**sustentacular** *adj.*

Sutures of the skull (internal surface of the vault)

suture 1. *n.* (in anatomy) a type of immovable joint, found particularly in the skull, that is characterized by a minimal amount of connective tissue between the two bones. The cranial sutures include the

coronal suture, between the frontal and parietal bones; the **lambdoidal suture**, –between the parietal and occipital bones; and the **sagittal suture**, between the two parietal bones (see illustration). **2.** *n.* (in surgery) the closure of a wound or incision with material such as silk or catgut, to facilitate the healing process. There is a wide variety of suturing techniques developed to meet the differing circumstances of injuries to and incisions in the body tissues (see illustration). **3.** *n.* the material – silk, catgut, nylon, any of various polymers, or wire – used to sew up a wound. **4.** *vb.* to close a wound by suture.

Types of surgical suture

suxamethonium *n.* a drug that relaxes voluntary muscle (*see* MUSCLE RELAXANT). It is administered by intravenous injection and is used mainly to produce muscle relaxation during surgery carried out under general anaesthesia and to reduce muscular movements occurring during *electroconvulsive therapy. Trade names: **Anectine, Scoline**.

Suzi *n.* *see* SUBZONAL INSEMINATION.

swab *n.* a pad of absorbent material (such as cotton), sometimes attached to a stick or wire, used for cleaning out or applying medication to wounds, operation sites, or body cavities. In operations, gauze swabs are used to clean blood from the site; such swabs are always carefully counted and contain a *radiopaque 'tag' to facilitate identification should it by mischance remain in the body after operation.

swallowing (deglutition) *n.* the process by which food is transferred from the mouth to the oesophagus (gullet). Voluntary raising of the tongue forces food backwards towards the pharynx. This stimulates reflex actions in which the larynx is closed by the epiglottis and the nasal passages are closed by the soft palate, so that food does not enter the trachea (windpipe). Lastly, food moves down the oesophagus by *peristalsis and gravity.

Swan-Ganz catheter a catheter with an inflatable balloon at its tip, which can be inserted into the pulmonary artery via the right chambers of the heart. Inflation of the balloon enables measurement of pressure in the left atrium and hence pulmonary artery pressure. [H. J. C. Swan (1922–), US cardiologist; W. Ganz (20th century), US engineer]

sweat *n.* the watery fluid secreted by the *sweat glands. Its principal constituents in solution are sodium chloride and urea. The secretion of sweat is a means of excreting nitrogenous waste; at the same time it has a role in controlling the temperature of the body – the evaporation of sweat from the surface of the skin has a cooling effect. Therefore an increase in body temperature causes an increase in sweating. Other factors that increase the secretion of sweat include pain, nausea, nervousness, and drugs (*diaphoretics). Sweating is reduced by colds, diarrhoea, and certain drugs. Anatomical name: **sudor**.

sweat gland a simple coiled tubular *exocrine gland that lies in the dermis of the *skin. A long duct carries its secretion

(*sweat) to the surface of the skin. Sweat glands occur over most of the surface of the body; they are particularly abundant in the armpits, on the soles of the feet and palms of the hands, and on the forehead.

sycosis *n.* inflammation of the hair follicles caused by infection with *Staphylococcus aureus*; it commonly affects the beard area (**sycosis barbae**) of men in their thirties or forties. The infection usually spreads unless treated by applying antibiotic ointments or giving antibiotics by mouth.

symbiosis *n.* an intimate and obligatory association between two different species of organism (**symbionts**) in which there is mutual aid and benefit. *Compare* COMMENSAL, MUTUALISM, PARASITE.

symblepharon *n.* a condition in which the eyelid adheres to the eyeball. It is usually the result of chemical (especially alkali) burns to the conjunctiva lining the eyelid and eyeball.

symbolism *n.* (in psychology) the process of representing an object or an idea by something else. Typically an abstract idea is represented by a simpler and more tangible image. Psychoanalytic theorists hold that conscious ideas frequently act as symbols for unconscious thoughts and that this is particularly evident in dreaming, in *free association, and in the formation of psychological symptoms. According to this theory, a symptom (such as difficulty in swallowing) might be a symbolic representation of an unconscious idea (such as a fantasy of oral intercourse). —**symbolic** *adj.*

symmelia *n.* a developmental abnormality in which the legs appear to be fused.

symmetry *n.* (in anatomy) the state of opposite parts of an organ or parts at opposite sides of the body corresponding to each other.

sympathectomy *n.* the surgical *division of sympathetic nerve fibres. It is done to minimize the effects of normal or excessive sympathetic activity. Most often it is used to improve the circulation to part of the body; less commonly to inhibit excess sweating or to relieve the *photophobia induced by an abnormally dilated pupil of the eye.

sympathetic nervous system one of the two divisions of the *autonomic nervous system, having fibres that leave the central nervous system, via a chain of ganglia close to the spinal cord, in the thoracic and lumbar regions. Its nerves are distributed to the blood vessels, heart, lungs, intestines and other abdominal organs, sweat glands, salivary glands, and the genitals, whose functions it governs by reflex action, in balance with the *parasympathetic nervous system.

sympathin n. the name given by early physiologists to the substances released from sympathetic nerve endings, now known to be a mixture of *adrenaline and *noradrenaline.

sympathoblast n. one of the small cells formed in the early development of nerve tissue that eventually become the neurones of the sympathetic nervous system.

sympatholytic n. a drug that opposes the effects of the sympathetic nervous system. Drugs such as *guanethidine and *methyldopa block the transmission of impulses along adrenergic nerves; they are used to treat high blood pressure. *Alpha blockers, such as *phentolamine, block alpha-adrenergic receptors, causing – in particular – dilatation of peripheral blood vessels; they are used for disorders of the circulation or to lower the blood pressure. *Beta blockers, such as *propranolol, selectively block the beta-adrenergic receptors and principally affect the heart.

sympathomimetic n. a drug that has the effect of stimulating the *sympathetic nervous system. The actions of sympathomimetic drugs are **adrenergic** (resembling those of *noradrenaline). **Alpha-adrenergic** stimulants, such as *phenylephrine, constrict blood vessels in the skin and intestine and are used in nasal decongestants; **beta-adrenergic** drugs, such as *salbutamol, *salmeterol, and *terbutaline, relax bronchial smooth muscle and are used as *bronchodilators. Some beta-adrenergic drugs, e.g. *ephedrine and *isoprenaline, are less selective and also stimulate beta receptors in the heart, producing an increased heart rate; if used as bronchodilators, these

drugs may have unwanted side-effects on the heart.

sympathy n. (in physiology) a reciprocal influence exercised by different parts of the body on one another.

symphysiotomy n. the operation of cutting through the front of the pelvis at the pubic *symphysis in order to enlarge the diameter of the pelvis and aid delivery of a fetus whose head is too large to pass through the pelvic opening. This procedure is now rarely employed.

symphysis n. **1.** a joint in which the bones are separated by fibrocartilage, which minimizes movement and makes the bony structure rigid. Examples are the **pubic symphysis** (the joint between the pubic bones of the pelvis) and the joints of the backbone, which are separated by intervertebral discs (see illustration). **2.** the line that marks the fusion of two bones that were separate at an early stage of development, such as the symphysis of the *mandible.

adjacent vertebrae

intervertebral disc

Symphysis between two vertebrae

sympodia (sirenomelia) n. a developmental abnormality in which there is fusion of the legs with absence of the feet.

symptom n. an indication of a disease or disorder noticed by the patient himself. A **presenting symptom** is one that leads a patient to consult a doctor. *Compare* SIGN.

symptomatology (semeiology) n. **1.** the branch of medicine concerned with the study of symptoms of disease. **2.** the symptoms of a disease, collectively.

syn- (sym-) *prefix denoting* union or fusion.

synaesthesia *n.* a condition in which a secondary subjective sensation (often colour) is experienced at the same time as the sensory response normally evoked by the stimulus. For example, the sound of the word 'cat' might evoke the colour purple.

synalgia *n. see* REFERRED PAIN.

synapse *n.* the minute gap across which *nerve impulses pass from one neurone to the next, at the end of a nerve fibre. Reaching a synapse, an impulse causes the release of a *neurotransmitter, which diffuses across the gap and triggers an electrical impulse in the next neurone. Some brain cells have more than 15,000 synapses. *See also* NEUROMUSCULAR JUNCTION.

synarthrosis *n.* an immovable joint in which the bones are united by fibrous tissue. Examples are the cranial *sutures. *See also* GOMPHOSIS, SCHINDYLESIS.

synchilia (syncheilia) *n.* congenital fusion of the lips.

synchondrosis *n.* a slightly movable joint (*see* AMPHIARTHROSIS) in which the surfaces of the bones are separated by hyaline cartilage, as occurs between the ribs and sternum. This cartilage may become ossified in later development, as between the *epiphyses and shaft of a long bone.

synchysis scintillans tiny refractile crystals of cholesterol suspended in the vitreous humour of the eye. They usually cause no symptoms.

syncope (fainting) *n.* loss of consciousness induced by a temporarily insufficient flow of blood to the brain. It commonly occurs in otherwise healthy people and may be caused by an emotional shock, by standing for prolonged periods, or by injury and profuse bleeding. An attack comes on gradually, with lightheadedness, sweating, and blurred vision. Recovery is normally prompt and without any persisting ill-effects.

syncytiotrophoblast *n. see* PLASMODITROPHOBLAST.

syncytium *n.* (*pl.* **syncytia**) a mass of *protoplasm containing several nuclei. Muscle fibres are syncytia. —**syncytial** *adj.*

syndactyly *n.* congenital webbing of the fingers. Adjacent fingers are joined along part or all of their length. They may be joined only by skin, or the bones of the fingers may be joined. Treatment is surgical separation of the fingers, and skin grafts may be required.

syndesm- (syndesmo-) *prefix denoting* connective tissue, particularly ligaments.

syndesmology *n.* the branch of anatomy dealing with joints and their components.

syndesmophyte *n.* a vertical outgrowth of bone from a vertebra, seen in ankylosing *spondylitis, *Reiter's syndrome, and *psoriatic arthritis. Fusion of syndesmophytes across the joints between vertebrae contributes to rigidity of the spine, seen in advanced cases of these diseases.

syndesmosis *n.* an immovable joint in which the bones are separated by connective tissue. An example is the articulation between the bases of the tibia and fibula (see illustration).

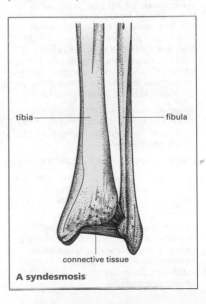

tibia ——————   ———— fibula

connective tissue

A syndesmosis

syndrome *n.* a combination of signs and/or symptoms that forms a distinct clinical picture indicative of a particular disorder.

synechia *n.* an adhesion between the iris and another part of the eye. An **anterior synechia** is between the iris and the endothelium of the cornea or the part of the sclera that normally hides the extreme outer edge of the iris from view. A **posterior synechia** is between the iris and the lens.

syneresis *n.* contraction of a blood clot. When first formed, a blood clot is a loose meshwork of fibres containing various blood cells. Over a period of time this contracts, producing a firm mass that seals the damaged blood vessels.

synergist *n.* **1.** a drug that interacts with another to produce increased activity, which is greater than the sum of the effects of the two drugs given separately. Some synergists may have dangerous effects, as when MAO inhibitors enhance the effects of antihistamine and anticholinergic drugs. **2.** a muscle that acts with an *agonist in making a particular movement. —**synergism** *n.*

synergistic gangrene gangrene of tissues produced by different bacteria acting together, usually a mixture of aerobic and anaerobic organisms. Particular forms are **Meleney's gangrene** (of the abdominal wall) and **Fournier's gangrene** (of the scrotal area). Synergistic gangrene has a pronounced tendency to spread along fascial planes, causing *necrotizing fasciitis.

syngeneic *adj.* describing grafted tissue that is genetically identical to the recipient's tissue, as when the donor and recipient are identical twins.

synoptophore *n. see* AMBLYOSCOPE.

synostosis *n.* the joining by ossification of two adjacent bones. It occurs, for example, at the *sutures between the bones of the skull.

synovectomy *n.* surgical removal of the synovium of a joint. This is performed in cases of chronic synovitis, when other measures have been ineffective, in order to reduce pain in the joint and prevent further destruction.

synovia (synovial fluid) *n.* the thick colourless lubricating fluid that surrounds a joint or a bursa and fills a tendon sheath. It is secreted by the synovial membrane.

synovial joint *see* DIARTHROSIS.

synovial membrane (synovium) the membrane, composed of mesothelium and connective tissue, that forms the sac enclosing a freely movable joint (*see* DIARTHROSIS). It secretes the lubricating synovial fluid.

synovioma *n.* a benign or malignant tumour of the synovial membrane. Benign synoviomas occur on tendon sheaths; malignant synoviomas (**synovial sarcomas**) may occur where synovial tissue is not normally found, e.g. in the oesophagus.

synovitis *n.* inflammation of the membrane (synovium) that lines a joint capsule, resulting in pain and swelling (arthritis). It is caused by injury, infection, or rheumatic disease. Treatment depends on the underlying cause; to determine this, samples of the synovial fluid or membrane are taken for examination.

synovium *n. see* SYNOVIAL MEMBRANE.

syphilide (syphilid) *n.* the skin rash that appears in the second stage of *syphilis, usually two months to two years after primary infection. Syphilides occur in crops that may last from a few days to several months. They denote a highly infectious stage of the disease.

syphilis *n.* a chronic sexually transmitted disease caused by the bacterium *Treponema pallidum*, resulting in the formation of lesions throughout the body. Bacteria usually enter the body during sexual intercourse, through the mucous membranes of the vagina or urethra, but they may rarely be transmitted through wounds in the skin or scratches. Bacteria may also pass from an infected pregnant woman across the placenta to the developing fetus, resulting in the disease being present at birth (**congenital syphilis**).

The primary symptom – a hard ulcer (*chancre) at the site of infection – forms 2–4 weeks after exposure. Neighbouring lymph nodes enlarge about two weeks later. Secondary stage symptoms appear about two months after infection and include fever, malaise, general enlargement of lymph nodes, and a faint red rash on the chest that persists for 1–2 weeks. After months, or even years, the disease enters its tertiary stage with widespread formation of tumour-like masses (*gummas). Tertiary syphilis may cause serious damage to the heart and blood vessels (**cardiovascular syphilis**) or to the brain and spinal cord (**neurosyphilis**), resulting in *tabes dorsalis, blindness, and *general paralysis of the insane.

Treatment with penicillin is fully effective if administered in the early weeks of the infection. Syphilis can be diagnosed by several tests. *Compare* BEJEL. —**syphilitic** *adj.*

syring- (syringo-) *prefix denoting* a tube or long cavity, especially the central canal of the spinal cord.

syringe *n.* an instrument consisting of a piston in a tight-fitting tube that is attached to a hollow needle or thin tube. A syringe is used to give injections, remove material from a part of the body, or to wash out a cavity, such as the outer ear.

syringobulbia *n.* *see* SYRINGOMYELIA.

syringoma *n.* multiple benign tumours of the sweat glands, which show as small hard swellings usually on the face, neck, or chest. They can be readily treated by *diathermy.

syringomyelia *n.* a disease of the spinal cord in which longitudinal cavities form within the cord in the cervical (neck) region. The centrally situated cavity (**syrinx**) is especially likely to damage the motor nerve cells and the nerve fibres that transmit the sensations of pain and temperature. Characteristically there is weakness and wasting of the muscles in the hands with a loss of awareness of pain and temperature. An extension of the cavitation into the lower brainstem is called **syringobulbia**. Cerebellar *ataxia, a partial loss of pain sensation in the face, and weakness of the tongue and palate may occur.

system *n.* (in anatomy) a group of organs and tissues associated with a particular physiological function, such as the *nervous system or *respiratory system.

systemic *adj.* relating to or affecting the body as a whole, rather than individual parts and organs.

systemic circulation the system of blood vessels that supplies all parts of the body except the lungs. It consists of the aorta and all its branches, carrying oxygenated blood to the tissues, and all the veins draining deoxygenated blood into the vena cava. *Compare* PULMONARY CIRCULATION.

systemic inflammatory response syndrome (SIRS) the general responses of the body, including mobilization of *leucocytes, to an injury (*see* INFLAMMATION). It is mediated by release of *cytokines.

systemic sclerosis a rare connective-tissue disease affecting many systems in the body, mainly in women (3–6:1) in their forties. Genetic and autoimmune factors may be implicated. Besides *scleroderma, there may be involvement of the lungs, with pulmonary *fibrosis; renal failure and gastrointestinal and myocardial disease also occur. *See also* CREST SYNDROME.

systole *n.* the period of the cardiac cycle during which the heart contracts. The term usually refers to **ventricular systole**, which lasts about 0.3 seconds. **Atrial systole** lasts about 0.1 seconds. —**systolic** *adj.*

systolic pressure *see* BLOOD PRESSURE.

tabes dorsalis (locomotor ataxia) a form of neurosyphilis occurring 5–20 years after the original sexually transmitted infection. The infecting organisms progressively destroy the sensory nerves. Severe stabbing pains in the legs and trunk, an unsteady gait, and loss of bladder control are common. Some patients have blurred vision caused by damage to the optic nerves. Penicillin is used to arrest the progression of this illness. *See also* SYPHILIS, GENERAL PARALYSIS OF THE INSANE.

tablet *n.* (in pharmacy) a small disc containing one or more drugs, made by compressing a powdered form of the drug(s). It is usually taken by mouth but may be inserted into a body cavity (*see* SUPPOSITORY).

tabo-paresis *n.* a late effect of syphilitic infection of the nervous system in which the patient shows features of *tabes dorsalis and *general paralysis of the insane.

TAB vaccine a combined vaccine used to produce immunity against the diseases typhoid, paratyphoid A, and paratyphoid B.

tachy- *prefix denoting* fast; rapid.

tachycardia *n.* an increase in the heart rate above normal. **Sinus tachycardia** may occur normally with exercise or excitement or it may be due to illness, such as fever. *Arrhythmias may also produce tachycardia (**ectopic tachycardia**).

tachyphylaxis *n.* a falling-off in the effects produced by a drug during continuous use or constantly repeated administration, common in drugs that act on the nervous system.

tachypnoea *n.* rapid breathing.

tacrolimus (FK506) *n.* a powerful *immunosuppressive drug used mainly to prevent rejection of transplanted organs. It has also been used to treat allergic skin conditions and psoriasis. Side-effects include damage to the kidneys, and there is an increased risk of developing certain cancers. Trade name: **Prograf**.

tactile *adj.* relating to or affecting the sense of touch.

taenia *n.* (*pl.* **taeniae**) a flat ribbon-like anatomical structure. The **taeniae coli** are the longitudinal ribbon-like muscles of the colon.

Taenia *n.* a genus of large tapeworms, some of which are parasites of the human intestine. The 4–10 m long beef tapeworm, *T. saginata*, is the commonest tapeworm parasite of man. Its larval stage (*see* CYSTICERCUS) develops within the muscles of cattle and other ruminants, and man becomes infected on eating raw or undercooked beef. *T. solium*, the pork tapeworm, is 2–7 m long. Its larval stage may develop not only in pigs but also in man, in whom it may cause serious disease (*see* CYSTICERCOSIS). *See also* TAENIASIS.

taeniacide (taenicide) *n.* an agent that kills tapeworms.

taeniafuge *n.* an agent, such as *niclosamide, that eliminates tapeworms from the body of their host.

taeniasis *n.* an infestation with tapeworms of the genus *Taenia*. Man becomes infected with the adult worms following ingestion of raw or undercooked meat containing the larval stage of the parasite. The presence of a worm in the intestine may occasionally give rise to increased appetite, hunger pains, weakness, and weight loss. Worms are expelled from the intestine using various anthelmintics, including *niclosamide. *See also* CYSTICERCOSIS.

Tagamet *n. see* CIMETIDINE.

Takayasu's disease (pulseless disease) progressive occlusion of the arteries arising from the arch of the aorta (including those to the arms and neck), resulting in the absence of pulses in the arms and neck. Symptoms include attacks of unconsciousness (syncope), paralysis of facial muscles, and transient blindness, due to an inadequate supply of blood to the head. [M. Takayasu (1860–1938), Japanese ophthalmologist]

tal- (talo-) *prefix denoting* the ankle bone (talus).

talampicillin *n.* a penicillin-type antibiotic chemically related to *ampicillin, effective against Gram-positive and many Gram-negative organisms (*see* GRAM'S STAIN). It is administered by mouth; a possible side-effect is a severe penicillin hypersensitivity reaction. Trade name: **Talpen.**

talc *n.* a soft white powder, consisting of magnesium silicate, used in dusting powders and skin applications. Talc used to dust surgical rubber gloves causes irritation of serous membranes, resulting in adhesions, if not washed off prior to an operation.

talipes *n. see* CLUB-FOOT.

talus (astragalus) *n.* the ankle bone. It forms part of the *tarsus, articulating with the tibia above, with the fibula to the lateral (outer) side, and with the calcaneus below.

tambour *n.* a recording drum consisting of an elastic membrane stretched over one end of a cylinder. It is used in various instruments for recording changes in air pressure.

tamoxifen *n.* a drug used in the treatment of *breast cancer: it combines with hormone receptors in the tumour to inhibit the effect of oestrogens (*see* ANTI-OESTROGEN). Side-effects are uncommon but include facial flushing, tumour pain, and hypercalcaemia. Tamoxifen is being investigated for its effects in preventing breast cancer in those women considered to be at risk of developing the disease. Trade name: **Nolvadex.**

tampon *n.* a pack of gauze, cotton wool, or other absorbent material used to plug a cavity or canal in order to absorb blood or secretions. A vaginal tampon is commonly used by women to absorb the menstrual flow.

tamponade *n.* **1.** the insertion of a tampon. **2.** abnormal pressure on a part of the body; for example, as caused by the presence of excessive fluid between the pericardium (sac surrounding the heart) and the heart.

tantalum *n.* a rare heavy metal used in surgery as it is easily moulded and does not corrode. For example, tantalum sutures and plates are used for repair of defects in the bones of the skull. Symbol: Ta.

tapetum *n.* **1.** a layer of specialized reflecting cells in the *choroid behind the retina of the eye. **2.** a band of nerve fibres that form the roof and wall of the lower posterior part of the *corpus callosum.

tapeworm *n.* any of a group of flatworms that have a long thin ribbon-like body and live as parasites in the intestines of man and other vertebrates. The body of a tapeworm consists of a head (**scolex**), a short neck, and a **strobila** made up of a chain of separate segments (**proglottides**). Mature proglottides, full of eggs, are released from the free end of the worm and pass out in the host's stools. Eggs are then ingested by an intermediate host, in whose tissues the larval stages develop (*see* PLEROCERCOID, CYSTICERCUS, HYDATID). Man is the primary host for some tapeworms (*see* TAENIA, HYMENOLEPIS). However, other genera are also medically important (*see* DIPHYLLOBOTHRIUM, DIPYLIDIUM, ECHINOCOCCUS).

tapotement *n.* a technique used in *massage in which a part of the body is struck rapidly and repeatedly with the hands. Tapotement of the chest wall in bronchitic patients often helps to loosen mucus within the air passages so that it can be coughed up.

tapping *n. see* PARACENTESIS.

target cell **1.** a cell that is the focus of attack by antibodies or killer cells or the object of the action of a specific hormone. **2.** (in haematology) an abnormal form of red blood cell (*erythrocyte) in which the cell assumes the ringed appearance of a 'target' in stained blood films. Target cells are a feature of several types of anaemia, including those due to iron deficiency, liver disease, and abnormalities in haemoglobin structure.

target organ the specific organ or tissue upon which a hormone, drug, or other substance acts.

tars- (tarso-) *prefix denoting* **1.** the ankle; tarsal bones. **2.** the edge of the eyelid.

tarsal **1.** *adj.* relating to the bones of the

ankle and foot (*tarsus). **2.** *adj.* relating to the eyelid, esp. to its supporting tissue (tarsus). **3.** *n.* any of the bones forming the tarsus.

tarsalgia *n.* aching pain arising from the tarsus in the foot.

tarsal glands *see* MEIBOMIAN GLANDS.

tarsectomy *n.* **1.** surgical excision of the tarsal bones of the foot. **2.** surgical removal of a section of the tarsus of the eyelid.

tarsitis *n.* inflammation of the eyelid.

tarsoplasty *n.* *see* BLEPHAROPLASTY.

tarsorrhaphy *n.* an operation in which the upper and lower eyelids are joined together, either completely or along part of their length. It is performed to protect the cornea or to allow a corneal injury to heal.

tarsus *n.* (*pl.* **tarsi**) **1.** the seven bones of the ankle and proximal part of the foot (see illustration). The tarsus articulates with the metatarsals distally and with the tibia and fibula proximally. **2.** the firm fibrous connective tissue that forms the basis of each eyelid.

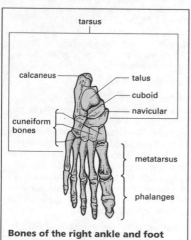

Bones of the right ankle and foot

tartar *n.* an obsolete term for *calculus, the hard deposit that forms on the teeth.

taste *n.* the sense for the appreciation of the flavour of substances in the mouth. The sense organs responsible are the *taste buds on the surface of the *tongue, which are stimulated when food dissolves in the saliva in the mouth. It is generally held that there are four basic taste sensations – sweet, bitter, sour, and salt – but two others – alkaline and metallic – are sometimes added to this list.

taste buds the sensory receptors concerned with the sense of taste (see illustration). They are located in the epithelium that covers the surface of the *tongue, lying in the grooves around the papillae, particularly the circumvallate papillae. Taste buds are also present in the soft palate, the epiglottis, and parts of the pharynx. When a taste cell is stimulated by the presence of a dissolved substance impulses are sent via nerve fibres to the brain. From the anterior two-thirds of the tongue impulses pass via the facial nerve. The taste buds in the posterior third of the tongue send impulses via the glossopharyngeal nerve.

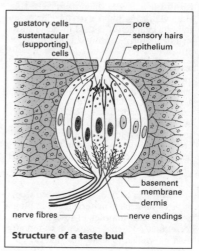

Structure of a taste bud

taurine *n.* an amino acid that is a constituent of the *bile salt taurocholate and also functions as a *neurotransmitter in the central nervous system.

taurocholic acid *see* BILE ACIDS.

taxis *n.* (in surgery) the returning to a

normal position of displaced bones, organs, or other parts by manipulation only, unaided by mechanical devices.

Taxol *n. see* PACLITAXEL.

Tay-Sachs disease (amaurotic familial idiocy) an inherited disorder of lipid metabolism (*see* LIPIDOSIS) in which abnormal accumulation of lipid in the brain leads to blindness, mental retardation, and death in infancy. The gene responsible for the disorder is *recessive, and the disease can now be largely prevented by genetic counselling in communities known to be affected. [W. Tay (1843–1927), British physician; B. Sachs (1858–1944), US neurologist]

tazarotene *n. see* RETINOID.

TCC transabdominal cervical cerclage: *see* CERVICAL CERCLAGE.

T-cell *n. see* LYMPHOCYTE, HELPER T-CELL, KILLER CELL, SUPPRESSOR T-CELL.

TCP *Trade name.* a solution of trichlorphenol: an effective *antiseptic for minor skin injuries and irritations. It may also be used as a gargle for colds and sore throats.

TCR T-cell receptor: an important component of the surface of T-*lymphocytes, by which antigen is recognized.

TCRE *see* TRANSCERVICAL RESECTION OF THE ENDOMETRIUM.

tear gas any of the several kinds of gas used in warfare and by the police to produce temporary incapacitation. Most tear gases produce stinging pain in the eyes and streaming from the eyes and nose. *See also* CS GAS.

tears *pl. n.* the fluid secreted by the lacrimal glands (*see* LACRIMAL APPARATUS) to keep the front of the eyeballs moist and clean. Tears contain *lysozyme, an enzyme that destroys bacteria. Irritation of the eye, and sometimes emotion, cause excessive production of tears. *See also* BLINKING.

technetium-99 *n.* an isotope of the artificial radioactive element technetium. It emits gamma radiation and is used as a *tracer for the examination of many organs in the technique of scintigraphy (*see* SCINTIGRAM).

tectospinal tract a tract that conveys nerve impulses from the midbrain, across the midline as it descends, to the spinal cord in the cervical (neck) region. It contains important *motor neurones.

tectum *n.* the roof of the *midbrain, behind and above the *cerebral aqueduct. From the nerve tissue protrude two pairs of rounded swellings called the **superior** and **inferior colliculi**, which contain cells concerned with reflexes involving vision and hearing, respectively.

teeth *pl. n. see* TOOTH.

tegmen *n.* (*pl.* **tegmina**) a structure that covers an organ or part of an organ. For example the **tegmen tympani** is the bony roof of the middle ear.

tegmentum *n.* the region of the *midbrain below and in front of the *cerebral aqueduct. It contains the nuclei of several cranial nerves, the *reticular formation, and other ascending and descending nerve pathways linking the forebrain and the spinal cord.

teichopsia *n.* shimmering coloured lights, accompanied by blank spots in the visual field (**transient scotomata**), often seen by sufferers at the beginning of an attack of migraine.

tel- (tele-, telo-) *prefix denoting* **1.** end or ending. **2.** distance.

tela *n.* any thin weblike tissue, particularly the **tela choroidea**, a folded double layer of *pia mater containing numerous small blood vessels that extends into several of the *ventricles of the brain.

telangiectasis *n.* (*pl.* **telangiectases**) a localized collection of distended blood capillary vessels. It is recognized as a red spot, sometimes spidery in appearance, that blanches on pressure. Telangiectases may be found in the skin or the lining of the mouth, gastrointestinal, respiratory, and urinary passages. The condition in which multiple telangiectases occur is termed **telangiectasia**. It may be seen as an inherited condition associated with a bleeding tendency (**haemorrhagic telangiectasia**). Accessible bleeding telangiectases (e.g. in the nose) may be obliterated by cauterization.

telangiitis *n.* inflammation of the smallest blood vessels (*see* ANGIITIS).

teleceptor *n.* a sensory *receptor that is capable of responding to distant stimuli. An example is the eye, which is capable of detecting changes and events at a great distance, unlike touch receptors, which depend on close contact.

telecurietherapy *n.* a form of *radiotherapy in which penetrating radiation is directed at a patient from a distance. Originally radium was used as the radiation source; today artificial radioactive isotopes, such as cobalt-60, are used.

telegony *n.* the unsubstantiated theory that mating with one male has an effect on the offspring of later matings with other males.

telencephalon *n.* see CEREBRUM.

teleradiology *n.* the process of transmitting and receiving medical images, to and from distant sites, using the telephone network. This requires a specialized link, such as an ISDN line, that has greater capacity for data transfer than standard telephone lines.

telocentric *n.* a chromosome in which the centromere is situated at either of its ends. —**telocentric** *adj.*

telodendron *n.* one of the branches into which the *axon of a neurone divides at its destination. Each telodendron finishes as a terminal **bouton**, which takes part in a *synapse or a *neuromuscular junction.

telogen *n.* see ANAGEN.

telomere *n.* the end of a chromosome, which consists of repeated sequences of DNA that perform the function of ensuring that each cycle of DNA replication has been completed. Each time a cell divides some sequences of the telomere are lost; eventually (after 60–100 divisions in an average cell) the cell dies. Replication of telomeres is directed by **telomerase**, an enzyme consisting of RNA and protein that is inactive in normal cells. Its presence in tumours is linked to the uncontrolled multiplication of cancer cells.

telophase *n.* the final stage of *mitosis and of each of the divisions of *meiosis, in which the chromosomes at each end of the cell become long and thin and the nuclear membrane reforms around them. The cytoplasm begins to divide.

temazepam *n.* a *benzodiazepine used for the treatment of insomnia associated with difficulty falling asleep, frequent nocturnal awakenings, or early morning awakening. It is given by mouth; common side-effects include drowsiness, dizziness, and loss of appetite. Trade name: **Normison**.

temple *n.* the region of the head in front of and above each ear.

temporal *adj.* of or relating to the temple.

temporal arteritis see ARTERITIS.

temporal artery a branch of the external carotid artery that supplies blood mainly to the temple and scalp.

temporal bone either of a pair of bones of the cranium. The **squamous** portion forms part of the side of the cranium. The **petrous** part contributes to the base of the skull and contains the middle and inner ears. Below it are the *mastoid process, *styloid process, and zygomatic process (see ZYGOMATIC ARCH). See also SKULL.

temporalis *n.* a fan-shaped muscle situated at the side of the head, extending from the temporal fossa to the mandible. This muscle lifts the lower jaw, thus closing the mouth.

temporal lobe one of the main divisions of the *cerebral cortex in each hemisphere of the brain, lying at the side within the temple of the skull and separated from the frontal lobe by a cleft, the **lateral sulcus**. Areas of the cortex in this lobe are concerned with the appreciation of sound and spoken language.

temporal lobe epilepsy see EPILEPSY.

temporo- *prefix denoting* **1.** the temple. **2.** the temporal lobe of the brain.

temporomandibular joint the articulation between the *mandible and the *temporal bone: a hinge joint (see GINGLYMUS).

temporomandibular joint syndrome a condition in which the patient has painful temporomandibular joints, tenderness in the muscles that move the jaw, clicking of the joints, and limitation of jaw movement. Stress, resulting in clenching the jaws and grinding the teeth, is thought to be a causal factor.

tenaculum *n.* **1.** a sharp wire hook with a handle. The instrument is used in surgical operations to pick up pieces of tissue or the cut end of an artery. **2.** a band of fibrous tissue that holds a part of the body in place.

tendinitis *n.* inflammation of a tendon. It occurs most commonly after excessive overuse but is sometimes due to bacterial infection (e.g. *gonorrhoea), or a generalized rheumatic disease (e.g. *rheumatoid arthritis or ankylosing spondylitis). Treatment is by rest, achieved sometimes by splinting the adjacent joint, and corticosteroid injection into the tender area around the tendon. Tendinitis at the insertion of the supraspinatus muscle is a frequent cause of pain and restricted movement in the shoulder. *See also* JUMPER'S KNEE, TENNIS ELBOW. *Compare* TENOSYNOVITIS.

tendon *n.* a tough whitish cord, consisting of numerous parallel bundles of collagen fibres, that serves to attach a muscle to a bone. Tendons are inelastic but flexible; they assist in concentrating the pull of the muscle on a small area of bone. Some tendons are surrounded by **tendon sheaths** – these are tubular double-layered sacs lined with synovial membrane and containing synovial fluid. Tendon sheaths enclose the flexor tendons at the wrist and ankle, where they minimize friction and facilitate movement. *See also* APONEUROSIS. **—tendinous** *adj.*

tendon organ (Golgi tendon organ) a sensory *receptor found within a tendon that responds to the tension or stretching of the tendon and relays impulses to the central nervous system. Like stretch receptors in muscle, tendon organs are part of the *proprioceptor system.

tendonosis *n.* a degenerative condition of a tendon, most commonly the patellar tendon. Overuse is a causal factor.

tendon transfer plastic surgery in which the tendon from an unimportant muscle is used to replace the damaged tendon of an important muscle.

tendovaginitis (tenovaginitis) *n.* inflammatory thickening of the fibrous

sheath containing one or more tendons, usually caused by repeated minor injury. It usually occurs at the back of the thumb (**de Quervain's tendovaginitis**) and results in pain on using the wrists. Treatment is by rest, injection of cortisone into the tendon sheath, and, if these fail, surgical incision of the sheath.

tenesmus *n.* a sensation of the desire to defecate, which is continuous or recurs frequently, without the production of significant amounts of faeces (often small amounts of mucus or blood alone are passed). This uncomfortable symptom may be due to *proctitis, prolapse of the rectum, rectal tumour, or *irritable bowel syndrome.

tennis elbow a painful inflammation of the tendon at the outer border of the elbow, caused by overuse of the forearm muscles. Treatment is by rest, massage, and local corticosteroid injection. *See also* TENDINITIS. *Compare* GOLFER'S ELBOW.

teno- *prefix denoting* a tendon.

Tenon's capsule the fibrous tissue that lines the orbit and surrounds the eyeball. [J. R. Tenon (1724–1816), French surgeon]

tenoplasty *n.* surgical repair of a ruptured or severed tendon.

tenoposide *n.* a drug used in the treatment of certain cancers, particularly in childhood. It is very similar to *etoposide.

tenorrhaphy *n.* the surgical operation of uniting the ends of divided tendons by suture.

tenosynovitis (peritendinitis) *n.* inflammation of a tendon sheath, producing pain, swelling, and an audible creaking on movement. It may result from a bacterial infection or occur as part of a rheumatic disease causing *synovitis.

tenotomy *n.* surgical *division of a tendon. This may be necessary to correct a joint deformity caused by tendon shortening or to reduce the imbalance of forces caused by an overactive muscle in a spastic limb. *See also* SCISSOR LEG.

tenovaginitis *n. see* TENDOVAGINITIS.

TENS *see* TRANSCUTANEOUS ELECTRICAL NERVE STIMULATION.

tensor *n.* any muscle that causes stretching or tensing of a part of the body.

tent *n.* **1.** an enclosure of material (usually transparent plastic) around a patient in bed, into which a gas or vapour can be passed as part of treatment. An **oxygen tent** is relatively inefficient as a means of administering oxygen; a face mask or intranasal oxygen are used where possible. **2.** a piece of dried vegetable material, usually a seaweed stem, shaped to fit into an orifice, such as the cervical canal. As it absorbs moisture it expands, providing a slow but forceful means of dilating the orifice.

tented diaphragm the radiological sign of a raised diaphragm, which is indicative of *peritonitis.

tentorium *n.* a curved infolded sheet of *dura mater that dips inwards from the skull and separates the cerebellum below from the occipital lobes of the cerebral hemispheres above.

terat- (terato-) *prefix denoting* a monster or congenital abnormality.

teratogen *n.* any substance, agent, or process that induces the formation of developmental abnormalities in a fetus. Known teratogens include such drugs as *thalidomide and alcohol; such infections as German measles and cytomegalovirus; and also irradiation with X-rays and other ionizing radiation. *Compare* MUTAGEN. —**teratogenic** *adj.*

teratogenesis *n.* the process leading to developmental abnormalities in the fetus.

teratology *n.* the study of developmental abnormalities and their causes.

teratoma *n.* a tumour composed of a number of tissues not usually found at that site. Teratomas most frequently occur in the testis and ovary, possibly derived from remnants of embryological cells that have the ability to differentiate into many types of tissue. **Malignant teratoma of the testis** is found in young men: it is most common in the undescended testis. Like *seminoma, it frequently occurs as a painless swelling of one testis (pain is not a good indication that the swelling is benign). Treatment is by *orchidectomy avoiding an incision

into the scrotum. The tumour can spread to lymph nodes, lungs, and bone, treatment of which may involve the use of radiotherapy and drugs such as vinblastine, bleomycin, cisplatin, and etoposide. Teratomas often produce *alpha-fetoprotein, beta human chorionic gonadotrophin, or both; the presence of these substances (*tumour markers) in the blood is a useful indication of the amount of tumour and the effect of treatment.

teratospermia *n.* *see* OLIGOSPERMIA.

terbinafine *n.* an antifungal drug used to treat severe ringworm. It is administered by mouth; possible side-effects include nausea, abdominal pain, and allergic skin rashes. Trade name: **Lamisil**.

terbutaline *n.* a *bronchodilator drug (*see* SYMPATHOMIMETIC) used in the treatment of asthma, bronchitis, and other respiratory disorders. It may be given by mouth, injection, or inhalation; common side-effects include nervousness and dizziness. Trade name: **Bricanyl**.

teres *n.* either of two muscles of the shoulder, extending from the scapula to the humerus. The **teres major** draws the arm towards the body and rotates it inwards; the **teres minor** rotates the arm outwards.

terfenadine *n.* an antihistamine for the treatment of the symptoms of hay fever, such as sneezing, itching, and watering of the eyes. It is administered by mouth; commonest side-effects are drowsiness, headache, and gastrointestinal upsets. Trade name: **Triludan**.

terlipressin *n.* a drug that releases *vasopressin over a period of hours. It is used to help to control bleeding from *oesophageal varices by constricting the small arteries in the intestinal tract.

terpene *n.* any of a group of unsaturated hydrocarbons many of which are found in plant oils and resins and are responsible for the scent of these plants (e.g. mint). Larger terpenes include vitamin A, squalene, and the carotenoids.

Terramycin *n.* *see* OXYTETRACYCLINE.

tertian fever *see* MALARIA.

tertiary health care the services provided by specialized hospitals equipped with diagnostic and treatment facilities not available at general hospitals or by doctors who are uniquely qualified to treat unusual disorders that do not respond to therapy that is available at secondary care centres. *Compare* PRIMARY HEALTH CARE, SECONDARY HEALTH CARE.

tesla *n.* the *SI unit of magnetic flux density, equal to a density of 1 weber per square metre. Symbol: T.

testicle *n.* either of the pair of male sex organs within the scrotum. It consists of the *testis and its system of ducts (the vasa efferentia and epididymis).

Testicular Tumour Panel the body that is responsible for identifying the main types of testicular tumours and their subvarieties.

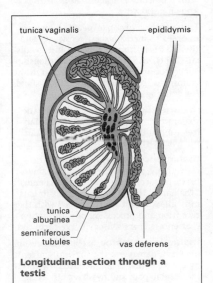

tunica vaginalis — epididymis

tunica albuginea

seminiferous tubules

vas deferens

Longitudinal section through a testis

testis *n.* (*pl.* **testes**) either of the pair of male sex organs that produce spermatozoa and secrete the male sex hormone *androgen under the control of *gonadotrophins from the pituitary gland. The testes of the fetus form within the abdomen but descend into the *scrotum in order to maintain a lower temperature that favours the production and storage of spermatozoa.

The bulk of the testis is made up of long convoluted **seminiferous tubules** (see illustration), in which the spermatozoa develop (*see* SPERMATOGENESIS). The tubules also contain *Sertoli cells, which may nourish developing sperm cells. Spermatozoa pass from the testis to the *epididymis to complete their development. The **interstitial (Leydig) cells**, between the tubules, are the major producers of androgen.

test meal a standard meal given to stimulate secretion of digestive juices, which can then be withdrawn by tube and measured as a test of digestive function. A **fractional test meal** was a gruel preparation to stimulate gastric secretion, whose acid content was measured. This has been replaced by tests using histamine or pentagastrin as secretory stimulants. The **Lundh test meal** is a meal of oil and protein to stimulate pancreatic secretion, which is withdrawn from the duodenum and its trypsin content measured as a test of pancreatic function.

testosterone *n.* the principal male sex hormone (*see* ANDROGEN).

test-tube baby a baby born to a woman as a result of fertilization of one of her ova by her partner's sperm outside her body. *See* IN VITRO FERTILIZATION.

tetan- (tetano-) *prefix denoting* **1.** tetanus. **2.** tetany.

tetanolysin *n.* a toxin produced by tetanus bacilli in an infected wound, causing the local destruction of tissues.

tetanospasmin *n.* a toxin produced by tetanus bacilli in an infected wound. The toxin diffuses along nerves, causing paralysis, and may reach the spinal cord and brain, when it causes violent muscular spasms and the condition of lockjaw.

tetanus (lockjaw) *n.* an acute infectious disease, affecting the nervous system, caused by the bacterium *Clostridium tetani*. Infection occurs by contamination of wounds by bacterial spores. Bacteria multiply at the site of infection and produce a toxin that irritates nerves so that they cause spasmodic contraction of muscles. Symptoms appear 4–25 days after infection and consist of muscle stiffness, spasm, and subsequent rigidity, first in the jaw and neck then in the back, chest, abdomen, and limbs; in severe cases the spasm may affect the whole body, which is arched backwards (*see* OPISTHOTONOS). High fever, convulsions, and extreme pain are common. If respiratory muscles are affected, a *tracheostomy or intubation and ventilation is essential to avoid death from asphyxia. Mortality is high in untreated cases but prompt treatment is effective. An attack does not necessarily confer complete immunity. Immunization against tetanus is effective but temporary. —**tetanic** *adj.*

tetany *n.* spasm and twitching of the muscles, particularly those of the face, hands, and feet. Tetany is caused by a reduction in the blood calcium level, which may be due to underactive parathyroid glands, rickets, or *alkalosis.

tetra- *prefix denoting* four.

tetracycline *n.* **1.** one of a group of *antibiotic compounds derived from cultures of *Streptomyces* bacteria. These drugs, which include *chlortetracycline, *doxycycline, *oxytetracycline, and tetracycline, are effective against a wide range of bacterial infections. They are usually given by mouth to treat various conditions, including respiratory-tract infections, syphilis, and acne. Side-effects such as nausea, vomiting, and diarrhoea are fairly common. In addition, suppression of normal intestinal bacteria may make the patient susceptible to infection with tetracycline-resistant organisms. Tetracyclines should not be administered after the fourth month of pregnancy and their use should be avoided in young children to prevent unsightly staining of the permanent teeth. **2.** a particular antibiotic of the tetracycline group. Trade names: **Achromycin, Tetrabid.**

tetrad *n.* (in genetics) **1.** the four cells resulting from meiosis after the second telophase. **2.** the four chromatids of a pair of homologous chromosomes (*see* BIVALENT) in the first stage of meiosis.

tetradactyly *n.* a congenital abnormality in which there are only four digits on a hand or foot.

tetrahydrocannabinol *n.* a derivative of marijuana that has antiemetic activity

and also produces euphoria. These two properties are utilized in the prevention of chemotherapy-induced sickness.

tetrahydrozoline *n.* a drug that constricts blood vessels and is used as a nasal decongestant. *See* VASOCONSTRICTOR.

tetralogy of Fallot a form of congenital heart disease in which there is *pulmonary stenosis, enlargement of the right ventricle, a *ventricular septal defect, and in which the origin of the aorta lies over the septal defect. The affected child is blue (cyanosed) and frequently squats. The defect is corrected surgically. [E. L. A. Fallot (1850–1911), French physician]

tetraplegia *n. see* QUADRIPLEGIA.

tetrodotoxin *n.* puffer-fish toxin, one of the most powerful known nerve toxins with a mortality of about 50%. There is no known antidote.

T-group *n.* a group of people who meet in order to increase their sensitivity and their skills in human relationships by discussing themselves and their relationships. Such groups are sometimes formed in the training of psychiatric staff (the 'T' stands for training).

thalam- (thalamo-) *prefix denoting* the thalamus. Example: **thalamolenticular** (relating to the thalamus and lenticular nucleus of the brain).

thalamencephalon *n.* the structures, collectively, at the anterior end of the brainstem, comprising the *epithalamus, *thalamus, *hypothalamus, and subthalamus, all of which are concerned with the reception and processing of information that enters from sensory nerve pathways.

thalamic syndrome a condition resulting from damage to the thalamus, often by a stroke, that is characterized by severe intractable pain and hypersensitivity in the area of the body served by the damaged brain region. It is extremely resistant to treatment.

thalamotomy *n.* an operation on the brain in which a lesion is made in a precise part of the *thalamus. It has been used to control psychiatric symptoms of severe anxiety and distress, in which cases the lesion is made in the dorsomedial nucleus of the thalamus, which connects with the frontal lobe. *See also* PSYCHO-SURGERY.

thalamus *n.* (*pl.* **thalami**) one of two egg-shaped masses of grey matter that lie deep in the cerebral hemispheres in each side of the forebrain. The thalami are relay stations for all the sensory messages that enter the brain, before they are transmitted to the cortex. All sensory pathways, except that for the sense of smell, are linked to nuclei within the thalamus, and it is here that the conscious awareness of messages as sensations – temperature, pain, touch, etc. – probably begins.

thalassaemia (Cooley's anaemia) *n.* a hereditary blood disease, widespread in the Mediterranean countries, Asia, and Africa, in which there is an abnormality in the protein part of the *haemoglobin molecule. The affected red cells cannot function normally, leading to anaemia. Other symptoms include enlargement of the spleen and abnormalities of the bone marrow. Individuals inheriting the disease from both parents are severely affected (**thalassaemia major**), but those inheriting it from only one parent are usually symptom-free. Patients with the major disease are treated with repeated blood transfusions. The disease can be detected by prenatal diagnosis.

thalassotherapy *n.* treatment by means of remedial bathing in sea water.

thalidomide *n.* a drug that was formerly used as a sedative. If taken during the first three months of pregnancy, it was found to cause fetal abnormalities involving limb malformation and has now been withdrawn.

thallium *n.* a leadlike element that has several dangerously poisonous compounds. The poison is cumulative and causes liver and nerve damage and bone destruction. The victim's hair is likely to fall out and does not grow again. Treatment is by administration of *chelating agents. Symbol: Tl.

thallium scan a method of studying blood flow through the heart muscle (myocardium) and diagnosing myocardial *ischaemia using an injection of the radioisotope thallium-201. Defects of perfusion,

such as a recent infarct, emit little or no radioactivity and are seen as 'cold spots' when an image is formed using a *gamma camera and computer. Exercise may be used to provoke 'cold spots' in the diagnosis of ischaemic heart disease.

thallium-technetium isotope subtraction imaging an accurate method (90%) used for the identification of thyroid adenomas.

theca *n.* a sheathlike surrounding tissue. For example, the **theca folliculi** is the outer wall of a *Graafian follicle.

theine *n.* the active volatile principle found in tea (*see* CAFFEINE).

thelarche *n.* the process of breast development, which occurs as a normal part of *puberty. Isolated premature breast development in girls is not uncommon and is almost always benign.

thenar *n.* **1.** the palm of the hand. **2.** the fleshy prominent part of the hand at the base of the thumb. *Compare* HYPOTHENAR. —**thenar** *adj.*

theobromine *n.* an alkaloid, occurring in cocoa, coffee, and tea, that has a weak diuretic action and dilates coronary and other arteries. It was formerly used to treat angina.

theophylline *n.* an alkaloid, occurring in the leaves of the tea plant, that has a diuretic effect and relaxes smooth muscles, especially of the bronchi. Theophylline preparations, particularly *aminophylline, are used mainly to control bronchial asthma. Trade names: **Lasma**, **Pro-Vent**.

therapeutic index the ratio of a dose of a therapeutic agent that produces damage to normal cells to the dose that is necessary to have a defined level of anticancer activity. It indicates the relative efficacy of a treatment against tumours.

therapeutics *n.* the branch of medicine that deals with different methods of treatment and healing (**therapy**), particularly the use of drugs in the cure of disease.

therm *n.* a unit of heat equal to 100,000 British thermal units. 1 therm = 1.055×10^8 joules.

therm- (thermo-) *prefix denoting* **1.** heat. **2.** temperature.

thermoalgesia (thermalgesia) *n.* an abnormal sense of pain that is felt when part of the body is warmed. It is a type of *dysaesthesia and is a symptom of partial damage to a peripheral nerve or to the fibre tracts conducting temperature sensation to the brain.

thermoanaesthesia *n.* absence of the ability to recognize the sensations of heat and coldness. When occurring as an isolated sensory symptom it indicates damage to the spinothalamic tract in the spinal cord, which conveys the impulses of temperature to the thalamus.

thermocautery *n.* the destruction of unwanted tissues by heat (*see* CAUTERIZE).

thermocoagulation *n.* the coagulation and destruction of tissues by cautery.

thermography *n.* a technique for measuring and recording the heat produced by different parts of the body: by using photographic film sensitive to infrared radiation. The picture produced is called a **thermogram**. The heat radiated from the body varies in different parts according to the flow of blood through the vessels; thus areas of poor circulation produce less heat. On the other hand a tumour with an abnormally increased blood supply may be revealed on the thermogram as a 'hot spot'. The technique was formerly used in the diagnosis of tumours of the breast (**mammothermography**) before the development of more sensitive techniques (*see* MAMMOGRAPHY).

thermoluminescent dosimeter (TLD) a radiation *dosimeter that utilizes the ability of activated sodium fluoride to luminesce in proportion to the radiation dose to which it is exposed. It is now the commonest form of radiation dosimeter for personnel.

thermolysis *n.* (in physiology) the dissipation of body heat by such processes as the evaporation of sweat from the skin surface.

thermometer *n.* a device for registering temperature. A **clinical thermometer** consists of a sealed narrow-bore glass tube with a bulb at one end. It contains mercury, which expands when heated and rises up the tube. The tube is calibrated in degrees, and is designed to register temperatures between 35°C (95°F) and 43.5°C (110°F). An **oral thermometer** is placed in the mouth; a **rectal thermometer** is inserted into the rectum.

thermophilic *adj.* describing organisms, especially bacteria, that grow best at temperatures of 48–85°C. *Compare* MESOPHILIC, PSYCHROPHILIC.

thermophore *n.* any substance that retains heat for a long time, such as kaolin, which is often used in hot poultices.

thermoreceptor *n.* a sensory nerve ending that responds to heat or to cold. Such *receptors are scattered widely in the skin and in the mucous membrane of the mouth and throat.

thermotaxis *n.* the physiological process of regulating or adjusting body temperature.

thermotherapy *n.* the use of heat to alleviate pain and stiffness in joints and muscles and to promote an increase in circulation. *Diathermy provides a means of generating heat within the tissues themselves.

thiabendazole *n.* an *anthelmintic used to treat infestations of threadworms and other intestinal worms. It is administered orally and may cause vomiting, vertigo, and gastric discomfort. Trade name: **Mintezol**.

thiacetazone (thioparamizone) *n.* a drug that can be used in the treatment of tuberculosis (in combination with *isoniazid). It is administered by mouth. Toxic effects, though infrequent, are severe and include anorexia, hepatitis, and exfoliative dermatitis.

thiamin *n. see* VITAMIN B$_1$.

thiazide diuretic *see* DIURETIC.

Thiersch's graft (split-skin graft) a type of skin graft in which thin partial thicknesses of skin are cut in narrow strips or sheets and placed onto the wound area to be healed. [K. Thiersch (1822–95), German surgeon]

thioguanine *n.* a drug that prevents the growth of cancer cells and is used in the treatment of leukaemia. It is given by mouth and commonly reduces the numbers of white blood cells and platelets. Other side-effects include nausea, vomiting, loss of appetite, and jaundice. Trade name: **Lanvis**.

thioparamizone *n. see* THIACETAZONE.

thiopentone *n.* a short-acting *barbiturate. It is given by intravenous injection to produce general *anaesthesia or as a premedication prior to surgery. Possible complications of thiopentone anaesthesia can include respiratory depression, laryngeal spasm, and thrombophlebitis. The drug is not used when respiratory obstruction is present. Trade names: **Intraval, Pentothal**.

thiophilic *adj.* growing best in the presence of sulphur or sulphur compounds. The term is usually applied to bacteria.

thioridazine *n.* a phenothiazine *antipsychotic drug used in the treatment of a wide range of mental and emotional disturbances, including schizophrenia and senile dementia. The drug is given by mouth; side-effects include faintness, dizziness, dry mouth, and impairment of sexual function. Trade name: **Melleril**.

thioxanthene *n. see* ANTIPSYCHOTIC.

thorac- (thoraco-) *prefix denoting* the thorax or chest.

thoracentesis *n. see* PLEUROCENTESIS.

thoracic cavity the chest cavity. *See* THORAX.

thoracic duct one of the two main trunks of the *lymphatic system. It receives lymph from both legs, the lower abdomen, left thorax, left side of the head, and left arm and drains into the left innominate vein.

thoracic vertebrae the 12 bones of the *backbone to which the ribs are attached. They lie between the cervical (neck) and lumbar (lower back) vertebrae and are characterized by the presence of facets for articulation with the ribs. *See also* VERTEBRA.

thoracocentesis *n. see* PLEUROCENTESIS.

thoracoplasty *n.* a former treatment for pulmonary tuberculosis involving surgical removal of parts of the ribs, thus allowing the chest wall to fall in and collapse the affected lung.

thoracoscope *n.* an instrument used to inspect the *pleural cavity. —**thoracoscopy** *n.*

thoracotomy *n.* surgical opening of the chest cavity to inspect or operate on the heart, lungs, or other structures within.

thorax *n.* the chest: the part of the body cavity between the neck and the diaphragm. The skeleton of the thorax is formed by the sternum, costal cartilages, ribs, and thoracic vertebrae of the backbone. It encloses the lungs, heart, oesophagus, and associated structures. *Compare* ABDOMEN. —**thoracic** *adj.*

thorium-X *n.* the radioactive isotope radium-224, which emits alpha radiation and was formerly used in *radiotherapy. *See also* RADIUM.

thought-stopping *n.* a technique of *behaviour therapy used in the treatment of obsessional thoughts. Attention is voluntarily withdrawn from these thoughts and focused on some other vivid image or engrossing activity.

threadworm (pinworm) *n.* a parasitic nematode worm of the genus *Enterobius* (*Oxyuris*), which lives in the upper part of the large intestine of man. The threadlike female worm, some 12 mm long, is larger than the male; it emerges from the anus in the evening to deposit its eggs, and later dies. If the eggs are swallowed by man and reach the intestine they develop directly into adult worms. Threadworms cause *enterobiasis, a disease common in children throughout the world.

threonine *n.* an *essential amino acid. *See also* AMINO ACID.

threshold *n.* (in neurology) the point at which a stimulus begins to evoke a response, and therefore a measure of the sensitivity of a system under particular conditions. A *thermoreceptor that responds to an increase in temperature of only two degrees is said to have a much lower threshold than one that will only respond to a change in temperature of ten degrees or more. In this example the threshold can be measured directly in terms of degrees.

thrill *n.* a vibration felt on placing the hand on the body. A heart murmur that is felt by placing the hand on the chest wall is said to be accompanied by a thrill.

-thrix *suffix denoting* a hair or hairlike structure.

thromb- (thrombo-) *prefix denoting* **1.** a blood clot (thrombus). **2.** thrombosis. **3.** blood platelets.

thrombasthenia *n.* a hereditary blood disease in which the function of the *platelets is defective although they are present in normal numbers. The manifestations are identical to those of thrombocytopenic *purpura.

thrombectomy *n.* a surgical procedure in which a blood clot (thrombus) is removed from an artery or vein (*see* ENDARTERECTOMY, PHLEBOTHROMBOSIS).

thrombin *n.* a substance (*coagulation factor) that acts as an enzyme, converting the soluble protein fibrinogen to the insoluble protein fibrin in the final stage of *blood coagulation. Thrombin is not normally present in blood plasma, being derived from an inactive precursor, **prothrombin**.

thromboangiitis obliterans *see* BUERGER'S DISEASE.

thrombocyte *n.* *see* PLATELET.

thrombocythaemia *n.* a disease in which there is an abnormal proliferation of the cells that produce blood *platelets (*megakaryocytes), leading to an increased number of platelets in the blood. This may result in an increased tendency to form clots within blood vessels (thrombosis); alternatively the function of the platelets may be abnormal, leading to an increased tendency to bleed. Treatment is by radiotherapy or by *cytotoxic drugs.

thrombocytopenia *n.* a reduction in the number of *platelets in the blood. This results in bleeding into the skin (*see* PURPURA), spontaneous bruising, and prolonged bleeding after injury. Thrombocytopenia may result from failure of platelet production or excessive

destruction of platelets. —**thrombocytopenic** *adj.*

thrombocytosis *n.* an increase in the number of *platelets in the blood. It may occur in a variety of diseases, including chronic infections, cancers, and certain blood diseases and is likely to cause an increased tendency to form blood clots within vessels (thrombosis).

thromboembolism *n.* the condition in which a blood clot (thrombus), formed at one point in the circulation, becomes detached and lodges at another point. It is most commonly applied to the association of phlebothrombosis and *pulmonary embolism (**pulmonary thromboembolic disease**).

thromboendarterectomy *n.* *see* ENDARTERECTOMY.

thromboendarteritis *n.* thrombosis complicating *endarteritis, seen in temporal *arteritis, *polyarteritis nodosa, and syphilis. It may cause death of part of the organ supplied by the affected artery.

thrombokinase *n.* *see* THROMBOPLASTIN.

thrombolysis *n.* the dissolution of a blood clot (thrombus) by the infusion of an enzyme, such as *streptokinase, into the blood (*see also* TISSUE PLASMINOGEN ACTIVATOR). It may be used in the treatment of *phlebothrombosis, *pulmonary embolism, and coronary thrombosis.

thrombolytic *adj.* describing an agent that breaks up blood clots (thrombi). *See* FIBRINOLYTIC, TISSUE PLASMINOGEN ACTIVATOR.

thrombophlebitis *n.* inflammation of the wall of a vein (*see* PHLEBITIS) with secondary thrombosis occurring within the affected segment of vein. Pregnant women are more prone to thrombophlebitis because of physiological changes in the blood and the effects of pressure within the abdomen. It may involve superficial or deep veins of the legs (the latter being less common in pregnancy than the former). Thrombophlebitis of the femoral vein may produce **phlegmasia alba dolens** (painful white leg), which was a common accompaniment to puerperal fever (now fortunately rare). Deep-vein thrombosis may precede *pulmonary embolism.

thromboplastin (thrombokinase) *n.* a substance formed during the earlier stages of *blood coagulation. It acts as an enzyme, converting the inactive substance prothrombin to the enzyme *thrombin.

thrombopoiesis *n.* the process of blood *platelet production. Platelets are formed as fragments of cytoplasm shed from giant cells (*megakaryocytes) in the bone marrow by a budding process.

thrombosis *n.* a condition in which the blood changes from a liquid to a solid state and produces a blood clot (**thrombus**). Thrombosis may occur within a blood vessel in diseased states. Thrombosis in an artery obstructs the blood flow to the tissue it supplies: obstruction of an artery to the brain is one of the causes of a *stroke and thrombosis in an artery supplying the heart – *coronary thrombosis – results in a heart attack (*see* MYOCARDIAL INFARCTION). Thrombosis can also occur in a vein (**deep vein thrombosis**; *see* PHLEBOTHROMBOSIS), and it may be associated with inflammation (*see* THROMBOPHLEBITIS). The thrombus may become detached from its site of formation and carried in the blood to lodge in another part (*see* EMBOLISM).

thrombus *n.* a blood clot (*see* THROMBOSIS).

thrush *n.* *see* CANDIDOSIS.

thym- (thymo-) *prefix denoting* the thymus.

thymectomy *n.* surgical removal of the thymus gland.

-thymia *suffix denoting* a condition of the mind. Example: **cyclothymia** (alternations of mood).

thymic aplasia failure of development of the *thymus gland. This was formerly thought to predispose to *hypersensitivity reactions and to infection and so to death in childhood (*see* STATUS LYMPHATICUS), a concept no longer held.

thymidine *n.* a compound containing thymine and the sugar ribose. *See also* NUCLEOSIDE.

thymine *n.* one of the nitrogen-containing bases (*see* PYRIMIDINE) occurring in the nucleic acids DNA and RNA.

thymitis *n.* inflammation of the thymus gland (the mass of lymphatic tissue behind the breastbone).

thymocyte *n.* a lymphocyte within the *thymus.

thymoma *n.* a benign or malignant tumour of the *thymus gland. It is sometimes associated with *myasthenia gravis, a chronic disease in which muscles tire easily. Surgical removal of the tumour may result in improvement of the muscle condition, but the response is often slow.

thymoxamine *n.* an *alpha blocker drug that causes peripheral blood vessels to dilate (*see* VASODILATOR). It is administered by mouth in the treatment of Raynaud's disease and similar conditions. Side-effects include mild nausea, diarrhoea, headache, and flushing. The drug should be used with caution in patients with diabetes mellitus or heart disease. Trade name: **Opilon**.

thymus *n.* a bilobed organ in the root of the neck, above and in front of the heart. The thymus is enclosed in a capsule and divided internally by cross walls into many lobules, each full of T-*lymphocytes (white blood cells associated with antibody production). In relation to body size the thymus is largest at birth. It doubles in size by puberty, after which it gradually shrinks, its functional tissue being replaced by fatty tissue. In infancy the thymus controls the development of *lymphoid tissue and the immune response to microbes and foreign proteins (accounting for allergic response, autoimmunity, and the rejection of organ transplants). T-lymphocytes migrate from the bone marrow to the thymus, where they mature and differentiate until activated by antigen. —**thymic** *adj.*

thyro- *prefix denoting* the thyroid gland. Example: **thyroglossal** (relating to the thyroid gland and tongue).

thyrocalcitonin *n.* *see* CALCITONIN.

thyrocele *n.* a swelling of the thyroid gland. *See* GOITRE.

thyroglobulin *n.* a protein in the thyroid gland from which the *thyroid hormones (thyroxine and triiodotyrosine) are synthesized.

thyrohyoid *adj.* relating to the thyroid cartilage and hyoid bone. The **thyrohyoid ligaments** form part of the *larynx; contraction of the **thyrohyoid muscle** raises the larynx.

thyroid antibodies autoantibodies against the thyroid gland, which cause *Hashimoto's disease. They are of two types: **microsomal**, against thyroid cytoplasm; and **anti-thyroglobulin**, against thyroid colloid (*see* THYROID GLAND).

thyroid cartilage the main cartilage of the *larynx, consisting of two broad plates that join at the front to form a V-shaped structure. The thyroid cartilage forms the **Adam's apple** in front of the larynx.

thyroidectomy *n.* surgical removal of the thyroid gland. In **partial thyroidectomy**, only the diseased part of the gland is removed; in **subtotal thyroidectomy**, a method of treating *thyrotoxicosis, the surgeon removes 90% of the gland.

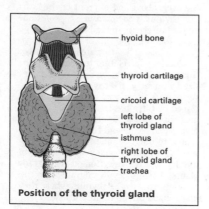

hyoid bone

thyroid cartilage

cricoid cartilage

left lobe of thyroid gland

isthmus

right lobe of thyroid gland

trachea

Position of the thyroid gland

thyroid gland a large *endocrine gland situated in the base of the neck (see illustration). It consists of two lobes, one on either side of the trachea, that are joined by an **isthmus** (sometimes a third lobe extends upwards from the isthmus). The thyroid gland consists of a large number of closed follicles inside which is a jellylike **colloid**, which contains *thyroglobulin and the principal active substances that are secreted by the gland.

The thyroid gland is concerned with regulation of the metabolic rate by the secretion of *thyroid hormone, which is stimulated by *thyroid-stimulating hormone from the pituitary gland and requires trace amounts of iodine. The *C cells of the thyroid gland secrete *calcitonin.

Thyroid extract is used in the treatment of thyroid deficiency diseases.

thyroid hormone an iodine-containing substance, synthesized and secreted by the thyroid gland, that is essential for normal metabolic processes and mental and physical development. There are two thyroid hormones, **triiodothyronine** and **thyroxine**, which are formed from *thyroglobulin. Lack of these hormones gives rise to *cretinism in infants and *myxoedema in adults. Excessive production of thyroid hormones gives rise to *thyrotoxicosis.

thyroiditis *n.* inflammation of the thyroid gland. **Acute thyroiditis** is due to bacterial infection; **chronic thyroiditis** is commonly caused by an abnormal immune response (*see* AUTOIMMUNITY) in which lymphocytes invade the tissues of the gland. *See* HASHIMOTO'S DISEASE, STRUMA.

thyroid-stimulating hormone (TSH, thyrotrophin) a hormone, synthesized and secreted by the anterior pituitary gland under the control of *thyrotrophin-releasing hormone, that stimulates activity of the thyroid gland. Defects in TSH production lead to over- or under-secretion of *thyroid hormones. TSH may be given by injection to test thyroid gland function.

thyroplasty *n.* a surgical procedure performed on the thyroid cartilage of the larynx to alter the characteristics of the voice.

thyrotomy *n.* surgical incision of either the thyroid cartilage in the neck or of the thyroid gland itself.

thyrotoxicosis *n.* the syndrome due to excessive amounts of thyroid hormones in the bloodstream, causing a rapid heartbeat, sweating, tremor, anxiety, increased appetite, loss of weight, and intolerance of heat. Causes include simple overactivity of the gland, a hormone-secreting benign tumour or carcinoma of the thyroid, and

Graves's disease (exophthalmic goitre), in which there are additional symptoms including swelling of the neck (**goitre**) due to enlargement of the gland and protrusion of the eyes (**exophthalmos**). Treatment may be by surgical removal of the thyroid gland, administration of radioactive iodine to destroy part of the gland, or by the use of drugs (such as *carbimazole or *propylthiouracil) that interfere with the production of thyroid hormones. —**thyrotoxic** *adj*.

thyrotrophin *n*. *see* THYROID-STIMULATING HORMONE.

thyrotrophin-releasing hormone (TRH) a hormone from the hypothalamus (in the brain) that acts on the anterior pituitary gland to stimulate the release of *thyroid-stimulating hormone. TRH is given by intravenous injection to test thyroid gland function and to estimate reserves of thyroid-stimulating hormone in the pituitary.

thyroxine *n*. one of the hormones synthesized and secreted by the thyroid gland (*see* THYROID HORMONE). Thyroxine can be administered by mouth to treat underactivity of the thyroid gland (*see* CRETINISM, MYXOEDEMA).

TIA *see* TRANSIENT ISCHAEMIC ATTACK.

tibia *n*. the shin bone. the inner and larger bone of the lower leg (see illustration). It articulates with the *femur above, with the *talus below, and with the *fibula to the side (at both ends); at the lower end is a projection, the medial *malleolus, forming part of the articulation with the talus.

tibialis *n*. either of two muscles in the leg, extending from the tibia to the metatarsal bones of the foot. The **tibialis anterior** turns the foot inwards and flexes the toes backwards. Situated behind it, the **tibialis posterior** extends the toes and inverts the foot.

tibial torsion a normal variation in posture in which there is an in-toe gait due to mild internal rotation of the tibia. The condition is often apparent in infancy when the child starts walking and resolves spontaneously with time. Usually symmetrical it is associated with normal mobility and is pain-free.

tibio- *prefix denoting* the tibia. Example: **tibiofibular** (relating to the tibia and fibula).

tic *n*. a repeated and largely involuntary movement varying in complexity from the twitch of a muscle to elaborate well-coordinated actions. Simple tics occur in about a quarter of all children and usually disappear within a year. Tics most often become prominent when the individual is exposed to emotional stress. *See also* GILLES DE LA TOURETTE SYNDROME.

ticaricillin *n*. a *penicillin-type antibiotic useful for its action against the bacterium *Pseudomonas aeruginosa*.

tic douloureux *see* NEURALGIA.

Right tibia and fibula

tick *n*. a bloodsucking parasite belonging to the order of arthropods (the Acarina) that also includes the *mites. Tick bites can cause serious skin lesions and occasionally paralysis (*see* IXODES, AMBLYOMMA), and certain tick species transmit *typhus, *Lyme disease, and *relapsing fever. Dimethyl phthalate is used as a tick repellent. There are two families: Argasidae (soft ticks), which includes *Ornithodoros*, with mouthparts invisible from above and no hard shield (**scutum**) on the dorsal surface; and Ixodidae (hard ticks), including

Dermacentor, Haemaphysalis, and *Rhipicephalus,* with clearly visible mouthparts and a definite scutum.

tick fever any infectious disease transmitted by ticks, especially *Rocky Mountain spotted fever.

Tietze's syndrome (costochondritis) a painful swelling of a rib in the region of the chest, over the junction of bone and cartilage. The cause is unknown and the condition usually resolves without treatment, but in some cases local injections of corticosteroids are required. [A. Tietze (1864–1927), German surgeon]

time sampling (in psychology) a way of recording behaviour in which the presence or absence of particular kinds of behaviour is noted during each of several fixed prearranged periods of time. *See also* EVENT SAMPLING.

timolol *n.* a *beta blocker used in the treatment of high blood pressure (hypertension), long-term prophylaxis after an acute myocardial infarction, and *glaucoma. It is administered by mouth or in solution as eye drops; side-effects include decreased heart rate, hypotension, and dizziness. Trade names: **Betim, Blocadren, Timoptol**.

tincture *n.* an alcoholic extract of a drug derived from a plant.

tinea *n. see* RINGWORM.

Tinel's sign a method for checking the regeneration of a nerve: direct tapping over the sheath of the nerve elicits a distal tingling sensation (*see* PARAESTHESIAE), which indicates the beginning of regeneration. [J. Tinel (1879–1952), French neurosurgeon]

tinnitus *n.* the sensation of sounds in the ears or head in the absence of an external sound source. The commonest cause is ordinary age-related hair cell loss in the *cochlea. Other causes include wax (*cerumen) blocking the ear canal; damage to the eardrum; diseases of the inner ear, such as *Ménière's disease; drugs, such as aspirin and quinine; and abnormalities of the auditory nerve and its connections within the brain. Treatment includes the correction of any underlying condition, counselling, *cognitive therapy, relaxation techniques, white noise therapy (*see* WHITE NOISE INSTRUMENT), and use of *hearing aids.

tinnitus masker the former name for a *white noise instrument.

tintometer *n.* an instrument for measuring the depth of colour in a liquid. The colour can then be compared with those on standard charts so that the concentration of a particular compound in solution can be estimated.

TIPSS (transcutaneous intrahepatic porto-systemic shunt) *see* PORTAL HYPERTENSION.

tissue *n.* a collection of cells specialized to perform a particular function. The cells may be of the same type (e.g. in nervous tissue) or of different types (e.g. in connective tissue). Aggregations of tissues constitute organs.

tissue culture the culture of living tissues, removed from the body, in a suitable medium supplied with nutrients and oxygen. **Tissue engineering**, in which skin, cartilage, and other connective-tissue cells are cultured on a *fibronectin 'mat' to create new tissues, is being explored for use in tissue grafting for patients with burns, sports injuries, etc.

tissue plasminogen activator (tPA, TPA) a natural protein, found in the body and now able to be manufactured by genetic engineering (*see* ALTEPLASE), that can break up a thrombus (*see* THROMBOLYSIS). It requires the presence of *fibrin as a cofactor and is able to activate *plasminogen on the fibrin surface, which distinguishes it from the other plasminogen activators, *streptokinase and *urokinase.

tissue typing determination of the *HLA profiles of tissues to assess their compatibility. It is the most important predictor of success or failure of a transplant operation.

titre *n.* (in immunology) the extent to which a sample of blood serum containing antibody can be diluted before losing its ability to cause agglutination of the relevant antigen. It is used as a measure of the amount of antibody in the serum.

titubation *n.* a rhythmical nodding movement of the head, sometimes involving the trunk. Occasionally the use of this term is extended to include a stumbling gait.

TLD *see* THERMOLUMINESCENT DOSIMETER.

T-lymphocyte *n. see* LYMPHOCYTE.

TNM classification a classification defined by the American Joint Committee on Cancer for the extent of spread of a cancer. T refers to the size of the tumour, N the presence and extent of lymph node involvement, and M the presence of distant spread (metastasis).

tobacco *n.* the dried leaves of the plant *Nicotiana tabacum* or related species, used in smoking and as snuff. Tobacco contains the stimulant but poisonous alkaloid *nicotine, which enters the bloodstream during smoking. The volatile tarry material also released during smoking contains carcinogenic chemicals (*see* CARCINOGEN).

tobramycin *n.* an antibiotic used to treat septicaemia, external eye infections, and lower respiratory, urinary, skin, abdominal, and central nervous system infections. It is administered by intravenous or intramuscular injections or applied by ointment or solution to the eye. Kidney damage or hearing impairment may occur with high doses or prolonged use. Trade names: **Nebcin, Tobralex**.

tocainide *n.* an *anti-arrhythmic drug used to treat life-threatening cardiac arrest due to ventricular *fibrillation. It is administered by mouth. Possible side-effects include nausea, vomiting, dizziness, tremor, and reduced white blood cell production. Trade name: **Tonocard**.

toco- *prefix denoting* childbirth or labour.

tocopherol *n. see* VITAMIN E.

toddler's diarrhoea a disorder of young children characterized by the passage of frequent loose, offensive, and bulky stools in which partially digested or undigested food may be visible (the 'peas and carrot' stool). There is no other definable abnormality and the children gain weight normally. Management consists of excluding other causes of diarrhoea and reassurance that the disorder is benign and self-limiting (it resolves by school age).

Todd's paralysis (Todd's palsy) transient paralysis of a part of the body that has previously been involved in a focal epileptic seizure (*see* EPILEPSY). [R. B. Todd (1809–60), British physician]

Tofranil *n. see* IMIPRAMINE.

tolazamide *n.* a drug administered by mouth in the treatment of noninsulin-dependent diabetes. Side-effects include nausea, loss of appetite, diarrhoea, weakness, and lethargy. Trade name: **Tolanase**. *See also* SULPHONYLUREA.

tolbutamide *n.* a drug taken by mouth in the treatment of noninsulin-dependent diabetes mellitus. It acts directly on the pancreas to stimulate insulin production and is particularly effective in elderly patients with mild diabetes (*see* SULPHONYLUREA). Side-effects are similar to those of the *sulphonamides and include skin reactions and transient jaundice. Trade names: **Pramidex, Rastinon**.

tolerance *n.* the reduction or loss of the normal response to a drug or other substance that usually provokes a reaction in the body. **Drug tolerance** may develop after taking a particular drug over a long period of time. In such cases increased doses are necessary to produce the desired effect. Some drugs that cause tolerance also cause *dependence. *See also* GLUCOSE TOLERANCE TEST, IMMUNOLOGICAL TOLERANCE, TACHYPHYLAXIS.

tolnaftate *n.* an antiseptic applied topically as a cream, powder, or solution in the treatment of various fungal infections of the skin, including ringworm. It is not effective in candidosis. Trade names: **Tinactin, Tinaderm**.

toluidine blue a dye used in microscopy for staining *basophilic substances in tissue specimens.

-tome *suffix denoting* a cutting instrument. Example: **microtome** (instrument for cutting microscopical sections).

tomo- *prefix denoting* **1.** section or sections. **2.** surgical operation.

tomography *n.* the technique of using a rotating source of X-rays to produce an image of structures at a particular depth within the body, bringing them into sharp focus while deliberately blurring structures at other depths. The visual record of this technique is called a **tomogram** (*see also* DENTAL PANTOMOGRAM). *See* COMPUTERIZED TOMOGRAPHY, POSITRON EMISSION TOMOGRAPHY.

-tomy (-otomy) *suffix denoting* a surgical incision into an organ or part. Example: **gastrotomy** (into the stomach).

tone *n. see* TONUS.

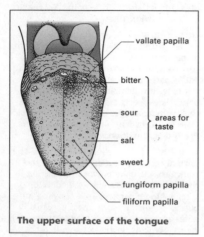

The upper surface of the tongue

(labels: vallate papilla, bitter, sour, salt, sweet, areas for taste, fungiform papilla, filiform papilla)

tongue *n.* a muscular organ attached to the floor of the mouth. It consists of a **body** and a **root**, which is attached by muscles to the hyoid bone below, the styloid process behind, and the palate above. It is covered by mucous membrane, which is continuous with that of the mouth and pharynx. On the undersurface of the tongue a fold of mucous membrane, the **frenulum linguae**, connects the midline of the tongue to the floor of the mouth. The surface of the tongue is covered with minute projections (**papillae**), which give it a furred appearance (see illustration). *Taste buds are arranged in grooves around the papillae, particularly the fungiform and circumvallate papillae. The tongue has three main functions. It helps in manipulating food during mastication and swallowing; it is the main organ of taste; and it plays an important role in the production of articulate speech. Anatomical name: **glossa**.

tongue-tie *n.* a disorder of young children in which the tongue is anchored in the floor of the mouth more firmly than usual. No treatment is required unless the condition is extreme and associated with forking of the tongue.

tonic 1. *adj.* **a.** relating to normal muscle tone. **b.** marked by continuous tension (contraction), e.g. a tonic muscle *spasm. **2.** *n.* a medicinal substance purporting to increase vigour and liveliness and produce a feeling of well-being: beneficial effects of tonics are probably due to their placebo action.

tonicity *n.* **1.** the normal state of slight contraction, or readiness to contract, of healthy muscle fibres. **2.** the effective osmotic pressure of a solution. *See* HYPERTONIC, HYPOTONIC, OSMOSIS.

tonic pupil (Adie's pupil) a pupil that is dilated as a result of damage to the nerves supplying the ciliary muscle and iris. It reacts poorly to light but contracts normally for near vision, with slow redilation of the pupil on refixation at a distance. The most common characteristic of the tonic pupil is its extreme sensitivity to dilute 0.1% pilocarpine drops, which cause marked constriction of a tonic pupil but have little effect on a normal pupil.

tono- *prefix denoting* **1.** tone or tension. **2.** pressure.

tonofibril *n.* a tiny fibre occurring in bundles in the cytoplasm of cells that lie in contact, as in epithelial tissue. Tonofibrils are concerned with maintaining contact between adjacent cells. *See* DESMOSOME.

tonography *n.* measurement of the pressure within the eyeball in such a way as to allow a record to be made on a chart of variations in pressure occurring over a period of several minutes.

tonometer *n.* an instrument for measuring pressure in a part of the body, e.g. the eye (*see* OPHTHALMOTONOMETER).

tonsil *n.* a mass of *lymphoid tissue on either side of the back of the mouth. It is concerned with protection against infection. The term usually refers to either of the **palatine tonsils**, but below the tongue is another pair, the **lingual**

tonsils. *See also* ADENOIDS (NASOPHARYNGEAL TONSIL).

tonsillectomy *n.* surgical removal of the tonsils.

tonsillitis *n.* inflammation of the tonsils due to bacterial or viral infection, causing a sore throat, fever, and difficulty in swallowing. If tonsillitis due to streptococcal infection is not treated (by antibiotics) it may lead to *rheumatic fever or *nephritis.

tonus (tone) *n.* the normal state of partial contraction of a resting muscle, maintained by reflex activity.

tooth *n.* (*pl.* **teeth**) one of the hard structures in the mouth used for cutting and chewing food. Each tooth is embedded in a socket in part of the jawbone (mandible or maxilla) known as the **alveolar bone** (or **alveolus**), to which it is attached by the *periodontal membrane. The exposed part of the tooth (**crown**) is covered with *enamel and the part within the bone (**root**) is coated with *cementum; the bulk of the tooth consists of *dentine enclosing the *pulp (see illustration). The group of embryological cells that gives rise to a tooth is known as the **tooth germ**.

There are four different types of tooth (*see* CANINE, INCISOR, PREMOLAR, MOLAR). *See also* DENTITION.

tooth extraction *see* EXTRACTION.

topagnosis *n.* inability to identify a part of the body that has been touched. It is a symptom of disease in the parietal lobes of the brain. The normal ability to localize touch is called **topognosis**.

tophus *n.* (*pl.* **tophi**) a hard deposit of crystalline uric acid and its salts in the skin, cartilage (especially of the ears), or joints; a feature of *gout.

topical *adj.* local: used for the route of administration of a drug that is applied directly to the part being treated (e.g. to the skin or eye).

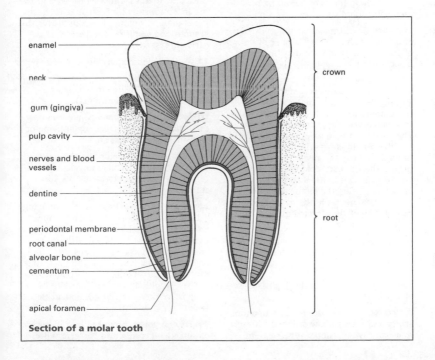

enamel

neck

gum (gingiva)

pulp cavity

nerves and blood vessels

dentine

periodontal membrane

root canal

alveolar bone

cementum

apical foramen

crown

root

Section of a molar tooth

topiramate *n. see* ANTICONVULSANT.

topo- *prefix denoting* place; position; location.

topography *n.* the study of the different regions of the body, including the description of its parts in relation to the surrounding structures. **—topographical** *adj.*

Torkildsen procedure an operation in which a *shunt is created between the lateral *ventricle of the brain and the *cisterna magna to bypass a block of the cerebral *aqueduct and thus relieve *hydrocephalus. Originally this was achieved by means of an external indwelling catheter, but later techniques use an internal catheter, which reduces the risk of septic complications. [A. Torkildsen (20th century), Norwegian neurosurgeon]

tormina *n. see* COLIC.

torpor *n.* a state of sluggishness and diminished responsiveness: a characteristic of certain mental disorders and a symptom of certain forms of poisoning or metabolic disorder.

torsion *n.* twisting. Abnormal twisting of a testis within the scrotum or of a loop of bowel in the abdomen may impair blood and nerve supplies to these parts and cause severe damage.

torticollis (wryneck) *n.* an irresistible turning movement of the head that becomes more persistent, so that eventually the head is held continually to one side. The spasm of the muscles is often painful and the patient is sensitive about his appearance. It may be caused by a birth injury to the sternomastoid muscle (*see* STERNOMASTOID TUMOUR). Relief may be obtained by cutting the motor nerve roots of the spinal nerves in the neck region or by injection of the affected muscles with *botulinum toxin.

toruloma *n.* a tumour-like lesion in the lungs resulting from *cryptococcosis.

torulosis *n. see* CRYPTOCOCCOSIS.

Tourette's syndrome (TS) *see* GILLES DE LA TOURETTE SYNDROME.

tourniquet *n.* a device to press upon an artery and prevent flow of blood through it, usually a cord, rubber tube, or tight bandage bound around a limb. Tourniquets are no longer recommended as a first-aid measure to stop bleeding from a wound because of the danger of reducing the supply of oxygen to other tissues (direct pressure on the wound itself is considered less harmful). However, a temporary tourniquet to increase the distension of veins when a sample of blood is being taken does no harm.

tow *n.* the teased-out short fibres of flax, hemp or jute, used in swabs for cleaning, in *packs or *stupes for the application of poultices, and for a variety of other purposes.

Towne's projection a *posteroanterior X-ray film to show the entire skull and mandible. [E. B. Towne (1883–1957), US otolaryngologist]

tox- (toxi-, toxo-, toxic(o)-) *prefix denoting* **1.** poisonous; toxic. **2.** toxins or poisoning.

toxaemia *n.* blood poisoning that is caused by toxins formed by bacteria growing in a local site of infection. It produces generalized symptoms, including fever, diarrhoea, and vomiting. *Compare* PYAEMIA, SAPRAEMIA, SEPTICAEMIA.

toxic *adj.* having a poisonous effect; potentially lethal.

toxicity *n.* the degree to which a substance is poisonous. *See also* LD_{50}.

toxicology *n.* the study of poisonous materials and their effects upon living organisms. **—toxicologist** *n.*

toxicosis *n.* the deleterious effects of a toxin; poisoning: includes any disease caused by the toxic effects of any substances.

toxic shock syndrome a state of acute *shock due to *septicaemia. The commonest cause is a retained foreign body (e.g. a tampon or IUCD) combined with the presence of staphylococci (*see also* STREPTOCOCCAL TOXIC SHOCK SYNDROME). The condition can be life-threatening if not treated aggressively with appropriate antibiotics and supportive care (including fluid and electrolyte replacement).

toxin *n.* a poison produced by a living organism, especially by a bacterium (*see*

ENDOTOXIN, EXOTOXIN). In the body toxins act as *antigens, and special *antibodies (**antitoxins**) are formed to neutralize their effects.

Toxocara *n.* a genus of large nematode worms that are intestinal parasites of vertebrates. *T. canis* and *T. cati*, the common roundworms of dogs and cats respectively, have life cycles similar to that of the human roundworm, *Ascaris lumbricoides*. *See* TOXOCARIASIS.

toxocariasis (visceral larva migrans) *n.* an infestation with the larvae of the dog and cat roundworms, *Toxocara canis* and *T. cati*. Man, who is not the normal host, becomes infected on swallowing eggs of *Toxocara* present on hands or in food and drink contaminated with the faeces of infected domestic pets. The larvae, which migrate around the body, cause destruction of various tissues; the liver becomes enlarged and the lungs inflamed (*see* PNEUMONITIS). Symptoms may include fever, joint and muscle pains, vomiting, an irritating rash, and convulsions. Larvae can also lodge in the retina of the eye where they cause inflammation and *granuloma. The disease, widely distributed throughout the world, primarily affects children. Severe cases are treated with thiabendazole.

toxoid *n.* a preparation of the poisonous material (toxin) that is produced by dangerous infective organisms, such as those of tetanus and diphtheria, and has been rendered harmless by chemical treatment while retaining its antigenic activity. Toxoids are used in *vaccines.

Toxoplasma *n.* a genus of crescent-shaped sporozoans that live as parasites within the cells of various tissues and organs of vertebrate animals, especially birds and mammals, and complete their life cycle in a single host, the cat. *T. gondii* infects sheep, cattle, dogs, and man, sometimes provoking an acute illness (*see* TOXO-PLASMOSIS).

toxoplasmosis *n.* a disease of mammals and birds caused by the protozoan *Toxoplasma gondii*, which is usually transmitted to humans through ingesting undercooked meat or cat faeces. Generally symptoms are mild (swollen lymph nodes and an influenza-like illness), but the dis-

ease can be serious in immunocompromised patients. Infection usually confers lifelong immunity. If caught during pregnancy it can cause **congenital toxoplasmosis** in the unborn baby. Although most babies are unaffected or have very mild disease, some can have severe malformations of the skull and eyes or active infection in the liver. It can also cause stillbirth. Infection can be detected by blood tests in the mother; if the diagnosis is confirmed, the mother can be treated with spiromycin.

tPA (TPA) *see* TISSUE PLASMINOGEN ACTIVATOR.

Tpot an acronym for the *p*otential doubling time, the time taken for a tumour to double its cells in the absence of cell loss (i.e. by radiation). It is related to the rate constant for cell production (kP), where $kP = log2/Tpot$, and enables direct measurement of the rate of cell proliferation by tumours.

trabecula *n.* (*pl.* **trabeculae**) **1.** any of the bands of tissue that pass from the outer part of an organ to its interior, dividing it into separate chambers. For example, trabeculae occur in the penis. **2.** any of the thin bars of bony tissue in spongy *bone. **3.** the hypertrophied bands of bladder-wall muscle that are found in bladder outflow obstruction —**trabecular** *adj.*

trabeculectomy *n.* an operation for glaucoma, one part of which is the removal of a small segment of tissue from part of the wall of *Schlemm's canal. This area is known as the **trabecular meshwork**. Trabeculectomy allows aqueous fluid to filter out of the eye under the conjunctiva, thus reducing the pressure inside the eye.

trabeculoplasty *n.* a method used to selectively destroy parts of the **trabecular meshwork** (*see* TRABECULECTOMY) and hence reduce intraocular pressure in the treatment of glaucoma. This may be achieved by means of a laser, as in **argon laser trabeculoplasty** (**ALT**).

trace element an element that is required in minute concentrations for normal growth and development. Trace elements include fluorine (*see* FLUORIDE), manganese, zinc, copper, *iodine, cobalt, *selenium, molybdenum, chromium, and silicon. They may serve as *cofactors or as constituents of complex molecules (e.g. cobalt in vitamin B_{12}).

tracer *n.* a substance that is introduced into the body and whose progress can subsequently be followed so that information is gained about metabolic processes. Radioactive tracers, which are substances labelled with *radionuclides, give off radiation that can be detected on a *scintigram or with a *gamma camera. They are used for a variety of purposes, such as the investigation of thyroid disease or possible brain tumours.

trache- (tracheo-) *prefix denoting* the trachea.

trachea *n.* the windpipe: the part of the air passage between the *larynx and the main *bronchi, i.e. from just below the Adam's apple, passing behind the notch of the *sternum (breastbone) to behind the angle of the sternum. The upper part of the trachea lies just below the skin, except where the thyroid gland is wrapped around it. —**tracheal** *adj.*

tracheal tugging a sign that is indicative of an *aneurysm of the aortic arch: a downward tug is felt on the windpipe when the finger is placed in the midline at the root of the neck.

tracheitis *n.* inflammation of the *trachea, usually secondary to bacterial or viral infection in the nose or throat. Tracheitis causes soreness in the chest and a painful cough and is often associated with bronchitis. In babies it can cause asphyxia, particularly in *diphtheria. Treatment includes appropriate antibacterial drugs, humidification of the inhaled air or oxygen, and mild sedation to relieve exhaustion due to persistent coughing.

tracheostomy (tracheotomy) *n.* a surgical operation in which a hole is made into the *trachea through the neck to relieve obstruction to breathing, as in diphtheria. A curved metal, plastic, or rubber tube is usually inserted through the hole and held in position by tapes tied round the neck. It may be possible for the patient to speak by occluding the opening with his fingers. The tube must be kept clean and unblocked. Tracheostomy is also used in conjunction with artificial respiration, when it serves not only to secure the airway but also provides a route for sucking out secretions and protects the airway against the inhalation of pharyngeal contents. *See also* MINITRACHEOSTOMY.

tracheotomy *n.* *see* TRACHEOSTOMY.

trachoma *n.* a chronic contagious eye disease – a severe form of *conjunctivitis – caused by the virus-like bacterium *Chlamydia trachomatis*; it is common in some hot countries. The conjunctiva of the eyelids becomes inflamed, leading to discharge of pus. If untreated, the conjunctiva becomes scarred and shrinks, causing the eyelids to turn inwards so that the eyelashes scratch the cornea (*trichiasis); blindness can be a late complication. Treatment with tetracyclines is effective in the early stages of the disease.

tract *n.* **1.** a group of nerve fibres passing from one part of the brain or spinal cord to another, forming a distinct pathway, e.g. the spinothalamic tract, pyramidal tract, and corticospinal tract. **2.** an organ or collection of organs providing for the passage of something, e.g. the digestive tract.

traction *n.* the application of a pulling force, especially as a means of counteracting the natural tension in the tissues surrounding a broken bone (*see* COUNTERTRACTION), to produce correct alignment of the fragments. Considerable force, exerted with weights, ropes, and pulleys, may be necessary to ensure that a broken femur is kept correctly positioned during the early stages of healing.

tractotomy *n.* a neurosurgical operation for the relief of intractable pain. The nerve fibres that carry painful sensation to consciousness travel from the spinal cord through the brainstem in the spinothalamic tracts. This procedure is designed to sever the tracts within the medulla oblongata. *See also* CORDOTOMY.

tragus *n.* the projection of cartilage in the *pinna of the outer ear that extends back over the opening of the external auditory meatus.

trance *n.* a state in which reaction to the environment is diminished although awareness is not impaired. It can be caused by hypnosis, meditation, catatonia, conversion disorder, drugs (such as hallucinogens), and religious ecstasy.

tranexamic acid a drug that prevents the breakdown of blood clots in the circulation (*fibrinolysis) by blocking the activation of plasminogen to form *plasmin, i.e. it is an **antifibrinolytic** drug. It is administered by mouth as an antidote to overdosage by *fibrinolytic drugs and to control severe bleeding, for example in haemophiliacs. Possible side-effects include nausea and vomiting. Trade name: **Cyklokapron**.

tranquillizer *n.* a drug that produces a calming effect, relieving anxiety and tension. *Antipsychotic drugs (formerly known as **major tranquillizers**) have this effect and are used to treat severe mental disorders (psychoses), including schizophrenia and mania. The **minor tranquillizers**, such as benzodiazepines (e.g. *chlordiazepoxide and *diazepam) and *meprobamate, are used to treat neuroses and to relieve anxiety and tension due to various causes. Common side-effects of these drugs are drowsiness and dizziness, and prolonged use may result in *dependence.

trans- *prefix denoting* through or across. Example: **transurethral** (through the urethra).

transaminase *n.* an enzyme that catalyses the transfer of an amino group from an amino acid to an α-keto acid in the process of *transamination. Examples include *glutamic oxaloacetic transaminase (GOT), which catalyses the transamination of glutamate and oxaloacetate to α-ketoglutarate and aspartate, and *glutamic pyruvic transaminase (GPT), converting glutamate and pyruvate to α-ketoglutarate and alanine.

transamination *n.* a process involved in the metabolism of amino acids in which amino groups ($-NH_2$) are transferred from amino acids to certain α-keto acids, with the production of a second keto acid and amino acid. The reaction is catalysed by enzymes (*see* TRANSAMINASE), which require pyridoxal phosphate as a coenzyme.

transcervical resection of the endo-

metrium (TCRE) an operation, which is performed under local anaesthetic, in which the membrane lining the uterus (*see* ENDOMETRIUM) is cut away by a form of *electrosurgery using a *resectoscope, which is introduced through the cervix. Like *endometrial ablation, TCRE is used as an alternative to hysterectomy to treat abnormally heavy menstrual bleeding as it results in fewer complications and shorter stays in hospital.

transcription *n.* the process in which the information contained in the *genetic code is transferred from DNA to RNA: the first step in the manufacture of proteins in cells. *See* MESSENGER RNA, TRANSLATION.

transcutaneous electrical nerve stimulation (TENS) the introduction of pulses of low-voltage electricity into tissue for the relief of pain. It is effected by means of a small portable battery-operated unit with leads connected to electrodes attached to the skin; the strength and frequency of the pulses, which prevent the passage of pain impulses to the brain, can be adjusted by the patient. TENS is used mainly for the relief of rheumatic pain; as a method of producing pain relief in labour, it is less frequently used than epidural anaesthesia (*see* SPINAL ANAESTHESIA), which has a much wider application for pain relief in obstetrics.

transducer *n.* a device used to convert one form of signal into another, allowing its measurement or display to be made appropriately. For example, an *ultrasound probe converts reflected ultrasound waves into electronic impulses, which can be displayed on a TV monitor.

transduction *n.* the transfer of DNA from one bacterium to another by means of a *bacteriophage (phage). Some bacterial DNA is incorporated into the phage. When the host bacterium is destroyed the phage infects another bacterium and introduces the DNA from its previous host, which may become incorporated into the new host's DNA.

transection *n.* **1.** a cross section of a piece of tissue. **2.** cutting across the tissue of an organ (*see also* SECTION).

transfection *n.* the direct transfer of DNA molecules into a cell.

transferase *n.* an enzyme that catalyses the transfer of a group (other than hydrogen) between a pair of substrates.

transference *n.* (in psychoanalysis) the process by which a patient comes to feel and act towards the therapist as though he or she were somebody from the patient's past life, especially a powerful parent. The patient's transference feelings may be of love or of hatred, but they are inappropriate to the actual person of the therapist. **Countertransference** is the reaction of the therapist to the patient, which is similarly based on past relationships.

transferrin (siderophilin) *n.* a *glycoprotein, found in the blood plasma, that is capable of binding iron and thus acts as a carrier for iron in the bloodstream.

transfer RNA a type of RNA whose function is to attach the correct amino acid to the protein chain being synthesized at a *ribosome. *See also* TRANSLATION.

transformation zone the area of the *cervix of the uterus where the squamous epithelium, which covers the vaginal portion of the cervix, joins with the columnar epithelium, which forms the lining (endocervix) of the cervical canal.

transfusion *n.* **1.** the injection of a volume of blood obtained from a healthy person (the **donor**) into the circulation of a patient (the **recipient**) whose blood is deficient in quantity or quality, through accident or disease. Direct transfusion from one person to another is rarely performed; usually bottles of carefully stored blood of different *blood groups are kept in *blood banks for use as necessary. During transfusion the blood is allowed to drip, under gravity, through a needle inserted into one of the recipient's veins. Blood transfusion is routine during major surgical operations in which much blood is likely to be lost. **2.** the administration of any fluid, such as plasma or saline solution, into a patient's vein by means of a *drip. *See also* AUTOTRANSFUSION.

transient ischaemic attack (TIA) the result of temporary disruption of the circulation to part of the brain due to *embolism, *thrombosis to brain arteries, or spasm of the vessel walls. The symptoms may be similar to those of a *stroke but patients recover within 24 hours.

transillumination *n.* the technique of shining a bright light through part of the body to examine its structure. Transillumination of the sinuses of the skull is a means of detecting abnormalities.

translation *n.* (in cell biology) the manufacture of proteins in a cell, which takes place at the ribosomes. The information for determining the correct sequence of amino acids in the protein is carried to the ribosomes by *messenger RNA, and the amino acids are brought to their correct position in the protein by *transfer RNA.

translocation *n.* (in genetics) a type of chromosome mutation in which a part of a chromosome is transferred to another part of the same chromosome or to a different chromosome. This changes the order of the genes on the chromosomes and can lead to serious genetic disorders, e.g. chronic myeloid leukaemia.

transmethylation *n.* the process whereby an amino acid donates its terminal methyl ($-CH_3$) group for the methylation of other compounds. Methionine is the principal methyl donor in the body and the donated methyl group may subsequently be involved in the synthesis of such compounds as choline or creatinine or in detoxification processes.

transmigration *n.* the act of passing through or across, e.g. the passage of blood cells through the intact walls of capillaries and venules (*see* DIAPEDESIS).

transmyocardial revascularization a form of laser surgery that is being evaluated in the treatment of coronary artery disease. At *diastole, a laser positioned over the left ventricle fires beams that create minute channels, about 1 mm in diameter, through the thickness of the ventricle. When the ventricle contracts, oxygenated blood is forced into the channels and supplies the damaged muscle; the blood clots at the surface of the heart, thus preventing leakage.

transplantation *n.* the implantation of

an organ or tissue (*see* GRAFT) from one part of the body to another or from one person (the donor) to another (the recipient). Success for transplantation depends on the degree of compatibility between donor and graft: it is greatest for *autografts (self-grafts), less for *homografts (between individuals of the same species), and least for *heterografts (between different species; *see* XENOTRANSPLANTATION). Skin and bone grafting are examples of transplantation techniques in the same individual. A kidney transplant involves the grafting of a healthy kidney from a donor to replace the diseased kidney of the recipient: renal transplantation is the second commonest example of human transplant surgery using homografts (after corneal grafts — *see* KERATOPLASTY). Heart, heart–lung, and liver transplants are also very successful, and pancreatic transplantation is now being done. Transplanting organs or tissues between individuals is a difficult procedure because of the natural rejection processes in the recipient of the graft. Special treatment (e.g. with *immunosuppresive drugs) is needed to prevent graft rejection.

transposition *n.* the abnormal positioning of a part of the body such that it is on the opposite side to its normal site in the body. For example, it may involve the heart (*see* DEXTROCARDIA).

transposition of the great vessels a congenital abnormality of the heart in which the aorta arises from the right ventricle and the pulmonary artery from the left ventricle. Life is impossible unless there is an additional abnormality, such as a septal defect, that permits the mixing of blood between the pulmonary and systemic (aortic) circulations. Few of those untreated survive infancy and childhood, but the defect may be improved or corrected surgically.

transsexualism *n.* the condition of one who firmly believes that he (or she) belongs to the sex opposite to his (or her) biological gender. The roots of such a belief usually go back to childhood. Children with such beliefs are treated with encouragement to engage in the activities appropriate to their biological sex and to work through their difficulties in psychotherapy. Adults with such beliefs can

seldom be persuaded to change them; surgical sex reassignment is sometimes justifiable, to make the externals of the body conform to the individual's view of himself (or herself). —**transsexual** *adj.*, *n.*

transudation *n.* the passage of a liquid through a membrane, especially of blood through the wall of a capillary vessel. The liquid is called the **transudate**.

transuretero-ureterostomy *n.* the operation of connecting one ureter to the other in the abdomen. The damaged/obstructed ureter is cut above the diseased or damaged segment and joined end-to-side to the other ureter.

transurethral resection of the prostate (TUR, TURP) *see* RESECTION.

transvaginal ultrasonography *ultrasonography using a vaginal probe instead of an abdominal transducer. It allows the use of a higher frequency, thus providing superior resolution and therefore a more detailed anatomy of the female pelvis and an earlier and more accurate identification of fetal structures.

transverse *adj.* (in anatomy) situated at right angles to the long axis of the body or an organ.

transverse process the long projection from the base of the neural arch of a *vertebra.

transvestism (cross-dressing) *n.* dressing in clothes normally associated with the opposite sex, which may occur in both heterosexual and homosexual people. Cross-dressing may be practised by transsexuals (*see* TRANSSEXUALISM), in whom it is not sexually arousing. Other transvestites are fetishistic, and in these cross-dressing is sexually arousing and may lead to masturbatory or other sexual behaviour. Treatment may be by behavioural techniques, such as *aversion therapy, but is not always needed. *See also* SEXUAL DEVIATION. —**transvestite** *n.*

Trantas dots slightly elevated greyish-white dots consisting of clumps of degenerating eosinophils and epithelial cells, seen on the conjunctiva at the junction of the cornea and sclera in cases of allergic conjunctivitis. [A. Trantas (1867–1960), Greek ophthalmologist]

tranylcypromine *n.* an antidepressant drug – one of the *MAO inhibitors – given by mouth for the treatment of severe mental depressive states. Common side-effects include restlessness, insomnia, giddiness, and a fall in blood pressure. Trade name: **Parnate**.

trapezium *n.* a bone of the wrist (*see* CARPUS). It articulates with the scaphoid bone behind, with the first metacarpal in front, and with the trapezoid and second metatarsal on either side.

trapezius *n.* a flat triangular muscle covering the back of the neck and shoulder. It is important for movements of the scapula and it also draws the head backwards to either side.

occipital bone

trapezius

insertion

scapula

origin

Left trapezius muscle

trapezoid bone a bone of the wrist (*see* CARPUS). It articulates with the second metatarsal bone in front, with the scaphoid bone behind, and with the trapezium and capitate bones on either side.

trauma *n.* **1.** a physical wound or injury, such as a fracture or blow. **Trauma scores** are numerical systems for assessing the severity and prognosis of serious injuries. **2.** (in psychology) an emotionally painful and harmful event. Theorists have speculated that some events (such as birth) are always traumatic. Symptoms of neurosis may follow an overwhelmingly stressful event, such as battle or serious injury. *See* POST-TRAUMATIC STRESS DISORDER. —**traumatic** *adj.*

traumatic fever a fever resulting from a serious injury.

traumatology *n.* accident surgery: the branch of surgery that deals with wounds and disabilities arising from injuries.

travel sickness *see* MOTION SICKNESS.

trazodone *n.* a drug used in the treatment of depression with and without anxiety. It is administered by mouth; side-effects include dry mouth, nausea, excitement, and skin rash. Trade name: **Molipaxin**.

Treacher Collins syndrome (Treacher Collins deformity) a hereditary disorder of facial development. It is characterized by underdevelopment of the jaw and zygomatic (cheek) bones and the precursors of the ear fail to develop, which results in a variety of ear and facial malformations. The ear abnormality may cause deafness. [E. Treacher Collins (1862–1919), British ophthalmologist]

trematode *n.* *see* FLUKE.

tremor *n.* a rhythmical and alternating movement that may affect any part of the body. The **physiological tremor** is a feature of the normal mechanism for maintaining posture. It may be more apparent in states of fatigue or anxiety. **Essential tremor** is slower and particularly affects the hands. It can be embarrassing and inconvenient but it is not accompanied by any other symptoms. A similar tremor may also occur in several members of one family and also in elderly people. Propranolol reduces the intensity of essential tremor. **Primary orthostatic tremor** affects the legs when standing still, causing unsteadiness if the position is maintained. **Resting tremor** is a prominent symptom of *parkinsonism. An **intention tremor** occurs when a patient with disease of the cerebellum tries to touch an object. The closer the object is approached the wilder become the movements.

trench foot (immersion foot) blackening of the toes and the skin of the foot due to death of the superficial tissues and caused by prolonged immersion in cold water or exposure to damp and cold.

Trendelenburg position a special operating-table posture for patients undergoing surgery of the pelvis or for patients suffering from shock. The patient is laid on his back with the pelvis higher than the head, inclined at an angle of about 45°. [F. Trendelenburg (1844–1924), German surgeon]

trephine *n.* a surgical instrument used to remove a circular area of tissue, usually from the cornea of the eye or from bone (the latter for microscopical examination). It consists of a hollow tube with a serrated cutting edge. It is used during the preliminary stages of craniotomy.

Treponema *n.* a genus of anaerobic spirochaete bacteria. All species are parasitic and some cause disease in animals and man: *T. carateum* causes *pinta, T. pallidum* *syphilis, and *T. pertenue* *yaws.

treponematosis *n.* any infection caused by spirochaete bacteria of the genus *Treponema. See* PINTA, SYPHILIS, YAWS.

tretinoin *n.* a *retinoid drug used in the treatment of acne. It is administered topically as a cream, gel, or liquid; side-effects include blistering, altered pigmentation, increased sensitivity to sunlight, and fetal abnormalities. Trade name: **Retin-A**.

triad *n.* (in medicine) a group of three united or closely associated structures or three symptoms or effects that occur together. A **portal triad** in a portal canal of the liver consists of a branch of the portal vein, a branch of the hepatic artery, and an interlobular bile tubule.

triage *n.* a system whereby a group of casualties or other patients is sorted according to the seriousness of their injuries or illnesses so that treatment priorities can be allocated between them. In emergency situations it is designed to maximize the number of survivors.

triamcinolone *n.* a synthetic corticosteroid hormone with uses similar to *cortisone; it reduces inflammation but does not cause salt and water retention. It is administered by mouth and common side-effects include headache, dizziness, somnolence, muscle weakness, and a fall in blood pressure, particularly on the sudden withdrawal of treatment. Trade names: **Adcortyl, Ledercort**.

triamterene *n.* a potassium-sparing *diuretic that is given by mouth and produces an effect within two hours. It causes the loss of sodium and chloride from the kidneys and is used in the treatment of various forms of fluid retention (oedema). Common side-effects include nausea, vomiting, weakness, reduced blood pressure, and digestive disorders. Trade name: **Dytac**.

triangle *n.* (in anatomy) a three-sided structure or area; for example, the *femoral triangle.

triangular bandage a piece of material cut or folded into a triangular shape and used for making an arm sling or holding dressings in position.

Triatoma *n.* a genus of bloodsucking bugs (*see* REDUVIID). *T. infestans* is important in transmitting *Chagas' disease in Argentina, Uruguay, and Chile.

triceps *n.* a muscle with three heads of origin, particularly the **triceps brachii**, which is situated on the back of the upper arm and contracts to extend the forearm. It is the *antagonist of the *brachialis.

trich- (tricho-) *prefix denoting* hair or hairlike structures.

trichiasis *n.* a condition in which the eyelashes rub against the eyeball, producing discomfort and sometimes ulceration of the cornea. It may result from inflammation of the eyelids, which makes the lashes grow out in abnormal directions, or when scarring of the conjunctiva (lining membrane) turns the eyelid inwards. It accompanies all forms of *entropion.

Trichinella *n.* a genus of minute parasitic nematode worms. The adults of *T. spiralis* live in the small intestine of man, where the females release large numbers of larvae. These bore through the intestinal wall and can cause disease (*see* TRICHINOSIS). The parasite can also develop in pigs and rats.

trichiniasis *n. see* TRICHINOSIS.

trichinosis (trichiniasis) *n.* a disease of cold and temperate regions caused by the larvae of the nematode worm *Trichinella spiralis*. Humans contract trichinosis after eating imperfectly cooked meat infected with the parasite's larval cysts. Larvae, released by females in the intestine, penetrate the intestinal wall and cause diarrhoea and nausea. They migrate around the body and may cause fever, vertigo, delirium, and pains in the limbs. The larvae eventually settle within cysts in the muscles, and this may result in pain and stiffness. Trichinosis, rarely a serious disease, is treated with thiabendazole.

trichloracetic acid an *astringent used in solution for a variety of skin conditions. It is also applied topically to produce sloughing, especially for the removal of warts.

trichobezoar n. hairball: a mass of swallowed hair in the stomach. It may be the patient's own hair or animal hairs. See BEZOAR.

Trichocephalus n. see WHIPWORM.

trichoglossia n. hairiness of the tongue, due to the growth of fungal organisms infecting its surface.

trichology n. the study of hair.

Trichomonas n. a genus of parasitic flagellate protozoans that move by means of a wavy membrane, bearing a single flagellum, projecting from the body surface. T. vaginalis often infects the vagina, where it may cause severe irritation and a foul-smelling discharge (see VAGINITIS), and sometimes also the male *urethra; it can be transmitted during sexual intercourse. T. hominis and T. tenax live in the large intestine and mouth respectively. See also TRICHOMONIASIS.

trichomoniasis n. **1.** an infection of the digestive system by the protozoan Trichomonas hominis, causing dysentery. **2.** an infection of the vagina due to the protozoan Trichomonas vaginalis, causing inflammation of genital tissues with vaginal discharge (see VAGINITIS). It can be transmitted to males in whom it causes urethral discharge. Treatment is with *metronidazole.

trichomycosis n. any hair disease that is caused by infection with a fungus.

Trichophyton n. a genus of fungi, parasitic to man, that frequently infect the skin, nails, and hair and cause *ringworm. See also DERMATOPHYTE.

trichorrhexis nodosa a condition in which the hairs break easily. It may be due to a hereditary condition or it may occur as a consequence of repeated physical or chemical injury. The latter condition may follow the use of heat or bleach on the hair or be caused by persistent rubbing.

Trichosporon n. a genus of fungi, parasitic to man, that infect the scalp and beard (see PIEDRA).

trichotillomania n. a pathologically strong impulse that causes a person to persistently rub or pull out his or her hair.

trichromatic adj. describing or relating to the normal state of colour vision, in which a person is sensitive to all three of the primary colours (red, green, and blue) and can match any given colour by a mixture of these three. Compare DICHROMATIC, MONOCHROMAT.

trichuriasis n. an infestation of the large intestine by the *whipworm, Trichuris trichiura; it occurs principally in humid tropical regions. Man acquires the infection by eating food contaminated with the worms' eggs. Symptoms, including bloody diarrhoea, anaemia, weakness, and abdominal pain, are evident only in heavy infestations. Trichuriasis can be treated with various anthelmintics, including thiabendazole and piperazine salts.

Trichuris n. see WHIPWORM.

tricuspid atresia a rare form of congenital heart disease in which there is no communication between the right atrium and the right ventricle. Affected babies present with *cyanosis, breathlessness, particularly on feeding, and *failure to thrive. Diagnosis is by *echocardiography. Treatment involves surgical intervention, but the prognosis is often poor.

tricuspid valve the valve in the heart between the right atrium and right ventricle. It consists of three cusps that channel the flow of blood from the atrium to the ventricle and prevent any backflow.

tricyclic antidepressant see ANTIDEPRESSANT.

tridactyly n. a congenital abnormality in

which there are only three digits on a hand or foot.

trifluoperazine n. an *antipsychotic drug (a phenothiazine) with uses and effects similar to those of *chlorpromazine. Common side-effects include drowsiness, dryness of mouth, dizziness, and muscular spasm and tremor. Trade name: **Stelazine**.

trifluridine n. see ANTIVIRAL DRUG.

trifocal lenses lenses in which there are three segments. The upper provides a clear image of distant objects; the lower is used for reading and close work; and the middle one for the intermediate distance. Musicians sometimes find the middle segment useful for reading the score during performance.

trigeminal nerve the fifth and largest *cranial nerve (V), which is split into three divisions: the ophthalmic, maxillary, and mandibular nerves (see illustration). The motor fibres are responsible for controlling the muscles involved in chewing, while the sensory fibres relay information about temperature, pain, and touch from the whole front half of the head (including the mouth) and also from the meninges.

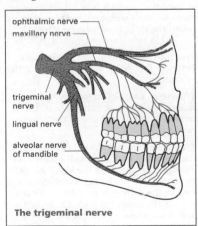

ophthalmic nerve
maxillary nerve
trigeminal nerve
lingual nerve
alveolar nerve of mandible

The trigeminal nerve

trigeminal neuralgia (tic doulour-eux) see NEURALGIA.

trigeminy n. a condition in which the heartbeats can be subdivided into groups

of three. The first beat is normal, but the second and third are premature beats (see ECTOPIC BEAT).

trigger finger an impairment in the ability to extend a finger, resulting either from a nodular thickening in the flexor tendon or a narrowing of the flexor tendon sheath. On unclenching the fist, the affected finger (usually the third or fourth) at first remains bent and then, on overcoming the resistance, suddenly straightens ('triggers'). Treatment is by incision of the tendon sheath or injection of steroid around the tendon.

triglyceride n. a lipid or neutral *fat consisting of glycerol combined with three fatty-acid molecules. Triglycerides are synthesized from the products of digestion of dietary fat: they are the form in which fat is stored in the body.

trigone n. a triangular region or tissue, such as the triangular region of the wall of the bladder that lies between the openings of the two ureters and the urethra.

trigonitis n. inflammation of the trigone (base) of the urinary bladder. This can occur as part of a generalized *cystitis or it can be associated with inflammation in the urethra, prostate, or cervix (neck) of the uterus. The patient experiences an intense desire to pass urine frequently; treatment includes the clearing of any underlying infection by antibiotic administration.

trigonocephaly n. a deformity of the skull in which the vault of the skull is sharply angled just in front of the ears, giving the skull a triangular shape. —**trigonocephalic** adj.

triiodothyronine n. one of the hormones synthesized and secreted by the thyroid gland. See THYROID HORMONE.

trimeprazine n. an *antihistamine drug (a *phenothiazine derivative) that also possesses sedative properties. Given by mouth, it is mainly used in the treatment of pruritus (itching) and urticaria (nettle rash). Common side-effects include drowsiness, dizziness, dryness of mouth, muscular tremor and incoordination, and confusion. Trade name: **Vallergan**.

trimester n. (in obstetrics) any one of

the three successive three-month periods (the **first**, **second**, and **third trimesters**) into which a pregnancy may be divided.

trimethoprim n. an antibacterial drug that is active against a range of microorganisms; taken by mouth or injection, it is used mainly in the treatment of chronic urinary-tract infections and respiratory-tract infections. Long-term treatment may cause anaemia due to deficiency of folic acid, with which the drug interacts. Trimethoprim has been administered in a combined preparation with sulphamethoxazole (*see* CO-TRIMOXAZOLE) but is now more usually prescribed alone, because of the severity of the side-effects of co-trimoxazole. Trade names: **Ipral**, **Trimopan**.

trimipramine n. a tricyclic *antidepressant drug that also possesses sedative properties. It is given by mouth or by injection for the treatment of acute or chronic mental depression. Common side-effects include drowsiness, dizziness, dry mouth, and a fall in blood pressure. Trade name: **Surmontil**.

trinitrophenol n. see PICRIC ACID.

triose n. a carbohydrate with three carbon units: for example, glyceraldehyde.

triple marker test a blood test used in the prenatal diagnosis of *Down's syndrome, which can be performed at about the 16th week of pregnancy. Levels of *alpha-fetoprotein (afp), unconjugated *oestriol (uE$_3$), and *human chorionic gonadotrophin in the serum are computed with maternal age to determine the statistical likelihood of the fetus being affected. If the risk is high, the diagnosis can be confirmed by chromosome analysis.

triploid *adj.* describing cells, tissues, or individuals in which there are three complete chromosome sets. *Compare* HAPLOID, DIPLOID. —**triploid** n.

triprolidine n. an *antihistamine drug used to treat allergy and, in combination with other drugs (e.g. dextromethorphan in **Actifed**), to relieve the symptoms of the common cold. Trade name: **Actidil**.

triquetrum (triquetral bone) n. a bone of the wrist (*see* CARPUS). It articulates with the ulna behind and with the pisiform, hamate, and lunate bones in the carpus.

trismus n. spasm of the jaw muscles, keeping the jaws tightly closed. This is the characteristic symptom of *tetanus but it also occurs less dramatically as a sensitivity reaction to certain drugs and in disorders of the *basal ganglia.

trisomy n. a condition in which there is one extra chromosome present in each cell in addition to the normal (diploid) chromosome set. A number of chromosome disorders are due to trisomy, including *Down's syndrome and *Klinefelter's syndrome. —**trisomic** *adj.*

tritanopia n. a rare defect of colour vision in which affected persons are insensitive to blue light and confuse blues and greens. *Compare* DEUTERANOPIA, PROTANOPIA.

tritium n. an isotope of hydrogen that emits beta particles (electrons) during its decay. It has been used as a *tracer in the investigation of diseases of the heart and the lungs. Symbol: T or ^{3}H.

trocar n. an instrument used combined with a *cannula to draw off fluids from a body cavity (such as the peritoneal cavity). It comprises a metal tube containing a removable shaft with a sharp three-cornered point; the shaft is withdrawn after the trocar has been inserted into the cavity.

trochanter n. either of the two protuberances that occur below the neck of the *femur.

troche n. a medicinal lozenge, taken by mouth, used to treat conditions of the mouth or throat and also of the alimentary canal.

trochlea n. an anatomical part having the structure or function of a pulley; for example the groove at the lower end of the *humerus or the fibrocartilaginous ring in the frontal bone (where it forms part of the orbit), through which the tendon of the superior oblique eye muscle passes. —**trochlear** *adj.*

trochlear nerve the fourth *cranial nerve (IV), which supplies the superior oblique muscle, one of the muscles responsible for movement of the eyeball in its socket. The action of the trochlear nerve is coordinated with that of the *oculomotor and the *abducens nerves.

trochoid joint (pivot joint) a form of *diarthrosis (freely movable joint) in which a bone moves round a central axis, allowing rotational movement. An example is the joint between the atlas and axis vertebrae.

Troisier's sign enlargement of the lymph node at the base of the neck on the left side (**Troisier's node**), which indicates metastatic spread from an abdominal malignant growth, usually a carcinoma of the stomach. [C. E. Troisier (1844–1919), French physician]

Trombicula *n.* a genus of widely distributed mites – the harvest mites. The six-legged parasitic larvae (chiggers) are common in fields during the autumn and frequently attack man, remaining attached to the skin for several days while feeding on the lymph and digested skin tissues. Their bite causes intense irritation and a severe dermatitis. Various repellents, e.g. benzyl benzoate, can be applied to clothing. *Trombicula* larvae transmit scrub typhus in southeast Asia.

troph- (tropho-) *prefix denoting* nourishment or nutrition.

trophoblast *n.* the tissue that forms the wall of the *blastocyst. At implantation it forms two layers, an inner cellular layer (**cytotrophoblast**) and an outer syncytial layer (**plasmoditrophoblast**), which forms the outermost layer of the placenta and attains direct contact with the maternal bloodstream.

Trophoblast sampling was the name originally given to the technique now known as *chorionic villus sampling.

trophozoite *n.* a stage in the life cycle of the malarial parasite (*Plasmodium*) that develops from a merozoite in the red blood cells. The trophozoite, which has a ring-shaped body and a single nucleus, grows steadily at the expense of the blood cell; eventually its nucleus and cytoplasm undergo division to form a *schizont containing many merozoites.

-trophy *suffix denoting* nourishment, development, or growth Example: **dystrophy** (defective development).

-tropic *suffix denoting* **1.** turning towards. **2.** having an affinity for; influencing. Example: **inotropic** (muscle).

tropical abscess (amoebic abscess) an abscess of the liver caused by infection with *Entamoeba histolytica*. *See* (AMOEBIC) DYSENTERY.

tropical medicine the study of diseases more commonly found in tropical regions than elsewhere, such as *malaria, *leprosy, *trypanosomiasis, *schistosomiasis, and *leishmaniasis.

tropical ulcer (Naga sore) a skin disease prevalent in wet tropical regions. A large open sloughing sore usually develops at the site of a wound or abrasion. The ulcer, commonly located on the feet and legs, is often infected with spirochaetes and bacteria and may extend deeply and cause destruction of muscles and bones. Treatment involves the application of mild antiseptic dressings and intramuscular doses of *penicillin. Skin grafts may be necessary in more serious cases. The exact cause of the disease has not yet been determined.

tropicamide *n.* a drug used in the form of eye drops to dilate the pupil so that the inside of the eye can more easily be examined or operated upon. Trade name: **Mydriacyl**

tropocollagen *n.* the molecular unit of *collagen. It consists of a helix of three collagen molecules: this arrangement confers on the fibres structural stability and resistance to stretching.

Trousseau's sign spasmodic contractions of muscles, especially the muscles of mastication, in response to nerve stimulation (e.g. by tapping). It is a characteristic sign of hypocalcaemia (*see* TETANY). [A. Trousseau (1801–67), French physician]

truncus *n.* a *trunk: a main vessel or other tubular organ from which subsidiary branches arise.

truncus arteriosus the main arterial trunk arising from the fetal heart. It develops into the aorta and pulmonary artery.

trunk *n.* **1.** the main part of a blood vessel, lymph vessel, or nerve, from which branches arise. **2.** the body excluding the head and limbs.

truss *n.* a device for applying pressure to a hernia to prevent it from protruding. It usually consists of a pad attached to a belt with straps or spring strips and it is worn under the clothing.

trust *n.* (in the NHS) a self-governing body that provides any of a range of health-care services, including *hospital services, *community health services, and services for the mentally ill and other groups. NHS trusts have their own budgets and the freedom to provide services of their own selection (within the framework of their contracts), without direction from Health Authorities.

trypanocide *n.* an agent that kills trypanosomes and is therefore used to treat infestations caused by these parasites (see TRYPANOSOMIASIS). The main trypanocides are arsenic-containing compounds.

Trypanosoma *n.* a genus of parasitic protozoans that move by means of a long trailing flagellum and a thin wavy membrane, which project from the body surface. Trypanosomes undergo part of their development in the blood of a vertebrate host. The remaining stages occur in invertebrate hosts, which then transmit the parasites back to the vertebrates. *T. rhodesiense* and *T. gambiense*, which are transmitted through the bite of *tsetse flies, cause *sleeping sickness in Africa. *T. cruzi*, carried by *reduviid bugs, causes Chagas' disease in South America.

trypanosomiasis *n.* any disease caused by the presence of parasitic protozoans of the genus *Trypanosoma*. The two most important diseases are *Chagas' disease (South American trypanosomiasis) and *sleeping sickness (African trypanosomiasis).

tryparsamide *n.* a drug used in the treatment of trypanosomiasis (sleeping sickness). Usually given by injection, it penetrates the cerebrospinal fluid and is highly active against the infective organism (*Trypanosoma gambiense*). Trade name: **Tryparsam**.

trypsin *n.* an enzyme that continues the digestion of proteins by breaking down

peptones into smaller peptide chains (see PEPTIDASE). It is secreted by the pancreas in an inactive form, trypsinogen, which is converted in the duodenum to trypsin by the action of the enzyme enteropeptidase.

trypsinogen *n.* see TRYPSIN.

tryptophan *n.* an *essential amino acid. *See also* AMINO ACID.

TSAB thyroid-stimulating antibody. TSABs are implicated in the causes of *thyroiditis.

tsetse *n.* a large bloodsucking fly of tropical Africa belonging to the genus *Glossina*. Tsetse flies, which have slender forwardly projecting biting mouthparts, feed during the day on man and other mammals. They transmit the blood parasites that cause *sleeping sickness. *G. palpalis* and *G. tachinoides*, which are found along river banks, transmit *Trypanosoma gambiense*; *G. morsitans*, *G. swynnertoni*, and *G. pallidipes*, which are found in savannah country, transmit *T. rhodesiense*.

TSH *see* THYROID-STIMULATING HORMONE.

tsutsugamushi disease *see* SCRUB TYPHUS.

tubal occlusion blocking of the Fallopian tubes. This is achieved by surgery as a means of *sterilization; it is also a result of *pelvic inflammatory disease.

tubal pregnancy *see* ECTOPIC PREGNANCY.

tube *n.* (in anatomy) a long hollow cylindrical structure, e.g. a *Fallopian tube.

tuber *n.* (in anatomy) a thickened or swollen part. The **tuber cinereum** is a part of the brain situated at the base of the hypothalamus, connected to the stalk of the pituitary gland.

tubercle *n.* **1.** (in anatomy) a small rounded protuberance on a bone. For example, there are two tubercles at the upper end of the humerus. **2.** the specific nodular lesion of *tuberculosis.

tubercular *adj.* having small rounded swellings or nodules, not necessarily caused by tuberculosis.

tuberculide *n.* an eruption of the skin that arises in response to an internal focus of tuberculosis.

tuberculin *n.* a protein extract from cultures of tubercle bacilli, used to test whether a person has suffered from or been in contact with tuberculosis. In the **Mantoux test** a quantity of tuberculin is injected beneath the skin and a patch of inflammation appearing in the next 48–72 hours is regarded as a positive reaction, meaning that a degree of immunity is present.

tuberculoma *n.* a mass of cheeselike material resembling a tumour, seen in some cases of *tuberculosis. Tuberculomas are found in a variety of sites, including the lung or brain, and a single mass may be the only clinical evidence of disease. Treatment is by surgical excision, together with antituberculous drugs.

tuberculosis *n.* an infectious disease caused by the bacillus *Mycobacterium tuberculosis* (first identified by Koch in 1882) and characterized by the formation of nodular lesions (**tubercles**) in the tissues.

In **pulmonary tuberculosis** – formerly known as **consumption** and **phthisis** (wasting) – the bacillus is inhaled into the lungs where it sets up a primary tubercle and spreads to the nearest lymph nodes (the **primary complex**). Natural immune defences may heal it at this stage; alternatively the disease may smoulder for months or years and fluctuate with the patient's resistance. Many people become infected but show no symptoms. Others develop a chronic infection and can transmit the bacillus by coughing and sneezing. Symptoms of the active disease include fever, night sweats, weight loss, and the spitting of blood. In some cases the bacilli spread from the lungs to the bloodstream, setting up millions of tiny tubercles throughout the body (**miliary tuberculosis**), or migrate to the meninges to cause tuberculous *meningitis. Bacilli entering by the mouth, usually in infected cows' milk, set up a primary complex in abdominal lymph nodes, leading to *peritonitis, and sometimes spread to other organs, joints, and bones (*see* POTT'S DISEASE).

Tuberculosis is curable by various combinations of the antibiotics *streptomycin, *ethambutol, *isoniazid (INH), *rifampicin, and *pyrazinamide. Preventive measures in the UK include the detection of cases by X-ray screening of vulnerable populations and inoculation with *BCG vaccine of those with no immunity to the disease (the *tuberculin test identifies which people require vaccination).

tuberose *adj. see* TUBEROUS.

tuberosity *n.* a large rounded protuberance on a bone. For example, there is a tuberosity at the upper end of the tibia.

tuberous (tuberose) *adj.* knobbed; having nodules or rounded swellings.

tuberous sclerosis (Bourneville's disease, epiloia) a hereditary disorder in which the brain, skin, and other organs are studded with small plaques or tumours; eye involvement includes retinal tumours, optic nerve gliomas, and eyelid neuromas. Symptoms include epilepsy, mental retardation, and behavioural disorders.

tubo- *prefix denoting* a tube, especially a Fallopian tube or Eustachian tube.

tuboabdominal *adj.* relating to or occurring in a Fallopian tube and the abdomen.

tubocurarine *n.* a drug given by intravenous injection to produce relaxation of voluntary muscles before surgery and in such conditions as tetanus, encephalitis, and poliomyelitis (*see* MUSCLE RELAXANT). Toxic side-effects are usually only seen with overdosage, when respiratory failure due to paralysis of respiratory muscles may occur. Trade names: **Jexin, Tubarine**.

tubo-ovarian *adj.* relating to or occurring in a Fallopian tube and an ovary.

tubotympanal *adj.* relating to the tympanic cavity and the *Eustachian tube.

tubule *n.* (in anatomy) a small cylindrical hollow structure. *See also* RENAL TUBULE, SEMINIFEROUS TUBULE.

tuftsin *n.* a tetrapeptide derived from IgG (*see* IMMUNOGLOBULIN), produced mainly in the spleen, that stimulates *neutrophil activity (phagocytosis). Levels of tuftsin are reduced after *splenectomy, resulting in diminished resistance to infection, especially by encapsulated organisms.

tularaemia (rabbit fever) *n.* a disease of rodents and rabbits, caused by the bacterium *Francisella tularensis*, that is transmitted to man by deer flies (*see* CHRYSOPS), by direct contact with infected animals, by contamination of wounds, or by drinking contaminated water. Symptoms include an ulcer at the site of infection, inflamed and ulcerating lymph nodes, headache, aching pains, loss of weight, and a fever lasting several weeks. Treatment with chloramphenicol, streptomycin, or tetracycline is effective.

tulle gras a soft dressing consisting of open-woven silk (or other material) impregnated with a waterproof soft paraffin wax.

tumbu fly a large non-bloodsucking fly, *Cordylobia anthropophaga*, widely distributed in tropical Africa. The female fly lays her eggs on ground contaminated with urine or excreta or on clothing tainted with sweat or urine. The maggots are normally parasites of rats, but if they come into contact with man they penetrate the skin, producing boil-like swellings (*see also* MYIASIS). The maggots can be gently eased out by applying oil to the swellings.

tumefaction *n.* the process in which a tissue becomes swollen and tense by accumulation within it of fluid under pressure.

tumescence *n.* a swelling, or the process of becoming swollen, usually because of an accumulation of blood or other fluid within the tissues.

tumid *adj.* swollen.

tumor *n.* swelling: one of the classical signs of *inflammation in a tissue, the other three being *calor (heat), *rubor (redness), and *dolor (pain). The swelling of an inflamed area is due to the leakage from small blood vessels of clear protein-containing fluid, which accumulates between the cells.

tumour *n.* any abnormal swelling in or on a part of the body. The term is usually applied to an abnormal growth of tissue, which may be *benign or *malignant. *Compare* CYST.

tumour-associated antigen a protein produced by cancer cells. Its presence in the blood can be revealed by means of a simple blood test, which could provide a basis for the diagnosis of malignant melanoma and other cancers at their earliest – and most treatable – stages of development.

tumour-infiltrating lymphocyte (TIL) a lymphoid cell that can infiltrate solid tumours. Such cells can be cultured in vitro, in the presence of *interleukin 2, and have been used as vehicles for *tumour-necrosis factor in gene therapy trials for cancer.

tumour marker a substance produced by a tumour that can be used to monitor the size of the tumour and the effects of treatment. An example is *alpha-fetoprotein, which is used to monitor treatment of testicular *teratomas.

tumour necrosis factor (TNF) either of two proteins, TNF-α or TNF-β, that function as *cytokines. Among their many actions is destruction of tumour cells. The gene encoding TNF has been used in gene therapy trials for cancer.

Tunga *n.* a genus of sand fleas found in tropical America and Africa. The fertilized female of *T. penetrans*, the chigoe or jigger, burrows beneath the skin of the foot, where it becomes enclosed in a swelling of the surrounding tissues and causes intense itching and inflammation. Surgical removal of the fleas is recommended.

tunica *n.* a covering or layer of an organ or part; for example, a layer of the wall of a blood vessel (*see* ADVENTITIA, INTIMA, MEDIA). The **tunica albuginea** is a fibrous membrane comprising one of the covering tissues of the ovary, penis, and testis.

tunnel *n.* (in anatomy) a canal or hollow groove. *See also* CARPAL TUNNEL.

TUR (TURP) transurethral resection (of the prostate): *see* RESECTION.

turbinate bone *see* NASAL CONCHA.

turbinectomy *n.* the surgical removal of one of the bones forming the nasal cavity (nasal conchae, or turbinate bones).

turgescence *n.* a swelling, or the process by which a swelling arises in tissues, usually by the accumulation of blood or other fluid under pressure.

turgor *n.* a state of being swollen or distended.

Turkel's needle a specially designed needle for purposes of transrectal prostatic biopsy.

Turner's syndrome a genetic defect in women in which there is only one X chromosome instead of the usual two. Affected women are infertile: they have female external genitalia but no ovaries and therefore no menstrual periods (*see* AMENORRHOEA). Characteristically they are short and have variable developmental defects, which may include webbing of the neck. [H. H. Turner (1892–1970), US endocrinologist]

turricephaly *n. see* OXYCEPHALY.

tussis *n.* the medical name for *coughing.

twilight state a condition of disturbed consciousness in which the individual can still carry out some normal activities but is impaired in his awareness and has no memory of what he has done. It is encountered after epileptic attacks, in alcoholism, and in organic states of confusion. It may be associated with other symptoms, such as physical and mental slowing, episodes of rage, and hallucinations. Twilight states last only for a short time, commonly a few hours.

twins *pl. n.* two individuals who are born at the same time and of the same parents. **Fraternal** (or **dizygotic**) **twins** are the result of the simultaneous fertilization of two egg cells; they may be of different sexes and are no more alike than ordinary siblings. **Identical** (or **monozygotic**) **twins** result from the fertilization of a single egg cell that subsequently divides to give two separate fetuses. They are of the same sex and otherwise genetically identical; any differences in their appearance are due to environmental influences. *See also* SIAMESE TWINS.

tylosis *n.* diffuse *keratosis occurring especially on the palms and soles. It occurs early in life and is inherited as an autosomal *dominant.

tympan- (tympano-) *prefix denoting* **1.** the eardrum. Example: **tympanectomy** (surgical excision of). **2.** the middle ear.

tympanic cavity *see* MIDDLE EAR.

tympanic membrane (eardrum) the membrane at the inner end of the external auditory meatus, separating the outer and middle ears. It is formed from the outer wall of the lining of the tympanic cavity and the skin that lines the external auditory meatus. When sound waves reach the ear the tympanum vibrates, transmitting these vibrations to the malleus – one of the auditory *ossicles in the middle ear – to which it is attached.

tympanites (meteorism) *n.* distension of the abdomen with air or gas: the abdomen is resonant (drumlike) on *percussion. Causes include intestinal obstruction, the *irritable bowel syndrome, and *aerophagy.

tympanoplasty *n.* surgical repair of defects of the eardrum and middle ear ossicles. *See* MYRINGOPLASTY.

tympanotomy *n.* a surgical operation to expose the middle ear and allow access to the ossicles. It is usually performed by incising around the eardrum and turning it forwards.

tympanum *n.* the *middle ear (tympanic cavity) and/or the eardrum (*tympanic membrane).

typhlitis *n. Obsolete* inflammation of the caecum: formerly a common diagnosis of the condition now recognized as appendicitis.

typhlosis *n.* an obsolete term for *blindness.

typho- *prefix denoting* **1.** typhoid fever. **2.** typhus.

typhoid fever an infection of the digestive system by the bacterium *Salmonella typhi*, causing general weakness, high fever, a rash of red spots on the chest and abdomen, chills, sweating, and in serious cases inflammation of the spleen and bones, delirium, and erosion of the intestinal wall leading to haemorrhage. It is transmitted through food or drinking water contaminated by the faeces or urine of patients or carriers. In most cases recovery occurs naturally but treatment with such antibiotics as ampicillin, amoxicillin, ciprofloxacin, or chloramphenicol reduces the severity of symptoms. Vaccination with *TAB provides temporary immunity. *Compare* PARATYPHOID FEVER.

typhus (spotted fever) *n.* any one of a group of infections caused by *rickettsiae and characterized by severe headache, a widespread rash, prolonged high fever, and delirium. They all respond to treatment with chloramphenicol or tetracyclines. **Epidemic typhus** (also known as **classical** or **louse-borne typhus**) is caused by infection with *Rickettsia prowazekii* transmitted by lice. It was formerly very prevalent in overcrowded insanitary conditions (as during wars and famines), with a mortality rate approaching 100%. **Endemic typhus** (**murine** or **flea-borne typhus**) is a disease of rats due to *Rickettsia mooseri*; it can be transmitted to man by rat fleas, causing a mild typhus fever. There are in addition several kinds of **tick typhus** (in which the rickettsiae are transmitted by ticks), including *Rocky Mountain spotted fever, and typhus transmitted by mites (*see* RICKETTSIAL POX, SCRUB TYPHUS).

tyramine *n.* an amine naturally occurring in cheese. It has a similar effect in the body to that of *adrenaline. This effect can be dangerous in patients taking *MAO inhibitors (antidepressants), in whom blood pressure may become very high. Cheese is therefore not advised when such drugs are prescribed.

Tyroglyphus *n. see* ACARUS.

tyrosine *n. see* AMINO ACID.

tyrosinosis *n.* an inborn defect of metabolism of the amino acid tyrosine that causes excessive excretion of parahydroxyphenylpyruvic acid in the urine, giving it abnormal reducing power.

tyrothricin *n.* an *antibiotic derived from the bacterium *Bacillus brevis*. It is used, alone or in combination with some other drugs (e.g. benzocaine in **Tyrozets**), in the form of skin applications and lozenges in the treatment of infections of the mouth, throat, and skin, and of wounds and burns.

ubiquinone *n.* a *coenzyme that acts as an electron transfer agent in the mitochondria of cells (*see* ELECTRON TRANSPORT CHAIN).

UICC *see* UNION INTERNATIONAL CONTRE LE CANCER.

UKCC United Kingdom Central Council for Nursing, Midwifery and Health Visiting: a statutory body that regulates the nursing, midwifery, and health visiting professions in the public interest. *See* NURSE.

ulcer *n.* a break in the skin extending to all its layers, or a break in the mucous membrane lining the alimentary tract, that fails to heal and is often accompanied by inflammation. Of the many types of skin ulcer, the most common is the **venous** (or **hypostatic**) **ulcer** of the leg, known incorrectly as a **varicose ulcer**, which is caused by increased venous pressure and usually occurs in older women. *See also* BEDSORE.

For ulcers of the alimentary tract, *see* APHTHA, DUODENAL ULCER, GASTRIC ULCER, PEPTIC ULCER. Ulcers may also affect the cornea (*see* DENDRITIC ULCER).

ulcerative colitis inflammation and ulceration of the colon and rectum. *See* COLITIS.

ulcerative gingivitis acute painful gingivitis with ulceration, in which the tissues of the gums are rapidly destroyed. Occurring mainly in debilitated patients, it is associated with anaerobic microorganisms (*see* FUSOBACTERIUM, BACTEROIDES) and is accompanied by an unpleasant odour. Treatment is with *metronidazole and a careful and thorough regime of oral hygiene supplemented with oxidizing mouthwashes. In the past ulcerative gingivitis has been called **Vincent's angina**; in its severe form it is known as *noma.

ule- (ulo-) *prefix denoting* **1.** scars; scar tissue. **2.** the gums.

ulna *n.* the inner and longer bone of the forearm (see illustration). It articulates with the humerus and radius above and with the radius and indirectly with the wrist bones below. At its upper end is the *olecranon process and *coronoid process; at the lower end is a cone-shaped **styloid process**. —**ulnar** *adj.*

Right ulna and radius (front view)

ulnar artery a branch of the brachial artery arising at the elbow and running deep within the muscles of the medial side of the forearm. It passes into the palm of the hand, where it unites with the arch of the radial artery and gives off branches to the hand and fingers.

ulnar nerve one of the major nerves of the arm. It originates in the neck, from spinal roots of the last cervical and first thoracic divisions, and runs down the inner side of the upper arm to behind the elbow. In the forearm it supplies the muscles with motor nerves; lower down it divides into branches that supply the skin of the palm and fourth and fifth fingers.

ultra- *prefix denoting* **1.** beyond. **2.** an extreme degree (e.g. of large or small size).

ultracentrifuge *n.* a *centrifuge that works at extremely high speeds of rotation: used for separating large molecules, such as proteins.

ultrafiltration *n.* filtration under pressure. In the kidney, blood is subjected to ultrafiltration to remove the unwanted water, urea, and other waste material that goes to make up urine.

ultramicroscope *n.* a microscope for examining particles suspended in a gas or liquid under intense illumination from one side. Light is scattered or reflected from the particles, which can be seen through the eyepiece as bright objects against a dark background.

ultramicrotome *n.* an instrument for cutting extremely thin sections of tissue (not more than 0.1 µm thick) for electron microscopy. *See also* MICROTOME.

ultrasonics *n.* the study of the uses and properties of sound waves of very high frequency (*see* ULTRASOUND). —**ultrasonic** *adj.*

ultrasonography (sonography) *n.* the use of *ultrasound, usually in excess of 1 MHz, to produce images of structures of the human body that may be observed on a TV screen and subsequently transferred to photographic film. It is based on the principle of detecting the reflected waves (echoes) occurring at interfaces within human organs, following a short pulse of ultrasound. This is repeated many times to build up a complete picture. Both the transmitter and detector are contained within the scanning probe (*see* TRANSDUCER). As far as is known, there are no adverse effects from the use of ultrasound and it has particular value in obstetrics (including the diagnosis of pregnancy, assessment of gestational age, diagnosis of *malpresentations and *hydatidiform moles, and detection of fetal abnormalities) and in examination of the biliary and urinary tract and the vas-

cular tree. More specialized techniques include *echocardiography, *transvaginal ultrasonography, and **intraoperative, transrectal,** and **transoesophageal ultrasound** (endoscopic ultrasound) examinations.

ultrasound (ultrasonic waves) *n.* sound waves of extremely high frequency (above 20,000 Hz), inaudible to the human ear. Ultrasound, usually in excess of 1 MHz, can be used to produce images of the interior of the human body, in the same way that X-rays can be used to build up pictures, but with the advantages that the patient is not submitted to potentially harmful radiation and that structures not opaque to X-rays can be seen (*see* ULTRASONOGRAPHY). The vibratory effect of ultrasound can also be used to break up stones in the kidney or elsewhere (*see* LITHOTRIPSY) and in the treatment of rheumatic conditions and cataract (*see* PHACOEMULSIFICATION). Ultrasonic instruments are used in dentistry to remove *calculus from the surfaces of teeth and to remove debris from the root canals of teeth in *root canal treatment.

ultrasound marker the appearance, on *ultrasound examination of a pregnant woman, of a particular physical abnormality in the fetus at a specific stage in fetal development. Such markers suggest the presence of specific chromosomal or developmental abnormalities. For example, the **nuchal marker** – a dark area in the neck region of the fetus – is one of the markers for Down's syndrome (*see* NUCHAL THICKNESS SCANNING).

ultraviolet rays invisible short-wavelength radiation beyond the violet end of the visible spectrum. Sunlight contains ultraviolet rays, which are responsible for the production of both suntan and – on overexposure – sunburn. The dust and gases of the earth's atmosphere absorb most of the ultraviolet rays in sunlight (*see* OZONE). If this did not happen, the intense ultraviolet radiation from the sun would be lethal to living organisms.

umbilical cord the strand of tissue connecting the fetus to the placenta. It contains two arteries that carry blood to the placenta and one vein that returns it to the fetus. It also contains remnants of the *allantois and *yolk sac and becomes ensheathed by the *amnion.

umbilicus (omphalus) *n.* the navel: a circular depression in the centre of the abdomen marking the site of attachment of the *umbilical cord in the fetus. —**umbilical** *adj.*

umbo *n.* a projecting centre of a round surface, especially the projection of the inner surface of the eardrum to which the malleus is attached.

unciform bone *see* HAMATE BONE.

uncinate fits a form of temporal lobe *epilepsy in which hallucinations of taste and smell and inappropriate chewing movements are prominent features.

unconscious *adj.* **1.** in a state of unconsciousness. **2.** describing those mental processes of which a person is not aware. **3.** (in psychoanalysis) denoting the part of the mind that includes memories, motives, and intentions that are not accessible to awareness and cannot be made conscious without overcoming resistances. *Compare* SUBCONSCIOUS.

unconsciousness *n.* a condition of being unaware of one's surroundings, as in sleep, or of being unresponsive to stimulation. An unnatural state of unconsciousness may be caused by factors that produce reduced brain activity, such as lack of oxygen, *head injuries, poisoning, blood loss, and many diseases, or it may be brought about deliberately during general *anaesthesia. *See also* COMA.

uncus *n.* any hook-shaped structure, especially a projection of the lower surface of the cerebral hemisphere that is composed of cortex belonging to the temporal lobe.

undecenoic acid an antifungal agent, applied to the skin in the form of powder, ointment, lotion, or aerosol spray for the treatment of such infections as athlete's foot. Trade name: **Mycota**.

undine *n.* a small rounded container, usually made of glass, for solutions used to wash out the eye. It has a small neck for filling and a long tapering spout with a narrow outlet to deliver a fine stream of fluid to the eye.

undulant fever *see* BRUCELLOSIS.

ungual *adj.* relating to the fingernails or toenails (ungues).

unguentum *n.* (in pharmacy) an ointment.

unguis *n.* a fingernail or toenail. *See* NAIL.

uni- *prefix denoting* one.

unicellular *adj.* describing organisms or tissues that consist of a single cell. Unicellular organisms include the protozoans, most bacteria, and some fungi.

unilateral *adj.* (in anatomy) relating to or affecting one side of the body or one side of an organ or other part.

union *n.* (in a fractured bone) the successful result of healing of a fracture, in which the previously separated bone ends have become firmly united by newly formed bone. Failure of union (**nonunion**) may result if the bone ends are not immobilized or from infection or bone diseases. *Compare* MALUNION.

Union international contre le cancer (UICC) an international body promoting cancer prevention and treatment. It produces respected texts on the most important types of cancer.

unipolar *adj.* (in neurology) describing a neurone that has one main process extending from the cell body. *Compare* BIPOLAR.

UPPP *n.* *see* UVULOPALATOPHARYNGOPLASTY.

urachus *n.* the remains of the cavity of the *allantois, which usually disappears during embryonic development. In the adult it normally exists in the form of a solid fibrous cord connecting the bladder with the umbilicus, but it may persist abnormally as a patent duct. —**urachal** *adj.*

uracil *n.* one of the nitrogen-containing bases (*see* PYRIMIDINE) occurring in the nucleic acid RNA.

uraemia *n.* the presence of excessive amounts of urea and other nitrogenous waste compounds in the blood. These waste products are normally excreted by the kidneys in urine; their accumulation in the blood occurs in kidney failure and results in nausea, vomiting, lethargy, drowsiness, and eventually (if untreated) death. Treatment may require *haemodialysis on a kidney machine. —**uraemic** *adj.*

uramustine *n.* a *cytotoxic drug used in the treatment of various forms of cancer, particularly chronic lymphatic leukaemia. Uramustine is administered by intravenous injection and it is highly toxic; common side-effects are nausea, vomiting and diarrhoea, and depression of bone marrow function.

uran- (urano-) *prefix denoting* the palate.

urataemia *n.* the presence in the blood of sodium urate and other urates, formed by the reaction of uric acid with bases. In *gout, urataemia leads to deposition of urates in various parts of the body.

uraturia *n.* the presence in the urine of urates (salts of uric acid). Abnormally high concentrations of urates in urine occur in *gout.

urea *n.* the main breakdown product of protein metabolism. It is the chemical form in which unrequired nitrogen is excreted by the body in the urine. Urea is formed in the liver from ammonia and carbon dioxide in a series of enzyme-mediated reactions (the **urea cycle**). Accumulation of urea in the bloodstream together with other nitrogenous compounds is due to kidney failure and gives rise to *uraemia.

urease *n.* an enzyme that catalyses the hydrolysis of urea to ammonia and carbon dioxide.

urecchysis *n.* the escape of uric acid from the blood into spaces in the connective tissue.

ureter *n.* either of a pair of tubes, 25–30 cm long, that conduct urine from the pelvis of kidneys to the bladder. The walls of the ureters contain thick layers of smooth muscle, which contract to force urine into the bladder, between an outer fibrous coat and an inner mucous layer. —**ureteral, ureteric** *adj.*

ureter- (uretero-) *prefix denoting* the ureter(s). Example: **ureterovaginal** (relating to the ureters and vagina).

ureterectomy *n.* surgical removal of a ureter. This usually includes removal of the associated kidney as well (*see* NEPHRO-URETERECTOMY). If previous nephrectomy has been performed to remove a kidney that has been destroyed by *vesicoureteric reflux or because of a tumour of the renal pelvis, subsequent ureterectomy may be necessary to cure reflux into the stump of the ureter or tumour in the ureter, respectively.

ureteritis *n.* inflammation of the ureter. This usually occurs in association with inflammation of the bladder (*see* CYSTITIS), particularly if caused by *vesicoureteric reflux. Tuberculosis of the urinary tract can also cause ureteritis, which progresses to *stricture formation.

ureterocele *n.* a cystic swelling of the wall of the ureter at the point where it passes into the bladder. It is associated with stenosis of the opening of the ureter and it may cause impaired drainage of the kidney with dilatation of the ureter and *hydronephrosis. If urinary obstruction is present, the ureterocele should be dealt with surgically.

ureteroenterostomy *n.* an artificial communication, surgically created, between the ureter and the bowel. In this form of urinary diversion, which bypasses the bladder, the ureters are attached to the sigmoid colon (*see* URETEROSIGMOIDOS-TOMY).

ureterolithotomy *n.* the surgical removal of a stone from the ureter (*see* CAL-CULUS). The operative approach depends upon the position of the stone within the ureter. If the stone occupies the lower portion of the ureter, it may be extracted by *cystoscopy, thus avoiding open surgery.

ureterolysis *n.* an operation to free one or both ureters from surrounding fibrous tissue causing an obstruction.

ureteroneocystostomy *n.* the surgical reimplantation of a ureter into the bladder. This is most commonly performed to cure *vesicoureteric reflux. The ureter is reimplanted obliquely through the bladder wall to act as a valve and prevent subsequent reflux. The operation is usually referred to as an **antireflux procedure** or simply **reimplantation of ureter**.

ureteronephrectomy *n. see* NEPHRO-URETERECTOMY.

ureteroplasty *n.* surgical reconstruction of the ureter using a segment of bowel or a tube of bladder (*see* BOARI FLAP). This is necessary if a segment of ureter is damaged by disease or injury.

ureteropyelonephritis *n.* inflammation involving both the ureter and the renal pelvis (*see* URETERITIS, PYELITIS).

ureteroscope *n.* a rigid or flexible instrument that can be passed into the ureter and up into the pelvis of the kidney. Usually, the ureter needs to be dilated before the instrument is passed. It is most commonly used to visualize a stone in the ureter and remove it safely under direct vision with a stone basket or forceps. Larger stones can be fragmented with an ultrasound or electrohydraulic *lithotripsy probe, passed through the instrument.

ureteroscopy *n.* the inspection of the lumen of the ureter with a *ureteroscope.

ureterosigmoidostomy *n.* the operation of implanting the ureters into the sigmoid colon (*see* URETERENTEROSTOMY). This method of permanent urinary diversion may be used after *cystectomy or to bypass a diseased or damaged bladder. The urine is passed together with the faeces, and continence depends upon a normal anal sphincter. The main advantage of this form of diversion is the avoidance of an external opening and appliance to collect the urine; the disadvantages include possible kidney infection and acidosis.

ureterostomy *n.* the surgical creation of an external opening into the ureter. This usually involves bringing the ureter to the skin surface so that the urine can drain into a suitable appliance (**cutaneous ureterostomy**). The divided dilated ureter can be brought through the skin to form a spout, but ureters of a normal size need to be implanted into a segment of bowel used for this purpose (*see* ILEAL CONDUIT) to avoid narrowing and obstruction.

ureterotomy *n.* surgical incision into the ureter. The commonest reason for performing this is to allow removal of a stone (*see* URETEROLITHOTOMY).

urethr- (urethro-) *prefix denoting* the urethra.

urethra *n.* the tube that conducts urine from the bladder to the exterior. The female urethra is quite short (about 3.5 cm) and opens just within the *vulva, between the clitoris and vagina. The male urethra is longer (about 20 cm) and runs through the penis. As well as urine, it receives the secretions of the male accessory sex glands (prostate and Cowper's glands and seminal vesicles) and spermatozoa from the *vas deferens; thus it also serves as the ejaculatory duct.

urethritis *n.* inflammation of the urethra. This may be due to gonorrhoea (**specific urethritis**), another sexually transmitted infection, often infection with *Chlamydia trachomatis* (**nongonococcal urethritis, NGU**; or **nonspecific urethritis, NSU**), or to the presence of a catheter in the urethra. The symptoms are those of urethral discharge with painful or difficult urination (*dysuria). Treatment of urethritis due to infection is by administration of appropriate antibiotics after the causative organisms have been isolated from the discharge. Untreated or severe urethritis results in a urethral *stricture.

urethrocele *n.* prolapse of the urethra into the vaginal wall causing a bulbous swelling to appear in the vagina, particularly on straining. The condition is associated with previous childbirth. Treatment usually involves surgical repair of the lax tissues to give better support to the urethra and the vaginal wall.

urethrography *n.* X-ray examination of the urethra, after the introduction of a *radiopaque fluid, so that its outline and any narrowing or other abnormalities may be observed in X-ray photographs (**urethrograms**). In **ascending urethrography** a radiopaque jelly is injected up the urethra using a special syringe and penile clamp. In **descending urethrography** (or **micturating cystourethrography, MCU**), X-rays of the urethra can be taken during the passing of water-soluble contrast material previously inserted into the bladder in order to demonstrate disorders of micturition, particularly bladder emptying.

urethroplasty *n.* surgical repair of the

urethra, especially a urethral *stricture. The operation entails the insertion of a flap or patch of skin from the scrotum or perineum into the urethra at the site of the stricture, which is laid widely open. The operation can be performed in one stage, although two stages are usual in the reconstruction of a posterior urethral stricture (*see* URETHROSTOMY). **Transpubic urethroplasty** is performed to repair a ruptured posterior urethra following a fractured pelvis. Access to the damaged urethra is achieved by partial removal of the pubic bone.

urethrorrhaphy *n.* surgical restoration of the continuity of the urethra. This may be required following laceration of the urethra.

urethrorrhoea *n.* a discharge from the urethra. This is a symptom of *urethritis.

urethroscope *n.* an *endoscope, consisting of a fine tube fitted with a light and lenses, for examination of the interior of the male urethra, including the prostate region. —**urethroscopy** *n.*

urethrostenosis *n.* a *stricture of the urethra.

urethrostomy *n.* the operation of creating an opening of the urethra in the perineum in men. This can be permanent, to bypass a severe *stricture of the urethra in the penis, or it can form the first stage of an operation to cure a stricture of the posterior section of the urethra (*urethroplasty).

urethrotomy *n.* the operation of cutting a *stricture in the urethra. It is usually performed with a **urethrotome**. This instrument, a type of *endoscope, consists of a sheath down which is passed a fine knife, which is operated by the surgeon viewing the stricture down an illuminated telescope.

-uria *suffix denoting* **1.** a condition of urine or urination. Example: **polyuria** (passage of excess urine). **2.** the presence of a specified substance in the urine. Example: **haematuria** (blood in).

uric acid a nitrogen-containing organic acid that is the end-product of nucleic acid metabolism and is a component of the urine. Crystals of uric acid are de-

posited in the joints of people suffering from *gout.

uricosuric drug a drug, such as *probenecid or *sulphinpyrazone, that increases the amount of *uric acid excreted in the urine. Uricosuric drugs are used to treat gout and other conditions in which the levels of uric acid in the blood are increased, as during treatment with some *diuretics. Uricosuric drugs are sometimes administered with certain antibiotics (such as penicillin) to maintain high blood levels since they inhibit their excretion.

uridine *n.* a compound containing uracil and the sugar ribose. *See also* NUCLEOSIDE.

uridrosis *n.* the presence of excessive amounts of urea in the sweat; when the sweat dries, a white flaky deposit of urea may remain on the skin. The phenomenon occurs in *uraemia.

urin- (urino-, uro-) *prefix denoting* urine or the urinary system.

urinalysis *n.* the analysis of *urine, using physical, chemical and microscopical tests, to determine the proportions of its normal constituents and to detect alcohol, drugs, sugar, or other abnormal constituents.

urinary bladder *see* BLADDER.

urinary diversion any of various techniques for the collection and diversion of urine away from its usual excretory channels, after the bladder has been removed (*see* CYSTECTOMY) or bypassed. These techniques include *ureterosigmoidostomy and the construction of an *ileal conduit. **Continent diversion**, usually after cystectomy, may be achieved by constructing a reservoir or pouch from a section of small or large intestine or a combination of both. This can be emptied by catheterization via a small *stoma and has the advantage over an ileal conduit in that a urinary drainage bag is not required.

urinary tract the entire system of ducts and channels that conduct urine from the kidneys to the exterior. It includes the ureters, the bladder, and the urethra.

urination (micturition) *n.* the periodic discharge of urine from the bladder through the urethra. It is initiated by voluntary relaxation of the sphincter muscle below the bladder and maintained by reflex contraction of the muscles of the bladder wall.

urine *n.* the fluid excreted by the kidneys, which contains many of the body's waste products. It is the major route by which the end-products of nitrogen metabolism – *urea, *uric acid, and *creatinine – are excreted. The other major constituent is sodium chloride. Over 100 other substances are usually present, but only in trace amounts. Biochemical analysis of urine is commonly used in the diagnosis of diseases (for example, there are high levels of urinary glucose in diabetes and of ketone bodies in ketonuria); immunological analysis of urine is the basis of most *pregnancy tests.

uriniferous tubule *see* RENAL TUBULE.

urinogenital (urogenital) *adj.* of or relating to the organs and tissues concerned with both excretion and reproduction, which are anatomically closely associated.

urinogenital sinus the duct in the embryo that receives the ureter and mesonephric and paramesonephric ducts and opens to the exterior. The innermost portion forms most of the bladder and the remainder forms the urethra with its associated glands. Part of it may also contribute towards the vagina.

urinometer *n.* a hydrometer for measuring the specific gravity of urine.

urobilinogen *n.* a colourless product of the reduction of the *bile pigment bilirubin. Urobilinogen is formed from bilirubin in the intestine by bacterial action. Part of it is reabsorbed and returned to the liver; part of it is excreted in the faeces (a trace may also appear in the urine). When exposed to air, urobilinogen is oxidized to a brown pigment, **urobilin**.

urocele *n.* a cystic swelling in the scrotum, containing urine that has escaped from the urethra. This may arise following urethral injury. Immediate treatment is to divert the urine by suprapubic *cystotomy, local drainage of the swelling, and antibiotic administration.

urochesia *n.* the passage of urine through the rectum. This may follow a penetrating injury involving both the lower urinary tract and the bowel.

urodynamics *n.* the recording of pressures within the bladder by the use of special equipment that can also record urethral sphincter pressures. It is an essential investigation in the study of urinary incontinence.

urogenital *adj. see* URINOGENITAL.

urogram *n.* an X-ray of the urinary tract or any part of it. It is usually obtained after the intravenous injection of a radioopaque substance, as in an *intravenous pyelogram (or urogram), but the contrast medium can also be introduced percutaneously or, in the case of the bladder, transurethrally (for a **cystogram**; *see* CYSTOGRAPHY).

urography *n.* radiological examination of the urinary tract or any part of it after the introduction of a contrast medium. *See* CYSTOGRAPHY, PYELOGRAPHY, URETHROGRAPHY.

urokinase *n.* an enzyme produced in the kidney that is capable of breaking up blood clots (*see* FIBRINOLYTIC). It activates *plasminogen directly to plasmin, which dissolves blood clots. When injected, it has a short half-life, which makes it more useful in certain cases. It is used in the treatment of pulmonary embolism, deep-vein thrombosis, acute myocardial infarction and other causes of thrombosis. Trade name: **Ukidan**.

urolith *n.* a stone in the urinary tract. *See* CALCULUS.

urology *n.* the branch of medicine concerned with the study and treatment of diseases of the urinary tract. —**urological** *adj.* —**urologist** *n.*

uroporphyrin *n.* a porphyrin that plays an intermediate role in the synthesis of *protoporphyrin IX. It is excreted in significant amounts in the urine in porphyria.

ursodeoxycholic acid a drug used to dissolve cholesterol gallstones; it is administered by mouth. Side-effects are infrequent but include diarrhoea and indigestion. Trade names: **Destolit**, **Ursofalk**.

urticaria (nettle rash, hives) *n.* an

itchy rash resulting from the release of *histamine by *mast cells. Individual swellings (weals) appear rapidly and resolve spontaneously within hours. **Acute urticaria** is common and represents an immediate response to such allergens as seafood or strawberries. **Chronic urticaria** is not an allergic condition and may persist for years. **Angio-oedema** occurs when the weals involve the lips, eyes, or tongue, which may swell alarmingly and constitute a medical emergency. Urticaria can be prevented by taking antihistamines regularly.

uter- (utero-) *prefix denoting* the uterus. Examples: **uterocervical** (relating to the cervix (neck) of the uterus); **uterovaginal** (relating to the uterus and vagina); **uterovesical** (relating to the uterus and bladder).

uterine *adj.* of or relating to the uterus.

uterography *n.* *radiography of the uterus.

uterosalpingography (hysterosalpingography) *n.* *radiography of the interior of the uterus and the Fallopian tubes following injection of a *radiopaque fluid.

uterus (womb) *n.* the part of the female reproductive tract that is specialized to allow the embryo to become implanted in its inner wall and to nourish the growing fetus from the maternal blood. The nonpregnant uterus is a pear-shaped organ, about 7.5 cm long. It is suspended in the pelvic cavity by means of peritoneal folds (ligaments) and fibrous bands. The upper part is connected to the two *Fallopian tubes and the lower part joins the vagina at the cervix. The uterus has an inner mucous lining (*endometrium) and a thick wall of smooth muscle (*myometrium). During childbirth the myometrium undergoes strong contractions to expel the fetus through the cervix and vagina. In the absence of pregnancy the endometrium undergoes periodic development and degeneration (*see* MENSTRUAL CYCLE). —**uterine** *adj.*

uterus didelphys (double uterus) a congenital condition resulting from the incomplete midline fusion of the two *paramesonephric (Müllerian) ducts dur-

ing early embryonic development. The usual result is a double uterus with one or two cervices and a single vagina. Complete failure of fusion results in a double uterus with double cervices and two separate vaginae.

utricle (utriculus) *n.* **1.** the larger of the two membranous sacs within the vestibule of the ear: it forms part of the membranous *labyrinth. It is filled with fluid (endolymph) and contains a *macula. This responds to gravity and relays information to the brain about the position of the head. **2.** a small sac (the **prostatic utricle**) extending out of the urethra of the male into the substance of the prostate gland.

uvea (uveal tract) *n.* the vascular pigmented layer of the eye, which lies beneath the outer layer (sclera). It consists of the *choroid, *ciliary body, and *iris. —**uveal** *adj.*

uveal tract *see* UVEA.

uveitis *n.* inflammation of any part of the uveal tract of the eye, either the iris (**iritis**), ciliary body (**cyclitis**), or choroid (**choroiditis**). Inflammation confined to the iris and ciliary body, which are commonly inflamed together, is called **anterior uveitis** or **iridocyclitis** (*see also* FUCHS' HETEROCHROMIC CYCLITIS); that confined to the choroid is termed **posterior uveitis**. In general, the causes of anterior and posterior uveitis are different; anterior uveitis (unlike choroiditis) is usually painful, with clusters of inflammatory cells (keratic precipitates) adhering to the inner surface of the cornea. All types may lead to visual impairment, and uveitis is an important cause of blindness. In most cases the disease appears to originate in the uveal tract itself, but it may occur secondarily to disease of other parts of the eye, particularly of the cornea and sclera.

Treatment consists of the use of drugs that suppress the inflammation, combined with measures to relieve the discomfort and more specific drug treatment if a specific cause of the uveitis is found. The drugs may be given as drops, injections, or tablets, often in combination.

uveoparotitis (uveoparotid fever) *n.* inflammation of the iris, ciliary body, and choroid regions of the eye (the uvea) and swelling of the parotid salivary gland: one of the manifestations of the chronic disease *sarcoidosis.

uvula *n.* a small soft extension of the soft palate that hangs from the roof of the mouth above the root of the tongue. It is composed of muscle, connective tissue, and mucous membrane.

uvulectomy *n.* surgical removal of the uvula.

uvulitis *n.* inflammation of the uvula.

uvulopalatopharyngoplasty (UPPP) *n.* a surgical operation to remove the uvula, part of the soft palate, and the tonsils in the treatment of snoring.

V

vaccination *n.* a means of producing immunity to a disease by using a *vaccine, or a special preparation of antigenic material, to stimulate the formation of appropriate antibodies. The name was applied originally only to treatment with vaccinia (cowpox) virus, which gives protection not only against cowpox itself but also against the related smallpox. However, it is now used synonymously with **inoculation** as a method of *immunization against any disease. Vaccination is often carried out in two or three stages, as separate doses are less likely to cause unpleasant side-effects. A vaccine is usually given by injection but may be introduced into the skin through light scratches; for some diseases, oral vaccines are available.

vaccine *n.* a special preparation of antigenic material that can be used to stimulate the development of antibodies and thus confer active *immunity against a specific disease or number of diseases. Many vaccines are produced by culturing bacteria or viruses under conditions that lead to a loss of their virulence but not of their antigenic nature. Other vaccines consist of specially treated toxins (*toxoids) or of dead bacteria that are still antigenic. Examples of live but attenuated (weakened) organisms in vaccines are those against tuberculosis, rabies, and smallpox. Dead organisms are used against cholera and typhoid; precipitated toxoids are used against diphtheria and tetanus. *See* IMMUNIZATION.

vaccinia *n. see* COWPOX.

vaccinoid *adj.* resembling a local infection with vaccinia (cowpox) virus. A vaccinoid reaction is one of the possible results of vaccination against smallpox in individuals who already have partial immunity. The swelling, reddening, and blistering are considerably less than the so-called primary reaction that occurs after the inoculation of a person with no immunity against smallpox.

vacuole *n.* a space within the cytoplasm of a cell, formed by infolding of the cell membrane, that contains material taken in by the cell. White blood cells form vacuoles when they surround and digest bacteria and other foreign material.

vacuum extractor (ventouse) a device to assist delivery consisting of a suction cup that is attached to the head of the fetus: traction is then applied slowly. Introduced in 1954, it has been widely used but has not been accepted as a substitute for obstetric forceps.

vagin- (vagino-) *prefix denoting* the vagina.

vagina *n.* the lower part of the female reproductive tract: a muscular tube, lined with mucous membrane, connecting the cervix of the uterus to the exterior. It receives the erect penis during coitus: semen is ejaculated into the upper part of the vagina and from there the sperms must pass through the cervix and uterus in order to fertilize an ovum in the Fallopian tube. The wall of the vagina is sufficiently elastic to allow the passage of the newborn child. —**vaginal** *adj.*

vaginismus *n.* sudden and painful contraction of the muscles surrounding the vagina, usually in response to the *vulva or vagina being touched. Sexual intercourse may be impeded, and the condition may be associated with fear of or aversion to coitus. Other causative factors include vaginal injury or ulceration, dryness or shrinkage of the lining membrane of the vagina, and inflammation of the vagina or bladder. *See also* DYSPAREUNIA.

vaginitis *n.* inflammation of the vagina, which may be caused by infection (most commonly with *Trichomonas vaginalis*), dietary deficiency, or poor hygiene. There is often itching (*see* PRURITUS), increased vaginal discharge, and pain on passing urine. Vaginitis may indicate the presence of sexually transmitted disease.
Postmenopausal (or **atrophic**) **vaginitis**

is caused by a deficiency of female sex hormones.

vaginoplasty (colpoplasty) *n.* a tissue-grafting operation on the vagina.

vaginoscope *n. see* COLPOSCOPE.

vago- *prefix denoting* the vagus nerve.

vagotomy *n.* the surgical cutting of any of the branches of the vagus nerve. This is usually performed to reduce secretion of acid and pepsin by the stomach in order to cure a peptic ulcer. **Truncal vagotomy** is the cutting of the main trunks of the vagus nerve; in **selective vagotomy** the branches of the nerve to the gall bladder and pancreas are left intact. **Highly selective** (or **proximal) vagotomy** is the cutting of the branches of the vagus nerve to the body of the stomach, leaving the branches to the outlet (pylorus) intact: this makes additional surgery to permit emptying of the stomach contents unnecessary. Following surgery, patients may experience **postvagotomy diarrhoea** after a meal (*compare* DUMPING SYNDROME).

vagus nerve the tenth *cranial nerve (X), which supplies motor nerve fibres to the muscles of swallowing and parasympathetic fibres to the heart and organs of the chest cavity and abdomen. Sensory branches of the vagus carry impulses from the viscera and the sensation of taste from the mouth.

valgus *adj.* describing any deformity that displaces the hand or foot away from the midline. *See* CLUB-FOOT (TALIPES VALGUS), HALLUX VALGUS, KNOCK KNEE (GENU VALGUM).

validity *n.* an indication of the extent to which a clinical sign or test is a true indicator of disease. Reduced validity can arise if the tests produce different results when conducted several times on the same person under identical conditions (i.e. **reduced reproducibility**, **reliability**, or **repeatability**). This may be because the same observer gets different results on successive occasions (**intraobserver error**) or because a series of different observers fail to obtain the same result (**interobserver error**). Such errors may arise because of a true difference in observation and/or interpretation or because of a preconceived notion (often unconscious) by the observer, which influences either his

judgment or the tone and manner with which he questions the patient. *Compare* INTERVENTION STUDY.

valine *n.* an *essential amino acid. *See also* AMINO ACID.

Valium *n. see* DIAZEPAM.

vallecula *n.* a furrow or depression in an organ or other part. On the undersurface of the cerebellum a vallecula separates the two hemispheres.

(A) cut vein showing the two cusps of a valve; (B) action of a venous valve

valve *n.* a structure found in some tubular organs or parts that restricts the flow of fluid within them to one direction only. Valves are important structures in the heart, veins, and lymphatic vessels. Such a valve consists of two or three *cusps fastened like pockets to the walls of the vessel. Blood flowing in the right direction flattens the cusps to the walls, but when flow is reversed the cusps become filled with blood or lymph and dilate to block the opening (see illustration). *See also* MITRAL VALVE, TRICUSPID VALVE, SEMILUNAR VALVE.

valvotomy (valvulotomy) *n.* surgical cutting through a valve. The term is usually used to describe the operation to relieve obstruction caused by stenosed valves in the heart. In **percutaneous balloon valvotomy** the narrowed valves are opened up by *balloon dilatation, the balloon being introduced on a catheter passed up a great vessel. In **mitral valvotomy** (*see* MITRAL STENOSIS) an **INOVE balloon** is commonly used.

valvula *n.* (*pl.* **valvulae**) a small valve. The **valvulae conniventes** are circular folds of mucous membrane in the small intestine.

valvulitis *n.* inflammation of one or more valves, particularly the heart valves. This may be acute or chronic and is most often due to rheumatic fever (*see* ENDOCARDITIS).

vancomycin *n.* an *antibiotic, derived from the bacterium *Streptomyces orientalis*, that is effective against most Gram-positive organisms (e.g. streptococci and staphylococci). It is given by intravenous infusion for infections due to strains that are resistant to other antibiotics. It usually has a low toxicity but may cause deafness or thrombophlebitis. Trade name: **Vancocin**.

van den Bergh's test a test to determine whether excess bilirubin in the blood is conjugated or unconjugated, and therefore whether jaundice in a patient is due to *haemolysis or to disease of the liver or bile duct. A sample of serum is mixed with sulphanilic acid, hydrochloric acid, and sodium nitrite. The immediate appearance of a violet colour is called a **direct reaction** and indicates that the jaundice is due to liver damage or obstruction of the bile duct. If the colour appears only when alcohol is added, this is an **indirect reaction** and points to haemolytic jaundice or a congenital unconjugated hyperbilirubinaemia (*see*

GILBERT'S SYNDROME). [A. A. H. van der Bergh (1869–1943), Dutch physician]

vaporizer *n.* a piece of equipment for producing an extremely fine mist of liquid droplets by forcing a jet of liquid through a narrow nozzle with a jet of air. Vaporizers are used to produce aerosols of various medications for use in inhalation therapy.

Vaquez-Osler disease *see* POLYCYTHAEMIA VERA. [L. H. Vaquez (1860–1936), French physician; Sir W. Osler (1849–1919), Canadian physician]

variable *n.* (in biostatistics) a characteristic (e.g. morbidity, lifestyle, or habit) relating to a single individual or group. **Qualitative variables** are descriptive characteristics, such as sex, race, or occupation; **quantitative variables** relate to a numerical scale and are subdivided into **discrete variables**, found only at fixed points (e.g. number of children), and **continuous variables**, found at any point on a scale (e.g. weight).

variance *n.* *see* STANDARD DEVIATION.

varicectomy *n.* *see* PHLEBECTOMY.

varicella *n.* *see* CHICKENPOX.

varices *pl. n.* *see* VARICOSE VEINS.

varicocele *n.* a collection of dilated veins in the spermatic cord, more commonly affecting the left side of the scrotum than the right. It usually produces no symptoms apart from occasional aching discomfort. In some cases varicocele is associated with a poor sperm count (*see* OLIGOSPERMIA) sufficient to cause infertility. Surgical correction of the varicocele in such patients (**varicocelectomy**) usually results in a considerable improvement in the quality and motility of the sperm.

varicose veins veins that are distended, lengthened, and tortuous. The superficial veins (saphenous veins) of the legs are most commonly affected; other sites include the oesophagus (*see* OESOPHAGEAL VARICES) and testes (*varicocele). There is an inherited tendency to varicose veins but obstruction to blood flow is responsible in some cases. Complications including thrombosis, *phlebitis, and haemorrhage may occur. Treatment includes elastic support and *sclerotherapy, but *avulsion (stripping) or excision (*phlebectomy) is required in some cases. Medical name: **varices**.

varicotomy *n.* incision into a varicose vein (*see* PHLEBECTOMY).

variola *n. see* SMALLPOX.

varioloid 1. *n.* a mild form of smallpox in people who have previously had smallpox or have been vaccinated against it. **2.** *adj.* resembling smallpox.

varix *n.* (*pl.* **varices**) a single *varicose vein.

varus *adj.* describing any deformity that displaces the hand or foot towards the midline. *See* BOWLEG (GENU VARUM), CLUB-FOOT (TALIPES VARUS), HALLUX VARUS.

vas *n.* (*pl.* **vasa**) a vessel or duct.

vas- (vaso-) *prefix denoting* **1.** vessels, especially blood vessels. **2.** the vas deferens.

vasa efferentia (*sing.* **vas efferens**) the many small tubes that conduct spermatozoa from the testis to the epididymis. They are derived from some of the excretory tubules of the *mesonephros.

vasa vasorum *pl. n.* the tiny arteries and veins that supply the walls of blood vessels.

vascular *adj.* relating to or supplied with blood vessels.

vascularization *n.* the development of blood vessels (usually capillaries) within a tissue.

vascular system *see* CARDIOVASCULAR SYSTEM.

vasculitis *n. see* ANGIITIS.

vas deferens (*pl.* **vasa deferentia**) either of a pair of ducts that conduct spermatozoa from the *epididymis to the *urethra on ejaculation. It has a thick muscular wall the contraction of which assists in ejaculation.

vasectomy *n.* the surgical operation of severing the duct (vas deferens) connecting the testis to the seminal vesicle and urethra. Vasectomy of both ducts causes sterility and is an increasingly popular means of birth control. Vasectomy does not affect sexual desire or potency.

vaso- *prefix. see* VAS-.

vasoactive *adj.* affecting the diameter of blood vessels, especially arteries. Examples of vasoactive agents are emotion, pressure, carbon dioxide, and temperature. Some exert their effect directly, others via the *vasomotor centre in the brain.

vasoconstriction *n.* a decrease in the diameter of blood vessels, especially arteries. This results from activation of the *vasomotor centre in the brain, which brings about contraction of the muscular walls of the arteries and hence an increase in blood pressure.

vasoconstrictor *n.* an agent that causes narrowing of the blood vessels and therefore a decrease in blood flow. Examples are *metaraminol and *phenylephrine. Vasoconstrictors are used to raise the blood pressure in disorders of the circulation, shock, or severe bleeding and to maintain blood pressure during surgery. Some vasoconstrictors (e.g. *xylometazoline) have a rapid effect when applied to mucous membranes and may be used to relieve nasal congestion. If the blood pressure rises too quickly headache and vomiting may occur. A vasoconstrictor is often added to local anaesthetic solutions used in dentistry to prolong their effectiveness.

vasodilatation *n.* an increase in the diameter of blood vessels, especially arteries. This results from activation of the *vasomotor centre in the brain, which brings about relaxation of the arterial walls and a consequent lowering of blood pressure.

vasodilator *n.* a drug that causes widening of the blood vessels and therefore an increase in blood flow. Vasodilators are used to lower blood pressure in cases of hypertension. **Coronary vasodilators**, such as *glyceryl trinitrate and *pentaerythritol, increase the blood flow through the heart and are used to relieve and prevent angina. Large doses of coronary vasodilators cause such side-effects as flushing of the face, severe headache, and fainting. **Peripheral vasodilators**, such as *alpha blockers and *nicotinyl, affect the blood vessels of the limbs and are used to treat conditions of poor circulation, such as acrocyanosis, chilblains, and Raynaud's disease.

vaso-epididymostomy *n.* the opera-tion of joining the vas deferens to the epi-didymis in a side-to-side manner in order to bypass an obstruction to the passage of sperm from the testis. The obstruction, which may be congenital or acquired, is usually present in the mid-portion or tail of the epididymis. Vaso-epididymostomy is therefore usually performed by anasto-mosing the head of the epididymis to a longitudinal incision in the lumen of the adjacent vas.

vasoligation *n.* the surgical tying of the vas deferens (the duct conveying sperm from the testis). This is performed to pre-vent infection spreading from the urinary tract and causing recurrent *epididymitis. It is sometimes performed at the same time as *prostatectomy to prevent the complication of epididymitis in the post-operative period.

vasomotion *n.* an increase or decrease in the diameter of blood vessels, particu-larly the arteries. *See* VASOCONSTRICTION, VASODILATATION.

vasomotor *adj.* controlling the muscular walls of blood vessels, especially arteries, and therefore their diameter.

vasomotor centre a collection of nerve cells in the medulla oblongata that re-ceives information from sensory receptors in the circulatory system (*see* BARO-RECEPTOR) and brings about reflex changes in the rate of the heartbeat and in the di-ameter of blood vessels, so that the blood pressure can be adjusted. The vasomotor centre also receives impulses from else-where in the brain, so that emotion (such as fear) may also influence the heart rate and blood pressure. The centre works through *vasomotor nerves of the sympa-thetic and parasympathetic systems.

vasomotor nerve any nerve, usually belonging to the autonomic nervous sys-tem, that controls the circulation of blood through blood vessels by its action on the muscle fibres within their walls or its ac-tion on the heartbeat. The *vagus nerve slows the heart and reduces its output, but sympathetic nerves increase the rate and output of the heart and increase blood pressure by causing the constriction of small blood vessels at the same time.

vasomotor symptoms subjective sen-sations experienced by women around the time of the *menopause, often described as explosions of heat, mostly followed by profuse sweating and sometimes preceded by an undetermined sensation with wak-ing at night. Objective signs are sudden reddening of the skin on the head, neck, and chest and profuse sweating. Physiological changes include peripheral vasodilatation, *tachycardia with normal blood pressure, and raised skin tempera-ture with normal body temperature.

vasopressin (antidiuretic hormone, ADH) *n.* a hormone, released by the pitui-tary gland, that increases the reabsorption of water by the kidney, thus preventing excessive loss of water from the body. Vasopressin also causes constriction of blood vessels. It is administered either nasally or by injection to treat *diabetes insipidus. Intravenous injections of vaso-pressin are used to control bleeding from *oesophageal varices by restricting arter-ial blood flow to the liver.

vasopressor *adj.* stimulating the con-traction of blood vessels and therefore bringing about an increase in blood pres-sure.

vasospasm *n.* *see* RAYNAUD'S DISEASE.

vasotomy *n.* a surgical incision into the vas deferens (the duct conveying sperm from the testis). This is usually under-taken to allow catheterization of the vas and the injection of radiopaque contrast material for X-ray examination (**vasogra-phy**), to test for patency of the duct in pa-tients with *azoospermia.

vasovagal *adj.* relating to the action of impulses to the *vagus nerve on the circu-lation. The vagus reduces the rate at which the heart beats, and so lowers its output.

vasovagal attack excessive activity of the vagus nerve, causing slowing of the heart and a fall in blood pressure, which leads to fainting. *See* SYNCOPE.

vasovasostomy *n.* the surgical opera-tion of reanastomosing the vas deferens after previous vasectomy: the reversal of vasectomy, undertaken to restore fertility.

vasovesiculitis *n.* inflammation of the

*seminal vesicles and *vas deferens. This usually occurs in association with *prostatitis and causes pain in the perineum, groin, and scrotum and a high temperature. On examination the vasa and seminal vesicles are thickened and tender. Treatment includes administration of antibiotics.

vastus *n.* any of three muscles (**vastus intermedius**, **vastus lateralis**, and **vastus medialis**) that form part of the *quadriceps muscle of the thigh.

vector *n.* **1.** an animal, usually an insect or a tick, that transmits parasitic microorganisms – and therefore the diseases they cause – from person to person or from infected animals to human beings. Mosquitoes, for example, are vectors of malaria, filariasis, and yellow fever. **2.** an agent used to insert a foreign gene or DNA fragment into a bacterial or other cell in *genetic engineering and *gene therapy. Viruses, especially retroviruses, are often used as vectors: once inside the host cell, the virus can replicate and thus produce copies (*clones) of the gene.

vectorcardiography *n.* see ELECTROCARDIOGRAPHY.

vegetation *n.* (in pathology) an abnormal outgrowth from a membrane, fancied to resemble a vegetable growth. In ulcerative endocarditis, such outgrowths, consisting of *fibrin with enmeshed blood cells, are found on the membrane lining the heart valves.

vegetative *adj.* **1.** relating to growth and nutrition rather than to reproduction. **2.** functioning unconsciously; autonomic.

vehicle *n.* (in pharmacy) any substance that acts as the medium in which a drug is administered. Examples are sterile water, isotonic sodium chloride, and dextrose solutions.

vein *n.* a blood vessel conveying blood towards the heart. All veins except the *pulmonary vein carry deoxygenated blood from the tissues, via the capillaries, to the vena cava. The walls of veins consist of three tissue layers, but these are much thinner and less elastic than those of arteries (see illustration). Veins contain *valves that assist the flow of blood back

to the heart. Anatomical name: **vena**. —**venous** *adj.*

lumen
endothelium
thin tunica media
tunica adventitia

Transverse section through a vein

velamen (velamentum) *n.* a covering membrane.

vellus *n.* the fine hair that occurs on the body before puberty is reached.

velum *n.* (in anatomy) a veil-like covering. The **medullary velum** is either of two thin layers of tissue that form part of the roof of the fourth ventricle of the brain.

vena *n.* (*pl.* **venae**) see VEIN.

vena cava (*pl.* **venae cavae**) either of the two main veins, conveying deoxygenated blood from the other veins to the right atrium of the heart. The **inferior vena cava**, formed by the union of the right and left common iliac veins, receives blood from parts of the body below the diaphragm. The **superior vena cava**, originating at the junction of the two innominate veins, drains blood from the head, neck, thorax, and arms.

vene- (veno-) *prefix denoting* veins.

veneer *n.* a facing of *composite resin or *porcelain applied to the surface of a tooth to give improved shape and/or colour. The tooth requires minimal preparation and the facing is retained by enamel that has been treated by the *acid-etch technique. Veneers are a more conservative way of treating discoloured teeth than by *crowns.

venene *n.* a mixture of two or more *venoms: used to produce antiserum against venoms (**antivenene**).

venepuncture (venipuncture) *n.* the puncture of a vein for any therapeutic purpose; for example, to extract blood for laboratory tests. See also PHLEBOTOMY.

internal jugular
external jugular
superior vena cava
suprarenal
renal
testicular (ovarian)
common iliac
external iliac
femoral
great saphenous

subclavian
cephalic
axillary
hepatic
brachial
inferior vena cava
median cubital
basilic
superficial palmar network
popliteal
small saphenous
anterior tibial
dorsal venous arch

The principal veins of the body

venereal disease (VD) *see* SEXUALLY TRANSMITTED DISEASE.

venesection *n. see* PHLEBOTOMY.

veno- *prefix. see* VENE-.

venoclysis *n.* the continuous infusion into a vein of saline or other solution.

venography (phlebography) *n.* X-ray examination to demonstrate the anatomy of veins in a particular region of the body. A *radiopaque contrast medium is injected into a vein and X-ray photographs (**venograms**) taken as the medium flows towards the heart. Damage, obstruction, or abnormal communication with other vessels can be demonstrated. *See also* ANGIOGRAPHY.

venom *n.* the poisonous material produced by snakes, scorpions, spiders, and other animals for injecting into their prey or enemies. Some venoms produce no more than local pain and swelling; others produce more general effects and can prove lethal.

venosclerosis *n. see* PHLEBOSCLEROSIS.

ventilation *n.* the passage of air into and out of the respiratory tract. The air that reaches only as far as the conducting airways cannot take part in gas exchange and is known as **dead space ventilation** – this may be reduced by performing a *tracheostomy. In the air sacs of the lungs (alveoli) gas exchange is most efficient when matched by adequate blood flow (*perfusion). Ventilation/perfusion imbalance (ventilation of underperfused alveoli or perfusion of underventilated alveoli) is an important cause of *anoxia and *cyanosis.

ventilator *n.* **1.** a device to ensure a supply of fresh air. **2.** equipment that is manually or mechanically operated to maintain a flow of air into and out of the lungs of a patient who is unable to breathe normally. *See also* RESPIRATOR.

ventouse *n. see* VACUUM EXTRACTOR.

ventral *adj.* relating to or situated at or close to the front of the body or to the anterior part of an organ.

ventricle *n.* **1.** either of the two lower chambers of the *heart, which have thick muscular walls. The left ventricle, which

is thicker than the right, receives blood from the pulmonary vein via the left atrium and pumps it into the aorta. The right ventricle pumps blood received from the venae cavae (via the right atrium) into the pulmonary artery. **2.** one of the four fluid-filled cavities within the brain (see illustration). The paired first and second ventricles (**lateral ventricles**), one in each cerebral hemisphere, communicate with the third ventricle in the midline between them. This in turn leads through a narrow channel, the **cerebral aqueduct**, to the fourth ventricle in the hindbrain, which is continuous with the spinal canal in the centre of the spinal cord. *Cerebrospinal fluid circulates through all the cavities. —**ventricular** *adj.*

— frontal lobe
— lateral ventricle

foramen of Monro (interventricular foramen)
third ventricle—
cerebral aqueduct

fourth ventricle

Ventricles of the brain (side view)

ventricul- (ventriculo-) *prefix denoting* a ventricle (of the brain or heart).

ventricular folds *see* VOCAL FOLDS.

ventricular septal defect (VSD) a congenital defect of the heart in which there is a hole in the partition (septum) separating the two ventricles (*see* SEPTAL DEFECT); it is the most common congenital heart disease. In 25% of patients there are other defects present. 50% of VSDs close spontaneously. If the hole is large, blood is diverted to the lungs at a greater pressure than usual and *pulmonary hypertension can occur, which becomes irreversible and progressive. Early surgical intervention can prevent this.

ventriculitis *n.* inflammation in the ventricles of the brain, usually caused by infection. It may result from the rupture of a cerebral abscess into the cavity of the ventricle or from the spread of a severe form of *meningitis from the subarachnoid space.

ventriculoatriostomy *n.* an operation for the relief of raised pressure due to the build-up of cerebrospinal fluid that occurs in *hydrocephalus. Using a system of catheters, the fluid is drained into the jugular vein in the neck.

ventriculography *n.* X-ray examination of the ventricles of the brain after the introduction of a contrast medium, such as air or radiopaque material. This procedure has been largely made redundant by CT and MRI scanning.

ventriculoscopy *n.* observation of the ventricles of the brain through a fibreoptic instrument. *See* ENDOSCOPE, FIBRE OPTICS.

ventriculostomy *n.* an operation to introduce a hollow needle (cannula) into one of the lateral ventricles (cavities) of the brain. This may be done to relieve raised intracranial pressure, to obtain cerebrospinal fluid from the ventricle for examination, or to introduce antibiotics or contrast material for X-ray examination.

ventro- *prefix denoting* **1.** ventral. **2.** the abdomen.

ventrofixation *n. see* VENTROSUSPENSION.

ventrosuspension (ventrofixation) *n.* surgical fixation of a displaced uterus to the anterior abdominal wall. This may be achieved by shortening the round ligaments at their attachment either to the uterus or to the abdominal wall.

venule *n.* a minute vessel that drains blood from the capillaries. Many venules unite to form a vein.

verapamil *n.* a *calcium antagonist used in the treatment of essential hypertension, angina, and arrhythmia. It is administered by mouth; side-effects include constipation, nausea, and hypotension. Trade names: **Cordilox, Securon, Univer**.

verbigeration *n.* repetitive utterances of the same words over and over again.

This is a kind of *stereotypy affecting speech and is most common in institutionalized schizophrenics.

vermicide *n.* a chemical agent used to destroy parasitic worms living in the intestine. *Compare* VERMIFUGE.

vermiform appendix *see* APPENDIX.

vermifuge *n.* any drug or chemical agent used to expel worms from the intestine. *See also* ANTHELMINTIC.

vermis *n.* the central portion of the *cerebellum, lying between its two lateral hemispheres and immediately behind the pons and the medulla oblongata of the hindbrain.

vermix *n.* the vermiform *appendix.

vernal conjunctivitis *conjunctivitis of allergic origin, often associated with hay fever or other forms of *atopy.

vernier *n.* a device for obtaining accurate measurements of length, to 1/10th, 1/100th or smaller fractions of a unit. It consists of a fixed graduated main scale against which a shorter vernier scale slides. The vernier scale is graduated into divisions equal to nine-tenths of the smallest unit marked on the main scale. The vernier scale is often adjusted by means of a screw thread. A reading is taken by observing which of the markings on the scales coincide.

vernix caseosa the layer of greasy material which covers the skin of a fetus or newborn baby. It is produced by the oil-secreting glands of the skin and contains skin scales and fine hairs.

verruca (plantar wart) *n.* (*pl.* **verrucae**) *see* WART.

verrucous carcinoma an *indolent preinvasive wartlike carcinoma of the oral cavity, which is associated with chewing tobacco.

version *n.* a manoeuvre to alter the position of a fetus in the uterus to facilitate delivery. For example, the fetus may be turned from a transverse to a longitudinal position or from a buttocks-first to a head-first presentation (*see* CEPHALIC VERSION).

vertebra *n.* (*pl.* **vertebrae**) one of the 33

bones of which the *backbone is composed. Each vertebra typically consists of a **body**, or **centrum**, from the back of which arises an arch of bone (the **neural arch**) enclosing a cavity (the **vertebral canal**, or **foramen**) through which the spinal cord passes. The neural arch bears one **spinous process** and two **transverse processes**, providing anchorage for muscles, and four **articular processes**, with which adjacent vertebrae articulate (see illustration). Individual vertebrae are bound together by ligaments and *intervertebral discs. —**vertebral** *adj.*

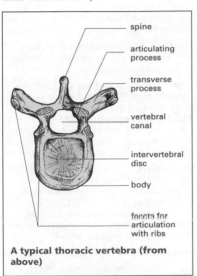

- spine
- articulating process
- transverse process
- vertebral canal
- intervertebral disc
- body
- facets for articulation with ribs

A typical thoracic vertebra (from above)

vertebral column *see* BACKBONE.

vertigo *n.* a disabling sensation in which the affected individual feels that either he himself or his surroundings are in a state of constant movement. It is most often a spinning sensation but there may be a feeling that the ground is tilting. It is a symptom of disease either in the *labyrinth of the inner ear or in the *vestibular nerve or its nuclei in the brainstem, which are involved in the sense of balance.

vesical *adj.* relating to or affecting an anatomical bladder, especially the urinary bladder.

vesicant *n.* an agent that causes blistering of the skin.

vesicle *n.* **1.** a very small blister in the skin, often no bigger than a pinpoint, that contains a clear fluid (serum). Vesicles occur in a variety of skin disorders, including eczema and herpes. **2.** (in anatomy) any small bladder, especially one filled with fluid. —**vesicular** *adj.*

vesico- *prefix denoting* the urinary bladder. Example: **vesicovaginal** (relating to the bladder and vagina).

vesicofixation *n. see* CYSTOPEXY.

vesicostomy *n.* the surgical creation of an artificial channel between the bladder and the skin surface for the passage of urine. It is sometimes combined with closure of the urethra.

vesicoureteric reflux the backflow of urine from the bladder into the ureters. This is due to defective valves (which normally prevent reflux). Infection is conveyed to the kidneys, causing recurrent attacks of acute *pyelonephritis and scarring of the kidneys in childhood. Children with urinary infection must be investigated for reflux by *cystoscopy; if the condition does not settle with antibiotic therapy corrective surgery must be performed.

vesicovaginal fistula an abnormal communication between the bladder and the vagina causing urinary incontinence. This may result from surgical damage to the bladder during a gynaecological operation (e.g. hysterectomy) or radiation damage following radiotherapy for pelvic malignancy. In Third World countries it is often caused by necrosis associated with prolonged obstructed labour.

vesicular breathing *see* BREATH SOUNDS.

vesiculectomy *n.* surgical removal of a *seminal vesicle. This operation, which is rarely undertaken, may be performed for a tumour of the seminal vesicles.

vesiculitis *n.* inflammation of the seminal vesicles. *See* VASOVESICULITIS.

vesiculography *n.* X-ray examination of the seminal vesicles. This is usually performed by injecting radiopaque contrast material into the exposed vasa deferentia.

It can also be undertaken by inserting a catheter into the ejaculatory duct (which discharges semen from the vesicle into the vas deferens) via an *endoscope. This examination is rarely undertaken for the specific purpose of outlining the seminal vesicles; it is more commonly performed to test for the patency of the vas deferens in patients with *azoospermia.

vessel *n.* a tube conveying a body fluid, especially a blood vessel or a lymphatic vessel.

vestibular glands the two pairs of glands that open at the junction of the vagina and vulva. The more posterior of the two are the **greater vestibular glands** (**Bartholin's glands**); the other pair are the **lesser vestibular glands**. Their function is to lubricate the entrance to the vagina during coitus.

vestibular nerve the division of the *vestibulocochlear nerve that carries impulses from the semicircular canals, utricle, and saccule of the inner ear to the brain, conveying information about the body's posture and movements in space and allowing coordination and balance.

vestibule *n.* (in anatomy) a cavity situated at the entrance to a hollow part. The vestibule of the ear is the cavity of the bony *labyrinth that contains the *saccule and *utricle – the organs of equilibrium.

vestibulocochlear nerve (acoustic nerve, auditory nerve) the eighth cranial nerve (VIII), responsible for carrying sensory impulses from the inner ear to the brain. It has two branches, the **vestibular nerve** and the **cochlear nerve**. The cochlear nerve carries impulses from the spiral *cochlea and is therefore the nerve of hearing, while the vestibular nerve serves equilibrium, carrying impulses from the semicircular canals, utricles, and saccules with information about posture, movement, and balance.

vestigial *adj.* existing only in a rudimentary form. The term is applied to organs whose structure and function have diminished during the course of evolution until only a rudimentary structure exists.

viable *adj.* capable of living a separate existence. The legal age of viability of a fetus is 24 weeks, but some fetuses now survive birth at an even earlier age.

Viagra *n.* *see* SILDENAFIL.

Vibramycin *n.* *see* DOXYCYCLINE.

vibrator *n.* a machine used to generate vibrations of different frequencies, which have a stimulating effect when applied to different parts of the body. A vibrator may also be used to loosen thick mucus in the sinuses or air passages.

Vibrio *n.* a genus of Gram-negative motile comma-shaped bacteria widely distributed in soil and water. Most species are saprophytic but some are parasites, including *V. cholerae*, which causes *cholera.

vibrissa *n.* (*pl.* **vibrissae**) a stiff coarse hair, especially one of the stiff hairs that lie just inside the nostrils.

vicarious *adj.* describing an action or function performed by an organ not normally involved in the function. For example, **vicarious menstruation** is a rare disorder in which monthly bleeding occurs from places other than the vagina, such as the sweat glands, breasts, nose, or eyes.

vidarabine *n.* an antiviral drug that inhibits DNA synthesis and is used to treat herpes simplex, herpes zoster (shingles), and *cytomegalovirus infections. It is administered by intravenous infusion. Possible side-effects include weakness and skin rashes. Trade name: **Vira-A**.

vigabatrin *n.* *see* ANTICONVULSANT.

villus *n.* (*pl.* **villi**) one of many short finger-like processes that project from some membranous surfaces. Numerous **intestinal villi** line the small *intestine. Each contains a network of blood capillaries and a *lacteal. Their function is to absorb the products of digestion and they greatly increase the surface area over which this can take place. **Chorionic villi** are folds of the *chorion (the outer membrane surrounding a fetus) from which the fetal part of the *placenta is formed. They provide an extensive area for the exchange of oxygen, carbon dioxide, nutrients, and waste products between maternal and fetal blood. *See also* ARACHNOID VILLUS, CHORIONIC VILLUS SAMPLING.

vinblastine *n.* a *cytotoxic drug that is

given by intravascular injection mainly in the treatment of cancers of the lymphatic system, such as Hodgkin's disease. It is highly toxic, since it also acts on normal tissues; common side-effects include nausea, vomiting, diarrhoea, and depression of bone marrow function. Trade name: **Velbe**.

vinca alkaloid one of a group of antimitotic drugs (see CYTOTOXIC DRUG) derived from the periwinkle (*Vinca rosea*). Vinca alkaloids, which are used especially to treat leukaemias and lymphomas, include *vinblastine, *vincristine, and *vindesine.

Vincent's angina an obsolete term for *ulcerative gingivitis. [H. Vincent (1862–1950), French physician]

vincristine *n.* a cytotoxic drug with uses and side-effects similar to those of vinblastine. Trade name: **Oncovin**.

vinculum *n.* (*pl.* **vincula**) a connecting band of tissue. The **vincula tendinum** are threadlike bands of synovial membrane that connect the flexor tendons of the fingers and toes to their point of insertion on the phalanges.

vindesine *n.* a cytotoxic drug with similarities to *vinblastine and vincristine. Additional side-effects include alopecia and peripheral neuropathy. Trade name: **Eldisine**.

VIP (vasoactive intestinal peptide) a protein produced by cells of the pancreas. Large amounts of this protein cause severe diarrhoea.

vipoma *n.* a tumour of islet cells of the pancreas that secrete *VIP.

viraemia *n.* the presence in the blood of virus particles.

viral pneumonia an acute infection of the lung caused by any one of a number of viruses, such as *respiratory syncytial virus, adenovirus, influenza and parainfluenza viruses, and enteroviruses. It is characterized by headache, fever, muscle pain, and a cough that produces a thick sputum. The pneumonia can often occur with or subsequent to a systemic viral infection. Treatment is by supportive care, but antibiotics are administered if a bacterial infection is superimposed.

virilism *n.* the development in a female of a combination of increased body hair, muscle bulk, and deepening of the voice (*masculinization) and male psychological characteristics.

virilization *n.* the most extreme result of excessive androgen production (*hyperandrogenism) in women. It is characterized by temporal balding, a male body form, muscle bulk, deepening of the voice, enlargement of the clitoris, and *hirsutism. Virilization in prepubertal boys may be caused by some tumours (see LEYDIG TUMOUR).

virology *n.* the science of viruses. See also MICROBIOLOGY.

virulence *n.* the disease-producing (pathogenic) ability of a microorganism. See also ATTENUATION.

virus *n.* a minute particle that is capable of replication but only within living cells. Viruses are too small to be visible with a light microscope and too small to be trapped by filters. They infect animals, plants, and microorganisms (see BACTERIOPHAGE). Each consists of a core of nucleic acid (DNA or RNA) surrounded by a protein shell. Some bear an outer lipid capsule. Viruses cause many diseases, including the common cold, influenza, measles, mumps, chickenpox, herpes, AIDS, polio, and rabies. *Antiviral drugs are effective against some of them, and many viral diseases are controlled by means of vaccines. —**viral** *adj.*

viscera *pl. n.* (*sing.* **viscus**) the organs within the body cavities, especially the organs of the abdominal cavities (stomach, intestines, etc.). —**visceral** *adj.*

visceral arch see PHARYNGEAL ARCH.

visceral cleft see PHARYNGEAL CLEFT.

visceral pouch see PHARYNGEAL POUCH.

viscero- *prefix denoting* the viscera.

viscus *n.* see VISCERA.

visual acuity sharpness of vision: the degree to which a person is able to distinguish and resolve detail. Visual acuity depends on how well objects are illuminated and upon such factors as practice and motivation, but the essential requirements are a healthy retina and the ability of the eye to focus incoming light to form a sharp image on the retina. The commonest way of assessing visual acuity is the *Snellen chart, which measures the **resolving power** of the eye.

visual field the area in front of the eye in any part of which an object can be seen without moving the eye. With both eyes open and looking straight forward it is possible to see well-illuminated objects placed anywhere in front of the eyes, although the eyebrows and eyelids reduce the extent of the field somewhat. This is the **binocular visual field**. With only one eye open the field is **uniocular** and is restricted inwards by the nose. If the object is small or poorly illuminated it will not be seen until it is moved closer to the point at which the eye is actually looking, i.e. nearer to the centre of the visual field. Similarly, coloured objects are not seen so far away from the centre as are white objects of the same size and brightness. This is because the retina is not uniformly sensitive to light of different colours or intensities (see ROD, CONE): retinal sensitivity increases towards its centre (the *macula). Thus, while there is an absolute visual field beyond which things cannot be seen, no matter how large or bright they are, a relative field exists for objects of different brightness, size, and colour. The most common visual field loss is due to *glaucoma. See also CAMPIMETRY, PERIMETER.

visual purple see RHODOPSIN.

vital capacity the maximum volume of air that a person can exhale afer maximum inhalation. It is usually measured on an instrument called a **spirometer**.

vital centre any of the collections of nerve cells in the brain that act as governing centres for different vital body functions – such as breathing, heart rate, blood pressure, temperature control etc. – making reflex adjustments according to the body's needs. Most lie in the hypothalamus and brainstem.

Vitallium n. Trademark. an alloy of chromium and cobalt that is used in instruments, prostheses, surgical appliances, and dentures.

vital staining (intravital staining) the process of staining a living tissue by injecting a stain into the organism. Compare SUPRAVITAL STAINING.

vital statistics see BIOSTATISTICS.

vitamin n. any of a group of substances that are required, in very small amounts, for healthy growth and development: they cannot be synthesized by the body and are therefore essential constituents of the diet. Vitamins are divided into two groups, according to whether they are soluble in water or fat. The water-soluble group includes the vitamin B complex and vitamin C; the fat-soluble vitamins are vitamins A, D, E, and K. Lack of sufficient quantities of any of the vitamins in the diet results in specific vitamin deficiency diseases.

vitamin A (retinol) a fat-soluble vitamin that occurs preformed in foods of animal origin (especially milk products, egg yolk, and liver) and is formed in the body from the pigment β-*carotene, present in some vegetable foods (for example cabbage, lettuce, and carrots). Retinol is essential for growth, vision in dim light, and the maintenance of soft mucous tissue. A deficiency causes stunted growth, *night blindness, *xerophthalmia, *keratomalacia, and eventual blindness. The recommended daily intake is 750 μg retinol equivalents for an adult (1 μg retinol equivalent = 1 μg retinol or 6 μg β-carotene).

vitamin B any one of a group of water-soluble vitamins that, although not chemically related, are often found together in the same kinds of food (milk, liver, cereals, etc.) and all function as *coenzymes. See VITAMINS B_1, B_2, B_6, B_{12}, BIOTIN, FOLIC ACID, NICOTINIC ACID, PANTOTHENIC ACID.

vitamin B_1 (thiamin, aneurine) a vitamin of the B complex that is active in the form of **thiamin pyrophosphate**, a coenzyme in decarboxylation reactions in carbohydrate metabolism. A deficiency of vitamin B_1 leads to *beriberi. Good sources of the vitamin are cereals, beans, meat, potatoes, and nuts. The recommended daily intake is 1 mg for an adult.

vitamin B_2 (riboflavin) a vitamin of the B complex that is a constituent of the coenzymes *FAD (flavine adenine dinucleotide) and *FMN (flavine mononucleotide). Riboflavin is therefore important in tissue respiration. A deficiency of riboflavin causes a condition known as *ariboflavinosis, which is not usually serious. Good sources of riboflavin are liver, milk, and eggs. The recommended daily intake for an adult is 1.7 mg.

vitamin B$_6$ (pyridoxine) a vitamin of the B complex from which the coenzyme *pyridoxal phosphate, involved in the transamination of amino acids, is formed. The vitamin is found in most foods and a deficiency is therefore rare.

vitamin B$_{12}$ (cyanocobalamin) a vitamin of the B complex. The form of vitamin B$_{12}$ with coenzyme activity is **5-deoxyadenosyl cobalamin**, which is necessary for the synthesis of nucleic acids, the maintenance of *myelin in the nervous system, and the proper functioning of *folic acid, another B vitamin. The vitamin can be absorbed only in the presence of **intrinsic factor**, a protein secreted in the stomach. A deficiency of vitamin B$_{12}$ affects nearly all the body tissues, particularly those containing rapidly dividing cells. The most serious effects of a deficiency are *pernicious anaemia and degeneration of the nervous system. Vitamin B$_{12}$ is manufactured only by certain microorganisms and is contained only in foods of animal origin. Good sources are liver, fish, and eggs. The daily recommended adult intake is 3–4 µg.

vitamin C (ascorbic acid) a water-soluble vitamin with *antioxidant properties that is essential in maintaining healthy connective tissues and the integrity of cell walls. It is necessary for the synthesis of collagen. A deficiency of vitamin C leads to *scurvy. The recommended daily intake is 30 mg for an adult; rich sources are citrus fruits and vegetables (the main source of the vitamin in the British diet is potatoes).

vitamin D a fat-soluble vitamin that enhances the absorption of calcium and phosphorus from the intestine and promotes their deposition in the bone. It occurs in two forms: **ergocalciferol** (**vitamin D$_2$, calciferol**), which is manufactured by plants when the sterol ergosterol is exposed to ultraviolet light, and **cholecalciferol** (**vitamin D$_3$**), which is produced by the action of sunlight on 7-dehydrocho-

lesterol, a sterol widely distributed in the skin. A deficiency of vitamin D, either from a poor diet or lack of sunlight, leads to decalcified bones and the development of *rickets and *osteomalacia. Good sources of vitamin D are liver and fish oils. The recommended daily intake is 10 µg for a child up to five years and 2.5 µg thereafter. Vitamin D is toxic and large doses must therefore be avoided.

vitamin E any of a group of chemically related fat-soluble compounds (**tocopherols** and **tocotrienols**) that have *antioxidant properties and are thought to stabilize cell membranes by preventing oxidation of their unsaturated fatty acid components. The most potent of these is α-**tocopherol**. Good sources of the vitamin are vegetable oils, eggs, butter, and wholemeal cereals. It is fairly widely distributed in the diet and a deficiency is therefore unlikely. There is evidence to suggest that vitamin E supplements (400–800 mg/day) reduce the risk of coronary thrombosis in patients with heart disease.

vitamin K a fat-soluble vitamin occurring in two main forms: **phytomenadione** (of plant origin) and **menaquinone** (of animal origin). It is necessary for the formation of *prothrombin in the liver, which is essential for blood clotting, and it also regulates the synthesis of other clotting factors. A dietary deficiency does not often occur as the vitamin is synthesized by bacteria in the large intestine and is widely distributed in green leafy vegetables and meat.

vitelliform degeneration (Best's disease) degeneration of the *macula of the eye that is inherited as a dominant characteristic and usually starts in childhood. There is widespread abnormality of retinal pigment epithelium (*see* RETINA) with the accumulation of a yellowish material, especially in the macular area.

vitellus *n.* the yolk of an ovum.

vitiligo *n.* a common disorder in which symmetrical white or pale *macules appear on the skin. It affects all races, but is more conspicuous in dark-skinned races. Vitiligo is an *autoimmune disease and may occur with other such diseases (e.g. thyroid disease or *alopecia areata). It is usually progressive, although spontaneous repigmentation may occur. Treatment with *PUVA may be effective in darker-skinned people; pale-skinned sufferers can best be helped by using potent sunscreens or by cosmetic camouflage.

vitrectomy *n.* the removal of the whole or part of the vitreous humour of the eye, including vitreous haemorrhage. **Anterior vitrectomy** is removal of the front portion of the vitreous humour. Vitrectomy is often necessary in surgery to repair a detached retina.

vitreous detachment the separation of the *vitreous humour from the underlying retina. This is a normal ageing process, but it is also more common in such conditions as diabetes and severe myopia. It can sometimes cause a tear in the retina and lead to *retinal detachment.

vitreous humour (vitreous body) the transparent jelly-like material that fills the chamber behind the lens of the eye.

vitritis *n.* inflammation within the vitreous humour of the eye.

viviparous *adj.* describing animal groups (including most mammals) in which the embryos develop within the body of the mother so that the young are born alive rather than hatch from an egg. —**viviparity** *n.*

vivisection *n.* a surgical operation on a living animal for experimental purposes.

vocal folds (vocal cords) the two folds of tissue which protrude from the sides of the *larynx to form a narrow slit (glottis) across the air passage (see illustration). Their controlled interference with the expiratory air flow produces audible vibrations that make up speech, song, and all other vocal noises. Alterations in the vocal folds themselves or in their nerve supply by disease interferes with phonation.

vocal fremitus *see* FREMITUS.

vocal resonance the sounds heard through the stethoscope when the patient speaks ("ninety nine"). These are normally just audible but become much louder (**bronchophony**) if the lung under the stethoscope is consolidated, when they resemble the sounds heard over the trachea and main bronchi. Vocal resonance is lost

over pleural fluid except at its upper surface, when it has a bleating quality and is called **aegophony**. *See also* PECTORILOQUY.

vocational training a period of supervised training for dentists and doctors in general practice before they are allowed to work independently in NHS practice.

volar *adj.* relating to the palm of the hand or the sole of the foot (the **vola**).

Volkmann's contracture fibrosis and shortening of muscles due to inadequate blood supply. It is a complication that arises if the blood supply is interrupted by pressure on the blood vessels from a fracture fragment, or from raised pressure due to *compartment syndrome, or by pressure from constricting bandages and plaster casts. *See also* COMPARTMENT SYNDROME. [R. von Volkmann (1830–89), German surgeon]

volsellum (vulsellum) *n.* surgical forceps with clawlike hooks at the ends of both blades.

volt *n.* the *SI unit of electric potential, equal to the potential difference between two points on a conducting wire through which a constant current of 1 ampere flows when the power dissipated between these points is 1 watt. Symbol: V.

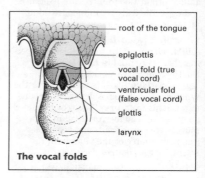

The vocal folds

voluntary admission entry of a patient into a psychiatric hospital with his (or her) agreement. *Compare* COMPULSORY ADMISSION.

voluntary muscle *see* STRIATED MUSCLE.

volvulus *n.* twisting of part of the digestive tract, usually leading to partial or complete obstruction and sometimes reducing the blood supply, causing gangrene. A volvulus may untwist spontaneously or by manipulation, but surgical exploration is usually performed. **Gastric volvulus** is a twist of the stomach, usually in a hiatus *hernia. **Small-intestinal volvulus** is twisting of part of the bowel around an *adhesion. **Sigmoid volvulus** is a twist of the sigmoid colon, usually when this loop is particularly long. **Compound volvulus** (or **ileosigmoid knotting**) involves both the small and the large bowel.

vomer n. a thin plate of bone that forms part of the nasal septum (*see* NASAL CAVITY). *See also* SKULL.

vomica n. **1.** an abnormal cavity in an organ, usually a lung, sometimes containing pus. **2.** the abrupt expulsion from the mouth of a large quantity of pus or decaying matter originating in the throat or lungs.

vomit 1. vb. to eject the contents of the stomach through the mouth (*see* VOMITING). **2.** n. the contents of the stomach ejected during vomiting. Medical name: **vomitus**.

vomiting n. the reflex action of ejecting the contents of the stomach through the mouth. Vomiting is controlled by a special centre in the brain that may be stimulated by drugs (e.g. *apomorphine) acting directly on it; or by impulses transmitted through nervous pathways either from the stomach (e.g. after ingesting irritating substances or in stomach diseases, such as peptic ulceration or pyloric stenosis), the intestine (e.g. in intestinal obstruction), or from the inner ear (in motion sickness). The stimulated vomiting centre sets off a chain of nerve impulses producing coordinated contractions of the diaphragm and abdominal muscles, relaxation of the muscle at the entrance to the stomach, etc., causing the stomach contents to be expelled. Medical name: **emesis**.

von Hippel-Lindau disease an inherited syndrome in which *haemangioblastomas, particularly in the cerebellum, are associated with renal and pancreatic cysts, *angiomas in the retina (causing blindness), cancer of the kidney cells, and red birthmarks. [E. von Hippel (1867–1939), German ophthalmologist; A. Lindau (1892–1958), Swedish pathologist]

von Recklinghausen's disease 1. a syndrome due to excessive secretion of *parathyroid hormone (hyperparathyroidism), characterized by loss of mineral from bones, which become weakened and fracture easily, and formation of kidney stones. Medical name: **osteitis fibrosa**. **2.** *see* NEUROFIBROMATOSIS. [F. D. von Recklinghausen (1833–1910), German pathologist]

Von Rosen's sign *see* BARLOW'S SIGN. [S. Von Rosen, Swedish orthopaedic surgeon]

von Willebrand's disease an inherited disorder of the blood that is characterized by episodes of spontaneous bleeding similar to *haemophilia. It may or may not be associated with deficiency of *Factor VIII and is inherited as an autosomal *dominant. [A. von Willebrand (1870–1949), Swedish physician]

voxel n. the volume of tissue in a body that is represented by a *pixel in a cross-sectional image.

voyeurism n. the condition of obtaining sexual pleasure by watching other people undressing or enjoying sexual relations. *See also* SEXUAL DEVIATION. **—voyeur** n.

VSD *see* VENTRICULAR SEPTAL DEFECT.

vulsellum n. *see* VOLSELLUM.

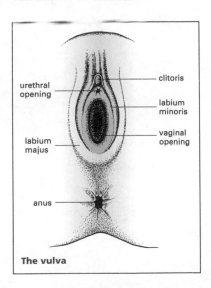

The vulva

urethral opening — clitoris — labium minoris — vaginal opening — labium majus — anus

vulv- (vulvo-) *prefix denoting* the vulva.

vulva *n.* the female external genitalia. Two pairs of fleshy folds – the **labia majora** and **labia minora** – surround the openings of the vagina and urethra and extend forward to the clitoris (see illustration). *See also* VESTIBULAR GLANDS.

vulvectomy *n.* surgical removal of the external genitals (*see* VULVA) of a woman. **Simple vulvectomy** involves excision of the labia majora, labia minora, and clitoris and is carried out for a nonmalignant growth. **Radical vulvectomy** is a much more extensive operation carried out for a malignant growth, e.g. cancer of the vulva. It involves wide excision of the labia majora and minora and the clitoris in addition to complete removal of all regional lymph nodes on both sides. The skin covering these areas is also removed, leaving an extensive raw area that is allowed to heal by *granulation.

vulvitis *n.* inflammation of the vulva, which is often accompanied by intense itching (*see* PRURITUS).

vulvovaginitis *n.* inflammation of the vulva and vagina (*see* PRURITUS, VAGINITIS).

Waardenburg's syndrome an inherited form of deafness accompanied by a characteristic white forelock of hair and multiple colours within the irises of the eyes. It is inherited as an autosomal *dominant disease, i.e. the children of an affected parent have a 50% chance of inheriting the disorder, although severity is variable. The gene responsible has recently been identified. [P. J. Waardenburg (1886–1979), Dutch ophthalmologist]

wafer *n.* a thin sheet made from moistened flour, formerly used to enclose a powdered medicine that is taken by mouth.

WAGR syndrome *see* ANIRIDIA.

waiting list a list of the names of patients who are awaiting admission to hospital after having been assessed either as an out-patient or on a *domiciliary consultation involving a specialist. In general the patients are offered places in the order in which their names were placed on the list, but in certain circumstances (e.g. if the condition is potentially dangerous or painful) the consultant may recommend urgent or even immediate admission. One of the facts recorded in relation to hospital admissions is the length of time between the name being placed on the list and the patient being admitted (**waiting time**). General practitioners may also request **direct admission** (immediate) for urgent cases who have not been seen by the consultant; such admission may be arranged by phone with the consultant or his or her deputy or channelled through the accident and emergency department of the hospital.

Waldeyer's ring the ring of lymphoid tissue formed by the tonsils. [H. W. G. von Waldeyer (1836–1921), German anatomist]

walking distance the measured distance that a patient can walk before he or she is stopped by pain in the muscles, usually the calf muscles. It is a useful estimate of the degree of impairment of the blood supply. *See* CLAUDICATION.

Wallerian degeneration fatty degeneration of a ruptured nerve fibre that occurs within the nerve sheath distal to the point of severance. [A. V. Waller (1816–70), British physician]

warfarin *n.* an *anticoagulant used mainly in the treatment of coronary or venous thrombosis to reduce the risk of embolism. It is given by mouth or injection. The principal toxic effect is local bleeding, usually from the gums and other mucous membranes. Warfarin has also been used as a rat poison. Trade name: **Marevan**.

wart *n.* a benign growth on the skin caused by infection with *human papillomavirus (a few of the many serotypes are *oncogenic). **Common warts** are firm horny papules, 1–10 mm in diameter, found mainly on the backs of the hands. Most will clear spontaneously within two years. **Plantar warts** (or **verrucae**) occur on the soles and are often tender. **Plane warts** are flat and skin-coloured – and therefore difficult to see; they are usually found on the face and may be present in very large numbers. **Genital warts** are frequently associated with other genital infections and affected women have an increased risk of developing cervical cancer. Treatment of warts is with OTC (over-the-counter) remedies, such as lactic and salicylic acids, but *cryotherapy with liquid nitrogen is probably more effective. Occasionally curettage and cautery are used: surgical excision is never indicated.

Warthin's tumour (adenolymphoma) a tumour of the parotid salivary glands, containing epithelial and lymphoid tissues with cystic spaces. [A. S. Warthin (1866–1931), US pathologist]

Wassermann reaction formerly, the most commonly used test for the diagnosis of *syphilis. A sample of the patient's blood is examined, using a *complement-fixation reaction, for the presence of antibodies to the organism *Treponema pallidum*. A positive reaction (WR+) indicates the presence of antibodies and therefore infection with syphilis. [A. P. von Wassermann (1866–1925), German bacteriologist]

water bed a bed with a flexible water-containing mattress. The surface of the bed adapts itself to the patient's posture, which leads to greater comfort and fewer bedsores.

waterbrash *n.* a sudden filling of the mouth with dilute saliva. This often accompanies dyspepsia, particularly if there is nausea.

Waterhouse-Friderichsen syndrome acute haemorrhage in the adrenal glands with haemorrhage into the skin associated with the sudden onset of acute bacteraemic *shock. It is usually caused by meningococcal septicaemia (*see* MENINGITIS). [R. Waterhouse (1873–1958), British physician; C. Friderichsen (20th century), Danish physician]

Waters' projection a *posteroanterior X-ray film to show the maxillae, maxillary sinuses, and zygomatic bones. [C. A. Waters (1888–1961), US radiologist]

watt *n.* the *SI unit of power, equal to 1 joule per second. In electrical terms it is the energy expended per second when a current of 1 ampere flows between two points on a conductor between which there is a potential difference of 1 volt. 1 watt = 10^7 ergs per second. Symbol: W.

weal *n.* a transient swelling, confined to a small area of the skin, that is characteristic of *urticaria and occurs following *dermographism.

weber *n.* the *SI unit of magnetic flux, equal to the flux linking a circuit of one turn that produces an e.m.f. of 1 volt when reduced uniformly to zero in 1 second. Symbol: Wb.

Weber-Christian disease *see* PANNICULITIS. [F. P. Weber (1863–1962), British physician; H. A. Christian (1876–1951), US physician]

Weber's test a hearing test in which a vibrating tuning fork is placed at the midpoint of the forehead. A normal individual hears it equally in both ears, but if one ear is affected by conductive *deafness the sound appears louder in the affected ear. [F. E. Weber (1832–91), German otologist]

web space the soft tissue between the bases of the fingers and toes.

Wechsler scales standardized scales for the measurement of *intelligence quotient (IQ) in adults and children. They are administered by a chartered psychologist. *See* INTELLIGENCE TEST. [D. Wechsler (1896–1981), US psychologist]

Wegener's granulomatosis an autoimmune disease predominantly affecting the nasal passages, lungs, and kidneys, characterized by *granuloma formation in addition to arteritis. Untreated the disease is usually fatal, but it can be controlled (sometimes for years) with steroids, cyclophosphamide, and azathioprine. [F. Wegener (1907–90), German pathologist]

Weil-Felix reaction a diagnostic test for typhus. A sample of the patient's serum is tested for the presence of antibodies against the organism *Proteus vulgaris*. Although this relatively harmless organism is not the cause of typhus, it possesses certain antigens in common with the causative agent of the disease and can therefore be used instead of it in laboratory tests. Typhus is suspected if antibodies are found to be present. [E. Weil (1880–1922), German physician; A. Felix (1887–1956), Czech bacteriologist]

Weil's disease *see* LEPTOSPIROSIS. [A. Weil (1848–1916), German physician]

Welch's bacillus *see* CLOSTRIDIUM. [W. H. Welch (1850–1934), US pathologist]

wen *n.* *see* SEBACEOUS CYST.

Werdnig-Hoffmann disease a hereditary disorder – a severe form of *spinal muscular atrophy – in which the cells of the spinal cord begin to die between birth and the age of six months, causing a symmetrical muscle weakness in affected infants that starts proximally. Respiratory and facial muscles become affected. Children usually die by the age of 20 months from respiratory failure and there is no treatment. *Genetic counselling is required for parents of an affected child as each of their subsequent children has a one in four chance of being affected. [G. Werdnig (1844–1919), Austrian neurologist; J. Hoffmann (1857–1919), German neurologist]

Werner's syndrome a rare genetic disorder resulting in premature ageing that starts at adolescence. Growth may be retarded and affected individuals may suffer from a thin skin, arterial disease, leg ulcers, and diabetes. Treatment is limited to the management of complications, such as diabetes. The gene responsible codes for an enzyme involved in the mechanisms of DNA replication and repair, which in affected individuals is defective. [C. W. O. Werner (1879–1936), German physician]

Wernicke's encephalopathy mental confusion or delirium occurring in combination with paralysis of the eye muscles, *nystagmus, and an unsteady gait. It is caused by a deficiency of vitamin B_1 (thiamin) and is most commonly seen in alcoholics and in patients with persistent vomiting. Treatment with thiamin relieves the symptoms. [K. Wernicke (1848–1905), German neurologist]

Wertheim's hysterectomy a radical operation performed for cervical cancer, in which the uterus, Fallopian tubes, ovaries, upper vagina, broad ligaments, and regional lymph nodes are removed. [E. Wertheim (1864–1920), Austrian gynaecologist]

Western blot analysis a technique for the detection of specific proteins. After separation by *electrophoresis, the proteins are bound to radioactively labelled antibodies and identified by X-ray. Compare NORTHERN BLOT ANALYSIS, SOUTHERN BLOT ANALYSIS.

wet-and-dry bulb hygrometer see HYGROMETER.

Wharton's duct the secretory duct of the submandibular *salivary gland. [T. Wharton (1614–73), English physician]

Wharton's jelly the mesoderm tissue of the umbilical cord, which becomes converted to a loose jelly-like *mesenchyme surrounding the umbilical blood vessels.

wheeze n. an abnormal high-pitched (sibilant) or low-pitched sound heard – either by the unaided human ear or through the stethoscope – mainly during expiration. Wheezes occur as a result of

narrowing of the airways, such as results from *bronchospasm or increased secretion and retention of sputum; they are commonly heard in patients with asthma or chronic bronchitis.

whiplash injury damage to the ligaments, vertebrae, or spinal cord, caused by sudden jerking back of the head and neck, often in occupants of a car hit from behind. Whiplash is an injury to the soft tissues causing pain and stiffness in the neck. Treatment is with a soft surgical collar for a short period, and physiotherapy can help. Symptoms occasionally last for many months.

Whipple's disease a rare disease, occurring only in males, in which absorption of digested food in the intestine is reduced. As well as symptoms and signs of *malabsorption there is usually skin pigmentation and arthritis. Diagnosis is made by *jejunal biopsy; microorganisms have been found in the mucosa, and the disease usually responds to prolonged antibiotic treatment. [G. H. Whipple (1878–1976), US pathologist]

Whipple's operation see PANCREATECTOMY. [A. O. Whipple (1881–1963), US surgeon]

Whipple's triad a combination of three clinical features that indicate the presence of an *insulinoma: (1) attacks of fainting, dizziness, and sweating on fasting; (2) severe hypoglycaemia present during the attacks; (3) relief from the attacks achieved by administering glucose. [A. O. Whipple]

whipworm n. a small parasitic whiplike nematode worm, *Trichuris trichiura* (*Trichocephalus dispar*), that lives in the large intestine. Eggs are passed out of the body with the faeces and human infection (see TRICHURIASIS) results from the consumption of water or food contaminated with faecal material. The eggs hatch in the small intestine but mature worms migrate to the large intestine.

Whitaker's test a direct percutaneous renal infusion test to investigate obstruction of the ureter causing *hydronephrosis.

white blood cell see LEUCOCYTE.

white finger the appearance of a finger

resulting from spasm of the vessels of the finger. It occurs in *Raynaud's disease but can also be attributed to the long-term use of percussion implements. In the latter case, it is a source of compensation claims.

white leg *see* THROMBOPHLEBITIS.

white matter nerve tissue of the central nervous system that is paler in colour than the associated *grey matter because it contains more nerve fibres and thus larger amounts of the insulating material *myelin. In the brain the white matter lies within the grey layer of cerebral cortex; in the spinal cord it is between the arms of the X-shaped central core of grey matter.

white noise instrument a device, resembling a small hearing aid, that produces sounds of many frequencies at equal intensities and is used in the treatment of tinnitus. It was formerly known as a **tinnitus masker**.

whitlow *n. see* PARONYCHIA.

WHO *see* WORLD HEALTH ORGANIZATION.

whoop *n.* a noisy convulsive drawing in of the breath following the spasmodic coughing attack characteristic of *whooping cough.

whooping cough an acute infectious disease, primarily of infants, caused by the bacterium *Bordetella pertussis*, which affects the respiratory tract. It often occurs in epidemics. After an incubation period of 1–2 weeks there is a catarrhal stage, in which the infant has signs of an upper respiratory-tract infection. A cough develops, which becomes increasingly severe and is accompanied by a *whoop; the child can become exhausted and may stop breathing. This stage lasts 4–6 weeks. The most common complication is pneumonia, but bronchiectasis and convulsions due to *asphyxia or bleeding into the brain tissue may also occur. Immunization offers protection and is usually given in the form of the *DPT vaccine. An attack usually confers lifelong immunity. Medical name: **pertussis**.

Widal reaction an *agglutination test for the presence of antibodies against the *Salmonella* organisms that cause typhoid

fever. It is thus a method of diagnosing the presence of the disease in a patient and also a means of identifying the organisms in infected material. [G. F. I. Widal (1862–1929), French physician]

Wilms' tumour *see* NEPHROBLASTOMA. [M. Wilms (1867–1918), German surgeon]

Wilson's disease an inborn defect of copper metabolism in which there is a deficiency of *caeruloplasmin (which normally forms a nontoxic complex with copper). The free copper may be deposited in the liver, causing jaundice and cirrhosis, or in the brain, causing mental retardation and symptoms resembling *parkinsonism. There is a characteristic brown ring in the cornea (the **Kayser-Fleischer ring**). If the excess copper is removed from the body by regular treatment with *penicillamine both mental and physical development may be normal. Medical name: **hepatolenticular degeneration**. [S. A. K. Wilson (1878–1936), British neurologist]

windigo *n.* a delusion of having been transformed into a windigo, a mythical monster that eats human flesh. It is often quoted as an example of a syndrome confined to one culture (that of some North American Indian tribes, such as the Cree).

windpipe *n. see* TRACHEA.

wisdom tooth the third *molar tooth on each side of either jaw, which erupts normally around the age of 20.

witch hazel (hamamelis) a preparation made from the leaves and bark of the tree *Hamamelis virginiana*, used as an *astringent, especially for the treatment of sprains and bruises.

withdrawal *n.* **1.** (in psychology) the removal of one's interest from one's surroundings. **Thought withdrawal** is the experience of one's thoughts being removed from one's head, which is characteristic of *schizophrenia. **2.** *see* COITUS INTERRUPTUS.

withdrawal symptoms *see* DEPENDENCE.

Wohlfahrtia *n.* a genus of non-blood-sucking flies. Females of the species *W. magnifica* and *W. vigil* deposit their parasitic maggots in wounds and the openings of the body. This causes *myiasis, particularly in children.

Wolffian body *see* MESONEPHROS. [K. F. Wolff (1733–94), German anatomist]

Wolffian duct the mesonephric duct (*see* MESONEPHROS).

Wolff-Parkinson-White syndrome a congenital abnormality of heart rhythm caused by the presence of an accessory conduction pathway between the atria and ventricles (*see* ATRIOVENTRICULAR BUNDLE). It results in premature excitation of one ventricle and is characterized by an abnormal wave (**delta wave**) at the start of the *QRS complex on the electrocardiogram. [L. Wolff (1898–1972), US cardiologist; Sir J. Parkinson (1885–1976), British physician; P. D. White (1886–1973), US cardiologist]

womb *n.* *see* UTERUS.

Wood's light ultraviolet light filtered through a nickel oxide prism, which causes fluorescence in skin and hair affected by some fungal and bacterial infections and is therefore useful in diagnosis. For example, *erythrasma fluoresces coral pink, while scalp ringworm caused by *Microsporon* species fluoresces green. [R. W. Wood (1868–1955), US physician]

woolsorter's disease *see* ANTHRAX.

word blindness *see* ALEXIA.

World Health Organization (WHO) an international organization, membership of which is open to every country, with subscription according to means; health issues are discussed and policies evolved mainly through working groups, including acknowledged authorities, and published reports. Staff are seconded by invitation to advise on self-help to solve problems (especially infectious disease control). WHO handles information on the internationally *notifiable diseases, pub-

lishes the *International Classification of Diseases, and awards fellowships to enable health staff from poorer countries to obtain further training.

worm *n.* any member of several groups of soft-bodied legless animals, including flatworms, nematode worms, earthworms, and leeches, that were formerly thought to be closely related and classified as a single group – Vermes.

wormian bone one of a number of small bones that occur in the cranial sutures.

wound *n.* a break in the structure of an organ or tissue caused by an external agent. Bruises, grazes, tears, cuts, punctures, and burns are all examples of wounds.

wrist *n.* **1.** the joint between the forearm and hand. It consists of the proximal bones of the *carpus, which articulate with the radius and ulna. **2.** the whole region of the wrist joint, including the carpus and lower parts of the radius and ulna.

wrist drop paralysis of the muscles that raise the wrist, which is caused by damage to the *radial nerve. This may result from compression of the nerve against the humerus in the upper arm or from selective damage to the nerve, which is a feature of *lead poisoning.

wryneck *n.* *see* TORTICOLLIS.

Wuchereria *n.* a genus of white threadlike parasitic worms (*see* FILARIA) that live in the lymphatic vessels. *W. bancrofti* is a tropical and subtropical species that causes *elephantiasis, lymphangitis, and chyluria. The immature forms concentrate in the lungs during the day. At night they become more numerous in the blood vessels of the skin, from which they are taken up by blood-sucking mosquitoes, acting as carriers of the diseases they cause.

xamoterol *n.* a drug that stimulates beta receptors in the heart (*see* SYMPATHO-MIMETIC) and used in the treatment of long-term mild heart failure. It is administered by mouth. Possible side-effects include headache, dizziness, muscle cramps, palpitations, and skin rashes. Trade name: **Corwin**.

xanthaemia (carotenaemia) *n.* the presence in the blood of the yellow pigment *carotene, from excessive intake of carrots, tomatoes, or other vegetables containing the pigment.

xanthelasma *n.* yellow *plaques occurring symmetrically around the eyelids. In elderly people it is quite common and of no more than cosmetic importance, but in some cases it may be a manifestation of disorders of fat metabolism (hyperlipidaemia).

xanthine *n.* a nitrogenous breakdown product of the purines adenosine and guanine. Xanthine is an intermediate product of the breakdown of nucleic acids to uric acid.

xanthinuria *n.* excess of the purine derivative *xanthine in the urine, usually the result of an inborn defect of metabolism. It is both rare and symptomless.

xantho- *prefix denoting* yellow colour.

xanthochromia *n.* yellow discoloration, such as may affect the skin (for example, in jaundice) or the cerebrospinal fluid (when it contains the breakdown products of haemoglobin from red blood cells that have entered it).

xanthoma *n.* (*pl.* **xanthomata**) a yellowish skin lesion associated with any of various disorders of lipid metabolism. There are several types of xanthomata. **Tuberous xanthomata** are found on the knees and elbows; **tendon xanthomata** involve the extensor tendons of the hands and feet and the Achilles tendon. Crops of small yellow papules at any site are known as **eruptive xanthomata**, while

larger flat lesions are called **plane xanthomata**.

xanthomatosis *n.* the presence of multiple xanthomata in the skin. *See* XANTHOMA.

xanthophyll *n.* a yellow pigment found in green leaves. An example of a xanthophyll is **lutein**.

xanthopsia *n.* yellow vision: the condition in which all objects appear to have a yellowish tinge. It is sometimes experienced in digitalis poisoning.

X chromosome the sex chromosome present in both sexes. Women have two X chromosomes and men one. Genes for some important genetic disorders, including *haemophilia, are carried on the X chromosomes; these genes are described as *sex-linked. *Compare* Y CHROMOSOME.

xeno- *prefix denoting* different; foreign; alien.

xenodiagnosis *n.* a procedure for diagnosing infections transmitted by insect carriers. Uninfected insects of the species known to carry the disease in question are allowed to suck the blood of a patient suspected of having the disease. A positive diagnosis is made if the disease parasites appear in the insects. This method has proved invaluable for diagnosing Chagas' disease, using reduviid bugs (the carriers), since the parasites are not always easily detected in blood smears.

xenogeneic *adj.* describing grafted tissue derived from a donor of a different species.

xenograft *n. see* HETEROGRAFT.

xenophobia *n.* excessive fear of strangers and foreigners. *See* PHOBIA.

Xenopsylla *n.* a genus of tropical and subtropical fleas, with some 40 species. The rat flea, *X. cheopis*, occasionally attacks man and can transmit plague from an infected rat population; it also transmits murine typhus and two tapeworms, *Hymenolepis nana* and *H. diminuta*.

xenotransplantation *n.* the *transplantation of organs from one species into another. Experimental work into the feasibility of transplanting pig organs into human beings is under way. It includes the genetic manipulation of pig embryos to produce animals whose organs produce a human cell-surface protein and would therefore not be rejected at transplantation.

xero- *prefix denoting* a dry condition.

xeroderma *n.* a mild form of the hereditary disorder *ichthyosis, in which the skin develops slight dryness and forms branlike scales. It is common in the elderly. **Xeroderma pigmentosum** is a rare genetically determined disorder (*see* GENODERMATOSIS) in which there is an inherited defect in the mechanism that repairs damage to DNA brought about by ultraviolet radiation (*see* DNA REPAIR); this leads to multiple skin cancers. Affected individuals must avoid any exposure to sunlight.

xerophthalmia *n.* a progressive nutritional disease of the eye due to deficiency of vitamin A. The cornea and conjunctiva become dry, thickened, and wrinkled. This may progress to *keratomalacia and eventual blindness.

xeroradiography *n.* X-ray imaging produced on photoconductive paper. This technique is no longer used in routine work.

xerosis *n.* abnormal dryness of the conjunctiva, the skin, or the mucous membranes. Xerosis affecting the conjunctiva is due not to decreased production of tears but to changes in the membrane itself, which becomes thickened and grey in the area exposed when the eyelids are open.

xerostomia *n.* *see* DRY MOUTH. *Compare* PTYALISM.

xiphi- (xipho-) *prefix denoting* the xiphoid process of the sternum. Example: **xiphocostal** (relating to the xiphoid process and ribs).

xiphisternum *n.* *see* XIPHOID PROCESS.

xiphoid process (xiphoid cartilage) the lowermost section of the breastbone (*see* STERNUM): a flat pointed cartilage that gradually ossifies until it is completely replaced by bone, a process not completed until after middle age. It does not articulate with any ribs. Also called: **ensiform process or cartilage**, **xiphisternum**.

X-linked disease *see* SEX-LINKED.

X-linked lymphoproliferative syndrome (XLP syndrome) a hereditary disorder of the immune system caused by a defective *sex-linked gene carried on an ^X-chromosome. There is uncontrolled proliferation of B-*lymphocytes in response to infection by the Epstein-Barr virus, which can lead to fulminating hepatitis or lymphoma.

XLP syndrome *see* X-LINKED LYMPHOPROLIFERATIVE SYNDROME.

X-rays *pl. n.* electromagnetic radiation of extremely short wavelength (beyond the ultraviolet), with great penetrating powers in matter opaque to light. X-rays are produced when high-energy beams of electrons strike matter. They are used in diagnosis in the techniques of *radiography and also in *radiotherapy. Great care is needed to avoid unnecessary exposure, because the radiation is harmful to all living things. *See* IONIZATION, RADIATION SICKNESS.

X-ray screening the use of a TV monitor to perform X-ray investigations under direct control by a radiologist or radiographer. It has replaced fluoroscopy using a fluorescent screen (*see* FLUOROSCOPE).

xylene (dimethylbenzene) *n.* a liquid used for increasing the transparency of tissues prepared for microscopic examination after dehydration. *See* CLEARING.

xylometazoline *n.* a drug that constricts blood vessels (*see* VASOCONSTRICTOR). It is rapidly acting and long lasting and is applied topically as a nasal decongestant in the relief of the common cold and sinusitis. Toxic effects are rare. Trade name: **Otrivine**.

xylose *n.* a pentose sugar (i.e. one with five carbon atoms) that is involved in carbohydrate interconversions within cells. It is used as a diagnostic aid for intestinal function.

YAG laser yttrium–aluminium–garnet laser: a type of *laser used for cutting tissue, for example in lens *capsulotomy or *iridotomy.

yawning *n.* a reflex action in which the mouth is opened wide and air is drawn into the lungs then slowly released. It is a result of drowsiness, fatigue, or boredom.

yaws (pian, framboesia) *n.* a tropical infectious disease caused by the presence of the spirochaete *Treponema pertenue* in the skin and its underlying tissues. Yaws occurs chiefly in conditions of poor hygiene. It is transmitted by direct contact with infected persons and their clothing and possibly also by flies of the genus *Hippelates*. The spirochaetes enter through abrasions on the skin. Initial symptoms include fever, pains, and itching, followed by the appearance of small tumours, each covered by a yellow crust of dried serum, on the hands, face, legs, and feet. These tumours may deteriorate into deep ulcers. The final stage of yaws, which may appear after an interval of several years, involves destructive and deforming lesions of the skin, bones, and periosteum (*see also* GANGOSA, GOUNDOU). Yaws, which commonly affects children, is prevalent in hot humid lowlands of equatorial Africa, tropical America, the Far East, and the West Indies. It responds well to treatment with *penicillin and other antibiotics.

Y chromosome a sex chromosome that is present in men but not in women; it is believed to carry the genes for maleness. *Compare* X CHROMOSOME.

yeast *n.* any of a group of fungi in which the body (mycelium) consists of individual cells, which may occur singly, in groups of two or three, or in chains. Yeasts reproduce by budding and by the formation of sexual spores (in the case of the perfect yeasts) or asexual spores (in the case of the imperfect yeasts). The group includes baker's yeast (*Saccharomyces*), which ferments carbohydrates to produce alcohol and carbon dioxide and is important in brewing and breadmaking. Some yeasts are a commercial source of proteins and of vitamins of the B complex. Yeasts that cause disease in man include *Candida, *Cryptococcus, and *Pityrosporum.

yellow fever an infectious disease, caused by an *arbovirus, occurring in tropical Africa and the northern regions of South America. It is transmitted by mosquitoes, principally *Aëdes aegypti*. The virus causes degeneration of the tissues of the liver and kidneys. Symptoms, depending on severity of infection, include chill, headache, pains in the back and limbs, fever, vomiting, constipation, a reduced flow of urine (which contains high levels of albumin), and *jaundice. The more serious cases may prove fatal, but recovery from a first attack confers subsequent immunity. The disease is treated by fluid replacement and can be prevented by vaccination.

yellow spot *see* MACULA (LUTEA).

Yersinia *n.* a genus of aerobic or facultatively anaerobic Gram-negative bacteria that are parasites of animals and man. The species *Y. pestis* causes bubonic *plague, and *Y. enterocolitica* causes intestinal infections.

yohimbine *n.* an alkaloid with *sympatholytic effects: it lowers blood pressure and controls arousal and anxiety and has been used to treat both physical and psychogenic impotence.

yolk (deutoplasm) *n.* a substance, rich in protein and fat, that is laid down within the egg cell as nourishment for the embryo. It is absent (or nearly so) from the eggs of mammals (including man) whose embryos absorb nutrients from their mother.

yolk sac (vitelline sac) the membranous sac, composed of mesoderm lined with endoderm, that lies ventral to the embryo. It is one of the *extraembryonic membranes. Its initially wide communication with the future gut is later reduced to a narrow duct passing through the *umbilicus. It probably assists in transporting nutrients to the early embryo and is one of the first sites where blood cells are formed.

yttrium-90 *n.* an artificial radioactive isotope of the element yttrium, used in *radiotherapy.

Z

zalcitabine (ddC) *n.* a drug, similar to *didanosine, that is used in attempts to prolong the lives of AIDS patients. It is administered by mouth. Possible side-effects include reversible nerve damage, ulceration of the gullet, skin rashes, severe pancreatitis, nausea, vomiting, and headache.

Zantac *n.* see RANITIDINE.

zein *n.* a protein found in maize.

zidovudine (AZT) *n.* an antiviral drug used in the treatment of AIDS and of AIDS-related complex. It is not approved for HIV-positive patients who are asymptomatic. The drug slows the growth of HIV infection in the body, but is not curative. It is administered by mouth and intravenously; the most common side-effects are nausea, headache, and insomnia, and it may damage the blood-forming tissues of the bone marrow. Trade name: **Retrovir.**

Ziehl-Neelsen stain an acid-fast *carbol fuchsin stain used specifically for identifying the tubercle bacillus. [F. Ziehl (1857–1926), German bacteriologist; F. K. A. Neelsen (1854–94), German pathologist]

zinc *n.* a *trace element that is a cofactor of many enzymes. Deficiency is rare with a balanced diet but may occur in alcoholics and those with kidney disease; symptoms include lesions of the skin, oesophagus, and cornea and (in children) retarded growth. Symbol: Zn.

zinc oxide a mild *astringent used in various skin conditions, usually mixed with other substances. It is applied as a cream, ointment, dusting powder, or as a paste, sometimes in the form of an impregnated bandage.

zinc sulphate a preparation used in the treatment of proven zinc deficiency. It is administered by mouth. Trade names: **Solvazinc, Z Span Spansule.**

zinc undecenoate (zinc undecylenate) an antifungal agent with uses similar to those of *undecenoic acid.

Zollinger-Ellison syndrome a rare disorder in which there is excessive secretion of gastric juice due to high levels of circulating *gastrin, which is produced by a pancreatic tumour (see GASTRINOMA) or an enlarged pancreas. The high levels of stomach acid cause diarrhoea and peptic ulcers, which may be multiple, in unusual sites (e.g. jejunum), or which may quickly recur after *vagotomy or partial *gastrectomy. Treatment with a histamine-blocking drug, by removal of the tumour (if benign); or by total gastrectomy is usually effective. [R. M. Zollinger (1903–92) and E. H. Ellison (1918–70), US physicians]

zona pellucida the thick membrane that develops around the mammalian oocyte within the ovarian follicle. It is penetrated by at least one spermatozoon at fertilization and persists around the *blastocyst until it reaches the uterus. *See* OVUM.

zonula *n.* see ZONULE.

zonule (zonula) *n.* (in anatomy) a small band or zone; for example the **zonule of Zinn** (**zonula ciliaris**) is the suspensory ligament of the eye. —**zonular** *adj.*

zonulolysis *n.* dissolution of the suspensory ligament of the lens of the eye (the **zonule of Zinn**) by means of an enzyme solution injected behind the iris, which facilitates removal of the lens in cases of cataract. This technique is not used for modern cataract surgery.

zoo- *prefix denoting* animals.

zoonosis *n.* an infectious disease of animals that can be transmitted to man. *See* ANTHRAX, BRUCELLOSIS, CAT-SCRATCH FEVER, COWPOX, GLANDERS, Q FEVER, RIFT VALLEY FEVER, RABIES, RAT-BITE FEVER, TOXOPLASMOSIS, TULARAEMIA, TYPHUS.

zoophilism *n.* sexual attraction to animals, which may be manifest in stroking and fondling animals or in sexual intercourse (**bestiality**). —**zoophilic** *adj.*

zoophobia *n.* excessively strong fear of animals. *See* PHOBIA.

zoopsia *n.* visual hallucinations of animals. These can occur in any condition causing hallucinations but are most typical of *delirium tremens.

zwitterion *n.* an ion that bears a positive and a negative charge. Amino acids can yield zwitterions.

zygoma *n. see* ZYGOMATIC ARCH, ZYGOMATIC BONE.

zygomatic arch (zygoma) the horizontal arch of bone on either side of the face, just below the eyes, formed by connected processes of the zygomatic and temporal bones. *See* SKULL.

zygomatic bone (zygoma, malar bone) either of a pair of bones that form the prominent part of the cheeks and contribute to the orbits. *See* SKULL.

zygote *n.* the fertilized ovum before *cleavage begins. It contains both male and female pronuclei.

zygotene *n.* the second stage of the first prophase of *meiosis, in which the homologous chromosomes form pairs (bivalents).

zym- (zymo-) *prefix denoting* **1.** an enzyme. **2.** fermentation.

zymogen *n. see* PROENZYME.

zymology *n.* the science of the study of yeasts and fermentation.

zymolysis *n.* the process of *fermentation or digestion by an enzyme.

zymosis *n.* **1.** the process of *fermentation, brought about by yeast organisms. **2.** the changes in the body that occur in certain infectious diseases, once thought to be the result of a process similar to fermentation. —**zymotic** *adj.*

zymotic disease an old name for a contagious disease, which was formerly thought to develop within the body following infection in a process similar to the fermentation and growth of yeast.

Appendix

TABLE 1 Base and supplementary SI units

Physical quantity	Name of unit	Symbol for unit
length	metre	m
mass	kilogram	kg
time	second	s
electric current	ampere	A
thermodynamic temperature	kelvin	K
luminous intensity	candela	cd
amount of substance	mole	mol
*plane angle	radian	rad
*solid angle	steradian	sr
*supplementary units		

TABLE 2 Derived SI units with special names

Physical quantity	Name of unit	Symbol for unit
frequency	hertz	Hz
energy	joule	J
force	newton	N
power	watt	W
pressure	pascal	Pa
electric charge	coulomb	C
electric potential difference	volt	V
electric resistance	ohm	Ω
electric conductance	siemens	S
electric capacitance	farad	F
magnetic flux	weber	Wb
inductance	henry	H
magnetic flux density (magnetic induction)	tesla	T
luminous flux	lumen	lm
illuminance (illumination	lux	lx
absorbed dose	gray	Gy
activity	becquerel	Bq
dose equivalent	sievert	Sv

TABLE 3 **Decimal multiples and submultiples to be used with SI units**

Submultiple	Prefix	Symbol	Multiple	Prefix	Symbol
10^{-1}	deci-	d	10^{1}	deca-	da
10^{-2}	centi-	c	10^{2}	hecto-	h
10^{-3}	milli-	m	10^{3}	kilo-	k
10^{-6}	micro-	μ	10^{6}	mega-	M
10^{-9}	nano-	n	10^{9}	giga-	G
10^{-12}	pico-	p	10^{12}	tera-	T
10^{-15}	femto-	f	10^{15}	peta-	P
10^{-18}	atto-	a	10^{18}	exa-	E
10^{-21}	zepto-	z	10^{21}	zetta-	Z
10^{-24}	yocto-	y	10^{24}	yotta-	Y

OXFORD

MORE OXFORD PAPERBACKS

This book is just one of nearly 1000 Oxford Paper-backs currently in print. If you would like details of other Oxford Paperbacks, including titles in the World's Classics, Oxford Reference, Oxford Books, OPUS, Past Masters, Oxford Authors, and Oxford Shakespeare series, please write to:

UK and Europe: Oxford Paperbacks Publicity Manager, Arts and Reference Publicity Department, Oxford University Press, Walton Street, Oxford OX2 6DP.

Customers in UK and Europe will find Oxford Paperbacks available in all good bookshops. But in case of difficulty please send orders to the Cash-with-Order Department, Oxford University Press Distribution Services, Saxon Way West, Corby, Northants NN18 9ES. Tel: 01536 741519; Fax: 01536 746337. Please send a cheque for the total cost of the books, plus £1.75 postage and packing for orders under £20; £2.75 for orders over £20. Customers outside the UK should add 10% of the cost of the books for postage and packing.

USA: Oxford Paperbacks Marketing Manager, Oxford University Press, Inc., 200 Madison Avenue, New York, N.Y. 10016.

Canada: Trade Department, Oxford University Press, 70 Wynford Drive, Don Mills, Ontario M3C 1J9.

Australia: Trade Marketing Manager, Oxford University Press, G.P.O. Box 2784Y, Melbourne 3001, Victoria.

South Africa: Oxford University Press, P.O. Box 1141, Cape Town 8000.

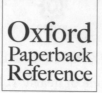

OXFORD PAPERBACK REFERENCE

From *Art and Artists* to *Zoology*, the Oxford Paperback Reference series offers the very best subject reference books at the most affordable prices.

Authoritative, accessible, and up to date, the series features dictionaries in key student areas, as well as a range of fascinating books for a general readership. Included are such well-established titles as Fowler's *Modern English Usage*, Margaret Drabble's *Concise Companion to English Literature*, and the bestselling science and medical dictionaries.

The series has now been relaunched in handsome new covers. Highlights include new editions of some of the most popular titles, as well as brand new paperback reference books on *Politics*, *Philosophy*, and *Twentieth-Century Poetry*.

With new titles being constantly added, and existing titles regularly updated, Oxford Paperback Reference is unrivalled in its breadth of coverage and expansive publishing programme. New dictionaries of *Film*, *Economics*, *Linguistics*, *Architecture*, *Archaeology*, *Astronomy*, and *The Bible* are just a few of those coming in the future.

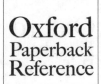

Oxford
Paperback
Reference

THE OXFORD DICTIONARY OF PHILOSOPHY

Edited by Simon Blackburn

* **2,500 entries covering the entire span of the subject including the most recent terms and concepts**

* **Biographical entries for nearly 500 philosophers**

* **Chronology of philosophical events**

From Aristotle to Zen, this is the most comprehensive, authoritative, and up to date dictionary of philosophy available. Ideal for students or a general readership, it provides lively and accessible coverage of not only the Western philosophical tradition but also important themes from Chinese, Indian, Islamic, and Jewish philosophy. The paperback includes a new Chronology.

'an excellent source book and can be strongly recommended . . . there are generous and informative entries on the great philosophers . . . Overall the entries are written in an informed and judicious manner.'
Times Higher Education Supplement

**Oxford
Paperback
Reference**

THE CONCISE OXFORD DICTIONARY OF POLITICS

Edited by Iain McLean

Written by an expert team of political scientists from Warwick University, this is the most authoritative and up-to-date dictionary of politics available.

* **Over 1,500 entries provide truly international coverage of major political institutions, thinkers and concepts**

* **From Western to Chinese and Muslim political thought**

* **Covers new and thriving branches of the subject, including international political economy, voting theory, and feminism**

* **Appendix of political leaders**

* **Clear, no-nonsense definitions of terms such as veto and subsidiarity**

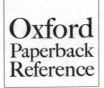

Oxford Paperback Reference

THE CONCISE OXFORD COMPANION TO ENGLISH LITERATURE

Edited by Margaret Drabble and Jenny Stringer

Derived from the acclaimed *Oxford Companion to English Literature*, the concise maintains the wide coverage of its parent volume. It is an indispensable, compact guide to all aspects of English literature. For this revised edition, existing entries have been fully updated and revised with 60 new entries added on contemporary writers.

* **Over 5,000 entries on the lives and works of authors, poets and playwrights**

* **The most comprehensive and authoritative paperback guide to English literature**

" **New entries include Peter Ackroyd, Martin Amis, Toni Morrison, and Jeanette Winterson**

* **New appendices list major literary prize-winners**

From the reviews of its parent volume:

'It earns its place at the head of the best sellers: every home should have one'
Sunday Times

**Oxford
Paperback
Reference**

CONCISE SCIENCE DICTIONARY

New edition

Authoritative and up to date, this bestselling dictionary is ideal reference for both students and non-scientists. Fully revised for this third edition, with over 1,000 new entries, it provides coverage of biology (including human biology), chemistry, physics, the earth sciences, astronomy, maths and computing.

* 8,500 clear and concise entries

* Up-to-date coverage of areas such as molecular biology, genetics, particle physics, cosmology, and fullerene chemistry

* Appendices include the periodic table, tables of SI units, and classifications of the plant and animal kingdoms

'handy and readable . . . for scientists aged nine to ninety'
Nature

'The book will appeal not just to scientists and science students but also to the interested layperson. And it passes the most difficult test of any dictionary—it is well worth browsing through.'
New Scientist

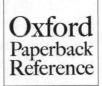

Oxford
Paperback
Reference

THE CONCISE OXFORD DICTIONARY OF MATHEMATICS

New Edition

Edited by Christopher Clapham

Authoritative and reliable, this is the ideal reference guide for students of mathematics at school or in the first year at university. Nearly 1,000 entries have been added for this new edition and the dictionary provides clear definitions, with helpful examples, of a wide range of mathematical terms and concepts.

* **Covers both pure and applied mathematics as well as statistics.**

* **Entries on the great mathematicians**

* **Coverage of mathematics of more general interest, including fractals, game theory, and chaos**

'the depth of information provided is admirable'
New Scientist

'the style encourages browsing and a desire to find out more about the topics discussed'
Mathematica

Oxford
Paperback
Reference

THE CONCISE OXFORD DICTIONARY OF OPERA

New Edition

Edited by Ewan West and John Warrack

Derived from the full *Oxford Dictionary of Opera*, this is the most authoritative and up-to-date dictionary of opera available in paperback. Fully revised for this new edition, it is designed to be accessible to all those who enjoy opera, whether at the opera-house or at home.

* **Over 3,500 entries on operas, composers, and performers**

* **Plot summaries and separate entries for well-known roles, arias, and choruses**

* **Leading conductors, producers and designers**

From the reviews of its parent volume:

'the most authoritative single-volume work of its kind'
Independent on Sunday

'an invaluable reference work'
Gramophone

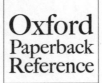

Oxford
Paperback
Reference

THE CONCISE OXFORD DICTIONARY OF MUSIC

New Edition

Edited by Michael Kennedy

Derived from the full *Oxford Dictionary of Music* this is the most authoritative and up-to-date dictionary of music available in paperback. Fully revised and updated for this new edition, it is a rich mine of information for lovers of music of all periods and styles.

* 14,000 entries on musical terms, works, composers, librettists, musicians, singers and orchestras.

* Comprehensive work-lists for major composers

* Generous coverage of living composers and performers

'clearly the best around . . . the dictionary that everyone should have'
Literary Review

'indispensable'
Yorkshire Post